AIDS in Africa

Second Edition

AIDS in Africa
Second Edition

Edited by

Max Essex, DVM, PhD

Chairman, Harvard AIDS Institute
Mary Woodard Lasker Professor of Health Sciences
Harvard University, Boston, Massachusetts, USA

Souleymane Mboup, PharmD, PhD

Professor of Microbiology, Laboratory of Bacteriology and Virology
CHU Le Dantec, Université Cheikh Anta Diop, Dakar, Senegal

Phyllis J. Kanki, DVM, DSc

Professor of Immunology and Infectious Diseases, Department of Immunology and Infectious Diseases and the Harvard AIDS Institute, Harvard School of Public Health, Boston, Massachusetts, USA

Richard G. Marlink, MD

Senior Research and Executive Director
Harvard AIDS Institute, Boston, Massachusetts, USA

and

Sheila D. Tlou, PhD

Associate Professor, Department of Nursing Education
University of Botswana, Gaborone, Botswana

Managing Editor

Molly Holme

Department of Immunology and Infectious Diseases and the Harvard AIDS Institute
Harvard School of Public Health, Boston, Massachusetts, USA

Springer Science+Business Media, LLC

Contributors

Quarraisha Abdool Karim, PhD, University of Natal Medical School, Durban, South Africa

Iain W. Aitken, MB BChir, DCMT, MPH, Lecturer on Maternal and Child Health, Harvard School of Public Health, Boston, Massachusetts, USA

Anthony Amoroso, MD, Assistant Professor of Medicine, Institute of Human Virology, Baltimore, Maryland, USA

Gabriel M. Anabwani, MBChB, MMed, MSc, Professor of Pediatrics, Senior Consultant Pediatrician, Princess Marina Hospital, Gaborone, Botswana

Ahidjo Ayouba, PhD, Centre Pasteur, Yaoundé, Cameroon

Francis R. Barin, PhD, Professor, Université François Rabelais, Tours, France

Augustine Barnaba, Queen Elizabeth Central Hospital, Blantyre, Malawi

Françoise Barré-Sinoussi, PhD, Professor, and Head, Retroviral Biology Unit, Institut Pasteur, Paris, France

Michael Bartos, MEd, Senior Policy Advisor, Joint United Nations Programme on HIV/AIDS, Geneva, Switzerland

Seth Berkley, MD, President and CEO, International AIDS Vaccine Initiative, New York, New York, USA

Gunnel Biberfeld, MD, PhD, Professor, Department of Immunology, Karolinska Institute, Stockholm, Sweden

Kelly Blanchard, MSc, Robert H. Ebert Program on Critical Issues in Reproductive Health, Population Council, Johannesburg, South Africa

Elisabeth Bouvet, MD, Infectious Disease Physician and Professor, Bichat Hospital, University and GERES, Paris, France

Bluma G. Brenner, PhD, McGill University AIDS Centre, Montréal, Québec, Canada

Carl H. Campbell, Jr., MPA, Senior Public Health Advisor, Global AIDS Program, Centers for Disease Control and Prevention, Atlanta, Georgia, USA

Robert Colebunders, MD, PhD, Professor of Infectious Diseases, Institute of Tropical Medicine and University of Antwerp, Antwerp, Belgium

Sylvie Corbet, PhD, Serum Statens Institute, Copenhagen, Denmark

Brian Coulter, MD, Senior Lecturer in Tropical Child Health, Liverpool School of Tropical Medicine, Liverpool, United Kingdom

Charles E. Davis, MD, Assistant Professor of Medicine, Institute of Human Virology, Baltimore, Maryland, USA

Martin Dedicoat, Liverpool School of Tropical Medicine and the Africa Centre, Hlabisa Hospital, Hlabisa, KwaZulu Natal, South Africa

Beth A. Dillon, MSW, MPH, Centers for Disease Control, Atlanta, Georgia, USA

Ousmane M. Diop, PhD, Institut Pasteur, Dakar, Sénégal

José Esparza, MD, PhD, WHO-UNAIDS HIV Vaccine Initiative, World Health Organization, Geneva, Switzerland

Max Essex, DVM, PhD, Chairman, Harvard AIDS Institute, and Mary Woodard Lasker Professor of Health Sciences, Harvard University, Boston, Massachusetts, USA

Eka Esu-Williams, PhD, Population Council, Horizons Program, Johannesburg, South Africa

Wafaie W. Fawzi, MD, DrPH, Associate Professor of International Nutrition and Epidemiology, Harvard School of Public Health, Boston, Massachusetts, USA

Geoff Foster, MBBS, DCH, MRCP, Consultant Pediatrician, Mutare Provincial Hospital, Mutare, Zimbabwe,

Stefan Germann, Masiye Camp, Bulawayo, Zimbabwe

Peter B. Gilbert, MS, PhD, Assistant Research Professor, Department of Biostatistics, University of Washington, Seattle, Washington, USA

Sofia Gruskin, JD, MIA, Assistant Professor of Health and Human Rights, Harvard School of Public Health, Boston, Massachusetts, USA

Aïssatou Guèye, Institut Pasteur, Paris, France

Aissatou Guèye-Ndiaye, PharmD, Assistant Professor of Microbiology, Centre Hospitalier Universitaire, Dakar, Senegal

Amar A. Hamoudi, Center for International Development, Harvard University, Cambridge, Massachusetts, USA

Keith E. Hansen, MPA, JD, Deputy Manager, AIDS Campaign Team for Africa, The World Bank, Washington, DC, USA

Samuel Kalibala, MD, Horizons Project, East and Southern Africa, Population Council, Nairobi, Kenya

Phyllis J. Kanki, DVM, DSc, Professor of Immunology and Infectious Diseases, Harvard School of Public Health, Boston, Massachusetts, USA

Saidi H. Kapiga, MD, MPH, ScD, Assistant Professor of Reproductive Health, Harvard School of Public Health, Boston, Massachusetts, USA

Elly T. Katabira, MD, World Health Organization, Harare, Zimbabwe

David A. Katzenstein, MD, Associate Professor of Medicine, Stanford University School of Medicine, Stanford, California, USA

Patrick K. Kayembe, MD, DrPH, Associate Professor of Medicine and Public Health, University of Kinshasa, Kinshasa, Democratic Republic of Congo

Poloko Kebaabetswe, RN, RM, MPH, CHES, Botswana-Harvard AIDS Institute Partnership, Gaborone, Botswana

Annamaria K. Kiure, MD, SM, Harvard School of Public Health, Boston, Massachusetts, USA

Mark W. Kline, MD, Professor of Pediatrics, Baylor College of Medicine, Houston, Texas, USA

Sibylle Kristensen, MPH, MSPH, Co-director, AIDS International Training and Research Program, University of Alabama at Birmingham, Birmingham, Alabama, USA

Marc Lallemant, MD, Perinatal HIV Prevention Trial, Thailand, Institut de Recherche pour le Développement, Chiang Mai, Thailand

Anne Laporte, MD, Institut de Veille Sanitaire, Saint-Maurice, France

Sophie Le Coeur, MD, PhD, Institut National d'Études Démographiques, Paris, France

Tun-Hou Lee, SD, Professor of Virology, Harvard School of Public Health, Boston, Massachusetts, USA

Shahin Lockman, MD, Harvard School of Public Health, Boston, Massachusetts, USA

Chewe Luo, MBChB, MMED, PhD, HIV/AIDS Officer, UNICEF, Gaborone, Botswana

Eligius Lyamuya, MD, PhD, Senior Lecturer and Head, Department of Microbiology and Immunology, Muhimbili University College of Health Sciences, Dar es Salaam, Tanzania

Miriam Maluwa, LLB, LLM, The Joint United Nations Programme on HIV/AIDS, Geneva, Switzerland

Indu Mani, DVM, Harvard School of Public Health, Boston, Massachusetts, USA

Richard G. Marlink, MD, Senior Research and Executive Director, Harvard AIDS Institute, Boston, Massachusetts, USA

Elizabeth Marum, PhD, Centers for Disease Control and Prevention, Nairobi, Kenya

Philippe Mauclère, MD, PhD, Director, Institut Pasteur de Madagascar, Antananarivo, Madagascar

Harriet Mayanja-Kizza, MBChB, MMed, MSc, Senior Lecturer and Head, Department of Medicine, Makerere University Medical School, Kampala, Uganda

Dorothy Mbori-Ngacha, MBChB, MMed, MPH, Senior Lecturer, Department of Pediatrics, University of Nairobi College of Health Sciences, Nairobi, Kenya

Souleymane Mboup, PharmD, PhD, Professor of Microbiology, CHU Le Dantec/Université Cheikh Anta Diop, Dakar, Senegal

Kenneth McIntosh, MD, Professor of Pediatrics, Children's Hospital/Harvard Medical School, Boston, Massachusetts, USA

Monty Montano, PhD, Assistant Professor of Medicine, Boston University School of Medicine, Boston, Massachusetts, USA

Gernard I. Msamanga, MD, ScD, Associate Professor, Department of Community Health, Muhimbili University College of Health Sciences, Dar es Salaam, Tanzania

Katawa Msowoya, MSc, Malawi AIDS Counseling and Resource Organization, Blantyre, Malawi

Michaela C. Müller-Trutwin, PhD, Institut Pasteur, Paris, France

Ruth Nduati, MBChB, MMed, MPH, Senior Lecturer, Department of Pediatrics, University of Nairobi College of Health Sciences, Nairobi, Kenya

Ann Marie Nelson, MD, Chief, AIDS Pathology Branch, Armed Forces Institute of Pathology, Washington, DC, USA

Eric Nerrienet, PhD, Head, Virology Laboratory, Centre Pasteur, Yaounde, Cameroon

Robert Newton, MBBS, DPhil, MFPHM, Radcliffe Infirmary, Oxford, United Kingdom,

Kathleen F. Norr, PhD, Associate Professor, University of Illinois at Chicago, College of Nursing, Chicago, Illinois, USA

Vlad Novitsky, MD, PhD, Harvard School of Public Health, Boston, Massachusetts, USA

Stephen J. O'Brien, PhD, Chief, Laboratory of Viral Carcinogenesis, National Cancer Institute-Frederick, Frederick, Maryland, USA

Churchill L. Onen, MBChB, MMed, Senior Consultant Physician and Head of Department of Medicine, Princess Marina Hospital, Gaborone, Botswana

Martine Peeters, PhD, Institut de Recherche pour le Développement, Montpelier, France

Peter Piot, MD, PhD, Executive Director, Joint United Nations Programme on HIV/AIDS, Geneva, Switzerland

Jean-Christophe Plantier, PhD, Assistant Professor, Laboratoire de Virologie, Hôpital Bretonneau, Tours, France

Kirthana Ramanathan, MD, MPH, Harvard AIDS Institute, Boston, Massachusetts, USA

Robert R. Redfield, MD, Professor of Medicine and Director of Clinical Care and Research, Institute of Human Virology, Baltimore, Maryland, USA

Boris Renjifo, MD, MS, PhD, Harvard School of Public Health, Boston, Massachusetts, USA

Renée Ridzon, MD, Centers for Disease Control and Prevention, Atlanta, Georgia, USA

Jeffrey Sachs, PhD, Galen L. Stone Professor of International Trade, and Director, Center for International Development, Harvard University, Cambridge, Massachusetts, USA

Jean-Louis Sankalé, PharmD, DSc, Harvard School of Public Health, Boston, Massachusetts, USA

Roger L. Shapiro, MD, Harvard School of Public Health, Boston, Massachusetts, USA

François Simon, MD, PhD, Head, Retrovirology Laboratory, Centre International de Recherche Médicales de Franceville, Franceville, Gabon

Moses Sinkala, MD, MPH, Director, Lusaka Urban District Health Management Board, Lusaka, Zambia

Freddy Sitas, PhD, Head, Cancer Epidemiology Research Group, National Cancer Registry, South African Institute for Medical Research, Johannesburg, South Africa

Karen A. Stanecki, MPH, Chief, Health Studies Branch, International Programs Center, U.S. Census Bureau, Washington, DC, USA

Zena A. Stein, MA, MB BCh, Professor of Public Health and Psychiatry Emeritus, Mailman School of Public Health, Columbia University, New York, New York, USA

Arnaud Tarantola, MD, GERES, Faculté Xavier Bichat, Paris, France

Daniel Tarantola, MD, Senior Policy Advisor, Director General's Office, World Health Organization, Geneva, Switzerland

Sheila D. Tlou, PhD, Associate Professor, Department of Nursing Education, University of Botswana, Gaborone, Botswana

Coumba Toure-Kane, PharmD, MD, Assistant Professor, Laboratoire de Virologie, Hôpital Le Dantec, Dakar, Senegal

Sten H. Vermund, MD, PhD, Professor and Director, Division of Geographic Medicine, University of Alabama at Birmingham, Birmingham, Alabama, USA

Mark A. Wainberg, PhD, Professor, McGill University AIDS Centre, Montréal, Québec, Canada

Neff Walker, AB, MA, PhD, Senior Advisor for Statistics and Modeling, United Nations Joint Programme on HIV/AIDS, Geneva, Switzerland

Carolyn Williamson, Associate Professor, Faculty of Health Sciences, University of Capetown, Capetown, South Africa

Anne Willoughby, MD, MPH, Director, Center for Research for Mothers and Children, National Institute of Child Health and Human Development, Rockville, Maryland, USA

Cheryl A. Winkler, PhD, National Cancer Institute-Frederick, Frederick, Maryland, USA

Debrework Zewdie, PhD, Manager, AIDS Campaign Team for Africa, The World Bank, Washington, DC, USA

John L. Ziegler, MD, MSc, Professor of Medicine, Emeritus, and Director, Cancer Risk Program, University of California at San Francisco Comprehensive Cancer Center, San Francisco, California, USA

Lynn S. Zijenah, PhD, Senior Lecturer, Department of Immunology, University of Zimbabwe Medical School, Harare, Zimbabwe

Foreword

The way we deal with AIDS in Africa will determine Africa's future. The devastation wrought by HIV/AIDS on the continent is so acute that it has become one of the main obstacles to development itself. AIDS threatens to unravel whole societies, communities, and economies. In this way, AIDS is not only taking away Africa's present—it is taking away Africa's future.

This crisis requires an unprecedented response. It requires communities, nations, and regions, the public and the private sector, international organizations and nongovernmental groups to come together in concerted, coordinated action. Only when all these forces join in a common effort will we be able to expand our fight against the epidemic to decrease risk, vulnerability, and impact. All of us must be open about HIV, and raise our voices against stigma and discrimination. All of us must rise above turf battles and doctrinal disputes. The only acceptable result is that we replace suffering with hope.

This is indeed a time of hope, for after years of slow and inadequate responses, we have seen a turning point in the fight against HIV/AIDS. For much of the international community, the magnitude of the crisis is finally beginning to sink in. At no time in dealing with this catastrophe has there been such a sense of common resolve and collective possibility. At no time have we seen such strength of purpose shown by African leaders themselves.

We have seen examples of effective prevention efforts across the continent. All of them were developed by actors inside the country; they were not imposed from outside. All of them take account of the local cultural context. But they all have something else in common: they stem from a political will to fight AIDS, and a recognition that facing up to the problem is the first step towards conquering it. I am convinced that, *given* that will, every society can do the same.

We have seen a growing understanding of the inextricable link between prevention and treatment, and a conviction that treatment can work even in the poorest societies. We have seen AIDS drugs become more available and affordable in poor countries, and scientific progress promises simplified treatment regimes. Above all, we have seen a growing understanding that the key is political commitment to providing treatment, backed up by community involvement.

Our challenge now is to build on the momentum that has been achieved. Practical medical education is a vital pillar in that process, and this book promises to be an invaluable tool. I am especially heartened that so many of its chapters are written by Africans—for the solutions to this crisis must come primarily from Africa itself, with support from the wider international community. Whether you are a practitioner, a policymaker, a public health expert, a person living with AIDS, or a concerned member of the public, I hope you will use this authoritative work to advance our fight against AIDS in Africa.

Kofi A. Annan
Secretary-General of the United Nations and Winner of the 2001 Nobel Peace Prize

Preface

Eight years ago the first edition of *AIDS in Africa* was published. Since then, many millions of Africans have died of AIDS and huge numbers of children have become orphans. In some countries, life expectancy has been reduced by more than a third, and more than a third of young women are HIV-infected.

The worldwide AIDS epidemic has now surpassed the former benchmark of infectious disease epidemics—the bubonic plague—in total deaths. That epidemic of the 14th century eliminated entire civilizations and changed the course of history. Numbers of annual deaths from AIDS also recently surged past those representing the burden of death from malaria. While the numbers for AIDS morbidity and mortality worldwide may seem astounding, they should be even more astounding when we consider that more than 70% of the world's burden is concentrated in sub–Saharan Africa, home to just 10% of the world's population.

During the 1980s most of the attention given to AIDS issues focused on the United States and Europe. Africa was largely ignored by the rest of the world and many African governments were in denial. Few political leaders remain in denial, but the devastation of AIDS in Africa is still largely ignored by governments of the affluent nations of the North. Even some countries that were previously considered models of success in Africa—those with expanding economies, lack of violence, and good governments—have been devastated by HIV and AIDS.

Over the last eight years, there has been a massive expansion of the AIDS epidemic in Africa. During the same period there have also been major milestones of progress. Perhaps the most dramatic of these has been the recognition that the lives of most AIDS patients can be saved with the use of combinations of antiretroviral drugs. However, with very few exceptions, Africans have not yet benefited from the fruits of research on AIDS treatment.

For more than 15 years, there have been statements of intent to develop a vaccine. Yet, such statements have never been backed by resource allocation for vaccine research that has matched the allocations for drug research. Preventive medicine has never been as popular as therapy to save the lives of those who are already ill, even when it is much more cost-effective. Those who cannot pay the cost of treatment are often left to die.

There is some good news. Some of the drugs designed for treatment have been shown to be remarkably effective and also cost-effective for preventing the transmission of HIV from mother to child. Some countries within Africa, such as Senegal and Uganda, have made impressive progress in controlling HIV epidemics. A few international agencies, especially the Bill and Melinda Gates Foundation, have made important commitments to the problem of AIDS in Africa. The United Nations has established the Global Fund.

The new edition of *AIDS in Africa* has been completely reorganized and revised to reflect the current and future epidemics of

AIDS in Africa. With the hope that we are on the edge of a new era of concern and commitment, more space has been devoted to vaccines and therapy. The new edition is divided into eight sections. The first section, Pathogenesis, now has a chapter on the effect of genetic variation on HIV transmission and progression to AIDS. Insufficient information was available to warrant a chapter on this topic eight years ago. The second section, on the detection and monitoring of infection and disease, contains five chapters as opposed to only one in the first edition. Topics concerning mother-to-child transmission and pediatric AIDS have been expanded from two chapters to six, to reflect the massive expansion of new knowledge and opportunities for chemoprophylaxis. Chapters have been added on access to care, tuberculosis, drug resistance, home-based care, nursing, and nutrition. In order to address new knowledge on prevention, chapters have been added on male condoms and circumcision, female condoms and microbicides, and post-exposure prophylaxis for occupational exposure and sexual assault. Vaccine development has been expanded from one chapter to three. The chapters of this book were written by 100 authors from 28 countries. Twenty-nine of the 46 chapters were authored or coauthored by Africans.

One objective of the book is to provide a single comprehensive source of information to those who are already addressing the problem of AIDS in Africa. A second objective is to try to recruit others to join the cause, including political leaders, public health experts, care providers, scientists, educators, and community leaders.

Perhaps the most sobering of all statistics about AIDS in Africa comes from Figure 4 of Chapter 12 in this volume. It estimates that 65% to 85% of teenagers in some countries will die of AIDS unless major changes occur now. Will we be able to tell future generations that we've done our best to save them from this scourge? We have become familiar with the annual death counts. We must now begin to address the numbers for HIV infections prevented and lives saved.

Max Essex, DVM, PhD
Souleymane Mboup, PharmD, PhD
Phyllis J. Kanki, DVM, DSc
Richard G. Marlink, MD
Sheila D. Tlou, PhD

Acknowledgments

The editors would like to thank the collaborative authors for their dedication to HIV research and for their dedication of time and effort to contribute to this publication. We are extremely grateful for Esmond Harmsworth's constant advice, expertise, advocacy, and other support. We are especially indebted to Ann Menting, whose hard work, experience, and skill were invaluable throughout the entire process.

We wish to thank Mr. Maurice Tempelsman and Mrs. William McCormick Blair, Jr., for their tireless support and devotion to responding to the AIDS epidemic, especially in Africa.

Others who have supported our AIDS research in Africa include the Oak Foundation, the Secure the Future Foundation of Bristol Myers Squibb, the Merck Foundation, The African Comprehensive HIV/AIDS Partnership, the Elton John Foundation, the Prince of Wales Foundation, the G. Harold and Leila Y. Mathers Charitable Trust, the Oliver Twist Charitable Trust, the Margaret T. Morris Foundation, the Archer Daniels Midland Foundation, the Arthur Loeb Foundation, the Overbrook Foundation, the Horace Goldsmith Foundation, the Niagra Trust, the Clarence and Anne Dillon Dunwalke Trust, the Annie Laurie Aitken Charitable Lead Trust, the Henry L. Hill Foundation, the Francis H. Curren, Jr. Charitable Trust, the Charles A. Dana Foundation, the Diller Foundation, the Coca-Cola Company, Agouron Pharmaceuticals, Mr. and Mrs. Arthur Altschul, Martha Bartlett, Douglas Bauer, Bruce Beal, David Beer, Pierre Berge, Scott Bessent, Bill Blass, Carl Brenner, Frances Brody, Joseph Brooks, Buffy Cafritz, Madison Cox, Douglas Cramer, Susan Curran, Pierre Durand, Alexander Forger, Cathy Graham, Lisa Henson, Marguerite Littman, Arthur Loeb, Sally and Ernest Marx, John McCaw, Nan Tucker McEvoy, John McFadden, Richard Menschel, Jim and Joanna Moore, Judy Peabody, Michael Perry, Sarah Peter, Patsy Preston, Brian Raffanelli, Nasser Al Rashid, Felix Robyns, Ardath Rodale, Mr. and Mrs. Joshua Ruch, Kate Sedgewick, Howard Slatkin, Spencer Stokes, Eric Weinmann, and the late Khalil Rizk.

We are delighted to acknowledge the contributions of Abbott Laboratories, Exxon Mobil Corporation, and others, whose support of this project will allow those who are working to minimize the AIDS crisis in the poorest countries to have access to this book.

Table of Contents

I: PATHOGENESIS

VIII: IMPACT AND RESPONSE

1

Introduction: The Etiology of AIDS

*Max Essex and †Souleymane Mboup

*Harvard AIDS Institute and the Department of Immunology and Infectious Diseases, Harvard School of Public Health, Boston, Massachusetts, USA.
†Laboratory of Bacteriology and Virology, School of Medicine and Pharmacy, Université Cheikh Anta Diop, Dakar, Senegal.

HISTORY

In 1981, the acquired immunodeficiency syndrome (AIDS) was identified as a new disease, initially in homosexual men in the United States (1–3). The initial syndrome was characterized by clusters of unusual diseases that had previously been extremely rare in young adults in the West. Kaposi's sarcoma, *Pneumocystis carinii* pneumonia, and *Mycobacterium avium* tuberculosis were the most frequently observed. Because these early AIDS cases were sometimes observed in men who knew each other, "clustered" by time and space, it was soon hypothesized that their disparate outcomes might have some common underlying cause. Soon after, similar AIDS cases were also described in entirely different groups in the United States and Europe. These groups included injection drug users (IDUs) (4), hemophiliacs (5–7), certain blood transfusion recipients (8,9), a few newborn infants (10,11), and a few travelers from central Africa who went to Europe for medical treatment (12).

Because men with multiple same-sex partners, presumed to be at high risk for AIDS, often reported taking drugs to enhance sexual performance, and IDUs were also apparently at high risk for AIDS, drugs were initially considered a potential cause. At the same time, some hypothesized that AIDS might be caused by immune reactions to tissue antigens present on sperm. The recognition that what was apparently AIDS was expanding beyond the communities in which it was originally identified, facilitated consideration that AIDS might be an infectious disease (13). However, even among those who initially endorsed an infectious etiology for AIDS, many did not include a retrovirus as a candidate causative agent (14).

INFECTIOUS ORIGIN

When a "new" disease syndrome, such as AIDS, is first recognized, it must be either completely new as a disease entity in people (i.e. one that has moved to people from an animal reservoir), or previously existing in the human species but formerly unrecognized. If the disease is truly new in people, the etiologic agent must also be new to the human species. Over the past several decades, many new infectious agents of people have been identified, including such ubiquitous viruses as hepatitis B, hepatitis C, human herpesviruses 7 and 8, HTLV-1, and various arthropod-borne viruses (15).

Often, but not always, "new" infectious agents appeared to enter the human population from some animal reservoir. In some instances, viruses were newly recognized in people for diseases that were not previously known to be of infectious origin, such as adult T-cell leukemia (16) or cancer of the uterine cervix (17). When a new infectious etiology is considered, however, viruses are often considered as more likely causes than bacteria or other microbes, simply because they are harder to detect.

At the time when AIDS was first identified in people, the first human retroviruses had only been described a year or two before (16), and most public health officials were unaware of their existence. Nevertheless, the first human retrovirus discovered, the human T-cell lymphotropic virus type 1 (HTLV-1), was known to preferentially infect human T4 lymphocytes, exactly the cell that appeared to be preferentially depleted in people with AIDS (18,19). Those who developed adult T-cell leukemia associated with HTLV-1 were also known to have an associated immunosuppression (20). This encouraged some to hypothesize that a virus related to HTLV-1 might be the cause of AIDS (21–25).

Most infectious diseases are known to have short incubation periods. While some occur only after chronic infections and/or long incubation periods, such infections usually have a low rate for induction of lethal disease. AIDS was unusual in that a lethal disease developed with high frequency, but only after a latent period of at least 4 to 5 years.

It was soon apparent that the actual cause of death from AIDS varied within and between geographic locations. Tuberculosis was a common outcome in all locations, for example, while *Penicillium marneffei* pneumonias were only common in Southeast Asia (26) and "slim disease" was typical in East Africa (27). Those who failed to appreciate that an irreversible destruction of the immune system was the specific disease entity were reluctant to accept HIV (or any other infectious agent) as the cause of AIDS. This sometimes led to confusion, controversy, and denial (28).

RETROVIRUSES

Prior to the identification of human retroviruses, including HIV, numerous retroviruses were known to exist in lower animals. These retroviral infections had certain common features, such as a tropism for lymphocytes and a long incubation period before disease development. Such retroviruses, common in species such as mice and cats, were clearly linked to outcomes such as lymphocytic leukemia (29) and subsequently neurologic disease (30) and immunosuppression (31). Because the viral incubation periods were so prolonged before disease development, and laboratory mice with retroviral infections were genetically inbred, it was often incorrectly assumed that retroviruses were only transmitted from mother to infant by genetic or epigenetic means (32). Studies with cats soon revealed that retroviruses were often transmitted among adults as classical infectious agents (33). Furthermore, such infections in cats were even more likely to cause immunosuppression than to cause leukemia or other cancers (31).

General features of retroviruses, including their manner of replication, help explain many of the characteristics of HIV and AIDS. First, because retroviral genomes are RNA, their mutation rate using an RNA template is much higher than for DNA viruses such as pox viruses or herpes (34,35). In the realm of pathogenesis and treatment, this translates into constant opportunities to generate drug-resistant variants, progeny viruses that can evade neutralizing antibodies or other immune responses, and viruses that can change their affinity for cell receptors or coreceptors. Second, because retroviruses undergo reverse transcription through a DNA proviral stage, they have an opportunity to stabilize such mutations when the provirus is integrated into chromosomal DNA (36). Third, as all retroviruses are diploid, they have constant opportunities to undergo recombination when different parental genomes are packaged in the same virus particle. Such recombination can occur at high efficiency when viruses of different parental origin happen to infect the same cell, since the assembly and release of progeny viruses would not be able to select against genetic changes in parental viruses that affected functions other than virus assembly (37). These features provide ample opportunity for HIV to rapidly evolve. While HIV recombinants are most often identified and appreciated when they occur between different parental subtypes (i.e. intersubtype recombinants), recombinants within subtypes (i.e. intrasubtype recombinants) are presumably generated at even higher rates.

Still another feature of retroviruses that contributes to their great ability to adapt is their property of latency. Latently infected cells may be protected from attack by immune cells and antibodies when no viral proteins are expressed. Lymphocytes with complete genomic copies of HIV DNA are activated whenever they undergo mitosis, or when antigenic stimulations or general cellular gene expression occurs. At such times, the HIV proviral DNA would produce RNA for both proteins and progeny virus particles, causing a wave of virus release in the environment of the activated cell.

The latency feature is also very important in protecting a subset of infected cells from elimination during drug therapy. All existing approaches for chemotherapy target viral proteins, particularly the protease and reverse transcriptase enzymes. Drugs for other HIV gene products are also under development. However, no therapeutic regimens based on current knowledge and reagents can target cells with proviral DNA that are not activated. Because such cells may live for years, it is not possible to eliminate all virus, or to eliminate the potential for making newly activated virus in the future. For this reason, a complete "cure" is essentially impossible for the HIV-infected individual, as it would require the excision of integrated provirus from the chromosomes of all latently infected cells.

VARIATION AMONG HUMAN LENTIVIRUSES

Although HIV-1 was the first lentivirus to be identified, related viruses were soon discovered in monkeys. The first simian immunodeficiency viruses (SIVs) were identified in experimental colonies of Asian macaques that had an immunodeficiency syndrome similar to human AIDS (38,39). Soon after, other SIVs were identified in several species of African monkeys (40–43). The infections in African monkeys often occurred in large fractions of the population of healthy adults, suggesting they were not causing lethal immunosuppression in the species for which they had a long period of evolutionary adaptation (44) (Figure 1A).

Soon after the identification of SIVs, the HIV-2 was identified in populations of female commercial sex workers in West Africa (45). HIV-2 was initially categorized as distinct from the HIV-1s identified earlier because HIV-2 was antigenically indistinguishable from the SIVs identified in macaques, whereas it was clearly distinguishable from HIV-1 (45,46) (Figure 1A).

After HIV-2–infected individuals were monitored for prolonged periods, it also

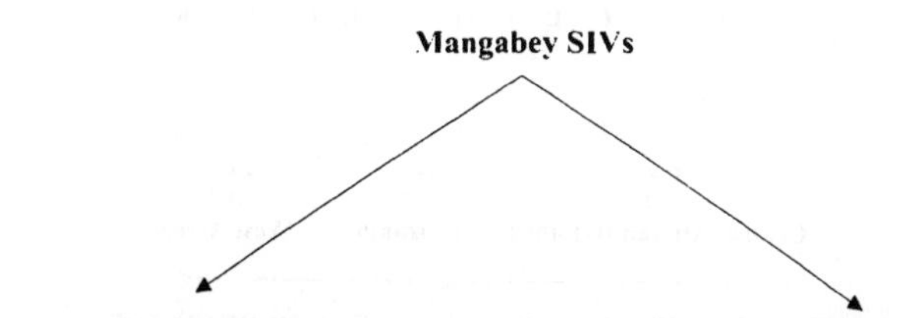

FIGURE 1A. Possible entry of HIV-2s into human species.

became apparent that HIV-2 was less virulent than HIV-1. Although HIV-2 could cause clinical AIDS that seemed similar or identical to AIDS caused by HIV-1, this outcome did not occur in the majority of HIV-2–infected adults, at least not within the same period of time (47). Similarly, HIV-2 did not spread as efficiently between people, either by sexual transmission (48), or by transmission from infected mothers to their infants (49,50). In retrospect, it seems likely that HIV-2 had moved into the human population before HIV-1, yet it has not expanded beyond West Africa, except perhaps for small numbers of infections in a few sites that were linked to West Africa by frequent travel (51).

After multiple HIV-1s were genotyped by nucleotide sequencing, it became apparent that some HIV-1s from Asia or Africa were easily categorized as different from the dominant HIV-1 of the West, now designated HIV-1B (52,53). At least 10 subtypes of HIV-1 were soon distinguishable on branches of a genetic tree, based on evolutionary variation (Figure 1B). Designated as subtypes A through K, each grouping had nucleotide variation that was generally less than 15% within a subtype, but more than 20% when compared between subtypes. The extent of variation, both between and within subtypes, also appeared to be related to host selection pressure. Regions of the envelope gene that were subjected to antibody neutralizing immunoselection pressure, for example, seemed to vary most. Genes that encoded for structural genes localized at the core of the virus showed the least amount of variation.

In a few people, other viruses were identified that were more related to HIV-1 than to HIV-2, but more distant from each of the known HIV-1 subtype groupings than the subtypes were from each other. These were called the HIV-1 "O" group for outliers (54,55), as the HIV-1 subtypes A–K were designated the "major" or "main" group (56). Subsequently, others were found that were similarly unrelated, designated the HIV-1 "N" group (57). To date, viruses of the HIV-1 "O" and "N" groups seem to be rare in people, with relatively few isolations, primarily linked to the West African region around Cameroon. However, isolations of viruses closely related to HIV-1 "O" were also detected in subhuman apes (58), allowing for the interpretation that such viruses entered the human species even more recently than other HIV-1s and HIV-2 (Figure 1B).

It was also soon learned that some of the subtypes, such as HIV-1E, were actually recombinants (59). In that case, one end of the viral genome is E, a distinct subtype, but the other end is A, clearly originating from the same "pure A" that currently exists in East Africa (56). The virus that predominates

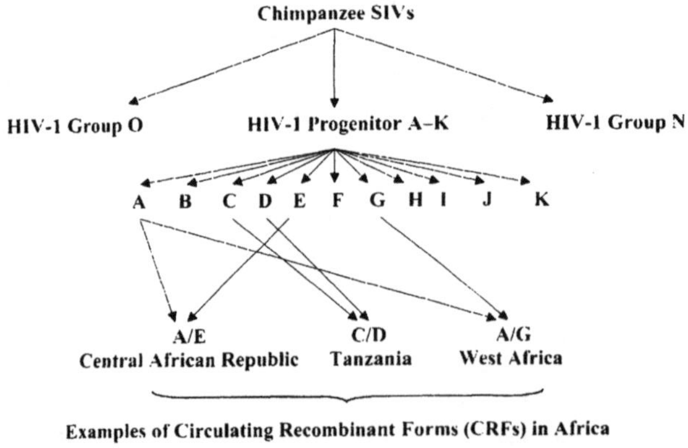

FIGURE 1B. Possible entry of HIV-1s into human species.

throughout West Africa is also a recombinant subtype, in this case A/G (60,61). As recombinants are being generated at high rates when regional epidemics from different HIV-1 subtypes converge and overlap, we may expect that more epidemics will be caused by "circulating recombinant forms" in future decades.

PHENOTYPIC DIFFERENCES

Along with the wide range of genotypic variation observed for types, subtypes, and particular isolates, it might be expected that phenotypic properties could be different for different genotypes. As mentioned already, this seemed apparent when HIV-2 was compared to HIV-1 in the same cohort (47,48). While viruses such as SIV may be highly virulent in some monkeys, such as Asian macaques, and apparently nonvirulent in indigenous mangabey monkeys, this is presumably due to genetic selection of the host for disease resistance. It is well known that chimpanzees ordinarily do not develop clinical disease when inoculated with HIV-1s taken from AIDS patients, presumably also because the chimpanzees have been evolutionarily selected for resistance (44).

One of the clear phenotypic differences observed for HIVs at the cellular level was the property of "lymphotropism" vs. tropism for fresh monocytes and macrophages. This was initially detected because some clinical isolates of HIV-1 were found to grow well in lymphoblastoid cell lines, while others grew poorly in such cells. The former were designated "rapid-high" viruses and the latter "slow-low" (62). This phenotypic property could be mapped to a few amino acid changes in the V3 region of the envelope gp120 protein (63), a property subsequently shown to be regulated through attachment to chemokine coreceptors during infection (64,65).

For patients infected in the West with HIV-1 subtype B, who provided the vast majority of clinical isolates analyzed in the laboratory, early infections were regularly "slow-low" or macrophage-tropic, but half or more of the patients gave rise to "lymphotropic" phenotypes by the time they developed clinical AIDS (66). This was subsequently found to hold for HIV-1s of some other subtypes, such as HIV-1A and HIV-1D, but not for HIV-1C (67–69). In the case of HIV-1C, even patients with late AIDS disease regularly have viremia with virus of the macrophage "slow-low" phenotype. In most or all cases of infection through sexual routes, the "macrophage-tropic" viruses appear to predominate for all subtypes (70).

DISEASE DEVELOPMENT AND PROGRESSION

Following infection by sexual routes, an acute disease syndrome may occur within 2 to 5 weeks. This syndrome is characterized by general lymphopenia and a high-level viremia (Figure 2). As the symptoms become resolved, the viremia is usually reduced by a hundred-fold or more, presumably due to an immune response that includes both viral neutralizing antibodies and cytolytic T-cells. The baseline level of virus replication that occurs immediately after the acute viremia resolves is often called the setpoint. A lower setpoint is thought to be associated with better prognosis; individuals with the lowest setpoints are more likely to survive for prolonged periods as "long-term nonprogressors."

The lymphopenia that occurs during both acute disease and several years later is presumably largely due to the formation of syncitia as well as the direct killing of T4 cells by HIV (71,72). Although virus envelope determinants seem important for cell killing as well as coreceptor tropism, other viral genetic determinants can also have a strong effect on virus activation and replication rates (73).

The amount of virus in the blood appears to be well correlated with disease development and progression. Although only 1% or less of the T4 lymphocytes in blood

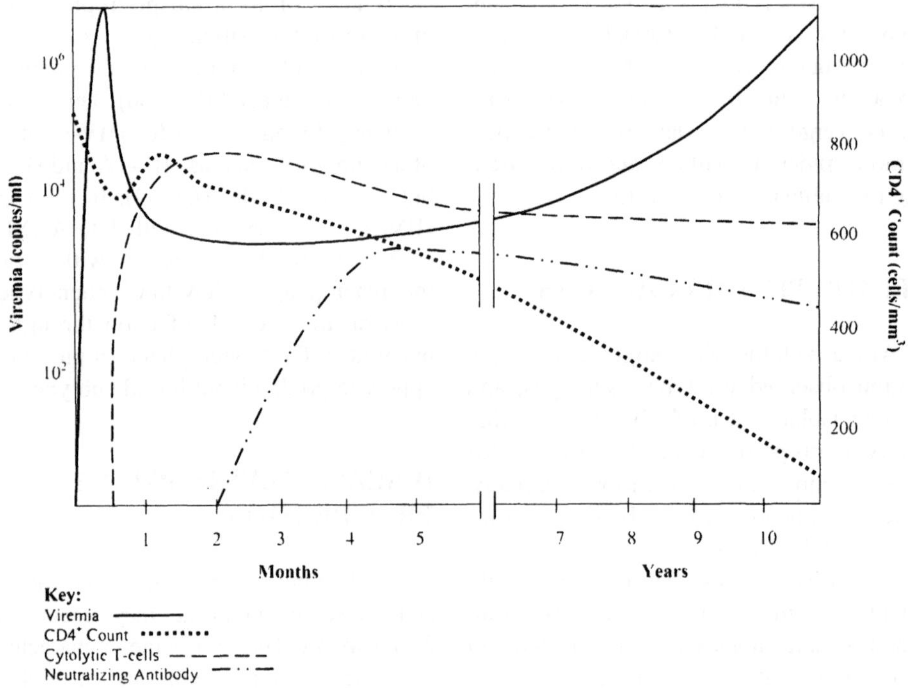

FIGURE 2. Kinetics of viremia, immune responsiveness, and immune cell deterioration in typical infection.

appear to be infected during most stages, 100-fold or more of the T4 cells in lymph nodes may be infected (74,75). This seems highly relevant because only a small fraction of lymphocytes are circulating at any given time. HIV made by lymph node cells spills over to show free virus and viral proteins in the blood. Although blood is the easiest source for sampling cells, it gives a misleading view of the percentage of lymphocytes that may be infected and thus killed by the infection.

Although a few infected individuals may become long-term nonprogressors, most progress to lymphocyte depletion and disease development within 8 to 12 years (76–78). A small fraction progress to disease within 2 to 3 years (79), but most remain disease-free for 5 to 6 years. Rapid progressors have the highest viral load at early stages (80,81), presumably because they fail to mount a significant immune response and harbor a higher fraction of infected T4 cells in the lymph nodes. Neutralizing antibodies are thought to be important in early infections (82–84), though they clearly fail to eliminate virus from the host. Both neutralizing antibodies and cytolytic T-cell responses are thought to be more robust in long-term nonprogressors (85, 86). The genetics of the infected individuals may also impact the rate of disease development, presumably through both immune responses and other mechanisms (see Chapter 4, *this volume*). Persistent antigenic stimulation of infected immune cells may also accelerate disease development by causing such cells to replicate and release HIV. Some of the same pathogens that cause AIDS-related diseases, such as cytomegalovirus and tuberculosis, may in turn accelerate virus replication and release (87). Such organisms may cause tissue damage, activating inflammatory cytokines such as tumor necrosis factor, which in turn activate HIV (88).

Virtually all of the studies to determine the natural history of HIV infection have been conducted with western populations infected with HIV-1B as homosexuals or injection drug users. Thus, whether some variation might occur with other viruses, heterosexual infection, or different genetic responses is unclear. Potential opportunistic infections may also occur at different rates in different environments, especially when comparing the tropical climate of Africa to the temperate climate of the West. One recent study suggested slight differences in rates of progression to clinical AIDS for Senegalese women according to subtype of HIV-1 (89). Another study showed differences in mother-to-infant transmission according to HIV-1 subtype in Tanzania, suggesting that differences in viral load or cell tropism may be present, at least in some body compartments (90). Many more studies must be done in African populations to determine whether significant differences in the natural history of disease may be present in different regions.

REFERENCES

1. Gottlieb MS, Schroff R, Schanker HM, et al. Pneumocystis carinii pneumonia and mucosal candidiasis in previously healthy homosexual men: evidence of a new acquired cellular immunodeficiency. *N Engl J Med*, 1981;305:1425–1431.
2. Masur H, Michelis MA, Greene JB, et al. An outbreak of community-acquired Pneumocystis carinii pneumonia: initial manifestation of cellular immune dysfunction. *N Engl J Med*, 1981;305:1431–1438.
3. Siegal FP, Lopez C, Hammer GS, et al. Severe acquired immunodeficiency in male homosexuals, manifested by chronic perianal ulcerative herpes simplex lesions. *N Engl J Med*, 1981;305:1439–1444.
4. Epidemiologic aspects of the current outbreak of Kaposi's sarcoma and opportunistic infections. *N Engl J Med*, 1982;306:248–252.
5. Davis KC, Horsburgh CR, Jr., Hasiba U, et al. Acquired immunodeficiency syndrome in a patient with hemophilia. *Ann Intern Med*, 1983;98:284–286.
6. Poon MC, Landay A, Prasthofer EF, et al. Acquired immunodeficiency syndrome with Pneumocystis carinii pneumonia and Mycobacterium avium-intracellulare infection in a previously healthy patient with classic hemophilia. Clinical, immunologic, and virologic findings. *Ann Intern Med*, 1983;98:287–290.
7. Elliott JL, Hoppes WL, Platt MS, et al. The acquired immunodeficiency syndrome and Mycobacterium avium-intracellulare bacteremia in a patient with hemophilia. *Ann Intern Med*, 1983;98:290–293.
8. Curran JW, Lawrence DN, Jaffe H, et al. Acquired immunodeficiency syndrome (AIDS) associated with transfusions. *N Engl J Med*, 1984;310:69–75.
9. Jaffe HW, Francis DP, McLane MF, et al. Transfusion-associated AIDS: serologic evidence of human T-cell leukemia virus infection of donors. *Science*, 1984;223:1309–1312.
10. Rubinstein A, Sicklick M, Gupta A, et al. Acquired immunodeficiency with reversed T4/T8 ratios in infants born to promiscuous and drug-addicted mothers. *JAMA*, 1983;249:2350–2356.
11. Oleske J, Minnefor A, Cooper R, Jr., et al. Immune deficiency syndrome in children. *JAMA*, 1983;249:2345–2349.
12. Clumeck N, Mascart-Lemone F, de Maubeuge J, et al. Acquired immune deficiency syndrome in Black Africans. *Lancet*, 1983;1:642.
13. Francis DP, Curran JW, Essex M. Epidemic acquired immune deficiency syndrome: epidemiologic evidence for a transmissible agent. *J Natl Cancer Inst*, 1983;71:1–4.
14. Rogers MF, Morens DM, Stewart JA. National case-control study of Kaposi's sarcoma and *Pneumo-cystis carinii* pneumonia in homosexual men: part 2, laboratory results. *Ann Intern Med*, 1983;99:151.
15. Essex M. The New AIDS Epidemic. *Harvard Magazine*, 1999;101:37–42.
16. Poiesz BJ, Ruscetti FW, Gazdar AF, et al. Detection and isolation of type C retrovirus particles from fresh and cultured lymphocytes of a patient with cutaneous T-cell lymphoma. *Proc Natl Acad Sci USA*, 1980;77:7415–7419.
17. Durst M, Gissmann L, Ikenberg H, et al. A papillomavirus DNA from a cervical carcinoma and its prevalence in cancer biopsy samples from different geographic regions. *Proc Natl Acad Sci USA*, 1983;80:3812–3815.
18. Ammann AJ, Abrams D, Conant M, et al. Acquired immune dysfunction in homosexual men: immunologic profiles. *Clin Immunol Immunopathol*, 1983; 27:315–325.
19. Fahey JL, Prince H, Weaver M, et al. Quantitative changes in T helper or T suppressor/cytotoxic lymphocyte subsets that distinguish acquired immune deficiency syndrome from other immune subset disorders. *Am J Med*, 1984;76:95–100.
20. Essex M, McLane MF, Tachibana N. Sero-epidemiology of HTLV in relation to immunosuppression and the acquired immunodeficiency syndrome. In: Gallo RC, Essex M, Gross L, eds. *Human T-cell Leukemia/Lymphoma Viruses*. Cold Spring Harbor: Cold Spring Harbor Press, 1984:355–362.

21. Essex M, McLane MF, Lee TH, et al. Antibodies to cell membrane antigens associated with human T-cell leukemia virus in patients with AIDS. *Science*, 1983;220:859–862.
22. Essex M, McLane MF, Lee TH, et al. Antibodies to human T-cell leukemia virus membrane antigens (HTLV-MA) in hemophiliacs. *Science*, 1983;221: 1061–1064.
23. Gelmann EP, Popovic M, Blayney D, et al. Proviral DNA of a retrovirus, human T-cell leukemia virus, in two patients with AIDS. *Science*, 1983;220: 862–865.
24. Gallo RC, Sarin PS, Gelmann EP, et al. Isolation of human T-cell leukemia virus in acquired immune deficiency syndrome (AIDS). *Science*, 1983;220: 865–867.
25. Barre-Sinoussi F, Chermann JC, Rey F, et al. Isolation of a T-lymphotropic retrovirus from a patient at risk for acquired immune deficiency syndrome (AIDS). *Science*, 1983;220:868–871.
26. Supparatpinyo K, Khamwan C, Baosoung V, et al. Disseminated Penicillium marneffei infection in southeast Asia. *Lancet*, 1994;344:110–113.
27. Serwadda D, Mugerwa RD, Sewankambo NK, et al. Slim disease: a new disease in Uganda and its association with HTLV-III infection. *Lancet*, 1985;2:849–852.
28. Duesberg P. HIV is not the cause of AIDS. *Science*, 1988;241:514–517.
29. Jarrett WFH, Crawford E, Martin WB, et al. A virus-like particle associated with leukaemia. *Nature (London)*, 1964;202:567–569.
30. Gardner MB. Neurotropic retroviruses of wild mice and macaques. *Ann Neurol*, 1988;23: S201–S206.
31. Essex M, Hardy WD, Jr., Cotter SM, et al. Naturally occurring persistent feline oncornavirus infections in the absence of disease. *Infect Immun*, 1975;11:470–475.
32. Huebner RJ, Todaro GJ. Oncogenes of RNA tumor viruses as determinants of cancer. *Proc Natl Acad Sci USA*, 1969;64:1087–1094.
33. Hardy WD, Jr., Old LJ, Hess PW, et al. Horizontal transmission of feline leukaemia virus. *Nature*, 1973;244:266–269.
34. Bebenek K, Abbotts J, Roberts JD, et al. Specificity and mechanism of error-prone replication by human immunodeficiency virus-1 reverse transcriptase. *J Biol Chem*, 1989;264:16948–16956.
35. Boyer JC, Bebenek K, Kunkel TA. Unequal human immunodeficiency virus type 1 reverse transcriptase error rates with RNA and DNA templates. *Proc Natl Acad Sci USA*, 1992;89:6919–6923.
36. Folks TM, Hart CE. The life cycle of human immunodeficiency virus type 1. In: DeVita VT, Hellman S, Rosenberg SA, Curran J, Essex M, Fauci AS, eds. *AIDS Etiology, Diagnosis, Treatment and Prevention*. Philadelphia: Lippincott Co., 1997:29–43.
37. Robertson DL, Sharp PM, McCutchan FE, et al. Recombination in HIV-1. *Nature*, 1995;374: 124–126.
38. Kanki PJ, McLane MF, King NW, Jr., et al. Serologic identification and characterization of a macaque T- lymphotropic retrovirus closely related to HTLV-III. *Science*, 1985;228:1199–1201.
39. Daniel MD, Letvin NL, King NW, et al. Isolation of T-cell tropic HTLV-III-like retrovirus from macaques. *Science*, 1985;228:1201–1204.
40. Kanki PJ, Kurth R, Becker W, et al. Antibodies to simian T-lymphotropic retrovirus type III in African green monkeys and recognition of STLV-III viral proteins by AIDS and related sera. *Lancet*, 1985;1:1330–1332.
41. Tsujimoto H, Hasegawa A, Maki N, et al. Sequence of a novel simian immunodeficiency virus from a wild-caught African mandrill. *Nature*, 1989;341: 539–541.
42. Muller MC, Saksena NK, Nerrienet E, et al. Simian immunodeficiency viruses from central and western Africa: evidence for a new species-specific lentivirus in tantalus monkeys. *J Virol*, 1993; 67:1227–1235.
43. Peeters M, Janssens W, Fransen K, et al. Isolation of simian immunodeficiency viruses from two sooty mangabeys in Cote d'Ivoire: virological and genetic characterization and relationship to other HIV type 2 and SIVsm/mac strains. *AIDS Res Hum Retroviruses*, 1994;10:1289–1294.
44. Essex M, Kanki PJ. The origins of the AIDS virus. *Sci Am*, 1988;259:64–71.
45. Barin F, M'Boup S, Denis F, et al. Serological evidence for virus related to simian T-lymphotropic retrovirus III in residents of West Africa. *Lancet*, 1985;2:1387–1389.
46. Kanki PJ, Barin F, M'Boup S, et al. New human T-lymphotropic retrovirus related to simian T-lymphotropic virus type III (STLV-IIIAGM). *Science*, 1986;232:238–243.
47. Marlink R, Kanki P, Thior I, et al. Reduced rate of disease development after HIV-2 infection as compared to HIV-1. *Science*, 1994;265:1587–1590.
48. Kanki PJ, Travers KU, Mboup S, et al. Slower heterosexual spread of HIV-2 than HIV-1. *Lancet*, 1994;343:943–946.
49. Andreasson PA, Dias F, Naucler A, et al. A prospective study of vertical transmission of HIV-2 in Bissau, Guinea-Bissau. *AIDS*, 1993;7:989–993.
50. Adjorlolo-Johnson G, De Cock KM, Ekpini E, et al. Prospective comparison of mother-to-child transmission of HIV-1 and HIV-2 in Abidjan, Ivory Coast. *JAMA*, 1994;272:462–466.
51. Kanki P. Epidemiology and natural history of human immunodeficiency virus type 2. In: DeVita VT, Hellman S, Rosenberg SA, Curran J, Essex M, Fauci AS, eds. *AIDS Etiology, Diagnosis,*

Treatment and Prevention. Philadelphia: Lippincott Co., 1997:127–135.

52. Louwagie J, McCutchan F, Van der Groen G, et al. Genetic comparison of HIV-1 isolates from Africa, Europe, and North America. *AIDS Res Hum Retroviruses*, 1992;8:1467–1469.
53. Louwagie J, McCutchan FE, Peeters M, et al. Phylogenetic analysis of gag genes from 70 international HIV-1 isolates provides evidence for multiple genotypes. *AIDS*, 1993;7:769–780.
54. Gurtler LG, Hauser PH, Eberle J, et al. A new subtype of human immunodeficiency virus type 1 (MVP-5180) from Cameroon. *J Virol*, 1994;68: 1581–1585.
55. Janssens W, Nkengasong JN, Heyndrickx L, et al. Further evidence of the presence of genetically aberrant HIV-1 strains in Cameroon and Gabon. *AIDS*, 1994;8:1012–1013.
56. McCutchan FE. Understanding the genetic diversity of HIV-1. *AIDS*, 2000;14:S31–S44.
57. Sullivan PS, Do AN, Ellenberger D, et al. Human immunodeficiency virus (HIV) subtype surveillance of African-born persons at risk for group O and group N HIV infections in the United States. *J Infect Dis*, 2000;181:463–469.
58. Huet T, Cheynier R, Meyerhans A, et al. Genetic organization of a chimpanzee lentivirus related to HIV-1. *Nature*, 1990;345:356–359.
59. Gao F, Robertson DL, Morrison SG, et al. The heterosexual human immunodeficiency virus type 1 epidemic in Thailand is caused by an intersubtype (A/E) recombinant of African origin. *J Virol*, 1996;70:7013–7029.
60. Carr JK, Salminen MO, Albert J, et al. Full genome sequences of human immunodeficiency virus type 1 subtypes G and A/G intersubtype recombinants. *Virology*, 1998;247:22–31.
61. Sankale JL, Hamel D, Woolsey A, et al. Molecular evolution of human immunodeficiency virus type 1 subtype A in Senegal: 1988–1997. *J Hum Virol*, 2000;3:157–164.
62. Asjo B, Morfeldt-Manson L, Albert J, et al. Replicative capacity of human immunodeficiency virus from patients with varying severity of HIV infection. *Lancet*, 1986;2:660–662.
63. Shioda T, Levy JA, Cheng-Mayer C. Small amino acid changes in the V3 hypervariable region of gp120 can affect the T-cell-line and macrophage tropism of human immunodeficiency virus type 1. *Proc Natl Acad Sci USA*, 1992;89:9434–9438.
64. Feng Y, Broder CC, Kennedy PE, et al. HIV-1 entry cofactor: functional cDNA cloning of a seven-transmembrane, G protein-coupled receptor. *Science*, 1996;272:872–877.
65. Alkhatib G, Combadiere C, Broder CC, et al. CC CKR5: a RANTES, MIP-1alpha, MIP-1beta receptor as a fusion cofactor for macrophage-tropic HIV-1. *Science*, 1996;272:1955–1958.
66. Tersmette M, Lange JM, de Goede RE, et al. Association between biological properties of human immunodeficiency virus variants and risk for AIDS and AIDS mortality. *Lancet*, 1989;1:983–985.
67. Tscherning C, Alaeus A, Fredriksson R, et al. Differences in chemokine coreceptor usage between genetic subtypes of HIV-1. *Virology*, 1998;241:181–188.
68. Peeters M, Vincent R, Perret JL, et al. Evidence for differences in MT2 cell tropism according to genetic subtypes of HIV-1: syncytium-inducing variants seem rare among subtype C HIV-1 viruses. *J Acquir Immune Defic Syndr Hum Retrovirol*, 1999;20:115–121.
69. Ping LH, Nelson JA, Hoffman IF, et al. Characterization of V3 sequence heterogeneity in subtype C human immunodeficiency virus type 1 isolates from Malawi: underrepresentation of X4 variants. *J Virol*, 1999;73:6271–6281.
70. Choe H, Farzan M, Sun Y, et al. The beta-chemokine receptors CCR3 and CCR5 facilitate infection by primary HIV-1 isolates. *Cell*, 1996;85:1135–1148.
71. Wei X, Ghosh SK, Taylor ME, et al. Viral dynamics in human immunodeficiency virus type 1 infection. *Nature*, 1995;373:117–122.
72. Ho DD, Neumann AU, Perelson AS, et al. Rapid turnover of plasma virions and CD4 lymphocytes in HIV-1 infection. *Nature*, 1995;373:123–126.
73. Montano MA, Novitsky VA, Blackard JT, et al. Divergent transcriptional regulation among expanding human immunodeficiency virus type 1 subtypes. *J Virol*, 1997;71:8657–8665.
74. Pantaleo G, Graziosi C, Demarest JF, et al. HIV infection is active and progressive in lymphoid tissue during the clinically latent stage of disease. *Nature*, 1993;362:355–358.
75. Embretson J, Zupancic M, Ribas JL, et al. Massive covert infection of helper T lymphocytes and macrophages by HIV during the incubation period of AIDS. *Nature*, 1993;362:359–362.
76. Lifson AR, Buchbinder SP, Sheppard HW, et al. Long-term human immunodeficiency virus infection in asymptomatic homosexual and bisexual men with normal CD4+ lymphocyte counts: immunologic and virologic characteristics. *J Infect Dis*, 1991;163:959–965.
77. Buchbinder SP, Katz MH, Hessol NA, et al. Long-term HIV-1 infection without immunologic progression. *AIDS*, 1994;8:1123–1128.
78. Schrager LK, Young JM, Fowler MG, et al. Long-term survivors of HIV-1 infection: definitions and research challenges. *AIDS*, 1994;8:S95.
79. Phair JP. Keynote address: variations in the natural history of HIV infection. *AIDS Res Hum Retroviruses*, 1994;10:883–885.
80. Gupta P, Kingsley L, Armstrong J, et al. Enhanced expression of human immunodeficiency virus type

1 correlates with development of AIDS. *Virology*, 1993;196:586–595.

81. Saksela K, Stevens C, Rubinstein P, et al. Human immunodeficiency virus type 1 mRNA expression in peripheral blood cells predicts disease progression independently of the numbers of CD4+ lymphocytes. *Proc Natl Acad Sci USA*, 1994;91: 1104–1108.
82. Matthews TJ, Langlois AJ, Robey WG, et al. Restricted neutralization of divergent human T-lymphotropic virus type III isolates by antibodies to the major envelope glycoprotein. *Proc Natl Acad Sci USA*, 1986;83:9709–9713.
83. Albert J, Abrahamsson B, Nagy K, et al. Rapid development of isolate-specific neutralizing antibodies after primary HIV-1 infection and consequent emergence of virus variants which resist neutralization by autologous sera. *AIDS*, 1990;4:107–112.
84. Moore JP, Cao Y, Ho DD, et al. Development of the anti-gp120 antibody response during seroconversion to human immunodeficiency virus type 1. *J Virol*, 1994;68:5142–5155.
85. Cao Y, Quin L, Zhang L, et al. Virologic and immunologic characterization of long-term survivors of human immunodeficiency virus type 1 infection. *N Engl J Med*, 1995;332:201–208.
86. Klein MR, van Baalen CA, Holwerda AM, et al. Kinetics of Gag-specific cytotoxic T lymphocyte responses during the clinical course of HIV-1 infection: a longitudinal analysis of rapid progressors and long-term asymptomatics. *J Exp Med*, 1995;181:1365–1372.
87. Rosenberg ZF, Fauci AS. Immunopathogenesis of HIV infection. *FASEB J*, 1991;5:2382–2390.
88. Montano MA, Nixon CP, Ndung'u T, et al. Elevated tumor necrosis factor-alpha activation of human immunodeficiency virus type 1 subtype C in Southern Africa is associated with an NF-kappaB enhancer gain-of-function. *J Infect Dis*, 2000;181:76–81.
89. Kanki PJ, Hamel DJ, Sankale JL, et al. Human immunodeficiency virus type 1 subtypes differ in disease progression. *J Infect Dis*, 1999;179:68–73.
90. Renjifo B, Fawzi W, Mwakagile D, et al. Differences in perinatal transmission among human immunodeficiency virus type 1 genotypes. *J Hum Virol*, 2001;4:16–25.

2

The Molecular Virology of HIV-1

*Monty Montano and †Carolyn Williamson

*Section of Infectious Diseases, Department of Medicine, Boston University School of Medicine, Boston, Massachusetts, 02118 USA.
†Division of Medical Virology, University of Capetown, Capetown, South Africa.

The human immunodeficiency virus type 1 (HIV-1) belongs to the genus *Lentivirus* of the family Retroviridae. Retroviruses derive their name from the Latin "retro" ("backwards") because they transcribe DNA from a viral RNA template, a process reverse to the usual flow of genetic information. It is this fundamental feature of their replication that provides the basis for their enormous adaptability: reverse transcriptase, the enzyme responsible for transcribing the viral RNA into DNA, has no proofreading function. As a result, errors introduced during replication remain uncorrected. Mutation, along with recombination, enables HIV-1 to rapidly respond to selection pressures within the environment. This chapter will describe features of HIV-1 within the context of other known retroviruses. The nonhuman primate origins and evolution of HIV-1 will be discussed, as well as the molecular basis for the viral life cycle, with an emphasis on each viral gene product in relation to viral replication within host cells. Finally, the concept of "adaptive landscape" will be introduced and the potential adaptive response within the human population will be discussed.

CLASSIFICATION OF RETROVIRUSES

Historically, retroviruses were classified into three subfamilies (Oncovirinae, Lentivirinae, Spumavirinae) based on pathogenic, morphologic and biologic features. However, as more information became available, particularly sequence data, it became apparent that this classification system was no longer relevant. Retroviruses are now classified into seven genera (Table 1) (1), with HIV falling into the *Lentivirus* group. Lentiviruses have been detected in a range of vertebrates including cattle (bovine immunodeficiency virus), horses (equine infectious anemia virus), cats (feline immunodeficiency virus), sheep (maedi–visna virus), goats (caprine arthritis-encephalitis virus), and primates. Human primate lentiviruses include HIV-1 and human immunodeficiency virus type 2 (HIV-2), which is less pathogenic than HIV-1. Nonhuman primate lentiviruses include the simian immmunodeficiency viruses (SIVs), which are widely distributed in African primates. Although SIV causes an AIDS-like disease in certain monkeys, it is usually nonpathogenic in its natural host (2).

TABLE 1. Retrovirus Classification

Genus*	Previous classification#	Type species*	Host	Comments§
Alpharetrovirus	Avian type C retroviruses	Avian leukosis virus (ALV)	Birds	Exogenous and endogenous viruses with simple genomes; "C" type morphology; many contain oncogenes; associated with malignancies and other disease.
Betaretrovirus	Mammalian type B oncoviruses, and "type D" retroviruses	Mouse mammary tumor virus (MMTV)	Mice, primates, sheep	Endogenous and exogenous viruses with simple genomes; "B-type" or "D-type" morphology; may be associated with mammary carcinoma, T-cell lymphomas or immunodeficiency.
Gammaretrovirus	Mammalian type C retroviruses	Murine leukaemia virus (MLV)	Mice, guineapigs, pigs, squirrel, snakes, chickens, ducks, cat, primates	Endogenous and exogenous viruses with simple genomes; "C-type" morphology; many contain oncogenes; associated with a variety of diseases including malignancies, immunosuppression, neurological disorders.
Deltaretrovirus	BLV-HTLV retroviruses	Bovine leukaemia virus (BLV)	Cattle, primates	Exogenous viruses with complex genomes; associated with B- or T- cell leukemias or lymphomas as well as neurological disease.
Epsilonretrovirus	Unclassified	Walleye dermal sarcoma virus (WDSV)	Fish	Exogenous viruses with complex genomes.
Lentivirus	Lentivirus	Human immunodeficiency 1 (HIV-1)	Primates, sheep, goats, horses, cats, cattle	Exogenous viruses with complex genomes. Associated with variety of diseases including immunodeficiencies, neurological disorders, arthritis and others.
Spumavirus	Spumavirus	Chimpanzee foamy virus (formerly called Human foamy virus)	Cattle, primates, cats (no natural human infections)	Exogenous viruses with complex genomes; no known disease association.

*Hunter E, Casey J, Hahn B, et al. Family Retroviridae in virus taxonomy. Seventh Report of the International Committee on Taxonomy of Viruses. In: van Regenmortel MHV, Fauquet CM, Bishop DHL, et al., eds., San Diego: Academic Press, 2000:369–387.

#1998 Retroviridae Study Group, ICTV.

§ Endogenous: provirus integrated into the germline and passed from parent to offspring.
Simple genomes: genomes encode for structural genes.
Complex genomes: encode for structural genes as well as a range of additional regulatory and accessory proteins which regulate expression and are essential for their life cycle.

GENERAL MORPHOLOGIC AND GENETIC CHARACTERISTICS OF RETROVIRUSES

Mature retrovirus particles are spherical with a diameter of 80 to 100 nm. Virions have an outer lipid bilayer that is cellular in origin. For simple retroviruses, such as murine leukemia virus (MLV), the viral gene organization includes *gag, pro, pol,* and *env. Gag* encodes the internal structural polyprotein of the virus and is proteolytically processed into mature proteins—MA (matrix), CA (capsid), NC (nucleocapsid)—and into other, less well characterized proteins. The viral core contains two identical copies of single-stranded, positive sense RNA bound to NC. *Pol* encodes the enzyme reverse transcriptase (RT), which contains both DNA polymerase and associated RNAseH activities, and integrase (IN), which mediates insertion of the provirus into the host genome. *Pro* encodes the viral protease (PR), which acts late in assembly of the viral particle to process proteolytically the proteins coded for by *gag, pro,* and *pol*, and, in some cases, *env. Env* encodes the surface (SU) glycoprotein and the transmembrane (TM) glycoprotein of the virion, which form a complex that interacts specifically with cellular receptor and coreceptor proteins. This interaction ultimately leads to fusion of the viral membrane with the cell membrane. Complex retroviruses, such as human T-lymphotropic virus (HTLV) and HIV also contain accessory genes. Accessory genes regulate and coordinate viral gene expression as well as other functions. These genes generally flank *env* or overlap portions of *env* and require splicing. Retroviruses have two distinct morphogenetic pathways known as C-type and A-type. C-type particles assemble at the plasma membrane in the form of an inverted C while A-type particles (immature virions) assemble in the cytoplasm. These immature particles then bud through the cell membrane to produce virions with a secondary B-type [mouse mammary tumor virus (MMTV)] or D-type morphology [Mason–Pfizer monkey virus (M-PMV)] according to the International Committee on Taxonomy of Viruses (ICTV) (3).

HIV-1 has a number of regulatory and accessory genes including *vif, vpr, tat, rev, vpu,* and *nef* that encode proteins that are essential to the viral life cycle (Figures 1,2). The virus maximizes use of the sequence by encoding overlapping reading frames. In addition, *tat* and *rev* consist of two exons with the second exon overlapping the *env* coding region. This basic genome organization holds for all primate lentiviruses, except HIV-1 and SIVcpz, which have an additional gene, *vpu*, upstream of *env*, and HIV-2 and SIVsm, which have an additional gene, *vpx*, also upstream of *env* (Figure 2). HIV-2 and HIV-1 also differ in that the HIV-2 *env* open reading frame overlaps the *nef* open reading frame, a situation which may constrain diversity.

PRIMATE LENTIVIRUSES

SIV is the closest relative to the HIVs and understanding the relationship between HIV-1, HIV-2, SIV, and their hosts, is important for a number of reasons: SIV is the animal model most commonly used in vaccine and pathogenicity studies (4); research of SIV contributes to our understanding of host protective mechanisms because SIV does not seem to cause disease in its natural host (although it does cause disease in Asian macaques) (5,2); understanding the origins of HIV-1, the reservoir of HIV-1 infection, and the mechanisms of zoonotic transmission will contribute to the prevention of similar epidemics in the future; and, analysis of HIV-1 ancestral sequences provides information researchers need to deduce viral rates of change and anticipate future variations that may be relevant to vaccine design.

The primate lentiviruses fall into six lineages based on phylogenetic analysis of nucleic acid sequences (6–8). It is hypothesized that both HIV-1 and HIV-2 originated

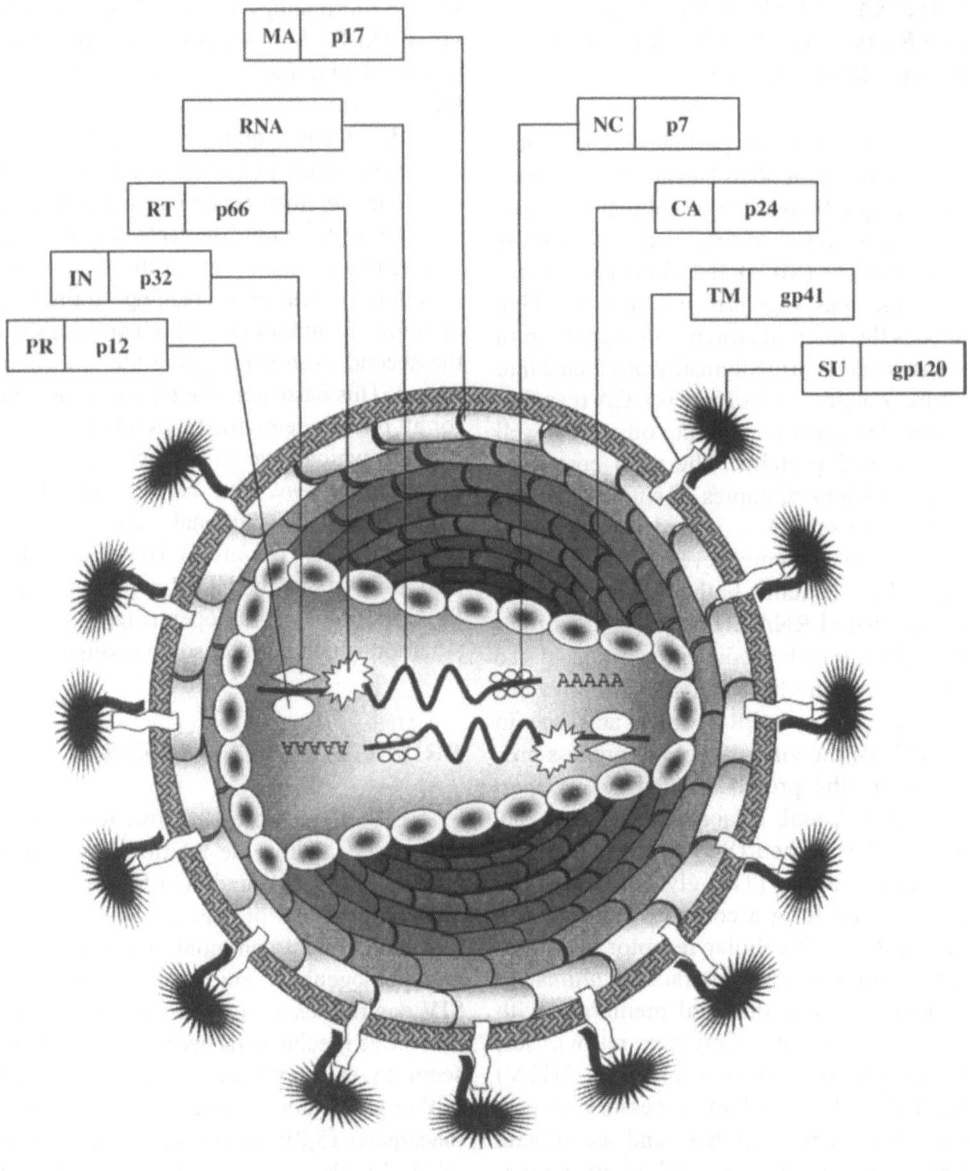

FIGURE 1. Organization of the mature HIV-1 virion. Component parts of the genome are indicated. PR indicates protease; IN, integrase; RT, reverse transcriptase; MA, matrix; NC, nucleocapsid; CA, capsid; TM, transmembrane; SU, surface.

in distinct primate species and were transmitted from primates to humans in a number of independent cross-species transmission events. The evidence that HIV-2 originated in sooty mangabeys *(Cercocebus atys)* rests on the knowledge that HIV-2 is indistinguishable from SIVsm both genomically and phylogenically (Figure 2), that West Africa is the epicenter of both the HIV-2 and SIVsm infections, that SIVsm has been detected in a large number of wild sooty mangabeys in West Africa and in sooty mangabeys kept as domestic pets (9,10), and that SIV has the capacity to replicate in humans, discovered as a result of the inadvertent infection of a laboratory worker (11). Because some HIV-2

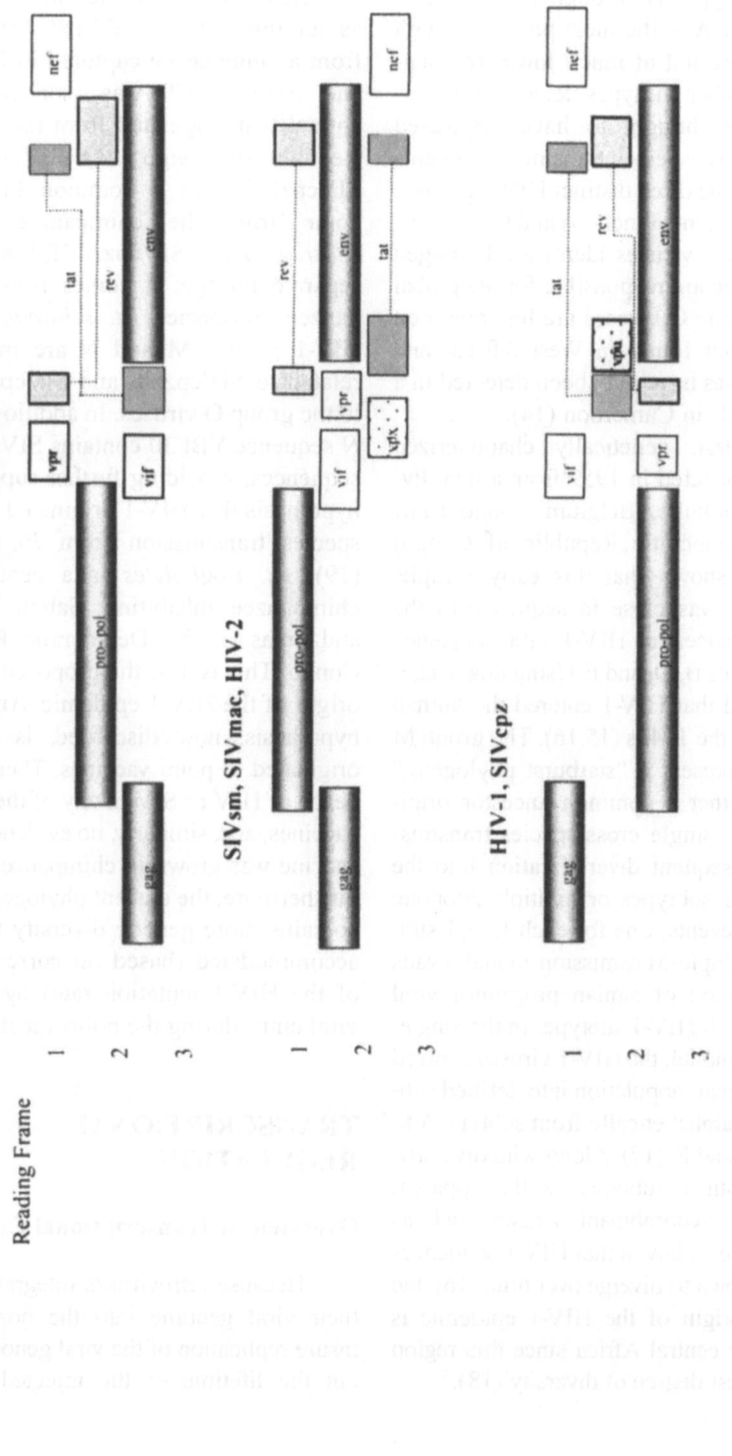

FIGURE 2. Primate lentivirus genome organization showing approximate size and position of genes. Representative isolates were used to indicate reading frames including SIVsyk for SIVagm, SIVsyk, SIVmnd, SIVl'hoest, SIVsun, and SIVcol; HIV-2 strain ben for SIVsm, SIVmac, and HIV-2; and HIV-1 strain HXB2 for HIV-1 and SIVcpz viruses. The reading frames may not be representative of all members of these groups.

subtypes are more closely related to SIVsm strains than to other HIV-2 subtypes, it is likely that SIVsm independently crossed the species barrier a number of times giving rise to HIV-2 subtypes A through F (10,12,13). HIV-2 subtype A is the most prevalent, with subtype B detected at much lower frequencies and the other subtypes detected rarely.

HIV-1 is thought to have originated from three cross-species transmission events giving rise to the three distinct HIV-1 groups: M (major), N (non-M, non-O) and O (outlier). The first HIV-1 viruses identified belonged to group M and are responsible for the global epidemic. Group O viruses are less common and most often found in West Africa, and group N viruses have only been detected in a few individuals in Cameroon (14).

The oldest, genetically characterized HIV-1 was collected in 1959 from a man living in Leopoldville, Belgium Congo (now Kinshasa, Democratic Republic of Congo) (15). It was shown that this early sample, called ZA59, was close in sequence to the hypothetical ancestral HIV-1 viral sequence for the subtypes B, D, and F. Using this data, it was estimated that HIV-1 entered the human population in the 1940s (15,16). The group M sequences represent a "starburst phylogeny," suggesting either a common ancestor originating from a single cross-species transmission and subsequent diversification into the distinct HIV-1 subtypes or multiple zoonotic transmission events, one for each HIV-1 subtype. The multiple-transmission model awaits the identification of simian progenitor viral isolates for each HIV-1 subtype. In the single-transmission model, the HIV-1 viruses evolved within the human population into defined subtypes named alphabetically from subtype A to D, F, G, H, J, and K (17). Along with diversification of distinct subtypes is the apparent emergence of recombinant viruses such as HIV-1 subtype E. Given that HIV-1 sequences have been shown to diverge over time (16), the geographic origin of the HIV-1 epidemic is thought to be central Africa since this region has the greatest degree of diversity (18).

The closest relatives to HIV-1 are SIV sequences isolated from members of the chimpanzee species *Pan troglodytes* (19,20). SIVcpzUS was isolated from a chimpanzee exported from Africa to the United States as an infant (19). SIVcpzGAB originated from a chimpanzee captured in Gabon (20), and SIVcpzANT was isolated from an animal that originated from the Democratic Republic of Congo (21). SIVcpzGAB and SIVcpzUS have a common lineage; both come from the chimpanzee subspecies *P.t. troglodytes*. SIVcpzANT, however, has a separate lineage; it comes from the chimpanzee subspecies *P.t. schweinfurthii* (19). HIV-1 groups M and N are more closely related to SIVcpzUS and SIVcpzGAB than to the group O viruses. In addition, the group N sequence YBF30 contains SIVcpzUS–like sequences, providing further support for the hypothesis that HIV-1 originated from cross-species transmission from *P.t. troglodytes* (19). *P.t. troglodytes* is a central African chimpanzee inhabiting Gabon, Cameroon, and areas of the Democratic Republic of Congo. This is also the proposed geographic origin of the HIV-1 epidemic. An alternative hypothesis, now discarded, is that HIV-1 originated in polio vaccines. There is no evidence of HIV or SIV in any of the early polio vaccines, and, similarly, no evidence that polio vaccine was grown in chimpanzee cells (22). Furthermore, the current phylogeny of HIV-1 contains more genetic diversity than can be accommodated (based on current estimates of the HIV-1 mutation rate) by a mode of viral entry during the polio vaccination.

TRANSCRIPTIONAL REGULATION

Overview of Transcriptional Control

Because retroviruses integrate a copy of their viral genome into the host cell, they insure replication of the viral genome throughout the lifetime of the infected cell. Once resident within the cellular genome, viral gene expression is initially dependent upon host-cell RNA polymerase II, which transcribes both cellular and viral genes. To influence the efficiency of RNA polymerase II transcription, the HIV-1 provirus has devised a set of *cis*-acting sequences within the long terminal repeat (LTR) that recruit transcription factors (that is, DNA-binding proteins that influence RNA transcription) to the HIV-1 promoter. Many cellular states can influence the nuclear location and activity of these transcription factors including the particular cell type, the differentiation state of the cell, the activation state of the cell brought about by extracellular signals (such as inflammatory cytokines), and the presence of other signaling coinfections. This potential variation in cellular states can yield considerable variation in the expression profile of HIV-1. However it is useful to view HIV-1 gene expression in two phases: early and late. In the early phase, relatively low levels of viral RNA are detected, while late in the cycle, virally encoded Tat mediates the production of higher levels of viral RNA.

HIV-1 transcription is influenced by two types of *cis*-acting control elements within the LTR: core and regulatory elements (Figure 3). Core elements are common to many, if not most, cellular and viral promoters and include DNA target sites for RNA polymerase II and transcription-associated factors (TAFs). Most core elements are proximal to the RNA start site (where RNA transcription begins). In general, a "TATA" sequence is the most common core promoter element, including for HIV-1. A complex HIV-1 initiator sequence (23–25), which overlaps the RNA transcription start site, also contributes to promoter activity.

For most promoters, the first step in transcription involves the assembly of a "preinitiation complex." This complex is formed by binding the transcription factor IID (TFIID) to the TATA box followed by the nucleation of the several TATA-binding-protein–(TBP) associated factors to form a holocomplex. This preinitiation complex is capable of mediating basal transcription of RNA (26).

Although core elements use factors common to most cell types, regulatory-enhancer elements provide the virus with the capacity for complex and variable expression based on the activity of cell-type-specific regulatory factors. Regulatory-control elements consist of an array of DNA sequences (that is, enhancers) generally located more distal to the RNA start site than core elements. Enhancers are short DNA sequences, 10 to 25 base pairs in length, that function as target binding sites for transcriptional regulators. The role of nuclear transcription factors within a specific cell type or at a particular developmental stage affects the relative activity of transcriptional control elements in the LTR. Cell signaling can alter the activity of transcription-changing viral expression as the physiologic state of the cell changes. Many immune-response cellular genes are regulated by enhancer elements similar to those present within HIV-1. This provides an efficient mechanism for coordinated response to cellular signals—viral quiescence when the cell is resting (for example, resting T-cell) and viral activation when the cell is stimulated (for example, activated T-cell).

The Cellular Activator NF-κB

Once a cell is infected, transcription of proviral DNA is influenced by an inducible class of cellular transcription factors encoded by the nuclear factor-kappaB (NF-κB)/Rel gene family (27,28). Proteins in this family form a variety of homodimers and heterodimers. The NF-κB heterodimer p50:p65 is found in the cytoplasm of non-activated lymphocytes bound to the negative regulator IκB. Binding of NF-κB to IκB prevents NF-κB from entering the nucleus (29). Multiple stimuli can lead to the release of NF-κB from IkB, allowing NF-κB to enter the nucleus to activate target genes that contain DNA sequences related to the κB enhancer site GGGACTTTCC.

Several lines of evidence have indicated NF-κB proteins are important in HIV transcription. HIV enhancer sites are present in all

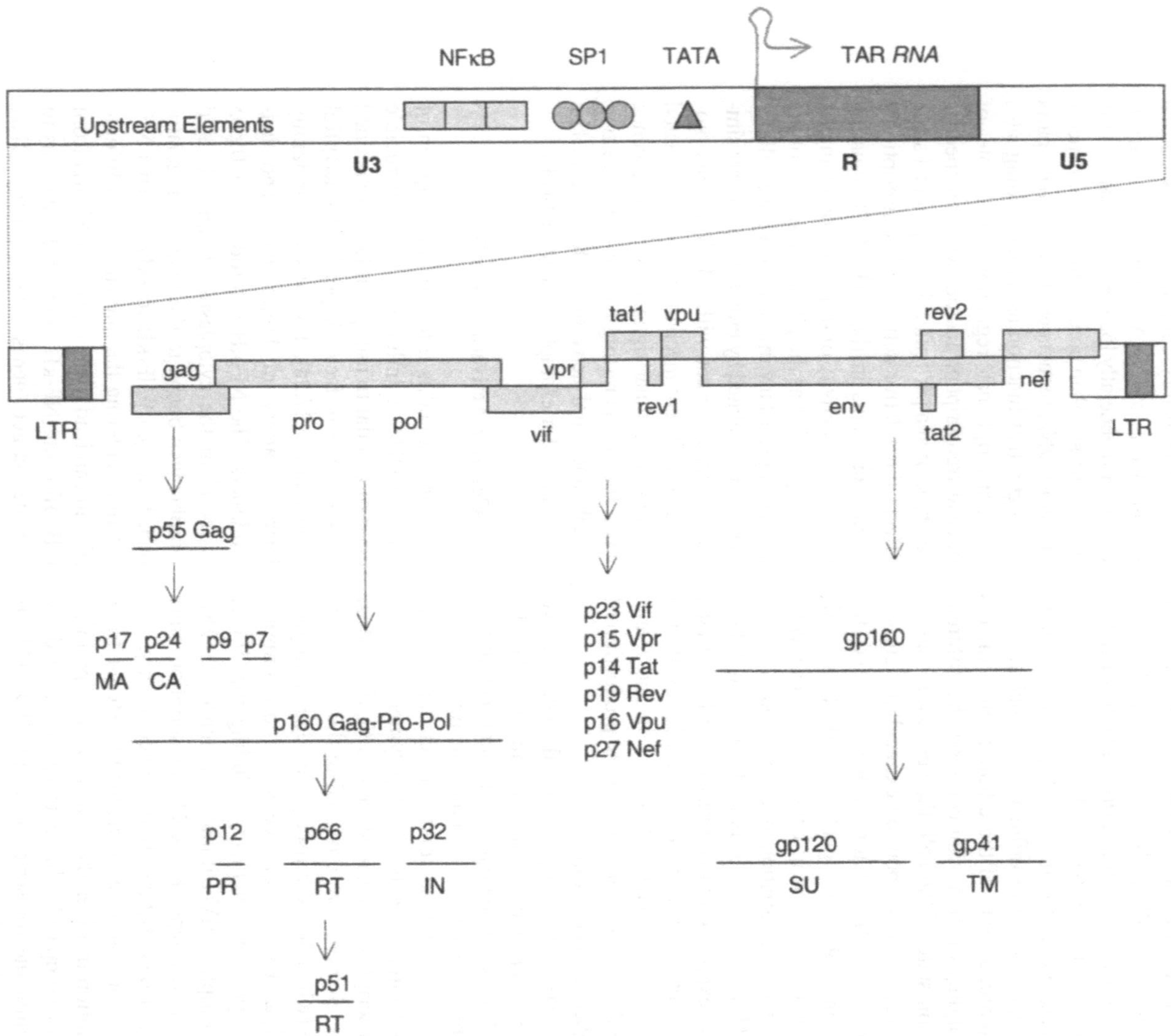

FIGURE 3. Organization of the HIV-1 long terminal repeat (LTR) and coding region of the genome in three open reading frames. All 15 proteins are indicated in stippled boxes. Polyprotein precursors are shown. NF-κB indicates nuclear factor-kappaB; TAR, transactivation response element; LTR, long terminal repeat; MA, matrix; CA, capsid; PR, protease; RT, reverse transcriptase; IN, integrase; SU, surface; TM, transmembrane.

HIV-1 isolates and are also found in HIV-2 isolates. It is interesting to note that HIV-1 subtype C isolates contain three, and sometimes four, copies of this critical enhancer (30–33). A variety of NF-κB homodimers and heterodimers have been shown to bind to the NF-κB sites in vitro. While transcription assays demonstrate that NF-κB proteins can function at these sites, various NF-κB species exert differential effects on HIV gene expression.

Strong support for a role of NF-κB in HIV-1 transcription comes from mutational analysis of the NF-κB binding sites. In transient-expression assays with reporter genes, a large number of stimuli that induce nuclear translocation of NF-κB have been shown to activate HIV-1 LTR-mediated transcription (27). Deletion of the NF-κB sites results in a loss of part or all of the LTR activation by these stimuli. Activation of latent HIV proviruses in T-cell lines and monocyte cell lines by cytokines such as tumor necrosis factor-alpha (TNF-α) and interleukin-1 (IL-1) correlates with the induction of nuclear NF-κB (34,35). TNF-α induction of HIV-1 gene expression has also been correlated with the copy number of NF-κB enhancer sites (36). T-cell lines containing an HIV provirus with deletions or mutations in the NF-κB binding sites do not undergo activation following cytokine treatment (37). Thus, HIV-1 transcription is influenced by the activation state of infected cells, and NF-κB proteins appear to be critical for the activation of silent integrated proviruses. An important evolutionary advantage conferred upon HIV-1 by the presence of NF-κB binding sites may be the capacity to activate integrated provirus following immune or cytokine stimulation of infected cells. The presence of this enhancer may provide a selective advantage by increasing the replication efficiency of HIV-1 under conditions of cellular stimulation.

The Retroviral Activator Tat

In contrast to simple retroviruses such as MLV, complex retroviruses such as HTLV and HIV have evolved regulatory mechanisms that employ virally encoded transcriptional activators in addition to core and regulatory elements for cellular activators. These *trans*-acting viral proteins establish a strong positive feedback loop that amplifies viral gene expression many-fold. In most cases, the expression of retroviral *trans*-activators has been associated with two distinct phases of retroviral infection (38,39). An early phase can be associated with gene expression restricted to multiply spliced regulatory genes, and a late phase can be associated with high-level expression of minimally spliced structural genes, enzymes, and genomic RNA.

The virally encoded transcriptional transactivator (Tat) is a small protein (86–102 amino acids) derived from the multiple splicing of two exons, one within the central region of the HIV-1 genome and one within *env* (40,41). Tat is a potent activator of HIV gene expression. The *tat* gene appears to be essential for HIV replication: mutations of *tat* introduced into infectious molecular clones of HIV-1 eliminate HIV-1 production (42,43). An interesting feature of Tat is its ability to be released from infected cells and to enter uninfected cells (44). Exogenous Tat can activate cellular gene expression by affecting cellular signal transduction pathways (45,46) and can influence the activity of transcription factors, for example, activator protein-1 (AP-1) (47,48); NF-κB (49,50), and NF-IL6 (51). Tat has also been shown to upregulate the expression of HIV-1 coreceptors, CCR5 and CXCR4, making cells potentially more susceptible to infection (52). The mechanism for Tat activation of cellular genes is unknown and requires further study.

Efforts to map the Tat-responsive region of the HIV LTR led to the unexpected discovery that Tat binds to an RNA element that forms a stable RNA stem-loop structure, referred to as the transactivation response element (TAR), present at the 5′ end of all HIV-1 RNAs (+1 to +59). The RNA secondary structure is highly conserved and required for Tat-mediated activation of HIV-1. A subdomain of Tat is sufficient for binding to TAR; arginine residues in the basic domain interact with a uridine residue (U23) at the base of the predicted bulge of TAR (53).

The biochemical mechanism by which Tat activates HIV-1 gene expression is not entirely resolved. There is strong evidence that Tat may enhance the efficiency of transcriptional elongation. HIV-1 RNA transcripts initiated in the absence of Tat tend to be truncated, suggesting inefficient elongation. Transcripts synthesized in the presence of Tat are more likely to be full length. Many cellular factors seem to interact with Tat to modulate HIV-1 transcription. One cellular complex, composed of the protein Cdk9 and cyclin-T, has been shown to bind to the activation domain of Tat and to promote phosphorylation of RNA polymerase II, resulting in an increase in transcription efficiency for HIV-1 RNA (54). Tat has also been shown to positively interact with the transcription factors NF-κB and Sp1, and with the oncoprotein Gli-2 (55), further indicating that many factors may converge upon Tat to influence HIV-1 expression.

Upstream Cellular Activators

Many sites have been identified in the upstream region of HIV-1 (56,57). Those for AP-1 and nuclear factor of activated T-cells (NFAT) will be discussed here.

AP-1 sites have been identified in upstream and downstream regions of the HIV-1 promoter and may play a role in cell-type-specific expression of HIV-1. AP-1 (a dimer composed of Jun and Fos protein subunits) is a member of the bZIP transcription-factor family, which also includes CREB/ATF and C/EBP families. These factors can form homodimers and heterodimers through a leucine zipper domain (58). A nonconsensus AP-1 site was recently identified in neurotropic strains of HIV-1 that interact with Jun and Fos (59). AP-1 binding in nuclear extracts from glial and HeLa cells has been observed but not in extracts from neuronal and Jurkat T-cells. AP-1 mediated transcriptional activation was also observed in glial but not neuronal cells.

In addition to AP-1, two sets of binding sites for NFAT have been identified in the HIV-1 LTR based on in-vitro footprinting. One of these sites overlaps with the NF-κB enhancer site. In cotransfection experiments, NFAT1 and NFATc (members of the NFAT family) are able to activate expression of HIV-1. This activation appears to be cyclosporin A-sensitive and it does not affect NF-κB–mediated HIV-1 activation but does require the NF-κB site (60). Thus, separate pathways of T-cell activation seem to converge on the NF-κB enhancer region to stimulate HIV-1 replication.

Collectively, these data support a capacity for alternative transcription complexes to form at the HIV-1 promoter. During latency, one type of promoter complex may mediate the formation of complexes that elongate inefficiently. Under cellular conditions of activation, however, many other potential promoter complexes may form that favor the formation of initiation complexes that elongate efficiently. The capacity for alternative transcription complexes to form at the same promoter underscores the variability in expression displayed by HIV-1 and necessitates an understanding of the context of HIV-1 infection. The multimode capacity for HIV-1 may allow for latency, perhaps to escape immune surveillance, or for vigorous replication within a short-lived activated lymphoid cell (61).

ASSEMBLY AND PROCESSING OF VIRAL PROTEINS

HIV-1 Replication

The HIV-1 life cycle can be viewed as a regulated sequential process that requires both viral and cellular proteins (Figure 4). The infection process can be viewed as beginning when SU envelope (Env) glycoprotein binds to the CD4 molecule on host cells and interacts with coreceptor. Following receptor binding, a

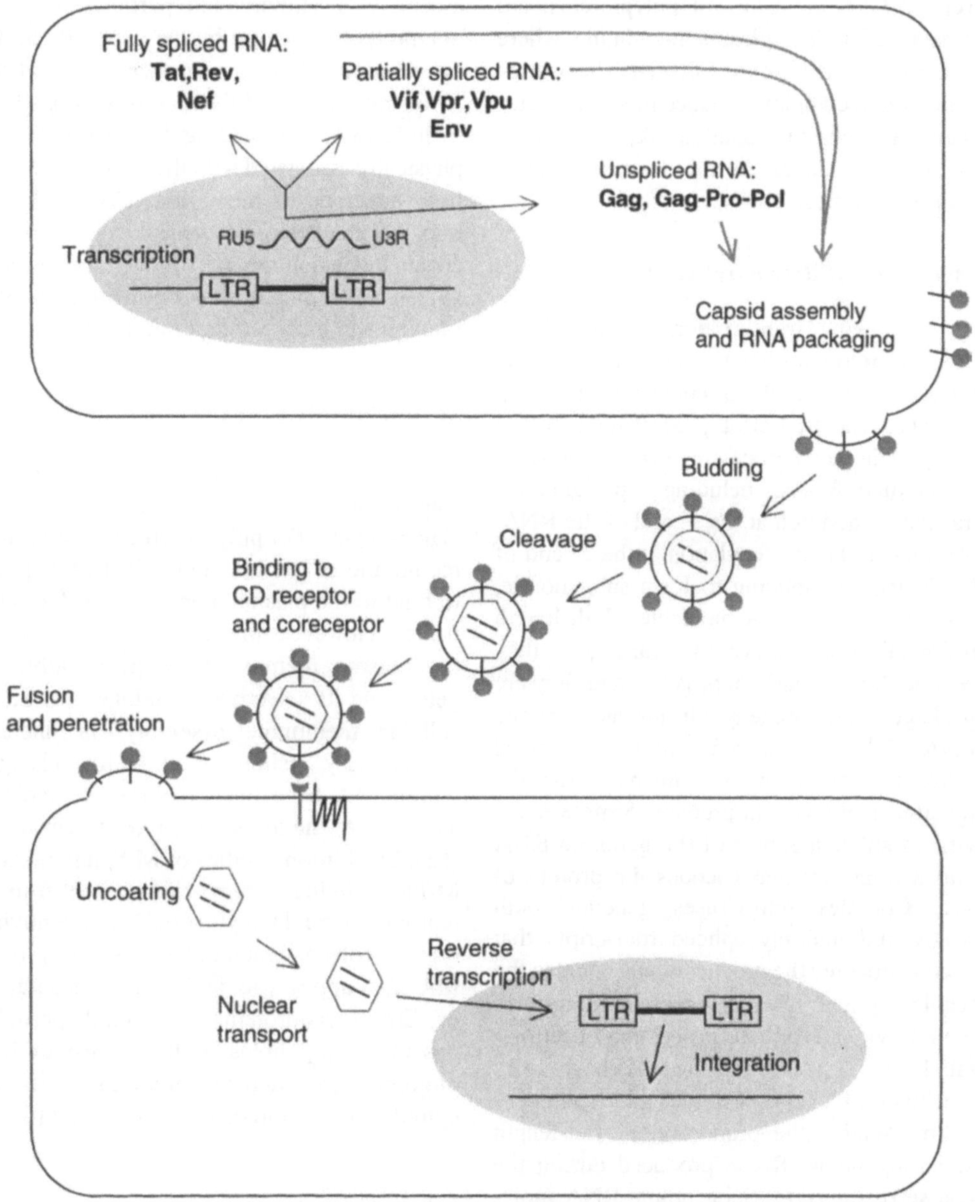

FIGURE 4. HIV-1 replication cycle.

fusion event, mediated by the gp41 TM protein, occurs between the viral and cellular lipid bilayer and results in the release of the viral core into the cytoplasm. An uncoating process begins and results in the reverse transcription of the viral RNA to generate a double-stranded DNA copy preintegration complex with a simultaneous loss of CA and MA proteins. The preintegration complex is then transported into the nucleus where integration of the viral DNA into the host chromosomal DNA is catalyzed by IN. The integrated provirus serves as the template for viral transcription of regulatory and structural components of the virus. Env, as well as Gag and Gag–Pol polyproteins, are transported to the plasma membrane where assembly of the virion is initiated. The assembled protein complexes induce membrane curvature and eventual budding. After budding, PR cleavage leads to the formation of a mature, infectious virion.

Processing of Retroviral RNA

Following transcription of the HIV-1 provirus, retroviral RNA is subject to variable processing to yield 15 currently identified proteins. The transcript processing involves many of the same processing events that occur for cellular RNAs, including cap signal for translation addition at the 5′ end of the RNA, cleavage and polyadenylation at the 3′ end of the RNA, and splicing to form subgenomic, variably spliced RNA molecules. Full-length retroviral RNAs serve two functions: they encode the Gag and Pol proteins, and they are packaged into progeny virions as genomic RNA. Variably spliced, subgenomic-sized RNA molecules provide mRNAs for the remainder of the viral proteins. Simple retroviruses splice a subset of the genomic RNA into a transcript that encodes the protein of *env*. Complex retroviruses generate both singly and multiply spliced transcripts that encode not only the product of *env* but also the regulatory and accessory proteins unique to the retrovirus. While the processing of retroviral RNA is controlled by the host cell's machinery, the virus exploits this machinery by modulating the proportion of full-length and subgenomic RNAs produced during the course of infection. Subgenomic RNA molecules are associated with regulatory and accessory functions while, with the exception of *env*, full-length transcripts yield structural proteins that incorporate the full-length genome.

The Gag Polyprotein MA-CA-NC-p6

As for other retroviruses, *gag* of HIV-1 is translated into a polyprotein that in the absence of other viral proteins, is sufficient for the assembly of retrovirus-like particles. The Gag polyprotein is cleaved by the viral PR shortly after budding from the host cell to yield the structural proteins of the mature virion, which include MA, CA, NC, and p6 (62). MA is physically associated with the host cell-derived lipid envelope of the virion, CA condenses into the characteristic conical core, and NC covers the genomic viral RNA within the core (62). The p6 protein may be involved in Vpr binding and incorporation into the virion.

MA (p17)

MA is the N-terminal component of Gag; it initiates virion assembly by targeting Gag and Gag–Pol polyproteins to the plasma membrane of the infected cell. MA appears to bind to the plasma membrane surface as a trimer. However, the mechanism by which the plasma membrane is specifically targeted, and its selective advantage over intracellular membrane assembly, is unclear. Interestingly, single-amino-acid changes within MA have been reported to redirect assembly to the intracellular Golgi apparatus (63). In addition, studies of MA mutations in M-PMV indicate they can switch from a lentiviral type D (cytosolic) to a lentiviral type C (plasma membrane) assembly (64). MA also appears to facilitate incorporation of Env glycoproteins into viral particles possibly using holes in the lattice of MA oligomers (65) and by interacting with the cytoplasmic region of full-length Env (65).

CA (p24)

CA forms the major core protein within the matrix shell of the viral particle and, like MA, is processed from Gag. The N-terminal domain appears to be important for infectivity and viral uncoating, apparently through an association with the enzyme cyclophilin A (66). Interestingly, cyclophylin A can also be bound by cyclosporin A, which also inhibits cellular NFAT-mediated HIV-1 activation.

However, treatment of viral cultures with cyclosporin A results in the rapid emergence of viral variants that are resistant to cyclosporin and related compounds (67). The C-terminal domain of CA appears to function in dimerization, the formation of Gag oligomers, and viral assembly. The C-terminal domain also contains the major homology region (MHR), a highly conserved region that contributes to membrane affinity by producing a hydrophobic core and that also appears to be essential for particle assembly by providing global conformational stability of Gag oligomers.

NC (p7) and p6

These two proteins represent the C-terminal portion of Gag. NC is a nucleic acid binding protein that recognizes the viral RNA packaging signal, psi, and mediates full-length viral RNA incorporation during virion assembly. NC contains zinc finger motifs, which are highly conserved motifs among retroviruses, as well as certain cellular DNA binding proteins. Protein:RNA interaction between NC and psi occurs through two specific zinc finger domains within NC. Inhibition studies suggest that zinc chelators that inhibit zinc binding to these fingers also inhibit retroviral replication (68,69). The p6 protein is the most C-terminal portion of HIV-1 Gag (a region that is variable among different retroviruses) and its role is less well understood.

The Pol Polyprotein PR-RT-IN

PR

Gag and Gag–Pol polyproteins that are incorporated into the virion are immature and must be cleaved by PR to produce mature infectious viruses. This maturation occurs during or shortly after the virus buds from the host cell. PR cleaves at several sites within the Gag–Pol polyprotein to produce the subunits MA, CA, NC, and p6 proteins. Similarly, PR, RT, and IN proteins are processed from the Pol polyprotein. Because PR is initially part of the Pol polyprotein, full PR activity requires autocleavage. Because cleavage efficiencies and accessibility to proteolysis can vary among sites, a sequential appearance of different, processed proteins occurs (70). PR functions as a dimer and the enzyme active site is apparently formed at the dimer interface. The active site resembles many other aspartyl proteases and contains a conserved, triad amino acid, sequence, Asp-Thr-Gly. PR has been a key target for drug design. Although many PR inhibitors are in clinical use, mutants resistant to multiple inhibitors have been observed (71).

RT

The conversion of viral RNA into proviral DNA is dependent upon RT. RT's enzymatic activity includes the catalysis of an RNA-dependent DNA synthesis step, and a DNA-dependent DNA polymerization step that includes RNAseH catalyzed degradation of the RNA within the newly formed RNA:DNA hybrid. RT is a heterodimer (p66:p51) composed of four polymerase subunits described as the fingers, palm, thumb, and connection domains, with the p66 monomer also containing the RNAseH domain. Like PR, RT is a major target for drug design, and many reverse transcription inhibitory drugs have been studied using a 3-D crystalline structure analysis of an RT complexed with an inhibitor. Two classes of RT inhibitors are in clinical use: nucleoside inhibitors, such as zidovudine and dideoxyinosine, that bind to the polymerase active site and nonnucleoside inhibitors, such as nevirapine, that bind outside the active site. HIV-1 isolates, gathered from patients on essentially all of the currently available antiretroviral drug regimens, have exhibited drug resistance. Whether the high rate for genetic variants is the result of the high rate of HIV-1 replication (72) or an intrinsically error-prone RT is unknown and requires further study. The lack of a proofreading function for RT may explain much of this high error rate. Recombination is frequent because of the packaging of two complete RNA genomes in each virion and because of the high replication rate of HIV (13,73–76). RT's tendency to switch templates coupled with its ability to extend mismatches would seem to indicate that genetic recombination may also be a significant source of error. Estimates suggest an error rate of 10^{-4} per nucleotide incorporated. This results in about one error per viral progeny genome, neglecting potential errors made by host RNA polymerase II. The consequent emergence of a population of highly related but genetically distinct viruses has been termed a "quasispecies" (77).

IN

Once synthesis of the proviral DNA is complete, its integration into the host genome occurs, catalyzed by IN. Integration can occur at various sites within the host genome. Potential interactions with DNA binding proteins may bias integration toward specific sites (78,79). IN appears to function as a tetramer. Each monomer contains a helix-turn-helix region, reminiscent of many nucleic acid binding proteins. The catalytic domain (residues 50–212) contains a triad of acidic residues (a DDE motif) that is highly conserved among INs and that appears to be essential for the processing and joining reactions during integration.

The Env Polyprotein gp120-gp41

All retroviruses contain two types of Env proteins, SU and TM, derived from a precursor Env polyprotein. The 160-kilodalton HIV-1 Env protein, known as gp160, is expressed from a singly spliced mRNA and is synthesized in the endoplasmic reticulum. Following synthesis, Env migrates through the Golgi complex where it undergoes glycosylation, adding 20–30 complex N-linked carbohydrate side chains on asparagine residues. Full Env glycosylation is important for infectivity, and partial glycosylation affects infectivity in various ways. A cellular protease distinct from viral PR cleaves gp160 to form gp120 and gp41.

Gp120 is located on the surface of the infected cell, while gp41 contains the transmembrane domain of Env. In all retroviruses, except the avian sarcoma and leukemia virus, SU is noncovalently associated with TM. In HIV-1, gp120 is complexed with gp41 through somewhat labile interactions that may often lead to the dissociation and the formation of defective viral particles. It has been suggested that such defective particles may direct the humoral response away from the infectious virion (80). Viral infection is initiated when Env glycoprotein on the outer shell of the mature virion binds to specific receptors on the surface of the host cell. Env most likely exists as a trimer on the surface of the virion. The binding of viral Env to the cellular surface receptor CD4 causes structural changes in Env and apparently exposes the V3 loop within Env, presumably allowing for coreceptor interaction (81).

TM(gp41)

Following virus–host cell binding, fusion of the viral and cellular membrane occurs, mediated by TM, known as gp41. An N-terminal glycine-rich region has been associated with this fusion event (82). Gp41 forms a trimer that contains a central, parallel a-helical coiled-coil and an outer, antiparallel α-helical layer. This structure is probably formed during the fusion process, in a manner analogous to that of the influenza hemagglutinin protein (83).

Viral Accessory Proteins

Although the basic steps of the HIV-1 life cycle are the same as those for other retroviruses, the presence of six virally encoded regulatory/accessory proteins—Tat,

Rev, Vif, Vpr, Vpu, and Nef—not found in other classes of retroviruses brings added complexity to HIV-1's replication process. Each of these regulators will be discussed, except for Tat, which was described earlier in this chapter.

Vpr

In contrast with oncogenic retroviruses, which require active cell division for a productive infection, HIV-1 can efficiently infect nondividing cells, such as terminally differentiated monocyte-derived macrophages. Vpr also appears to interfere with the host cell's cycle, potentially allowing for higher viral expression in short-lived cells. Vpr appears to be important to the transport of nucleoprotein complexes containing viral DNA, mediating this transport through its nuclear localizing signal. This protein has also been shown to interact with TFIIB and Sp1 (84, 85), and to act synergistically with coactivator CBP to activate HIV-1 transcription (86).

Vpu

Vpu facilitates transport of Env to the cell surface for assembly into viral particles, potentially by promoting the degradation of complexes formed between CD4 and viral Env within the endoplasmic reticulum. Coimmunoprecipitation experiments indicate that Vpu associates with CD4 (87), although it remains unclear whether direct contact is made between Vpu and CD4 or whether cofactors facilitate Vpu-mediated CD4 degradation.

Vif

The accessory protein Vif appears to be important to the production of highly infectious virions in certain cell types, based on the analysis of Vif mutants (88). Virions produced with mutations in Vif also appear to contain altered core structures, suggesting that this protein may play a role in viral maturation.

Rev

Early in viral gene expression, most viral mRNAs are multiply spliced to produce the viral regulatory proteins Tat, Rev, and Nef. As these regulatory products accumulate, a shift from multiply spliced to singly and unspliced transcripts occurs. The transcripts accumulate and are transported to the cytoplasm to produce structural proteins necessary for RNA packaging and virion assembly. Rev is important in this switch because it prevents the default process of multiple splicing, possibly by increasing the export of singly and unspliced products by binding to the viral RNA element, RRE, within unspliced transcripts (89). The RRE contains several RNA hairpins that function as binding elements for Rev monomers.

Nef

Nef appears to be associated with increased CD4 downregulation through degradation, as with Vpu. It also may enhance Env incorporation into virions and may participate in cell signaling pathways (90). Nef-mutant viruses exhibit decreased rates of viral DNA synthesis following infection. Nef contains a SH3 domain that allows for interaction and modulation of the activity of several tyrosine kinases in the Src family (91). Nef may also promote transcriptional activation of HIV-1 gene expression by modulating cell signaling (92,93).

CELLULAR RECEPTORS

HIV-1 enters cells by attaching to the target cell, then fusing its membrane with the cellular membrane. Both steps are mediated by specific receptors with the major host cell receptor being the CD4 molecule, an immunoglobulin-like protein expressed on the surface of a subset of T-lymphocytes,

TABLE 2. Chemokine Receptors Used for HIV-1 Entry

Coreceptor	Ligand	Expression pattern
Major receptors		
CCR5	MIP-1α, MIP1-β, RANTES	Monocytes, T-cells
CXCR4	SDF-1	Lymphocytes, macrophages, brain
Minor receptors		
CCR3	Eotaxin, MCP-3, MCP-4, RANTES	Eosinophils, microglia, Th2 cells
CCR2b	MCP-1, MCP-3	Monoctyes, T-cells
STRL33/Bonzo	?	T-cells, monocytes, placenta
GPR1	?	Macrophages
GPR15/Bob	?	T-cells, colon
CCR8	1-309	Monocytes, thymocytes
CCR1	MIP-1α, RANTES	Lymphocytes, monocytes and eosinophils
CX3CR1 (V28)	Fractalkine/Neurotactin	Lymphocytes, brain
APJ	Apelin	Brain

? orphan receptors, no ligands identified.
RANTES: Regulated-on-activation, normal T-cell expressed and secreted.
MIP: macrophage inflammatory protein.
MCP: monocyte chemoattractant protein.

monocytes, dendritic cells, and brain microglial cells. The Env glycoprotein binds CD4 with a high affinity. However, the Env–CD4 interaction alone is not sufficient for viral entry; HIV-1 requires a second receptor. This second receptor can be either of two proteins belonging to the chemokine coreceptor family (members of the transmembrane G-coupled receptor protein superfamily).

CXCR4 (formerly known as fusin) was the first coreceptor identified. It is associated with entry of T-cell-line–tropic or syncytium-inducing isolates (94). CCR5 has been shown to be the primary coreceptor for macrophage-tropic, nonsyncytium-inducing viruses (94,95).

A nomenclature, based on viral phenotype, designates viruses that use the CCR5 coreceptor as R5 and viruses that use CXCR4 as X4. Dual-tropic viruses, those that use both CCR5 and CXCR4, are designated R5X4 (96). Viruses that are transmitted almost invariably use the CCR5 receptor; the R5 phenotype dominates early in infection. There is evidence, at least with certain subtypes, that HIV-1 broadens its use of coreceptors during disease progression to include use of CXCR4 and perhaps some minor coreceptors. Minor coreceptors that have been proposed include CCR3, CCR2b, STRL33 (Bonzo), GPR15 (Bob), GPR1, CCR8, CCR9, CCR1, CCR4, CX3CR1 (formerly V28), APJ, and US28 (Table 2) (97–99). Of these, CCR3 appears to be of greatest relevance; it may play a role in infection of microglia cells and, presumably, the development of AIDS dementia (100).

The interaction between the virus and the cellular receptors results in sequential structural changes in the gp120/gp41 complex (101). Two conformations are thought to occur: the native or nonfusogenic form that occurs on free virions, and the fusogenic form that is induced when the complex binds to cellular coreceptors. The first interaction, between gp120 and CD4, results in structural changes in gp120 that apparently expose the V3 loop within gp120 presumably allowing for coreceptor interaction (81,99). The interaction with the coreceptor results in further changes to the fusion–active state. In this state, the fusion peptide becomes exposed and gp41 is thought to insert into the cellular membrane. This intermediate state is relatively stable with receptor-activated conformational changes occurring within 1 to 4 minutes of the binding of the receptor and fusion completed within 20 minutes. The fusion between the viral and cell membrane occurs by mechanisms not yet fully understood.

Two mechanisms that are being explored for therapeutic applications will inhibit entry of virus into cells. The first would prevent attachment of virus to CD4 and coreceptors, and the second would block fusion of the virus with the host cell. One group of molecules known to act as potent inhibitors are chemokines. These small molecules, about 70–90 amino acids in length, attract white blood cells to areas of inflammation. The chemokine SDF-1 (stromal-derived factor 1) blocks entry of X4 isolates into cells, while chemokines such as RANTES (regulated-on-activation, normal T-cell expressed-and-secreted), MIP-1α (macrophage inflammatory protein 1 alpha) and MIP-1β, inhibit viral entry through the CCR5 coreceptor (Table 2). These ligands also inhibit infection by down-regulating expression of the receptors on the surface of cells. Thus chemokine analogues may represent promising candidates for therapy (97). The second mechanism, blocking the fusion intermediate, is currently being explored. A number of peptides have been identified that bind to the prehairpin-like intermediate and inhibit fusion (102).

The central role that CCR5 coreceptor plays in transmission is demonstrated by the fact that individuals with defective CCR5, are largely, but not completely resistant to infection with HIV-1 (103). The most common deletion associated with resistance is the 32bp deletion (CCR5Δ32), which is largely restricted to Caucasian populations and rare among black African populations (103–105). Heterozygosity for this mutation is associated with a delay in disease progression presumably because of decreased levels of CCR5 expression in these individuals. Similarly, genetic polymorphism identified in the promoter region of CCR5 has been associated with altered disease outcomes (106). Other polymorphisms identified include a mutation in the untranslated region of the CXCR4 ligand, SDF1-3′A (107), and in the CCR2b-64I open reading frame. These polymorphisms occur in different frequencies in different populations and may contribute to the varying course of natural history of disease caused by HIV-1 infection.

THE ADAPTIVE LANDSCAPE

An interesting biochemical consequence of the quasispecies structure of HIV-1 is the existence of an error threshold (108), defined as a sharp transition from an organized mutant swarm to random sequences that lack sufficient information content for the virus to replicate (a condition described as error catastrophe). Replication near, but not beyond, this threshold allows HIV-1 to maximally navigate through sequence space as an adaptive strategy without losing the capacity to replicate. Because HIV-1 exists as a quasispecies rather than as a defined genomic sequence, it has the potential to adapt and to expand to a range of environments. However, any genetic changes that do occur may be restricted by the viral genome's initial position in sequence space (or the ensemble of sequence variants present in the population) and by biochemical constraints on replication competence (109,110). Any adaptive response to an environment may therefore be suboptimal; specialized adaptation to a single environment will often decrease the chances for adaptation to a broader range of alternative environments in the course of the viral life cycle. The pathway that the virus traverses through these selection bottlenecks can be considered an adaptive landscape. For the purposes of this review, adaptive landscape will be described for the cellular, physiologic, and population levels of HIV-1.

Responses to selective pressure at the cellular level can be detailed when viruses are exposed to strong driving forces such as antiretroviral drugs, and to a lesser extent, immunologic pressures. Small differences are likely to have a significant effect on reproductive advantage (111). For example, high-level resistance to lamivudine is associated with the rapid point substitution M184V (Met → Val) within the catalytic tyr-met-asp-asp core (YMDD core) motif of RT. During treatment, M184I (Met → Ile) appears initially and is then outgrown by M184V-containing viruses. Typically, in-vitro experiments indicate that mutants generally display a loss of fitness and tend to revert to the wild-type sequence in the absence of drug. One potentially interesting outcome of such studies is that a partial replication disadvantage could be used as a clinical advantage, since reduced viral replication may yield a viral population that has a lower overall capacity for generating diversity and that may, in turn, allow for better immune control of infection.

At the physiologic level, genetic evolution between biologic compartments may occur. Analysis of HIV-1's genetic diversity early after infection indicates that although a small number of viral variants are transmitted, an expansion of genetic diversity and distribution occurs within the body. For example, several studies have documented distinct viral populations in matched blood and genital secretions from the same individuals (112–114). Similarly, in a study of women infected with subtype A HIV-1, in which *env* sequences in peripheral blood and in cervical secretions were compared for about 2 years following seroconversion, the data showed different tissues harbored distinct genetic variants (115). Interestingly, the pattern of variation suggested repeated migration of viruses into the genital tract followed by a local expansion of those variants. Additionally, HIV-1 detected in the breast milk of infected women might also represent a distinct genetic variant when compared to the dominant viral genotype found in the blood of the same women (112,113,116). The genetic evolution of HIV-1 in distinct physiologic compartments may influence transmission likelihood and may also lead to distinct viral reservoirs.

At the population level, many risk factors are likely to influence the outcome in both transmission and epidemic spread of HIV subtypes. It is widely accepted that HIV-1 and HIV-2 occupy different positions within the adaptive landscape. For example, certain studies established that HIV-1 was transmitted 5- to10-fold more efficiently than HIV-2 in one cohort of female sex workers (117). Similarly, studies have also shown that mother-to-infant transmission was much less frequent with HIV-2 (118,119). Differences also have been observed in virulence between HIV-1 and HIV-2 (120). However, population differences between HIV-1 subtypes have been more difficult to prove, although certain data do suggest potential biologic and clinical differences (121–125). Although these observations need further verification, they underscore the need to determine the extent to which subtype can play a role in both transmission efficiency and natural history for the various HIV-1 subtypes. What is clear is that the HIV-1 epidemic is characterized by a substantial genetic diversity of subtypes that are themselves not uniformly distributed geographically. Among the five major subtypes of HIV-1 (A–E), subtype C appears to be associated with the largest number of infections in the world, with major epidemics fueled by heterosexual transmission occurring in western India, China, and, especially, southern Africa (126,127).

It is interesting to note that recent studies of HIV-1 subtype C suggest that this subtype displays a preferential use of CCR5 (121), maintains a higher viral load compared with cocirculating subtypes (128), and exhibits an apparent increase in TNF responsiveness (36,124,129); a comparative structure analysis is shown in Figure 5. However, because African individuals appear to have increased activation markers compared to European individuals (130), the predominant use of CCR5 in vivo is likely complicated by an immune-activated upregulation of CCR5 on cell surfaces that creates more target cells for infection, not solely by any intrinsic property of the virus.

A recent study comparing Ugandans living in rural Uganda with Italians living in Italy showed that chronic immune activation

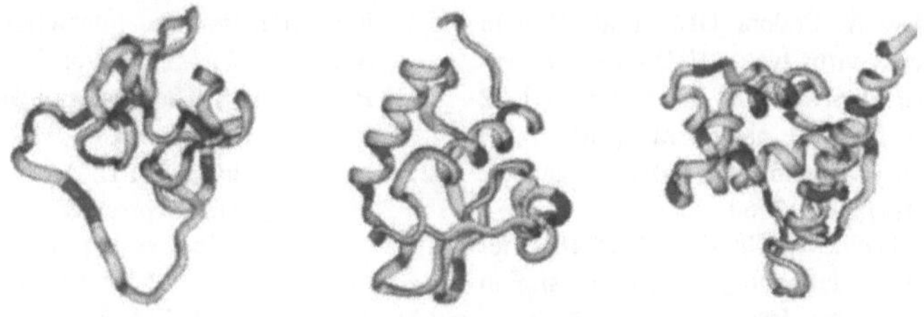

FIGURE 5. Structural amino acid sequence (signature) differences between HIV-1 Tat, Nef, and Matrix. The three-dimensional structures for these viral proteins were used to overlap differences in the signature of HIV-1 subtype C isolates (Russell M, Montano M: manuscript in preparation).

was environmentally induced, probably as a result of parasitic, viral, and bacterial infections, nutritional deficiencies, and possibly hygienic conditions (131). The dominance of R5 isolates throughout the course of disease may be especially significant when inflammatory sexually transmitted diseases (STDs) are also present (132–136). Ulcerative STDs not only make transmission easier, but localized infection results in recruitment of $CD4^+$ T-cells, monocytes, and dendritic cells—target cells for HIV-1 infection. Within Africa, there is also the aggravating presence of opportunistic infections such as tuberculosis (TB), which is associated with vigorous upregulation of a Th1-type cytokine response. Of particular relevance are high levels of TNF-α detected in TB-infected patients. TNF-α upregulates CCR5 and indirectly upregulates HIV-1 replication by activation of NF-κB. In addition, components of TB have been shown to directly stimulate virus replication. TB infection thus creates fertile territory for infection. It is possible, in fact, that subtype C viruses have taken advantage of this niche by duplicating NF-κB binding sites and by preferentially using CCR5 (137). Thus, each virus population at various selective levels, consisting of dynamic mutant spectra rather than a defined genomic sequence, may have the capacity to adapt and expand to a range of environments toward an improved local fitness. It remains to be determined what future pathogenetic global fitness HIV-1 will take within the epidemic.

REFERENCES

1. Hunter E, Casey J, Hahn B, et al. Family Retroviridae. *Virus Taxonomy- Seventh Periodical of the International Committee on Taxonomy of Viruses*, 2001:369–387.
2. Rey-Cuille MA, Berthier JL, Bomsel-Demontoy MC, et al. Simian immunodeficiency virus replicates to high levels in sooty mangabeys without inducing disease. *J Virol*, 1998;72(5):3872–3886.
3. Coffin JM. Retroviridae: The viruses and their replication. In: Fields BN, Knipe DM, Howley PM, et al., eds. *Fields Virology*. Philadelphia, New York: Lippincott-Raven Publishers, 1996:1767–1847.
4. Nathanson N, Hirsch VM, Mathieson BJ. The role of nonhuman primates in the development of an AIDS vaccine. *AIDS*, 1999;13(Suppl A):S113–S120.
5. Goldstein S, Ourmanov I, Brown CR, et al. Wide range of viral load in healthy African green monkeys naturally infected with simian immunodeficiency virus. *J Virol*, 2000;74(24):11744–11753.
6. Beer BE, Bailes E, Sharp P, et al. A compilation and analysis of nucleic acid and amino acid sequences. In: Kuiken CL, Foley B, Hahn B, et al., eds. *Diversity and Evolution of Primate Lentiviruses*. Los Alamos, NM: Theoretical Biology and Biophysics Group, Los Alamos National Laboratory, 1999:460–474.
7. Peeters M, Sharp PM. Genetic diversity of HIV-1: the moving target. *AIDS*, 2000;14(Suppl 3):S129–S1240.
8. Courgnaud V, Pourrut X, Bibollet-Ruche F, et al. Characterization of a novel simian immunodeficiency virus from guereza colobus monkeys (Colobus guereza) in Cameroon: a new lineage in the nonhuman primate lentivirus family. *J Virol*, 2001;75(2):857–866.
9. Chen Z, Telfier P, Gettie A, et al. Genetic characterization of new West African simian immunodeficiency virus SIVsm: geographic clustering of household-derived SIV strains with human immunodeficiency virus type 2 subtypes and genetically diverse viruses from a single feral sooty mangabey troop. *J Virol*, 1996;70(6):3617–3627.

10. Chen Z, Luckay A, Sodora DL, et al. Human immunodeficiency virus type 2 (HIV-2) seroprevalence and characterization of a distinct HIV-2 genetic subtype from the natural range of simian immunodeficiency virus-infected sooty mangabeys. *J Virol*, 1997;71(5):3953–3960.
11. Khabbaz RF, Heneine W, George JR, et al. Brief report: infection of a laboratory worker with simian immunodeficiency virus [see comments]. *N Engl J Med*, 1994;330(3):172–177.
12. Gao F, Yue L, White AT, et al. Human infection by genetically diverse SIVSM-related HIV-2 in West Africa. *Nature*, 1992;358(6386):495–499.
13. Sharp PM, Robertson DL, Hahn BH. Cross-species transmission and recombination of 'AIDS' viruses. *Philos Trans R Soc Lond B Biol Sci*, 1995;349 (1327):41–47.
14. Simon F, Mauclere P, Roques P, et al. Identification of a new human immunodeficiency virus type 1 distinct from group M and group O. *Nat Med*, 1998;9:1032–1037.
15. Zhu T, Korber BT, Nahmias AJ, et al. An African HIV-1 sequence from 1959 and implications for the origin of the epidemic [see comments]. *Nature*, 1998;391(6667):594–597.
16. Korber B, Theiler J, Wolinsky S. Limitations of a molecular clock applied to considerations of the origin of HIV-1. *Science*, 1998;280(5371): 1868–1871.
17. Robertson DL, Anderson JP, Bradac JA, et al. HIV-1 nomenclature proposal [letter]. *Science*, 2000;288(5463):55–56.
18. Vidal N, Peeters M, Mulanga-Kabeya C, et al. Unprecedented degree of human immunodeficiency virus type 1 (HIV-1) group M genetic diversity in the Democratic Republic of Congo suggests that the HIV-1 pandemic originated in Central Africa. *J Virol*, 2000;74(22):10498–10507.
19. Gao F, Bailes E, Robertson DL, et al. Origin of HIV-1 in the chimpanzee Pan troglodytes troglodytes [see comments]. *Nature*, 1999;397(6718):436–441.
20. Huet T, Cheynier R, Meyerhans A, et al. Genetic organization of a chimpanzee lentivirus related to HIV-1 [see comments]. *Nature*, 1990;345(6273): 356–359.
21. Vanden Haesevelde MM, Peeters M, Jannes G, et al. Sequence analysis of a highly divergent HIV-1-related lentivirus isolated from a wild captured chimpanzee. *Virology*, 1996;221(2):346–350.
22. Dickson D. Tests fail to support claims for origin of AIDS in polio vaccine [news]. *Nature*, 2000;407 (6801):117.
23. Roy AL, Malik S, Meisterernst M, et al. An alternative pathway for transcription initiation involving TFII-I. *Nature*, 1993;365(6444):355–359.
24. Smale ST, Baltimore D. The Initiator as a transcription control element. *Cell*, 1989;57:103–113.
25. Montano MA, Kripke K, Norina CD, et al. NF-kappa B homodimer binding within the HIV-1 initiator region and interactions with TFII-I. *Proc Natl Acad Sci USA*, 1996;93:12376–12381.
26. Buratowski S. The Basics of Basal Transcription by RNA Polymerase II. *Cell*, 1994;77:5–8.
27. Nabel G, Baltimore D. An inducible transcription factor activates expression of human immunodeficiency virus in T cells [published erratum appears in *Nature* 1990 Mar 8;344(6262):178]. *Nature*, 1987;326(6114):711–713.
28. Lenardo MJ, Baltimore D. NF-κB: a pleiotropic mediator of inducible and tissue-specific gene control. *Cell*, 1989;58:227–229.
29. Baeuerle PA, Baltimore D. IkB: A specific inhibitor of the NF-κB transcription factor. *Science*, 1988;242:540–546.
30. Montano MA, Novitsky VA, Blackard JT, et al. Divergent transcriptional regulation among expanding human immunodeficiency virus type 1 subtypes. *J Virol*, 1997;71(11):8657–8665.
31. Salminen MO, Johansson B, Sonnerborg A, et al. Full-length sequence of an ethiopian human immunodeficiency type 1 (HIV-1) isolate of genetic subtype C. *AIDS Res Hum Retrovirus*, 1996;12:1329–1339.
32. Gao F, Robertson DL, Morrison SG, et al. The heterosexual human immunodeficiency virus type 1 epidemic in Thailand is caused by an intersubtype (A/E) recombinant of African origin. *J Virol*, 1996; 70:7013–7029.
33. Montano M, Nixon C, Essex M. Dysregulation through the NF-κB enhancer and TATA box of the HIV-1 subtype E promoter. *J Virol*, 1998;72(10): 8446–8452.
34. Duh EJ, Maury WJ, Folks TM, et al. Tumor necrosis factor alpha activates human immunodeficiency virus type 1 through induction of nuclear factor binding to the NF-kappa B sites in the long terminal repeat. *Proc Natl Acad Sci USA*, 1989;86(15): 5974–5978.
35. Osborn L, Kunkel S, Nabel G. Tumor necrosis factor alpha and interleukin 1 stimulate the human immunodeficiency virus enhancer by activation of the nuclear factor kappa B. *Proc. Natl. Acad. Sci. USA*, 1989;86:2336–2340.
36. Montano MA, Nixon CP, Ndung'u T, et al. Elevated tumor necrosis factor-alpha activation of human immunodeficiency virus type 1 subtype C in southern Africa is associated with an NF-kappa B enhancer gain-of-function. *J Infect Dis*, 2000;181(1):76–81.
37. Antoni B, Rabson A, Kinter A, et al. NF-kappa B-dependent and -independent pathways of HIV activation in a chronically infected T cell line. *Virology*, 1994;202(2):684–694.
38. Cullen BR, Greene WC. Regulatory pathways governing HIV-1 replication. *Cell*, 1989;58(3):423–426.
39. Feinberg MB, Baltimore D, Frankel AD. The role of Tat in the human immunodeficiency virus life cycle indicates a primary effect on transcriptional

elongation. *Proc Natl Acad Sci USA*, 1991;88(9):4045–4049.

40. Arya SK, Guo C, Josephs SF, et al. Trans-activator gene of human T-lymphotropic virus type III (HTLV-III). *Science*, 1985;229:69–73.
41. Sodroski J, Rosen C, Wong-Staal F, et al. Trans-acting transcriptional regulation of human T-cell leukemia virus type III long terminal repeat. *Science*, 1985;227:171–173.
42. Dayton AI, Sodroski JG, Rosen CA, et al. The trans-activator gene of the human T cell lymphotropic virus type III is required for replication. *Cell*, 1986;44(6):941–947.
43. Fisher AG, Feinberg MB, Josephs SF, et al. The trans-activator gene of HTLV-III is essential for virus replication. *Nature*, 1986;320(6060):367–371.
44. Ensoli B, Buonaguro L, Barillari G, et al. Release, uptake, and effects of extracellular human immunodeficiency virus type 1 Tat protein on cell growth and viral transactivation. *J Virol*, 1993;67(1):277–287.
45. Borgatti P, Zauli G, Cantley LC, et al. Extracellular HIV-1 Tat protein induces a rapid and selective activation of protein kinase C (PKC)-alpha, and -epsilon and -zeta isoforms in PC12 cells. *Biochem Biophys Res Commun*, 1998;242(2):332–337.
46. Zauli G, Previati M, Caramelli E, et al. Exogenous human immunodeficiency virus type-1 Tat protein selectively stimulates a phosphatidylinositol-specific phospholipase C nuclear pathway in the Jurkat T cell line. *Eur J Immunol*, 1995;25(9):2695–2700.
47. Gibellini D, Caputo A, Capitani S, et al. Upregulation of c-Fos in activated T lymphoid and monocytic cells by human immunodeficiency virus-1 Tat protein. *Blood*, 1997;89(5):1654–1664.
48. Kumar A, Manna SK, Dhawan S, et al. HIV-Tat protein activates c-Jun N-terminal kinase and activator protein-1. *J Immunol*, 1998;161(2):776–781.
49. Conant K, Ma M, Nath A, et al. Extracellular human immunodeficiency virus type 1 Tat protein is associated with an increase in both NF-kappa B binding and protein kinase C activity in primary human astrocytes. *J Virol*, 1996;70(3): 1384–1389.
50. Ott M, Lovett JL, Mueller L, et al. Superinduction of IL-8 in T cells by HIV-1 Tat protein is mediated through NF-kappa B factors. *J Immunol*, 1998;160 (6):2872–2880.
51. Ambrosino C, Ruocco MR, Chen X, et al. HIV-1 Tat induces the expression of the interleukin-6 (IL6) gene by binding to the IL6 leader RNA and by interacting with CAAT enhancer-binding protein beta (NF-IL6) transcription factors. *J Biol Chem*, 1997;272(23):14883–14892.
52. Huang L, Bosch I, Hofmann W, et al. Tat protein induces human immunodeficiency virus type 1 (HIV-1) coreceptors and promotes infection with both macrophage-tropic and T-lymphotropic HIV-1 strains. *J Virol*, 1998;72(11):8952–8960.
53. Frankel AD. Peptide models of Tat-TAR protein-RNA interaction. *Protein Science*, 1992;1:1539–1542.
54. Wei P, Garber ME, Fang SM, et al. A novel CDK9-associated C-type cyclin interacts directly with HIV-1 Tat and mediates its high-affinity, loop-specific binding to TAR RNA. *Cell*, 1998;92(4):451–462.
55. Browning C, Smith M, Roeder R, et al. Transcriptional activation and synergy of Gl-2/THP proto-oncogene with HIV Tat. *J Virol*, 2001; in press.
56. Gaynor R. Cellular transcription factors involved in the regulation of HIV-1 gene expression. *AIDS*, 1992;6:347–363.
57. Pereira LA, Bentley K, Peeters A, et al. A compilation of cellular transcription factor interactions with the HIV-1 LTR promoter. *Nucleic Acids Res*, 2000;28(3):663–668.
58. Karin M, Liu Z, Zandi E. AP-1 function and regulation. *Curr Opin Cell Biol*, 1997;9(2):240–246.
59. Canonne-Hergaux F, Aunis D, Schaeffer E. Interactions of the transcription factor AP-1 with the long terminal repeat of different human immunodeficiency virus type 1 strains in Jurkat, glial, and neuronal cells. *J Virol*, 1995;69(11):6634–6642.
60. Kinoshita S, Chen B, Kaneshima H, Nolan G. Host control of HIV-1 parasitism in T cells by the nuclear factor of activated T cells. *Cell*, 1998;95:595–604.
61. Perelson AS, Neumann AU, Markowitz M, et al. HIV-1 dynamics in vivo: virion clearance rate, infected cell life-span, and viral generation time. *Science*, 1996;271(5255):1582–1586.
62. Freed EO. HIV-1 gag proteins: diverse functions in the virus life cycle. *Virology*, 1998;251(1):1–15.
63. Freed EO, Orenstein JM, Buckler-White AJ, et al. Single amino acid changes in the human immunodeficiency virus type 1 matrix protein block virus particle production. *J Virol*, 1994;68(8):5311–5320.
64. Rhee SS, Hunter E. A single amino acid substitution within the matrix protein of a type D retrovirus converts its morphogenesis to that of a type C retrovirus. *Cell*, 1990;63(1):77–86.
65. Hill CP, Worthylake D, Bancroft DP, et al. Crystal structures of the trimeric human immunodeficiency virus type 1 matrix protein: implications for membrane association and assembly. *Proc Natl Acad Sci USA*, 1996;93(7):3099–3104.
66. Luban J. Absconding with the chaperone: essential cyclophilin-Gag interaction in HIV-1 virions. *Cell*, 1996;87(7):1157–1159.
67. Aberham C, Weber S, Phares W. Spontaneous mutations in the human immunodeficiency virus type 1 gag gene that affect viral replication in the presence of cyclosporins. *J Virol*, 1996;70(6):3536–3544.
68. Rice WG, Supko JG, Malspeis L, et al. Inhibitors of HIV nucleocapsid protein zinc fingers as candidates for the treatment of AIDS. *Science*, 1995;270 (5239):1194–1197.

69. Ott DE, Hewes SM, Alvord WG, et al. Inhibition of Friend virus replication by a compound that reacts with the nucleocapsid zinc finger: anti-retroviral effect demonstrated in vivo. *Virology*, 1998;243(2): 283–292.
70. Dunn BM, Gustchina A, Wlodawer A, et al. Kay J. Subsite preferences of retroviral proteinases. *Methods Enzymol*, 1994;241:254–278.
71. Condra JH, Schleif WA, Blahy OM, et al. In vivo emergence of HIV-1 variants resistant to multiple protease inhibitors [see comments]. *Nature*, 1995; 374(6522):569–571.
72. Coffin JM. HIV population dynamics in vivo: Implications for genetic variation, pathogenesis and therapy. *Science*, 1995;267:483–489.
73. Robertson DL, Sharp PM, McCutchan FE, et al. Recombination in HIV-1 [letter]. *Nature*, 1995;374 (6518):124–126.
74. Robertson DL, Hahn BH, Sharp PM. Recombination in AIDS viruses. *Journal of Mol. Evol*, 1995;40:249–259.
75. Renjifo B, Chaplin B, Mwakagile D, et al. HIV-1 subtypes A,C,D and inter-subtype recombinant genotypes in newborns of Dar-es-Salaam, Tanzania. *AIDS Res Hum Retro*, 1998;14:635–638.
76. Blackard JT, Renjifo BR, Mwakagile D, et al. Transmission of human immunodeficiency type 1 viruses with intersubtype recombinant long terminal repeat sequences. *Virology*, 1999;254(2):220–225.
77. Wain-Hobson S. The fastest genome evolution ever described: HIV variation in situ. *Curr Opin Genet Dev*, 1993;3(6):878–883.
78. Miller MD, Bor YC, Bushman F. Target DNA capture by HIV-1 integration complexes. *Curr Biol*, 1995; 5(9):1047–1056.
79. Farnet CM, Bushman FD. HIV-1 cDNA integration: requirement of HMG I(Y) protein for function of preintegration complexes in vitro. *Cell*, 1997;88 (4):483–492.
80. Wyatt R, Kwong PD, Desjardins E, et al. The antigenic structure of the HIV gp120 envelope glycoprotein [see comments]. *Nature*, 1998;393(6686): 705–711.
81. Wyatt R, Sodroski J. The HIV-1 envelope glycoproteins: fusogens, antigens, and immunogens. *Science*, 1998;280(5371):1884–1888.
82. Hernandez LD, Hoffman LR, Wolfsberg TG, et al. Virus-cell and cell-cell fusion. *Annu Rev Cell Dev Biol*,1996;12:627–661.
83. Chan DC, Fass D, Berger JM, et al. Core structure of gp41 from the HIV envelope glycoprotein. *Cell*, 1997;89(2):263–273.
84. Agostini I, Navarro JM, Rey F, et al. The human immunodeficiency virus type 1 Vpr transactivator: cooperation with promoter-bound activator domains and binding to TFIIB. *J Mol Biol*, 1996;261(5): 599–606.
85. Wang L, Mukherjee S, Jia F, et al. Interaction of virion protein Vpr of human immunodeficiency virus type 1 with cellular transcription factor Sp1 and trans-activation of viral long terminal repeat. *J Biol Chem*, 1995;270(43):25564–25569.
86. Felzien LK, Woffendin C, Hottiger MO, et al. HIV transcriptional activation by the accessory protein, VPR, is mediated by the p300 co-activator. *Proc Natl Acad Sci USA*, 1998;95(9):5281–5286.
87. Bour S, Schubert U, Strebel K. The human immunodeficiency virus type 1 Vpu protein specifically binds to the cytoplasmic domain of CD4: implications for the mechanism of degradation. *J Virol*, 1995;69(3):1510–1520.
88. Cohen EA, Subbramanian RA, Gottlinger HG. Role of auxiliary proteins in retroviral morphogenesis. *Curr Top Microbiol Immunol*, 1996;214: 219–235.
89. Hope TJ. Viral RNA export. *Chem Biol*, 1997;4(5): 335–344.
90. Mangasarian A, Trono D. The multifaceted role of HIV. *Nef Res Virol*, 1997;148(1):30–33.
91. Moarefi I, LaFevre-Bernt M, Sicheri F, et al. Activation of the Src-family tyrosine kinase Hck by SH3 domain displacement [see comments]. *Nature*, 1997;385(6617):650–653.
92. Manninen A, Herma Renkema G, Saksela K. Synergistic activation of NFAT by HIV-1 nef and the Ras/MAPK pathway. *J Biol Chem*, 2000;275 (22):16513–16517.
93. Wang JK, Kiyokawa E, Verdin E, et al. The Nef protein of HIV-1 associates with rafts and primes T cells for activation. *Proc Natl Acad Sci USA*, 2000;97(1):394–399.
94. Feng Y, Broder CC, Kennedy PE, et al. HIV-1 entry cofactor: functional cDNA cloning of a seven transmembrane, G protein-coupled receptor. *Science*, 1996;272:872–877.
95. Alkhatib G, Combadiere C, Broder CC, et al. CC CKR5: a RANTES, MIP-1alpha, MIP-1beta receptor as a fusion cofactor for macrophage-tropic HIV-1. *Science*, 1996;272(5270):1955–1958.
96. Berger EA, Doms RW, Fenyo EM, et al. A new classification for HIV-1 [letter]. *Nature*, 1998;391 (6664):240.
97. Clapham PR, Reeves JD, Simmons G, et al. HIV coreceptors, cell tropism and inhibition by chemokine receptor ligands. *Mol Membr Biol*, 1999;16(1):49–55.
98. Berger EA, Murphy PM, Farber JM. Chemokine receptors as HIV-1 coreceptors: roles in viral entry, tropism, and disease. *Annu Rev Immunol*, 1999; 17:657–700.
99. Littman DR. Chemokine receptors: keys to AIDS pathogenesis? *Cell*, 1998;93(5):677–680.
100. He J, Chen Y, Farzan M, et al. CCR3 and CCR5 are co-receptors for HIV-1 infection of microglia. *Nature*, 1997;385(6617):645–649.

101. Chan DC, Kim PS. HIV entry and its inhibition. *Cell*, 1998;93(5):681–684.
102. Furuta RA,Wild CT, Weng Y, et al. Capture of an early fusion-active conformation of HIV-1 gp41 [published erratum appears in *Nat Struct Biol* 1998 Jul;5(7):612]. *Nat Struct Biol*, 1998;5(4): 276–279.
103. Samson M, Libert F, Doranz BJ, et al. Resistance to HIV-1 infection in caucasian individuals bearing mutant alleles of the CCR-5 chemokine receptor gene [see comments]. *Nature*, 1996;382(6593): 722–725.
104. Williamson C, Loubser SA, Brice B, et al. Allelic frequencies of host genetic variants influencing susceptibility to HIV-1 infection and disease in South African populations. *AIDS*, 2000;14(4):449–451.
105. Martinson JJ, Chapman NH, Rees DC, et al. Global distribution of the CCR5 gene 32-basepair deletion. *Nat Genet,* 1997;16(1):100–103.
106. McDermott DH, Zimmerman PA, Guignard F, et al. CCR5 promoter polymorphism and HIV-1 disease progression. Multicenter AIDS Cohort Study (MACS). *Lancet*, 1998;352(9131): 866–870.
107. Winkler C, Modi W, Smith MW, et al. Genetic restriction of AIDS pathogenesis by an SDF-1 chemokine gene variant. ALIVE Study, Hemophilia Growth and Development Study (HGDS), Multicenter AIDS Cohort Study (MACS), Multicenter Hemophilia Cohort Study (MHCS), San Francisco City Cohort (SFCC) [see comments]. *Science*, 1998;279(5349):389–393.
108. Eigen M, Biebricher C. Sequence space and quasispecies distribution. In: Domingo E, Holland, J.J, and Ahlquist, P., ed. *RNA Genetics*. Vol. 3. Boca Raton, FL: CRC Press; 1988:211–245.
109. Simpson GG. The meaning of evolution. New Haven, CT: Yale University Press; 1949.
110. Maynard Smith J, Burian R, Kauffman Sea. Developmental constraints and evolution. *Quarterly Review of Biology,* 1985;60:265–287.
111. Goudsmit J, de Ronde A, de Rooij E, et al. Broad spectrum of in vivo fitness of human immunodeficiency virus type 1 subpopulations differing at reverse transcriptase codons 41 and 215. *J Virol*, 1997;71(6):4479–4484.
112. Overbaugh J, Anderson RJ, Ndinya-Achola JO, et al. Distinct but related human immuniodeficeincy virus type 1 variant populations in genital secretions and blood. *AIDS Res. Human Retroviruses*, 1996;12:107–115.
113. Poss M, Martin HL, Kreiss JK, et al. Diversity in virus populations from genital secretions and peripheral blood from women recently infected with human immumodeficiency virus type 1. *J Virol*, 1995;69:8118–8122.
114. Zhu T, Wang N, Carr A, et al. Genetic characterization of human immunodeficiency virus type 1 in blood and genital secretions: evidence for viral compartmentalization and selection during sexual transmission. *J Virol*, 1996;70:3098–3107.
115. Poss M, Rodrigo AG, Gosink JJ, et al. Evolution of envelope sequences from the genital tract and peripheral blood of women infected with clade A human immunodeficiency virus type 1. *J Virol*, 1998;72(10):8240–8251.
116. Kampinga G, Simonon A, Van de Perre P, et al. Primary infections with HIV-1 of women and their offspring in Rwanda: findings of heterogeneity at seroconversion, coinfection, and recombinants of HIV-1 subtypes A and C. *Virology*, 1997;227:63–76.
117. Kanki PJ, Travers K, MBoup S, et al. Slower het*erosexual* spread of HIV-2 than HIV-1. *Lancet, 1994*;343:943–946.
118. Adjorlolo-Johnson G, De Cock KM, Ekpini E, et al. Prospective comparison of mother-to-child transmission of HIV-1 and HIV- 2 in Abidjan, Ivory Coast. *JAMA*, 1994;272(6):462–466.
119. Del Mistro A, Chotard J, Hall AJ, et al. HIV-1 and HIV-2 seroprevalence rates in mother-child pairs living in The Gambia (West Africa). *J Acquir Immune Defic Syndr*, 1992;5(1):19–24.
120. Marlink R, Kanki P, Thior K, et al. Reduced rate of disease development after HIV-2 infection as compared to HIV-1. *Science*, 1994;265:1587–1590.
121. Tscherning C, Alaeus A, Fredrikson R, et al. Differences in chemokine coreceptor usage between genetic subtypes of HIV-1. *Virology*, 1998; 241:181–188.
122. Björnal Å, Sönnerborg A, Tschering C, et al. Phenotypic Characteristics of Human Immunodeficiency Virus Type 1 Subtype C Isolates of Ethiopian AIDS Patients. *AIDS* Research Hum Retroviruses, 1999;15(7):647–653.
123. Neilson JR, John GC, Carr JK, et al. Subtypes of HIV-1 and Disease Stage among Women in Nairobi, Kenya. *J. Virol*, 1999;73(5):4393–4403.
124. Verhoef K, Sanders R, Fontaine V, et al. Evolution of the Human Immunodeficiency Virus Type 1 Long Terminal Repeat Promoter by Conversion of an NF-κB Enhancer Element into a GABP Binding Site. *J. Virol*, 1999;73(2):1331–1340.
125. Kanki PJ, Hamel DG, Sankale J-L, et al. HIV-1 subtypes differ in disease progression. *J. Infect. Dis.*, 1999;179(1):68–73.
126. Weniger BG, Takebe Y, Ou CY, et al. The molecular epidemiology of HIV in Asia. *AIDS*, 1994;8: S13–S28.
127. Stanecki KA, and Way PO. The Dynamic HIV/AIDS Pandemic. In: Tarantola D, Mann J, eds. *AIDS in the World II*. New York: Oxford Press, 1996:41.
128. Neilson JR, John GC, Carr JK, et al. Subtypes of human immunodeficiency virus type 1 and disease stage among women in Nairobi, Kenya. *J Virol*, 1999:73(5):4393–4403.
129. Naghavi M, Schwartz S, Sonerborg A, et al. Long terminal repeat promoter/enhancer activity of

different subtypes of HIV type 1. *AIDS Res Hum Retroviruses*, 1999;15(14):1293–1303.
130. Clerici M, Butto S, Lukwiya M, et al. Immune activation in Africa is environmentally-driven and is associated with upregulation of CCR5. Italian-Ugandan AIDS Project [In Process Citation]. *AIDS*, 2000;14(14):2083–2092.
131. Rizzardini G, Trabattoni D, Saresella M, et al. Immune activation in HIV-infected African individuals. Italian-Ugandan AIDS cooperation program. *AIDS*, 1998;12(18):2387–2396.
132. Sha BE, D'Amico RD, Landay AL, et al. Evaluation of immunological markers in cervicovaginal fluid of HIV-infected and uninfected women: implications for the immunological response to HIV in the female genital tract. *J AIDS and Human Retrovirol*, 1997;16:161–169.
133. Anderson DJ, Politch JA, Tucker LD, et al. Quantitation of mediators of inflammation and immunity in genital tract secretions and their relevance to HIV type 1 transmission. *AIDS Res Hum Retroviruses*, 1988;14:43–49.
134. Ho JL, He S, Hu A, et al. Neutrophils from human immunodeficiency virus (HIV)-seronegative donors induce HIV replication from HIV-infected patients' mononuclear cells and cell lines: an in vitro model of HIV transmission facilitated by Chlamydia trachomatis [published erratum appears in *J Exp Med* 1999 Nov 1;190(9):following 1362]. *J Exp Med*, 1995;181(4):1493–1505.
135. Plummer F, Simonsen J, Cameron D, et al. Cofactors in male-female sexual transmission of human immunodeficiency virus type 1. *J Infect Dis*, 1991;163(2):233–239.
136. Plummer FA. Heterosexual transmission of HIV-1: Interactions of conventional sexually transmitted diseases, hormone contraception and HIV-1. *AIDS Res Hum Retroviruses*, 1998;14(Supplement 1):5–10.
137. Bentwich Z, Maartens G, Torten D, et al. Concurrent infections and HIV pathogenesis [In Process Citation]. *AIDS*, 2000;14(14):2071–2081.

3

Immunopathogenesis of AIDS

*Lynn S. Zijenah and †David A. Katzenstein

**Department of Immunology, University of Zimbabwe Medical School, Harare, Zimbabwe.*
†AIDS Research Center, Stanford University School of Medicine, Stanford, California 94305-5107, USA.

Human immunodeficiency virus (HIV) infection results in an antibody response that is an early demonstration of the viral infection. Progressively, $CD4^+$ cells decrease, and the weakened immune system becomes unable to control a range of endogenous and environmental pathogens (1). The immunopathogenesis of acquired immunodeficiency syndrome (AIDS) includes the cellular and humoral immune responses to

HIV-1 infection. HIV infection causes AIDS through the depletion and eventual exhaustion of immune responses, leading to clinical illness and, eventually, death in most individuals.

The period for progression from primary HIV infection to terminal-stage AIDS ranges from 1 year to more than 20 years, with a median time to onset of AIDS of nearly 10 years after HIV infection. This variable time to onset may depend upon host susceptibility, viral virulence, immune responses against the virus, and endogenous and exogenous copathogens (2,3). These factors have emerged from studies comparing rapid progressors (RPs)—individuals who generally have developed AIDS within 7 years of initial infection—with long-term nonprogressors (LTNPs)—individuals who have $CD4^+$ cell counts greater than $500/mm^3$ more than 10 years after initial infection and/or have no AIDS-related symptoms (4–8). The HIV replication rate in vivo, as determined by measuring plasma levels of viral RNA (viral load), differs significantly in RPs and LTNPs (9–11). Higher viral load and lower $CD4^+$ counts correlate with increased likelihood for onset of clinical disease (12–17), while low levels of viral load have been associated with a low likelihood for disease onset (18,19).

The hallmark of immunodeficiency caused by HIV infection is the depletion of cells of the immune system: $CD4^+$ T-lymphocytes, macrophages, monocytes, and dendritic cells that express the CD4 receptors. In addition, apoptosis of uninfected $CD8^+$ cells has been observed in HIV-1–infected individuals (20,21). HIV infection can be divided into three phases: primary infection, a chronic asymptomatic period, and overt AIDS. Each phase is associated with distinct changes in the number of immune cells and accessory molecules involved in the generation and regulation of the immune response to HIV. The gradual decrease in the number of cells of the immune system and the functional decline of these cells lead to the breakdown of the immune system, exposing infected individuals to a wide variety of viral, bacterial, fungal, and parasitic infections that result in full-blown AIDS. An infected individual's increasing susceptibility to specific pathogens and decreasing $CD4^+$ cell count have been ascribed to the depletion of memory T-cells specific for epitopes expressed by opportunistic pathogens.

The humoral markers of HIV-1 infection include B-cell activation (22,23), hypergammaglobulinemia (24–26), and an increase in circulating β_2-microglobulin (27–30) and neopterin (27,31–33). The dynamics of $CD4^+$ and $CD8^+$ cell production and death (34,35) and cytokines are intense areas of research. There are early, potent, cytotoxic-T-lymphocyte (CTL) immune responses directed against HIV-1 epitopes. However, because HIV infects the cells that develop cellular immune responses, these responses may wane with progressive infection (8).

In Africa, tuberculosis, as an opportunistic infection, is the most significant clinical manifestation of HIV infection (36,37) and Kaposi's Sarcoma is the most common neoplasm associated with HIV infection. Endemic parasitic infections, which are prevalent throughout Africa, may play a role triggering either T-helper 1 (Th1) cellular or Th2 humoral responses. In HIV infection, Th1 immune responses may be associated with resistance to and control of HIV infection, while Th2 responses may be less effective in controlling virus replication (38). Chronic parasitic infections may determine the type of initial immune response to HIV infection and its ability to control viral replication (39–45). Recently, studies in Uganda demonstrated an increased frequency of clinical malaria and parasitemia in individuals infected with HIV-1 as compared to uninfected individuals (46,47).

Immunologic function is sensitive to nutritional deficiencies and malnutrition, both of which are common problems in Africa (48–53). A substantial proportion of individuals with advanced HIV disease and low $CD4^+$ cell counts have clinical evidence of wasting and malnutrition (54).

Knowledge of immune responses to HIV infection is critical to the design of a vaccine that will effectively prevent or ameliorate the pathogenicity of this infection. Studies involving exposed uninfected individuals in Africa have demonstrated a range of immune responses against viral antigens including Th-cell activity (55), CTL responses (56,57), and mucosal secretion of IgA antibodies (58). Human lymphocyte antigen (HLA) genes also appear to play a role in the immunopathogenesis of AIDS (59–62). The diversity of HLA types and alleles is significantly associated with a broader HIV-1 immune-response capability and a slower rate of disease progression.

$CD4^+$ AND $CD8^+$ LYMPHOCYTES

The measurement most widely used to determine immunodeficiency in HIV infection is the number and percentage of $CD4^+$ (helper) and $CD8^+$ (cytotoxic and suppressor) T-lymphocytes in the blood (63). T-cell depletion in HIV infection may be the result of direct killing of mature T-cells with the rapid replication of HIV-1 (64,65). A reduction in the rate of production of T-cell precursors or in the maturation of T-cells from progenitor cells may also explain the progressive immunodeficiency found in HIV infection (66,67). New studies, particularly those that involve patients receiving highly active antiretroviral therapy (HAART), provide information about immune restoration in HIV infection. These studies demonstrate that a reduction in viral replication results in an increase in the number of circulating $CD4^+$ T-cells and in a return of functional T-cell immunity (68,69). Additional studies using deuterated glucose to label $CD4^+$ T-cells among treated patients show that both the half-life and the rate of production of mature $CD4^+$ T-cells increase with suppression of virus (35). $CD4^+$ T-lymphocytes, which differentiate into memory and naïve (uncommitted) cells, originate in the bone marrow, spleen, and lymph nodes; mature in the thymus, and then move in and out of the circulatory system and the tissues of the solid organs and lymph system. Studies of HIV infection and $CD4^+$ T-cell dynamics may provide insight into the complex multi-staged life of $CD4^+$ and $CD8^+$ T-lymphocytes (70).

The dynamics of $CD4^+$ lymphocytes in HIV infection demonstrate a precipitous drop in their number within 1 to 2 weeks of infection, followed by a rapid rebound in the number of $CD4^+$ cells as immune responses against HIV are detected. Ultimately there is a variable rate of decline in their number over several years. The depletion of $CD4^+$ lymphocytes has recently been shown to result from a decrease in the average circulating half-life of $CD4^+$ lymphocytes that is not compensated for by an increase in production (35).

$CD4^+$ lymphocytes in the circulation usually number more than 1,000/mm^3, although a normal range for $CD4^+$ cell counts in some individuals may extend to 500–600/mm^3. $CD8^+$ lymphocyte counts in the absence of HIV are usually <500/mm^3 and typically the $CD4^+$:$CD8^+$ ratio is >2. $CD4^+$ lymphocytes are recognized as a heterogenous population that includes naïve cells and memory/effector cells with differing half-lives, functions, and circulation patterns. The organization of lymphoid follicles in the gut, lymph nodes, and spleen is distinct and includes different ratios and types of $CD4^+$ and $CD8^+$ cells in different tissue compartments.

There is a clear relationship between the number of circulating $CD4^+$ cells and disease progression and mortality in HIV infection that is consistent worldwide. In the United States and Europe, individuals who respond to antiretroviral therapy with increased numbers of circulating $CD4^+$ cells are able to cease prophylactic medications for opportunistic infections; their risk for these infections and for death decreases in direct proportion to the increase in $CD4^+$ cells (71). Limited studies of $CD4^+$ cell counts among HIV-infected individuals in Africa suggest that, in the absence of treatment, individuals with $CD4^+$ counts <50/mm^3 have a 50%

annual mortality rate, while individuals with a count of <200/mm^3 have mortality rates of 10% to 15% per year (72,73). The risk for tuberculosis, *Pneumocystis carinii* pneumonia, and wasting increases abruptly as CD4$^+$ cell counts decline to <200/mm^3.

HUMORAL (ANTIBODY) IMMUNE RESPONSES

Studies of HIV infection indicate that antibody responses to the proteins encoded by the envelope (*env*), group specific antigen (*gag*), polymerase (*pol*), and regulatory (*tat, rev*) genes of HIV are detectable 2 to 4 weeks after exposure and infection (74,75). While there is some evidence for an initial IgM response, IgG and IgA antibodies are detectable early and there is an exponential increase in their titer, particularly for IgG1 antibodies, over the first 3 to 6 months of infection.

New antibody testing formats may provide more convenient diagnostic tools. The rapid test kits that have been developed, and that are being used in counseling and testing centers, do not require electricity or sophisticated laboratory equipment. Enzyme-linked immunosorbent assay (ELISA) tests of urine, and saliva give results that approach the sensitivity and specificity of the standard ELISA test, which detects HIV antibodies from serum or plasma. These assays have also been used to detect antibodies eluted from dried blood spots (76–78). One of the more interesting epidemiologic and surveillance tools developed in the past few years, is the "detuned" or sensitive/less sensitive ELISA test. A rapid increase in antibody titer and antibody maturation occurs within the first 5 to 6 months of HIV infection. Janssen and colleagues (79) have shown that among individuals who have recently seroconverted, most will have low-affinity antibodies, that is, they will measure positive for HIV on the sensitive test and below a cut-off optical density (OD) on the less sensitive test. Thus, seroconverters can be distinguished from individuals in later stages of infection, based on their low-affinity antibodies. Using this detuned assay in African seroconverters, about 80% of those with recent infection will detune, and very few individuals with prevalent infections of longer than 1 year will demonstrate low-affinity antibodies (Katzenstein and Zijenah: personal communication). Our preliminary data indicate the utility of this methodology. However, because the standard HIV ELISAs are formatted with subtype B antigen, further evaluation will be required to determine their applicability across Africa, where other subtypes and circulating recombinant forms are prevalent. The value of this test, however, does not rest in establishing an individual diagnosis, rather it can be used as an epidemiologic tool to estimate community incidence from screening tests that identify prevalent infection.

Neutralizing antibody (NA) responses increase in titer and breadth over the course of infection. In the envelope glycoprotein, continuous and discontinuous epitopes that mediate neutralization have been identified. Antibodies that neutralize HIV by preventing effective CD4$^-$ and chemokine-receptor binding have also been identified. Some potent NAs do not prevent binding of gp120 to CD4, rather they interact with the viral envelope–receptor complex to prevent the necessary conformational change that allows viral entry to be mediated by gp41 (80), the transmembrane glycoprotein (81). A broad range of monoclonal antibodies that bind gp120 and gp41 to specific sites also have been characterized. The *env* glycoprotein varies by as much as 5% within a given individual and shows as much as 30% variation in its amino acid sequence across the different subtypes of HIV-1. In addition, cross-reactivity between NAs produced in individuals infected with different subtypes of HIV-1 has been demonstrated (82).

Although some in-vitro investigations have demonstrated "enhancing antibodies," immunologlobulins that at very high dilutions increase the infectivity of HIV, the significance of these in infected individuals is uncertain (83). The identification of the phenomena of antibody enhancement does suggest caution in the application of experimental vaccines that may elicit low titers of envelope-binding antibodies. Such vaccines might then be expected to increase infectivity via enhancement, rather than protect against HIV.

In longitudinal studies of infected individuals, autologous NAs that neutralize the concomitant virus isolated from an individual have been examined to determine their relationship to disease progression. Autologous NAs are detected more readily when macrophages, rather than lymphocytes, are the target cells for infection (84). Autologous NAs in macrophages are associated with reduced viral load and decreased mother-to-infant transmission (85). Studies comparing LTNPs and RPs suggest that the titer and breadth of NAs against heterologous and autologous clinical isolates is significantly greater in LTNPs than RPs (86–90). Escape mutations, which allow virus to resist autologous NAs in early HIV infection, suggest that the evolution of viral quasispecies may be directed by mutation and by the selection pressure of humoral responses (91–93). In longitudinal studies of HIV-infected individuals in Denmark, autologous NA responses were associated with decreases in the rates of disease progression (94). The concept of immunoselection is consistent with autologous NAs that are usually detected against previous, but rarely against current, virus isolates in individuals followed over years of infection (95). Small studies in our laboratory suggest that NA responses wane with antiretroviral drug therapy, suggesting that continued antigenic exposure is required to maintain vigorous NA response (Mary Kate Morris: personal communication).

CELLULAR IMMUNE RESPONSES

Cell-mediated immune responses, predominantly by $CD8^+$ major histocompatibility complex (MHC) class I restricted CTLs, are detected before an antibody response is measured in acute HIV infection. These $CD8^+$ CTL responses to peptide "T-cell" epitopes of HIV may be measured using the classic chromium-release assay, where EBV-transformed autologous target cells, infected with vaccinia recombinants or coated with antigenic peptides, are lysed by $CD8^+$ effector lymphocytes. The number and percentage of cells that respond to a peptide antigen can be determined by the release of interferon gamma (IFN-γ) measured in ELISPOT assays, which enumerate the cells secreting IFN-γ as single-cell ELISA spots. Cells that recognize specific peptide epitopes have been cloned by limiting-dilution culture with interleukin 2 (IL-2) and by antigen stimulation to identify the number and percentage of CTL precursors that respond to a specific peptide. Among patients with the appropriate HLA haplotype, it is possible to determine the number of CTL effector cells that recognize a peptide-MHC molecular complex by using a fluorescence-activated cell sorting (FACS) analysis in a tetramer assay in which MHC complex–antigenic-peptide binding activity is directly measured. Each of these techniques has shown there is an increase in cellular responses triggered by antigen exposure and by the presentation of T-cell epitopes by class I MHC processing. In a small number of cases of acute infection where it has been possible to follow the course of early infections, a decline in the early peak viremia has been associated with the emergence of CTL responses against epitopes encoded by the *gag*, negative regulator factor (*nef*), and *env* genes. Among individuals with established HIV infection, it is possible to demonstrate CTL responses using chromium-release assay, ELISPOT, or tetramer assays for peptides derived from sequences of structural genes of the virus. Among LTNPs, cellular immune responses can be demonstrated in peripheral blood cells by each of these assays (96).

Cell-mediated (Th1) responses have also been detected in exposed, uninfected sexual partners of infected individuals and in commercial sex workers in Africa, suggesting that Th1 responses to HIV antigens may provide protection against infection. This has focused vaccine strategies on candidate vaccines engineered to present multiple peptides identified as HLA-specific T-cell epitopes. The presence of mucosal antibodies and cellular immunity in the genital tract of some exposed uninfected individuals (55–58) provides evidence for a potential protective effect that might be useful for future vaccine strategies that elicit cellular and mucosal immunity. On the other hand, the frequency of recombinant viruses among some serially exposed and recently infected individuals suggests that natural infection and the induced immunity may not provide a high barrier against "superinfection" (97).

Further evidence for the importance of HLA-specific cellular immunity can be found in the association between the alleles of the class I and class II MHC genes, and clinical progression. In well-characterized cohorts in the United States, specific HLA types and supergroups have been identified in a statistically significant fraction of LTNPs and RPs. One of the more compelling demonstrations of the role of HLA genes can be found in an analysis by Carrington and O'Brien of the rate of progression among seroconverting individuals in cohorts in U. S. studies (61). Among HIV-infected individuals in this study, homozygosity at any of the three class I HLA loci was shown to be associated with a two-fold increase in risk for AIDS. In addition, specific HLA-C and -B alleles were shown to be associated with more rapid progression. Similarly, a study of mother-to-infant transmission in Kenya provides evidence that shared maternal–infant alleles represent an independent risk factor for such transmission (98).

CYTOKINES IN HIV INFECTION

Cytokines play a critical role in the regulation of both innate and acquired immune responses and can therefore affect several steps of the viral life cycle. Like studies carried out in developed countries where HIV-1 subtype B predominates, studies conducted in Africa have reported elevated levels of proinflammatory cytokines, particularly TNF-α in plasma or serum of HIV-1–infected individuals (30,38,43,99–101). Interestingly, in some of the studies that sought to compare in-vitro cytokine levels between HIV-1–negative Caucasians and Africans, members of the latter group showed higher immune activation (38,43,100). This difference may reflect the chronic activation of the immune system of Africans owing to the prevalence of infections by microorganisms such as *Mycobacterium tuberculosis*, helminths, and other parasites.

Cytokines affect every step of the viral life cycle, from cell entry to the budding of progeny virions. In vitro, the proinflammatory cytokines, tumor necrosis factor-alpha (TNF-α) and TNF-β upregulate HIV infection (102–107). Nuclear factor-kappaB (NF-κB) binding to a consensus sequence in the core enhancer region of HIV's long terminal repeat (LTR), in proximity to the transcription start site, triggers or potentiates HIV expression (108). A cascade of events in the signaling pathways that arise from HIV–host receptor interactions culminate in the dissociation of the NF-κB from an inhibitory molecule in the cytoplasm. Activated NF-κB then migrates into the nucleus and binds to consensus sequences in the promoter region of several cellular genes as well as to consensus sequences in the viral LTR, leading to potentiation for viral transcription (108). Recent studies have shown that the NF-κB–enhancer configuration and copy number differ among HIV-1 subtypes. Thus, in the subtype B and E viruses, one or two NF-κB consensus sequences are present in the core enhancer region of the viral LTR in proximity to the transcription start site (30,109,110). In contrast, three or more NF-κB consensus sequences have been reported in subtype C isolates, with an NF-κB–enhancer configuration that has been shown to correlate with an elevated TNF-α activation (30,110). The significance of this subtype-specific variation in the number and configuration of NF-κB binding sites remains to be established. Several other proinflammatory cytokines, such as IL-1α, IL-1β (104,105,111), IL-2 (112), IL-3 (113), IL-6 (110,114), IL-7 (115), IL-15 (116,117), IL-18 (118), macro-phage colony-stimulating factor (119), and granulocyte macrophage-colony stimulating factor (113,120) have been reported to upregulate HIV replication. The precise mechanism by which these other proinflammatory cytokines upregulate HIV expression/replication has not been elucidated; however, a similar mechanism to that exerted by TNF-α has been reported in some studies. The anti-inflammatory cytokines, IFN-α, IFN-β, IL-13, and IL-16, have been shown to inhibit HIV replication in vitro (121–125). However, some anti-inflammatory cytokines, such as IL-4, IL-10, IL-12, transforming growth factor-β, IFN-γ, and chemokines (a group of chemotactic cytokines), have been shown to either suppress or activate HIV-1 replication depending on the conditions in vitro (112,113,126–134).

Several studies have quantified levels of cytokines, their receptors, and receptor antagonists in HIV-1–infected patients in Africa and in AIDS patients in Africa. A comparative study in the Democratic Republic of the Congo (formerly Zaire) of women with HIV-1 infection and women with AIDS reported high plasma levels of IL-1β, TNF-α, and an excess of IL-1β receptor antagonist and TNF-α soluble p55 receptor in HIV-infected women who were clinically asymptomatic but not in women with AIDS or in seronegative controls (99). The researchers concluded that circulating antagonists may play a clinical role in modulating cytokine-associated symptoms in early HIV infection. HIV-1–infected Africans living in Sweden were shown to have higher levels of TNF-α than their Caucasian counterparts living in Sweden, suggesting that factors other than the immediate environment may contribute to elevated levels of TNF-α in seropositive patients in Africa (100).

Studies comparing immune activation in HIV-1–infected/uninfected Ugandans and Italians have revealed some interesting differences. In-vitro activation of freshly isolated peripheral blood mononuclear cells showed that Ugandan patients infected with HIV had higher levels of TNF-α, IFN-γ, IL-10, and Th2-associated markers than did Italian patients infected with HIV. These differences in the degree of immune activation are also reflected in comparisons of the Ugandan HIV-negative controls with the Italian negative controls, leading the researchers to conclude that HIV disease in Africa is associated with abnormal immune activation, a feature that is also present in HIV-negative Africans (42). In contrast, a comparison of immune activation between subtype B- and subtype C-infected individuals from Israel and Ethiopia, respectively, showed similar immune activation profiles with decreases in the levels of IL-2, IL-4, IL-10, and IL-12 despite the distinct immune backgrounds of the two populations (44). However, in the same study, the researchers reported that the Ethiopians who were seronegative had exceedingly high levels of p75 TNF receptors, IL-4 and IL-10, relative to those measured in their Israeli counterparts (44).

Other studies in Africa have investigated the cytokine network in seropositive individuals who are also infected with tropical microorganisms or who have disorders associated with defective immune systems. A study conducted in Kenya reported an increase in the levels of IL-4, IL-6, IL-10, and TNF-α in HIV-infected individuals with gonococcal cervicitis followed by a return to baseline levels after gonorrheal treatment. Similar changes were noted among women with acute pelvic inflammatory disease (101). In Ghana, treatment of tuberculosis (TB) in patients infected with HIV-1 and TB did not reduce the high levels of TNF-α and IL-6 observed in these patients before treatment (102). In a similar study in Burkina Faso, the rate of production of IL-5 in patients infected with HIV-1 and TB was not significantly different than that found in HIV-1–negative, TB-positive patients (135).

Chemokines have recently been shown to inhibit HIV-1 replication by competing with the virus for members of the seven-transmembrane-spanning chemokine receptor family (136,137). Chemokines are classified into two subfamilies: CXC or α-chemokines and CC or β-chemokines. HIV-1 uses the CD4 receptor together with several members of a given chemokine coreceptor to gain entry into target cells (138–143). The T-tropic HIV-1 viruses that use the CX receptor 4 (CXR4) as their chemokine coreceptor have also been characterized as syncytium-inducing (SI) viruses (138), while the HIV-1 viruses characterized as nonsyncytium-inducing (NSI) (known as macrophage tropic or M-tropic viruses) have been shown to use the CC receptor 5 (CCR5) as their major coreceptor and CCR2b, CCR3, and CCR8 as minor coreceptors (138–142). The beta-chemokines, macrophage inflammatory protein (MIP)-1α, MIP-1β, and regulated-on-activation-normal-T-cell expressed-and-secreted (RANTES), which are the physiologic ligands for CCR5, inhibit CD4/CCR5-mediated HIV-1 entry into target cells (144). Stromal derived factor (SDF)-1, the natural ligand for CXCR4, inhibits target-cell entry of T-tropic HIV-1 viruses (145,146). Recently, CCR3 has been shown to promote HIV-1 infection of the central nervous system (147). Other HIV-1 chemokine coreceptors, CCR1, CCR2, CCR3, and CCR4, have also been reported to play a role in HIV-1 entry into target cells (148).

Although coreceptor use in subtype B viruses has been studied extensively, there are a limited number of studies of chemokine coreceptor use in other HIV-1 subtypes. Zhang and colleagues tested 14 non-B subtype isolates (three A, three C, three D, three E, and two O) and found that use of the CXR4 coreceptor appeared to correlate with biologic phenotype rather than viral genotype (149). A larger study of 81 viral isolates representing nine genetic subtypes (A–J, except I) reported that chemokine receptor use appeared to be subtype-dependent (150). For each of the HIV-1 subtypes investigated in this study, there was a correlation between the ability to infect using the CXCR4 coreceptor and the ability to induce syncytium formation. These researchers also noted that among subtype C isolates, 94% only used CCR5 coreceptor entry while one isolate, taken from a patient with stage A2 AIDS (based on staging guidelines of the Centers for Disease Control and Prevention in the United States) used the CXCR4 coreceptor. In addition, the investigators also noted that subtype D isolates did not show dual tropism for the CXCR4 and CCR5 coreceptors. The subtype-specific differences observed in coreceptor use in this study were not the result of differences in clinical status, $CD4^+$ cell counts, or treatment (150). In a subsequent study, the same team of investigators reported that subtype C isolates obtained from Ethiopian AIDS patients used the CCR5 coreceptor exclusively (151). Although M-tropic viruses use CCR5 for entry into target cells, the subtype C isolates from the Ethiopian AIDS patients failed to establish productive infection in primary monocytes-macrophages (151). The use of CCR5 as the sole receptor by subytpe C isolates was further supported by a study of subtype C isolates from patients in Malawi (152).

The ability of the most extensively studied subtype B virus to use a chemokine coreceptor and to switch from the use of one coreceptor to another has been largely attributed to the sequence variation in the variable third region (V3) domain of the envelope protein, particularly to basic amino acid substitutions in this region (153,154). In contrast, sequence variability in the V3 loop of the subtype C isolates from Malawi was not associated with the presence of basic amino acid substitutions (152). A study of 22 subtype C isolates from patients in Zimbabwe demonstrated that three of these isolates were

SIs while 19 were NSIs, and that the viral phenotypes of those isolated were associated with CXCR4 and CCR5 coreceptor use, respectively (155). However, subsequent investigations have shown that two of the SI isolates use CCR5 coreceptor, although the reason for the genotype/phenotype discordance is not clear (Katzenstein et al.: unpublished observations). In agreement with other studies, the SI phenotype observed with the three subtype C isolates from patients in Zimbabwe was associated with low $CD4^+$ cell count and high viral load (156–158).

Mutations in some of the chemokine receptors are associated with resistance to HIV-1 infection or with a slower rate of AIDS progression among Caucasians in the United States (159). Deletion of a 32-base-pair (CCR5D32) in the CCR5 gene is associated with resistance to infection by CCR5-tropic viruses in 15% to 20% of those Caucasians who are heterozygous for the mutation but only in 1% or less of those who are homozygous for the mutation (159). The homozygous genotype is associated with high resistance to HIV-1 infection while the heterozygous genotype, commonly found in LTNPs is associated with slower rates of AIDS progression (160). There are contradictory reports on the influence of the 64I allele of CCR2 on disease progression with some studies claiming decreased HIV-1 disease progression (161–163) and one study reporting that this allele had no influence on disease progression (164). Polymorphisms in the gene that encodes SDF-1, the natural ligand for CXCR4, are significantly associated with an accelerated progression in advanced disease (165). There are very few studies, however, that have investigated the role of chemokine polymorphisms in patients in Africa who are infected with HIV-1 or who have AIDS. In studies in Kenya in a cohort of commercial sex workers who showed resistance to infection despite repeated exposure to HIV-1, resistance was not rela-ted to any of the above polymorphisms in HIV-1 coreceptors or chemokine receptors (58,166,167).

T-CELLS AND ANTIGEN RESPONSE

T-lymphocytes are involved in both innate and specific immunity, playing a role in both humoral- and cell-mediated immune responses. CTLs are usually associated with antiviral immunosurveillance. Consequently, the role of CTLs, especially in HIV-1 subtype B infection, has been an intensive field of research (168). The majority of investigations of CTL responses to proteins formed by HIV-1 subtype B viruses have argued that HIV-specific CTL responses are important to controlling HIV-1 replication and consequently act to slow the progression to AIDS (169). There are several studies that assess CTL responses in HIV-1–infected individuals in Africa. In a report of two HIV-exposed but uninfected female commercial sex workers in Gambia, vigorous, specific CTL responses to HIV-1, and HIV-2 cross-reactive peptides presented by HLA-B35, the most common HLA class I molecule in Gambia, led the researchers to conclude that this specific CTL activity may represent protective immunity against HIV infection (170). In another study, this one conducted in Kenya, investigators reported CTL responses to novel epitopes presented by HLA-A*6802 and by HLA-B18 in uninfected commercial sex workers exposed for up to 12 years to HIV-1 subtypes A, C, and D, leading the researchers to speculate that cross-clade CTL activity may protect this group of women against persistent infection (57). A recent study of adults and children that compared CTL responses in black South Africans infected with subtype C and Caucasoids from the United States infected with subtype B showed that three out of 46 Gag peptides tested (spanning p17- and p24-*gag* sequences) contained two-thirds of the dominant Gag-specific CTL epitopes irrespective of infecting subtype or an individual's ethnicity or age. However, there were differences in the regions of immunodominance within the p17 and p24 regions between the two racial groups (169). In Caucasians, dominant immune responses were found in the p17 *gag* peptide amino acid residues 16–30, while in black South Africans, the dominant responses were located in the p24 Gag peptide amino acid residues 41–60. Recently, a study to assess CTL responses in 17 HIV-1–infected individuals from Uganda, where subtypes A and D are endemic, reported a broad-based CTL response to antigens to subtypes A, B, and D with the most robust CTL response directed at subtype D epitopes. In some cases, the degree of recognition of subtype B epitopes by subtype D infected individuals was greater than that elicited for local coendemic subtype A epitopes, results that underpin decisions to conduct clinical trials of a subtype B-based vaccine in Uganda (171).

DELAYED-TYPE HYPERSENSITIVITY

Delayed-type hypersensitivity (DTH) reactions involve antigen sensitization of T-lymphocytes and the subsequent proliferation and differentiation of these lymphocytes into effector cells at the intradermal site of inoculation (172). Th1 or $CD8^+$ CTLs are involved in DTH reactions. DTH testing was used early in the HIV epidemic, in situations where anergy was considered a functional measure of immunodeficiency, and skin-test responses were used as part of the staging of HIV infection (173,174). Increased DTH to common antigens such as candida, streptokinase, streptodornase, and tetanus toxoid is associated with early responses to antiretroviral therapy (175). Increasing anergy to common skin-test antigens is associated with progression of HIV disease (176,177). One study of DTH testing of HIV-infected and uninfected individuals in Tanzania demonstrated an increase in the frequency of anergy among infected individuals (178). DTH testing is employed in clinical settings largely confined to determine whether an individual has previously been infected with *M. tuberculosis,* although this test has been found to be a poor tool for assessing immunity to tuberculosis in both vaccinated and unvaccinated populations (179,180). Because Th1 cells that release chemokines, proinflammatory cytokines, and cytotoxins are essential for protective immunity to *M. tuberculosis*, the tuberculin test may be a better choice for evaluating both the *M. tuberculosis* exposure status and the cytokine profile (Th1 or Th2) of an HIV-infected or AIDS patient.

A study in Uganda to determine the relationship between responses to tuberculin skin tests and cytokine profiles in HIV-positive and HIV-negative individuals showed that the Th1/Th2 balance was, in part, correlated with the skin-test results. In the HIV-negative cohort, a positive skin test was associated with type 1 or mixed cytokine production. In the HIV-positive cohort, by comparison, IFN-γ (Th1) production was profoundly impaired; IL-2 (Th1), IL-5, and TNF-α (Th2) levels were relatively sustained; and IL-10 (Th2) production was increased or sustained (181).

HLA DIVERSITY, IMMUNE-RESPONSE GENES AND DISEASE PROGRESSION

HLA molecules are important determinants of susceptibility and resistance to HIV-1 infection and disease progression. Several associations have been identified between HLA alleles and disease progression in individuals infected with HIV-1 subtype B (182–184). Recently, a longitudinal study of a cohort of repeatedly HIV-1–exposed female commercial sex workers in Pumwani, Kenya, reported that decreased susceptibility to HIV-1 infection was associated with the presence of HLA-A2/6802 supertype (185). In the same study, resistance to HIV-1 infection was independently associated with

HLA-DRB*01. It is interesting to note that earlier studies of the same Pumwani cohort reported that resistance to HIV-1 infection correlated with Th responses, CTL responses to HIV-1 peptide epitopes, and the presence of HIV-1–specific IgA in genital tract secretions (185). It would appear that both humoral and cell-mediated immunity are required for protection against HIV-1 infection, a conclusion relevant to efforts to develop a vaccine. An ongoing study of seronegative commercial sex workers in South Africa recently reported the clustering of HLA-A24, a characteristic not found in HIV-1–infected women, leading the researchers to speculate that this allele may confer protection against HIV-1 infection (186).

Th1 AND Th2 RESPONSES

T-helper cells are broadly classified as Th1, Th2, or Th0 based on the profile of cytokines they produce. Th1 cells, which are responsible for DTH reactions and for the activation of macrophages, produce IFN-γ, IL-2, TNF-β, and IL-12. Th2 cells, which are primarily associated with humoral immune responses, produce IL-4, IL-5, IL-6, IL-10 and IL-13. Th0 cells coexpress Th1 and Th2 cytokines in various combinations. In-vitro studies involving subtype B viruses have suggested a positive association between disease progression and the production of Th2 cytokines (187,188). Th1 cytokines have been shown to protect against disease progression (189), and Th2/Th0 cytokines have been shown to support replication of HIV-1 (190). The role of the Th1 to Th2 cytokine production switch, defined largely for subtype B viruses, is complicated by chronic infections in HIV-infected and AIDS patients in Africa. Helminthic infection has been shown to induce a predominantly Th2 effective response (191). Subsequent infection with mycobacteria was found to shift the immune response from the protective Th1 to the deleterious Th2 response (192). In contrast, Th1 and Th2 responses are found in malaria and each confers protection.

Several studies of HIV-infected individuals in Africa have documented high production of IFN-γ and IL-2 (Th1 cytokines) and of TNF-α, IL-4, and IL-10 (Th2 cytokines) (29,36,38,106–109), data that appear to refute the hypothesis that Th2 cytokines predominate in HIV-1–infected individuals. Comparisons of Th1 and Th2 cytokine levels in HIV-uninfected Africans and Caucasians have shown higher levels of both to be present in Africans, leading some investigators to speculate that hyperimmune activation observed in Africans is a major contributory factor in the pathogenesis of AIDS in Africa (193).

CONCLUSION

The immunopathogenesis of AIDS is a product of host and viral genetics, immune activation, and environmental conditions. Exposed individuals either become infected or resist infection based on the interactions of these factors. Among those infected, their capacity to transmit the virus, their rate of disease progression, and their clinical prognosis also depend upon multiple factors. We have come to understand that HLA alleles and their cognate T-cell epitopes; cellular and humoral immune responses; and chemokine receptor polymorphisms and mutations each play a role in the immunopathogenesis of HIV-1 infection. The immune response within an individual and a population may select for the transmission, replication, and the relative success of certain viral subtypes and circulating recombinant forms (194). Immune responses, conditioned by HLA alleles inherited from each parent and chemokine receptor genes, exert negative and positive selection pressures on viruses for their expression of antigens and their susceptibility to various arms of the immune system. In Africa, these interactions between host and pathogen take place in individuals and populations who may be more vulnerable to infection due to nutritional deficiencies and chronic parasitic infections with concomitant immune hyperactivation.

REFERENCES

1. Fauci AS. The human immunodeficiency virus: infectivity and mechanisms of pathogenesis. *Science*, 1988;239:617–622.
2. Fauci AS. Multifactorial nature of human immunodeficiency virus disease implications for therapy. *Science*, 1993;262:1011–1018.
3. Fauci AS. Host factors and the pathogenesis of HIV-1 induced disease. *Nature*, 1996;384:529–534.
4. Cao Y, Qin L, Zhang L, et al. Virologic and immunologic characterization of long term survivors of human immunodeficiency virus type 1 infection. *N Engl J Med*, 1995;332:301–330.
5. Pantaleo G, Menzo S, Vaccarezza M, et al. Studies in subjects with long-term nonprogressive HIV infection. *N Engl J Med*, 1995;332:209–216.
6. Pantaleo G, Graziosi C, Demarest JF, et al. HIV Infection is active and progressive in lymphoid tissue during the clinically latent stage of disease. *Nature*, 1993;362:355–358.
7. Alexander L, Weiskopf E, Greenough TC, et al. Unusual polymorphisms in human immunodeficiency virus type 1 associated with nonprogressive infection. *J Virol*, 2000;74:4361–4376.
8. Greenough TC, Brettler DB, Somasundaran DL. Human immundoeficiency virus type 1-specific cytotoxic T lymphocytes (CTL) virus load and CD4 cell loss: evidence supporting a protective role of CTL in vivo. *J Infect Dis*, 1997;176:118–125.
9. Rivets H, Marissens D, De Wit S, et al. Comparative Evaluation of NASBA HIV-1 RNA QT, AMPLICOR-HIV Monitor, and QUANTIPLEX HIV RNA Assay, Three Methods for Quantification of Human Immunodeficiency Virus Type 1 RNA in Plasma. *J Clin Microbiol*, 1996;34:1058–1064.
10. Piatak M, Saag MS, Yang LC, et al. High levels of HIV-1 in plasma during all stages of infection determined by competitive PCR. *Science*, 1993; 259:1749–1754.
11. Henrard DR, Daar E, Farzadegan H, et al. Virologic and immunologic characterizations of symptomatic and asymptomatic primary HIV-1 infection. *J Acq Imm Def Synd Hum Retro*, 1995;9:305–310.
12. Mellors JW, Muanoz A, Giorgi JV, et al. Plasma viral load and $CD4^+$ lymphocytes as prognostic markers of HIV-1 infection. *Ann Intern Med*, 1997;126: 946–954.
13. Miller V, Mocroft A, Reiss P, et al. Relations among CD4 lymphocyte count nadir, antiretroviral therapy, and HIV-1 disease progression: results from the EuroSIDA study. *Ann Intern Med*, 1999;130: 570–577.
14. Morgan D, Rutemberwa A, Malamba S, et al. HIV-1 RNA levels in an African population-based cohort and their relation to CD4 lymphocyte counts and World Health Organization clinical staging. *J Acquir Immune Defic Syndr*, 1999;22: 167–173.
15. Taha TE, Kumwenda NI, Hoover DR, et al. Association of HIV-1 load and CD4 lymphocyte count with mortality among untreated African children over one year of age. *AIDS*, 2000;10;14: 453–459.
16. Kassa E, Rinke de Wit TF, Hailu E, et al. Evaluation of the World Health Organization staging system for HIV infection and disease in Ethiopia: association between clinical stages and laboratory markers. *AIDS*, 1999;13:381–389.
17. van der Ryst E, Kotze M, Joubert G, et al. Correlation among total lymphocyte count, absolute CD4+ count, and CD4+ percentage in a group of HIV-1–infected South African patients. *J Acquir Immune Defic Syndr Hum Retrovirol*, 1998;19: 238–244.
18. Rinaldo C, Huang XL, Fan ZF, et al. High levels of anti-human immundoeficiency virus type 1 memory cytotoxic T-lymphocyte activity and low virus load are associated with lack of disease in HIV-1–infected long-term non-progressors. *J Virol*, 1995;69:5838–5842.
19. Rosenberg ES, Billingsley JM, Caliendo AM, et al. Vigorous HIV-1 specific $CD4^+$ T cell responses associated with control of viremia. *Science*, 1997;278:1447–1450.
20. Gourgeon ML, Montagnier L. Apoptosis in AIDS [published erratum in *Science*, 1993;260:1709]. *Science*, 1993;260:1269–1270.
21. Finkel TH, Tudor-Williams G, Banda NK, et al. Apoptosis occurs predominantly in bystander cells and not in productively infected cells of HIV- and SIV-infected lymph nodes. *Nat Med*, 1995; 129–134.
22. Lane HC, Masur H, Edgar LC, et al. Abnormalities of B-cell activation and immunoregulation in patients with the acquired immunodeficiency syndrome. *N. Engl J Med*, 1983;309:453–458.
23. Martinez-Maza O, Crabb E, Mitsyuasu RT, et al. Infection with human immunodeficiency virus (HIV) is associated with an *in vivo* increase in B lymphocyte activation and immaturity. *J Immunol*, 1987;138:3720–3724.
24. Katzenstein DA, Latif AS, Grace A, et al. Clinical and laboratory characteristics of HIV-1 infection in Zimbabwe. *J Acquir Immune Defic Syndr Hum Retrovirol*, 1990;3:701–701.
25. Wilcock G, Grace S, De Villiers D, et al. Karposi's sarcoma in Zimbabwe. II. Peripheral lymphocytes,

immunoglobulin G levels, and HIV positivity. *J Clin Lab Immunol*, 1998;27:25028.

26. Munoz A, Carey V, Saah AJ, et al. Predictors of decline in CD4 lymphocytes in a cohort of homosexual men infected with human immunodeficiency virus. *J Acquir Immune Defic Syndr Hum Retrovirol*, 1988;1:396–404.
27. Fahey JL, Taylor JMG, Detels R, et al. The prognostic value of cellular and serologic markers in infection with human immunodeficiency virus type I. *N. Engl J Med*, 1990;322:166–172.
28. Moss AR, Bacchetti P, Osmond D, et al. Seropositivity for HIV and the development of AIDS or AIDS related condition: three year follow up of the San Francisco cohort. *Br Med J*, 1988;296:745–750.
29. Lacey JN, Forbes MA, Waugh MA, et al. Serum beta2-microglobulin and human immunodeficiency virus infection. *AIDS*,1997;1:123–127.
30. Hofmann B, Wang Y, Cumberland WG, et al. Immune activation by HIV: seroconversion and progression in serum beta2-microglobulin. *AIDS*, 1990;4:207–214.
31. Fuchs D, Hausen A, Reignegger G, et al. Neopterin as a marker for activated cell mediated immunity: application in HIV infection. *Immunol Today*,1988; 9:150–155.
32. Ziegler I, Rokos H. Pteridines and the immune response. *J Immunol Immunopharm*, 1986;6: 169–177.
33. Melmed RN, Taylor JM, Detels R, et al. Serum neopterin changes in HIV-infected subjects: indicator of significant pathology, CD4 T cell change, and the development of AIDS. *J Acquir Immune Defic Syndr*, 1989;2:70–76.
34. Dyer JR, Eron JJ, Hoffman IF, et al. Association of CD4 cell depletion and elevated blood and seminal plasma human immunodeficiency virus type 1 (HIV-1) RNA concentrations with genital ulcer disease in HIV-1–infected men in Malawi. *J Infect Dis*, 1998;177:224–227.
35. McCune JM, Hanley MB, Cesar D, et al. Factors influencing T-cell turnover in HIV-1 seropositive patients. *J Clin Invest*, 1999;105:R1–R8.
36. Grant AD, Djomand G, De Cock KM. Natural history and spectrum of disease in adults with HIV/AIDS in Africa. *AIDS*, 1997;11 Suppl B:S43–S54.
37. Wood R, Maartens G, Lombard CJ. Risk factors for developing tuberculosis in HIV-1–infected adults from communities with a low or very high incidence of tuberculosis. *J Acquir Immune Defic Syndr*, 2000;23:75–80.
38. Bentwich Z, Kalinkovich A, Weisman Z. Immune activation is a dominant factor in the pathogenesis of African AIDS. *Immunol Today*, 1995;16: 187–91.
39. Migot F, Ouedraogo JB, Diallo J, et al. Selected *P. falciparum* specific immune responses are maintained in AIDS adults in Burkina Faso. *Parasite Immunol*, 1996;18:333–339.
40. Gopinath R, Ostrowski M, Justement SJ, et al. Filarial infections increase susceptibility to human immunodeficiency virus infection in peripheral blood mononuclear cells in vitro. *J Infect Dis*, 2000;182: 1804–1808.
41. Berneir RS, Turco J, Olivier M, Tremblay M. Acitvation of human immunodeficiency virus type 1 in monocytoid cells by the protozoan parasite Leishmania donovani. *J Virol*, 1995;69: 7282–7285.
42. Rizzardini G, Trabattoni D, Saresella M, et al. Immune activation in HIV-infected African individuals. Italian-Ugandan AIDS cooperation program. *AIDS*, 1998;12:2387–2396.
43. Messele T, Abdulkadir M, Fontanet AL et al. Reduced naive and increased activated CD4 and CD8 cells in healthy adult Ethiopians compared with their Dutch counterparts. *Clin Exp Immunol*, 1999;115: 443–450.
44. Weisman Z, Kalinkovich A, Borkow G et al. Infection by different HIV-1 subtypes (B and C) results in a similar immune activation profile despite distinct immune backgrounds. *J Acquir Immune Defic Syndr*, 1999;21:157–163.
45. Weissman D, Barker TD, Fauci AS. The efficiency of acute infection of $CD4^+$ T cells is markedly enhanced in the setting of antigen-specific immune activation. *J Exp Med*, 1996;183:687–692.
46. Whitworth J, Morgan D, Quigley M et al. Effect of HIV-1 and increasing immunosuppression on malaria parasitaemia and clinical episodes in adults in rural Uganda: a cohort study. *Lancet*, 2000;356: 1051–1056.
47. French N, Gilks CF. Royal Society of Tropical Medicine and Hygiene meeting at Manson House, London, 18 March 1999. Fresh from the field: some controversies in tropical medicine and hygiene. HIV and malaria, do they interact? *Trans Royal Soc Trop Med Hyg*, 2000;94: 233–237.
48. Antelman G, Msamanga GI, Spiegelman D, et al. Nutritional factors and infectious disease contribute to anemia among pregnant women with human immunodeficiency virus in Tanzania. *J Nutr*, 2000;130:1950–1957.
49. Tsegaye A, Messele T, Tilahun T, Immunohematological reference ranges for adult Ethiopians. *Clin Diagn Lab Immunol*, 1999;6:410–414.
50. Bogden JD, Kemp FW, Han S, et al. Status of selected nutrients and progression of human immunodeficiency virus type 1 infection. *Am J Clin Nutr*, 2000;2:809–815.
51. Baum MK, Shor-Posner G, Campa A. Zinc status in human immunodeficiency virus infection. *J Nutr*, 2000;130(5S Suppl):1421S-1423S.

52. Dannhauser A, van Staden AM, van der Ryst E, et al. Nutritional status of HIV-1 seropositive patients in the Free State Province of South Africa: anthropometric and dietary profile. *Eur J Clin Nutr*, 1999;53:165–173.
53. Fawzi WW, Msamanga GI, Spiegelman D. Randomised trial of effects of vitamin supplements on pregnancy outcomes and T cell counts in HIV-1-infected women in Tanzania. *Lancet*, 1998;351: 1477–1482.
54. Kelly P, Musonda R, Kafwembe E, Micronutrient supplementation in the AIDS diarrhoea-wasting syndrome in Zambia: a randomized controlled trial. *AIDS*, 1999;13:495–500.
55. Ng TT, Pinching AJ, Guntermann C, et al. Molecular immunopathogenesis of HIV infection. *Genitourin Med*, 1996;72(6):408–18.
56. Kaul R, Plummer FA, Kimani J, et al. HIV-1 specific $CD8^+$ lymphocyte responses in the cervix of HIV-1–resistant prostitutes in Nairobi. *J Immunol*, 2000;164:1602–1611.
57. Rowland-Jones S, Dong T, Fowke KR, et al. Cytotoxic T cell responses to multiple conserved HIV epitopes in HIV-resistant prostitutes in Nairobi. *J Clin Invest*, 1998;102:1758–1765.
58. Kaul R, Trabattoni D, Bwayo JJ, et al. HIV-specific mucosal IgA in a cohort of HIV-1 resistant Kenyan sex workers. *AIDS*, 1999;13:23–29.
59. MacDonald KS, Keith R, Kimani FJ, et al. Influence of HLA supertypes on susceptibility and resistance to human immunodeficiency virus type 1 infection. *J Infect Dis*, 200;181:1581–1589.
60. Roger M. Influence of Host genes on HIV-1 progression. *FASEB J*, 1998;12:625–632.
61. Carrington M, Nelson GW, Martin MP, et al. HLA and HIV-1: Heterozygote advantage and B*35-Cw*04 disadvantage. *Science*, 1999;283: 1748–1752.
62. Autran B, Haidida F, Haas G. Evolution and plasticity of CTL responses against HIV. *Curr Opin Immunol*, 1996;8:546–553.
63. French N, Mujugira A, Nakiyingi J, et al. Immunologic and clinical stages in HIV-1–infected Ugandan adults are comparable and provide no evidence of rapid progression but poor survival with advanced disease. *J Acquir Immune Defic Syndr*, 1999;22: 509–516.
64. Ho DD, Neuman AU, Perleson AS, et al. Rapid turnover of plasma virions and CD4+ lymphocytes in HIV infection. *Nature*, 1995;373:123–126.
65. Wei X, Ghosh, Talylor ME, et al. Viral dymanics in HIV-1 infection. *Nature*, 1995;373:117–122.
66. Hellerstein MK, McCune JM. T cell turnover in HIV-1 disease. *Immunity*, 1997;7:583–598.
67. Clark DR, de Boer RJ, Wolters KC and Miedma F. T cell dynamics in HIV-1 infection *Adv Immunol*, 1999;73:301–332.
68. Autran B, Carcelain G, Li TS, et al. Positive effects of combined antiretroviral therapy on CD4+ T-cell homeostasis and function in advanced HIV disease. *Science*, 1997;227:112–116.
69. Lederman MM, Connick E, Landay A, et al. Immunologic responses associated with 12 weeks of combination antiretroviral therapy consisting of zidovudine, lamivudine and ritonavir. *J Infect Dis*, 1998;178:70–79.
70. Richman DD, Normal physiology and HIV pathophysiology of human T-cell dynamics. *J Clin Invest*, 2000;105:565–566.
71. Lederman MM, Valdez H. Immune restoration with antiretroviral therapies. *JAMA*, 2000;284:223–228.
72. Katzenstein DA, Mbizvo M, Zijenah L, et al. Serum level of maternal human immunodeficiency virus (HIV) RNA, infant mortality, and vertical transmission of HIV in Zimbabwe. *J Infect Dis*, 1999; 179:1382–1387.
73. Nunn PP, Brindle R, Carpenter L, et al. Cohort study of HIV infection in patients with tuberculosis in Nairobi, Kenya. Analysis of early (6 mo) mortality. *Am Rev Respir Dis*, 1992;146:849–854.
74. Sloand E, Pitt E, Chiarello RJ, Nemo GJ. HIV testing state of the art. *JAMA*, 1991;266:2861–2866.
75. van Binsbergen J, de Rijk D, Peels H, et al. Evaluation of a new third generation anti-HIV-1/anti-HIV-2 assay with increased sensitivity for HIV-1 group O. *J Virol Methods*, 1996;60:131–137.
76. Frank AP, Wandell MG, Headings MD, et al. Anonymous HIV testing using home collection and telemedicine counseling. A multicenter evaluation. *Archives of Int Med*, 1997;157:309–314.
77. Gallo D, George JR, Fitchen JH, et al. Evaluation of a system using oral mucosal transudate for HIV-1 antibody screening and confirmatory testing. *JAMA*, 1997;277:254–258.
78. Urnovitz HB, Sturge JC, Gottfried TD, Murphy WH. Urine antibody tests: new insights into the dynamics of HIV-1 infection. *Clin Chem*, 1999;45; 1602–1613.
79. Janssen RS, Satten GA, Stramer, SL, et al. New testing strategy to detect early HIV-1 infection for use in incidence estimates and for clinical and prevention purposes. *JAMA*, 1998;280;42–48.
80. LaCasse RA, Follis KE, Trahey M, et al. Fusion-competent vaccines: broad neutralization of primary isolates of HIV. *Science*, 1999;283:357–362.
81. Park EJ, Gorny MK, Zolla-Pazner S, Quinnan GV Jr. A global neutralization resistance phenotype of human immunodeficiency virus type 1 is determined by distinct mechanisms mediating enhanced infectivity and conformational change of the envelope complex. *J Virol*, 2000;74:4183–4191.
82. Beirnaert E, Nyambi P, Willems B, et al. Identification and characterization of sera from HIV-infected individuals with broad cross-neutralizing

activity against group M (env clade A-H) and group O primary HIV-1 isolates. *J Med Virol,* 2000;62: 14–24.

83. Fust G. Enhancing antibodies in HIV infection. *Parasitology,* 1997;115 Suppl:S127–S140.
84. Ruppach H, Nara P, Raudonat I, et al. Human immunodeficiency virus (HIV)-positive sera obtained shortly after seroconversion neutralize autologous HIV type1 isolates on primary macrophages but not on lymphocytes. *J Virol,* 2000;74:5403–5411.
85. Lathey JL, Tsou J, Brinker K, et al. Lack of autologous neutralizing antibody to human immunodeficiency virus type 1 (HIV-1) and macrophage tropism are associated with mother-to-infant transmission. *J Infect Dis,* 1999;180:344–350.
86. Carotenuto P, Looij D, Keldermans L, de Wolf F, Goudsmit J. Neutralizing antibodies are positively associated with $CD4^+$ T-cell counts and T-cell function in long-term AIDS-free infection. *AIDS,* 1998;12:1591–1600.
87. Cecilia D, Kleeberger C, Munoz A, Giorgi JV, Zolla-Pazner S. A longitudinal study of neutralizing antibodies and disease progression in HIV-1–infected subjects. *J Infect Dis,* 1999;179: 1365–1374.
88. Barker E, Mackewicz CE, Reyes-Teran G, et al. Virological and immunological features of long-term human immunodeficiency virus-infected individuals who have remained asymptomatic compared with those who have progressed to acquired immunodeficiency syndrome. *Blood,* 1998;92: 3105–3114.
89. Jolly PE, Weiss HL. Neutralization and enhancement of HIV-1 infection by sera from HIV-1 infected individuals who progress to disease at different rates. *Virology,* 2000;273:52–59.
90. Nokta M, Turk P, Loesch K, Pollard RB. Neutralization profiles of sera from human immunodeficiency virus (HIV)-infected individuals: relationship to HIV viral load and CD4 cell count. *Clin Diagn Lab Immunol,* 2000;7:412–416.
91. Lewis J, Balfe P, Arnold C, et al. Development of a neutralizing antibody response during acute primary human immunodeficiency virus type 1 infection and the emergence of antigenic variants. *J Virol,* 1998;72:8943–8951.
92. Ciurea A, Hunziker L, Klenerman P, et al. Impairment of $CD4^+$ T cell responses during chronic virus infection prevents neutralizing antibody response against virus escape mutants. *J Exp Med,* 2001;193:297–305.
93. Poignard P, Sabbe R, Picchio GR. Neutralizing anti-bodies have limited effects on the control of established HIV-1 infection in vivo. *Immunity,* 1999; 10:431–438.
94. Schonning K, Joost M, Gram GJ, et al. Chemokine receptor polymorphism and autologous neutralizing antibody response in long-term HIV-1 infection. *J Acquir Immune Defic Syndr Hum Retrovirol,* 1998;18:195–202.
95. Bradney AP, Scheer S, Crawford JM, et al. Neutralization escape in human immunodeficiency virus type 1–infected long-term nonprogressors. *J Infect Dis,* 1999;179:1264–1267.
96. Gea-Banacloche JC, Migueles SA, Martino L, et al. Maintenance of large numbers of virus-specific CD8+ T cells in HIV-infected progressors and long-term nonprogressors. *J Immunol,* 2000;165: 1082–1092.
97. Salminen MO, Carr JK, Robertson DL, et al. Evolution and probable transmission of intrasubtype recombinant human immunodeficiency virus type 1 in a Zambian couple. *J Virol,* 1997;71: 2647–2655.
98. MacDonald KS, Embree J, Njenga S, et al. Mother-child class I HLA concordance increases perinatal human immunodeficiency virus type 1 transmission. *J Infect Dis,* 1998;177:551–556.
99. Thea DM, Porat R, Nagimbi K, et al. Plasma cytokines, cytokine antagonists, disease progression in African women infected with HIV-1. *Ann Intern Med,* 1996;124:757–762.
100. Sonnerborg A, Ayehunie S, Julander I. Elevated levels of circulating tumor necrosis factor alpha in human immunodeficiency virus type 1–infected Africans living in Sweden. *Clin Diagn Lab Immunol,* 1995;2:118–119.
101. Anzala A, Simonsen J, Kimani J, et al. Acute sexually transmitted infections increase HIV-1 plasma viremia, increase plasma type 2 cytokines, and decrease CD4 counts. *J Infect Dis,* 2000; 182:459–466.
102. Lawn SD, Shattock RJ, Acheampong JW, et al. Sustained plasma TNF-alpha and HIV-1 load despite resolution of other parameters of immune activation during treatment of tuberculosis in Africans. *AIDS,* 1999;12:2231–2237.
103. Clouse KA, Powell D, Washington I, et al. Monokine regulation of human immunodeficiency virus-1 expression in a chronically infected human T cell clone. *J. Immunol,* 1989;142:431–438.
104. Osborn L, Kunkel S, Nabel GJ. Tumour necrosis factor alpha and interleukin 1 stimulate the human immunodeficiency virus enhancer by activation of the nuclear factor kB. *Proc Natl Acad Sci USA,* 1989;2336–2340.
105. Duh EJ, Maury WJ, Folks TM, et al. Tumour necrosis factor a activates human immunodeficiency virus type 1 through induction of nuclear factor binding to the NF-kB sites in the long terminal repeat. *Proc Natl Acad Sci USA,* 1989;86: 5974–5978.
106. Griffin GE, Leung K, Folks TM, et al. Activation of HIV gene expression during monocyte differentiation by induction of NF-kappa B. *Nature,* 1989;339:70–73.

107. Franzoso G, Biswas P, Poli G, et al. A family of serine proteases expressed exclusively in myelo-monocytic cells specifically processes the nuclear factor kappa B subunit p65 in vitro and may impair human immunodeficiency virus replication in these cells. *J Exp Med,* 1994;180: 1445–1456.
108. Siebenlist U, Franzoso G, Brown K. Structure, regulation and function of NF-kB. *Ann Rev Cell Biol,* 1994;10:405–455.
109. Gao F, Roberton DL, Morrison SG, et al. The heterosexual human immunodeficiency virus type 1 epidemic in Thailand is caused by an intersubtype (A/E) recombinant of African origin. *J Virol,* 1996;70:7013–7029.
110. Montano MA, Novitsky VA, Blackard JT, et al. Divergent transcriptional regulation among expanding human immunodeficiency type 1 subtypes. *J Virol,* 1997;71:8657–8665.
111. Poli G, Kinter AL, Fauci AS. Interleukin 1 induces expression of the human immunodeficiency virus alone and in synergy with interleukin 6 in chronically infected U1 cells: inhibition of inductive effects by the interleukin 1 receptor antagonist. *Proc Natl Acad Sci USA,* 1994;91;108–112.
112. Kinter AL, Poli G, Fox L, et al. HIV replication in IL-2 stimulated peripheral blood mononuclear cells is driven in an autocrine/paracrine manner by endogenous cytokines. *J Immunol,* 1995; 2448–2459.
113. Koyanagi Y, O'Brien WA, Zhao JQ, et al. Cytokines alter production of HIV-1 from primary mononuclear phagocytes. *Science,* 1988;241: 1673–1675.
114. Poli G, Bressler P, Kinter A, et al. Interleukin 6 induces human immunodeficiency virus expression in infected monocytic cells alone and in synergy with tumor necrosis factor alpha by transcriptional and post-transcriptional mechanism. *J Exp Med,* 1990; 172:151–158.
115. Moran PA, Diegel ML, Sias JC, et al. Regulation HIV production by blood mononuclear cells from HIV-infected donors: I. Lack of correlation between HIV-1 production and T cell activation. *AIDS Res Hum Retroviruses,* 1993;9:455–464.
116. Al-Harthi L, Roebuck KA, Landay A. Induction of HIV-1 replication by type 1-like cytokines, IL-12 and IL-15:effect on viral transcriptional activation, cellular proliferation and endogenous cytokine production. *J Clin Immunol,* 1998;18:124–131.
117. Bayard-McNeeley M, Doo H, He S, Hafner A, et al. Differential effects of interleukin-12, interleukin 15, and interleukin 2 on human immunodeficiency virus type 1 replication in vitro. *Clin Diag Lab Immunol,* 1996;3:547–553.
118. Shapiro L, Puren AJ, Barton HA, et al. Interleukin 18 stimulate HIV type 1 in monocytic cells. *Proc Natl Acad Sci USA,* 1998;95:12550–12555.
119. Gendelman HE, Orenstein JM, Martin MA, et al. Efficient isolation and propagation of human immunodeficiency virus on recombinant colony-stimulating factor 1-treated monocytes. *J Exp Med,* 1988;167:1428–1441.
120. Folks TM, Justement J, Kinter A, et al. Cytokine-induced expression of HIV-1 in a chronically infected promonocyte cell line, *Science,* 1987; 238: 800–802.
121. Ho DD, Hartshorn KL, Rota TR, et al. Recombinant human interferon alpha-A suppresses HTLV-III interferon alpha-A suppresses HTLV-III replication in vitro. *Lancet,* 1985;I:1602–604.
122. Poli G, Orenstein JM, Kinter A, et al. Interferon-alpha but not AZT suppresses HIV expression in chronically infected cell lines. *Science,* 1989;244: 575–577.
123. Shirazi Y, Pitha PM. Interferon alpha-mediated inhibition of human immunodeficiency virus type 1 provirus synthesis in T-cells. *Virology,* 1993;193: 303–312.
124. Maciaszek JW, Parada NA, Cruikshank WW, et al. IL-16 represses HIV-1 promoter activity. *J Immunol,* 1997;158:5–8.
125. Scala E, D'Offizi G, Rossi R, Tirriziani O, et al. C-C chemokines, IL-16, and soluble antiviral factor activity are increased in cloned T cells from subjects with long-term nonprogressive HIV infection. *J Immunol,* 1997;158:4485–4492.
126. Schuitemaker H, Kootstra NA, Koppelman MH, et al. Proliferation-depended HIV-1 infection of monocytes occurs during differentiation into macro-phages. *J. Clin Invest,* 1992;89:1154–1160.
127. Kazazi F, Mathijs JM, Chang J, et al. Recombinant interleukin 4 stimulated human immunodeficiency virus production by infected monocytes and macrophages. *J Gen Virol,* 1992;73:941–949.
128. Foli A, Saville MW, Baseler MW, Yarchoan R. Effects of the Th1 and Th2 stimulatory cytokines interleukin 12 and interleukin 4 on human immunodeficiency virus replication. *Blood,* 1995;85: 2114–2123.
129. Weissman D, Poli G, Fauci AS. IL-10 synergizes with multiple cytokines in enhancing HIV production in cells of monocytic lineage. *J Acquir Immune Defic Syndr Hum Retrovirol,* 1995; 9442–9449.
130. Akridge RE, Reed SG. Interleukin-12 decreases human immunodeficiency virus type 1 replication in human macrophage cultures reconstituted with autologous peripheral blood mononuclear cells. *J Infect Dis,* 1996;173:559–564.
131. Poli G, Kinter AL, Justement JS, et al. Transforming growth factor beta suppresses human immunodeficiency virus expression and replication in infected cells on the monocyte/macrophage lineage. *J Exp Med,* 1991;173:559–564.
132. Poli G, Kinter AL, Justement JS, et al. Retinoic acid mimics transforming growth factor beta in the regulation of human immunodeficiency virus

expression in monocytic cells. *Proc Natl Acad Sci USA* 1992; 89:2689–2693.
133. Biswas P, Poli G, Kinter AL, et al. Interferon gamma induces the expression of human immunodeficiency virus in persistently infected promonocytic cells (U1) and redirects the production of virions to intracytoplasmic vacuoles in phorbol myristate acetate-differentiated U1 cells. *J Exp Med*, 1992;176:739–750.
134. Vicenzi E, Biswas P, Mengozzi M, Poli G. Role of proinflammatory cytokines and beta chemokines in controlling HIV replication. *J Leukoc Biol*, 1997;62:34–40.
135. Diagbouga S, Albert D, Fumoux F, et al. Relationship between IL-5 production and variations in eosino-phil during HIV infection in West Africa: influence of Mycobacterium tuberculosis infection. *Scand J Immunol*, 1999;49:203–209.
136. Dimitrov DS. How do viruses enter cells? The HIV coreceptors teach us a lesson of complexity. *Cell*, 1997;91:721–730.
137. Litman DR. Chemokine receptors — keys to AIDS pathogenesis. *Cell*, 1998;93:677–680.
138. Feng Y, Broder CC, Kennedy PE, Berger EA. HIV-1 entry cofactor: Function cDNA cloning of a seven-transmembrane G- protein-coupled receptor. *Science*, 1996;272:872–877.
139. Deng HK, Liu W, Ellmeier S, et al. Identification of a major co-receptor for primary isolates of HIV-1. *Nature*, 1996;381:661–666.
140. Dragic T. HIV-1 entry into CD+ cells is mediated by the chemokine receptor CC-CKR-5. *Nature*, 1996; 381:667–673.
141. Alkahatib G, Combadiere C, Broder CC, et al. CC-CK5: A RANTES, MIP-1, MPI-1 receptor as a fusion cofactor for macrophage-tropic HIV-1. *Science*, 1996;272:1955–1958.
142. Choc H, Farzan M, Sun Y, et al. The Beta-chemokine receptors CCR3 and CCR5 facilitate infection by primary HIV-1 isolates. *Cell*, 1996;85:1135–1148.
143. Doranz BJ, Rucker J, Yi Y, et al. A dual-tropic primary HIV-1 isolate that uses fusin and the beta-chemokine receptos CKR-5, CKR-3, and CKR-2b as fusion cofactors. *Cell*, 1996;85:1149–1158.
144. Cocchi F, DeVico AL, Garzine-Demo A, et al. Identification of RANTES, MPI-1 alpha and MIP-beta as the major HIV-suppressive factors produced by $CD8^+$ T cells. *Science*, 1995;270: 1811–1815.
145. Bleul C, Farzan M, Choe H, et al. The lymphocyte chemoattractant SDF-1 is a ligand for LESTR/fusin and blocks HIV-1 entry. *Nature*, 1996;382:829–833.
146. Nagasawa T, Hirota S, Tachibana K, et al. Defects of B-cell lymphopoiesis and bone-marrow myelopoiesis in mice lacking the CXC chemokine PBSF/SDF-1. *Nature*, 1996;382:635–638.
147. He J, Chen Y, Farzan M, et al. CCR3 and CCR5 are coreceptors for HIV-1 infection of microglia. *Nature*, 1997;385:645–649.
148. Poli G. Cytokines and the human immunodeficiency virus:from bench to bedside. *Europ J Clin Invest*, 1999;29:723–732.
149. Zhang P, Huang Y, He T, et al. HIV-1 subtype and second-receptor use. *Nature*, 1996;383:768.
150. Tscherning C, Alaeus A, Fredriksson R, et al. Difference in chemokine coreceptor usage between genetic subtypes of HIV-1. *Virol*, 1998;241: 181–189.
151. Bjorndal A, Sonnerborg A, Tscherning C, et al. Phenotypic characteristics of human immunodeficiency type 1 subtype C isolates from Ethiopian AIDS patients. *AIDS Res Human Retro*, 1999;15: 647–653.
152. Ping L-H, Nelson JAE, Hoffman F, et al. Characterization of V3 sequence heterogeneity in subtype C human immunodeficiency virus type 1 isolates from Malawi: underrepresentation of X4 variants. *J Virol*, 1999;73:6271–628.
153. Milich L, Margolin BH, Swanstrom. Patterns of amino acid variability in NSI-like and SI-like V3 sequences and a linked change in the CD4–binding domain of the HIV-1 entry Env protein. *Virol*, 1997;239:108–118.
154. Chesebro MW, Wehrly K, Nishio J, et al. Mapping of independent V3 envelope determinants of human immunodeficiency virus type 1 macrophage tropism and syncytium formation in lymphocytes. *J Virol*, 1996;7:9055–9059.
155. Tien PC, Chiu T, Latif A, et al. Primary subtype C HIV-1 infection in Harare, Zimbabwe. *J Acquir Immune Def Synd Human Retrovirol*, 1999; 20:147–153.
156. Balachandran R, Thampatty P, Enrico A, et al. Human immunodeficiency virus isolates from asymptomatic homosexual men and from AIDS patients have distinct biologic and genetic properties. *Virol*, 1991;180:229–238.
157. Tersmette M de Goede REY, Al BJM, et al. Differential syncytium-inducing capacity of human immuno-deficiency virus isolates: frequent detection of syncytium-inducing isolates in patients with acquired immunodeficiency syndrome (AIDS) and AIDS-related complex. *J Virol*, 1988;62:2026–2032.
158. Koot M, Keet IPM, Vos AHV, et al. Prognostic value of HIV-1 syncytium-inducing phenotype for rate of CD+ cell depletion and Progression of AIDS. *Ann Intern Med*, 1993;118:681–688.
159. Dean M, Carrington M, Winkler C, et al. Genetic restriction of HIV-1 infection and progression to AIDS by a deletion allele of the CKR5 structural gene. *Science*, 1996;273:1856–1862.
160. Morawetz RA, Rizzardi GP, Glauser D, et al. Genetic polymophism of CCR5 gene and HIV disease: the heterozygous (CCR5/Dccr5) genotype is neither

essential nor sufficient for protection against disease progression. *Europ J Immunol*, 1997;3223–3227.

161. Kostrikis LG, Huang Y, Moore JP, et al. A chemokine receptor *CCR2* allele delays HIV-1 disease progression and is associated with a CCR5 promoter mutation. *Nat Med*, 1998;4:350–353.
162. Lee B, Doranz BJ, Rana S, et al. Influence of the *CCR2–V64I* polymorphism on human immunodeficiency virus type 1 coreceptor activity and on chemokine receptor function of *CCR2b, CCR3, CCR5*, and *CXCR4*. *J Virol*, 1998;72:7450–7458.
163. van Rij RP, de Roda Husman AM, Brouwer M. Role of *CCR2* genotype in the clinical course of synctium-inducing (SI) or non-SI human immunodeficiency virus type 1 infection and in the time to conversion to SI virus variants. *J Infect Dis*, 1998;178:1806–1811.
164. Michael NL, Louie LG, Rohrbauch AL, et al. The role of CCR5 and CCR2 polymorphism in HIV-1 transmission and disease progression. *Nat Medicine*, 1997;3:1160–1162.
165. Brambila A, Villa C, Rizzardi GP, et al. Shorter survival of *SDF1–3'A/3'A* homozygotes linked to CD4+ T cell decrease in advanced human immunodeficiency virus type 1 infection. *J Infect Dis*, 2000; 182:311–315.
166. Fowke KR, Dong T, Rowland-Jones SL, et al. HIV-1 resistance in Kenyan sex workers is not associated with altered cellular susceptibility to HIV-1 infection or enhanced β-chemokine production. *AIDS Res Hum Retroviruses*, 1998;14:1521–1530.
167. Anzala AO, Ball TB, Roston T, et al. CCR2–641 allele and genotype association with delayed AIDS progression in African women. University of Nairobi Collaboration for HIV Research. *Lancet*, 1998;102:1758–1765.
168. Brander C, Walker BD. T lymphocytes responses in HIV-1 infection: implications for vaccine development. *Current Opin Immunol*, 1999;11:451–549.
169. Goulder PJR, Brander C, Annamalai K, et al. Differential Narrow focusing of immunodominant human immunodeficiency virus gag-specific cytotoxic T-lymphocyte responses in infected African and Caucasoid Adults and children. *J Virol*, 2000;74:5679–5690.
170. Rowland-Jones S, Sutton J, Ariyoshi K, et al. HIV-1 specific cytotoxic T cells in HIV-exposed but uninfected Gambian women. *Nat Med*, 1995; 1:59–64.
171. Cao H, Mani I, Vincet R, et al. Cellular immunity to human immunodeficiency virus type (HIV-1) clades: relevance to HIV-1 vaccine trials in Uganda. *J Infect Dis*, 2000;182:1350–1356.
172. Ahmed AT, Blose DA. Delayed type hypersensitivity skin testing. A review. *Arch Derm*, 1983;199: 934–945.
173. Blatt SP Hendrix CW, Butzin CA, et al. Delayed-type hypersensitivity skin testing predicts progression to AIDS in HIV infected patients. *Ann Int Med*, 1993;119:185–193.
174. Dolan MJ, Clerici M, Blatt SP, et al. In vitro T cell function, delayed type hypersensitivity skin testing and CD4 T cell subset phenotyping independently predict survival time in patients infected with HIV. *J Infect Dis*, 1995;172:79–87.
175. French MAH, Cameron PU, Grimsley G, Smith LA, Dawkins RL. Correction of human immunodeficiency virus-associated depression of delayed-type hypersensitivity (DTH) after zidovudine therapy: DTH, $CD4^+$ T cell numbers, and epidermal Langerhans cell density are independent variables. *Clin Immunopathol* 1990;55:86–96.
176. Brown AE, Markowitz L, Nitayaphan S. DTH responsiveness of HIV-infected Thai adults. *J Med Assoc Thai*, 2000;83:633–639.
177. Klein RS, Sobel J, Flanigan T, Smith D, Margolick JB. Stability of cutaneous anergy in women with or at risk for HIV infection. HIV Epidemiology Research Study Group. *J Acquir Immune Defic Syndr Hum Retrovirol*, 1999;20:238–244.
178. Miller WC, Thielman NM, Swai N, et al. Delayed type hypersensitivity testing in Tanzanian adults with HIV infection. *J Acquir Immune Defic Syndr Hum Retrovirol*, 1996;12:303–308.
179. Fine PEM, Sterne JA, Penninghaus JM, et al. Delayed-type hypersensitivity, mycobacterial vaccines and protective immunity. *Lancet*, 1994; 3344: 1245–1249.
180. Selwyn PA, Sckell BM, Alcabes P, et al. High risk of tuberculosis in HIV-infected drug users with cutaneous anergy. *JAMA*, 1992;268:504–509.
181. Elliot AM, Hurst TJ, Balyeku MN, et al. Immune response to *Mycobacterium tuberculosis* in HIV-infected and uninfected adults in Uganda: application of a whole blood cytokine assay in an epidemeological study. *Int J Tuberc Lung Dis*, 1998;239–246.
182. Kaslow RA, Carrington MN, Apple R, et al. Influence of combinations of human major histocompatibility complex genes on the course of HIV-1 infection. *Nat Med*, 1996;2:405–410.
183. Carrington M, Nelson GW, Martin MP, et al. HLA and HIV-1: Heterozygote advantage and B*35–Cw*04 disadvantage. *Science*, 1999;283: 1748–1752.
184. Ireneus P, Keet M, Tang J, et al. Consistent associations of HLA class I and II and transporter gene products with progression of human immunodeficiency virus type infection in homosexual men. *J Infect Dis*, 1999;188:299–309.
185. MacDonald KS, Fowke KR, Kimani J, et al. Influence of HLA supertypes on susceptibility and resistance to human immunodeficiency virus type I infection. *J Infect Dis*, 2000;181: 1581–1589.

186. Puren AJ, Ramjee G, Abdool-Karim S, Gray CM. HLA association with HIV-1 seronegative sex workers from KwaZulu-Natal, South Africa. In Program and abstracts of the XIII International Conference on AIDS; July 9–14, 2000, Durban, South Africa.
187. Clerici M, Shearer GM. The Th1–Th2 hypothesis of HIV infection: new insights. *Immunol Today*, 1994;15:575–581.
188. Hyjiek E, Lischner HW, Hyslop T. Cytokine patterns during progression to AIDS in children with perinatal HIV infection. *J Immunol* 1995;155: 4060–4071.
189. Maggi E, Mazzeti M, Ravina A, Annunziato F, de Carli M, Piccinni MP, et al. Ability of HIV to promote a TH1 to TH0 shift and to replicate preferentially in TH2 and TH0. *Science*, 1994;265:244–248.
190. Meyaard L, Otto SA, Keet PM, et al. Changes in cytokine secretion patterns of CD4+ T cell clones in human immunodeficiency virus infection. *Blood*, 1994;12:4265–4268.
191. Maizels RM, Bundy DA, Selkirk ME, et al. Immuno-logical modulation and evasion by helminth parasites in human population. *Nature*, 1993;365: 797–805.
192. Pearlman E, Kazura F, Hazlet F, Boom W. Modulation of murine cytokine responses to mycobacterium antigens by helminth-induced T helper 2 cell
193. Bentwich Z, Maartens G, Torten D, et al. Concurrent infections and HIV pathogenesis. *AIDS*, 2000;14: 2071–2081.
194. Wodarz D, Nowak MA. CD8 memory, immunodominance, and antigenic escape. *Eur J Immunol*, 2000;30:2704–2712.

4

Effect of Genetic Variation on HIV Transmission and Progression to AIDS

*Cheryl A. Winkler and †Stephen J. O'Brien

**Intramural Research Support Program, Science Applications International Corporation Frederick, National Cancer Institute, Frederick, MD, USA.*
†Laboratory of Genomic Diversity, National Cancer Institute, Frederick, MD, USA.

A critical challenge of human genetics research is to identify genes that interact with environmental components so as to point the way toward therapeutic and prevention strategies. The development of AIDS requires exposure to and infection by HIV-1; but, factors such as HIV-1 biologic phenotype (1), coreceptor use (2), HIV-1 subtype (3), coinfection with other infectious agents (4), and environmental pressures also contribute to HIV-1 transmission and disease progression. Thus, the genetic makeup of the host is only one of many factors that affect HIV-1 pathogenesis. Remarkably, variant alleles for at least 10 genetic loci have been shown to have marked effects on susceptibility to HIV-1 infection, rate of $CD4^{+}$ T-cell depletion, progression to AIDS-defining conditions, and/or specific AIDS-associated malignancies (Table 1) (5–18). The identification of the host's genetic determinants has pointed to factors required for HIV-1's life cycle and for the host's successful immune response, and to those possibly useful as therapeutic targets. These studies thus provide a model for the genetic analysis of a human disease that requires an environmental trigger or a pathogenic agent (16–18).

With few exceptions, associations between genetics and the rate of progression to AIDS have been identified and established through cohort studies in developed countries, not through similar studies conducted in developing nations where HIV-1 infection is highest. The unusual occurrence of opportunistic infections and Kaposi's sarcoma in European and American risk groups—men who have sex with men (MSM) and hemophiliacs and other recipients of blood or blood products—led to the organization of prospective, longitudinal AIDS cohorts to study the natural history of the syndrome (19,20). Unfortunately, this early demographic bias has had a profound and enduring effect on the investigation of the role of host genetic factors in HIV and AIDS. Most genetics studies have been conducted in male-dominated cohorts established in the early to mid-1980s in Europe or the United States. These early cohorts are highly informative because they include seroincident (also called seroconverter) individuals who develop HIV-1 antibodies after enrollment in the study (allowing their date of infection to be estimated) and have very long clinical follow-up intervals, conditions that are both necessary to assess the effects of host genetic factors on rates of AIDS progression (17).

However, these cohorts do not reflect the global patterns of infection in at least three important ways. First, although the earliest cohort studies enrolled MSM at risk for HIV-1 infection through sexual exposure and male hemophiliacs at risk through their use of HIV-1–contaminated clotting factors prior to 1984, UNAIDS estimates that women now make up 47% of those living with HIV-1 or AIDS globally (21). Second, the primary HIV-1 clade or subtype in North America, South America, and Europe is subtype B, while in sub–Saharan Africa, Central Asia, and Southeast Asia, subtypes A, C, and E are predominant (22,23). Third, these studies tend to identify genetic risk or protective factors in people of northern European descent; however, more than 75% of people living with HIV-1 or AIDS are of African origin or descent, and the HIV-1 epidemic is growing most rapidly in sub–Saharan Africa and developing nations in Asia (21). Because of population-specific differences in allele and haplotype frequency distributions (24–31), genetic factors found to influence HIV-1 infection or rates of AIDS progression in one ethnic or racial group may have different, perhaps even no, effects in other populations. Although the study of African Americans (a group having approximately 80% to 90% African admixture) as a surrogate population representing black Africans is useful, this population is unlikely to represent the genetic diversity found throughout Africa (32). It is imperative that genetics studies be performed in nonwestern populations so as to account for differences in gene frequencies between populations and for other confounding factors, such as endemic HIV-1 subtypes, coinfection with non-HIV-1 pathogens, gender, and routes of transmission.

OVERALL GENETIC RISKS

Of the 733,000 cases of AIDS reported in the United States, more than 37% occur in African Americans, a group representing just

TABLE 1. Genetic Variants Affecting HIV Progression to AIDS and AIDS Outcomes in European Americans and African Americans

Genetic variant	Effect	European Americans Genetic mode (ref.)	African Americans Genetic mode (ref.)[a]
Protective			
CCR5-Δ32	Overall 2–4 year delay of progression to AIDS	Dominant (6)	ND
CCR5-Δ32	Prevents lymphoma	Dominant (5)	ND
SDF1-3'A	Protective in first 10 years of infection	Recessive (8)	ND
CCR5-64I	Overall 2–4 year delay of progression to AIDS	Dominant (7)	Dominant (11)
RANTES-403A	No effect to moderate delay of progression to AIDS	Recessive (9)	No effect (An et al.)[b]
Detrimental			
CCR5-P1	Accelerates progression to AIDS	Recessive (12)	Dominant (11,60,111)
IL10-5'A	Accelerates progression to AIDS	Dominant (15)	No effect (15)
HLA class 1 homozygosity	Accelerates progression to AIDS	Codominant (13)	Codominant (13)
HLA-B*35/ -Cw*04	Accelerates progression to AIDS	Dominant (13)	Dominant (13)
RANTES In1.1C	Accelerates progression to AIDS	Dominant (An et al.)[b]	Dominant (An et al.)[b]

[a]ND indicates not determined. The CCR5-Δ32 allele is too rare to assess its epidemiologic effect with confidence in African Americans.
[b]An and Winkler: unpublished data.

12% of the U.S. population (33). Among U.S. women reported to have AIDS, nearly two-thirds are African American. In every risk group for HIV infection, African Americans are disproportionately represented (33). Globally, more than 74% of all HIV-1 infections and 84% of all AIDS-related deaths occur in sub–Saharan Africa (21). Rates for mother-to-infant HIV-1 transmission tend to be higher in African countries and Haiti (25% to 30%) than in Europe or the United States (14% to 25%) (34). However, it is probably a misconception that HIV-1 progression is more rapid in Africa than in developed countries (35–38); natural history studies suggest that progression rates in Africa are quite similar to those in developed countries (39–42). In developing countries, precise estimates of the time interval for progression from HIV-1 infection to clinical AIDS are confounded by long asymptomatic periods, uncertainty concerning the time of HIV-1 infection, differences in rate of transmission for HIV-1 subtypes (3), prevalence of endemic pathogens other than HIV-1 (4), infections with other sexually transmitted diseases (43), and limited access to health care (4,44).

An important concept to investigate is the relative contributions of genetic, viral, and environmental factors to the geographic and racial differences observed in infection rates and progression to AIDS. The similar rates of AIDS-free survival between cohorts predominantly made up of white seroincident homosexual men and those made up of predominantly African-American injection drug users (45) suggest that risk group and race may have only minor effects on the rates of HIV-1 progression to disease (Figure 1) (46).

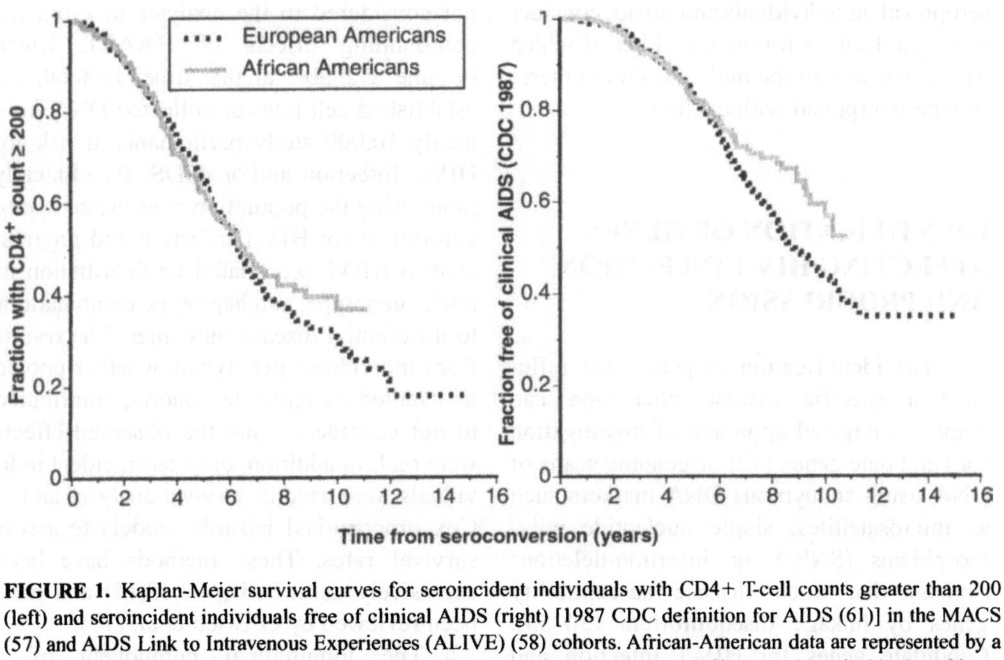

FIGURE 1. Kaplan-Meier survival curves for seroincident individuals with CD4+ T-cell counts greater than 200 (left) and seroincident individuals free of clinical AIDS (right) [1987 CDC definition for AIDS (61)] in the MACS (57) and AIDS Link to Intravenous Experiences (ALIVE) (58) cohorts. African-American data are represented by a solid line and European-American data by a dotted line. After six years, the rates of increased survival in the African-American cohort were not significant. African-American cohort data became sparse at this time because of a shorter follow-up interval; the ALIVE and MACS cohort studies began recruitment in 1988–89 and 1984–85, respectively. Relative hazard (RH) and p values for each graph (Cox model analyses) illustrate the statistically identical survival of the two groups: $CD4^+$ count < 200, RH=1.04, $p=0.73$; AIDS, RH=0.92, $p=0.62$.

Similarly, a large, London-based study of seroprevalent (infected by HIV-1 before enrolling in study) black sub–Saharan Africans, likely infected with subtypes A or C, and HIV-1 infected individuals born in developed countries and infected with subtype B, showed no significant differences in decreases in $CD4^+$ T-cell counts, AIDS-free survival rates, or survival rates between the two groups, after adjusting for age at infection (47,48). These results are in agreement with an earlier report showing no statistically significant differences in the rates of $CD4^+$ and $CD8^+$ T-cell depletion between seropositive Ethiopian immigrants infected with subtype C and non-Ethiopian Israeli men infected with subtype B (49). These studies suggest that geographic or racial differences in disease progression rates and AIDS-defining outcomes may be the result of factors other than population-specific racial differences. However, these studies are based on seroprevalent individuals and do not consider losses to death or follow-up, either of which would bias toward the null, and should therefore be interpreted with caution.

IDENTIFICATION OF GENES AFFECTING HIV-1 INFECTION AND PROGRESSION

The identification of genes that influence a specific disease phenotype can employ a targeted approach of investigation for candidate genes (17) or genome scans of DNA using anonymous DNA markers such as microsatellites, single nucleotide polymorphisms (SNPs), or insertion-deletions (indels) that track disease susceptibility genes by linkage disequilibrium (50–53). Candidate genes for HIV-1 infection and AIDS progression may include any gene that encodes a product that HIV-1 uses during its life cycle or that may be involved in the host's defense against invading viral pathogens. These genes are screened for polymorphisms using a combination of methods that detect genetic variation. The genotypes of SNPs, microsatellite markers, or indels may be determined in populations of at-risk individuals enrolled in prospective natural history studies (19,20,45,54–59).

The approach taken by our group was to identify genetic variants in candidate genes using B-cell lines (as a renewable DNA source) established from samples taken from participants in cohorts for a prospective natural history study. The risk groups included hemophiliacs exposed to HIV-1 in blood products received prior to the initiation of heat treatment in 1995, injection drug users, and MSM. The study population included more than 600 Europeans and 260 African Americans who, at enrollment, were seronegative and became seropositive during the study. The mean clinical follow-up for the two groups was 12 years and 7 years, respectively (60); events after January 1, 1996 were not considered in the analysis to avoid the confounding effects of HAART, which became available at this time. In total, we established cell lines or collected DNA from nearly 10,000 study participants at risk for HIV-1 infection and/or AIDS. By clinically monitoring the population over the course of enrollment for HIV-1 infection and progression to AIDS, we related its distribution of allele, genotype, and haplotype combinations to differential disease outcomes. The results from individuals genotyped, whether pooled or handled as replicate cohorts, contributed to our confidence that the observed effects were real. In addition, only seroincident individuals were used in survival analyses and in Cox proportional hazards models to assess survival rates. These methods have been extensively described (6–8,12,15) and have been reviewed by O'Brien et al. (17).

The longitudinal component of a prospective natural history study provides a dynamic and temporal epidemiologic and clinical view of HIV-1's pathogenesis. Chronic HIV-1 infection leads to a profound depletion in $CD4^+$ T-cells, generalized immune dysfunction, and the eventual collapse of the host's immune system. We have focused our efforts on identifying genetic variants in candidate genes affecting the host's capacity to control HIV-1 infection and transmission; rate of progression to clinical $CD4^+$ T-cell depletion; rate of progression to AIDS (using the 1987 and 1993 surveillance definitions of the Centers for Disease Control and Prevention) (61,62) and AIDS-related death; and cellular and humoral immune response to HIV-1. The host's genetic factors may also be important in control of HIV-1 replication, the evolution of HIV-1 diversity and biologic phenotype, and the efficacy and side effects of HAART. Finally, the genetic background of the host may serve to confound analyses of the efficacy of treatment for participants in therapeutic antiviral drug or vaccine trials.

Chemokine Receptors and Their Ligands

The demonstration that HIV-1 required CD4 plus a coreceptor to gain cell entry and establish a productive infection was further elucidated by the discoveries that the chemokines MIP-1α, MIP-1β, and RANTES (63), ligands for CCR5 (64), and stromal-derived factor 1-alpha (SDF1α), ligand for the CXCR4 receptor (65,66), inhibited the replication of nonsynctium-inducing (NSI) and synctium-inducing (SI) HIV-1 strains, respectively (67,68). R5 strains of HIV-1 use CCR5 while the more cytopathogenic X4 strains mainly use the CXCR4 coreceptor for cell entry (1,69–72). A few dual-tropic HIV-1 strains are able to use both CXCR4 and CCR5 as entry portals, and at least 12 other chemokine receptors have been shown to bind HIV-1 envelope proteins in vitro (73, 74). The importance of the minor chemokine receptors in vivo has not been resolved; however, there are reports that HIV-1 isolates that can use a range of receptors may follow a more rapid clinical course (2,75).

The *CCR5-Δ32* mutation, independently discovered by four research groups in 1996, contains a 32-base pair (bp) deletion in the first exon resulting in a codon frameshift that introduces a premature stop codon (6,76–78). The truncated protein thus produced is unable to leave the endoplasmic reticulum and is therefore not expressed on the cell surface (79,80). Homozygous individuals inheriting two *CCR-Δ32* alleles express no CCR5 receptors on their cell surfaces but apparently have few clinical abnormalities (81). In vitro, *CCR5-+/Δ32* cells express detectable levels of CCR5 on their cell membranes and both *CCR5-+/Δ32* heterozygous cells and individuals can be infected by HIV-1, although attenuated (6,82).

The limited geographic distribution of the *CR5-Δ32* allele (24–26) is consistent with its recent origin in northern Europe, probably within the last 10,000 years. Correspondingly, the allele is seen only in regions that have received migration from Europe in the past 5,000 years (26). The rapid increase of the allele from a single event on one chromosome to a frequency ranging from 8% to 17% in northern European descendents suggests that the *CCR5-Δ32* mutation is under strong and persistent positive selection, possibly from other infectious agents that may also use CCR5 to gain cell entry (25,83,84).

It is a rare event for a *CCR5-Δ32/Δ32* homozygote to become infected with HIV-1, suggesting that HIV-1 strains that use CXCR4 rarely establish productive infections. Possibly either X4 HIV-1–infected $CD4^+$ T-cells are rapidly eliminated by the immune system or X4 strains are rarely transmitted. Genetic association analysis of more than 12,000 individuals at risk for infection has shown that *CCR5-Δ32/Δ32* individuals show near complete resistance to infection by R5-tropic HIV-1 (Table 2) (6,17,26,77,78, 84–86). In those few cases where *CCR5-Δ32/Δ32* homozygotes have become infected, the biologic phenotype and

TABLE 2. Genetic Risk Factors for HIV Infection and HIV Maternal Transmission

Gene	Mode	Risk[a]	*p* value	Ethnicity	Risk group[b]	References
Susceptibility						
CCR5-Δ32[c]	Recessive	OR = 0.03	< 0.00001	European American	Hemophiliac, MSM	(6, 17, 76–78)
CCR5-Δ32	Recessive	HWE[d]	0.04	European American	Mother-child	(97)
CCR5-Δ32	Recessive	HWE	< 0.001	Latino American	Mother-child	(97)
CCR5-59356T	Recessive	RR = 5.9	< 0.001	African American	Mother-child	(123)
IL10-3'A	Dominant	OR = 1.75	0.03	European American	MSM	(15)
SDF1-3'A	Dominant	OR = 0.44	0.002	European American	MSM	(8)
CCR2-64I	Dominant	HWE	0.03	Argentinean	Mother-child	(102)
HLA=A2/6802*	Dominant	OR = 0.17	0.005	East African	Mother-child	(150)
HLA=A2/6802*	Dominant	IRR = 0.45	0.0003	East African	FSW	(149)
*HLA=A*2301*	Dominant	IRR = 3.62	0.001	East African	FSW	(149)
*HLA=DRB1*01*	Dominant	IRR = 0.22	0.003	East African	FSW	(149)
Transmission[e]						
SDF1-3'A	Dominant	OR = 1.8	0.05	East African	Mother-child	(125)

[a]OR indicates odds ratio; HWE, Hardy-Weinberg Equilibrium; RR, relative risk; IRR, incident rate ratio.
[b]Children are exposed to HIV-1 when mothers are infected. MSM indicates men who have sex with men; FSW, female sex workers.
[c]Heterosexual transmission is underrepresented in this category.
[d]Distortion in Hardy-Weinberg equilibrium, in each case, an excess of homozygotes for the variant allele was observed.
[e]Mothers with this factor were more likely to transmit HIV-1 to their children.

genotype of the HIV-1 isolates suggest that the infecting virus was an X4-tropic strain (87–91).

Although *CCR5-Δ32* homozygosity is highly protective against HIV-1 infection, *CCR5-Δ32* heterozygosity affords little or no protective advantage against HIV-1 infection (6). A study of 54 pairs of discordant sexually active couples found that *CCR5-+/Δ32* heterosexual partners were less likely to be infected by HIV-1 ($p = 0.03$), but this association was not observed in homosexual couples (92). Partial resistance to HIV-1 infection by *CCR5-+/Δ32* heterozygotes, however, has not been observed in other studies of adults exposed to HIV-1 (6,84,93) or in children born to women infected by HIV-1 (94–98).

While *CCR5-Δ32* heterozygosity does not protect against HIV-1 infection in either children or adults, some studies have shown that *CCR5-Δ32* heterozygotes enjoy a weak but statistically significant protection against progression to AIDS. In children, *CCR5-Δ32* heterozygosity has been shown in some studies (96,99,100)—but not others (94,101, 102)—to delay AIDS progression. *CCR5-+/Δ32* heterozygous children also have been found to have significantly lower viral burdens compared to those found in *CCR5-+/+* children (103). The cohorts where *CCR5-+/Δ32* protection was not observed tended to be statistically underpowered because of small sample size or a low frequency of *CCR2-+/Δ32* heterozygotes. A multicenter study in France of 512 non-black children found that while heterozygosity for *CCR5-Δ32* did not protect them from infection, it did significantly delay depletion of $CD4^+$ T-cells (99). Likewise, no protective association was observed in a study of 397 HIV-1–infected children in Argentina, probably because the study was underpowered since only 8% of its participants were *CCR5-+/Δ32* heterozygotes (101,102).

It is possible that the *CCR5-Δ32* mutation has significant effects on the dynamics of the AIDS epidemic. Although only 1% of individuals of northern European ancestry (*CCR5-Δ32/Δ32* homozygotes) are protected from infection, approximately 20% are *CCR5-Δ32* carriers. The influence of *CCR5-Δ32* heterozygosity may affect the spread of HIV-1 in two antagonistic ways: heterozygotes can live, on average, 2 to 4 years longer than HIV-1–infected noncarriers and thus may have a longer period during which they can transmit HIV-1 (6), and *CCR5-+/Δ32* heterozygotes may transmit the virus less frequently because, as a group, their viral load is lower (104–107). Higher viral load in a donor has been shown to be a significant risk factor for HIV-1 transmission (108–110).

Other mutations in chemokine receptor genes, occurring in the promoter region of *CCR5* and the open reading of *CCR2*, are more equally distributed among global populations and racial groups (Figure 2) (12,111, 112). A common mutation in *CCR2*, *CCR2-64I*, replaces valine with isoleucine at position 64 within the region encoding the first transmembrane domain of the *CCR2* receptor (7). Although the amino acid replacement is conservative and the mutation occurs within the transmembrane domain, the effects of *CCR2-64I* on progression to AIDS are nearly identical to those for *CCR5-Δ32*, each results in a 2 to 4 year delay in the development of AIDS-defining conditions (7,11,113). Moreover, *CCR2-64I* is protective in individuals of African and European descent. A study in Kenya of female sex workers compared rapid progressors to slow or nonprogressors to AIDS and reported that slow or nonprogressors had a significant increase in *CCR2-+/64I* and *CCR2-64I/64I* genotypes (114). The frequency of *CCR2-64I* was reported to be approximately 20% in blacks from Kenya (114) and 13% in blacks from South Africa (115), higher percentages than those reported in populations of European origin or descent (7,24,27).

Interestingly, the *CCR2-64I* mutation may not be protective for all risk groups. We failed to demonstrate a protective effect in a

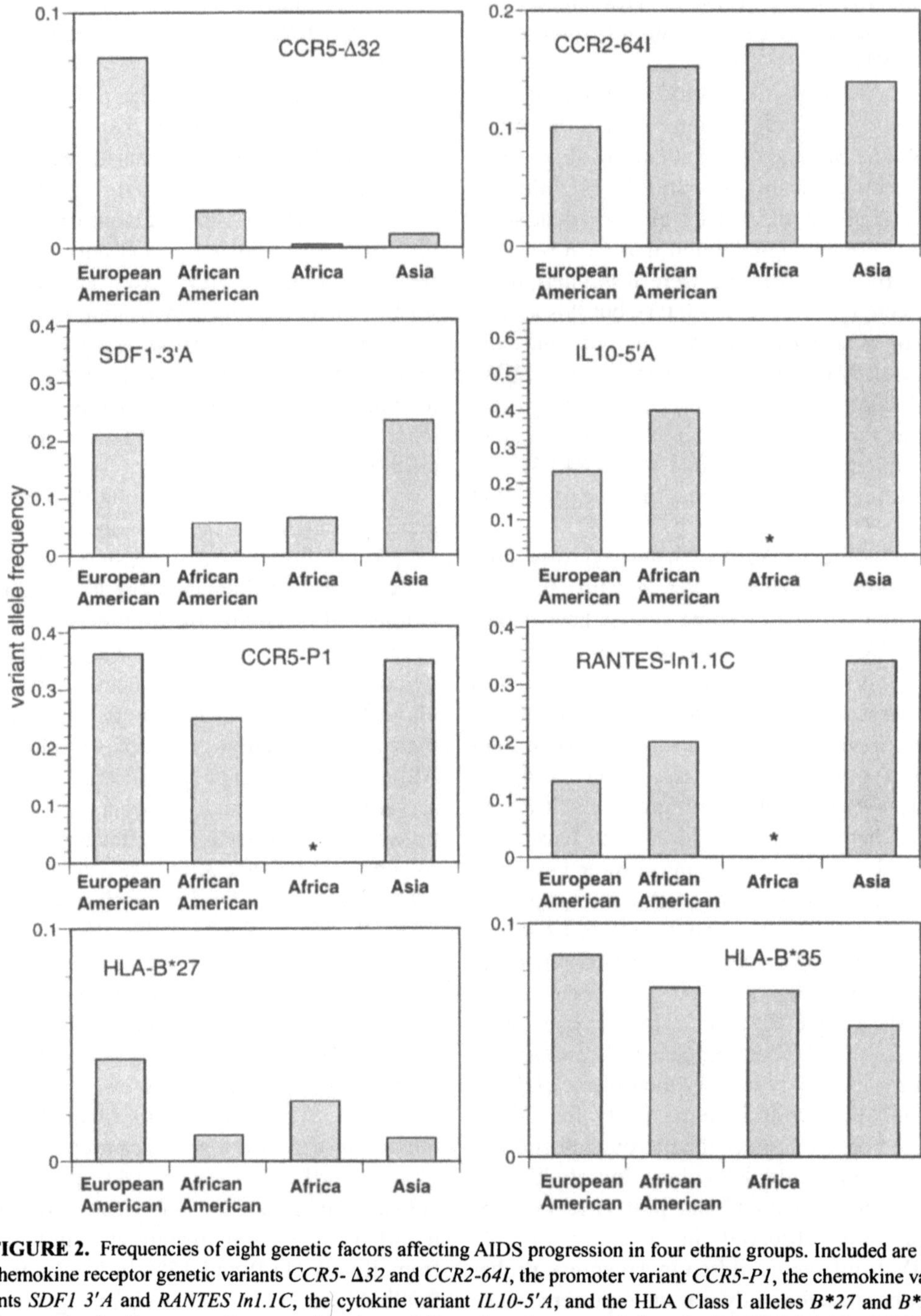

FIGURE 2. Frequencies of eight genetic factors affecting AIDS progression in four ethnic groups. Included are the chemokine receptor genetic variants *CCR5- Δ32* and *CCR2-64I*, the promoter variant *CCR5-P1*, the chemokine variants *SDF1 3'A* and *RANTES In1.1C*, the cytokine variant *IL10-5'A*, and the HLA Class I alleles *B*27* and *B*35*. Frequencies for Europeans, European-Americans, African-Americans, and Asians for *RANTES In1.1C, CCR5-P1*, and *IL10-5'A*, are compiled from various sources (8,12,15), and include our own unpublished data. African and Asian frequencies for *CCR5-Δ32*, SDF1-3'A, *CCR2-64I* are from Su and Martinson (26–28); we have referenced Clayton et al. (29) for *HLA B*27* and *B*35*. African and Asian frequencies from published sources are averages of reported frequencies from different African and Asian populations.

seroincident cohort composed primarily of African-American injection drug users (7), as did a study of injection drug users in the Amsterdam cohort (116). However, in a group of HIV-1–infected African-American service men with unknown HIV-1 risk factors (11) and in MSM enrolled in the Multicenter AIDS Cohort Study (MACS), *CCR2-64I* was significantly protective (7,113). In a seroprevalent cohort of children with hemophilia, *CCR2-64I* was associated with lower HIV-1 viral load and higher $CD4^+$ T-cell count (117). While differences in cohort design, power, analytical methods, or selection bias may account for the discordant effects of *CCR2-64I* found in various studies (118,119), these data also suggest that the route of infection may be a cofactor.

CCR2-64I was also highly protective in the Argentinean study that enrolled children who had been infected as infants. In a group of 329 children who were primarily of indigenous South American ancestry or Italian heritage, *CCR2-+/64I* heterozygotes had a median survival time of 87 months compared with 38 months for *CCR2-+/+* homozygotes (102). In contrast, a study in France of 101 black and 275 non-black children, with a mean observation period of 5.1 years and 6.4 years, respectively, failed to identify a protective role for *CCR2-64I*, although *CCR5-Δ32* was found to be strongly protective in the non-black children (120). The discordant results of these studies may result from differences in the ethnic backgrounds of the children, analytical methods, or sampling bias. Further testing of the effects of *CCR2-64I* in different ethnic and racial groups, and particularly in African cohorts where the *CCR2-64I* allele is common and protective (114,115), is needed.

Studies of the role of *CCR2-64I* in mother-to-infant transmission of HIV-1 suggest either no role (120) or a weak, beneficial role for *CCR2-64I* (102). No differences in *CCR2-64I* allele or genotype frequencies were reported between infected and uninfected infant groups in a mother-infant study conducted in France (120). A study in Argentina of 446 seropositive and 437 seronegative but perinatally exposed children also reported no differences in genotype frequencies of *CCR5-Δ32* or *SDF 1-3'A*. However, an increase in frequency of *CCR2-64I* was observed in the seronegative children compared to the seropositive group (17.5% and 14%, respectively, FET = 0.03), along with a significant ($p = 0.01$) departure from Hardy-Weinberg equilibrium for *CCR2-64I* in the seronegative group. However, care is needed in interpreting these results, since the cohort included both children of European and of indigenous South American ancestry, and allele frequency differences between these populations could account for the departure from Hardy-Weinberg equilibrium (102).

CCR5 Promoter Variants

Thirteen SNPs have been identified within a 1,000-bp segment upstream of the *CCR5* coding exons that contains regulatory and promoter elements (12,121–123). The SNPs in this region fall into 4 common (*CCR5-P1*, *-P2*, *-P3* and *-P4*) and 9 rare haplotypes in both African- and European-Americans (11,12,60,111–113,123). The haplotype structure and population distribution of *CCR2-64I*, *CCR5-Δ32*, and *CCR5-P1* reveals that the *CCR2-64I* mutation invariably occurs on a chromosome carrying the *CCR5-P1* haplotype (11,12,111). The *CCR5-Δ32* mutation also occurs on a chromosome containing the *CCR5-P1* haplotype as well as the wild type *CCR2-+* allele. Table 3 lists the three AIDS-influencing composite haplotypes, their frequency distribution in Caucasians and African Americans, and their relative hazards for AIDS progression.

The effect of the *CCR5* promoter haplotypes on progression to AIDS has been assessed in European-American and African-American seroconverters (Table 3, Figure 3).

TABLE 3. Common Haplotypes for ***CCR2***, ***CCR5*** Promoter Region,[a] the ***CCR5*** Structural Gene and Their Effects on Progression to AIDS (CDC, 1993 definition [62])

	African Americans			European Americans		
[CCR2.CCR5(P).CCR5(5)] haplotype[a]	Genotype frequency[b]	Mode frequency	RH[c]	Genotype	Mode	RH
[+.+.+]	0.35	Reference group		0.33	Reference group	
[+.P1.+]	0.37	Dominant	2.31	0.13	Recessive	1.52
[64I.P1.+]	0.25	Dominant	0.31	0.17	Dominant	1.56
[+.P1.Δ32]	< 0.01	NT[d]	NT	0.20	Dominant	1.38

[a]The *CCR5-P1* haplotype may be identified by the *CCR5-2459A* variant allele (60). The genetic epidemiologic effects of *CCR5-P2*, *-P3*, and *-P4* are indistinguishable and *CCR5-P2–4* are identified by the presence of the *CCR5-2459T* allele (60).
[b]Genotype frequency is the frequency of the effective genotypes for the genetic mode specified (12, 60, 111).
[c]RH indicates relative hazard.
[d]NT indicates not tested.

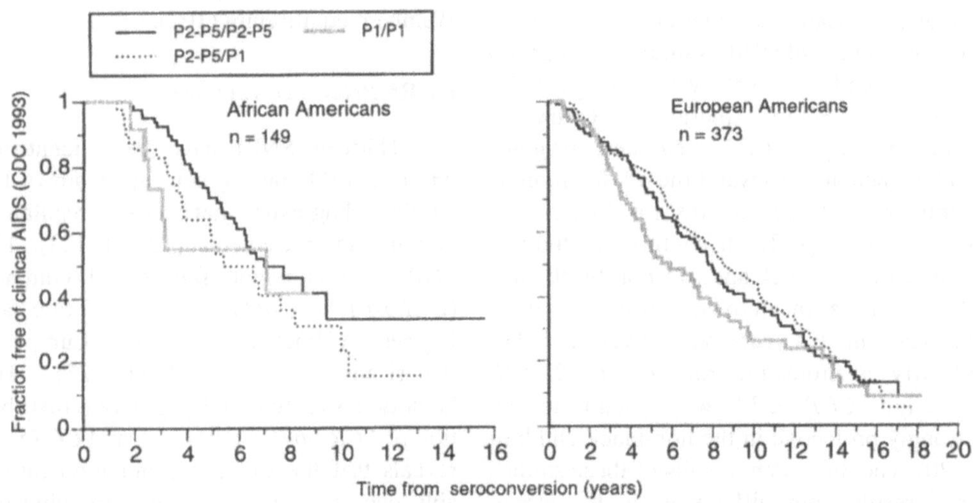

FIGURE 3. Kaplan-Meier survival curves showing effect of the *CCR5-P1* promoter variant on AIDS-free survival using the 1993 CDC definition of AIDS (62) (clinical AIDS, or CD4 T cell count < 200). Curves compare individuals carrying two (gray line) or one (dotted) *P1* haplotype with those carrying no *P1* haplotype (black line). Individuals carrying either *CCR5 -Δ32* or *CCR2-64I* are omitted from the analysis. Relative hazards (RH) and *p* values were determined by Cox model analyses for dominant (*P1/P1* and *P1/P2-P5* versus *P2-P5/P2-P5* individuals) and recessive (*P1/P1* versus *P1/P2-P5* and *P2-P5/P2-P5*) models. No significant effect of *P1* was observed in African Americans or European Americans for the dominant model (RH = 1.40, 1.08, p = 0.19, 0.57, respectively). In the recessive model, an effect was observed in European Americans (RH = 1.40, p = 0.04) but not in African Americans (RH = 1.14, p = 0.76). When the influence of *P1* was examined within the first 4 years following seroconversion, a dominant effect was observed for African Americans (RH = 2.31, p = 0.02), with a recessive effect again observed for European Americans (RH = 1.79, p = 0.02).

In each group, the [+.P1.+] haplotype (the composite allele genotype for *CCR2*, *CCR5P*, *CCR5*, respectively) is associated with more rapid progression to AIDS, possibly because an increase in gene transcription results in more *CCR5* coreceptors available on the cell surface for HIV-1 binding (10, 12). The accelerating effect of the [+.P1.+] haplotype on AIDS progression in European Americans is observed only among homozygous individuals (Table 3, Figure 3) (12). In a study of Italian children, the [+.P1.+]/[+.P1.+] haplotype was also associated with rapid progression to AIDS and a higher viral load (112). Among seroincident African Americans, primarily injection drug users, the effect of the [+.P1.+] haplotype is dominant (Figure 3) (60), possibly because of influences of population-specific modifying alleles. No differences in epidemiologic effects were observed among the *CCR5-P2*, *-P3*, or *-P4* haplotypes (12,60).

Homozygosity for a variant, *CCR5-59356T*, in the 5′ untranslated region of *CCR5* is associated with an increased risk of perinatal HIV-1 infection (123). The *CCR5-59356T* allele frequency is 21% in African Americans and 3% in European Americans, while the protective *CCR5-Δ32* allele is effectively absent in African Americans. These *CCR5* regulatory genetic factors, along with other influences, may contribute to the higher HIV-1 transmission rates observed among blacks in Africa and, in the United States, among African Americans.

Determining the *CCR5* promoter haplotypes and testing the epidemiologic effects of these haplotypes has been hampered by the difficulties inherent in using single-strand conformational polymorphism and heteroduplex assays to assign *CCR5P* genotypes. These methods are labor intensive and may discourage assessments of *CCR5*-promoter haplotypes in other cohorts. Recently, An et al. (60) reported that the *CCR5* promoter *–2459A* allele (position 59029) (10) is in nearly complete linkage disequilibrium with the *CCR5-P1* haplotypes in both African Americans and European Americans and can therefore be used as a marker for the *CCR5-P1* haplotype (60). Conversely, the common allele, *CCR5-2459T*, is invariably found with the *CCR5-P2*, *-P3*, and *-P4* haplotypes. The use of standard SNP genotyping assays to identify *CCR5* promoter haplotypes should facilitate the genetic analysis of *CCR5* promoter haplotypes in other ethnic and racial groups.

SDF1-3′A and Its Possible Role in HIV-1 Pathogenesis

SDF-1 is the primary natural ligand for CXCR4, the coreceptor for X4 HIV-1 strains. SDF-1 has been shown to potently inhibit cell-adapted X4 HIV-1 replication in vitro by both competitively binding to the CXCR4 receptor and by inducing an internalization of the CXCR4 protein (65,66). The X4 HIV-1 strains that emerge in the latter stages of HIV-1 infection in about 50% of the people infected with HIV-1 subtype B are frequently associated with a poor prognosis (69,70). The *SDF1-3′A* variant in the 3′ untranslated region of the SDF1β transcript was reported to be highly protective against progression to AIDS and death in the first 10 years of infection (8). Among individuals with the *SDF1-3′A/3′A* genotype plus a *CCR5-Δ32* or *CCR2-64I* allele, the protection is particularly strong. Remarkably, in our study of 603 HIV-1–infected individuals, no one who was protected by both *SDF1-3′A* and either *CCR5-Δ32* or *CCR2-64I* heterozygosity progressed to AIDS in the first 10 years following infection. Although *SDF1-3′A/3′A* is highly protective in the first 10 years of infection, it apparently confers no late protection, possibly because viral replication of R5 strains continues unabated and eventually leads to $CD4^+$ T-cell depletion and immune dysregulation. In other cohort studies, *SDF1-3′A* has been associated with rapid progression to AIDS or with prolonged survival after a diagnosis of AIDS (11,102,124).

Recently, a study in Kenya of 318 mothers reported that the maternal *SDF1-+/3'A* genotype is associated with an increase in mother-to-infant transmission but there was no difference in *SDF1-3'A* genotype frequencies between infected and uninfected infants (Table 2) (125). Viral load between transmitting and nontransmitting *SDF1-3'A* heterozygous mothers was similar, leading to the speculation that the *SDF1-+/3'A* genotype was limiting viral phenotype or cell tropism of the maternal HIV-1 and thereby influencing the kinetics of transmission to the infants. *SDF1-3'A* may slow the replication of the nontransmissible X4 strains by limiting the availability of the CXCR4 receptor in local tissue compartments, thus favoring R5 strains.

RANTES Regulatory Variants

The chemokine ligand, *RANTES*, inhibits R5 HIV-1 replication by competitively binding to CCR5 and by downregulating surface expression of CCR5 (63,64). Either mechanism would possibly stem R5 HIV-1 replication by limiting the portals available to the virus for cell entry.

Two single nucleotide polymorphisms, at G→A at -403 and C→G at -28, have been identified in the *RANTES* promoter region (126,127). The *RANTES–28G* allele upregulates *RANTES* transcription in in-vitro reporter assays (14), but the regulatory role of the *RANTES–403A* promoter allele on transcription is unclear. In one report, constructs containing *–403A* were shown to potently upregulate *RANTES* transcription (128) but *–403A* had no effect on transcription in other studies (An, Winkler: unpublished data, 14). In an analysis of a case-controlled study of seroprevalent individuals in Japan, the *–28G* allele was associated with higher $CD4^+$ T-cell counts, as might be expected from a promoter variant that upregulates *RANTES* transcription (14). In a study of European Americans, the *RANTES* [*–403A.-28C*] haplotype was associated with protection against progression to AIDS but, paradoxically, was also associated with increased susceptibility to infection (9).

Linkage disequilibrium between *RANTES–403A* and additional genetic variants in the *RANTES* gene may resolve this paradox. We have recently identified a regulatory element in the first intron of the *RANTES* gene that potently upregulates *RANTES* transcription levels in reporter assays. A newly discovered variant within the enhancer element, *In1.1C*, abrogates much of the enhancer activity, thus downregulating *RANTES* transcription. The variant is quite common in African Americans and Caucasians (f = 42% and 18%, respectively). The effect of the *In1.1C* allele is dominant since both the *In1.1T/C* and *In1.1C/C* genotypes are strongly associated with accelerated progression to AIDS in African Americans (RH = 2.01, $p < 0.008$). Thus it is quite possible that the *In1.1C* allele may also affect HIV-1 progression and possibly HIV-1 transmission among Africans (An et al., submitted).

IL10-5'A Is a Late-Acting Risk Factor for Progression

IL-10, produced by lymphoid cells, is a powerful anti-inflammatory cytokine that inhibits macrophage and T-cell replication (129,130) and cytokine secretion by T-helper cells (131). High levels of IL-10 have been shown in vitro to reduce HIV-1 replication in macrophages (132,133). A promoter variant in the 5′ untranslated region of *IL10* specifies a DNA sequence that differentially binds to certain ETS transcriptional factors and downregulates *IL10* transcription by 2- to 4-fold (15,134–136). In European Americans, the downregulating *IL10-5'A* allele was found to be dominant and associated with more rapid progression to AIDS, but the acceleration became apparent only 5 or more years after HIV-1 infection (15). The *IL10-5'A* allele was also associated with a slightly increased risk for HIV-1 infection in a group of highly exposed uninfected men enrolled in the MACS study (15). The effect of the *IL10-5'A* allele on progression to AIDS was not observed in a cohort of African-American injection drug users, possibly because the cohort underwent a shorter observation period than the European-American cohorts, and the effect of the *IL10-5'A* allele only becomes apparent 5 or more years after seroconversion (15). Because the allele frequency of *IL10-5'A* is almost 2-fold higher in African Americans (40%) than in European Americans (24%), the effects of this allele on infection and progression in black Africans or people of African ancestry should be evaluated. The differential allele frequency in ethnic and racial groups may be of consequence for selective pressure since *IL10* has been shown to affect other immune disorders, including asthma and diabetes (137–139).

HLA AND AIDS

HLA class I and class II alleles were probably the first human genetic factors to be examined for an effect on AIDS. The presentation of peptide fragments from pathogen proteins by class I and II receptors plays a central part in the immune response against pathogens, and different class I and II alleles vary in their capacity to present peptides from specific pathogens. It is both theoretically and empirically established that individuals with different HLA Class I and II alleles can have varying susceptibilities to infectious diseases (140–142).

Numerous associations between HLA class I and II alleles have been reported but only a few have consistently been observed (143). Notable among these are those for the class I alleles *B*27* (144) and *B*35* (13, 144), which are associated with resistance and susceptibility, respectively, to disease progression in HIV-1–infected individuals. While *B*27* is relatively rare in individuals not of European ancestry, *B*35* is frequent globally (Figure 2). However, the pattern of alleles of the *B*35* allele group varies between different groups (145), a fact that explains the lack of association of *B*35* observed for African Americans (13). A recent study of *B*35* subtypes indicates that susceptibility is associated with only certain subtypes (collectively termed *B*35Px*) (145). Two *B*35Px* subtype alleles, *B*3502* and *B*3503*, are common in European Americans but are rare in African Americans. However *B*53*, which is common in black Africans, is structurally equivalent to *B*35Px* subtypes and also shows association with susceptibility to AIDS progression (145).

As a consequence of the extreme polymorphism of HLA class I alleles, most people are heterozygous at all of the three main class I loci. However, certain individuals are homozygous for one, two, or, in rare cases, all three of these loci. These individuals have less variety in available class I alleles. Class I homozygotes will present a smaller range of peptides from pathogens and are potentially more susceptible to infectious diseases (140,141,146). Consistent with this idea are data showing a profound increase in the rate of AIDS progression among individuals homozygous for class I loci with the effect being cumulative, that is, individuals homozygous for two or three loci progress to AIDS even more rapidly than those homozygous for one locus (144). The HLA homozygosity acceleration is observed equally in African Americans and European Americans (Figure 4).

Several studies have looked specifically at the effect of HLA class I and class II alleles on susceptibility to HIV-1 infection among black Africans (Table 3). Among sex workers in Nairobi Kenya who resisted HIV-1 infection in spite of extremely high levels of exposure, resistance to infection was correlated with high levels of cytotoxic T-lymphocytes (CTLs), a cell type that responds to antigens

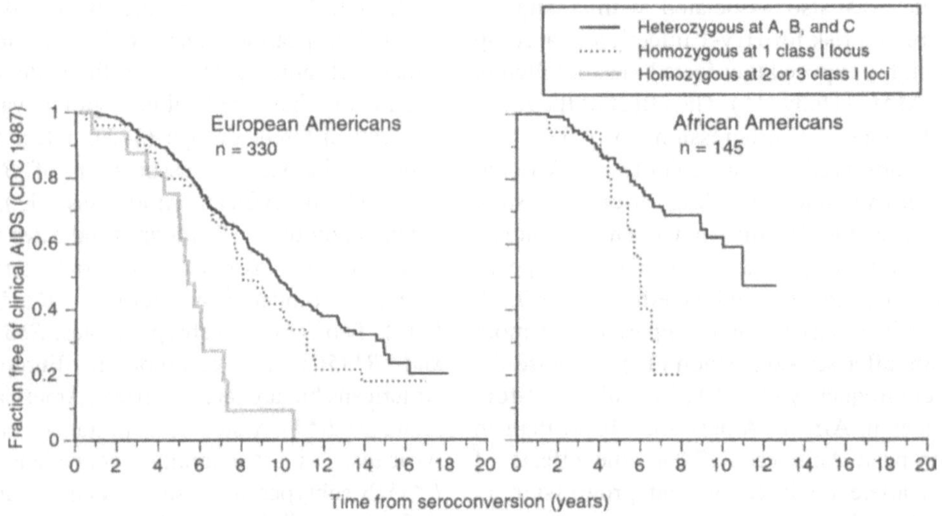

FIGURE 4. Effect of homozygosity at *HLA* Class I *A*, *B*, and *C* loci on survival in European Americans and African Americans using 1987 CDC definition of clinical AIDS (61). Curves compare individuals homozygous at one Class I locus (dotted line) or two or three Class I loci (gray line) with individuals heterozygous at all three loci (black line). No individuals homozygous at 2 or 3 loci were observed in this group of African American seroincident individuals. RH and p values (Cox model analyses) compare the singly and multiply homozygous groups with the fully heterozygous group (13). The effect of single and multiple locus homozygosity is associated with acceleration to AIDS-defining conditions: one locus homozygosity, RH = 1.6, 3.54, p = 0.02, 0.001, for European (number homozygotes [n] = 50) and African Americans (n = 19), respectively; two or three loci homozygosity, RH = 4.8, $p = 10 \times 10^7$ for European Americans (n = 16).

presented on infected cells by the class I receptor (147,148). For this cohort, resistance to HIV-1 infection was strongly correlated with the presence of alleles from the *A2/6802* supertype (149). In addition, the HLA class II allele *DRB1*01* was associated with resistance to infection. A second study demonstrated that infants carrying alleles of the *A2/6802* supertype were strongly protected against perinatal HIV-1 transmission (150). These studies affirm the importance of HLA alleles in differential susceptibility to HIV-1 infection and highlight the importance of an effective CTL response against invading pathogens.

WHY INCONSISTENCIES EXIST BETWEEN STUDIES

Differences in associations among genetic epidemiologic studies are common, particularly genetic associations with HIV-1 infection and progression to AIDS. HIV-1 infection is caused by exposure to the virus by a variety of routes (sexual intercourse, blood, breast milk) from individuals with quantitative differences in viral load and immunodeficiency. With the exception of mother-to-infant exposure, it is difficult to pinpoint the time of infection, determine the viral load and disease stage of the individual, or identify the individual(s) transmitting HIV-1. In sexual transmission, the HIV-1–infected individual may be unknown or unavailable, making it impossible to quantify the viral load of the transmitting partner, and determination of HIV-1 exposure by number of sexual partners or duration of high-risk behavior may be unreliable. In addition, it has been shown that other sexually transmitted diseases may increase both risk of infection in the susceptible partner and rate of progression (43,151). In the case of *CCR5-Δ32* homozygosity, the absence of a required cofactor for cell entry provides almost complete resistance to HIV-1 infection, but it is much more difficult to assess genetic factors that provide partial resistance. Selection of the correct HIV-1–infected control group is also critical. If a genetic factor that increases risk of infection is also associated with rapid progression, the genetic factor will be underrepresented in a seroprevalent control group because rapid progressors are underrepresented (118,119, 152,153). This unintended survival (also called frailty) bias is avoided by using an HIV-1 seroincident control group for infection tests.

Inconsistencies among studies have also been noted for associations between *CCR4-64I*, *SDF1-3'A*, and *CCR5-Δ32* and rate of progression to AIDS. The association between rate of progression to AIDS and a specific genetic factor depends on a reliable estimate of the time of HIV-1 infection and the length of clinical follow-up. Seroprevalent cohorts are likely to underrepresent rapid progressors and present difficulties for precisely estimating participants' time of HIV-1 infection. Both of these factors may introduce considerable bias and severely reduce the power of the cohort for detection of genetic association (118,119,153). In seroincident cohorts, survival bias may also be introduced because genetic testing depends on DNA availability. Natural history cohort studies that collected DNA or established cell lines sometime after HIV-1 infection of the study participants were nonrandomly depleted of rapid progressors who, by death or morbidity, were unavailable to provide a blood sample (17). Finally, the association between genetic factors and rate of progression requires both a substantial observation period and statistical power. Several of the studies failing to detect association between progression and a reported genetic factor were both underpowered and had mean observation times of 5 or fewer years, much less than the 10 years estimated to be the mean time to clinical AIDS in developed countries. Thus, effects may be slight and difficult to quantify.

CONCLUSION

The identification of genetic factors that regulate HIV-1 infection and AIDS kinetics has clarified our view of viral pathogenesis by illuminating the importance of host–virus interactions at virtually every stage of infection. Genetic studies often point to unexpected roles for host factors, providing insights into immune regulation of HIV-1 replication and possible selective forces that may influence HIV-1 quasispecies evolution. Host genetic factors have been shown to affect susceptibility to infection, the rate of $CD4^+$ T-cell depletion, and the rate of progression to AIDS. Thus, it is important to consider the genetic background of the host when assessing the efficacy of antiretroviral agents and vaccines in clinical trials.

Unfortunately, as a consequence of inadequate funding, political barriers, and lack of resolve for confronting diseases in developing nations, there are far too few natural history cohort studies conducted in Africa. Many of the ones that are available have been established late in the epidemic, thus limiting their prospective longitudinal component. Human populations are evolving under varying selective pressures including infectious agents. Genetic variants that have a selective advantage in one situation sometimes have a selective disadvantage in others. Over time, selective pressures and genetic drift cause allele frequencies and haplotype structures to differ among populations. A definition of genetic factors influencing HIV-1 infection, pathogenesis, and rate of progression in individuals in Africa and Asia is essential to understanding geographic differences in HIV-1 epidemic dynamics and the interaction between host genetic factors, specific viral subtypes, and other environmental correlates of this disease.

REFERENCES

1. Schuitemaker H, Koot M, Kootstra NA, et al. Biological phenotype of human immunodeficiency virus type 1 clones at different stages of infection: progression of disease is associated with a shift from monocytotropic to T-cell-tropic virus population. *J Virol*, 1992;66:1354–1360.
2. Connor RI, Sheridan KE, Ceradini D, et al. Change in coreceptor use correlates with disease progression in HIV-1–infected individuals. *J Exp Med*, 1997;185:621–628.
3. Kanki PJ, Hamel DJ, Sankale JL, et al. Human immunodeficiency virus type 1 subtypes differ in disease progression. *J Infect Dis*, 1999;179:68–73.
4. Morgan D, Maude GH, Malamba SS, et al. HIV-1 disease progression and AIDS-defining disorders in rural Uganda. *Lancet*, 1997;350:245–250.
5. Dean M, Jacobson LP, McFarlane G, et al. Reduced risk of AIDS lymphoma in individuals heterozygous for the CCR5-delta32 mutation. *Cancer Res*, 1999;59:3561–3564.
6. Dean M, Carrington M, Winkler C, et al. Genetic restriction of HIV-1 infection and progression to AIDS by a deletion allele of the CKR5 structural gene. *Science*, 1996;273:1856–1862.
7. Smith MW, Dean M, Carrington M, et al. Contrasting genetic influence of CCR2 and CCR5 variants on HIV-1 infection and disease progression. *Science*, 1997;277:959–965.
8. Winkler C, Modi W, Smith MW, et al. Genetic restriction of AIDS pathogenesis by an SDF-1 chemokine gene variant. *Science*, 1998;279:389–393.
9. McDermott DH, Beecroft MJ, Kleeberger CA, et al. Chemokine RANTES promoter polymorphism affects risk of both HIV infection and disease progression in the Multicenter AIDS Cohort Study. *AIDS*, 2000;14:2671–2678.
10. McDermott DH, Zimmerman PA, Guignard F, et al. CCR5 promoter polymorphism and HIV-1 disease progression. Multicenter AIDS Cohort Study (MACS). *Lancet*, 1998;352:866–870.
11. Mummidi S, Ahuja SS, Gonzalez E, et al. Gene-alogy of the CCR5 locus and chemokine system gene variants associated with altered rates of HIV-1 disease progression. *Nat Med*, 1998; 4:786–793.
12. Martin MP, Dean M, Smith MW, et al. Genetic acceleration of AIDS progression by a promoter variant of CCR5. *Science*, 1998;282:1907–1911.
13. Carrington M, Nelson GW, Martin MP, et al. HLA and HIV-1: heterozygote advantage and B*35-Cw*04 disadvantage. *Science*, 1999;283: 1748–1752.
14. Liu H, Chao D, Nakayama EE, et al. Polymorphism in RANTES chemokine promoter affects HIV-1 disease progression. *Proc Natl Acad Sci USA*, 1999;96:4581–4585.
15. Shin HD, Winkler C, Stephens JC, et al. Genetic restriction of HIV-1 pathogenesis to AIDS by promoter alleles of IL10. *Proc Natl Acad Sci USA*, 2000;97:14467–14472.
16. O'Brien SJ, Dean M, Smith M, et al. The Human Genes that Limit AIDS. In: Boulyjenkov V, Berg K, Christen Y, eds. Genes and Resistance to Diseases. 1st ed. Berlin Heidelberg: Springer-Verlag, 2000:9–17.
17. O'Brien SJ, Nelson GW, Winkler CA, et al. Polygenic and multifactorial disease gene association in man: Lessons from AIDS. *Annu Rev Genet*, 2000;34:563–591.
18. O'Brien SJ, Moore J. The effect of genetic variation in chemokines and their receptors on HIV transmission and progression to AIDS. *Immunol Rev*, 2000;177:99–111.
19. Kaslow RA, Ostrow DG, Detels R, et al. The Multicenter AIDS Cohort Study: rationale, organization, and selected characteristics of the participants. *Am J Epidemiol*, 1987;126:310–318.
20. Goedert JJ, Kessler CM, Aledort LM, et al. A prospective study of human immunodeficiency virus type 1 infection and the development of AIDS in subjects with hemophilia. *N Engl J Med*, 1989;321:1141–1148.
21. Pisani E, Schwartlander B, Cherney S, et al. *Report on the global HIV/AIDS epidemic*. Geneva: Joint United Nations Programme on AIDS, June 2000.
22. Burke D, McCutchan F. Global distribution of human immunodeficiency virus-1 clades. In: DeVita J, Hellman S, Rosenberg S, eds. *AIDS: Biology, Diagnosis, Treatment and Prevention.* Philadelphia: Lipincott-Raven, 1997:119–126.
23. Myers G, Korber B, Hahn B. *A compilation and analysis of nucleic acid and amino acid sequences.* Los Alamos, New Mexico: Los Alamos National Laboratory, Theoretical Biology and Biophysics Group, 1995.
24. Su B, Sun G, Lu D, et al. Distribution of three HIV-1 resistance-conferring polymorphisms (SDF1-3′A, CCR2-64I, and CCR5-Delta32) in global populations. *Eur J Hum Genet*, 2000;8:975–979.
25. Stephens JC, Reich DE, Goldstein DB, et al. Dating the origin of the CCR5-Delta32 AIDS-resistance allele by the coalescence of haplotypes. *Am J Hum Genet*, 1998;62:1507–1515.
26. Martinson JJ, Chapman NH, Rees DC, et al. Global distribution of the CCR5 gene 32-basepair deletion. *Nat Genet*, 1997;16:100–103.

27. Martinson JJ, Hong L, Karanicolas R, et al. Global distribution of the CCR2-64I/CCR5-59653T HIV-1 disease-protective haplotype. *AIDS*, 2000;14: 483–489.
28. Su, B, Jin L, Hu, F, et al. Distribution of two HIV-1 resistant polymorphisms (SDF1-3′A and CCR2-64I) in East Asian and world populations and its implication in AIDS epidemiology. *Am J Hum Genet*, 1999;65:1047–1053.
29. Clayton J, Lonjou C. Allele and haplotype frequencies for HLA loci in various ethnic groups. In: Charron D, ed. *Genetic Diversity of HLA: Functional and Medicinal Implication*. Paris: Medical and Scientific International, 1997: 665–776.
30. Weber W, Nash DJ, Motulsky AG, et al. Phylogenetic relationships of human populations in sub-Saharan Africa. *Hum Biol*, 2000;72:753–772.
31. Goddard KA, Hopkins PJ, Hall JM, et al. Linkage disequilibrium and allele-frequency distributions for 114 single-nucleotide polymorphisms in five populations. *Am J Hum Genet*, 2000; 66:216–234.
32. Shriver MD, Smith, MW, Jin L, et al. Ethnic-affiliation estimation by use of population-specific DNA markers. *Am J Hum Genet*, 1997;60:957–964.
33. HIV/AIDS Surveillance Report. Atlanta: Centers for Disease Control, 2001.
34. The Working Group on Mother-to-Child Transmission of HIV. Rates of mother-to-child transmission of HIV-1 in Africa, America, and Europe: results from 13 perinatal studies. *J Acquir Immune Defic Syndr Hum Retrovirol*, 1995;8:506–510.
35. Colebunders RL, Latif AS. Natural history and clinical presentation of HIV-1 infection in adults. *AIDS*, 1991;5:S103–S112.
36. Whittle H, Egboga A, Todd J, et al. Clinical and laboratory predictors of survival in Gambian patients with symptomatic HIV-1 or HIV-2 infection. *AIDS*, 1992;6:685–689.
37. Anzala OA, Nagelkerke NJ, Bwayo JJ, et al. Rapid progression to disease in African sex workers with human immunodeficiency virus type 1 infection. *J Infect Dis*, 1995;171:686–689.
38. Bwayo JJ, Nagelkerke NJ, Moses S, et al. Comparison of the declines in CD4 counts in HIV-1-seropositive female sex workers and women from the general population in Nairobi, Kenya. *J Acquir Immune Defic Syndr Hum Retrovirol*, 1995; 10:457–461.
39. Mann JM, Bila K, Colebunders RL, et al. Natural history of human immunodeficiency virus infection in Zaire. *Lancet*, 1986;2:707–709.
40. Leroy V, Msellati P, Lepage P, et al. Four years of natural history of HIV-1 infection in african women: a prospective cohort study in Kigali (Rwanda), 1988–1993. *J Acquir Immune Defic Syndr Hum Retrovirol*, 1995;9:415–421.
41. Morgan D, Malamba SS, Maude GH, et al. An HIV-1 natural history cohort and survival times in rural Uganda. *AIDS*, 1997;11:633–640.
42. Morgan D, Whitworth J. The natural history of HIV-1 infection in Africa. *Nat Med*, 2001; 7: 143–145.
43. Anzala AO, Simonsen JN, Kimani J, et al. Acute sexually transmitted infections increase human immunodeficiency virus type 1 plasma viremia, increase plasma type 2 cytokines, and decrease CD4 cell counts. *J Infect Dis*, 2000;182:459–466.
44. Hu DJ, Fleming PL, Castro KG, et al. How important is race/ethnicity as an indicator of risk for specific AIDS-defining conditions? *J Acquir Immune Defic Syndr Hum Retrovirol*, 1995;10:374–380.
45. Vlahov D, Polk BF. Perspectives on infection with HIV-1 among intravenous drug users. *Psychopharmacol Bull*, 1988;24:325–329.
46. Galai N, Vlahov D, Margolick JB, et al. Changes in markers of disease progression in HIV-1 seroconverters: a comparison between cohorts of injecting drug users and homosexual men. *J Acquir Immune Defic Syndr Hum Retrovirol*, 1995;8:66–74.
47. Low N, Paine K, Clark R, et al. AIDS survival and progression in black Africans living in south London, 1986–1994. *Genitourin Med*, 1996;72: 12–16.
48. O'Farrell N, Lau R, Yoganathan K, et al. AIDS in Africans living in London. *Genitourin Med*, 1995;71:358–362.
49. Galai N, Kalinkovich A, Burstein R, et al. African HIV-1 subtype C and rate of progression among Ethiopian immigrants in Israel. *Lancet*, 1997;349: 180–181.
50. Lander ES, Schork NJ. Genetic dissection of complex traits. *Science*, 1994;265:2037–2048.
51. Collins A, Lonjou C, Morton NE. Genetic epidemiology of single-nucleotide polymorphisms. *Proc Natl Acad Sci USA*, 1999;96:15173–15177.
52. Kruglyak L. Prospects for whole-genome linkage disequilibrium mapping of common disease genes. *Nat Genet*, 1999;22:139–144.
53. Huttley GA, Smith MW, Carrington M, et al. A scan for linkage disequilibrium across the human genome. *Genetics*, 1999;152:1711–1722.
54. Goedert JJ, Biggar RJ, Winn DM, et al. Decreased helper T lymphocytes in homosexual men. II. Sexual practices. *Am J Epidemiol*, 1985;121: 637–644.
55. Buchbinder SP, Katz MH, Hessol NA, et al. Long-term HIV-1 infection without immunologic progression. *AIDS*, 1994;8:1123–1128.
56. Detels R, Liu Z, Hennessey K, et al. Resistance to HIV-1 infection: the Multicenter AIDS Cohort Study. *J Acquir Immune Defic Syndr*, 1994;7: 1263–1269.
57. Phair J, Jacobson L, Detels R, et al. Acquired immune deficiency syndrome occurring within 5

years of infection with human immunodeficiency virus type-1: the Multicenter AIDS Cohort Study. *J Acquir Immune Defic Syndr*, 1992;5:490–496.

58. Vlahov D, Graham N, Hoover D, et al. Prognostic indicators for AIDS and infectious disease death in HIV-infected injection drug users: plasma viral load and CD4+ cell count. *JAMA*, 1998;279:35–40.
59. Hilgartner MW, Donfield SM, Willoughby A, et al. Hemophilia growth and development study: Design, methods, and entry data. *Am J Pediatr Hematol Oncol*, 1993;15:208–218.
60. An P, Martin MP, Nelson GW, et al. Influence of CCR5 promoter haplotypes on AIDS progression in African-Americans. *AIDS*, 2000;14:2117–2122.
61. Revision of the CDC surveillance case definition for acquired immunodeficiency syndrome. *MMWR*, 1987;36(suppl. 1):1S–15S.
62. 1993 revised classification system for HIV infection and an expanded surveillance case definition for AIDS among adolescents and adults. *MMWR*, 41:1992.
63. Cocchi F, DeVico AL, Garzino-Demo A, et al. Identification of RANTES, MIP-1 alpha, and MIP-1 beta as the major HIV-suppressive factors produced by CD8+ T cells. *Science*, 1995;270: 1811–1815.
64. Alkhatib G, Combadiere C, Broder CC, et al. CC CKR5: a RANTES, MIP-1alpha, MIP-1beta receptor as a fusion cofactor for macrophage-tropic HIV-1. *Science*, 1996;272:1955–1958.
65. Bleul CC, Farzan M, Choe H, et al. The lymphocyte chemoattractant SDF-1 is a ligand for LESTR/fusin and blocks HIV-1 entry. *Nature*, 1996;382:829–833.
66. Bleul CC, Wu L, Hoxie JA, et al. The HIV coreceptors CXCR4 and CCR5 are differentially expressed and regulated on human T lymphocytes. *Proc Natl Acad Sci USA*, 1997;94:1925–1930.
67. Dragic T, Litwin V, Allaway GP, et al. HIV-1 entry into CD4+ cells is mediated by the chemokine receptor CC- CKR-5. *Nature*, 1996;381:667–673.
68. Feng Y, Broder CC, Kennedy PE, et al. HIV-1 entry cofactor: functional cDNA cloning of a seven-transmembrane, G protein-coupled receptor. *Science*, 1996;272:872–877.
69. Richman DD, Bozzette SA. The impact of the syncytium-inducing phenotype of human immunodeficiency virus on disease progression. *J Infect Dis*, 1994;169:968–974.
70. Roos MT, Lange JM, de Goede RE, et al. Viral phenotype and immune response in primary human immunodeficiency virus type 1 infection. *J Infect Dis*, 1992;165:427–432.
71. Zhang YJ, Dragic T, Cao Y, et al. Use of coreceptors other than CCR5 by non-syncytium-inducing adult and pediatric isolates of human immunodeficiency virus type 1 is rare in vitro. *J Virol*, 1998; 72:9337–9344.
72. Zhu T, Mo H, Wang N, et al. Genotypic and phenotypic characterization of HIV-1 patients with primary infection. Science, 1993;261:1179–1181.
73. Choe H, Farzan M, Sun Y, et al. The beta-chemokine receptors CCR3 and CCR5 facilitate infection by primary HIV-1 isolates. *Cell*, 1996;85:1135–1148.
74. Berger EA, Murphy PM, Farber JM. Chemokine receptors as HIV-1 coreceptors: roles in viral entry, tropism, and disease. *Annu Rev Immunol*, 1999;17:657–700.
75. Xiao L, Rudolph DL, Owen SM, et al. Adaptation to promiscuous usage of CC and CXC-chemokine coreceptors in vivo correlates with HIV-1 disease progression. *AIDS*, 1998;12:F137–F143.
76. Liu R, Paxton WA, Choe S, et al. Homozygous defect in HIV-1 coreceptor accounts for resistance of some multiply-exposed individuals to HIV-1 infection. *Cell*, 1996;86:367–377.
77. Samson M, Libert F, Doranz BJ, et al. Resistance to HIV-1 infection in Caucasian individuals bearing mutant alleles of the CCR-5 chemokine receptor gene. *Nature*, 1996;382:722–725.
78. Zimmerman PA, Buckler-White A, Alkhatib G, et al. Inherited resistance to HIV-1 conferred by an inactivating mutation in CC chemokine receptor 5: studies in populations with contrasting clinical phenotypes, defined racial background, and quantified risk. *Mol Med*, 1997;3:23–36.
79. Wu L, Paxton WA, Kassam N, et al. CCR5 levels and expression pattern correlate with infectability by macrophage-tropic HIV-1, in vitro. *J Exp Med*, 1997;185:1681–1691.
80. Benkirane M, Jin DY, Chun RF, et al. Mechanism of transdominant inhibition of CCR5-mediated HIV-1 infection by ccr5del32. *J Biol Chem*, 1997;272:30603–30606.
81. Nguyen GT, Carrington M, Beeler JA, et al. Phenotypic expressions of CCR5-delta32/del32 homozygosity. *J Acquir Immune Defic Syndr*, 1999;22:75–82.
82. Paxton WA, Liu R, Kang S, et al. Reduced HIV-1 infectability of CD4+ lymphocytes from exposed-uninfected individuals: association with low expression of CCR5 and high production of beta-chemokines. *Virology*, 1998;244:66–73.
83. Maayan S, Zhang L, Shinar E, et al. Evidence for recent selection of the CCR5-delta 32 deletion from differences in its frequency between Ashkenazi and Sephardi Jews. Genes *Immun*, 2000;1:358–361.
84. Libert F, Cochaux P, Beckman G, et al. The delta CCR5 mutation conferring protection against HIV-1 in Caucasian populations has a single and recent origin in Northeastern Europe. *Hum Mol Genet*, 1998;7:399–406.
85. Michael NL, Louie LG, Rohrbaugh AL, et al. The role of CCR5 and CCR2 polymorphisms in HIV-1

transmission and disease progression. *Nat Med*, 1997;3:1160–1162.

86. Huang Y, Paxton WA, Wolinsky SM, et al. The role of a mutant CCR5 allele in HIV-1 transmission and disease progression. *Nat Med*, 1996;2:1240–1243.
87. Theodorou I, Meyer L, Magierowska M, et al. HIV-1 infection in an individual homozygous for CCR5 delta 32. *Lancet*, 1997;349:1219–1220.
88. O'Brien TR, Winkler C, Dean M, et al. HIV-1 infection in a man homozygous for CCR5 delta 32. *Lancet*, 1997;349:1219.
89. Biti R, French R, Young J, et al. HIV-1 infection in an individual homozygous for the CCR5 deletion allele. *Nat Med*, 1997;3:252–253.
90. Balotta C, Bagnarelli P, Violin M, et al. Homozygous delta 32 deletion of the CCR-5 chemokine receptor gene in an HIV-1-infected patient. *AIDS*, 1997;11:67–71.
91. Michael NL, Nelson JA, Kewal Ramani VN, et al. Exclusive and persistent use of the entry coreceptor CXCR4 by human immunodeficiency virus type 1 from a subject homozygous for CCR5 delta32. *J Virol*, 1998; 72:6040–6047.
92. Hoffman TL, MacGregor RR, Burger H, et al. CCR5 genotypes in sexually active couples discordant for human immunodeficiency virus type 1 infection status. *J Infect Dis*, 1997;176: 1093–1096.
93. Ioannidis JP, O'Brien TR, Rosenberg PS, et al. Genetic effects on HIV disease progression. *Nat Med*, 1998;4:536.
94. Rousseau CM, Just JJ, Abrams EJ, et al. CCR5del32 in perinatal HIV-1 infection. *J Acquir Immune Defic Syndr Hum Retrovirol*, 1997;16:239–242.
95. Edelstein RE, Arcuino LA, Hughes JP, et al. Risk of mother-to-infant transmission of HIV-1 is not reduced in CCR5/delta32ccr5 heterozygotes. *J Acquir Immune Defic Syndr Hum Retrovirol*, 1997; 16:243–246.
96. Misrahi M, Teglas JP, N'Go N, et al. CCR5 chemokine receptor variant in HIV-1 mother-to-child transmission and disease progression in children. *JAMA*, 1998;279:277–280.
97. Philpott S, Burger H, Charbonneau T, et al. CCR5 genotype and resistance to vertical transmission of HIV-1. *J Acquir Immun Defic Syndr*, 1999; 21: 189–193.
98. Shearer WT, Kalish LA, and Zimmerman PA. CCR5 HIV-1 Vertical Transmission. *J Acquir Immune Defic Syndr Hum Retrovirol*, 1998;17(2):180–181.
99. Mas A, Espanol T, Heredia A, et al. CCR5 genotype and HIV-1 infection in perinatally-exposed infants. *J Infect Dis*, 1999;38:9–11.
100. Barroga CF, Raskino C, Fangon MC, et al. The CCR5Delta32 allele slows disease progression of human immunodeficiency virus-1-infected children receiving antiretroviral treatment. *J Infect Dis*, 2000;182:413–419.
101. Mangano A, Prada F, Roldan A, et al. Distribution of CCR-5 delta32 allele in Argentinian children at risk of HIV-1 infection: its role in vertical transmission. *AIDS*, 1998;12:109–110.
102. Mangano A, Kopka J, Batalla M, et al. Protective effect of CCR2-64I and not of CCR5-delta32 and SDF1-3′A in pediatric HIV-1 infection. *J Acquir Immune Defic Syndr*, 2000;23:52–57.
103. Buseyne F, Janvier G, Teglas JP, et al. Impact of heterozygosity for the chemokine receptor CCR5 32-bp-deleted allele on plasma virus load and CD4 T lymphocytes in perinatally human immunodeficiency virus-infected children at 8 years of age. *J Infect Dis*, 1998;178:1019–1023.
104. Meyer L, Magierowska M, Hubert JB, et al. Early protective effect of CCR-5 delta 32 heterozygosity on HIV-1 disease progression: relationship with viral load. *AIDS*, 1997;11:F73–F78.
105. Michael NL, Louie LG, Rohrbaugh AL, et al. The role of CCR5 and CCR2 polymorphisms in HIV-1 transmission and disease progression. *Nat Med*, 1997;3:1160–1162.
106. Katzenstein TL, Eugen-Olsen J, Hofmann B, et al. HIV-infected individuals with the CCR delta32/CCR5 genotype have lower HIV RNA levels and higher CD4 cell counts in the early years of the infection than do patients with the wild type. *J Acquir Immune Defic Syndr Hum Retrovirol*, 1997;16:10–14.
107. Walli R, Reinhart B, Luckow B, et al. HIV-1-infected long-term slow progressors heterozygous for delta32-CCR5 show significantly lower plasma viral load than wild-type slow progressors. *J Acquir Immune Defic Syndr Hum Retrovirol*, 1998;18:229–233.
108. Ioannidis JP, Contopoulos-Ioannidis DG. Maternal viral load and the risk of perinatal transmission of HIV-1. *N Engl J Med*, 1999;341: 1698–1700.
109. Contopoulos-Ioannidis DG, Ioannidis JP. Maternal cell-free viremia in the natural history of perinatal HIV-1 transmission: a meta-analysis. *J Acquir Immune Defic Syndr Hum Retrovirol*, 1998; 18:126–135.
110. John GC, Nduati RW, Mbori-Ngacha DA, et al. Correlates of mother-to-child human immunodeficiency virus type 1 (HIV-1) transmission: association with maternal plasma HIV-1 RNA load, genital HIV-1 DNA shedding, and breast infections. *J Infect Dis*, 2001;183:206–212.
111. Gonzalez E, Bamshad M, Sato N, et al. Race-specific HIV-1 disease-modifying effects associated with CCR5 haplotypes. *Proc Natl Acad Sci USA*, 1999;96:12004–12009.

112. Ometto L, Bertorelle R, Mainardi M, et al. Polymorphisms in the CCR5 promoter region influence disease progression in perinatally human immunodeficiency virus type 1-infected children. *J Infect Dis*, 2001;183:814–818.
113. Kostrikis LG, Huang Y, Moore JP, et al. A chemokine receptor CCR2 allele delays HIV-1 disease progression and is associated with a CCR5 promoter mutation. *Nat Med*, 1998;4:350–353.
114. Anzala AO, Ball TB, Rostron T, et al. *CCR2-64I* allele and genotype association with delayed AIDS progression in African women. *Lancet*, 1998;351: 1632–1633.
115. Williamson C, Loubser SA, Brice B, et al. Allelic frequencies of host genetic variants influencing susceptibility to HIV-1 infection and disease in South African populations. *AIDS*, 2000;14: 449–451.
116. Schinkel J, Langendam MW, Coutinho RA, et al. No evidence for an effect of the CCR5 delta32/+ and CCR2b 64I/+ mutations on human immunodeficiency virus (HIV)-1 disease progression among HIV-1-infected injecting drug users. *J Infect Dis*, 1999;179:825–831.
117. Daar ES, Lynn H, Donfield S, et al. Effects of plasma HIV RNA, CD4+ T lymphocytes, and the chemokine receptors CCR5 and CCR2b on HIV disease progression in hemophiliacs. *J Acquir Immune Defic Syndr*, 1999;21:317–325.
118. Donfield SM, Lynn HS, Hilgartner MW. Progression to AIDS. *Science*, 1998;280:1819–1820.
119. Smith MW, Dean M, Carrington M, et al. Progression to AIDS response. *Science*, 1998; 280:1821.
120. Teglas JP, N'Go N, Burgard M, et al. CCR2B-64I chemokine receptor allele and mother-to-child HIV-1 transmission or disease progression in children. *J Acquir Immune Defic Syndr*, 1999;22:267–271.
121. Mummidi S, Ahuja SS, McDaniel BL, et al. Multiple transcripts with 5′end heterogeneity, dual promoter usage, and evidence for polymorphisms within the regulatory regions and noncoding exons. *J Biol Chem*, 1997;272:30662–30671.
122. Carrington M, Dean M, Martin MP, et al. Genetics of HIV-1 infection: Chemokine receptor CCR5 polymorphism and its consequences. *Hum Mol Genet*, 1999;8:1939–1945.
123. Kostrikis LG, Neumann AU, Thomson B, et al. A polymorphism in the regulatory region of the CC-chemokine receptor 5 gene influences perinatal transmission of human immunodeficiency virus type 1 to African-American infants. *J Virol*, 1999; 73:10264–10271.
124. Van Rij RP, Broersen S, Goudsmit J, et al. The role of a stromal cell-derived factor-1 chemokine gene variant in the clinical course of HIV-1 infection. *AIDS*, 1998;12:F85–F90.
125. John GC, Rousseau C, Dong T, et al. Maternal SDF1 3′A polymorphism is associated with increased perinatal human immunodeficiency virus type 1 transmission. *J Virol*, 2000;74:5736–5739.
126. Al Sharif F, Ollier WE, Hajeer AH. A rare polymorphism at position -28 in the human RANTES promoter. *Eur J Immunogenet*, 1999;26:373–374.
127. Hajeer AH, al Sharif F, Ollier WE. A polymorphism at position -403 in the human RANTES promoter. *Eur J Immunogenet*, 1999;26:375–376.
128. Nickel RG, Casolaro V, Wahn U, et al. Atopic dermatitis is associated with a functional mutation in the promoter of the C-C chemokine RANTES. *J Immunol*, 2000;164:1612–1616.
129. Fiorentino DF, Zlotnik A, Mosmann TR, et al. IL-10 inhibits cytokine production by activated macrophages. *J Immunol*, 1991;147:3815–3822.
130. Fiorentino DF, Zlotnik A, Vieira P, et al. IL-10 acts on the antigen-presenting cell to inhibit cytokine production by Th1 cells. *J Immunol*, 1991;146: 3444–3451.
131. Fiorentino DF, Bond MW, Mosmann TR. Two types of mouse T helper cell. IV. Th2 clones secrete a factor that inhibits cytokine production by Th1 clones. *J Exp Med*, 1989;170:2081–2095.
132. Kollmann TR, Pettoello-Mantovani M, Katopodis NF, et al. Inhibition of acute in vivo human immunodeficiency virus infection by human interleukin 10 treatment of SCID mice implanted with human fetal thymus and liver. *Proc Natl Acad Sci, USA*, 1996;93:3126–3131.
133. Schols D, De Clercq E. Human immunodeficiency virus type 1 gp120 induces anergy in human peripheral blood lymphocytes by inducing interleukin-10 production. *J Virol*, 1996;70: 4953–4960.
134. Turner DM, Williams DM, Sankaran D, et al. An investigation of polymorphism in the interleukin-10 gene promoter. *Eur J Immunogenet*, 1997; 24:1–8.
135. Crawley E, Kay R, Sillibourne J, et al. Polymorphic haplotypes of the interleukin-10 5′ flanking region determine variable interleukin-10 transcription and are associated with particular phenotypes of juvenile rheumatoid arthritis. *Arthritis Rheum*, 1999;42:1101–1108.
136. Gibson AW, Edberg JC, Wu J, et al. Novel single nucleotide polymorphisms in the distal IL-10 promoter affect IL-10 production and enhance the risk of systemic lupus erythematosus. *J Immunol*, 2001;166:3915–3922.
137. Lalani I, Bhol K, Ahmed AR. Interleukin-10: biology, role in inflammation and autoimmunity. *Ann Allergy Asthma Immunol*, 1997;79:469–483.
138. Lee MS, Mueller R, Wicker LS, et al. IL-10 is necessary and sufficient for autoimmune diabetes in conjunction with NOD MHC homozygosity. *J Exp Med*, 1996;183:2663–2668.

139. Llorente L, Zou W, Levy Y, et al. Role of interleukin 10 in the B lymphocyte hyperactivity and autoantibody production of human systemic lupus erythematosus. *J Exp Med*, 1995;181,:839–844.
140. Zinkernagel RM, Dunlop MB, Doherty PC. Cytotoxic T cell activity is strain-specific in outbred mice infected with lymphocytic choriomeningitis virus. *J Immunol*, 1975;115:1613–1616.
141. Zinkernagel RM, Doherty PC. Virus-immune cytotoxic T cells are sentized to by virus specifically altered structures coded for in H-2K or H-2D: a biological role for major histocompatibility antigens. *Adv Exp Med Biol*, 1976;66:387–389.
142. Hill AV. The immunogenetics of human infectious diseases. *Annu Rev Immunol*, 1998;16:593–617.
143. Just JJ. Genetic predisposition to HIV-1 infection and acquired immune deficiency virus syndrome: a review of the literature examining associations with HLA. *Hum Immunol*, 1995;44:156–169.
144. Kaslow RA, Carrington M, Apple R, et al. Influence of combinations of human major histocompatibility complex genes on the course of HIV-1 infection. *Nat Med*, 1996;2:405–411.
145. Gao X, Nelson GW, Karacki P, et al. Effect of a single amino acid substitution in MHC class I molecules on the rate of progression to AIDS. *N Engl J Med*, 2001;344:1668–1675.
146. Hughes, A, Yeager, M. Natural selection at major histocompatibility complex loci vertebrates. *Annu Rev Genet*, 1999;32:415–435.
147. Rowland-Jones SL, Dong T, Dorrell L, et al. Broadly cross-reactive HIV-specific cytotoxic T-lymphocytes in highly-exposed persistently seronegative donors. *Immunol Lett*, 1999;66:9–14.
148. Rowland-Jones SL, Dong T, Fowke KR, et al. Cytotoxic T cell responses to multiple conserved HIV epitopes in HIV-resistant prostitutes in Nairobi. *J Clin Invest*, 1998;102:1758–1765.
149. MacDonald KS, Fowke KR, Kimani J, et al. Influence of HLA supertypes on susceptibility and resistance to human immunodeficiency virus type 1 infection. *J Infect Dis*, 2000;181:1581–1589.
150. MacDonald KS, Embree JE, Nagelkerke NJ, et al. The HLA A2/6802 supertype is associated with reduced risk of perinatal human immunodeficiency virus type 1 transmission. *J Infect Dis*, 2001;183:503–506.
151. Plummer FA, Simonsen JN, Cameron DW, et al. Cofactors in male-female sexual transmission of human immunodeficiency virus type 1. *J Infect Dis*, 1991;163:233–239.
152. Eskild A, Jonassen TO, Heger B, et al. The estimated impact of the CCR-5 delta32 gene deletion on HIV disease progression varies with study design. *AIDS*, 1998;12:2271–2274.
153. Smith MW, Dean M, Carrington M, et al. CCR5-delta 32 gene deletion in HIV-1 infected patients. *Lancet*, 1997;350:741.

5

Biology of Human Immunodeficiency Virus Type 2 (HIV-2)

*Phyllis J. Kanki, *Jean-Louis Sankalé, and †Souleymane Mboup

*Department of Immunology and Infectious Diseases, Harvard School of Public Health, Harvard AIDS Institute, Boston, Massachusetts 02115, USA.
†Department of Bacteriology and Virology, Cheikh Anta Diop University, Dakar, Senegal.

Human immunodeficiency virus type 2 (HIV-2) is the second immunodeficiency virus in the class of human retroviruses. Currently, it is known to be the virus most closely related to the prototype AIDS-causing virus, HIV-1. HIV-2 was discovered because of its close serologic and antigenic relationship to simian immunodeficiency virus (SIV), in addition to its weak cross-reactivity with HIV-1 antigens (1). Most HIV-2 isolates are virtually indistinguishable from the SIVs isolated from species of nonhuman primates such as mangabeys and macaques, indicating that some SIVs and most HIV-2s are essentially the same virus (2,3). In vivo, this relationship is substantiated by evidence of HIV-2's ability to infect and replicate in monkeys (4,5). By contrast, HIV-1 readily infects chimpanzees and gibbon apes, (6–9) but not most other monkey species.

Early evidence of HIV-2's similarities to SIV and cross-reactivity to HIV-1 was found in data from analyses of serum samples gathered in the mid-1980s from female commercial sex workers in West Africa (1,10,11). When these samples were screened for antibodies to HIV-1 antigens, they showed extensive cross-reactivity for HIV-1's core antigens but minimal antibody-binding reactivity for viral envelope proteins (1). Yet, when the same sera samples were assayed against SIV antigens, they reacted strongly with SIV's envelope proteins as well as its core antigens, suggesting infection with a virus that was more closely related to SIV than to HIV-1.

HIV-2, however, does share many virologic and biologic features with HIV-1. HIV-2 and HIV-1 are transmitted by the same routes, infect the same cells, and exhibit considerable genetic variation in their respective outer envelope gene. Like other retroviruses, both HIVs induce lifelong infection with permanent integration of viral genetic material into host cell DNA. Despite these similarities, research studies conducted in the laboratory and with people infected with HIV-2 have highlighted distinct biologic differences between these related viruses (12–14). Compared with HIV-1, HIV-2 has a discrete global distribution with limited spread, significantly lower rates of perinatal and sexual transmission, slower rates of progression to AIDS and, among those infected with it, a potentially protective effect against subsequent HIV-1 infection (14). Although a complete review of all aspects of HIV-2 infection are beyond the scope of this chapter, we have

TABLE 1. Characteristics of HIV-2 Compared to HIV-1

Characteristic	HIV-2	HIV-1	Magnitude difference (x-fold)
Evolutionary age	Older	Early 1900s	Unknown
Geographic distribution	West Africa, former colonial ties	Worldwide	
Age-specific prevalence	Older		
Vertical transmission	Lower		10–20
Heterosexual transmission	Lower		2–9
Induction of immunity	Robust	Variable	
Proviral load	Similar	Similar	
Plasma viral load	Lower		30–40
Genetic diversity	Lower		5–10
Time to AIDS	20–30 yrs	6–8 yrs	2–4

chosen to highlight some of the biologic aspects of HIV-2 that are interesting when compared with those of HIV-1 (Table 1). Based on our current understanding, the distinct biologic differences between these related viruses suggest that viral rather than host determinants may be responsible for the pathogenic mechanisms employed by HIV viruses. It is hoped that further characterization of such determinants will be useful in the design of effective HIV interventions.

GENETIC PEDIGREE OF HIV-2

It has been estimated that the HIV-1 and HIV-2/SIV groups of viruses may have diverged genetically from each other 50 or 60 years ago (15,16). The SIVs of mangabeys and macaques are the closest relatives of HIV-2s (2,3,17). As a group, the SIVs vary more between different species and subspecies of monkey than the different HIV subtypes vary from each other (2,17–19) (Figure 1). Because the HIV-2s appear to be found primarily in West Africa, it is not surprising that they are most closely related to SIVs originating from monkeys in that region (2,3,17). The only exception may be the macaque SIV, which is also closely related to both HIV-2 and mangabey SIV (*Cercocebus atys*). Because SIVs have never been observed in wild Asian monkeys, such as macaques, it appears likely that infection of this species occurred accidentally during captivity with African monkeys originating from West Africa (2).

Forty to forty-five percent of the nucleotide sequence of the HIV-2 genome is related to HIV-1 (20). The degree of antigenic relatedness of both SIV and HIV-2 to the prototype HIV-1 prompted the discovery and further classification of these related viruses (1,21,22). Similar to the variability found in strains of HIV-1, restriction site polymorphism and sequence data also indicate significant genetic variability among HIV-2 strains (20,23). As more sequence data on various HIV-2 and SIV strains have become available, it has become apparent that no branching order of divergence can be specified and that these viral types may in fact share a common ancestor (3,24).

The genetic diversity of HIV-2 is less extensive than that found for HIV-1. Only two of its subtypes (A and B) have been well characterized. Some studies have reported the existence of four other subtypes (C, D, E, and F) but attempts to isolate these subtypes or to obtain additional samples of them for sequencing have been unsuccessful (25). An unusual HIV-2 isolate, Abt96, found in a blood sample drawn from an asymptomatic individual from Côte d'Ivoire has been

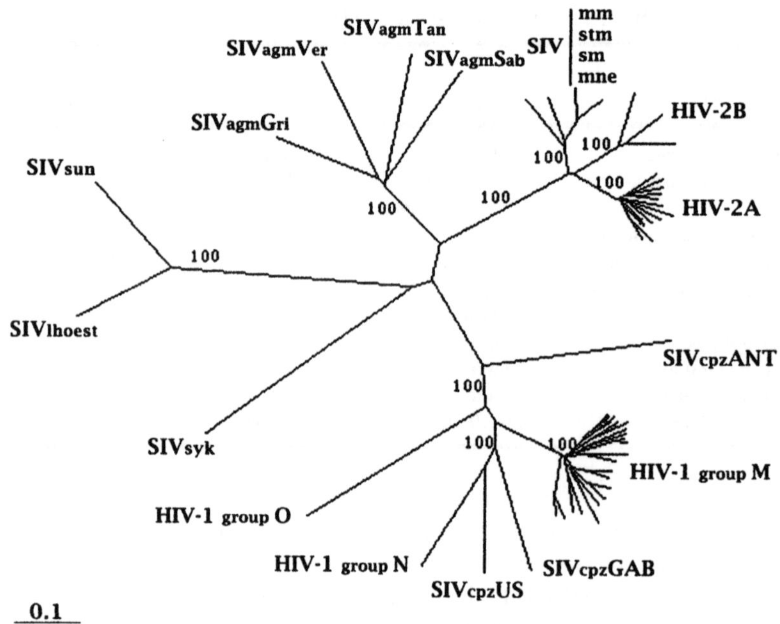

FIGURE 1. Phylogenetic tree of viruses representative of HIV-2, HIV-1, and SIV.

sequenced and its phylogenetic data suggest a novel HIV-2 subtype, preliminarily designated as G (26).

Thus far, A is the most characterized subtype of HIV-2 and appears to be the major strain circulating in West Africa (27–31). Subtype B isolates from individuals in Ghana (32,33) are thought to be most distant from the prototype HIV-2/mangabey/macaque virus (2). Only data from a recent study from Côte d'Ivoire suggest that HIV-2B is predominant in this country (34). Similar to the situation with HIV-1 subtypes, the potential effect of subtype differences on the epidemiology, pathogenicity, and transmissibility of HIV-2 is not yet well appreciated.

EPIDEMIOLOGY AND GLOBAL DISTRIBUTION

The isolation of HIV-2 led to fears that a second AIDS epidemic would occur, similar in scope and magnitude to that caused by HIV-1. However, the specific biologic properties of HIV-2—namely its comparatively lower transmissibility through both sexual and vertical routes—contributed to its more regionalized, ultimately endemic, distribution. Studies conducted in the late 1980s and early 1990s found significant rates of HIV-2 in a number of West African countries, but only low to absent rates of HIV-1 in these nations (35,36). In the late 1980s in West African countries such as Guinea Bissau, Gambia, Cape Verde, and Senegal, the prevalence of HIV-2 infection exceeded that of infection with HIV-1. However, HIV-1 infection rates in these countries have increased and now exceed such rates for HIV-2 (35,37–39). Rates of HIV-2 infection are highest in sexually active populations such as commercial sex workers, sexually transmitted disease (STD) patients, incarcerated individuals, or people hospitalized with other infectious diseases (35,38,40–42). Such risk groups usually have seroprevalence rates that are 5- to 10-fold higher than those of lower risk populations, usually represented by blood donors and pregnant women.

In 1985, the discovery of HIV-2 in West Africa prompted numerous serologic studies to determine its geographic distribution. Since that time, significant HIV-2 infection has been well documented in most West African countries, showing a distinctly different worldwide distribution than that of HIV-1 (14). It has been difficult to compare the prevalence rates of HIV-2 and HIV-1 owing to differences in study design, diagnostic methodologies, and HIV-2's comparatively low prevalence rates. Often, serosurveys were conducted using methods that failed to distinguish HIV-1 from HIV-2, resulting in erroneous reports of type-specific prevalence rates, or erroneous diagnoses of dual infections (HIV-1 and HIV-2), circumstances that may reflect a lack of HIV specificity in the serologic or nucleic acid-based assays used.

In other countries of West Africa—Burkina Faso, Ghana, Côte d'Ivoire, Nigeria, and Mali—infection rates for HIV-1 range from 3- to 24-fold higher than those for HIV-2 (14,42–46). For example, in a study conducted in Bamako, Mali, in the late 1990s, 3.9% of 176 commercial sex workers were infected with HIV-2 compared with 20.45% infected with HIV-1. Comparison of HIV-1 and HIV-2 seroprevalence data with earlier data from Mali showed a significant increase in HIV-1 prevalence and a significant decrease in HIV-2 prevalence, confirming similar trends observed in studies conducted in neighboring countries (30).

The existence of significant rates of HIV-1 and HIV-2 in many countries of West Africa raises the question of what will happen once these viruses interact at a population level. Anderson and May analyzed the available biologic and epidemiologic data on the pathogenicity, transmissibility, and antigenic similarity of HIV-1 and HIV-2 and used simple mathematical models to study the competition between the two viral types. Their model of concomitant transmission of the two viruses within the same sexually active population indicated a positive association between pathogenicity and reproductive success, suggesting that HIV-1 would competitively displace HIV-2 in the longer term (47).

This analysis is supported by comparison studies of the rates of sexual and perinatal transmission of the two viruses, as well as by temporal trends showing a decrease in HIV-2

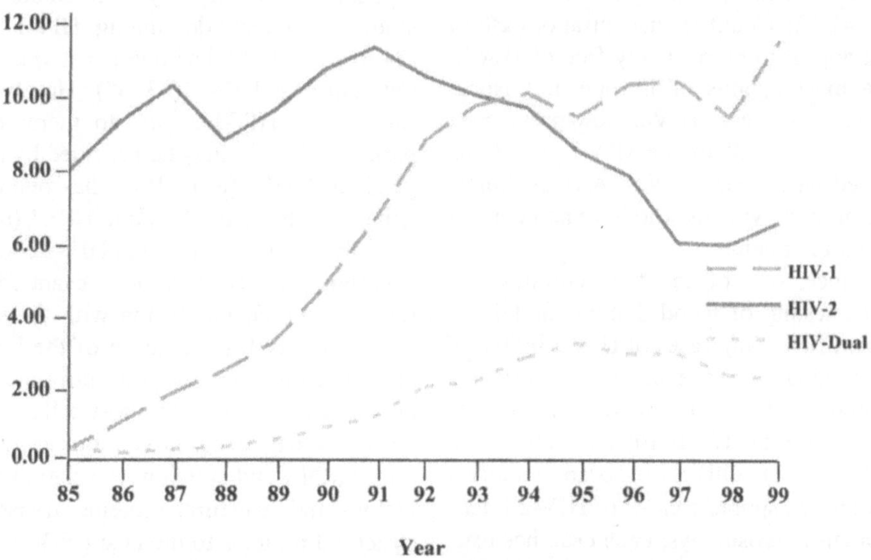

FIGURE 2. HIV prevalence in registered female sex workers in Dakar, Senegal.

prevalence throughout the region (48–51). Thus, current data suggest that HIV-2 has been present in certain populations long enough to have established endemic infection and that its spread outside of these endemic areas has been limited by its low transmission potential. It therefore seems unlikely that this virus will cause a global epidemic similar to that being caused by HIV-1.

A second epidemiologic pattern of HIV-2 infection has been suggested from reports of HIV-2 in Portugal and in areas with previous ties to Portugal—Mozambique, Angola, southwestern India, and Brazil (52–55)—where resident populations appear to have low but stable rates of HIV-2 infection (42,53,54). HIV-2 has been detected in the large cities of southwestern India, perhaps related to exchange with the former Portuguese colonies of Africa (55). Studies in Goa, a former Portuguese colony situated south of Bombay on the western coast of India, have reported a 4.9% infection rate of HIV-2 and a 9.8% infection rate of HIV-1 among patients with STDs (56). In contrast, significant HIV-2 infection has yet to be reported in other parts of Asia.

Geographically, the distribution of HIV-2 seems to be independent of that for HIV-1 (14,35,42,52). Countries in central or eastern Africa appear to be relatively free of HIV-2, as are most regions of Europe and North America. In these HIV-2 low-prevalence regions, almost all of the HIV-2 infections observed have been in West African immigrants or in individuals who have had contact with West Africans.

France, one of the first countries to institute testing of blood donors for HIV-2, has identified many cases of HIV-2 infection (57). Of 75 HIV-2–infected persons followed in a study in Paris, 58 individuals were of African origin, 12 European, and five Caribbean (58). Other European countries have reported sporadic cases of HIV-2 infection in large serosurveys; each case has usually had a link to West Africa (43,52,59). The first cases of HIV-2 infection in Spain were identified in 1988, in three African immigrants living in Barcelona. By 1999, 92 cases had been reported (60). For 22 individuals of this group of 92, HIV-2 subtyping was performed on their proviral DNA. Results showed 16 were infected with HIV-2: eight Spanish-born and eight African immigrants. The remaining six were infected with HIV-2B: two Spanish born and four African immigrants from Equatorial Guinea (60).

LIFE CYCLE OF HIV-2

The various subtypes of HIV-2 are morphologically similar to the subtypes of HIV-1. The virions are spherical with diameters between 100–120 nanometers (nm). The length of the HIV-2 genome is about 9 kilobases (kb), similar to that of HIV-1. The open reading frames of HIV-2 are also similar to those of HIV-1 (Figure 3). For different strains of HIV-1, HIV-2, and SIV, genes may be in different reading frames, but the level of conservation within each gene remains high. The *gag* and *pol* messages are unspliced, the *env* is singly spliced, and the major regulatory genes are doubly spliced. The regulatory gene sequences appear to vary more among HIV-2 strains than they do among HIV-1 strains (24,61,62). HIV-1 has one gene, *vpu*, that is not found in HIV-2 (63–65). However, the function of HIV-1's *vpu*—to increase viral particle release—may be provided by the *env* gene for HIV-2 (66). HIV-2 has one unique gene, *vpx*, that is not found in HIV-1 (67–70).

The replication cycle of HIV-2 comprises adsorption to CD4 and the relevant coreceptor with subsequent fusion with the surface of the host cell, penetration of the host cell and uncoating, reverse transcription, transport of viral DNA to the host cell's nucleus, chromosomal integration, transcription of viral mRNA and splicing, translation of regulatory and structural proteins, transport of structural proteins to the host cell's cytoplasmic membrane for viral assembly, and budding, maturation, and release of new virions.

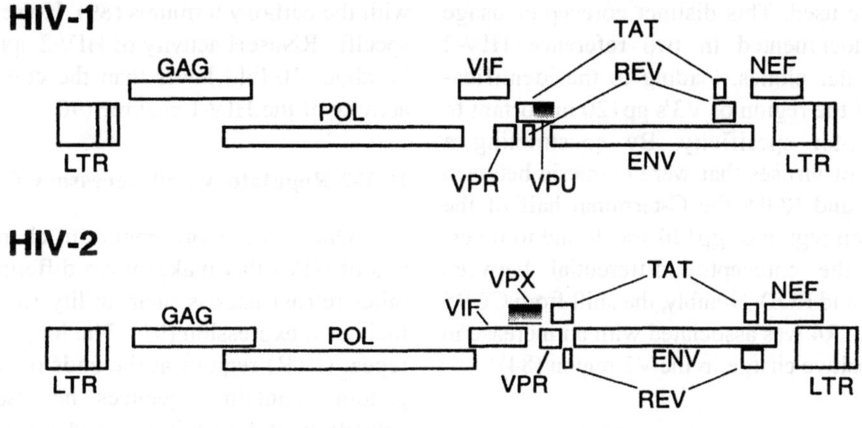

FIGURE 3. Genomic structures of HIV-1 and HIV-2.

Receptors and Coreceptors

HIV-2 infects the same types of cells that HIV-1 infects: CD4-bearing helper lymphocytes, monocytes, macrophages, and microglia cells in the central nervous system. Although HIV-2 uses the same CD4 receptor for infection of the host cell, it apparently does so with a 10- to 100-fold lower affinity than HIV-1 (71–73). Although the HIV-2 envelope protein (Env) appears to be slightly less glycosylated than the same protein for HIV-1, this difference does not appear to account for the difference in binding efficiencies (73). It is believed that HIV-2 infection is inhibited more efficiently by soluble CD4 than is HIV-1 infection (74).

Several members of the chemokine-receptor family have been shown to function in association with CD4 to facilitate HIV-1's entry and infection of various types of cells (74–76). Similar to HIV-1, certain strains of HIV-2 have been shown to use fusin/CXCR4 as both a coreceptor (in the presence of CD4) and as an alternative receptor (in the absence of CD4) (75,77). HIV-2 viruses appear to be more promiscuous than HIV-1 viruses in their use of coreceptors, successfully using CXCR4, CCR5, and the coreceptors designated BONZO/STRL33 and BOB/GPR15 (75,77,78). Most HIV-2 isolates that used CCR5 were nonsyncytium-inducing viruses, whereas isolates that used multiple coreceptors were syncytium-inducing viruses. However, the efficiency at which various HIV-2 isolates use coreceptors appeared to vary widely (79).

A number of in-vitro studies of HIV-2 isolates have described differences in the cytopathicity of HIV-2 and HIV-1 (80–83). Compared with isolates of HIV-1, HIV-2 isolates demonstrate lower rates of cell killing, less syncytial cell formation, lower rates of viral replication, and differences in interaction with CD4, the latter of which is related to the clinical stage of the HIV-2–infected individual (83).

The V3 loop (envelope) of rapid–high HIV-2 isolates, those that induce syncytium formation and cause a high load of virus in blood and blood cells, differs significantly from slow–low isolates, those that do not induce syncytia and cause only low loads of virus in blood and blood cells, in that its sequence is more heterogeneous and has a higher net charge. Mutations to positively charged amino acids at positions 313 and 314 have been significantly associated with the rapid/high phenotype, similar to that found for HIV-1 (83). Such amino acid changes in the V3 loop of HIV-2 also appear to determine whether coreceptor CXCR4 or CCR5 will be used. This distinct coreceptor usage was documented in two reference HIV-2 molecular clones, leading to the identification of the region of V3's gp120 important to coreceptor specificity. By constructing a series of viruses that were chimeric between GH-1 and ROD, the C-terminal half of the V3 loop region of gp120 was found to determine the coreceptor differential between GH-1 and ROD. Notably, the shift from CCR5 to CXCR4 was associated with an increase in net positive charge in the V3 region (84).

HIV-2 Polymerase Gene (POL)

The HIV *pol* encodes three proteins: protease (PR); reverse transcriptase (RT), which also has RNaseH activity; and endonuclease/integrase (IN). The HIV-2 protease, as expressed in yeast, has been shown to be efficient at hydrolyzing HIV-1 peptide junctions (85). This suggests that the substrate specificities of both viral proteins are analogous.

The RT/RNaseH molecule of HIV-2 is similar in size to HIV-1's RT and is serologically cross-reactive with human antibodies (86). The HIV-2 *pol* appears to be as error prone as that of HIV-1 (87). In studies of the fidelity of misinsertion and mispair extension exhibited by RT mutants resistant to nucleoside analogs, the Val74 mutant of HIV-1's RT has been shown to display a substantially enhanced fidelity, whereas the comparable RT mutant of HIV-2 has exhibited a fidelity similar to that of wild-type RT. Depending on the assay employed and the DNA sequences extended, most other mutants of HIV-2 RT displayed moderate effects on the enzyme, leading to mild increases in fidelity of DNA synthesis. These data imply a more complex and less distinctive correlation between drug resistance, misinsertion, and mispair extension in HIV-2's RT than in HIV-1's RT, providing evidence for potential biochemical differences between these two related RTs (88).

As for other retroviral RTs, the DNA polymerase is associated with the amino terminus of the molecule and RNaseH is associated with the carboxy terminus (89). However, the specific RNaseH activity of HIV-2 appears to be about 10-fold lower than the comparable activity of the HIV-1 enzyme (90).

HIV-2 Regulatory and Accessory Genes

One of the more important characteristics of HIVs that makes them different from other retroviruses is their ability to regulate their own expression (91). The long terminal repeat (LTR) regions at the ends of the viral genome contain sequences necessary for activation of transcription and for termination of the transcripts, but an important element of control for these viruses occurs through RNA processing or splicing. The 5′ LTR is the initiation region for transcription, which terminates at the 3′ LTR (92). The expression of HIVs can be activated by cellular transcription factors, such as NF-kappa B (NF-κB) and T-cell mitogens, that bind to the LTR. The LTR of HIV-1 is more responsive to cellular activation signals than HIV-2 LTR, and HIV-2 has different response elements (93,94). Whereas HIV-1 has two NF-κB enhancer binding sites, only one can be identified for HIV-2 or most SIVs (95). This may be of biologic significance; studies of two different strains of SIV having dramatic differences in virulence in vivo have demonstrated that duplication of the NF-κB binding sites occurs in the more virulent strain (96).

For HIV-1, the NF-κB transcription factor may be sufficient for inducible transcriptional activation (97). For HIV-2, additional factors are necessary (93,94,98). One that appears to bind to purine-rich motifs in the HIV-2 enhancer is Elf1, a transcription factor related to the *ets* cellular oncogene, and a novel peri-*ets* (pets) site (99). Studies also indicate that activation of the HIV-2 enhancer may require four or more *cis*-acting elements, most of which are not in HIV-1 (100). Such differences in sensitivity to cellular transcription factors may correlate with differences in viral load and cell tropism at the host level. Combined with the lower CD4 affinity seen with HIV-2's gp120, these differences may also help explain why HIV-2–infected individuals apparently have lower levels of virus than individuals infected with HIV-1 (101).

The *tat* and *rev* products, both made from doubly spliced messages, are the most important viral regulators of transcription (92). Tat is a 16-kDa protein that acts early in viral infection to enhance expression of regulatory genes. *Rev* expression occurs later and acts to enhance expression of structural genes. When Tat binds to a *tat* response element (TAR) in viral RNA, it can increase mRNA expression and protein synthesis more than 100-fold (91). For HIV-2, *tat* transactivation may be more complex than for HIV-1. HIV-2 appears to have two stem-loop TAR structures, whereas HIV-1 has only one (102). The *tat* of HIV-1 (*tat*-1) has a high degree of homology with the *tat* of HIV-2 (*tat*-2). However, *tat*-1 activates the LTRs of HIV-1 TAR (TAR-1) and HIV-2 TAR (TAR-2) equally, while *tat-2* activates TAR-1 less efficiently (103).

Rev is a 19-kDa protein that acts to increase transcription of RNA for *gag*, *pol*, *env*, *vif*, and *vpr* and to transport the messages for these genes out of the nucleus (104–106). Rev acts through a *rev* response element (RRE) stem-loop structure in the envelope open reading frame (104,107). The *rev* of HIV-2 appears to act similarly, although it appears to be less phosphorylated (108). Although HIV-1's *rev* functions on both the HIV-1 RRE and the HIV-2 RRE, HIV-2's *rev* functions only on RRE of HIV-2 (109,110). It has been hypothesized that the low level of function for HIV-2 *rev* on HIV-1 RRE may be because HIV-2's *rev* is inhibited from polymerization after binding the HIV-1 RRE (111).

TAR decoys have been developed for use in gene therapy for people infected with HIV-1. When a TAR RNA decoy is overexpressed, it binds Tat, thus leaving less of this crucial protein to bind to and activate the natural transcriptional promoter of HIV. Recent work developing an HIV-2 TAR decoy has demonstrated potent inhibition of both HIV-2 and HIV-1 gene expression, suggesting that the HIV-2 TAR decoy may prove useful for combating HIV-1 infection (112).

The *nef* product is a 27-kDa myristoylated protein that is highly cross-reactive between HIV-1 and HIV-2 (113,114). Genetic analysis of the *nef* of HIV-infected individuals has shown a correlation between *nef* truncation and long-term nonprogression. In a study in which proviral *nef* sequences from 60 HIV-2–infected persons were amplified from peripheral blood lymphocytes and *nef* open-reading frames were screened for the presence of full-length (32- to 36-kDa) or truncated (<32 kDa) Nef, six (10%) of the 60 persons had truncated Nef. Of these six, five were among the 36 asymptomatic individuals (13.9%) in the study, and only one was among the 24 symptomatic subjects (4.2%; $p=0.23$) (115). These results indicate that the strains of HIV-2 infecting these individuals contain defective *nef* genes but fail to demonstrate a significant association of *nef* truncation with disease status.

The *vif* gene encodes a 23-kDa protein (116). It was initially thought to enhance the spread of free virus (117), but more recent studies suggest a role in cellular tropism and viral core stability (118,119). The two remaining genes, *vpr* (found in HIV-1, HIV-2, and SIVs) and *vpx* (found in HIV-2 and SIVs), are related to each other, perhaps demonstrating an ancient evolutionary relationship (120). Studies show that *vpr* encodes a protein of about 13 kDa (121–123) and *vpx* a protein of about 12 kDa (68,69). Both proteins are packaged in virus particles (69, 121–123). Vpr is thought to enhance growth of HIV-2 in macrophages (124) and to inhibit the progression of infected cells from the G2 phase to the M phase of the cell cycle (125,126).

The observation that Vpx is packaged in amounts equimolar to Gag has been used to argue that it is essential to HIV-2 (69) with studies finding 2,000 to 3,000 copies of Vpx per virus particle with a half-life of

36 hours (127). However, Vpx appears to be dispensable; its absence has negligible effects on established T-cell lines (128–130). Vpx mutants grow poorly, however, in fresh lymphocytes, showing a reduction of 10-fold or more in early DNA synthesis (128,129, 131,132).

A significant proportion of people infected with HIV-2 produce antibodies to Vpx (68,133). When present, these antibodies can be used to discriminate between infection with HIV-2 or HIV-1. It has also been suggested that anti-Vpx antibodies may be predictive of a more rapid disease course in HIV-2 infection, based on longitudinal cohort studies (133). A minority of people infected with HIV-2 also make antibodies to Vpr (Ndung'u et al.: unpublished data, 123). The relevance of this observation to the function of these genes in HIV-2 is still not known.

HIV-2 Structural Genes: *gag* and *env*

The products of *gag* are essentially the same for HIV-1 and HIV-2 (134) and are highly conserved. A 55-kDa precursor is myristoylated and cleaved by the viral protease to form the matrix protein, p17 (MA); the capsid protein, p24 (CA); p2; the nucleocapsid protein, p7 (NC); p1; and p6. MA is at the amino terminus and, in its cleaved form, surrounds the nucleocapsid. CA is slightly larger for HIV-2 or SIV and is sometimes described as p26/p27 (1,135). It provides the structure for the core that contains the genome and the polymerase and integrase enzymes (92). Researchers have identified NC (p7-8) as a nucleic acid binding protein (136), and both zinc finger motifs are involved with the specificity of packaging the genomic viral RNA into the virions (137).

Compared with HIV-1, HIV-2's envelope glycoprotein precursor is slightly smaller, as are its external glycoprotein and transmembrane protein. Although usually described using the terminology for HIV-1 (gp160, gp120, and gp41, respectively), the HIV-2 glycoproteins are sometimes designated with lower sizes (that is, gp140–145, gp105–110, and gp32–40 respectively). Analyses of the primary amino acid sequences for the N-linked glycosylation sites of HIV-2 and SIV gp120s show significantly fewer conserved sites than for HIV-1. This could account for the lower molecular weight of HIV-2's gp120, since carbohydrates make up 50% or more of HIV-1's gp120 (138–140).

HIV-2 envelope sequences vary to approximately the same degree as HIV-1 envelope sequences (23,61,67,141–146). Although the V3 regions correspond in both viral types, HIV-2 does not have the conserved glycine-proline-glycine-arginine amino acid sequence at the tip of the V3 loop (23,67). External glycosylation sites appear to be conserved between HIV-1 and HIV-2 as are the sites for CD4 binding (20,24), precursor processing (147), fusion (147), principal neutralizing domain at V3 (23,148,149) cytolytic T-cell activity (150,151), and, perhaps, antibody-dependent cell cytotoxicity (149,152,153). With HIV-1, much of the envelope glycoprotein appears to generate binding antibodies. Antibodies from individuals infected with HIV-2 show binding activity concentrated in the middle of gp120, including the V3 loop (154,155), as well as in the amino terminus of the transmembrane protein (154,156). Another region, at the carboxy terminus of gp120, may be slightly less immunogenic, but it appears to be the most cross-reactive between HIV-1 and HIV-2 (156).

The most type-specific region of HIV-2's gp120, the V3 loop region, is also the principal neutralizing domain, as it is for HIV-1 (23,148,149). Two distinct antigenic sites in the V3 region of HIV-2 appear to correspond to the principal neutralizing determinant of HIV-1. Based on computer simulation modeling, the conserved phenylalanine-histidine-serine-glutamine and tryptophan-cysteine-arginine motifs (positions 315–318 and 329–331) may interact to form a discontinuous antigenic site (157). However, other neutralizing regions of lower activity have been described, including a linear epitope in V2 and one conformational epitope outside V1, V2, and V3 (149,158). Some investigators have described cross-neutralization between HIV-1 and HIV-2 with human antibodies (159,160). Although weakly bidirectional, they appear stronger for sera from HIV-2–infected people for cross-neutralization of HIV-1 (159,160).

Although the fusion domains for syncytia induction have been mapped to the hydro-phobic amino terminus of the transmembrane protein, loss of syncytium-inducing ability does not appear to have much of an effect on the infectivity of HIV-2 (147). Both HIV-1 and HIV-2 have a long cytoplasmic domain on the transmembrane protein. This often becomes truncated, at least when the virus is cultured in T-cell lines. Even small truncations of this sort appear to enhance fusion activity (81,161). It is unclear whether this has any importance in vivo.

HIV-2 DIAGNOSIS

Studies of HIV-2 epidemiology and natural history depend on accurate HIV-2 diagnoses. The same procedures for serologic testing, virus culture, and polymerase chain reaction (PCR) diagnostics that were developed for HIV-1 have been modified for HIV-2 diagnosis and have been improved through the years. The close relationship of HIV-2 and HIV-1 on genetic and antigenic levels has necessitated the development and implementation of type-specific diagnostic assays. Because most such tests were developed for HIV-1 using HIV-1 antigens, the degree of cross-reactivity and specificity for HIV-2 was variable. Most of the first generation tests used whole virus antigens, where core antigens such as p24 and *pol*'s p66/p51 are well represented. These antigens are more strongly cross-reactive than envelope antigens, especially gp120 (1,35,162,163).

Following the lead of many European nations, the United States instituted screening for HIV-2 in blood banks in 1990. As a result, the majority of commercial HIV enzyme-linked immunosorbent assays (ELISAs) use a combined antigen source that includes HIV-2–specific antigens. Confirmation of HIV-2 serostatus requires HIV-2–specific immunoblot assay or specific peptide assays. Immunoblots that recognize a profile of major structural gene products are typically used to confirm HIV-1 and HIV-2 diagnosis using standard criteria. HIV-2–specific diagnosis by immunoblot requires antibody reactivity to Env ± Gag ± Pol antigens. In the absence of reactivity to Gag or Pol antigens, the presence of reactivity to two envelope antigens is required (gp120 and gp32, the transmembrane protein) (164).

Various investigations have focused on identifying type-specific antigens to allow confirmatory tests that will distinguish between HIV-1 and HIV-2. Most have been made as synthetic peptides (165–168), but some have been made as larger bacterially expressed peptides (169,170). These antigens vary in sensitivity and specificity. Because most are selected for specificity, it might seem that sensitivity would be compromised. Thus, although appropriate for type-specific confirmation, they may not be as useful as larger HIV-2–specific antigens for initial screening.

For HIV investigators working in Africa where HIV-1 and HIV-2 infections are prevalent, it has been critical to identify cost-efficient, alternative, antibody-testing strategies for screening, confirmation, and discrimination of HIV-1 and HIV-2 infections. These strategies have included rapid simple tests (RSTs) as well as ELISAs. In a study of 1,110 consecutive sera from individuals in Bissau, Guinea Bissau, 198 (17.8%) were found to be seropositive for HIV: 52 (4.7%) for HIV-1, 120 (10.8%) for HIV-2, and 26 (2.3%) dually reactive for HIV-1 and HIV-2. Western blot analysis was used to confirm the reactivity of the specimens. The sensitivity of each assay was 100%. The specificity of each screening assay at initial testing was 98.0% for Enzygnost and 99.8% for Capillus. The various combinations of two or three assays showed specificities of 99.2% to 100%. Serodiagnostic strategies for HIV can be based on RST alone, and differentiation between HIV-1 and HIV-2 can be achieved as part of these strategies. However, there is considerable variability in the capacity of individual assays to discriminate between HIV-1 and HIV-2, a fact that needs to be considered in the design and interpretation of such data (171).

When serum samples have been tested in places such as Côte d'Ivoire, Senegal, and Burkina Faso, a disproportionately large fraction of the samples tested as "dual positive" because they appeared reactive on both HIV-1 and HIV-2 confirmatory tests (35,38, 170,171). These countries have significant infection rates for both HIV-1 and HIV-2, and a distinction between viruses in designations of dual reactivity remains a diagnostic challenge for the typical HIV laboratory. The HIV dual-antibody profile is characterized by antibodies with strong reactivity to the Env antigens of both HIV-1 and HIV-2 by immunoblot and/or radioimmunoprecipitation analysis (RIPA) (1,163,169,173–175). Several possible biologic explanations for this phenomenon can be entertained including extensive cross-reactivity by either of the HIVs, dual infection, or infection with a recombinant virus.

Isolation of both HIV-1 and HIV-2 has been reported from selected cases of dual reactivity and PCR evidence of both viruses has ranged from 30% to 80%, in serologically defined dual reactives reported from similar populations (176–178). It is unclear whether the low and variable rate of concordance between serology and PCR is the result of extensive HIV-1 cross-reactivity, misclassification of samples based on serodiagnosis, or insensitivity of the PCR assays. Improvement of PCR assays with Southern blot detection of the amplified product has maximized the sensitivity and specificity for HIV-2 provirus detection (179,180). Further development of such assays will be critical to studies that seek to characterize HIV-2 biology and its interaction with HIV-1 in vivo. Largely because of such problems, it has been difficult to predict from the published literature what the interactions of these two distinct HIV-type viruses would be in human populations. It seems clear that reports from Africa and elsewhere of dual infection, in the absence of HIV-2 infection alone, were more likely misinterpreted laboratory data than true biologic entities.

TRANSMISSION OF HIV-2

Although HIV-2, like HIV-1, is transmitted in blood and certain other body fluids, the rate of infection in West Africa appears more stable than that for HIV-1. In Senegal, during an 8-year period, there was a 26-fold increase in HIV-1 infections, while infections of HIV-2 remained relatively constant (48,181). This implies that HIV-2 may have been in the human population in Africa at least as long as HIV-1, and, in West Africa, for considerably longer. The relative lack of significant HIV-2 prevalence in Europe, North America, and Asia in the face of HIV-1 expansion also supports the general observation that HIV-2 is spread less efficiently than HIV-1 (35,47,48,52,182–185,186–188).

Although there have been case reports of HIV-2 transmitted in blood and blood products, widespread HIV testing in blood banks has limited the risk of this mode of transmission (189,190). The most common modes of transmission in HIV-2 endemic areas are perinatal and heterosexual transmission. Because most West African countries have incidence rates for both HIV-1 and HIV-2, direct comparison of transmission rates between the two viruses has been possible. Among female commercial sex workers in Senegal followed over an 11-year period, the incidence of HIV-1 dramatically increased, with a 1.18-fold increase in risk per year and a 13-fold increase in risk over the entire study period. The incidence of HIV-2 remained stable, despite higher HIV-2 prevalence

(48,191). In this high-risk group, the rate of heterosexual transmission of HIV-2 was significantly lower than that of HIV-1, which strongly suggests differences in the infectivity potential of these two related immunodeficiency viruses (48,191). Using mathematical modeling techniques, the efficiency of heterosexual transmission of HIV-2 per sexual act with an infected partner has been estimated to range from five to nine times less than that of HIV-1 (181) This has been recently corroborated using newer methods with fewer assumptions (192).

The sexual transmission of HIV-2, like that of HIV-1, appears to be enhanced by the presence of other sexually transmitted diseases such as chancroid or syphilis (193). In one study, enhanced risk for infection with HIV-2 was also associated with an increase in years of sexual activity, non-Senegalese nationality, and older age (194). Similarly, in a cross-sectional discordant couple study of HIV-2 transmission, older women were more likely to have a seropositive spouse than younger women (195).

Maternal or neonatal transmission of HIV-2 also occurs (196), but it appears to be less efficient than that for HIV-1 (197–199). Prospective studies of perinatal transmission of HIV-2 have been conducted in Guinea Bissau, Côte d'Ivoire, France, and Senegal, each demonstrating extremely low rates of perinatal transmission of HIV-2 (<3.7%) compared with that of HIV-1 (15% to 45% transmission) (49–51,200,201). In studies that measured perinatal transmission of both viruses, the rate of HIV-1 transmission was 10- to 20-fold higher than that of HIV-2.

In a study of HIV-2 and HIV-1 perinatal transmission in the Gambia, the mean antenatal plasma viral load of 94 HIV-1–infected women was 15,100 copies per ml (95% CI, 10,400 to 19,000), much higher than that for 60 randomly selected HIV-2–infected women, which was 410 copies per ml (95% CI, 150 to 910; $p < 0.001$). The estimated transmission rate of HIV-1 was 24.4% (95% CI, 14.6 to 33.9) and that of HIV-2 was 4.0% (95% CI, 1.9 to 7.4). Five of 17 HIV-1–positive babies and three of eight HIV-2–positive babies were infected after 2 months of age, presumably through breast milk. Birth in the rainy season (odds ratio [OR], 2.9; 95% CI, 1.2 to 7.2), a low postnatal $CD4^+$ cell percentage (OR for a 10% drop, 2.4; 95% CI, 1.1 to 5.1), and a high maternal plasma viral load (OR for a 10-fold increase, 2.9; 95% CI, 1.1 to 7.8) were risk factors for transmission that applied equally to both viruses. Low maternal HIV-2 RNA levels, which, on average, were 37-fold lower than for HIV-1 infections, were thought to explain the low rates of mother-to-infant transmission in HIV-2 infections (202).

HIV-2 PATHOGENESIS

During the late 1980s and early 1990s, natural history studies of HIV-1 infection conducted in the developed world provided important data on the pathogenesis of HIV-1 infection in vivo. Although numerous cross-sectional studies of HIV-2 infection were conducted in the late 1980s, they were intrinsically limited in their ability to describe the natural history of HIV-2 infection, an effort that required prospective studies (40). Studies of the natural histories of chronic infections such as HIV are difficult, particularly ones achieving minimal loss to follow-up. Not surprisingly, such studies have been rare in developing countries, where viruses such as HIV-2 can best be studied. Very few studies have assessed the deterioration of the immune system and/or changes in the viral load over time in HIV-2–infected individuals.

In cross-sectional studies, T4 lymphocyte counts and T4 : T8 ratios appear to be decreased in HIV-2–infected individuals, but less dramatically than that found in HIV-1–infected individuals (203–206). Alterations in T-cell subsets evaluated prospectively have shown similar changes, where immunosuppression in individuals infected with HIV-2 occurred at a significantly slower rate than that among individuals infected with HIV-1 and could not be demonstrated in all individuals in the studies (207,208). Skin-test anergy to various antigens is also less pronounced in individuals infected with HIV-2 (203,206).

Degree of immune activation and apoptosis in lymphocytes were compared in healthy West African patients infected with HIV-1 or HIV-2. The lower decline of $CD4^+$ T-cells in individuals infected with HIV-2 compared with those infected with HIV-1 was associated with lower levels of immune activation, evaluated by HLA-DR expression on lymphocytes and serum concentrations of IgG and β_2-microglobulin (205,206,209). Ex-vivo apoptosis was found in both viral infections in all lymphocyte subsets, including $CD4^+$ and $CD8^+$ T-cells, as well as in B cells, but was less in HIV-2 than in HIV-1 (210). These observations support the hypothesis that long-term activation of the immune system, which is weaker in HIV-2 infection, significantly contributes to T-cell apoptosis and disease progression (210). The HIV-2 envelope has also been shown to have an inhibitory effect on T-cell proliferation and on the upregulation of CD40L and OX40, which are costimulatory molecules important in the activation and differentiation of the T-cell response. This effect was accompanied by a decreased level of apoptosis (211).

HIV-2 Replication and Genetic Diversity

It is now well established that new genotypes of HIV-1 evolve over time in an individual after infection. The earliest isolates generally grow in macrophages as well as lymphocytes, these are generally slow–low viruses that do not induce syncytium. As disease develops, viruses with changes in their envelope V3 loop evolve; these are rapid–high viruses that are syncytium inducing (212,213).

The ability of HIV-2 to induce syncytia formation may be less than that for HIV-1 (214). HIV-2 is more difficult to isolate from asymptomatic people than is HIV-1, but, when it is isolated, it appears to show the slow–low pattern (82,215). Similarly, the rapid–high isolates are more likely to be isolated from HIV-2–infected individuals with disease. The determinants of cell tropism and replication capacity for HIV-2 have not yet been mapped. However, a correlation between the number of charged residues in the V3 loop, the nature of the residues at positions 18 and 19 of the V3 loop, and the phenotype of HIV-2 isolates has been described (83,146).

As with HIV-1, the polymerase activity of HIV-2 is error prone, and, as a result, extensive variation occurs between isolates (87). This variation is primarily exhibited in *env* against which much of the selective pressure of the immune system is exerted. This selective pressure results in differences in *env* of as much as 1% per year for evolutionary selection (23,91). Limited studies on the interpatient variability of HIV-2 have shown that the range of variability in the V3 loop sequence is similar to the interpatient variability of HIV-1 (23,27). Tissue-specific quasispecies have been identified in HIV-1 infection in vivo and in an analysis of the viral sequences from the blood and brain of an HIV-2–infected individual (146,216). Evaluation of intrapatient variation in the V3 loop region of HIV-2 in asymptomatic and symptomatic individuals followed over time has shown less variation than that found for a like group of HIV-1–infected individuals (27). This lower intrapatient variation appears to be a distinctive feature of HIV-2 infection that may result from decreased viral burden and that also may contribute to lower rates of transmission and disease development.

In an evaluation of paired blood and cervical lavage samples, the rate of viral shedding was 36.4% for HIV-1 and 16.0% for HIV-2, after repeat PCRs (216). In most cases, phylogenetic analysis showed that the viral sequences from blood and genital secretions were intermingled and subclusters did not segregate according to sample site. In rare cases, however, tissue-specific sequences were observed, suggesting a complex relationship between quasispecies in the two sites, where preferential transmission of HIV variants may occur because of multiple factors.

Evidence for a lower viral burden in HIV-2–infected individuals has been reported from both virus isolation and PCR studies (101,179,180,217–219). The isolation rate of HIV-2 from peripheral blood mononuclear cells (PBMCs) or plasma of asymptomatic individuals infected with HIV-2 was lower than the isolation rate of HIV-1 (217). At lower CD4$^+$ lymphocyte counts, virus isolation was equally efficient for either virus. Studies in Gambia and Senegal suggest that proviral HIV-2 copies increase with disease progression and the drop in CD4$^+$ lymphocyte counts (180,218).

In our studies comparing the HIV-2 proviral loads in singly (HIV-2) and dually infected individuals, we found that median proviral loads differed significantly, with those in the HIV-2 group ranging from 63.2 to 669.8 copies/10^5 CD4$^+$ cells, and demonstrated an inverse correlation with CD4$^+$ lymphocyte counts. The dually infected individuals showed less variation in viral load, ranging from 9.9 to 43.3 copies/10^5 CD4$^+$ cells. In contrast, among the dually infected individuals, low HIV-2 proviral load was correlated with low CD4$^+$ lymphocyte counts. The HIV-2 proviral loads in dually infected individuals were significantly lower than those in individuals infected with HIV-2 only ($p < 0.0001$) despite comparable CD4$^+$ lymphocyte counts. These results suggest that different HIV-2 proviral dynamics prevail in dual infections (180).

HIV-2 is less pathogenic than HIV-1, but the mechanisms underlying this difference have not yet been defined. We developed an internally controlled, quantitative RT PCR to measure HIV-2 viral load and used it to determine levels of plasma virus in a cohort of registered commercial sex workers in Dakar, Senegal (101). The assay has a lower limit of detection of 100 copies per ml and is linear over 4 logs. HIV-2 RNA was detected in 56% of the samples tested; the median load was 141 copies per ml. Levels of viral RNA in the plasma were inversely correlated to CD4$^+$ cell counts. HIV-2 and HIV-1 viral loads were compared among seroincident women in the cohort. The median viral load was 30-fold lower among the HIV-2–infected women ($p < 0.001$, Wilcoxon rank sum test), regardless of length of time infected. This suggests that plasma viremia is linked to the differences in the pathogenicities of the two types of virus (101).

Using an LTR-based RT PCR assay, Berry et al. reported a cross-sectional study of HIV-infected patients stratified according to their percentage of CD4$^+$ T-lymphocytes (CD4%) (219). Individuals infected with HIV-2 had lower plasma RNA levels than those infected with HIV-1 at lower CD4%, but had similar plasma RNA levels at higher CD4%. Similarly, in studies of HIV-2–infected patients in Portugal, plasma viremia could be detected in only 10 of 30 patients (33%), a rate much lower than that seen in HIV-1 infection. Virus was isolated from 16 of 30 patients (53.3%). A significant correlation was found between CD4$^+$ counts, clinical status, rate of virus isolation, and plasma viral load (220). In a study of known seroconverters, HIV-2–infected individuals demonstrated a viral setpoint approximately 28-fold lower than HIV-1–infected individuals (221).

Levels of virus in the plasma are closely related to the pathogenicity of HIV-1 and infection with HIV-2 produces significantly lower plasma viral load. To further identify the source of this difference, we measured both viral RNA and proviral DNA in matched samples from 34 HIV-2–infected individuals. The median level of HIV-2 RNA for the group was 189 copies per ml. Levels of HIV-2 RNA were below the limit of detection in nearly half the women, a result consistent with what we had previously reported for this population (222). Levels of HIV-2 proviral DNA were similar to those for HIV-1 but failed to correlate with levels of viral RNA.

It therefore appears that significant differences occur upon expression, release, and/or maintenance of virions in the bloodstream. It is possible that shifts in splicing patterns could be responsible for the differences in virion production, but further studies would be required to verify such an explanation for the current data. Comparative studies of both viral and host factors that may affect expression would be useful for understanding the differences between HIV-1 and HIV-2 pathogenesis.

CLINICAL OUTCOME

Early surveys included various case reports of AIDS in HIV-2–infected individuals (40,223,224). The disease characteristics, including tuberculosis, chronic diarrhea, and *Candida* infections, seemed similar to diseases seen in HIV-1–associated AIDS (40, 225,226). Central nervous system involvement was also occasionally seen in individuals infected with HIV-2 (227,228). However, diseases in Africa that are associated with AIDS, such as tuberculosis, often showed only a weak epidemiologic association with HIV-2, even in HIV-2 endemic areas (14,203,229).

Our prospective studies conducted in a registered female commercial sex worker cohort in Dakar, Senegal, have provided us the opportunity to measure infection and progression rates for both HIV-1 and HIV-2 infections (203,208,229). Importantly, these prospective studies have compared disease progression in individuals based on known times of infection in a cohort that has been studied for more than 15 years, representing one of the longest HIV natural history studies in the field. A Kaplan–Meier analysis of HIV-2–infected individuals indicated 85% (95% CI, 50% to 96%) remained AIDS-free after 8 years of HIV-2 infection (Figure 4) (172). These differences in survival probabilities between HIV-2 and HIV-1 were also seen in stage IV disease (Centers for Disease Control and Prevention) and $CD4^+$ lymphocyte counts below 400 cells/mm^3 and $CD4^+$ lymphocyte counts below 200 cells/mm^3 as outcomes.

In our prospective study of individuals infected with HIV-2, we have also identified individuals who can be considered long-term nonprogressors and have determined a rate of this phenotype in the study population (203,208, Traore et al., unpublished data). Using a definition of long-term nonprogression as the absence of AIDS or related symptoms for 8 or more years after infection and the maintenance of stable $CD4^+$ lymphocyte counts >500 cells/mm^3, we have found 39 of 41 (95%) of the women in this cohort could be classified as long-term nonprogressors.

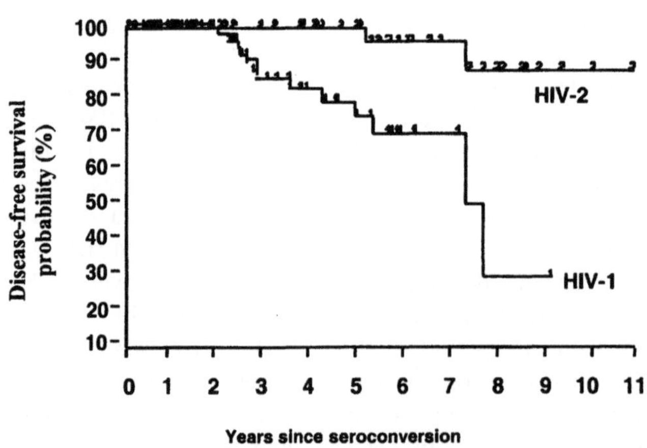

FIGURE 4. Comparison of Kaplan-Meier AIDS-free survival probability of incident HIV-1– and HIV-2–infected individuals, Wilcoxon-Gehan, $p<0.01$. (Traore et al., unpublished data.)

This dramatic difference in pathogenicity provides an unparalleled opportunity to identify viral and host immune mechanisms involved in a closely related and relevant virus system that is predicted to have a significantly slower course of progression.

Since a slower disease course appears to be common in HIV-2 infection, we reasoned that certain individuals in the population would possess characteristics that might predispose them to a more rapid disease course. We conducted a case-control study investigating possible associations between HLA and the risk of disease progression in HIV-2 (230). The HLA class I status was molecularly typed in 62 female commercial sex workers from the Dakar, Senegal, cohort. The absence of antibodies to the HIV-2 antigen, p26, was used as the surrogate marker for risk of disease progression (133). Statistical analysis showed that the *B*35* allele of HLA was associated with absence of p26 antibodies ($p < 0.05$) and with a higher risk of disease progression. The same association was found for the class I haplotypes *B*35Cw4* and *A*23Cw7* ($p < 0.05$) similar to the association with HIV-1 (231). Our data show that certain HLA molecules are associated with risk of disease progression in HIV-2, and that some of the alleles and haplotypes involved in susceptibility to disease are similar for both HIV-1 and HIV-2.

HIV-2 IMMUNITY

The attenuated phenotype of HIV-2 infection in vivo has sparked considerable interest in understanding the immunopathogenesis of this particular HIV infection. Although certain viral determinants appear to be central to the lower in-vivo replicative capacity, the virus appears unusually immunogenic inducing significant immunity, which may be central to the explanation of the weaker, more attenuated phenotype of HIV-2. As with HIV-1, the antibody response to most viral structural proteins occurs shortly after infection and is thought to persist. In HIV-2 infection, more than 90% of seropositives evaluated in the cohort in Senegal demonstrated strong antibodies to *gag*-, *pol*,- and *env*-encoded antigens (232, 233). As already noted, the cross-reactive response to analogous HIV-1 antigens is significant in highly conserved gene products such as Gag and Pol and less so with Env antigens.

Circulating p24 antigen of HIV-1 has been useful as a marker of viral replication in vivo, although this measure has been somewhat replaced with more direct measurements of concentrations of virion particles using PCR technology. Analogous studies with HIV-2 have not been described, perhaps because antibodies to p26 are found in the majority of sera taken from HIV-2–infected individuals and, therefore, it has been assumed that complexing by free, circulating p26 is less frequent. In our studies, we have found that the absence of antibodies to p26 is a fixed phenotype, not the result of the complexing of free p26, and is predictive of a more rapid disease course (133,230).

HIV-2 neutralizing antibodies have been described (148,159,160,234,235), and in studies with fresh isolates, the broadness of the neutralizing antibody response to HIV-2 has been unusual and distinct from the neutralizing antibody response to HIV-1 (236). Virus neutralization studies have shown that a proportion of HIV-2 isolates are also capable of cross-neutralizing HIV-1 isolates in addition to HIV-2 isolates (159,162). The degree to which HIV-1–positive sera can cross-neutralize HIV-2 isolates continues to be debated. It is still not known whether some of the conserved domains of *env* will be capable of eliciting a cross-protective response to both viruses.

Studies of HIV-2 humoral immunity have now been extended to evaluate the highly related mucosal immune response. Evaluation of HIV-2 antibody responses in the cervicovaginal secretions have shown that only one-third of infected women generate IgA responses to HIV-2 envelope antigens in this compartment, suggesting lower levels of viral replication compared to HIV-1. Of interest, the cross-reactivity by IgG and IgA to heterologous envelope antigens is more frequently found in HIV-2 infection (237). Cervicovaginal cross-reactivity is more pronounced for HIV-2–specific antibodies to HIV-1 epitopes than is conversely true. Such features could help explain differences in heterosexual transmission rates for one type of HIV in an individual infected by the other type, an interpretation that would support epidemiologic studies that show that HIV-2 infection protects against subsequent HIV-1 infection but that HIV-1 infection does not appear to protect significantly against subsequent HIV-2 infection.

Knowledge of immune mechanisms responsible for the cross-protection between highly divergent viruses such as HIV-1 and HIV-2 may contribute to an understanding of whether viral variability can be overcome in the design of vaccine candidates that are broadly protective across HIV subtypes. In early cytotoxic T-lymphocyte (CTL) studies of HIV-2, responses against HIV-2's Gag, Pol and Nef were described. HLA-*B*53*–restricted, HIV-2 Gag-specific CTLs did not recognize target cells expressing HIV-1's Gag suggesting the absence of a cross-protective cellular response (238). More recently, Bertoletti and colleagues working in Gambia, have shown that the majority of HIV-2–infected individuals with different HLA molecules possess a dominant CTL response that can recognize HIV-1 Gag (239). Furthermore, HLA-B*5801–positive individuals have shown a broad cross-recognition of HIV-1 subtypes after they mounted a T-cell response that tolerated extensive amino acid substitutions within HLA-B*5801– restricted HIV-1 and HIV-2 epitopes. These results suggest that HLA-B*5801–positive individuals infected with HIV-2 have an enhanced ability to react with HIV-1 that could play a role in cross-protection (239).

We have used the sensitive Elispot technique to further quantify the HIV-2–specific CTL response in HIV-2–infected individuals (240). To assess the antigen delivery system using the modified nontoxic form of the anthrax toxin, we fused the HIV-2 Gag (p26) to the terminal domain of the lethal factor (LFn, 255 aa). The LFn–HIV-2 recombinant proteins were expressed and used as antigens to stimulate CTL in a ELISPOT assay, compared to the classic delivery system using recombinant vaccinia virus expressing HIV-2 Gag. We found that 87.5% of the individuals in our study showed a specific Gag CTL response. Our results have shown that priming cells with the LFn–p26 gave better sensitivity and resolution when patients had a low frequency of CTL precursors. Interestingly, we found that the group with strong cellular immune response had no detectable HIV-2 plasma load.

PROTECTIVE IMMUNITY—IMPLICATIONS FOR VACCINE

Global statistics of the HIV epidemic continue to underscore the urgency for an effective HIV vaccine. The developing world, particularly regions of Africa, continue to bear a significant portion of the global HIV burden. These regions are unlikely to benefit from recent advances in therapeutic regimes in the foreseeable future. Important to vaccine design is the understanding of pathogenic mechanisms of HIV infection and the potential immunologic responses or correlates necessary for HIV containment. The identification of such correlates has been hampered by the relatively few instances of natural immunity that have withstood the challenge of viral exposure. In the early 1800s, Jenner's identification of the protected milkmaids provided the characterization of cowpox, information that was later used to produce a vaccine against the antigenically related smallpox, leading to its ultimate eradication.

Demonstrated differences in the infectivity and disease potential of HIV-2 and

HIV-1 support the notion that the mechanism for protection might be analogous to the attenuated virus vaccine model. In our studies of the female commercial sex worker cohort in Dakar, Senegal, we tested the hypothesis that the attenuated phenotype of HIV-2 infection might protect against subsequent HIV-1 infection (241). HIV-1 infection in individuals previously negative for HIV, along with superinfection in individuals infected with HIV-2, was documented over the study period with both serology and PCR assays. A Poisson regression model was used to estimate the independent effect of demographic, behavioral, and biologic variables on the risk of HIV-1 infection. Despite higher incidence of other STDs, HIV-2–infected women had lower incidence of HIV-1 infection than seronegatives with an incidence rate ratio of 0.32 (p=0.008). This analysis led to the conclusion that HIV-2 infection conferred a significant reduction in the risk of subsequent HIV-1 infection. Continued analysis of the Dakar cohort has extended the observation period from the first published report to more than 13 years, with HIV-2 protection ranges from 52% to 74%, depending on method of analysis (14,241,242).

The generalizability of these findings has been questioned by studies from other West African sites. In Côte d'Ivoire, Guinea Bissau, and Gambia, studies originally designed as cross-sectional surveys were analyzed for short periods of longitudinal observation (243–245). As a result of their design, they failed to possess sufficient statistical power, capable only of detecting an extremely high protected fraction (>99%) of HIV-1 infection due to HIV-2 infection (242). In addition, a mixture of serologic methods employed by these studies failed to meet the PCR-based standard for diagnosis of dual infection, a standard critical to any objective evaluation of HIV-2 protection in vivo (243–245). In a longitudinal study conducted in police officers in Guinea Bissau, Norrgren et al. failed to report a statistically significant result; however, only a portion of the samples were diagnosed by PCR technology (246). Unbiased, powerful studies using sensitive and specific classification methods will effectively address the generalizability of the observation of HIV-2's protective efficacy against subsequent HIV-1 infection. The observation of the Dakar cohort continues to document a protective effect. The long person-time of observation with few losses to follow-up and rigorous PCR testing has supported these important findings (172).

Studies from other research groups, including our own, have described in-vitro interactions of HIV-1 and HIV-2 that support our in-vivo observations, which range from virus–virus interactions to potential immune-mediated mechanisms for HIV-2 protection. Arya et al. have reported that HIV-2 inhibits the replication of HIV-1 at the molecular level. This inhibition was determined to be selective, dose-dependent, and nonreciprocal. Although the exact mechanism remains to be defined, the inhibition appeared to be the result of an intracellular molecular event;

TABLE 2[a]. Protective Effect of HIV-2 on Risk of Subsequent HIV-1 Infection in Dakar, Senegal

Incidence rate ratio	Fraction protected	Observation period (years)	p value
0.23–0.32	68%–77%	9	<0.05
0.26–0.36	64%–74%	11	<0.05
0.33–0.42	58%–67%	12	<0.03
0.34–0.44	56%–66%	13	<0.03

[a]The range of incidence rate ratios and associated fraction protected (Sources: 14,241,242, Travers et al., unpublished data).

it could not be explained solely on the basis of cell surface receptor-mediated interference. The results support the notion that the inhibition likely occurred at the level of viral RNA, possibly involving competition between viral RNAs for some transcriptional factor essential for viral replication (247,248).

We also suspected that viral determinants might play a role in HIV-2 protection, from which it could be hypothesized that HIV-2 would protect differentially against HIV-1 subtypes. To investigate the HIV-1 subtypes involved in dual infections, we sequenced the *env* region from 29 dually infected female commercial sex workers from Senegal (249,250). The majority of women (23 of 29) were infected by HIV-1 subtype A. Within the HIV-1A sequences, 14 of 23 (60.8%) clustered with the A/G recombinant form (A/G_{IbNG}) found in West Africa, and 9 of 23 (39.2%) formed a separate cluster distinct from A/G_{IbNG}. By contrast, in individuals infected by HIV-1 alone, non-IbNG subtype A was found in only 13 of 98 (13.3%). Therefore, the lack of protection and/or interaction with HIV-2 was associated with a distinct HIV-1A genotype. These results suggest differences in the biologic properties of HIV-1 genotypes and their in vivo interactions with HIV-2 (250).

β-chemokines have now been identified as potent soluble suppressors of macrophage-tropic HIV infection in vitro. Studies of multiply exposed, uninfected individuals have implicated the role of elevated β-chemokines in HIV resistance, in many cases, independent of genetic mutations in the chemokine receptor (251–253). Studies in macaques have also suggested a role for β-chemokines in vaccine-induced protective immunity using a variety of vaccine candidates and live virus challenges (254). We used an HIV-1 in vitro challenge system to determine if PBMCs from HIV-2–infected individuals showed altered susceptibility to HIV-1 infection (255). PBMCs were stimulated and infected with either R5 or X4 HIV-1 viruses. Fourteen of 28 (50%) HIV-2 PBMCs demonstrated more than 90% inhibition of R5/HIV-1 infection compared with 0 of 19 HIV-negative controls (Fisher exact test, $p = 0.0002$). In contrast, HIV-2–positive and HIV-negative control cells were equally susceptible to X4/HIV-1 infection. RANTES, MIP-1α, and MIP-1β, the natural ligands of the CCR5 receptor, were measured in culture supernatant by ELISA, and supernatant levels of MIP-1α ($r = -0.56$, $p = 0.03$) and MIP-1β ($r = -0.69$, $p = 0.004$) were inversely correlated with HIV-1 replication. Using polyclonal antibodies to RANTES, MIP-1α and MIP-1β, resistance was neutralized. A significant proportion of HIV-2–infected PBMCs demonstrated HIV-1 resistance in vitro; this resistance was β-chemokine dependent (255). Further studies are needed to characterize this potent antiviral activity and to determine its potential contribution to in-vivo protection.

HIV-2 infection might dramatically influence β-chemokine production by enhancing its magnitude and duration, thus enabling HIV-2–infected individuals to cope favorably with subsequent exposure to HIV-1. This is supported by studies demonstrating that binding of the HIV-2 envelope to the alpha chain of CD8 stimulates dramatic levels of β-chemokine production in comparison to HIV-1 gp120 activity (256). Not only does this implicate a novel viral suppressive mechanism but one that may be adapted for immunoprophylaxis. Antiretroviral vaccine strategies that incorporate β-chemokine induction or other receptor-blocking functions raise some encouraging possibilities for vaccine design and development.

HIV-2 infected baboons (*Papio cynocephalus*) provide a valuable animal model for the study of HIV pathogenesis since many features of disease progression resemble HIV-1 infection in humans. In some HIV-2–infected baboons that were clinically healthy, a $CD8^+$ cell antiviral response that was partly mediated by a soluble factor appeared to control viral replication in vitro. A soluble factor was found to be active against the chemokine-resistant, syncytium-inducing HIV-1 isolates and was relatively heat stable. Therefore, the soluble suppressing activity of $CD8^+$ cells in HIV-2–infected baboons may be analogous to the $CD8^+$ cell antiviral factor described in asymptomatic, HIV-infected humans (257).

HIV-2 infects between 1 and 2 million people in West Africa. It spreads less efficiently than HIV-1, making projections for future infections much lower than for HIV-1. Thus, development of an HIV-2 vaccine has not been a high research priority. However, HIV-2 infects monkeys, whereas HIV-1 does not, and the SIV vaccine model uses viruses that are closer to HIV-2 than to HIV-1. The development and testing of an HIV-2 vaccine might therefore be simpler than the development of an HIV-1 vaccine. A few reports with HIV-2 have described experimental studies with limited vaccine protection (258,259), although immune correlates of protection have not been identified (260–262). Nonetheless, the data from human studies indicates that HIV-2 may afford protection from HIV-1, suggesting that a candidate vaccine based on HIV-2 might provide necessary cross-immunity for HIV-1 protection, a possibility that may be worthy of further consideration.

THERAPY

Drugs that have efficacy against HIV-1 are generally assumed to be effective against HIV-2. However, with a few exceptions of in vitro analysis (263), most HIV-1 drugs have not been tested for activity against HIV-2. A case can therefore be made that HIV-2 infection in monkeys also provides a valuable in-vivo model for drug testing that is not readily available for HIV-1 (264). Use of antiretroviral therapy has been infrequently reported for HIV-2 infection. A recent report of two HIV-2 AIDS patients undergoing zidovudine treatment in the Netherlands demonstrated mutations in the RT genes similar to those associated with zidovudine resistance in HIV-1 (265).

Unlike HIV-1, there is limited clinical experience with antiretroviral therapy in HIV-2 infection. This is at least partly because the virus is found in Africa and partly because there are few related cases in developed countries. Furthermore, treatment decisions have been difficult in the absence of a commercially available assay to measure HIV-2 plasma viral load. From the limited situations where HIV-2 patients were treated in the United States, it appears that standard highly active antiretroviral therapy can readily reduce viral load levels below detection (266,267).

The RT and PR genes from 12 HIV-2–infected individuals who had been exposed to antiretroviral drugs were examined for the presence of mutation that could be involved in drug resistance. Four individuals carried viral genotypes with amino acid substitutions potentially associated with resistance to nucleoside analogues: two at codon 70 (lysine→ arginine) and two at codon 184 (methionine →valine). The latter two individuals harbored a codon 151 mutation (glutamine → methionine) that has been associated with multidrug resistance in HIV-1. Substitutions associated with resistance to protease inhibitors at codon 46 were observed in all individuals. Moreover, minor resistance mutations, as well as new ones, were often seen in the PR gene. Thus, amino acid changes in HIV-2's RT and PR genes, which could be associated with drug resistance, seem to occur at positions identical to those responsible for drug resistance in HIV-1 (268).

CONCLUSION

Since the discovery of HIV-2 in 1985, considerable progress has been made in understanding its virology and epidemiology. The data suggest differences between HIV-2 and HIV-1 in geographic distribution, distinct epidemic trends, perinatal transmission rates, and incubation periods to the development of

AIDS. The virologic determination and mechanisms for these apparent biologic differences are still unknown. However, understanding how HIV-2 differs from HIV-1 is essential to interpretations of comparative virologic studies. We hope such comparative studies will yield important information on the pathogenic mechanisms employed by HIV viruses and will lead the way to the development of effective interventions for the prevention of AIDS. This is best exemplified in studies indicating that this close relative of HIV-1 infection, via its attenuated phenotype, may confer significant protection from subsequent infection by HIV-1. This further suggests that understanding HIV-2 immunity and cross-immunity may be useful for HIV vaccine design and development.

REFERENCES

1. Barin F, Mboup S, Denis F, et al. Serological Evidence for Virus Related to Simian T-Lymphotropic Retrovirus III in Residents of West Africa. *Lancet.* 1985;2(8469–70):1387–1390.
2. Essex M, Kanki P. The Origins of the AIDS Virus. *Sci Amer.* 1988;259:64–71.
3. Gao F, Yue L, White A, et al. Human infection by genetically diverse SIVSM-related HIV-2 in West Africa. *Nature.* 1992;358:495–499.
4. Stahl Hennig C, Herchenroder O, Nick S, et al. Experimental infection of macaques with HIV-2ben, a novel HIV-2 isolate. *AIDS.* 1990;4:611–617.
5. Castro BA, Nepomuceno M, Lerche NW, et al. Persistent infection of baboons and rhesus monkeys with different strains of HIV-2. *Virology.* 1991; 184(1):219–226.
6. Alter HJ, Eichberg JW, Masur H, et al. Transmission of HTLV-III from human plasma to chimpanzees: an animal model for AIDS. *Science.* 1984;226:549–552.
7. Francis DP, Feorino PM, Broderson JR, et al. Infection of chimpanzees with lymphadenopathy-associated virus. *Lancet.* 1984;2(8414):1276–1277.
8. Gajdusek DC, Amyx HL, Gibbs CJJ, et al. Infection of chimpanzees by human T-lymphotropic retroviruses in brain and other tissues from AIDS patients. *Lancet.* 1985;1(8419):55–56.
9. Fultz PN, McClure HM, Swenson RB, et al. Persistent infection of chimpanzees with human T-lymphotropic virus type III/lymphadenopathy-associated virus: a potential model for acquired immunodeficiency syndrome. *J Virol.* 1986;58(1): 116–124.
10. Kanki P, McLane MF, King NWJ, et al. Serologic Identification and Characterization of a Macaque T-Lymphotropic Retrovirus Closely Related to HTLV-III. *Science.* 1985;228:1199–1201.
11. Kanki PJ, Kurth R, Becker W, et al. Antibodies to simian T-lymphotropic retrovirus type III in African green monkeys and recognition of STLV-III viral proteins by AIDS and related sera. *Lancet.* 1985;1(8441):1330–1332.
12. Essex M, Kanki P. Human Immunodeficiency Virus Type 2 (HIV-2). In: Broder S, Merigan T, Bologenesi D, eds. *Textbook of AIDS Medicine.* Baltimore: Williams & Wilkins; 1994:873–886.
13. Markovitz DM. Infection with the human immunodeficiency virus type-2. *Ann Intern Med.* 1993; 118:211–218.
14. Kanki PJ. Human Immunodeficiency Virus Type 2, (HIV-2). *AIDS Reviews.* 1999;1(20):101–108.
15. Smith TF, Srinivasan A, Schochetman G, et al. The phylogenetic history of immunodeficiency viruses. *Nature.* 1988;333:573–575.
16. Myers G, MacInnes K, Korber B. The emergence of simian/human immunodeficiency viruses. *AIDS Res Hum Retroviruses.* 1992;8(3):373–386.
17. Marx P, Li Y, Lerche N, et al. Isolation of a simian immunodeficiency virus related to human immunodeficiency virus type 2 from a west African pet sooty mangabey. *J Virol.* 1991;65:4480–4485.
18. Emau P, McClure HM, Isahakia M, et al. Isolation from African Sykes' monkeys (Cercopi-thecus mitis) of a lentivirus related to human and simian immunoeficiency viruses. *J Virol.* 1991;65(4): 2135–2140.
19. Allan JS, Kanda P, Kennedy RC, et al. Isolation and characterization of simian immunodeficiency viruses from two subspecies of African green monkeys. *AIDS Res Hum Retroviruses.* 1990;6:275–285.
20. Franchini G, Collalti E, Arya SK, et al. Genetic Analysis of a New Subgroup of Human and Simian T-Lymphotropic Retroviruses: HTLV-IV, LAV-2, SBL6669, and STLV-III$_{AGM}$. *AIDS Res Hum Retroviruses.* 1987;3:11–17.
21. Kanki P, Barin F, Mboup S, et al. Relationship of Simian T-Lymphotropic Virus Type III to Human Retroviruses in Africa. *Antibiot Chemother.* 1987;38:21–27.
22. Biberfeld G, Brown F, Esparza J, et al. Meeting Report, WHO working group on characterization of HIV-related, retroviruses: Criteria for characterization and proposal for a nomenclature system. *AIDS.* 1987;1:189–190.
23. Boeri E, Giri A, Lillo F, et al. In vivo genetic variability of the human immunodeficiency virus type 2 V3 region. *J Virol.* 1992;66:4546–4550.
24. Kirchhoff F, Jentsch KD, Bachmann B, et al. A novel proviral clone of HIV-2: biological and

phylogenetic relationship to other primate immunodeficiency viruses. *Virology.* 1990;177:305–311.
25. Gao F, Yue L, Robertson DL, et al. Genetic diversity of human immunodeficiency virus type 2: evidence for distinct sequence subtypes with differences in virus biology. *J Virol.* 1994;68:7433–7447.
26. Yamaguchi J, Devare S, Brennan C. Identification of a new HIV-2 subtype based on phylogenetic analysis of full-length genomic sequence. *AIDS Res Hum Retroviruses.* 2000;16(9):925–930.
27. Sankalé JL, Sallier de la Tour R, Renjifo B, et al. Intra-patient Variability of the Human Immunodeficiency Virus Type-2 (HIV-2) Envelope V3 Loop. *AIDS Res Hum Retroviruses.* 1995;11(5): 617–623.
28. Sarr AD, Sankale JL, Gueye-Ndiaye A, et al. Genetic analysis of HIV type 2 in monotypic and dual HIV infections. *AIDS Res Hum Retroviruses.* 2000;16(3):295–298.
29. Norrgren H, Marquina S, Leitner T, et al. HIV-2 genetic variation and DNA load in asymptomatic carriers and AIDS cases in Guinea-Bissau. *JAIDS.* 1997;16(1):31–38.
30. Peeters M, Koumare B, Mulanga C, et al. Genetic subtypes of HIV type 1 and HIV type 2 strains in commercial sex workers from Bamako, Mali. *AIDS Res Hum Retroviruses.* 1998;14(1):51–58.
31. Xiang Z, Ariyoshi K, Wilkins A, et al. HIV type 2 pathogenicity is not related to subtype in rural Guinea Bissau. *AIDS Res Hum Retroviruses.* 1997;13(6):501–505.
32. Dietrich U, Adamski M, Kreutz R, et al. A highly divergent HIV-2-related isolate. *Nature.* 1989;342: 948–950.
33. Kawamura M, Katahira J, Fukasawa M, et al. Isolation and characterization of a highly divergent HIV-2[GH-2]: generation of an infectious molecular clone and functional analysis of its rev-responsive element in response to primate retrovirus transactivators (Rev and Rex). *Virology.* 1992; 188(2): 850–853.
34. Pieniazek D, Ellenberger D, Janini L, et al. Predominance of Human Immunodeficiency Virus Type 2 Subtype B in Abidjan, Ivory Coast. *AIDS Res Hum Retroviruses.* 1999;15:603–608.
35. Kanki P. West African Human Retroviruses Related to STLV-III. *AIDS.* 1987;1:141–145.
36. Harrison LH, José da Silva AP, Gayle HD, et al. Risk factors for HIV-2 infection in Guinea-Bissau. *JAIDS.* 1991;4(11):1155–1160.
37. Naucler A, Albino P, Da Silva AP, et al. HIV-2 infection in hospitalized patients in Bissau, Guinea-Bissau. *AIDS.* 1990;5:301–304.
38. Denis F, Barin F, Gershy-Damet G, et al. Prevalence of Human T-Lymphotropic Retroviruses Type III (HIV) and Type IV in Ivory Coast. *Lancet.* 1987;1(8530):408–411.
39. Pepin J, Dunn D, Gaye I, et al. HIV-2 infection among prostitutes working in The Gambia: association with serological evidence of genital ulcer diseases and generalized lymphadenopathy. *AIDS.* 1991;5:69.
40. Romieu I, Marlink R, Kanki P, et al. HIV-2 link to AIDS in West Africa. *JAIDS.* 1990;3:220–230.
41. Naucler A, Andreasson PA, Costa CM, et al. HIV-2–associated AIDS and HIV-2 seroprevalence in Bissau, Guinea-Bissau. *JAIDS.* 1989;2:88–93.
42. Kanki P, DeCock KM. Epidemiology and Natural History of HIV-2. *AIDS.* 1994;8(supp.):S1–S9.
43. Kanki P, Marlink R, Siby T, et al. Biology of HIV-2 Infection in West Africa. In: Papas TS, ed. *Gene Regulation and AIDS.* Houston: Portfolio Publishing Company of Texas; 1990:255–271.
44. Ankrah T, Roberts M, Antwi P, et al. The African AIDS case definition and HIV serology in medical in-patients at Komfo Anokye Teaching Hospital, Kumasi, Ghana. *West Afr J Med.* 1994;13:98.
45. Olaleye O, Bernstein L, Ekweozor C, et al. Prevalence of human immunodeficiency virus types 1 and 2 infections in Nigeria. *J Infect Dis.* 1993;167:710.
46. Maiga Y, Sissoko Z, Maiga M. Etude de la seroprevalence de l'Infection a VIH dans les 7 regions economiques du Mali. VIIIth International Conference on AIDS in Africa/VIIIth African Conference on Sexually Transmitted Diseases. Marrakech; 1993.
47. Anderson RM, May RM. The population biology of the interaction between HIV-1 and HIV-2: coexistence or competitive exclusion? *AIDS.* 1996;10(14): 1663–1673.
48. Kanki P, Travers K, Hernandez-Avila M, et al. Slower Heterosexual Spread of HIV-2 Compared with HIV-1. *Lancet.* 1994;343:943–946.
49. Andreasson P, Dias F, Naucler A, et al. A prospective study of vertical transmission of HIV-2 in Bissau, Guinea-Bissau. *AIDS.* 1993;7:989.
50. Ngagne M, Diouf A, Kebe F, et al. Histoire Naturelle de la transmission verticale VIH1 et VIH 2 a Dakar. IXth International Conference on AIDS and Associated Cancers in Africa; 1995: Kampala, Uganda.
51. Adjorlolo-Johnson G, DeCock K, Ekpini E, et al. Prospective comparison of mother-to-child transmission of HIV-1 and HIV-2 in Abidjan, Ivory Coast. *JAMA.* 1994;272:462–466.
52. Smallman-Raynor M, Cliff A. The Spread of Human Immunodeficiency Virus Type 2 into Europe: A Geographical Analysis. *Intl J of Epi.* 1991;20:480.
53. Santos-Ferreira M, Cohen T, Lourenco M, et al. A study of seroprevalence of HIV-1 and HIV-2 in six provinces of People's Republic of Angola: clues to the spread of HIV infection. *JAIDS.* 1990;3:780.

54. Victorino RMM, Guerreiro D, Lourenço MH, et al. Prevalence of HIV-2 infection in a family planning clinic in Libson. *Intl J STD AIDS.* 1992;3:281–284.
55. Rubsamen-Waigmann H, Briesen H, Maniar J, et al. Spread of HIV-2 in India. *Lancet.* 1991;337: 550–551.
56. Rubsamen-Waigmann H, Maniar J, Gerte S, et al. High proportion of HIV-2 and HIV-1/2 double-reactive sera in two Indian states, Maharashtra and Goa: first appearance of an HIV-2 epidemic along with an HIV-1 epidemic outside of Africa. *Int J Med Microbiol Virol Parasitol Infect Dis.* 1994;280:398–402.
57. Courouce AM, Barin F, Baudelot J, et al. HIV-2 infection among blood donors and other subjects in France. *Transfusion.* 1989;29:368.
58. Matheron S, Simon F, Sassi G, et al. Infection HIV-2 chez l'adulte; etude de cohorte; Paris:1986–1993. VIIIth International Conference on AIDS in Africa and VIIIth African Conference on Sexually Transmitted Diseases; December 1993;Marrakech.
59. De Cock K, Brun-Vezinet F. Epidemiology of HIV-2 Infection. *AIDS.* 1989;3(supp 1):S89–S95.
60. Machuca A, Soriano V, Gutierrez M, et al. Human immunodeficiency virus type 2 infection in Spain. The HIV-2 Spanish Study Group. *Intervirology.* 1999;42(1):37–42.
61. Zagury JF, Franchini G, Reitz M, et al. Genetic variability between isolates of human immunodeficiency virus (HIV) type 2 is comparable to the variability among HIV type 1. *Proc Natl Acad Sci USA.* 1988;85:5941–5945.
62. Tristem M, Mansinho K, Champalimaud JL, et al. Six new isolates of human immunodeficiency virus type 2 (HIV-2) and the molecular characterization of one (HIV-2CAM2). *J Gen Virol.* 1989;70:479–484.
63. Matsuda Z, Chou MJ, Matsuda M, et al. Human immunodeficiency virus type 1 has an additional coding sequence in the central region of the genome. *Proc Natl Acad Sci USA.* 1988;85: 6968–6972.
64. Strebel K, Klimkait T, Maldarelli F, et al. Molecular and biochemical analyses of human immunodeficiency virus type 1 vpu protein. *J Virol.* 1989;63: 3784–3791.
65. Cohen EA, Terwilliger EF, Sodroski JG, et al. Identification of a protein encoded by the vpu gene of HIV-1. *Nature.* 1988;334:532–534.
66. Bour S, Strebel K. The human immunodeficiency virus (HIV) type 2 envelope protein is a functional complement to HIV type 1 Vpu that enhances particle release of heterologous retroviruses. *J Virol.* 1996;70(12):8285–8300.
67. Franchini G, Fargnoli KA, Giombini F, et al. Molecular and biological characterization of a replication competent human immunodeficiency type 2 (HIV-2) proviral clone. *Proc Natl Acad Sci USA.* 1989;86:2433–2437.
68. Yu XF, Ito S, Essex M, et al. A naturally immunogenic virion-associated protein specific for HIV-2 and SIV. *Nature.* 1988;335:262–265.
69. Henderson L, Sowder R, Copeland T, et al. Isolation and characterization of a novel protein (X-ORF product) from SIV and HIV-2. *Science.* 1988;241:199–201.
70. Kappes J, Morrow C, Lee S, et al. Identification of a novel retroviral gene unique to human immunodeficiency virus type 2 and simian immunodeficiency virus SIVMAC. *J Virol.* 1988;62:3501–3505.
71. Moore JP. Simple methods for monitoring HIV-1 and HIV-2 gp120 binding to soluble CD4 by enzyme-linked immunosorbent assay: HIV-2 has a 25–fold lower affinity than HIV-1 for soluble CD4. *AIDS.* 1990;4:297–305.
72. Morikawa Y, Moore JP, Fenouillet E, et al. Complementation of human immunodeficiency virus glycoprotein mutations in trans. *J Gen Virol.* 1992;73(Pt 8):1907–1913.
73. Bahraoui E, Benjouad A, Guetard D, et al. Study of the interaction of HIV-1 and HIV-2 envelope glycoproteins with the CD4 receptor and role of N-glycans. *AIDS Res Hum Retroviruses.* 1992;8(5): 565–573.
74. Looney DJ, Hayashi S, Nicklas M, et al. Differences in the interaction of HIV-1 and HIV-2 with CD4. *JAIDS.* 1990;3:649–657.
75. Feng Y, Broder CC, Kennedy PE, et al. HIV-1 entry cofactor: functional cDNA cloning of a seven-transmembrane, G protein-coupled receptor. *Science.* 1996;272(5263):872–877.
76. Clapham P, McKnight A, Weiss RA. Human immunodeficiency virus type 2 infection and fusion of CD4–negative human cell lines: induction and enhancement by soluble CD4. *J Virol.* 1992; 66:3531–3537.
77. Endres MJ, Clapham PR, Marsh M, et al. CD4–independent infection by HIV-2 is mediated by fusin/CXCR4. *Cell.* 1996;87(4):745–756.
78. Bron R, Klasse PJ, Wilkinson D, et al. Promiscuous Use Of Cc and Cxc Chemokine Receptors In Cell-to-Cell Fusion Mediated By a Human Immunodeficiency Virus Type 2 Envelope Protein. *J Virol.* 1997;71(11):8405–8415.
79. Heredia A, Vallejo A, Soriano V, et al. Chemokine receptors and HIV-2 [letter]. *AIDS.* 1997;11(9): 1198–1199.
80. Evans L, Moreau J, Odehouri K, et al. Characterization of a Noncytopathic HIV-2 Strain with Unusual Effects on CD4 Expression. *Science.* 1988;240:1522–1525.
81. Kong L, Lee S, Kappes J, et al. West African HIV-2–related human retrovirus with attenuated cytopathicity. *Science.* 1988;240:1525–1529.
82. Albert J, Naucler A, Bottiger B, et al. Replicative capacity of HIV-2, like HIV-1, correlates with

severity of immunodeficiency. *AIDS.* 1990;4(4): 291–295.

83. Albert J, Stalhandske P, Marquina S, et al. Biological phenotype of HIV type 2 isolates correlates with V3 genotype. *AIDS Res Hum Retroviruses.* 1996;12(9):821–828.
84. Isaka Y, Sato A, Miki S, et al. Small amino acid changes in the V3 loop of human immunodeficiency virus type 2 determines the coreceptor usage for CXCR4 and CCR5. *Virology.* 1999;264(1):237–243.
85. Pichuantes S, Babe LM, Barr PJ, et al. Recombinant HIV2 protease processes HIV1 Pr53gag and analogous junction peptides in vitro. *J Bio Chem.* 1990;265:13890–13898.
86. Allan JS, Coligan JE, Lee TH, et al. Immunogenic Nature of a *pol* Gene Product of HTLV-III/LAV. *Blood.* 1987;69:331–333.
87. Bakhanashvili M, Hizi A. Fidelity of the RNA-dependent DNA synthesis exhibited by the reverse transcriptases of human immunodeficiency virus types 1 and 2 and of murine leukemia virus: mispair extension frequencies. *Biochemistry.* 1992; 31(39):9393–9398.
88. Taube R, Avidan O, Hizi A. The fidelity of misinsertion and mispair extension throughout DNA synthesis exhibited by mutants of the reverse transcriptase of human immunodeficiency virus type 2 resistant to nucleoside analogs. *Euro J Biochem.* 1997;250(1):106–114.
89. Hizi A, Tal R, Hughes SH. Mutational analysis of the DNA polymerase and ribonuclease H activities of human immunodeficiency virus types 2 reverse transcriptase expressed in Escherichia coli. *Virology.* 1991;180(1):339–346.
90. Hizi A, Tal R, Shaharabany M, et al. Catalytic properties of the reverse transcriptase of human immunodeficiency viruses type 1 and type 2. *J Bio Chem.* 1991;266(10):6230–6239.
91. Myers G, Pavlakis GN. Evolutionary potential of complex retroviruses. In: Levy JA, ed. *The retroviridae.* New York: Plenum Press; 1992:1–37.
92. Haseltine WA. The Molecular Biology of HIV-1. In: DeVita VT, Jr., Hellman S, Rosenberg SA, et al., eds. *AIDS, Etiology, Diagnosis, Treatment and Prevention.* 3rd ed. Philadelphia: J.B. Lippincott Co.; 1992:39–59.
93. Markovitz DM, Hannibal M, Perez VL, et al. Differential regulation of human immunodeficiency viruses (HIVs): a specific regulatory element in HIV-2 responds to stimulation of the T-cell antigen receptor. *Proc Natl Acad Sci USA.* 1990;87(23):9098–9102.
94. Tong-Starksen S, Welsh T, Peterlin M. Differences in transcriptional enhancers of HIV-1 and HIV-2 response to T-cell activation signals. *J Immunol.* 1990;145:4348–4354.
95. Arya S, Gallo C. Human immunodeficiency virus type 2 long terminal repeat: Analysis of regulatory elements. *AIDS.* 1988;85:9753–9757.
96. Courgnaud V, Laure F, Fultz PN, et al. Genetic differences accounting for evolution and pathogencity of simian immunodeficiency virus from a sooty mangabey after cross-species transmission to a pig-tailed macaque. *J Virol.* 1992;66:414–419.
97. Nabel G, Baltimore D. An inducible transcription factor activates expression of human immunodeficiency virus in T cells. *Nature.* 1987;326:711–713.
98. Arya SK. Human immunodeficiency virus type-2 gene expression: two enhancers and their activation by T-cell activators. *New Biologist.* 1990;2(1): 57–65.
99. Fu GK, Markovitz DM. Purification of the pets factor. A nuclear protein that binds to the inducible TG-rich element of the human immunodeficiency virus type 2 enhancer. *J Biol Chem.* 1996; 271(32):19599–19605.
100. Markovitz DM, Smith MJ, Hilfinger J, et al. Activation of the human immunodeficiency virus type 2 enhancer is dependent on purine box and kappa B regulatory elements. *J Virol.* 1992; 66(9):5479–5484.
101. Popper SJ, Dieng-Sarr A, Travers KU, et al. Lower HIV-2 viral load reflects the difference in pathogenicity of HIV-1 and HIV-2. *J Infect Dis.* 1999;180:1116–1121.
102. Arya SK. Human and simian immunodeficiency retroviruses: activation and differential transactivation of gene expression. *AIDS Res Hum Retroviruses.* 1988;4:175–186.
103. Chang Y, Jeang KT. The basic RNA-binding domain of HIV-2 Tat contributes to preferential transactivation of a TAR 2–containing LTR. *Nucleic Acids Res.* 1992;20:5465–5472.
104. Malim MH, Hauber J, Le SY, et al. The HIV-1 rev transactivator acts through a structured target sequence to activate nuclear export of unspliced viral mRNA. *Nature.* 1989;338:254–257.
105. Hammarskjold ML, Heimer J, Hammarskjold B, et al. Regulation of human immunodeficiency virus env expression by the rev gene product. *J Virol.* 1989;63:1959–1966.
106. Emerman M, Vazeux R, Peden K. The rev gene product of the human immunodeficiency virus affects envelope-specific RNA localization. *Cell.* 1989;57(7):1155–1165.
107. Dayton AI, Terwilliger EF, Potz J, et al. Cis-acting sequences responsive to the rev gene product of the human immunodeficiency virus. *JAIDS.* 1988; 1:441–452.
108. Dillon P, Nelbock P, Perkins A, et al. Structural and functional analysis of the human immunodeficiency virus type 2 *rev* protein. *J Virol.* 1991;65:445–449.
109. Sakai H, Siomi H, Shida H, et al. Functional comparison of transactivation by human retrovirus rev and rex genes. *J Virol.* 1990;64(12):5833–5839.
110. Dillon PJ, Nelbock P, Perkins A, et al. Function of the human immunodeficiency virus types 1 and 2

Rev proteins is dependent on their ability to interact with a structured region present in env gene mRNA. *J Virol.* 1990;64:4428–4437.
111. Garrett ED, Cullen BR. Comparative analysis of Rev function in human immunodeficiency virus types 1 and 2. *J Virol.* 1992;66(7):4288–4294.
112. Browning CM, Cagnon L, Good PD, et al. Potent inhibition of human immunodeficiency virus type 1 (HIV-1) gene expression and virus production by an HIV-2 tat activation-response RNA decoy. *J Virol.* 1999;73(6):5191–5195.
113. Allan JS, Coligan J, Lee TH, et al. A new HTLV-III/LAV encoded antigen detected by antibodies from AIDS patients. *Science.* 1985;230:810–813.
114. Arya SK, Gallo RC. Three novel genes of human T-lymphotropic virus type III: immune reactivity of their products with sera from acquired immune deficiency syndrome patients. *Proc Natl Acad Sci USA.* 1986;83:2209–2213.
115. Switzer WM, Wiktor S, Soriano V, et al. Evidence of Nef truncation in human immunodeficiency virus type 2 infection. *J Infect Dis.* 1998; 177(1):65–71.
116. Lee TH, Coligan J, Allan J, et al. A New HTLV-III/LAV protein encoded by a gene found in cytopathic retroviruses. *Science.* 1986;231:1546–1549.
117. Fisher AG, Ensoli B, Ivanoff L, et al. The sor gene of HIV-1 is required for efficient virus transmission in vitro. *Science.* 1987;237:888–893.
118. Gabuzda D, Lawrence K, Langhoff E, et al. Role of *vif* in replication of human immunodeficiency virus type 1 in CD4+ T lymphocytes. *J Virol.* 1992; 66:6489–6495.
119. Ohagen A. Role of Vif in stability of HIV-1 core. *J Virol.* 2000;74:11055–11066.
120. Tristem M, Marshall C, Karpas A, et al. Origin of vpx in lentiviruses. *Nature.* 1990;347:341–342.
121. Yuan X, Matsuda Z, Matsuda M, et al. Human immunodeficiency virus vpr gene encodes a virion-associated protein. *AIDS Res Hum Retroviruses.* 1990;6(11):1265–1271.
122. Cohen EA, Dehni G, Sodroski JG, et al. Human immunodeficiency virus vpr product is a virion-associated regulatory protein. *J Virol.* 1990;64: 3097–3099.
123. Yu X-F, Matsuda M, Essex M, et al. Open reading frame vpr of simian immunodeficiency virus encodes a virion-associated protein. *J Virol.* 1990;64:5688–5693.
124. Hattori N, Michaels F, Fargnoli K, et al. The human immunodeficiency virus type 2 *vpr* gene is essential for productive infection of human macrophages. *Proc Natl Acad Sci USA.* 1990;87:8080–8084.
125. Fletcher TM, Brichacek B, Sharova N, et al. Nuclear import and cell cycle arrest functions of the HIV-1 Vpr protein are encoded by two separate genes in HIV-2/SIV(SM). *EMBO Journal.* 1996; 15(22):6155–6165.
126. Kewalramani VN, Park CS, Gallombardo PA, et al. Protein stability influences human immunodeficiency virus type 2 Vpr virion incorporation and cell cycle effect. *Virology.* 1996;218(2):326–334.
127. Kewalramani VN, Emerman M. Vpx association with mature core structures of HIV-2. *Virology.* 1996;218(1):159–168.
128. Marcon L, Michaels F, Hattori N, et al. Dispensable role of the human immunodeficiency virus type 2 Vpx protein in viral replication. *J Virol.* 1991;65(7):3938–3942.
129. Hu W, Vander Heyden N, Ratner L. Analysis of the function of viral protein X (VPX) of HIV-2. *Virology.* 1989;173:624–630.
130. Shibata R, Miura T, Hayami M, et al. Mutational analysis of the human immunodeficiency virus type 2 (HIV-2) genome in relation to HIV-1 and simian immunodeficiency virus SIVagm. *J Virol.* 1990;64:742–747.
131. Yu XF, Yu QC, Essex M, et al. The vpx gene of simian immunodeficiency virus facilitates efficient viral replication in fresh lymphocytes and macrophage. *J Virol.* 1991;65(9):5088–5091.
132. Kappes J, Conway J, Lee S, et al. Human immunodeficiency virus type 2 *vpx* protein augments viral infectivity. *Virology.* 1991;184:197–209.
133. Popper S, Sankalé JL, Thior I, et al. Vpx reactivity as a predictor of disease progression in HIV-2 infection. *AIDS Res Hum Retroviruses.* 1998; 14(13):1157–1162.
134. Voss G, Kirchhoff F, Nick S, et al. Morphogenesis of recombinant HIV-2 gag core particles. *Virus Research.* 1992;24(2):197–210.
135. Henderson L, Sowder R, Copeland T, et al. Gag precursors of HIV and SIV are cleaved into six proteins found in the mature virions. *J Med Primatol.* 1990;19:411–419.
136. Gorelick RJ, Nigida SM, Bess JW, et al. Noninfectious human immunodeficiency virus type 1 mutants deficient in genomic RNA. *J Virol.* 1990;64(7):3207–3211.
137. Komatsu H, Tsukahara T, Tozawa H. Viral RNA binding properties of human immunodeficiency virus type-2 (HIV-2) nucleocapsid protein-derived synthetic peptides. *Biochem Molec Bio Intern.* 1996;38(6):1143–1154.
138. Lee WR, Syu WJ, Du B, et al. Nonrandom distribution of gp120 N-linked glycosylation sites important for infectivity of human immunodeficiency virus type 1. *Proc Natl Acad Sci USA.* 1992; 89(6):2213–2217.
139. Lee WR, Yu XF, Syu WJ, et al. Mutational analysis of conserved N-linked glycosylation sites of human immunodeficiency virus type 1 gp41. *J Virol.* 1992;66(3):1799–1803.
140. Leonard CK, Spellman MW, Riddle L, et al. Assignment of intrachain disulfide bonds and characterization of potential glycosylation sites of

the type 1 recombinant human immunodeficiency virus envelope glycoprotein (gp120) expressed in Chinese hamster ovary cells. *J Bio Chem*. 1990; 265(18):10373–10382.

141. Guyader M, Emerman M, Sonigo P, et al. Genome organization and transactivation of the human immunodeficiency virus type 2. *Nature*. 1987; 326:662–669.
142. Kuhnel H, von Briesen H, Dietrich U, et al. Molecular cloning of two west African human immunodeficiency virus type 2 isolates that replicate well in macrophages: a Gambian isolate, from a patient with neurologic acquired immunodeficiency syndrome, and a highly divergent Ghanian isolate. *Proc Natl Acad Sci USA*. 1989;86:2383–2387.
143. Hasegawa A, Tsujimoto H, Maki N, et al. Genomic divergence of HIV-2 from Ghana. *AIDS Res Hum Retroviruses*. 1989;5(6):593–604.
144. Kumar P, Hui HX, Kappes JC, et al. Molecular characterization of an attenuated human immunodeficiency virus type 2 isolate. *J Virol*. 1990; 64:890–901.
145. Klemm E, Schneweis KE, Horn R, et al. HIV-2 infection with initial neurological manifestation. *J Neurol*. 1988;235:304–307.
146. Sankalé JL, De La Tour RS, Marlink RG, et al. Distinct quasi-species in the blood and the brain of an HIV-2–infected individual. *Virology*. 1996; 226(2):418–423.
147. Steffy K, Kraus G, Looney D, et al. Role of the fusogenic peptide sequence in syncytium induction and infectivity of human immunodeficiency virus type 2. *J Virol*. 1992;66:4532–4535.
148. Robert-Guroff M, Aldrich K, Muldoon R, et al. Cross-neutralization of human immunodeficiency virus type 1 and 2 and simian immunodeficiency virus isolates. *J Virol*. 1992;66(6):3602–3608.
149. Bjorling E, Broliden K, Bernardi D, et al. Hyperimmune antisera against synthetic peptides representing the glycoprotein of human immunodeficiency virus type 2 can mediate neutralization and antibody-dependent cytotoxic activity. *Proc Natl Acad Sci USA*. 1991;88:6082–6086.
150. Nixon DF, Huet S, Rothbard J, et al. An HIV-1 and HIV-2 cross-reactive cytotoxic T-cell epitope. *AIDS*. 1990;4(9):841–845.
151. Cao H, Kanki P, Sankale J-L, et al. Cytotoxic T-lymphocyte cross-reactivity among different human immunodeficiency virus type 1 clades: implication for vaccine development. *J Virol*. 1997;71(11):8615–8623.
152. Norley SG, Mikschy U, Werner A, et al. Demonstration of cross-reactive antibodies able to elicit lysis of both HIV-1– and HIV-2–infected cells. *J Immunol*. 1990;145:1700–1705.
153. Ljunggren K, Chiodi F, Biberfeld G, et al. Lack of cross-reaction in antibody-dependent cellular cytotoxicity between human immunodeficiency virus (HIV) and HIV-related West African strains. *J Immunol*. 1988;140(2):602–605.
154. Huang M, Essex M, Lee TH. Localization of immunogenic domains in the human immunodeficiency virus type 2 envelope. *J Virol*. 1991;65: 5073–5079.
155. Mannervik M, Putkonen P, Ruden U, et al. Identification of B-cell antigenic sites on HIV-2 gp125. *JAIDS*. 1992;5(2):177–187.
156. Norrby E, Putkonen P, Bottiger B, et al. Comparison of linear antigenic sites in the envelope proteins of human immunodeficiency virus (HIV) type 2 and type 1. *AIDS Res Hum Retroviruses*. 1991;7(3):279–285.
157. Bjorling E, von Garrelts E, Morner A, et al. Human neutralizing human immunodeficiency virus type 2–specific Fab molecules generated by phage display. *J Gen Virol*. 1999;80(Pt 8):1987–1993.
158. McKnight A, Shotton C, Cordell J, et al. Location, exposure, and conservation of neutralizing and nonneutralizing epitopes on human immunodeficiency virus type 2 SU glycoprotein. *J Virol*. 1996;70(7):4598–4606.
159. Weiss RA, Clapham PR, Weber JN, et al. HIV-2 antisera cross-neutralize HIV-1. *AIDS*. 1988;2:95–100.
160. Bottiger B, Karlsson A, Andreasson PA, et al. Cross-neutralizing antibodies against HIV-1 (HTLV-IIIB and HTLV-IIIRF) and HIV-2 (SBL-6669 and a new isolate SBL-K135). *AIDS Res Hum Retroviruses*. 1989;5:525–533.
161. Mulligan MJ, Ritter GD, Chaikin MA, et al. Human immunodeficiency virus type 2 envelope glycoprotein: differential CD4 interactions of soluble gp120 versus the assembled envelope complex. *Virology*. 1992;187:233–241.
162. Bottiger B, Karlsson A, Andreasson PA, et al. Envelope cross-reactivity between human immunodeficiency virus types 1 and 2 detected by different serological methods: correlation between cross-neutralization and reactivity against the main neutralizing site. *J Virol*. 1990;64:3492–3499.
163. Holzer T, Allen R, Heynen C, et al. Discrimination of HIV-2 infection from HIV-1 infection by western blot and radioimmuno-precipitation analysis. *AIDS Res Hum Retroviruses*. 1990;6:515–524.
164. AIDS: Recommendations for interpretation of HIV-2 western blot results. *WHO Weekly Epidemiol Rec*. 1990;65:74–5.
165. Baillou A, Janvier B, Mayer R, et al. Site-Directed Serology Using Synthetic Oligopeptides Representing the C-terminus of the External Glycoproteins of HIV-1, HIV-2, or SIV_{mac} May Distinguish Subtypes Among Primate Lentiviruses. *AIDS Res Hum Retroviruses*. 1991;7:767–772.
166. Baillou A, Janvier B, Leonard G, et al. Fine serotyping of human immunodeficiency virus

serotype 1 (HIV-1) and HIV-2 infections by using synthetic oligopeptides representing an immunodominant domain of HIV-1 and HIV-2/simian immunodeficiency virus. *J Clin Microbiol.* 1991;29(7):1387–1391.

167. Ayres L, Avillez F, Garcia Benito A, et al. Multicenter evaluation of a new recombinant enzyme immunoassay for the combined detection of antibody to HIV-1 and HIV-2. *AIDS.* 1990;4: 131–138.
168. Broliden PA, Ruden U, Ouattara AS, et al. Specific synthetic peptides for detection of and discrimination between HIV-1 and HIV-2 infection. *JAIDS.* 1991;4(10):952–958.
169. Gueye-Ndiaye A, Clark R, Samuel K, et al. Cost-Effective Diagnosis of HIV-1 and HIV-2 By Recombinant-Expressed env Peptide (566/966) Dot Blot Analysis. *AIDS.* 1993;7:481–495.
170. Zuber M, Samuel KP, Lautenberger JA, et al. Bacterially produced HIV-2 env polypeptides specific for distinguishing HIV-2 from HIV-1 infections. *AIDS Res Hum Retroviruses.* 1990;6:525–534.
171. Andersson S, da Silva Z, Norrgren H, et al. Field evaluation of alternative testing strategies for diagnosis and differentiation of HIV-1 and HIV-2 infections in an HIV-1 and HIV-2–prevalent area. *AIDS.* 1997;11(15):1815–1822.
172. Kanki PJ, Hamel DJ, Sankalé J-L, et al. Human Immunodeficiency Virus Type 1 Subtypes Differ in Disease Progression. *J Infect Dis.* 1999;179:68–73.
173. Kanki PJ, Barin F, M'Boup S, et al. New human T-lymphotropic retrovirus related to simian T-lymphotropic virus type III (STLV-IIIAGM). *Science.* 1986;232(4747):238–243.
174. Tedder R, O'Connor T, Hughs A, et al. Envelope cross-reactivity in western blot for HIV-1 and HIV-2 may not indicate dual infection. *Lancet.* 1988; 2(8617):927–930.
175. Kanki P, Mboup S, Barin F, et al. The Biology of HIV-1 and HIV-2 in Africa. In: Giraldo G, Beth-Giraldo E, Klumeck N, et al., eds. *AIDS and Associated Cancers in Africa.* Basel: S. Karger; 1988:230–236.
176. Evans L, Moreau J, Odehouri K, et al. Simultaneous isolation of HIV-1 and HIV-2 from an AIDS patient. *Lancet.* 1988;2(8625):1389–1391.
177. Peeters M, Gershy-Damet GM, Fransen K, et al. Virological and polymerase chain reaction studies of HIV-1/HIV-2 dual infection in Cote d'Ivoire. *Lancet.* 1992;340(8815):339–340.
178. Rayfield M, De Cock K, Heyward W, et al. Mixed human immunodeficiency virus (HIV) infection in an individual: demonstration of both HIV type 1 and type 2 proviral sequences by using polymerase chain reaction. *J Infect Dis.* 1988;158:1170–1176.
179. Dieng-Sarr A, Thior I, Kokkotou E, et al. HIV-1 and HIV-2 dual infection: lack of HIV-2 provirus correlates with low CD4+ lymphocyte counts. *AIDS.* 1998;12(2):131–137.
180. Dieng-Sarr A, Popper S, Thior I, et al. Relationship between HIV-2 proviral load and CD4+ lymphocytes differs in HIV monotypic and dual infection. *J Hum Virol.* 1999;2(1):45–51.
181. Donnelly C, Leisenring W, Kanki P, et al. Comparison of transmission rates of HIV-1 and HIV-2 in a cohort of prostitutes in Senegal. *Bull Math Biol.* 1993;55(4):731–743.
182. Hendry R, Parks D, Campos Mello D, et al. Lack of evidence for HIV-2 infection among at-risk individuals in Brazil. *JAIDS.* 1991;4:623.
183. Kvinesdal BB, Worm AM, Lindhardt BO, et al. HIV-2 infection in Denmark. *Scand J Inf Dis.* 1992;24(4):419–421.
184. Georgoulias V, Agelakis A, Fountouli P, et al. Seroprevalence of HIV-2 infection in Greece (Crete). *JAIDS.* 1990;3(12):1188–1192.
185. Costigliola P, Ricchi E, Manfredi R, et al. No evidence of HIV-2 infection amongst HIV-1 Ab positive people in the largest cities of north-eastern Italy. *Euro J Epid.* 1992;8(1):140–141.
186. Estebanez P, Sarasqueta C, Rua-Figueroa M, et al. Absence of HIV-2 in Spanish groups at risk for HIV-1 infection. *AIDS Res Hum Retroviruses.* 1992;8(4):423–424.
187. Downing RG, Biryahwaho B. No evidence for HIV-2 infection in Uganda. *Lancet.* 1990; 336(8729):1514–1515.
188. O'Brien TR, George JR, Epstein JS, et al. Testing for antibodies to human immunodeficiency virus type 2 in the United States. *MMWR.* 1992;41(RR-12):1–9.
189. Recommendations for the prevention of human immunodeficiency virus (HIV) transmission by blood and blood products. Food and Drug Administration, Center for Biologics Evaluation and Research, Bethesda, MD; 1990.
190. Dufoort G, Courouce A, Ancelle-Park R, et al. No Clinical Signs 14 years after HIV-2 transmission via Blood Transfusion. *Lancet.* 1988;2:510.
191. Kanki P. Epidemiology and Natural History of HIV-2. In: DeVita VJ, Hellman S, Rosenberg S, eds. *In AIDS: Etiology, Diagnosis, Treatment, and Prevention.* 4th Edition ed. Philadelphia, PA: J. B. Lippincott Co; 1997:127–135.
192. Gilbert P, McKeague I, Eisen G, et al. Comparison of HIV-1 and HIV-2 infectivity from a prospective cohort study in Senegal. 2001 (*in press*).
193. Pepin J, Quigley M, Todd J, et al. Association between HIV-2 infection and genital ulcer diseases among male sexually transmitted disease patients in The Gambia. *AIDS.* 1992;6(5):489–493.
194. Kanki P, Mboup S, Marlink R, et al. Prevalence and Risk Determinants of Human Immunodeficiency Virus Type 2 (HIV-2) and Human Immunodeficiency Virus Type 1 (HIV-1) in West African

Female Prostitutes. *Amer J Epidemiol.* 1992;136: 895–907.

195. Aaby P, Ariyoshi K, Buckner M, et al. Age of wife as a major determinant of male-to-female transmission of HIV-2 infection: a community study from rural West Africa. *AIDS.* 1996;10(13): 1585–1590.
196. Morgan G, Wilkins HA, Pepin J, et al. AIDS following mother-to-child transmission of HIV-2. *AIDS.* 1990;4(9):879–882.
197. Gayle H, Gnaore E, Adjorlolo G, et al. HIV-1 and HIV-2 infection in children in Abidjan, Cote D'Ivoire. *JAIDS.* 1992;5:513.
198. Del Mistro A, Chotard J, Mali A, et al. HIV-1 and HIV-2 seroprevalence rates in mother-child pairs living in The Gambia, West Africa. *JAIDS.* 1992;5:19–24.
199. Poulsen AG, Kvinesdal BB, Aaby P, et al. Lack of evidence of vertical transmission of human immunodeficiency virus type 2 in a sample of the general population in Bissau. *JAIDS.* 1992; 5:25–30.
200. Comparison of vertical human immunodeficiency virus type 2 and human immunodeficiency virus type 1 transmission in the French prospective cohort. The HIV Infection in Newborns French Collaborative Study Group. *Pediatr Infect Dis J.* 1994;13:502.
201. Abbott RC, Ndour-Sarr A, Diouf A, et al. Risk Determinants for HIV Infection and Adverse Obstetrical Outcomes in Pregnant Women in Dakar, Senegal. *JAIDS.* 1994;7:711–717.
202. O'Donovan D, Ariyoshi K, Milligan P, et al. Maternal plasma viral RNA levels determine marked differences in mother-to-child transmission rates of HIV-1 and HIV-2 in The Gambia. *AIDS.* 2000;14(4):441–448.
203. Marlink R, Kanki P, Thior I, et al. Reduced Rate of Disease Development with HIV-2 Compared to HIV-1. *Science.* 1994;265:1587–1590.
204. Lisse IM, Poulsen A-G, Aaby P, et al. Immunodeficiency in HIV-2 infection: a community study from Guinea-Bissau. *AIDS.* 1990;4: 1263–1266.
205. Kestens L, Brattegard K, Adjorlolo G, et al. Immunological comparison of HIV-1, HIV-2 and dually-reactive women delivering in Abidjan, Cote d'Ivoire. *AIDS.* 1992;6:803–807.
206. Pepin J, Morgan G, Dunn D, et al. HIV-2–induced immunosuppression among asymptomatic West African prostitutes: evidence that HIV-2 is pathogenic, but less so than HIV-1. *AIDS.* 1991; 5:1165–1172.
207. Lisse IM, Poulsen AG, Aaby P, et al. Serial CD4 and CD8 T-lymphocyte counts and associated mortality in an HIV-2–infected population in Guinea-Bissau. *JAIDS.* 1996;13(4):355–362.
208. Traore I, Marlink R, Thior I, et al. HIV-2 as a model for long term non-progression. XI International Conference on AIDS; 1996;Vancouver, Canada.
209. Victorino R, Guerreiro D, Pinto L, et al. Clinical, immunological and epidemiological assessment of women with indeterminate western blots for HIV antibodies. International Conference on AIDS. 1992;8(3):160 (abstract no. PuC 8046).
210. Michel P, Balde AT, Roussilhon C, et al. Reduced immune activation and T cell apoptosis in human immunodeficiency virus type 2 compared with type 1: correlation of T cell apoptosis with beta2 microglobulin concentration and disease evolution. *J Infect Dis.* 2000;181(1):64–75.
211. Cavaleiro R, Sousa A, Loureiro A, et al. Marked immunosuppressive effects of the HIV-2 envelope protein in spite of the lower HIV-2 pathogenicity. *AIDS.* 2000;14:2679–2686.
212. Asjo B, Albert J, Karlsson A, et al. Replicative capacity of human immunodeficiency virus from patients with varying severity of HIV infection. *Lancet.* 1986;ii:660–662.
213. Fenyo E, Albert J, Asjo B. Replicative capacity, cytopathic effect and cell tropism of HIV. *AIDS.* 1989;3(supp 1):S5–S12.
214. Mulligan MJ, Kumar P, Hui HX, et al. The env protein of an infectious noncytopathic HIV-2 is deficient in syncytium formation. *AIDS Res Hum Retroviruses.* 1990;6:707–720.
215. Schulz T, Whitby D, Hoad J, et al. Biological and molecular variability of human immunodeficiency virus type 2 isolates from The Gambia. *J Virol.* 1990;64:5177–5182.
216. Sankalé JL, MBoup S, Marlink R, et al. HIV-2 and HIV-1 Quasispecies in Cervical Secretions and Blood. *AIDS Res Hum Retroviruses.* 1998; 14(16): 1473–1481.
217. Simon F, Matheron S, Tamalet C, et al. Cellular and Plasma Viral Load in Patients Infected with HIV-2. *AIDS.* 1993;7:1411–1417.
218. Berry N, Ariyoshi K, Jobe O, et al. HIV Type 2 Proviral Load measured by Quantitative Poly-merase Chain Reaction correlates with CD4+ Lymphopenia in HIV Type 2–Infected Individuals. *AIDS Res Hum Retroviruses.* 1994;10:1031–1037.
219. Berry N, Ariyoshi K, Jaffar S, et al. Low peripheral blood viral HIV-2 RNA in individuals with high CD4 percentage differentiates HIV-2 from HIV-1 infection. *J Hum Virol.* 1998;1(7):457–468.
220. Soriano V, Gomes P, Holguin A, et al. HIV-2 in Portugal: circulating subtypes, virus isolation, plasma viral load, and clinical spectrum (The HIV-2 Iberian Project). International Conference on AIDS. 1998;12:269 (abstract no. 21154).
221. Andersson S, Norrgren H, da Silva Z, et al. Plasma viral load in HIV-1 and HIV-2 singly and dually infected individuals in Guinea Bissau,

West Africa: significantly lower plasma virus set point in HIV-2 infection than in HIV-1 infection. *ArchInternal Med.* 2000;160:3286–3293.

222. Popper SJ, Dieng-Sarr A, Guèye-NDiaye A, et al. Low Plasma HIV-2 viral load is independent of proviral load: low virus production in vivo. *J Virol.* 2000;74(3):1554–1557.
223. Clavel F, Guetard D, Brun-Vezinet F, et al. Isolation of a new human retrovirus from West African patients with AIDS. *Science.* 1986;233:343–346.
224. Saimot AG, Coulaud JP, Mechali D, et al. HIV-2/LAV-2 in Portuguese man with AIDS (Paris, 1978) who had served in Angola in 1968–74. *Lancet.* 1987;i:688.
225. De Cock K, Odehouri K, Colebunders R, et al. A comparison of HIV-1 and HIV-2 infections in hospitalized patients in Abidjan, Cote d'Ivoire. *AIDS.* 1990;4:443.
226. Le Guenno BM, Barabe P, Griffet PA, et al. HIV-2 and HIV-1 AIDS Cases in Senegal: Clinical patterns and immunological perturbations. *JAIDS.* 1991;4(4):421–427.
227. Schneider J, Luke W, Kirchhoff F, et al. Isolation and characterization of HIV-2 obtained from a patient with predominantly neurological defects. *AIDS.* 1990;4:455.
228. Dwyer D, Matheron S, Bakchine S, et al. Detection of human immunodeficiency virus type 2 in brain tissue. *J Infect Dis.* 1992;166:888.
229. Marlink RG, Ricard D, M'Boup S, et al. Clinical, hematologic, and immunologic cross-sectional evaluation of individuals exposed to human immunodeficiency virus type 2 (HIV-2). *AIDS Res Hum Retroviruses.* 1988;4:137–148.
230. Diouf K, Dieng-Sarr A, Popper S, et al. HIV-2 and HLA: associations with rate of disease progression. 2001 (*in press*).
231. Carrington M, Nelson GW, Martin MP, et al. HLA and HIV-1: heterozygote advantage and B*35-Cw*04 disadvantage. *Science.* 1999;283: 1748–1752.
232. Kanki P, Essex M, Barin F. Antigenic Relationships Between HTLV-3/LAV, STLV-3, and HTLV-4. In: Chanock RM, Lerner RA, Brown F, et al., eds. *Vaccines 87: Modern Approaches to New Vaccines.* Cold Spring Harbor: Cold Spring Harbor Laboratory; 1987:185–187.
233. Essex M, Kanki P, Barin F, et al. Immunogenicity of HIV-1 and HIV-2 Antigens and Relationship to Disease Development. In: Girard M, Vallette L, eds. *2e Colloque des «Cent Gardes»: Retroviruses of Human A.I.D.S. and Related Animal Diseases.* Paris: Marnes-la-Coquette; 1988:219–220.
234. Bjorling E, Scarlatti G, von Gegerfelt A, et al. Autologous neutralizing antibodies prevail in HIV-2 but not in HIV-1 infection. *Virology.* 1993;193(1): 528–530.
235. Bjorling E, Chiodi F, Utter G, et al. Two neutralizing domains in the V3 region of the envelope glycoprotein gp125 of HIV-2 type 2. *J Immunol.* 1994;152:1952–1959.
236. Fenyo EM, Putkonen P. Broad cross-neutralizing activity in serum is associated with slow progression and low risk of transmission in primate lentivirus infections. *Immunology Letters.* 1996;51(1–2):95–99.
237. Belec L, Tevi-Benissan C, Dupre T, et al. Comparison of cervicovaginal humoral immunity in clinically asymptomatic (CDC A1 and A2 category) patients with HIV-1 and HIV-2 infection. *J Clin Immunol.* 1996;16(1):12–20.
238. Gotch F, McAdam SN, Allsopp CE, et al. Cytotoxic T cells in HIV2 seropositive Gambians. Identification of a virus-specific MHC-restricted peptide epitope. *J Immunol.* 1993;151(6):3361–3369.
239. Bertoletti A, Cham F, McAdam S, et al. Cytotoxic T cells from human Immunodeficiency virus type 2 infected patients frequently cross-react with different human immunodeficiency virus type 1 clades. *J Virol.* 1998;72(3):2439–2448.
240. Dieng Sarr A, Lu Y, Sankalé J-L, et al. Robust HIV-2 cellular immune response measured by a modified Anthrax toxin-based ELISPOT assay. *AIDS Res Hum Retroviruses.* 2001;17(13):1257–1264.
241. Travers K, MBoup S, Marlink R, et al. Natural Protection Against HIV-1 Infection Provided by HIV-2. *Science.* 1995;268:1612–1615.
242. Travers K, Eisen G, Marlink, R, et al. Protection from HIV-1 infection by HIV-2. *AIDS.* 1998; 12:224–225.
243. Wiktor SZ, Nkengasong JN, Ekpini ER, et al. Lack of protection against HIV-1 infection among women with HIV-2 infection. *AIDS.* 1999;13(6):695–699.
244. Aaby P, Poulsen AG, Larsen O, et al. Does HIV-2 protect against HIV-1 infection? [letter] [see comments]. Comment in: AIDS 1998 Jan 22; 12(2):224–5. *AIDS.* 1997;11(7):939–940.
245. Ariyoshi K, van der Loeff M, Sabally S, et al. Does HIV-2 infection provide cross-protection against HIV-1 infection? (letter). *AIDS.* 1997; 11(1053–1054).
246. Norrgren H, Andersson S, Biague AJ, et al. Trends and interaction of HIV-1 and HIV-2 in Guinea-Bissau, West Africa: no protection of HIV-2 against HIV-1 infection. *AIDS.* 1999;13:701–707.
247. Arya SK, Gallo RC. Human immunodeficiency virus (HIV) type 2–mediated inhibition of HIV type 1: a new approach to gene therapy of HIV-infection. *Proc Natl Acad Sci USA.* 1996;93(9): 4486–4491.
248. Rappaport J, Arya SK, Richardson MW, et al. Inhibition of HIV-1 expression by HIV-2. *J Mole Med.* 1995;73(12):583–589.
249. Dieng-Sarr A, Sankalé J-L, Hamel DJ, et al. Genetic Analysis of HIV Type 2 in Monotypic and

Dual HIV Infections. *AIDS Res Hum Retroviruses*. 2000;16(3):297–300.
250. Dieng-Sarr A, Sankalé J-L, Hamel DJ, et al. Interaction with Human Immunodeficiency Virus (HIV) Type 2 Predicts HIV Type 1 Genotype. *Virology*. 2000;268:402–410.
251. Paxton WA, Martin SR, Tse D, et al. Relative resistance to HIV-1 infection of CD4 lymphocytes from persons who remain uninfected despite multiple high-risk sexual exposure. *Nature Medicine*. 1996;2(4):412–417.
252. Cocchi F, DeVico AL, Garzino-Demo A, et al. Identification of RANTES, MIP-1 alpha, and MIP-1 beta as the major HIV-suppressive factors produced by CD8+ T cells. *Science*. 1995; 270(5243):1811–1815.
253. Zagury D LA, Chams V, Fall L, et al. C–C chemokines, pivotal in protection against HIV type 1 infection. *Proc Natl Acad Sci USA*. 1998;95: 3857–3861.
254. Lehner T, Wang Y, Cranage M, et al. Protective mucosal immunity elicited by targeted iliac lymph node immunization with a subunit SIV envelope and core vaccine in macaques. *Nature Medicine*. 1996;2(7):767–775.
255. Kokkotou EG, Sankalé J-L, Mani I, et al. In vitro correlates of HIV-2 mediated HIV-1 protection. *Proc Natl Acad Sci USA*. 2000;97(12):6797–6802.
256. Neoh LP, Akimoto H, Kaneko H, et al. The production of beta-chemokines induced by HIV-2 envelope glycoprotein [letter]. *AIDS*. 1997;11(8): 1062–1063.
257. Locher CP, Blackbourn DJ, Barnett SW, et al. Superinfection With Human Immunodeficiency Virus Type 2 Can Reactivate Virus Production In Baboons But Is Contained By a Cd8 T Cell Antiviral Response. *J Infect Dis*. 1997;176(4):948–959.
258. Putkonen P, Thorstensson R, Albert J, et al. Infection of cynomolgus monkeys with HIV-2 protects against pathogenic consequences of a subsequent simian immunodeficiency virus infection. *AIDS*. 1990;4(8):783–789.
259. Putkonen P, Thorstensson R, Walther L, et al. Vaccine protection against HIV-2 infection in cynomolgus monkeys. *AIDS Res Hum Retroviruses*. 1991;7(3):271–277.
260. Andersson S, Makitalo B, Thorstensson R, et al. Immunogenicity and protective efficacy of a human immunodeficiency virus type 2 recombinant canarypox (ALVAC) vaccine candidate in cynomolgus monkeys. *J Inf Dis*. 1996;174(5):977–985.
261. Biberfeld G, Thorstensson R, Putkonen P. Protection against human immunodeficiency virus type 2 and simian immunodeficiency virus in macaques vaccinated against human immunodeficiency virus type 2. *AIDS Res Hum Retroviruses*. 1996;12(5):443–446.
262. Myagkikh M, Alipanah S, Markham PD, et al. Multiple immunizations with attenuated poxvirus HIV type 2 recombinants and subunit boosts required for protection of rhesus macaques. *AIDS Res Hum Retroviruses*. 1996;12(11):985–992.
263. De Clercq E, Yamamoto N, Pauwels R, et al. Potent and selective inhibition of human immunodeficiency virus (HIV)-1 and HIV-2 replication by a class of bicyclams interacting with a viral uncoating event. *Proc Natl Acad Sci USA*. 1992; 89(12):5286–5290.
264. Bottiger D, Putkonen P, Oberg B. Prevention of HIV-2 and SIV infections in cynomolgus macaques by prophylactic treatment with 3′-fluorothymidine. *AIDS Res Hum Retroviruses*. 1992;8(7):1235–1238.
265. Schutten M, van der Ende ME, Osterhaus AD. Antiretroviral therapy in patients with dual infection with human immunodeficiency virus types 1 and 2 [letter]. *N Eng J Med*. 2000;342(23):1758–1760.
266. Ayanian JZ, Maguire JH, Marlink R, et al. HIV-2 Infection in the United States. *N Engl J Med* 1989;320:1422–1423.
267. Clark NM, Dieng-Sarr A, Sankale JL, et al. Immunologic and virologic response of HIV-2 infection to antiretroviral therapy [letter]. *AIDS*. 1998;12(18):2506–2507.
268. Rodes B, Holguin A, Soriano V, et al. Emergence of drug resistance mutations in human immunodeficiency virus type 2–infected subjects undergoing antiretroviral therapy. *J Clin Microbio*. 2000;38(4): 1370–1374.

6

Simian Immunodeficiency Viruses and the Origin of HIVs

[*]Ousmane M. Diop, [†]Aïssatou Guèye, [‡]Ahidjo Ayouba, [‡]Eric Nerrienet, [†]Sylvie Corbet, [‡§]Philippe Mauclère, [||]François Simon, [†]Françoise Barré-Sinoussi, and [†]Michaela C. Müller-Trutwin

[*]*Laboratoire des Rétrovirus Simiens, Institut Pasteur, Dakar, Senegal.*
[†]*Unité de Biologie des Rétrovirus, Institut Pasteur, Paris, France.*
[‡]*Laboratoire de Virologie, Centre Pasteur, Yaoundé, Cameroon.*
[§]*Institut Pasteur, Antananarivo, Madagascar.*
[||]*Centre International de Recherche Médicales de Franceville, Franceville, Gabon.*

To date, three retroviruses have been isolated in humans: human T-lymphotropic virus (HTLV), human immunodeficiency virus (HIV), and human foamy virus (HFV). Each has a simian counterpart: simian T-lymphotropic virus (STLV), simian immunodeficiency virus (SIV), and simian foamy virus (SFV).

STLV-1, the simian form of HTLV-1, is present in at least 19 species of Old World primates living in Africa and Asia. Similar to HTLV-1, the seroprevalence rate for STLV-1 increases with the age of the host and is higher among females. Mother-to-infant transmission, occurring mainly through breastfeeding, and male-to-female sexual transmission are predominant. However, an investigation of STLV-1 transmission among mandrills in a semi-free colony showed an exception to this rule: Transmission was shown to be primarily male-to-male, the result of adult male fighting (1).

Phylogenetic analysis of STLV-1 *env* sequences from several species revealed 10 molecular aggregates reflecting the geographic origins of the animals rather than those of the host species. This implies that several cross-species transmissions occurred in the wild (2,3). The evolutionary history shared by the majority of HTLV-1 and STLV-1 subtypes isolated from wild-caught nonhuman primates also supports the hypothesis that these subtypes arose from interspecific transmissions (4). In summary, there is compelling evidence in support of the hypothesis that the origin and actual distribution of HTLV/STLV is the result of at least four running and/or concomitant events: (*i*) STLV-1 transmission to humans, (*ii*) STLV-1 transmission among different simian species in nature, (*iii*) HTLV-1 persistence in isolated human populations, and (*iv*) migration of HTLV-1–infected human populations (5).

As in humans infected with HTLV-1, adult T-cell leukemia/lymphoma (ATLL) disease has been described in some STLV-1–infected primates, with clonal integration of provirus in tumoral cells (6,7). However these pathologies are infrequent; about 10 cases have been reported in only a few species, that is, African green monkeys (AGMs) (*Chlorocebus* spp.), macaques (*Macaca* spp.), gorillas (*Gorilla gorilla*), and baboons (*Papio* spp.). No tropical spastic paralysis/HTLV-1 associated myelopathy (TSP/HAM) has yet been described in nonhuman primates.

EPIDEMIOLOGY OF SIV

In the mid-1980s, the first simian lentivirus closely related to HIV was isolated from a captive rhesus macaque (*Macaca mulatta*) presenting clinical signs of an AIDS-like immunodeficiency (8,9). Soon thereafter, several cases of SIV infection were described in various macaque species held in captivity in primate centers in the United States: SIVcyn from the crab-eating macaque (*Macaca fascicularis)* (10), SIVmne from the pigtailed macaque (*Macaca nemestrina*) (11), and SIVstm from the stumptailed macaque (*Macaca arctoïdes*) (12). Molecular analyses of the causative agent of those infections showed it to be a new SIV now named SIVmac. It is noteworthy that seroepidemiologic studies conducted in Asia, where macaques are indigenous, show that these monkeys are not infected in the wild (13,14) suggesting that they are not a natural host for SIV (Figure 1).

In contrast, studies of AGMs and sooty mangabeys (*Cercocebus atys*) reveal that these animals are infected in their natural habitats in Africa by SIVagm and SIVsm, respectively (15,16). In several hundred wild-born AGMs, regardless of species and geographic location [the vervet monkey (*Chlorocebus pygerythrus*) and the grivet monkey (*C. aethiops*) in East Africa, the green monkey (*C. ṣabaeus*) in West Africa, or the tantalus monkey (*C. tantalus*) in Central Africa], seroprevalence rates of about 40% to 50% were described (14,17–19). However, it appears that AGMs living on Caribbean islands, captured and brought from Africa during the seventeenth and eighteenth centuries, were not infected by SIVagm (17,20,21). The absence of SIVagm in these animals might suggest that SIV was not present in AGMs at the time of their migration. However, another possible explanation for this difference is that the Caribbean population of AGMs originated from a few very young monkeys that were not infected with SIV. Indeed, we did a retrospective analysis of samples of sabaeus monkey sera taken between 1967 and 2000 in Senegal and showed that the infection rate correlated with the age of the animals (22). In the adult monkeys the seroprevalence rate was 80%, a rate that was at least fourfold higher than that found for young monkeys between 1–3 years of age. Indeed, it is not unusual to find a lack of infection in very young monkeys as described in studies of some vervet colonies in East Africa (23). Similarly, in sooty mangabeys, adults seem to be infected more frequently than young animals (24). Exact seroprevalence rates, however, are unknown (25) owing to the limited amount of data available for animals in the wild.

Other species of the Cercopithecinae family are also natural hosts of SIV: SIVsyk in Sykes monkeys (*Cercopithecus albogularis*) (26), SIVrcm in red-capped mangabeys (*Cercocebus torquatus*) (27), SIVtal in talapoin monkeys (*Miopithecus talapoin*) (28), SIVdrl in drills (*Mandrillus leucophaeus*) (29), SIVlhoest in l'hoest monkeys (*Cercopithecus l'hoesti*) (30), SIVsun in suntailed monkeys (*Cercopithecus solatus*) (31), and SIVmnd in mandrills (*Mandrillus sphinx*) (Figure 1) (32). Mandrills, in fact, have recently been found to harbor two types of SIVmnd (33).

Among apes, the chimpanzee (*Pan troglodytes* spp.) has been found to be infected by a specific lentivirus (SIVcpz) (34). Chimpanzees have been classified into distinct subspecies (35,36): the Western common chimpanzee (*P.t. verus* and *P.t. vellerosus)* of West Africa, the Central common chimpanzee (*P.t. troglodytes)* of Central

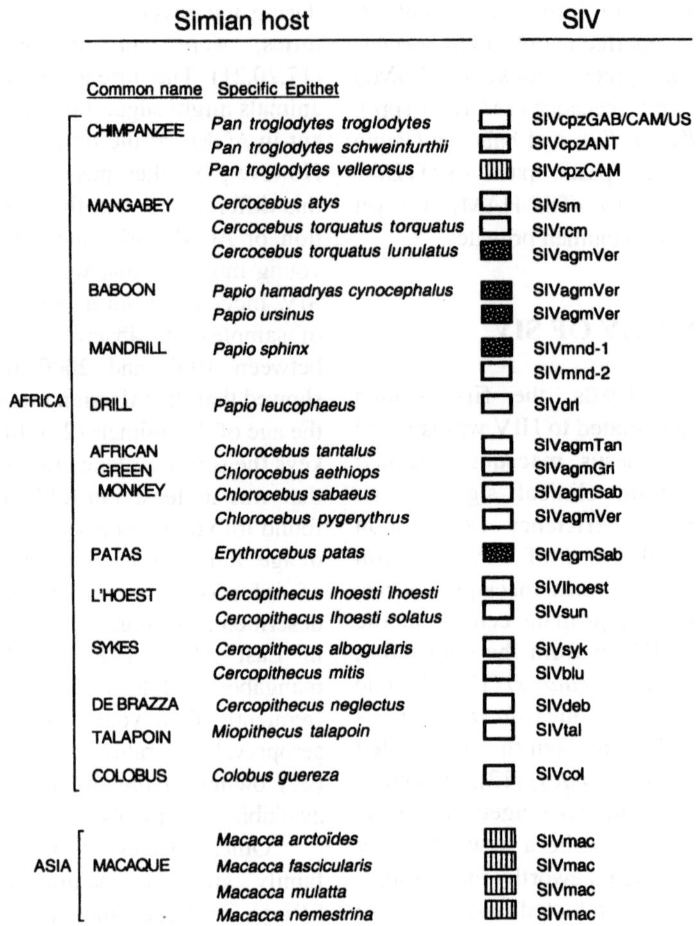

FIGURE 1. Simian host species for SIV. Simian species that correspond to natural host species for SIV are marked by a white box. Infection by SIV has been demonstrated in all cases by serology and sequence analysis. Those that do not carry a species-specific SIV, but that have been shown to occasionally harbor SIV, probably as a result of cross-species transmission in the wild, are indicated by a box with black points. All cited cross-species transmissions have been confirmed by sequence analysis (38,43,47–49,62). Simian species that harbor SIV only in captivity, that is, chimpanzees of the *P.t. vellerosus* subspecies and macaques, are indicated by a box with vertical lines. Indeed, no wild macaques or vellerosus chimpanzees have been found to be seropositive for SIV (13,14,37,38,62).

Africa, and the Eastern common chimpanzee (*P.t. schweinfurthii)* of East Africa. Until now, only members of the latter two subspecies have been found to harbor SIVcpz in nature (37,38). Of six known natural SIVcpz infections, five (SIVcpzGAB1, SIVcpzGAB2, SIVcpzUS, SIVcpzCAM3, and SIVcpzCAM5) have been found in members of the *P.t. troglodytes* subspecies, and one (SIVcpzANT) has been identified in a *P.t. schweinfurthii* animal (34). Interestingly, SIVcpzCAM5 was isolated from a wild-born chimpanzee immediately after its rescue, providing proof of SIVcpz infection in wild chimpanzees (39). Seroprevalence rates in wild adult chimpanzees are still unknown. Out of 125 wild-born animals that were captured at a young age (in Gabon, in the Democratic Republic of Congo, in Cameroon, or in Côte d'Ivoire), five were SIV seropositive (34,38,40). Of 98 chimpanzees held in U.S. primate centers, only one was infected by SIVcpz (37). However, a higher seroprevalence rate in wild adults versus captured young chimpanzees cannot be excluded.

SIV infections in guereza colobus monkeys (*Colobus guereza)* (41) and in three *Cercopithecus* species (42) have recently been reported (Figure 1). Finally, it is not unusual to find antibodies cross-reacting with HIV/SIV antigens in several other species of African monkeys including baboons (43) and patas (*Erythrocebus patas)* (our unpublished results). To date, however, all attempts to isolate lentivirus specific for these species have failed (13,14). It is likely that additional species harboring SIV will be identified in the future. In conclusion, most African apes and genera of monkeys, such as *Pan*, *Cercocebus*, *Chlorocebus*, *Cercopithecus*, *Colobus*, and *Miopithecus*, harbor SIV naturally. Among them, the AGMs, which have habitats in sub-Saharan regions with high SIV seroprevalence rates, represent the largest natural reservoir of SIVs.

MODES OF TRANSMISSION

Seroepidemiologic studies conducted thus far in AGMs, sooty mangabeys, and mandrills have shown that seroprevalence rates are higher in adults than in young animals and higher in males than in female monkeys, suggesting preferential horizontal transmission. In AGMs, we and others have shown that horizontal transmission probably occurs by sexual intercourse and through biting (44–46). Seropositivity was rare or absent in animals before behavioral adulthood despite high prevalence in adult females, suggesting a lack of mother-to-infant transmission (23). This scheme may not be applicable to all species and situations; in a study of members of a semi-free colony of mandrills, SIV transmission was found to occur primarily among males through male-on-male biting rather than among females through sexual intercourse. Interestingly, one case of mother-to-infant transmission was also described in this mandrill colony (1). Interspecies SIV transmission through biting may be an important route of infection in the wild, a conclusion to some extent substantiated by the presence of SIVagm in patas monkeys in West Africa (47) and in baboons in East and South Africa (48,49). Both groups share ecologic regions with AGMs.

CLASSIFICATION AND EVOLUTION OF PRIMATE LENTIVIRUSES

Genomic Organization

Primate lentiviruses share a complex genomic organization that differs from that of other retroviruses. Like HIV, SIVs possess three major structural genes common to all retroviruses (*gag*, *pol*, and *env*), in addition to regulatory elements [long terminal repeats (LTRs)] located at the extremities of the SIV genome. SIVs also contain several accessory genes (*vif*, *rev*, *tat*, *nef*, *vpr*, *vpx*, and *vpu*). These accessory genes, located in the genome's central region and at its 3′ end, encode proteins also implicated in the viral replication process. While all primate lentiviruses contain the regulatory genes *vif*, *rev*, *tat*, *vpr*, and *nef*, the presence of *vpu* and *vpx* is virus-specific. Therefore, primate lentiviruses have been grouped into at least three types: the HIV-1 and SIVcpz group of viruses, which contain *vpu* (50,51); the HIV-2, SIVsm, and SIVmac group of viruses, which is characterized by the presence of *vpx* (52–54); and the SIVagm, SIVmnd, SIVsyk, and SIVlhoest group, which contain neither *vpx* nor *vpu* (31,55,56) (see Chapter 2, Figure 2, *this volume*). Based on high-sequence homology, it is generally thought that *vpr* served as the ancestor to *vpx*, which resulted from duplication of *vpr* during its evolution. The general organization described for the HIV-1 genome is similar to that for SIVcpz, and the organization described for the HIV-2 genome is similar to that for SIVsm.

Phylogenetic Relationships

When full-length genomic sequences of certain nonhuman primate lentiviruses in the three groups are available, they are found to fall into at least six approximately equidistant lineages represented by: SIVcpz, SIVsm, SIVagm, SIVsyk, SIVcol, and SIVlhoest. Nucleotide divergence between two lineages is approximately 50% in *pol* and 70% in *env*. Within SIVs belonging to the same lineage, maximal variations reach 30% in *pol* and 45% in *env*.

Characterization of SIVcpz and HIV-1 genomes show they have the same genomic organization and the same phylogenetic lineage (Figure 2a). However, these viruses are highly divergent in their *pol* and *env* genes (30% and 45% of nucleotide difference, respectively). The five strains derived from *P.t. troglodytes* (SIVcpzGAB1, SIVcpzUS, SIVcpzCAM3, -CAM4, and -CAM5) cluster separately from the *P.t. schweinfurthii* virus (SIVcpzANT).

SIVsm, SIVmac, and HIV-2 likewise have the same genomic organization and the same phylogenetic lineage (Figure 2a). The human and simian viruses from this lineage show a higher degree of genetic identity when compared with that of viruses in the HIV-1–SIVcpz lineage.

The SIVagm lineage consists of four distinct monophyletic clusters (Figure 2a), which are generally more closely related to

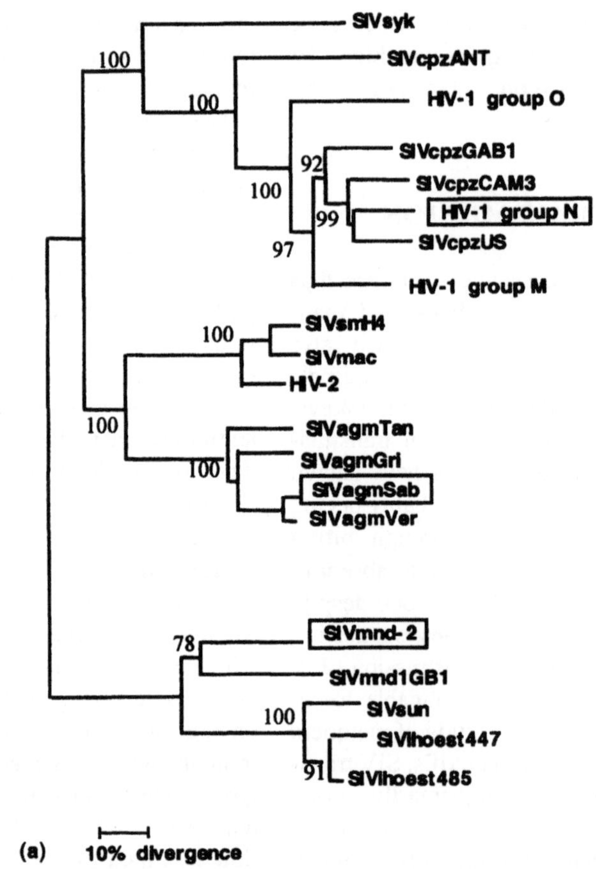

FIGURE 2a. Phylogenetic relationships among primate lentiviruses: Phylogenetic relationships of HIV and SIV prototypes in *env*. Viruses that have a mosaic genome, probably as a result of recombination between two distinct SIVs, are boxed.

each other than to other SIVs (19). Genetic diversity among these subtypes is similar to that found in HIV-1 groups. SIVagm viral variants have been designated SIVagmVer, SIVagmGri, SIVagmSab, and SIVagmTan according to their host species (vervet, grivet, sabaeus, and tantalus monkeys, respectively) (19). Clustering of SIVagm variants is host-specific and not geographically based; viruses from vervets in East Africa are much more closely related to viruses from vervets in South Africa than to viruses from grivets at nearby sites in East Africa (48). These observations are best explained by the assumption that the common ancestor of the four AGM species was infected with the common ancestor of the SIVagm group several thousand years ago, followed by coevolution of the virus and the host (19,58).

The SIVlhoest lineage comprises SIVlhoest and SIVsun viruses isolated from l'hoest and suntailed monkeys, respectively, and SIVmnd-1GB1 indicates virus from a mandrill (Figure 2a). Suntailed and l'hoest monkeys, which have geographically distinct habitats, are classified within the same superspecies. Genetic analysis of the two viruses revealed that SIVsun was more closely related to SIVlhoest than to SIVmnd or any other SIV, with an amino acid identity of 71% for *gag*, 73% for *pol* and 67% for *env* (30,31). These observations also include an indication of host-dependent virus evolution from a common ancestor within the l'hoest superspecies, suggesting that the SIVmndGB1–like viruses resulted from a SIVlhoest cross-species transmission to mandrills. Thus the lineage previously thought to originate in mandrills should be redesignated as belonging to the SIVlhoest lineage (30). This misdesignation emphasizes the problems of defining viral lineage solely on the basis of the species of origin.

The genetic variability of the SIVsyk and the SIVcol lineages have not been clearly defined because, to date, only one full-length genome of each has been characterized (41,55).

The phylogenetic position and genetic variability of other viruses, such as SIVrcm and SIVdrl, remain to be fully resolved. It is quite likely that further evidence of long-term coevolution of SIV and host lineages will emerge as more viruses from more primate species are fully characterized.

Thus far the number of phylogenetic lineages is higher than the number of genomic organization types, possibly a result of the accumulation of distinct substitutions within these genomes over time. Thus, infection of two distinct species by the same virus could lead to divergent host-specific viruses produced in response to the selective pressure exerted by the host. However, this hypothesis seems inadequate to explain either the close relationship between two viruses infecting two distinct species, such as the relationship between SIVsm and HIV-2, which are found in mangabeys and humans respectively, or why one virus, such as SIVagmSab, can appear to belong to two distinct phylogenetic lineages (depending on which of its gene fragments is analyzed). There is increasing evidence that cross-species transmissions are involved in the diversification of primate lentiviruses.

Cross-Species Transmissions

AGMs are the largest SIV reservoir in nature, based on the animals' high seroprevalence rate for SIVs and its wide geographic distribution in Africa. These features could explain in part the relatively high frequency of SIVagm transmission to other species sharing the same ecologic area (Figure 1). Indeed, such reported cases fulfill the five criteria used to substantiate cross-species transmissions (37): (*i*) similarities in viral genome organization, (*ii*) phylogenetic relatedness, (*iii*) prevalence in the natural host, (*iv*) geographic coincidence, and (*v*) plausible routes of transmission. In all cases, the SIVagm subtype isolated from a heterologous host was the same as that isolated from an AGM subspecies living in the same geographic region. Thus, SIVs identified in a yellow baboon (*Papio cynocephalus*) living in Tanzania and in a chacma baboon (*Papio ursinus*) living in South Africa are very closely related to the local form of SIVagm (SIVagmVer) (Figure 1) (48,49).

In the same way, SIVagmSab was isolated from a patas monkey in Senegal, a natural habitat of sabaeus monkeys (47). This is the only molecular evidence of SIVagm transmission to patas in nature, even though approximately 4% of wild patas monkeys harbor antibodies that cross-react with SIVagm antigens (our unpublished results). Moreover, patas monkeys have been shown to be highly susceptible to experimental SIVagm infection in vivo (77). The low frequency of SIVagm-infected patas in nature is, however, somewhat surprising since these species share habitat in Senegal and since some researchers (60) have observed regular contact and exchange of bodily fluids between the species. Another proposed case of SIV cross-species transmission in nature is that of SIVlhoest transmission to mandrills (Figure 1) (30).

Finally, it is notable that SIV cross-species transmission between AGMs and mangabeys in captivity has been described; specifically, a white-crowned mangabey (*C.t. lunulatus*) from Kenya infected with SIVagmVer from an AGM from Kenya (43). Two other instances of SIV transmission across species lines among animals in captivity are the SIVsm transmission from mangabey to macaques and the SIVcpzCAM transmission from *P.t. troglodytes* to *P.t. vellerosus* (Figure 1) (38). Cross-species transmissions of primate lentiviruses can occur between species belonging to distinct genera, although this is thought to be rare in nature.

Recombinations

Recombination events are frequent during the retrovirus life cycle but can only occur when a single cell is infected by two distinct viruses. In nonhuman primates, lentiviral coinfection has not been described to date. However it is likely that such events occur, even though scarce, since recombinant SIVs have been identified.

The first documented case was SIVagmSab (61), for which phylogenetic analysis revealed significant discordant branching patterns for different parts of the genome (Figure 2a). Indeed, in the central and 3′ regions of the genome (5′ *pol, vif, vpx, env*, and *nef*) SIVagmSab clusters with other SIVagm subtypes. However, in other parts of the genome [transactivation response element (TAR) in the LTR, 3′ *gag*, and 5′ *pol*], it clusters with viruses in the SIVsm lineage. The natural hosts of SIVagmSab and SIVsm, the sabaeus monkey and the sooty mangabey, respectively, inhabit the same geographic region in Africa. Thus the most likely explanation for the presence of this genetic mosaic virus is a recombination event between SIVagm and SIVsm viral ancestors that have coinfected cells within their sabaeus monkey hosts.

SIVrcm from red-capped mangabeys also appears to derive from a recombination event between two distinct lentiviruses. Indeed, in its *polgene*, SIVrcm is phylogenetically more related to HIV-1–SIVcpz than to other HIV–SIVs, whereas for its other genes, SIVrcm is more related to viruses such as SIVagm or SIVsm. The SIVrcm *pol* therefore seems to have the same ancestor as *pol* from the SIVcpz–HIV-1 lineage. The reservoirs of the ancestor viruses, however, have not yet been defined.

The second type of SIVmnd that is specific for mandrills, SIVmnd-2, also shows a discordant branching pattern for different parts of the viral genome. Thus, SIVmnd-2 is close to SIVrcm in *pol*, but related to SIVmnd-1 in *env* (Figure 2a). This discordance might be explained by a recombination event between the ancestors of SIVrcm, SIVmnd-2, and SIVmnd-1 (33).

Finally, recombination between two viral subtypes infecting the same species has been documented in SIVsm-infected sooty mangabeys (24).

In summary, cross-species transmissions among simians and coinfection of a simian species by two lentiviruses followed by recombination of these two viruses appears to occur in parallel to host-specific SIV evolution. These findings indicate that the emergence of new SIVs cannot be totally excluded from consideration. These new SIVs would, of course, increase the potential for human exposure to a wider range of transmission-competent lentiviruses.

ORIGIN OF HIV-1 AND HIV-2

SIVsm, SIVmac, and HIV-2 viral strains cannot be distinguished from each other at the genetic level (54). Since macaques, unlike mangabeys, are not infected in their natural habitat, it was assumed that SIVmac originated from SIVsm accidentally transmitted to captive macaques (62). For SIVsm and HIV-2, however, the similarities are phylogenetic and geographic. A substantial number of SIVsm-infected mangabeys are found in West Africa, from the Casamance River in Senegal to the Sassandra River in Côte d'Ivoire, a geographic region in which HIV-2 is endemic and where sooty mangabeys are hunted or kept as pets. Phylogenetic analysis of these viruses shows striking similarities between SIVsm and HIV-2 (54), and, in fact, some SIVsm variants are more closely related to HIV-2 variants from the same geographic region than to SIVsm variants from outside regions (Figure 2b) (24,63). The phylogenetic relatedness between SIVsm and at least three HIV-2 subtypes (D, E, and F), along with their overlapping geographic distribution, indicate that in at least three instances, SIVsm transmission to humans resulted in HIV-2 infection and suggest three further transmission events to explain HIV-2 A, B, and C. (24). Most of these events seem to be dead-ends as human-to-human transmission of HIV-2C, D, E, and F is rare; only subtypes A and B of HIV-2 are spreading within the human population.

Genetic similarities are less striking between HIV-1 and SIVcpz compared with HIV-2 and SIVsm (51), a fact that makes it more difficult to elucidate HIV-1's origin (64). Nevertheless, a chimpanzee origin of HIV-1 has been suggested based on the similarity of genomic organization between HIV-1 and SIVcpz (51). Recent studies appear to support this hypothesis. Indeed, HIV-1 viruses representative of a new group N were recently identified in Cameroon (65). Analysis of their *env* genes surprisingly showed them to be more related to the *env* of SIVcpzGAB1 than to the *envs* of either HIV-1 group M or HIV-1 group O (Figure 2c). At the time of this discovery, SIVcpzGAB1 was the only virus from a Central African chimpanzee (*P.t. troglodytes*) to have had a full-length sample analyzed. Shortly after this, however, a new SIVcpz (SIVcpzUS) was isolated from samples taken from a captive *P.t. troglodytes*. This virus was more closely related to HIV-1 group N than SIVcpzGAB1 (Figure 2c) (37).

While SIVcpzGAB1 originates from Gabon and HIV-1 group N was identified in Cameroon, SIVcpzUS is of unknown geographic origin. To determine whether the geographic distribution of HIV-1 group N and other related SIVcpz viruses overlap, 29 wild-born chimpanzees that had been rescued at a young age in Cameroon were screened. Three SIVcpz-infected animals were identified. Two of them (SIVcpzCAM3 and SIVcpzCAM5), both of the troglodytes subspecies (*P.t.t.*), had been infected in the wild (38,39). Genetic analysis showed them to be more closely related (in the *env* region) to SIVcpzUS and HIV-1 group N (Figure 2c) than to any other virus within the HIV-1–SIVcpz cluster (38). These data thus reveal a close geographic linkage between human and chimpanzee viruses and provide the strongest evidence to date for SIVcpz transmission from chimpanzees to humans.

Phylogenetic studies suggest at least three distinct zoonotic events for HIV-1 groups N, M, and O (65). However, the primate/ape reservoir for groups M and O is still unknown. In addition, the close phylogenetic

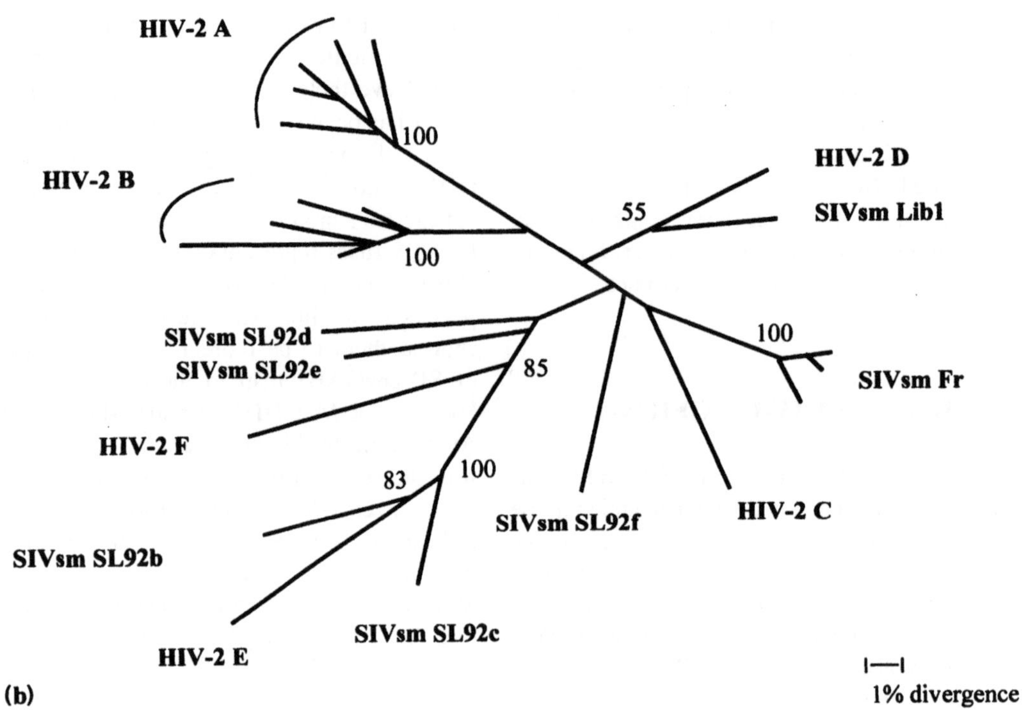

FIGURE 2b. Phylogenetic relationships among primate lentiviruses: Phylogenetic relationships of HIV-2 and SIVsm based on data from (24).

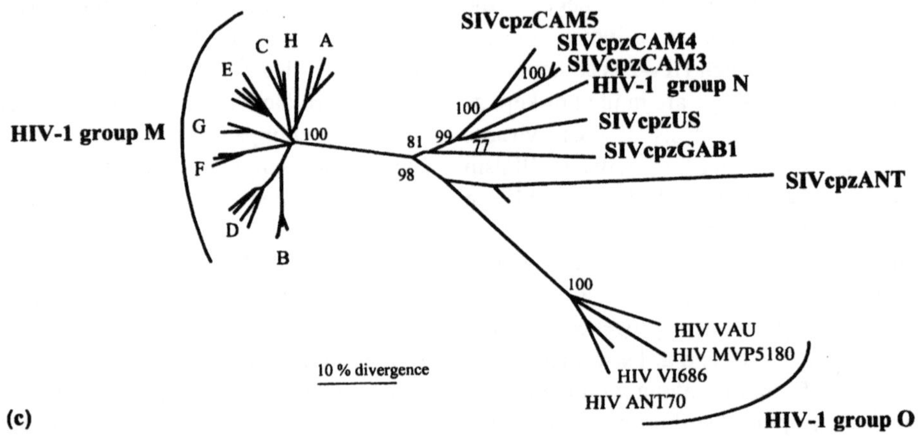

FIGURE 2c. Phylogenetic relationship of HIV-1 and SNcpz in *env* (1332bp).

relationship between SIVcpz and HIV-1 group N is limited primarily to *env* (37–39,65). Given the limited number of SIVcpz sequences available, the possibility exists that there are SIVs more closely related to HIV-1 present in chimpanzees of different geographic locales or in other simian species. Indeed, the presence of HIV-1–related SIVs in other central–African species cannot be totally excluded.

A distinction, however, must be made between the introduction of HIV-1–like viruses into humans and the beginning of the HIV-1 pandemic. Modeling of the HIV-1 evolution has produced an estimated period for the last common ancestor of

HIV-1 group M viruses of 1910–1950 (66). Currently, the most compelling hypothesis to explain the AIDS outbreaks is that human contact with blood of infected chimpanzees and sooty mangabeys resulted in the zoonotic transmission of SIVcpz and SIVsm. Since then, social, economic and behavioral changes, urbanization, and use of nonsterilized needles for large-scale immunizations in the early and mid-twentieth century might have provided the circumstances under which these viruses could expand and reach epidemic proportions. However, the role of viral characteristics must also be considered in this evolution scenario, since the AIDS epidemic attributed to HIV-1 is much more significant when compared to that attributed to HIV-2, despite common modes of entry into people.

CELLULAR TROPISM AND SIV RECEPTORS

The target cell populations for HIV and SIV viruses are $CD4^+$ lymphocytes and antigen-presenting cells. Entry to these cells is dependent on the interaction of the viral envelope protein with the main $CD4^+$ receptors and coreceptors, which are comprised of specific chemokine receptors or orphan receptors that are like chemokine receptors. SIVs resemble HIVs in their cellular tropism; they primarily use the cell-surface $CD4^+$ molecule to enter target cells.

Although in-vitro studies using SIVmac show it targets the same cells (or cell receptors) as HIV-1, the cellular tropism of SIVs in their natural hosts is less well explored. The preponderance of SIVmac and other in vitro-passaged SIVs (SIVagm, SIVcpz, SIVmac, and SIVsm) tested thus far appear to use the CCR5 coreceptor (67,68). Blood-derived SIVsm, SIVcpz, and SIVagm from naturally infected monkeys also use the CCR5, not the CXCR4, coreceptor (39,68; Diop OM, Gueye A, Ayouba A, et al.: unpublished data). SIVmac derived from four macaques with AIDS also did not use the macaque CXCR4 coreceptor, showing that X4 tropism did not develop during progression to disease (68). SIVrcm, however, is an exception. It uses the CCR2b coreceptor apparently as an adaptation; its natural host frequently shows a deletion in its CCR5 receptor (69).

In contrast to HIV, most SIVs do not use CXCR4 as a coreceptor. However, some primary SIV isolates (one SIVmac, one SIVagm, and four SIVsm) and a cell-line-adapted SIVmnd-1GB1 have been shown to use CXCR4 for entry into human cells (70,71). Since most SIV strains are unable to use CXCR4 but have demonstrated the ability to replicate in human T-cell lines that do not express significant levels of CCR5, it is apparent that additional SIV-specific coreceptors might exist. In addition, the frequent use of other coreceptors (BONZO, BOB, GPR1, APJ, and CCR8) by SIVs has been described in vitro (67). It is of interest that these SIV coreceptors were also found to be functional for some HIV-1 and HIV-2 viral isolates. Their exact role in the infection of target cells in vivo is less well understood.

RESISTANCE TO AIDS IN NATURALLY SIV-INFECTED AFRICAN MONKEYS

Although simian lentiviruses are called immunodeficiency viruses because of their genetic similarity to their human counterparts (HIV) and because SIVmac has been shown to induce AIDS in macaques, the main characteristic of SIV infections in their natural host is the lack of disease (Table 1). While long-term follow-up of infections has been performed only in AGMs, sooty mangabeys, and mandrills, the nonpathogenic outcome of such infections cannot be dismissed as viral attenuation. It has been shown that transmission of SIVs from African monkeys to Asian monkeys can lead to AIDS in the latter (Table 1). Similarly, SIVsm can induce AIDS in macaques. This experimental

TABLE 1. Simian Models for Lentiviral Infections[a]

Virus	Simian model	AIDS
HIV-1	Chimpanzee[b]	− (+)
HIV-2	Macaque[b]	+/−
	Baboon[b]	+/−
SHIV[c]	Macaque[b]	+/−
SIVmac		
— isolate	Macaque[b]	+
— attenuated clone	Macaque[b]	(−)
SIVsm	Mangabey[d]	−
	Macaque[b]	+
SIVagm	African green monkey[d]	−
	Patas[b]	−?
	Macaque[b]	+/−
SIVlhoest	L'hoest monkey[d]	−?
	Macaque[b]	+
SIVcpz	Chimpanzee[d]	−?
SIVmnd-1	Mandrill[d]	−
SIVmnd-2	Mandrill[d]	−

[a]SIV infections in macaques generally progress to AIDS in a manner similar to HIV-1's progression to AIDS in humans. SIV infections in macaques, therefore, represent the major animal model for AIDS. Macaques are, however, not susceptible to HIV-1 infection. Recently, recombinant viruses between SIV and HIV-1, known as SHIVs, have been shown to induce AIDS in macaques. The study of nonpathogenic infections has been undertaken in macaques using SIVmac-attenuated molecular clones. Such infections cause AIDS in newborn macaques and can progress to AIDS in adult monkeys, whereas SIVagm, SIVsm, and SIVmnd infections in their natural hosts are always nonpathogenic. The studies of natural SIV infections in other host species have involved few animals, and the nonpathogenicity of these infections has yet to be demonstrated.
[b]Experimental host.
[c]SHIV is a recombinant virus between SIVmac and HIV-1 constructed in vitro.
[d]Natural host.

construct now serves as a valuable animal model for HIV disease (54,62). Likewise, infection by a SIVagmVer isolate in a pigtailed macaque has also resulted in AIDS (72).

In some cases, serial passage of a virus in a heterologous host can increase its pathogenicity (73). It is likely that SIV transmission from one species to another disrupts the long-standing equilibrium between the virus and its natural host (19). For example, SIVsm infection in a pigtailed macaque resulted in the emergence of a highly pathogenic viral variant in both the macaque and the natural host, the sooty mangabey (74). These observations suggest that SIVs may retain their potential to be pathogenic in simians (75). It would seem then, that studies of AIDS resistance in naturally SIV-infected African monkeys would provide valuable information about virus–host relationships and their link to pathogenicity.

African Green Monkeys

The early phases of SIVagm infection in AGMs are characterized by high viral loads, both in the peripheral blood and tissues, about 10 days after infection. These load levels then decrease rapidly and significantly (76). This replicative capacity of SIVagm in its natural host correlates with its genetic evolution in vivo and indicates a rapid, continuous replication similar to that which occurs in HIV-infected humans and SIV-infected macaques (77). Thus, the nonpathogenic outcome of SIVagm infection in AGMs is associated with a rapidly induced equilibrium between virus and host rather than with a poorly replicating virus or with a constitutive host's genetic resistance to virus replication. In many AGMs, the chronic phase of SIVagm infection is characterized by low viral loads in plasma and tissues. In other AGMs, the viral load remains high (76,78,79). However in all AGMs, there is no dichotomy between the cell-associated viral loads in lymph nodes and in peripheral blood. Productive cells are found only in T areas of the lymph nodes and the spleen, and no trapping of virus particles by follicular dendritic cells has been found in either the lymph nodes or the spleen germinal centers (80,81). Thus, viral replication patterns in these organs are different from those that occur during pathogenic infections in humans and macaques. Factors underlying the control of viral replication in lymph nodes remain to be fully elucidated.

The correlation between mutations in receptors and coreceptors and AIDS resistance in African monkeys has been investigated. Analysis of $CD4^+$ and CCR5 genes in AGMs revealed high polymorphism (59,82, 83) but no deletions in their coding regions. Moreover, tests of $CD4^+$ and three CCR5 variants from AGMs showed them to be fully functional (83–85) and corroborated data from similar tests for other African monkeys (68,85). However, a possible role of $CD4^+$ in the down-regulation of its expression subsequent to the activation of immune cells by SIVagm cannot be excluded (86). Mutations in other known SIVagm coreceptors (BONZO and BOB) have not yet been studied.

Studies of humoral immune responses in infected AGMs revealed few differences with HIV-1–infected individuals. In AGMs, seroconversion occurs about five weeks postinfection (76) and neutralizing antibodies are difficult to detect, especially against homologous isolates (87,88). However, a recent study shows that levels of neutralizing antibodies are high in some animals and that this neutralization is strain-dependent (89). It is noteworthy that SIVagms become more sensitive to some neutralizing antibodies after exposure to soluble $CD4^+$, probably because of the cryptic nature of the conformational B epitope recognized by these antibodies (90). To summarize, it is unlikely that neutralizing antibodies play a major role in AIDS resistance in AGMs. One of the main differences with pathogenic lentiviral infection is the low p28 antibody titer in naturally infected AGMs (20,91). The biologic significance of the lack of an anti-major core protein response, which seems to be usual in the natural SIV hosts (32,92) but unusual in SIV-infected heterologous hosts, is unclear at present (72,93).

The cell-mediated immune responses in infected AGMs urgently require detailed investigations since it may contribute to AIDS resistance. Although cytotoxic T-cell responses during the chronic phase of infection may be weak (87), the use of new techniques (tetramer staining and Elispot) will help determine more fully the role of cytotoxic T-lymphocytes (CTLs) and natural killer cells during the course of SIVagm infection. Thus far it has not been possible to establish the immortal autologous AGM B-cell lines necessary for the use of classic CTL detection methods. In contrast, it is well known that AGM $CD8^+$ cells secrete soluble factors that inhibit viral replication in vitro. Some researchers suggest use of interleukin-16 to control viral dissemination (94) but, as for HIV-1 infection (95), the involvement of other factors such as CAF ($CD8^+$ T-cell antiviral factor) or β-chemokines (Rantes, MIP1-α, and MIP1-β) cannot be excluded (96).

In conclusion, nonpathogenic SIVagm infection in its natural host is characterized by a delicate balance between high viral replication and a moderate host immune response. This hypothesis of a low activation of immune cells in response to SIVagm infection correlates with previous findings on the absence of an abnormal rate of peripheral $CD4^+$ lymphocyte loss from chronically infected AGMs undergoing apoptosis following ex-vivo stimulation (97) and the absence of follicular hyperplasia and $CD8^+$ cell infiltration in lymph node germinal centers in early and late phases of SIVagm infection (76,78,81). Such a lack of chronic high immune system activation might lead to low $CD4^+$ T-cell destruction and/or compromise of the renewal capacity of the immune system. A greater number of directed immunologic studies are required to substantiate this hypothesis.

Sooty Mangabeys

SIVsm infection in mangabeys shares many characteristics with the AGM model. It seems that this infection is not associated with a chronic activation of immune responses. T-cell cytotoxic activity is weak, (98) and infected peripheral blood mononuclear cells are not highly susceptible to apoptosis (99). There also is no evidence of morphologic changes, follicular hyperplasia, or trapping of virus particles by follicular dendritic cells in lymph nodes of infected mangabeys (92).

Other features SIVsm infection in mangabeys has in common with SIVagm-infected AGMs are a weak humoral response against the p28 core antigen (92), weak or undetectable neutralizing antibodies (100), and secretion by $CD8^+$ cells of soluble factors that inhibit SIVsm replication in vitro (101).

In mangabeys chronically infected with SIVsm, plasma viral loads are particularly high (92)—above the threshold values associated with disease progression in macaques (102). Despite these high viral-load levels during the chronic phase of SIVsm infection, sooty mangabeys maintain a normal T-cell turnover rate (103). It could be instructive to conduct further studies, in particular during the early phases of infection in this model, for use as comparison with data from studies of pathogenic SIVsm infection in macaques.

Chimpanzees

In comparison to AGM and mangabeys, little is known about the virologic and immunologic characteristics of SIVcpz infection in chimpanzees; there are few naturally infected animals that can be studied. SIVcpz infection in chimpanzees has been shown to be persistent and, in two, long-term infected chimpanzees, without clear indications of immune dysfunction (38,104). However, one animal showed a slow decline in $CD4^+$ cell counts. It remains to be seen whether the levels of these cells remain within normal limits (105). In one animal that was naturally infected with SIVcpzANT, the viral load was higher than the viral load in HIV-1–inoculated chimpanzees and comparable to that in chronically HIV-1–infected humans (106). In one chimpanzee intentionally infected with SIVcpzANT, peak viral load was 10 times higher than peak load in HIV-1–inoculated chimpanzees (104). As in humans, viral load fluctuated over time. This variability could reflect viral escape subsequent to the generation of neutralizing antibodies (106), but such a hypothesis would require further testing. As in AGMs and mangabeys, no virus trapping by follicular dendritic cells was noted. But interestingly, and, in contrast to AGMs, follicular hyperplasia and $CD8^+$ cells infiltration in lymph node germinal centers were described (104). These infiltrating $CD8^+$ cells expressed the β-chemokine RANTES, however the specific function of these $CD8^+$ cells has not been determined.

Other Models of Nonpathogenic SIV Infection

Other natural SIV infections, such as SIVmnd-1 and -2, SIVsyk, SIVtal, SIVrcm, SIVdrl, and SIVlhoest, are also potential nonpathogenic models. Very little is known about these infections however, since few studies on them have been conducted.

CONCLUSION

Reconstruction of the phylogenetic relationships between the human lentiviruses responsible for the AIDS epidemic and lentiviruses from African nonhuman primates can help clarify the origin of the AIDS pandemic. These studies have several scientific—and public health—implications, although the detailed circumstances of such zoonotic events are still not fully understood. As the potential for simian-to-simian, simian-to-human, and human-to-human transmission of lentiviruses becomes better understood, the emergence of new and/or more virulent lentiviral strains, capable of causing new epidemics, needs to be considered. Multidisciplinary field studies remain important. It also appears clear that studies of simian lentiviral infections can advance our understanding of HIV's pathogenesis, an understanding necessary for the development of effective AIDS vaccines and therapeutics.

REFERENCES

1. Nerrienet E, Amouretti X, Müller-Trutwin MC, et al. Phylogenetic analysis of SIV and STLV type I in mandrills (mandrillus sphinx): indications that intracolony transmissions are predominantly the result of male-to-male aggressive contacts. *AIDS Res. & Hum. Retroviruses* 1998;14(9):785–796.
2. Saksena NK, Herve V, Durand JP, et al. Seroepidemiologic, molecular and phylogenetic analyses of simian T-cell leukemia viruses (STLV-I) from

various naturally infected monkey species from central and western Africa. *J. Virol.* 1994;198:297–310.

3. Koralnik IJ, Boeri E, Saxinger WC, et al. Phylogenetic associations of human and simian T-Cell Leukemia/Lymphotropic Virus type I strains: Evidence for interspecies transmissions. *J. Virol.* 1994;68:2693–2707.
4. Pecon Slattery J, Franchini G and Gessain A. Genomic evolution, patterns of global dissemination, and interspecies transmission of human and simian T-cell leukemia/lymphotropic viruses. *Genome Research* 1999;9(6):525–540.
5. Gessain A and Mahieux R. Genetic diversity and molecular epidemiology of primate T-cell lymphotropic viruses: human T-cell leukemia/lymphoma viruses types 1 and 2 and related simian retroviruses (STLV-1, STLV-2 Pan-P and PTLV-L). In: Dalgleish AG, Weiss RA, eds. *HIV and the New Viruses Second Edition.* London: Academic Press, 1999:281–327.
6. Homma T, Kanki PJ, King NW, et al. Lymphoma in macaques: association with virus of human T lymphotrophic family. *Science.* 1985;225:716–718.
7. Tsujimoto H, Noda Y, Ishikawa K, et al. Development of adult T-cell leukemia-like disease in African green monkey associated with clonal integration of simian T-cell leukemia virus type I. *Cancer Res.* 1987;47:269–274.
8. Daniel MD, Letvin NL, King NW, et al. Isolation of T-cell tropic HTLV-III-like retrovirus from macaques. *Science* 1985;228:1201–1204.
9. Kanki PJ, McLane MF, King NW, et al. Serologic identification and characterization of a macaque T-lymphotropic retrovirus closely related to HTLV-III. *Science.* 1985;228(4704):1199–1201.
10. Benveniste RE, Arthur L, Tsai CC, et al. Isolation of a lentivirus from a macaque with lymphoma: comparison with HTLV-III/LAV and other lentiviruses. *J. Virol.* 1986;60:483–490.
11. Gardner MB and Luciw P. Simian immunodeficiency viruses and their relationship to the human immunodeficiency viruses. *AIDS* 1988;2:S3–S10.
12. Kestler HW, Li Y, Naidu YM, et al. Comparison of simian immunodeficiency virus isolates. *Nature* 1988;331:619–622.
13. Lowenstine L, Pederson N, Higgins J, et al. Seroepidemiologic survey of captive old-world primates for antibodies to human and simian retroviruses, and isolation of a lentivirus from sooty mangabeys (*Cercocebus atys*). *Int. J. Cancer* 1986;38:563–574.
14. Ohta Y, Masuda T, Tsujimoto H, et al. Isolation of simian immunodeficiency virus from African green monkeys and seroepidemiological survey of the virus in various non-human primates. *Int. J. Cancer* 1988;41:155–122.
15. Kanki PJ, Alroy J, Essex M. Isolation of T-lymphotropic retrovirus related to HTLV-III/LAV from wild caught African green monkeys. *Science* 1985;230:951–954.
16. Fultz PN, McClure HM, Anderson DC, et al. Isolation of a T-lymphotropic retrovirus from naturally infected sooty mangabey monkeys (*Cercocebus atys*). *Proc. Natl. Acad. Sci. USA* 1986; 83:5286–5290.
17. Hendry RM, Wells MA, Phelan MA, et al. Antibodies to simian immunodeficiency virus in African green monkeys in Africa in 1957–1962. *Lancet* 1986;2(8504):455.
18. Kanki PJ, Kurth R, Becker W, et al. Antibodies to simian T-lymphotropic retrovirus type III in African green monkeys and recognition of STLV-III viral proteins by AIDS and related sera. *Lancet* 1985; 1(8441):1330–1332.
19. Müller MC, Saksena NK, Nerrienet E, et al. Simian immunodeficiency viruses from Central and Western Africa: evidence for a new species-specific lentivirus in tantalus monkeys. *J. Virol.* 1993; 67: 1227–1235.
20. Daniel MD, Li Y, Naidu Y, et al. Simian immunodeficiency virus from African green monkeys. *J. Virol.* 1988;62:4123–4128.
21. Denham WW. History of Green Monkeys in the West Indies: Part I. Migration from Africa. *The Journal of the B.M.H.S.* 1981;36(3):210–229.
22. Diop, OM. Epidémiologie des Infections SIV et STLV-I chez les singes d'Afrique et contributions à la mise en place d'un modèle d'étude de la protection naturelle contre le SIDA. Th: Sci. Paris 7, 1999. Université Denis Diderot.
23. Jolly C, Phillips-Conroy J, Turner T, et al. SIVagm incidence over two decades in a natural population of Ethiopian grivet monkeys (*Cercopithecus aethiops aethiops*). *J Med Primatol* 1996;25:78–83.
24. Chen Z, Telfier P, Gettie A, et al. Genetic characterization of new West African simian immunodeficiency virus SIVsm: geographic clustering of household-derived SIV strains with human immunodeficiency virus type 2 subtypes and genetically diverse viruses from a single feral sooty mangabey troop. *J. Virol.* 1996;70(6):3617–3627.
25. Benveniste RE, Raben D, Hill RW, et al. Molecular characterization and comparison of simian immunodeficiency virus isolates from macaques, mangabeys and African green monkeys. *J. Med. Primatol.* 1989;18:287–303.
26. Emau P, McClure HM, Isahakia M, et al. Isolation from African Sykes' monkeys (*Cercopithecus mitis*) of a lentivirus related to human and simian immunodeficiency viruses. *J. Virol.* 1991;65: 2135–2140.
27. Georges-Courbot MC, Lu CY, Makuwa M, et al. Natural infection of a household pet red-capped mangabey (*Cercocebus torquatus torquatus*) with a new simian immunodeficiency virus. *J. Virol.* 1998;72(1):600–608.
28. Osterhaus ADME, Pedersen N, Van Amerongen G, et al. Isolation and partial characterization of a

lentivirus from talapoin monkeys (*Miopithecus talapoin*). *Virology* 1999;260:116–124.

29. Clewley JP, Lewis JCM, Brown DWG and Gadsby EL. A novel simian immunodeficiency virus (SIVdrl) pol sequence from the drill monkey, *Mandrillus leucophaeus*. *J. Virol.* 1998;72: 10305–10309.
30. Beer BE, Bailes E, Goeken R, et al. Simian immunodeficiency virus (SIV) from sun-tailed monkeys (*Cercopithecus solatus*): evidence for host-dependent evolution of SIV within the C. lhoesti superspecies. *J. Virol.* 1999;72:7734–7744.
31. Hirsch VM, Campbell BJ, Bailes E, et al. Characterization of a novel simian immunodeficiency virus (SIV) from L'Hoest monkeys (*Cercopithecus l'hoesti*): Implications for the origins of SIVmnd and other primate lentiviruses. *J. Virol.* 1999;73:1036–1045.
32. Tsujimoto H, Cooper RW, Cooper T, et al. Isolation and characterization of simian immunodeficiency virus from mandrills in Africa and its relationship to other human and simian immunodeficiency viruses. *J. Virol.* 1988;62:4044–4050.
33. Souquière S, Bibollet-Ruche F, Robertson DL, et al. Wild *Mandrillus sphinx* are carriers of two types of lentiviruses. *J. Virol.* 2002;75: 7080–7090.
34. Peeters M, Honore C, Huet T, et al. Isolation and partial characterization of an HIV-related virus occurring naturally in chimpanzees in Gabon. *AIDS* 1989;3:625–630.
35. Morin PA. Kin selection, social structure, gene flow, and the evolution of chimpanzees. *Science* 1994;265:1193–1201.
36. Gonder MK, Oates JF, Disotell T, et al. A new west African chimpanzee subspecies? *Nature* 1997; 388:337.
37. Gao F, Bailes E, Robertson DL, et al. Origin of HIV-1 in the chimpanzee Pan troglodytes troglodytes. *Nature* 1999;397:436–440.
38. Corbet S, Müller-Truwin MC, Versmisse P, et al. SIVcpz from chimpanzee in Cameroon are related in env to human immunodeficiency virus group N from the same geographic area. *J. Virol.* 2000; 74(1):529–534.
39. Müller-Trutwin MC, Corbet S, Souquière S, et al. SIVcpz from a naturally infected Cameroonian chimpanzee: Biological and genetic comparison with HIV-N. *J. Med. Primatol.* 2000;29:166–172.
40. Peeters M, Fransen K, Delaporte E, et al. Isolation and characterization of a new chimpanzee lentivirus (simian immunodeficiency virus isolate cpz-ant) from a wild captured chimpanzee. *AIDS* 1992;6:447–451.
41. Courgnaud V, Pourrut X, Bibollet-Ruche F, et al. Characterization of a novel SIV from guereza colobus monkeys (Colobus guereza) in Cameroon: a new lineage in the nonhuman primate lentivirus family. *J. Virol.* 2001;75:857–866.
42. Bibollet-Ruche F, et al. Paper presented at: 7th Conference on Retroviruses and Opportunistic Infections; Jan. 30-Feb. 2, 2000; San Francisco, CA.
43. Tomonaga K, Katahira J, Fukasawa M, et al. Isolation and characterization of simian immunodeficiency virus from African white-crowned mangabey monkeys *(Cercocebus torquatus lunulatus)*. *Arch. Virol.* 1993;129:79–92.
44. Diop OM, Gogovor H, Galat-Luong A, et al. Transmission sexuelle et par morsure de SIVagm chez des singes verts, cercopithecus aethiops sabaeus, captifs. *5e Colloque de la Société Française de Primatologie (SFDP), Station Biologique de Paimont* 1993.
45. Phillips-Conroy JE, Jolly CJ, Petros B, et al. Sexual transmission of SIVagm in wild grivet monkeys. *J. Med. Primat.* 1994;23:1–7.
46. Otsyula M, Yees J, Jennings M, et al. Prevalence of antibodies against simian immunodeficiency virus (SIV) and simian T-lymphotropic virus (STLV) in a colony of non-human primates in Kenya, East Africa. *Ann. Trop. Med. Parasit.* 1996;90(1):65–70.
47. Bibollet-Ruche F, Galat-Luong A, Cuny G, et al. Simian immunodeficiency virus infection in a patas monkey (*Erythrocebus patas*): evidence for a cross-species transmission from African green monkeys (*Cercopithecus aethiops sabaeus*) in the wild. *J. Virol.* 1996;77:773–781.
48. Jin MJ, Rogers J, Philips-Conroy JE, et al. Infection of a yellow baboon with simian immunodeficiency virus from African green monkeys: evidence for cross-species transmission in the wild. *J. Virol.* 1994;68:8454–8460.
49. Van Rensburg EJ, Engelbrecht S, Mwenda J, et al. Simian immunodeficiency viruses (SIVs) from eastern and southern Africa: detection of a SIVagm variant from a chacma baboon. *J. Gen. Virol.* 1998;79(Pt 7):1809–1814.
50. Wain-Hobson S, Sonigo P, Danos O, et al. Nucleotide sequence of the AIDS virus LAV. *Cell* 1985;40:9–17.
51. Huet T, Chenyier R, Meyerhans A, et al. Genetic organization of a chimpanzee lentivirus related to HIV-1. *Nature* 1990;345:356–359.
52. Chakrabarti L, Guyader M, Alizon M, et al. Sequence of simian immunodeficiency virus from macaque and its relationship to other human and simian retroviruses. *Nature* 1987;328:543–547.
53. Guyader M, Emerman M, Sonigo P, et al. Genome organization and transactivation of the human immunodeficiency virus type 2. *Nature* 1987;326: 662–669.

54. Hirsch VM, Olmsted RA, Murphey-Corb M, et al. An African primate lentivirus (SIVsm) closely related to HIV-2. *Nature* 1989;339:389–392.
55. Hirsch VM, Dapolito GA, Goldstein S, et al. A distinct African lentivirus from sykes' monkeys. *J. Virol.* 1993;67:1517–1528.
56. Tsujimoto H, Hasegawa A, Maki N, et al. Sequence of a novel simian immunodeficiency virus from a wild caught African Mandrill. *Nature* 1989;341: 539–541.
57. Tristem M, Marshall C, Karpas A and Hill F. Evolution of the primate lentiviruses: evidence from vpx and vpr. *EMBO J.* 1992;11:3405–3412.
58. Allan JS, Short M, Taylor ME, et al. Species-specific diversity among simian immunodeficiency viruses from African green monkeys. *J. Virol.* 1991;65:2816–2828.
59. Müller-Trutwin MC, Corbet S, Hansen J, et al. Mutations in CCR5 coding sequences are not associated with SIV carrier status in African nonhuman primates. *AIDS Res. and Hum. Retroviruses.* 1999; 15(10);931–939.
60. Galat-Luong A. Observation de contacts interindividuels interspecifiques avec échanges de fluides corporels entre singes verts, *Cercopithecus aethiops*, et patas, *Erythrocebus patas*. Paper presented at: 6th International Conference on AIDS in Africa. Dakar, Sénégal 1991:T.A.124.
61. Jin MJ, Hui H, Robertson DL, et al. Mosaic genome structure of simian immunodeficiency virus from West African monkeys. *EMBO J.* 1994;13: 2935–2947.
62. Murphey-Corb M, Martin LN, Rangan SRS, et al. Isolation of an HTLV-III—related retrovirus from macaques with simian AIDS and its possible origin in asymptomatic mangabeys. *Nature (London)* 1986;321:435–437.
63. Gao F, Yue L, White AT, et al. Human infection by genetically diverse SIVsm-related HIV-2 in West Africa. *Nature* 1992;358:495–499.
64. Barré-Sinoussi F, Chermann J-C, Rey F, et al. Isolation of a T-lymphotropic retrovirus from a patient at risk of acquired immunodeficiency syndrome. *Science* 1983;220:868–871.
65. Simon F, Mauclère P, Roques P, et al. Identification of a new Human Immunodeficiency Virus type 1 distinct from group M and group O. *Nature Medicine* 1998;4(9):1032–1037.
66. Korber B, Muldoon M, Theiler J, et al. Timing the ancestor of the HIV-1 pandemic strains. *Science* 2000;288:1789–1796.
67. Edinger AL, Clements JE and Doms RW. Chemokine and orphan receptors in HIV-2 and SIV tropism and pathogenesis. *Virology* 1999;260: 211–221.
68. Chen Z, Gettie A, Ho DD, et al. Primary SIVsm isolates use the CCR5 coreceptor from sooty mangabeys naturally infected in West Africa: A comparison of coreceptor usage of primary SIVsm, HIV-2, and SIVmac. *Virology* 1998;246:113–124.
69. Chen Z, Kwon D, Jin Z, et al. Natural infection of a homozygous delta24 CCR5 red-capped mangabey with an R2b-tropic simian immunodeficiency virus. *J. Exp. Med.* 1998;188(11):2057–2065.
70. Owen SM, Masciota S, Novembre F, et al. Simian immunodeficiency viruses of diverse origin can use CXCR4 as a coreceptor for entry into human cells. *J. Virol.* 2000;74(12):5702–5708.
71. Schols D and De Clercq E. The simian immunodeficiency virus mnd(GB-1) strain uses CXCR4, not CCR5, as coreceptor for entry in human cells. *J. Gen. Virol.* 1998;79:2203–2205.
72. Hirsch V, Dapolito G, Johnson PR, et al. Induction of AIDS by simian immunodeficiency virus from an African green monkey: species-specific variation in pathogenicity correlates with the extent of *in vivo* replication. *J. Virol.* 1995;69:955–967.
73. Hirsch VM and Johnson PR. Pathogenic diversity of simian immunodeficiency viruses. *Virus Research* 1994;32:183–203.
74. Fultz PN, McClure HM, Anderson DC and Switzer WM. Identification and biologic characterization of an acutely lethal variant of simian immunodeficiency virus from sooty mangabeys (SIV/SMM). *AIDS Res. Hum. Retroviruses* 1989;5:397–409.
75. Courgnaud V, Lauré F, Fultz PN, et al. Genetic differences accounting for evolution and pathogenicity of simian immunodeficiency virus from sooty mangabey monkey after cross-species transmission to a pig-tailed macaque. *J. Virol.* 1992;66:414–419.
76. Diop OM, Guèye A, Dias-Tavares M, et al. High levels of viral replication during primary simian immunodeficiency virus SIVagm infection are rapidly and strongly controlled in African green monkeys. *J. Virol.* 2000;74:7538–7547.
77. Müller-Trutwin MC, Corbet S, Dias Tavares M, et al. The evolutionary rate of non-pathogenic simian immunodeficiency viruses (SIVagm) indicates a rapid and continuous replication *in vivo*. *Virology* 1996;223:89–102.
78. Guèye A, Diop OM, Kornfeld C, et al. High levels of viral replication in lymph nodes during primary SIVagm infection contrasts with lack of morphological changes. Proceedings of the Fifth European Conference on Experimental AIDS Research; *Nonduzzi Editore* 2000; 61–67.
79. Goldstein S, Ourmanov I, Brown CR, et al. Wide range of viral load in healthy African green monkeys naturally infected with Simian immunodeficiency virus. *J. Virol.* 2000;74(24):11744–11753.
80. Beer B, Scherer J, Megede JZ, et al. Lack of Dichotomy between Virus Load of Peripheral Blood and Lymph Nodes during Long-Term Simian Immunodeficiency Virus Infection of African Green Monkey. *Virology* 1996;219: 367–375.

81. Dias Tavares M, Müller-Trutwin MC, Avé P, et al. Non-pathogenic SIVagm infections of African mokeys correlate with a low viral burden associated with a lack of alterations in lymphoid tissues. Paper presented at: *14th Annual Symposium on non-human primate models for AIDS* 1996; Portland, OR, USA:141.
82. Fomsgaard A, Müller-Trutwin MC, Diop O, et al. Relation between phylogeny of African Green Monkey CD4 genes and their respective simian immunodeficiency virus. *J. Med. Primatol.* 1997; 26:120–128.
83. Kuhmann S, Platt EJ, Kozak SL, Kabat D. Polymorphisms in the CCR5 genes of African Green Monkeys and mice implicate specific amino acids in infections by simian and human immunodeficiency viruses. *J. Virol.* 1997;71:8642–8656.
84. Fomsgaard A, Johnson PR, Nielsen C, et al. Receptor function of CD4 structures from African green monkey and pig-tail macaque for simian immunodeficiency virus, SIVsm, SIVagm, and Human Immunodeficiency Virus type 1. *Viral Immunol.* 1995;8:121–133.
85. Edinger AL, Amedee A, Miller K, et al. Differential utilization of CCR5 by macrophage and T cell tropic simian immunodeficiency virus strains. *Proc. Natl. Acad. Sci.* 1997;94:4005–4010.
86. Murayama Y, Amano A, Mukai R, et al. CD4 and CD8 expressions in African green monkey helper T lymphocytes: implication for resistance to SIV infection. *Int. Immunol.* 1997;9(6):843–851.
87. Norley SG, Kraus G, Ennen J, et al. Immunological studies of the basis for the apathogenicity of simian immunodeficiency virus from African green monkeys. *Proc. Natl. Acad. Sci. USA* 1990;87: 9067–9071.
88. Robert-Guroff, Aldrich MK, Muldon R, et al. Cross-neutralizaion of human immunodeficiency virus type 1 and 2 and simain immunodeficiency virus isolates. *J. Virol.* 1992;66:3602–3608.
89. Gicheru MM, Otsyula M, Spearman P, et al. Neutralizing antibody responses in African green monkeys naturally infected with simian immunodeficiency virus (SIVagm). *J. Med. Primatol.* 1999;28:97–104.
90. Allan JS, Whitehead E, Strout K, et al. Cryptic neutralizing epitopes on SIVagm gp120; role in viral entry. *10th Annual symposium on nunhuman primate models for AIDS, San Juan* 1992:12.
91. Kraus G, Werner A, Baier M, et al. Isolation of human immunodeficiency viruses from African green monkeys. *Proc. Natl. Acad. Sci. USA* 1989; 86:2892–2896.
92. Rey-Cuille MA, Berthier JL, Bomsel-Demontoy MC, et al. Simian immunodeficiency virus replicates to high levels in sooty mangabeys without inducing disease. *J. Virol.* 1998;72(5):3872–3886.
93. Kodama T, Silva DP, Daniel MD, et al. Prevalence of antibodies to SIV in baboons in their native habitat. *AIDS Res. Hum. Retroviruses* 1989;3:337–343.
94. Baier M, Werner A, Bannert N, et al. HIV suppression by Interleukin-16. *Nature* 1995;378:563–564.
95. Cocchi F, De Vico AL, Garzino-Demo A, et al. Identification of RANTES, MIP-1a, and MIP-1b as the major HIV-suppressive factors produced by CD8+ cells. *Science* 1995;270(5243):1811–1815.
96. Levy JA, Mackewicz CE, Barker E. Controlling HIV pathogenesis: the role of noncytotoxic anti-HIV response of CD8+ cells. *Immunology Today* 1996;17(5):217–224.
97. Estaquier J, Idziorek T, De Bels F, et al. Programmed cell death and AIDS : significance of T-cell apoptosis in pathogenic and nonpathogenic primate lentiviral infections. *Proc. Natl. Acad. Sci. USA* 1994;91:9431–9435.
98. Kaur A, Grant RM, Means RE, et al. Diverse host responses and outcomes following simian immuno-deficiency virus SIVmac239 infection in sooty mangabeys and rhesus macaques. *J. Virol.* 1998; 72(12):9597–9611.
99. Villinger F, Folks TM, Lauro S, et al. Immunological and virological studies of natural SIV infection of disease-resistant nonhuman primates. *Immunology Letters* 1996;51(1–2):59–68.
100. Fultz PN, Stricker RB, McClure HM, et al. Humoral response to SIV/SMM infection in macaque and mangabey monkeys. *J. Acquir. Immune Defic. Syndr.* 1990;3:319–329.
101. Powell JD, Yehuda-Cohen T, Villinger F, et al. Inhibition of SIV/SMM replication in vitro by CD8+ cells from SIV/SMM infected seropositive clinically asymptomatic sooty mangabeys. *J. Med. Primatol.* 1990;19:239–249.
102. Ten Haaft P, Verstrepen B, Überla K, et al. A pathogenic threshold of virus load defined in SIV or SHIV-infected macaques. *J. Virol.* 1998;72: 10281–10285.
103. Chakrabarti LA, Lewin SR, Zhang L, et al. Normal T-cell turnover in sooty mangabeys harboring active Simian immunodeficiency virus infection. *J. Virol.* 2000;74(3):1209–1223.
104. Koopman G, Haaksma AGM, Ten Velden J, et al. The relative resistance of HIV–1-infected chimpanzees to AIDS correlates with the maintenance of follicular architecture and the absence of infiltration by CD8+ cytotoxic T lymphocytes. *AIDS Res. Hum. Retroviruses* 1999;15(4):365–373.
105. Kestens L, Peeters M, Vanham G, et al. Phenotypic and functional parameters of cellular immunity in a chimpanzee with a naturally acquired SIV infection. *J. Infect. Dis.* 1995;172:957–963
106. Peeters M, Janssens W, Vanden-Haesevelde M, et al. Virologic and serologic characteristics of a natural chimpanzee lentivirus infection. *Virology* 1995;211:315–315.

7

Serodiagnosis of HIV Infection

Aissatou Guèye-Ndiaye

Laboratoire de Bacteriologie-Virologie, Centre Hospitalier Universitaire, Dakar, Senegal.

Serologic assays have been an established method for the clinical diagnosis of HIV infection since the early 1980s. These techniques for detecting HIV infection have also been fundamental to the screening of blood donations and blood products, and to the epidemiologic monitoring of the severity and extent of the AIDS epidemic worldwide. The first laboratory methods to screen for HIV were developed shortly after the discovery of HIV (1).

HIV detection methods are based on the identification of various markers. Indirect, or serologic, detection is based on the identification of specific antibodies to HIV, while direct detection is based on the identification of whole viral particles, circulating antigens, or viral nucleic acids in biologic samples. Examples of assays that utilize each of these detection methods include the enzyme-linked immunosorbent assay (ELISA), the most common serologic or indirect assay; and the polymerase chain reaction (PCR), the most common direct detection assay.

The genetic variability of HIVs can reduce the efficiency of various HIV assays, including that of antibody tests and viral nucleic acid tests (2). In fact, HIV-1 group O was initially identified because it was not detected by certain serologic screening assays and it produced indeterminate Western blot results (3,4). In addition, assays that utilize antigen derived from HIV-1 subtype B have demonstrated a significantly lower sensitivity for screening some non-B subtypes (5–8). This reduced sensitivity is particularly problematic in Africa where multiple non-B subtypes are predominant, and the co-circulation of HIV-1 and HIV-2 in some areas further complicates HIV diagnosis (2). Non-B subtypes have also been documented recently in the United States and Europe (9,10). Most commercial HIV tests now appear to be able to detect most HIV-1 group M subtypes, although genetic variants, such as recombinant viruses, newly identified subtypes, or highly divergent viruses may still go undetected. Because diagnosis of acute infection relies heavily on these serologic assays rather than on clinical manifestations of HIV infection, the genetic variation of HIVs is of particular concern for recent seroconverters. Many third-generation assays incorporate subtype B antigens and perform well in narrowing the seroconversion window period during which infection with HIV is often difficult to detect. However, their accuracy in detecting early seroconversion with non-B subtypes has not been rigorously tested and requires extensive evaluation (11). Such serologic assays will need to be continually updated and tested to incorporate antigens from new subtypes and novel viral variants.

HIV TESTING STRATEGIES

Although advancements in molecular biology have provided alternative methods (12), serologic antibody testing remains the most commonly used method to diagnose HIV infection. The conventional algorithm for HIV testing consists of using a screening assay followed by a supplementary or confirmatory assay (13). Screening assays are designed to detect all potentially infected individuals, whereas confirmatory assays are used to distinguish true infections from nonspecific reactions that are not indicative of infection. Accordingly, screening tests should be highly sensitive, while confirmatory tests should be highly specific (14,15).

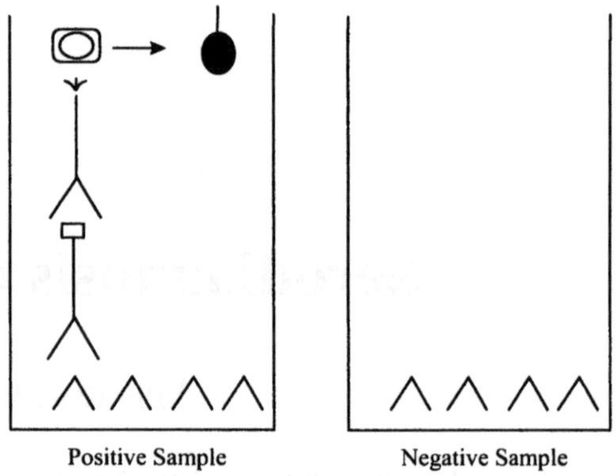

FIGURE 1. Indirect ELISA.

Key:

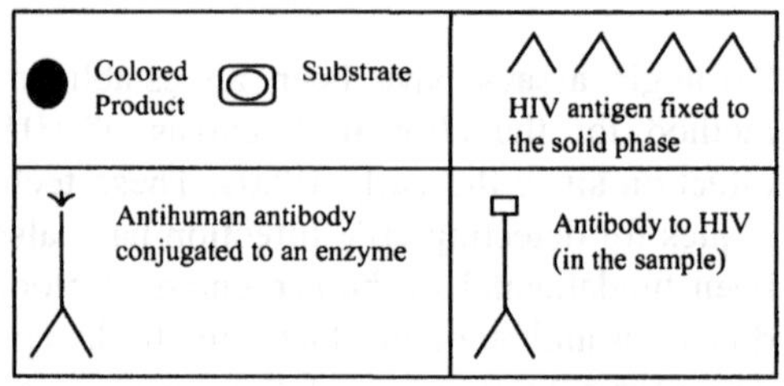

HIV Screening Assays

Serum or plasma samples are screened with an immunoenzymatic assay such as the ELISA, a rapid test, or a simple test.

Enzyme-linked Immunosorbent Assays

ELISAs are useful in many settings because they are relatively simple to perform, relatively inexpensive, standardized, highly reproducible, highly sensitive, and able to test large numbers of samples simultaneously. First-generation tests used antigens based on disrupted whole virus, obtained by purification of HIV grown in cell culture. Second-generation tests currently use recombinant proteins or synthetic peptides for higher specificity. Third-generation tests are based on the sandwich format. All varieties of ELISA use enzyme conjugates bound to HIV-specific antibodies. These, in turn, are bound to substrates that produce color in a reaction catalyzed by the bound enzyme conjugate.

The indirect method (Figure 1) is sensitive and varies in specificity. Serum is allowed to react with antigen fixed to the solid phase in a 96-well microtiter plate or beaded-well format. After 30 minutes of reaction at 37°C to 40°C, HIV antibodies present in the sample will bind to the antigen. Anti-human immunoglobulin (IgG) conjugated to an enzyme (such as peroxidase) is then added, followed by the addition of the appropriate substrate. The intensity of the resulting colorimetric reaction is approximately proportional to the amount of HIV antibody in the sample tested.

The competitive method is highly specific, but less sensitive. Serum or plasma sample from a potentially infected person and an enzyme-conjugated antibody to HIV made in a different species are added together on a solid phase containing the HIV antigen. The animal enzyme-conjugated antibody competes with the more avid human HIV-specific antibody in the sample for antigen sites on the solid phase. Because the human antibody binds more tightly than the enzyme-conjugated animal antibody, the human sample antibody will preferentially bind to the antigen sites. Incubation time is followed by a washing step to eliminate any unbound product (containing enzyme-conjugated antibody). Thus, when the substrate is added, there will be no enzyme bound to the solid phase to react, and a positive reaction will not be colored. With a negative sample, there will be no competition; the enzyme-conjugated animal antibody will bind to the antigen sites and react with the substrate, showing a colored signal.

In the sandwich method, multivalent antibody in the sample from a potentially infected person is captured between the antigen attached on the solid phase and a newly added antigen reagent bound to an enzyme. The colored signal is approximately proportional to the amount of antibody in the sample. The sandwich method is the most sensitive screening method, allowing detection of all types of antibodies, especially IgM (16).

The colored signal obtained in each of these methods (indirect, competitive, and sandwich) is interpreted with regard to a cutoff value that is calculated from controls' optical density (OD) based on a method specified in the test instructions and controls.

Rapid Tests

Rapid tests are based on immunofiltration or immunochromatography techniques and can generally be performed in less than 30 minutes. One such method, the dot blot, utilizes recombinant proteins or synthetic peptides absorbed onto nitrocellulose paper. Dilutions of test sera are then spotted onto the areas containing bound antigens and allowed to react. After incubation, the nitrocellulose is washed and incubated with enzyme-linked goat anti-human IgG antibody followed by the appropriate substrate for the bound enzyme. A positive reaction will show a spot. In another test, a dipstick method in which viral antigens are attached to the "teeth" of comb-like devices has been developed. Rapid tests can be performed easily without any instrumentation and some of them allow differentiation of HIV-1 and HIV-2.

Simple Tests

Simple tests are often based on agglutination and can be performed easily without any instrumentation, but can take longer than 30 minutes to perform. The solid phase can be red blood cells, latex particles, or gelatin. Simple tests cost less than rapid tests.

Confirmatory Assays

Because screening assays are highly sensitive, most testing algorithms require the use of very specific assays such as the Western blot, the indirect immunofluorescence assay (IFA), the radioimmunoprecipitation assay (RIPA), or the line immunoassay (LIA) to ensure that uninfected individuals are not falsely diagnosed with HIV infection (14).

Western Blot

Western blot, the gold standard of HIV testing, is based on electrophoretic migration of a viral lysate on a denaturing polyacrylamide gel to separate viral proteins according to their molecular weight. Proteins are then transferred onto nitrocellulose membranes, cut into strips, and incubated with a sample serum to be tested. Antigen–antibody complexes are visualized with an anti-human immunoglobulin conjugated to an enzyme. A colored band appears for every viral protein on which a specific antibody is bound. Western blots are extremely specific, allowing for identification of specific antibodies bound to their corresponding proteins.

Lee et al. have shown that Western blot immunoreactivity varies according to the viral isolate (17). For instance, the gp120 of isolates utilizing the chemokine receptor 5 (CCR5) has higher Western blot immunoreactivity to antibodies elicited against the protein in virus-infected human patients, compared with that of isolates utilizing the CXCR4 chemokine receptor, or dual isolates that utilize both receptors. These data have

TABLE 1. Interpretation Criteria for Western Blot Results (18)

Entities with developed criteria	HIV-1			HIV-2		
	Positive	Negative	Indeterminate	Positive	Negative	Indeterminate
WHO	At least 2 *env* bands (precursor gp160[a], mature gp120, or TM[b] gp41) +/− *pol* bands +/− *gag* bands	No HIV-1–specific bands or p17 only	Other profiles that are not considered positive or negative	At least 2 *env* bands (precursor gp140, mature gp125, or TM gp36) +/− *pol* bands +/− *gag* bands	No HIV-2–specific bands or p16 only	Other profiles that not considered positive or negative
U.S. FDA/Paul Erlich Institute, RDA/Bénélux	p24 and p31 and 1 *env* band (gp41, gp120 or gp 160)	No HIV-1–specific bands	Other profiles that are not considered positive or negative	Not defined	Not defined	Not defined
America Red Cross	1 band of every gene: 1 *gag* (p17, p24, p55) 1 *env* (gp41/120/160) 1 *pol* (p34, p51, p66)	No HIV-1–specific bands	Other profiles that are not considered positive or negative	Not defined	Not defined	Not defined
Japan	p24 and gp41 or gp160	No HIV-1–specific bands	Other profiles that are not considered positive or negative	Not defined	Not defined	Not defined
France	2 *env* bands (gp 120 and gp160) plus 1 *gag* band or 1 *pol* band	No HIV-1–specific bands or p17 only	gp160 only, p24 only	Not defined	Not defined	gp36 only

[a]gp indicates glycoprotein.
[b]TM indicates transmembrane.

shown that supplementing HIV-1 Western blot diagnostic kits with purified gp120 of CCR5 isolates could improve their sensitivity and facilitate early diagnosis.

Interpretation of Western Blot. The Western blot procedure is highly technical and requires well-trained personnel. Western blot results are interpreted by criteria that vary according to the lab performing the test. However, the World Health Organization (WHO), among other institutions, has made efforts to standardize the interpretation criteria for Western blots (Table 1) (18). Criteria for positive Western blot results vary according to institutions. It is now universally accepted that a negative result is the absence of reactivity on all bands/antigens (viral proteins). However, some institutions, including the WHO, suggest that results can also be reported as negative if there is only a very weak p17 band. Any Western blot reactivity that is neither positive nor negative according to the criteria being used must be classified as indeterminate.

Radioimmunoprecipitation Assay

The RIPA is a research technique confined to laboratories capable of propagating HIV in cell culture. HIV is grown in cells and then exposed to a radiolabeled amino acid, or another substance that allows isotopic incorporation or transfer to viral proteins. Cells are subsequently lysed, thereby releasing labeled viral proteins. Cell lysates are exposed to test serum, the IgG content of which has been previously bound to the "Fc" receptors of protein-A–coated Sepharose beads. The immunoprecipitates are then eluted from the beads and separated electrophoretically on polyacrylamide gels. The HIV antigen–antibody complexes are detected in the gel by autoradiography. The bands are similar to those of Western blot. RIPA is more sensitive than Western blot for the detection of antibodies to proteins of higher molecular weight, such as gp160 and gp120. These viral proteins may be detected with RIPA before anti-p24 or anti-gp41, thereby allowing confirmation of recent

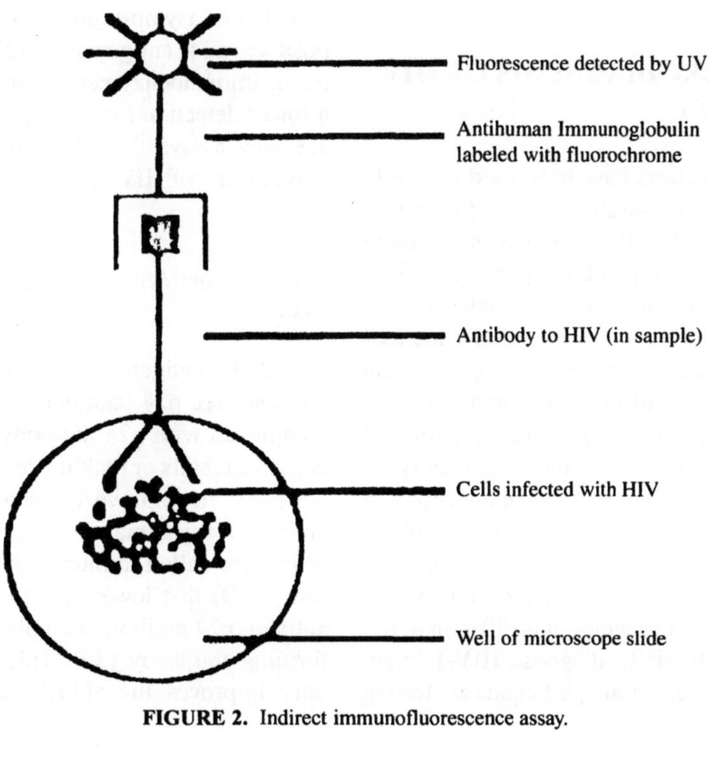

FIGURE 2. Indirect immunofluorescence assay.

seroconversion. RIPA has been found to be less sensitive than Western blot at detecting antibodies to p24 (19).

Indirect Immunofluorescence Assay

In the IFA, cells (usually lymphocytes) infected with HIV are fixed to a microscope slide. Serum containing HIV antibodies is added and reacts with the intracellular HIV. The slide is washed and then allowed to react with anti-human immunoglobulin antibodies with a covalently bound fluorescent label attached. The reaction is visualized using a fluorescent microscope (Figure 2).

Line Immunoassay

In the LIA, recombinant or synthetic peptide antigens are applied in lines on nitrocellulose, rather than electrophoresed as in a Western blot. The use of "artificial" (genetically engineered) antigens decreases the presence of contaminating substances derived from cell culture that in Western blots can cause interference, false reactions, or indeterminate results.

EARLY SERODIAGNOSIS OF HIV INFECTION

Serologic tests have been used primarily to monitor seroprevalence—the proportion of people with HIV antibodies—without distinguishing those with early infection from those with chronic infection. However, the ability to detect early HIV infection is increasingly important for prevention and treatment efforts. Measurements of incidence—the number of new infections within a period of time—offer researchers the opportunity to better evaluate recent changes in transmission rates. Furthermore, it is critical to be able to identify new infections among participants of vaccine trials. However, because viral components are used in vaccines, it is difficult to use serologic methods to diagnose HIV-1 infection in vaccine trial participants. Testing vaccine trial participants therefore requires the use of an antibody-based diagnostic test or a viral nucleic acid detection method that is capable of differentiating between immunization and true infection (20).

Detection of p24 Antigen

The core protein p24, which surrounds the viral ribonucleic acid, forms much of the internal structure of HIV-1. Antigenemia with p24 is a direct marker of viral replication (Figure 3). In plasma or cerebrospinal fluid, p24 antigen can be found in free form or complexed with immune cells. Only the free p24 is directly quantified by immunoenzymatic assays (21). The sensitivity of the assay used to detect p24 antigen varies according to the kit, but is generally higher in kits that use a monoclonal antibody with a detection limit of 10 to 40 pg/ml of p24 antigen. However, this quantity of antigen may not be present in the serum of infected individuals, even when the virus is actively replicating. In fact, only about 50% to 60% of AIDS patients, 30% to 40% of patients with AIDS-related complex, and 10% of asymp-tomatic patients will show positive p24 antigenemia (22). Some kits using immunoenzymatic amplification have a lower detection limit (1 pg/ml) (23). There are now assays that allow detection of the p26 antigen of HIV-2.

Improved Sensitivity of p24 Antigen Capture Assays

P24 antigen tests lack sensitivity because free p24 0antigen in serum may be complexed with p24 antibody, causing false negative results or making detection impossible (24). To improve the sensitivity of p24 antigen assays, manufacturers developed a procedure called immune complex dissociation (ICD) that lowers pH to dissociate p24 antigen–p24 antibody complexes before performing the assay (25). This procedure not only improves the ability of the assay to

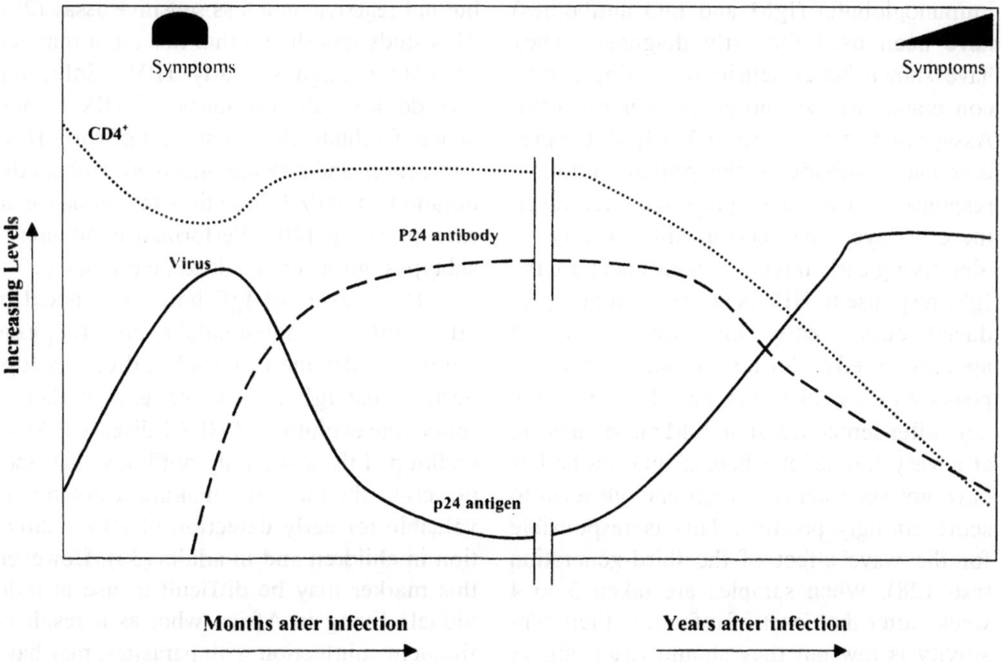

FIGURE 3. Comparison of p24 antigenemia, p24 antibody, $CD4^+$ count, and clinical symptoms during HIV infection.

detect p24 antigen in positive individuals (epidemiologic sensitivity), but also enables the detection of lower amounts of p24 antigen (analytical sensitivity). Nonetheless, p24 antigen tests are also subject to false positive reactions; specimens that are reactive by the p24 antigen test should be confirmed using a more specific method, such as an antigen neutralization assay (22).

According to Schupbach et al., boiling diluted samples for 5 minutes also abolishes all antigen binding by antibodies and leaves the p24 antigen reactive (26). This procedure increased the sensitivity of the p24 antigen test for pediatric diagnosis of HIV infection (27). The p24 antigen assay can also be boosted by a tyramide-based signal amplification step (26). In combination, these improvements led to a procedure that was as sensitive as the Roche Amplicor HIV-1 Monitor, an assay currently used to measure viral RNA levels. Finally, a combination of kinetic and endpoint evaluation of ELISA reactions has allowed quantification from about 0.5 pg/ml to more than 6 ng/ml. Several studies were undertaken to compare the optimized p24 antigen assays with PCR-based methods and have shown that p24 antigen assays, if assessed by proper methodology, are comparable to viral RNA assays with respect to sensitivity and specificity, monitoring antiretroviral treatment, and predicting disease progression (26).

Other Markers for Early Diagnosis of HIV Infection

During the seroconversion window period, antibodies to HIV may be present at low levels, but not up to the detection limits of some assays. Several components of the serologic response have been used to identify early infection in an individual when antibody titer is increasing but peak and persistently high antibody response has not yet occurred. In particular, the third-generation tests that allow detection of total immunoglobulin (IgM and IgG antibodies) have been used for early diagnosis. They have shown better sensitivity during seronconversion than second-generation tests (28). Assays to detect specific HIV-1 IgM, the predominant antibody in the primary immune response, have been proposed. However, these assays have shown little utility in identifying early infection in part because the IgM response to HIV is not consistently produced during early infection. Rather, it appears briefly during primary infection, peaks 2 to 3 weeks later, and then falls. Ten days after seroconversion, IgM antibodies are at a very low level whereas IgG antibodies have not yet reached a high enough level to score strongly positive. This is responsible for the wave effect of the third-generation tests (28). When samples are taken 3 to 4 weeks after the onset of infection, their sensitivity is low but they should reach higher reactivity levels later on.

The IgG antibody response to HIV-1 in infants born to HIV-1–infected mothers is obscured by persistent maternal HIV-specific IgG antibodies. Isotypes such as IgA and IgM have been proposed as alternative markers for early diagnosis in newborns. However, although IgA seems to be more sensitive than IgM, most studies have shown that these markers are not 100% accurate (20–27,29–33).

During early infection, the sandwich format tests, which allow detection of IgM and IgG, often appear to be more accurate than those that only detect IgG antibodies. To improve the lack of sensitivity and specificity of assays used to detect IgG antibodies, several improvements have been proposed. Andres et al. developed a new assay for HIV-1 and HIV-2 based entirely on correctly folded viral antigens (ectodomains of gp41 and gp36), which has demonstrated high sensitivity and specificity (34). Janssen et al. have proposed the use of a sensitive/less sensitive testing algorithm called a detuned assay, in which a blood specimen from a person with early infection is reactive on a sensitive assay but not reactive on a less sensitive assay (20). This study has shown that this algorithm can accurately diagnose early HIV-1 infection, provide accurate estimates of HIV-1 incidence, facilitate clinical studies of early HIV-1 infection, and provide information about the duration of HIV-1 infection for guidance in care planning (20). Performance on non-B subtypes, however, needs to be evaluated.

High levels of IgE have been noted in HIV-1-infected individuals in the early phase before the decline of $CD4^+$ cell counts suggesting that IgE may serve as a marker to reflect the evolution of HIV-1 disease (35). In addition, IgE is the only antibody that does not cross the placenta, making it potentially valuable for early detection of HIV-1 infection in children and in adults (36). However, this marker may be difficult to use in individuals living in Africa who, as a result of frequent coinfection with parasites, may have high levels of IgE.

Diagnostic Issues for HIV-2

Although strong serologic cross-reaction occurs between HIV-1 and HIV-2, particularly in viral structural proteins such as Gag and Pol (2,37,38), HIV-2 infection may not be detected when screening is done exclusively with HIV-1–specific serologic assays. Even though screening assays may be combined to detect both HIV-1 and HIV-2 infections, they are incapable of distinguishing HIV types.

The HIV-2 Western blot is required to specifically confirm HIV-2 infection. The specific antibody reactivity to envelope antigens in infected individuals has been used to distinguish between HIV-1 and HIV-2 infection (2,39).

Dual infection, most common in West Africa (Senegal, Gambia, Côte d'Ivoire, Guinea Bissau, and Ghana) and in India (40–44), is characterized by strong reactivity to the *env* antigens of both HIV-1 and HIV-2 by immunoblot and/or RIPA.

PCR is used to distinguish between HIV-1 and HIV-2 infection; however, PCR evidence of both viruses has been detected in as few as 30%, and up to 80%, of serologically defined dual reactive persons (2).

Evaluation and implementation of type-specific assays has been difficult, particularly in developing countries where the price per sample tested often exceeds the budget of many laboratories. It is unclear whether the low and variable concordance between serology and PCR is due to extensive HIV-1 cross-reactivity with HIV-2, misclassifications of samples based on serodiagnosis, or insensitivity of current PCR assays (4). Refinement of PCR assays with Southern blot detection has maximized their sensitivity and specificity for HIV-2 provirus detection (45,46).

Limitations of Current HIV Tests

Despite the high sensitivity and specificity of ELISAs and Western blots, they are prone to false positive and false negative results (47–49). Furthermore, although the Western blot is the most accepted confirmatory assay, it is not easily interpreted, and frequently produces indeterminate results. The significance of an indeterminate Western blot result varies depending on the patient's risk behaviors and clinical status (14,50). Indeterminate Western blot results may be observed as a result of cross-reactivity between antibodies to other HIV types and groups, or nonspecific reactions. They may also occur during the seroconversion window period, episodes of hypergammaglobulinemia in patients with late-phase AIDS, or infection with syphilis or malaria (51–53). The WHO recommends the following steps after obtaining indeterminate results: (i) sera from individuals with clinical signs of HIV infection who fit the WHO staging system criteria for stage III or IV and have an indeterminate result due to a decrease in antibodies, do not need to be retested (54); (ii) a second blood sample should be obtained from asymptomatic individuals after a minimum of 2 weeks following the first indeterminate sample. It is important to test both samples simultaneously to obtain a clear indication of changes in reactivity. If the second sample also produces an indeterminate result, it should be tested with another confirmatory assay. If these results are also indeterminate, longer follow-up may be required. Results that remain indeterminate for 1 year should be considered HIV-antibody–negative.

There are additional drawbacks to the use of Western blot assays. Confirmatory test results may be weakly reactive during early infection when antibody levels are low. Moreover, sera from some uninfected individuals may produce weakly reactive results, requiring follow-up after several weeks. Inconsistent results when testing specimens from the same individual or performing repeat tests may occur as a result of mislabeled specimens, technical errors in the laboratory, or the use of different assays. Technical errors can be minimized through the institution of a quality assurance program and documented preventive measures (18). Because HIV is diagnosed with serologic tests that are based on specific antigen–antibody reactions, subtle changes in antigenic structure may affect their sensitivity. Therefore, it is important to identify and further characterize divergent viruses in order to incorporate their antigens into successive generations of serologic assays (52).

Alternative Confirmatory Strategies

In addition to the drawbacks previously described, the Western blot is expensive and therefore not feasible in all laboratories in developing countries. One way to reduce the cost of HIV antibody testing is to select efficient, but simple, rapid, and inexpensive methods to monitor HIV infection (55). Because some developing countries are faced with overlapping HIV-1 and HIV-2 epidemics (44), assays for simultaneous detection of antibodies to HIV-1 and HIV-2 in a single run are now commonly used.

The WHO has recommended alternatives to the classic testing strategies (56,57). Alternative strategies utilize various combinations of screening assays without confirmatory

TABLE 2. UNAIDS and WHO Recommendations for HIV Testing Strategies According to Test Objective and Prevalence of Infection in Sample Population (57)

Objective of testing		Prevalence of infection	Testing strategy[a]
Transfusion and transplant safety		Any prevalence	I
Surveillance		>10%	I
		≤10%	II
Diagnosis	Patients with clinical signs/ symptoms of HIV infection	>30%	I
		≤30%	II
	Asymptomatic patients	>10%	II
		≤10%	III

[a]Each testing strategy is outlined in Table 3.

tests, to diagnose or rule out HIV infection. Their objectives are to obtain positive or negative predictive values equal to those of the classic strategy that uses confirmatory assays. Three testing strategies aimed at maximum accuracy for minimum cost have been recommended, including ELISA and/or rapid/simple assays instead of the ELISA plus Western blot strategy (57) (Tables 2, 3). The choice of the most appropriate strategy for a particular setting will depend on the testing objective, the prevalence of HIV in the population, and the sensitivity and specificity required. It is important to select appropriate assays and to use the most sensitive one for initial testing. The initial and second assays must be of different formats (beads vs. microtiter) and/or use a different antigen source (lysate vs. recombinant or synthetic peptides).

These alternatives strategies have been evaluated in many developing countries (58–61) and have shown that combinations of ELISA with rapid/simple assays provide results as reliable as those for ELISA plus Western blot, but at a much lower cost (62–70).

NEW TECHNOLOGIES

Since 1985, tremendous progress has been made in the field of HIV testing. However, much work remains to be done to develop and evaluate the next effective diagnostic tools in varied settings. The ideal diagnostic assay would be able to detect all HIV variants during the earliest phase of infection. It would be inexpensive and very simple to perform and interpret. It would also be highly specific and sensitive for us as an efficient prevention and control tool (28).

The use of body fluids other than blood, such as saliva or urine, for detecting antibodies to HIV is an attractive alternative for several reasons (71–73). Saliva specimens can be collected anywhere (at home, on the street, or in bars) and are easy to store. Sample collection methods that are not invasive are safer for the donors and for the health care workers because there is no danger of blood transmission through unsterilized syringes or needlestick injuries. Furthermore, the infectivity of saliva and urine seems to be very low. The collection of saliva and urine samples instead of blood may increase patient compliance, and is acceptable to those who experience difficulty giving blood.

The main technical problem in the use of saliva and urine samples for HIV testing is caused by the fact that IgG and IgA levels in saliva and urine are considerably lower than those in serum or plasma. A minimal concentration of IgG of 0.1 mg/L is needed to detect antibodies to HIV (74). Testing saliva or urine therefore requires an extremely sensitive test that is able to detect the small

TABLE 3. Schematic Representation of the UNAIDS and WHO HIV Testing Strategies (57)

Strategy I: One assay only	Strategy II: Sequential application of two assays
Objectives: • Transfusion/transplant safety • Surveillance in populations with >10% prevalence • Diagnosis of patients with clinical signs/ symptoms in populations with >30% prevalence	Objectives: • Surveillance in populations with ≤ 10% prevalence • Diagnosis of patients with clinical signs/symptoms in populations with ≤ 30% prevalence • Diagnosis of asymptomatic patients in populations with >10% prevalence

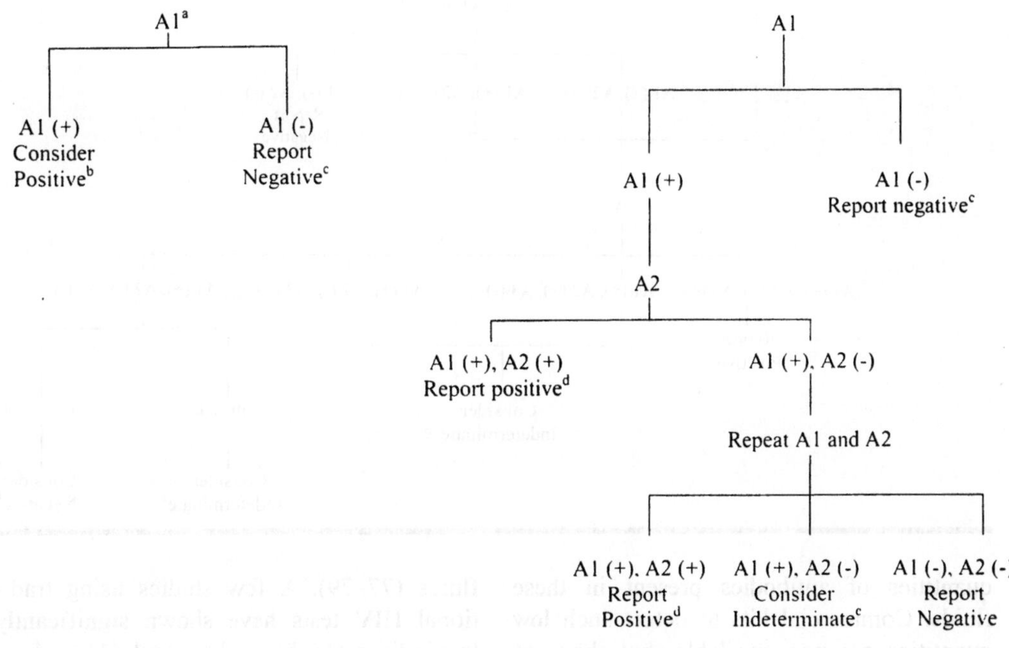

[a]A1, A2, and A3 indicate three different assays.
[b]This result is not adequate for diagnostic purposes. Use strategies II or III. Whatever the final diagnosis, donations that were initially reactive should not be used for transfusion or transplants.
[c]Result may be reported.
[d]For newly diagnosed individuals, a positive result should be confirmed on a second sample.
[e]Testing should be repeated on a second sample taken after 14 days.
[f]In absence of any risk for HIV infection.

Continued

TABLE 3. *Continued*

Strategy III: Sequential application of three assays

Objectives:
- Diagnosis of patients with clinical signs/symptoms in populations with >30% prevalence

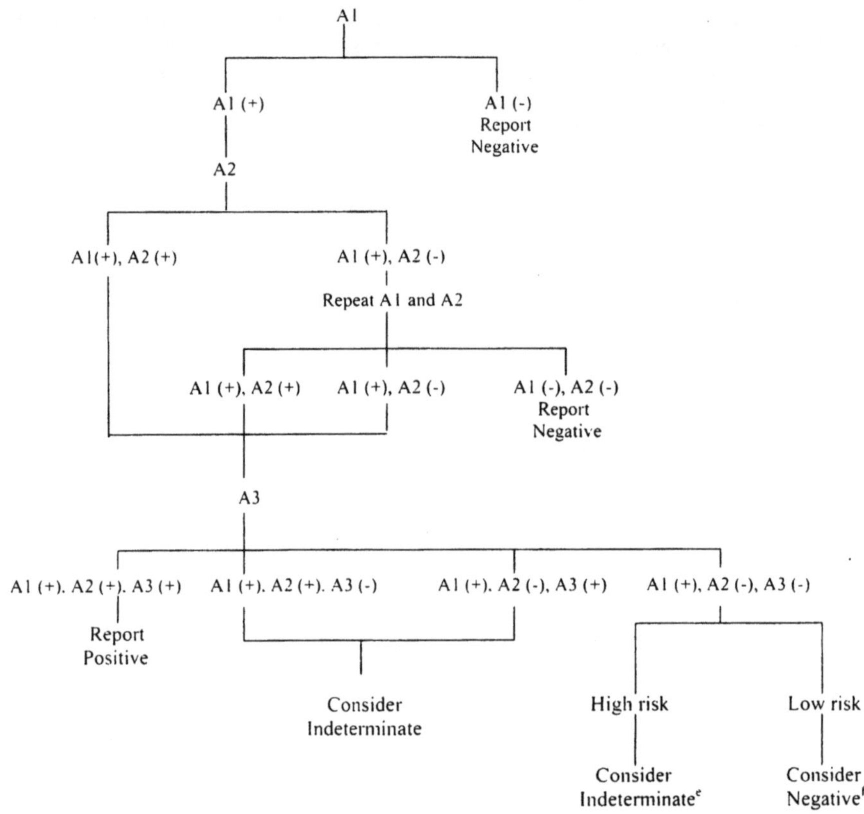

quantities of antibodies present in these fluids. Commercial kits to detect such low quantities are now available, but they are intended for use with blood samples only (14). When using these commercial kits to detect antibodies in saliva or urine, the volume of sample must be increased or concentrated before testing (71).

Saliva

Since 1986, several studies have shown that antibodies to HIV can be detected in the oral fluids of seropositive subjects (75,76). However, there have been conflicting reports on the sensitivity of HIV testing with these fluids (77–79). A few studies using traditional HIV tests have shown significantly low indices. Confusion has resulted largely in part from a failure to recognize that antibody concentrations in oral fluids are heavily influenced by collection methods. Saliva should be collected into a receptacle or with the aid of a commercial oral fluid kit. Several antibody-testing systems are commercially available in the United States. One system is used to collect and stabilize oral mucosal transudate (OMT), a fluid with increased levels of IgG. An enzyme immunoassay (EIA) screening test has been optimized for OMT, and a Western blot confirmatory test has also been designed for use with OMT. Several studies have shown that results obtained with these systems are substantially better than those obtained with systems using whole saliva (80).

Urine

The collection of urine samples, like that of saliva, is a simple procedure. However, there are several advantages to using urine samples for HIV antibody testing. Antibodies are stable in urine for 55 days when stored at room temperature (81). There is little risk of exposure to HIV as the presence of free virus in urine has not been described to date. In contrast, the saliva of some HIV-infected individuals may contain a small amount of infectious virions (82). Some screening assays can detect HIV antibodies in urine before an individual tests seropositive (83).

Unfortunately, there is not an approved confirmatory assay for HIV in urine. The classic confirmatory assay (Western blot) may be used, but its sensitivity to detect antibodies in urine requires improvement (84). According to Schopper and Vercauteren, the sensitivity and specificity of various methods using urine specimens has ranged from 77% to 100%, and 69.7% to 100%, respectively (71). This level of sensitivity in specimens other than sera or plasma would be inappropriate for diagnostic purposes, but acceptable for a surveillance program (71).

Dried Blood Spots

The collection of dried blood spots (DBS) on filter paper is another sampling method that has proven useful. In general, capillary blood is obtained by finger or heel prick. Quantities sufficient to saturate at least 2 spots on absorbent filter paper are obtained, air-dried, stored in a sealed plastic bag with desiccant, and mailed to the appropriate laboratory for testing. Little formal training is required for the collection of DBS, and the necessary supplies are inexpensive. Samples are easily transported because they do not require cold storage and can be stored for several months without loss of antibody reactivity. Large numbers of field specimens can be collected and shipped to centralized reference laboratories for genetic and/or serologic analysis. DBS methods are particularly useful in developing countries and isolated rural regions where resources are limited. However, DBS technology has been reported to have low sensitivity for HIV-2 infection (71,85).

Although new data suggest a need for technologies that detect antibodies in biologic fluids other than serum or plasma, their accuracy and reliability compared to established assays must be evaluated extensively before they are utilized in routine testing.

Home Tests

The potential for use of alternative specimens that are easily collected through noninvasive methods, and the development of the rapid and simple HIV tests may allow researchers to move toward a new concept in HIV diagnosis: the home test. There are two different concepts in HIV home testing: (i) the collection of samples in an individual's home for HIV testing at a laboratory location, and (ii) the use of an HIV test performed by the individual at home without any link to a medical setting or laboratory.

The first concept was implemented in the United States. In May 1996, the U.S. Food and Drug Administration (FDA) approved Confide (manufactured by Direct Access Diagnosis), the first HIV testing system not entirely linked to the medical setting (86). The FDA later licensed a different home HIV-1 testing system, manufactured by Home Access Health Corporation of Chicago. To use this test, an individual pricks his or her finger and puts a drop of blood on a piece of absorbent paper. The individual then mails the specimen, which is labeled with an anonymous code number, directly to a laboratory for HIV antibody testing.

Approximately 7 days later, he or she calls for the result. According to the test result, appropriate counseling is given either by voice mail (for a negative result) or person-to-person (for a positive result) (86,87). Considerable debate preceded the approval of home sample collection for HIV testing. Proponents maintained that its availability would increase testing (88), but opponents raised concerns about the negative consequences of receiving results by telephone and the possible effect on public health surveillance and control (86).

The second home-test concept has not yet been implemented. To perform this type of test, an individual could collect blood (obtained by finger prick), saliva, or urine for a self-administered test at home. Some of the rapid tests used in laboratories provide results in 10 to 15 minutes and could be used as true home tests (89). However, their future use in developing countries is uncertain.

CONCLUSION

An arsenal of laboratory methods is available to screen blood, diagnose infection, and monitor disease progression in individuals infected with HIV. However, antibody testing is currently the most widely used and most effective way to identify HIV infection. Due to the high cost and sensitivity of molecular genotyping assays, serologic methods will remain the first-line tools for detecting HIV infection in the foreseeable future.

In developing countries, the high cost of HIV diagnosis has been reduced by the replacement of the classic testing algorithm with an alternative that uses ELISA and/or rapid/simple tests. While this alternative does allow cost savings of up to 82%, savings vary according to the prevalence of HIV infection in the population being tested (55). For example, in settings with very low HIV prevalence and a small proportion of initially reactive serum samples (whether truly or falsely positive), little cost saving could be achieved by avoiding Western blot testing (55). A format has been described using recombinant antigen from both HIV-1 and HIV-2 that can be readily implemented in developing country laboratory settings and that will greatly reduce the time and the cost of HIV diagnosis (90).

Serodiagnosis has shown little utility for detecting HIV shortly after infection. Researchers must prioritize the development of accurate assays to identify early infection. Mathematical models suggest that 56% to 92% of all HIV infections may be transmitted during acute primary infection. Thus, reducing transmission from persons with acute primary infection may be one of the best ways to reduce the overall spread of HIV. Diagnosing primary infection is therefore key to both treatment and prevention (91). Diagnostic tools that are capable of identifying early infection and can be implemented in developing countries where all HIV subtypes are present and high rates of infection occur, will be useful in vaccine trials as well.

Alternative methods for blood sampling may be very useful in facilitating the use of HIV testing as a control and prevention tool. The United States is the only country where an oral fluid test system has been approved for initial diagnosis of HIV infection, although other countries have used such systems for surveillance purposes (28). Most European countries have cautioned against saliva tests for diagnostic purposes because their performance is still inferior to that of conventional specimens and their sensitivity for detecting seroconversion is unknown (71).

No countries yet envisage the approval of over-the-counter home self-test kits for HIV. Nevertheless, because the technology exists, manufacturers of these products may seek markets in some parts of the world where regulations are not restrictive. The use of home tests could increase the numbers of individuals being tested for HIV. However, no information exists on the potential impact of their widespread availability on individuals, on population groups that are at high risk or more vulnerable to HIV infection, or on society at large (14).

Programs of quality assurance, quality control and quality assessment should be largely promoted in African HIV testing settings, in order to be sure that HIV results obtained are accurate (92). Similarly, more voluntary counseling and testing centers should be established. It is also necessary to create institutions to regulate HIV reagents in developing countries, such as the FDA in the United States, the Agence du Medicament in France, or the Paul Erlich Institute in Germany.

REFERENCES

1. Weiss SH, Goedert JJ, Sarngadharan M, et al. Screening test for HTLV-III (AIDS agent) antibodies. Specificity, sensitivity, and applications. *JAMA*, 1985;253:221–225.
2. Kanki PJ, Peeters M and Guèye-Ndiaye A. Virology of HIV-1 and HIV-2: implication for Africa. *AIDS*, 1997;11(suppl B):S33–S42.
3. Loussert-Ajakat I, Ly TD, Chaix ML, et al. HIV-1/HIV-2 seronegativity in HIV-1 subtype O infected patients. *Lancet*, 1994;343:1393–1394.
4. Schabble C, Zekeng L, Pau CP, et al. Sensitivity of United States HIV antibody tests for detection of HIV-1 group O infections. *Lancet*, 1994;344:1333–1334.
5. Apetrei C, Loussert-Ajaka I, Descamps D, et al. Lack of screening test sensitivity during HIV-1 non-subtype B seroconversions. *AIDS*, 1996; 10:F57–F60.
6. Simon F, Ly TD, Baillou-Beaufils A, et al. Sensitivity of screening kits for anti-HIV-1 group O antibodies. *AIDS*, 1994;8:1628–1629.
7. Centers for Disease Control and Prevention. Persistent lack of detectable HIV-1 antibody in a person with infection. *MMWR*, 1996;45:181–185.
8. Soriano V, Dronda F, Gonzalez-Lopez A, et al. HIV-1 causing AIDS and death in a seronegative individual. *Voxsang*, 1994;7:410–411.
9. Simon F, Loussert-Ajaka I, Damond F, et al. HIV type 1 diversity in northern Paris, France. *AIDS Res Hum Retroviruses*, 1996;12:1427–1433.
10. Broodine SK, Mascola JR, Weiss PJ, et al. Detection of diverse HIV-1 genetic subtypes in the USA. *Lancet*, 1995;346:1198–1199.
11. Janssens W, Buve A, Nkengasong JN. The puzzle of HIV-1 subtypes in Africa. *AIDS*, 1997;11:705–712.
12. Nicoot T, Rogez S, Denis F. Application en virology humaine des différentes techniques de bilogie moléculaire (Hybridation, amplification génique). *Spectra Biol*, 1995;95/6:33–51.
13. Schochetmann G, Epstein J, Zuch T, et al. Serodiagnosis of infection with AIDS virus and other retroviruses. *Annu Rev Microbiol*, 1989; 43:629–659.
14. Constantine NT. HIV Antibody Testing. In: Cohen PT, Sande MA, Volberding PA, eds. *The AIDS Knowledge Base*, 3rd Ed., Philadelphia: Lippincott Williams & Wilkins, 1999;105–112.
15. Couroucé et le groupe de travail Rétrovirus de la société française de transfusion sanguine: Sensibilité des trousses de dépistage des anticorps anti-VIH. Réévaluation 1999. *Transfus Clin Biol*, 1999;6:381–394.
16. Constantine NT, Van Der Groen G, et al. Sensitivity of HIV antibody assays as determined by seroconversion panels. *AIDS*, 1994;16:1715–1720.
17. Lee MK, Martin MA, Cho MW. Higher western blot immunoreactivity of glycoprotein 120 from R5 HIV type 1 isolates compared with X4 and X4R5 isolates. *AIDS Res Hum Retroviruses*, 2000;8:765–775.
18. World Health Organization. Acquired immunodeficiency syndrome (AIDS): proposed WHO criteria for interpreting results from Western blot Assays for HIV-1, HIV-2 and HTLV-I/HTLV-II. *Wkly Epidemiol Rec*, 1990;65:281–283.
19. Schleupner CJ. Detection of HIV-1 infection. In: Mandel, Douglas, Bennett, eds. *Principles and Practice of Infectious Diseases*, 3rd Ed. New York: Churchill Livingstone, 1990;1097.
20. Janssen RS, Satten GA, Stramer SI et al. New testing strategy to detect early HIV-1 infection for use of incidence estimates and for clinical and prevention purposes. *JAMA*, 1998;280:42–48.
21. Bélec L. Antigénémie p24 et anticorps anti-p24. In: *Techniques virologiques et pratiques cliniques dans le domaine du SIDA*, Bristol-Meyers-Squibb, 1995;17–28.
22. Constantine NT. Tests to detect HIV Antigen. In: Cohen PT, Sande MA, Volberding PA, eds. *The AIDS Knowledge Base*, 3rd Ed., Philadelphia: Lippincott Williams & Wilkins, 1999;105–112.
23. Bélec L, Ripoli L, Matta F, al. Marqueurs biologiques prévionnels d'évolution au cours de l'infection par le virus d'immunodéficience humaine. *Ann Biol Clin*, 1992;50:621–637.
24. Nishanian P, Huskins KR, Stehn S, et al. A simple method for improved assay demonstrates that HIV p24 antigen is present as immune complexes in most sera from HIV-infected individuals. *J Infect Dis*, 1990;162:21–28.
25. Guay LA, Hom DL, Kabengera SR et al. HIV-1 ICD p24 antigen detection in Ugandan infants: use in early diagnosis of infection and as a marker of disease progression. *J Med Virol*, 2000; 62:426–434.

26. Schüpbach J, Varnier OE. HIV-1 p24 Antigen–a sensitive and precise, yet inexpensive alternative to PCR for viral DNA or RNA. *IAS Newsletter*, 2000;15:9–10.
27. Schüpbach J, Boni J, Tomasisik Z, et al. Sensitive detection and early prognostic significance of p24 antigen in heat-denatured plasma of human immunodeficiency virus type 1–infected infants: Swiss neonatal HIV study group. *J Infect Dis*, 1994;170:318–324.
28. Ataman-Önal Y, Biron F, Verrier B. Evolution des réactifs de détection des anticorps anti-VIH. *Méd Mal Infect*, 1998;28:496–504.
29. Schüpbach J, Boni I. Quantitative and sensitive detection of immune-complexes and free HIV antigen after boiling of serum. *J Virol Methods*, 1993;43:247–569.
30. Srugo I, Yogev R, Brunell P. Antigen requirement for an IgM ELISA to detect early HIV infection. In: Program and abstracts of the International Conference on AIDS; June 16–21, 1991;7:187; Abstract W.B. 2060.
31. Schüpbach J, Tomasik Z, Boni J, et al. Specificity of HIV-reactive IgM and IgA antibodies in pediatric HIV infection and their diagnostic usefulness. In: Program and abstracts of the Int Conf AIDS; June 16–21, 1991;7:349; Abstract W.C. 3212).
32. Schüpbach J, Tomasik Z, Jendis J, et al. IgG, IgM, and IgA: Response to HIV in infants born to HIV infected mothers. *JAIDS*, 1994;7:421–427.
33. McIntosh K, Comeau AM, Wara D, et al. The utility of IgA antibody to human immunodeficiency virus type 1 in early diagnosis of vertically transmitted infection. *Arch Pediatr Adolesc Med*, 1996;150:598–602.
34. Andres H, Boeck C, Brodeck H, et al. The new Cobas Core anti-HIV-1/2 EIA DAGS.II: A highly sensitive assay based entirely on correctly folded HIV antigens. In: Program and abstracts of the Int Conf AIDS; 1998;12:794; Abstract 42108.
35. Pletcher M, Miguez-Burrbano MJ, Shor-Posner, et al. Diagnosis of human immunodeficiency virus infection using an immunoglobulin E-based assay. *Clin Diagn Lab Immunol*, 2000;7:55–57.
36. Miguez-Burbano MJ, Shor-Posner G, Fletcher MA, et al. Immunoglobulin E levels in relationship to HIV-1 disease, route of infection, and vitamin E status. *Allergy*, 1995;50:157–161.
37. Kanki PJ, Marlink R, Siby T, et al. Biology of HIV-2 infection in West Africa. In: Papas T, ed. *Gene Regulation and AIDS*. Saratoga: Portfolio Publishing Company, Incorporated, 1990;255–272.
38. Essex M, Kanki P. Human immunodeficiency virus type 2 (HIV-2). In: Broder S, Merigan T, Bologenesi D, eds. *Textbook of AIDS Medicine*. Baltimore: Williams & Wilkins, 1994;873–886.
39. Tedder R, O'Connor T, Hughs A, et al. Envelope cross-reactivity in western blot for HIV-1 and HIV-2 may not indicate dual infection. *Lancet*, 1988;2:927–930.
40. Ghys PD, Diallo MO, Ettiegne-Traore V, et al. Dual seroreactivity to HIV-1 and HIV-2 in female sex workers in Abijdan, Côte d'ivoire. *AIDS*, 1995;9:955–988.
41. Hishida O, Ayisi NK, Aidoo M, et al. Serological survey of HIV-1, HIV-2 and human T-cell Leukemia virus type 1 for suspected AIDS cases in Ghana. *AIDS*, 1994;8:1257–1261.
42. Pfutzner A, Dietrich U, Von EU, et al. HIV-1 and HIV-2 infections in a high-risk population in Bombay, India: evidence for the spread of HIV-2 and presence of a divergent HIV-1 subtype. *JAIDS*, 1992;5:972–977.
43. Poulsen AG, Aaby P, Larsen O, et al. 9-year HIV-2 associated mortality in urban community in Bissau, West Africa. *Lancet*, 1997;349:911–914.
44. Kanki P, Mboup S, Barin F, et al. The biology of HIV-1 and HIV-2 in Africa. In: Giraldo G, Beth-Girado E, Klumeck N, Gharbi MDR, Kyalwazi SK, Dethé G, eds. *AIDS and Associated Cancers in Africa*. Basel: Karger, 1988;230–236.
45. Dieng-Sarr A, Hamel D, Thior I, et al. HIV-1 and HIV-2 dual infection: lack of HIV-2 provirus correlates with low CD4+ lymphocyte counts. In: Program and abstracts of the IX International Conference on AIDS in Africa; December 10–14, 1995; Kampala, Uganda. Abstract TuA137.
46. Ishika K, Fransen K, Ariyoshi K, et al. Improved detection of HIV-2 proviral DNA in dually seroreactive individuals by PCR. *AIDS*, 1998;12: 1419–1424.
47. Kleinman S, Busch MP, Hall L, et al. False-positive HIV-1 results in a low-risk screening setting of voluntary blood donation: Retrovirus Epidemiology Donor Study. *JAMA*, 1998;280:1080–1085.
48. Dwip K, et al. Estimated rate of HIV-1 infection but seronegative blood donations in Bangkok, Thailand. *AIDS*, 1996;10:1157–1162.
49. Mortimer PP. Antibody tests: progress and pitfalls. *Clin Diagn Virol*, 1996;5:131–136.
50. Tarjan V, Ujhelyi E, Kellner R, et al. Three cases of transient HIV-1 seropositivity observed in 10 years of practice of a national HIV confirmatory laboratory. *AIDS*, 1998;12:120–121.
51. Phair J, Hoover D, Huprikar J, et al. The significance of Western blot assays indeterminate for antibody to HIV in a cohort of homosexual/bisexual men. *JAIDS*, 1992;5:988–992.
52. Lutz G. Difficulties and strategies of HIV diagnosis. *Lancet*, 1996;348:176–179.
53. Cordes RJ, Ryan ME. Pitfalls in HIV testing. Applications and limitations of current tests. *Postgrad Med*, 1995;98:177–180, 185–186, 189. Review.

54. World Health Organization. Interim proposed for a WHO staging system for HIV infection and disease. *Wkly Epidemiol Rec*, 1990;65: 221–228.
55. Tamashiro H, Maskill W, Emmanuel A, et al. Reducing the cost of HIV antibody testing. *Lancet*, 1993;342:87–90.
56. World Health Organization. WHO recommendations for selection and use of HIV antibody tests. *Wkly Epidemiol Rec*, 1992;20:145–149.
57. World Health Organization–Joint United Nations program on HIV/AIDS (UNAIDS): WHO revised recommendations for selection and use of HIV antibody tests. *Wkly Epidemiol Rec*, 1997;72: 81–86.
58. Gresenguet G, Tevi-Benissan C, Payan C et al. Stratégie alternative pour le Diagnostic de l'infection par le VIH en Afrique Sub-Saharienne. Intérçet de la combinaison séquentielle d'un test Elisa et d'un test rapide de 2ème génération. *Bull Soc Path Exo*, 1993;86:236–242.
59. Urassa W, Matunda S, Bredberg-Raden U, et al. Evaluation of the WHO Human Immunodefiency Virus (HIV) antibody testing strategy for the diagnosis of HIV infection. *Clin Diagn Virol*, 1994;2:1–6.
60. Carvalho MB, Hamerschlak N, Vaz RS, et al. Risk factor analysis and serological diagnosis of HIV-1/HIV-2 infection in Brazilian blood donor population: Validation of the World Health Organization strategy for HIV testing. *AIDS*, 1996;10: 1135–1140.
61. Stetler HC, Granada TC, Nunez CA, et al. Field evaluation of rapid HIV serologic tests for screening and confirming HIV-1 infection in Honduras. *AIDS*, 1997;11:369–375.
62. Laleman G, Kambale M, Van Kerckhven I, et al. A simplified and less expensive strategy for confirming anti-HIV-1 screening results in a diagnostic laboratory in Lumbumshi, Zaire. *Ann Soc Belge Med Trop*, 1991;71:287–294.
63. Nkengasong J, Van Kerckhven I, Vercauteren G, et al. Alternative confirmatory strategy for anti-HIV antibody detection. *J Virol Methods*, 1992;36:159–170.
64. Brattegaard K, Kouadio J, Adom ML, et al. Rapid and simple screening and supplemental testing for HIV-1 and HIV-2 infections in west Africa. *AIDS*, 1993;7(6):883–885.
65. Blaxhult A, Anagrius A, Arneborn M, et al. Evaluation of HIV in Sweden, 1985–1991. *AIDS*, 1993;7:1625–1631.
66. Nunn AJ, Biryahwaho B, Downing RG, et al. Algorithms for detecting antibodies to HIV-1: results from a rural Ugandan Cohort. *AIDS*, 1993;7:1057–1061.
67. Anderson S, Da Silva Z, Norrgren H, et al. Field evaluation of alternative testing strategies for diagnosis and differentiation of HIV-1 and HIV-2 infections in an HIV-1 and HIV-2 prevalent area. *AIDS*, 1997;11:1815–1822.
68. Urwijitaroon Y, Barusrux S, Romphruk A, et al. Anti-HIV antibody titer: an alternative supplementary test for diagnosis of HIV-1 infection. *Asian Pac J Allergy Immunol*, 1997;15:193–198.
69. Nkengasong JN, Maurice C, Koblvi S, et al. Field evaluation of a combination of monospecific Enzyme-Linked-Immunosorbent Assays for type-specific diagnosis of human immunodeficiency virus type 1 (HIV-1) and HIV-2 infections in HIV-seropositive persons in Abidjan, Ivory Coast. *J Clin Microbiol*, 1998;36:123–127.
70. Nkengasong JN, Maurice C, Koblvi S, et al. Evaluation of HIV serial and parallel serologic testing algorithms in Abidjan, Côte d'Ivoire. *AIDS*, 1999;13:109–117.
71. Schopper D, Vercauteren G. Testing at Home: What are the issues? *AIDS*, 1996;10:1455–1456.
72. Hoelscher M, Riedner G, Hemed Y, et al. Estimating the number of HIV transmissions though reused syringes and needles in the Mbeya region, Tanzania. *AIDS*, 1994;8:1609–1615.
73. Major CJ, Read SE, Coates RA, et al. Comparison of saliva and blood for human immunodeficiency virus prevalence testing. *J Infect Dis*, 1991;163: 699–702.
74. Connell JA, Parry JV, Mortimer PP, et al. Novel assay for the detection of immnoglobulin G anti-human immunodeficiency virus in untreated saliva and urine. *J Med Virol*, 1993;41:159–164.
75. Coates R, Millson M, Myers T, et al. The benefits of HIV antibody testing of saliva in field research. *Can J Public Health*, 1991;82:397–398.
76. Schramm W, Angulo GB, Torres PC, et al. A simple saliva-based test for detecting antibodies to human immunodeficiency virus. *Clin Diagn Lab Immunol*, 1999;6(4):577–580.
77. Archibald DW, Zon L, Groopman JE, et al. Antibodies to human T-lymphotropic virus type III (HTLV-III) in saliva of Acquired Immunodeficiency Syndrome (AIDS) patients and in persons at risk for AIDS. *Blood*, 1986;67:831–834.
78. Major CJ, Read SE, Coates RA, et al. Comparison of saliva and blood for human immunodeficiency virus prevalence testing. *J Infect Dis*, 1991;163: 699–702.
79. King A, Marison SA, Cook D, et al. Accuracy of a saliva test for HIV antibody. *J Acquir Immune Defic Syndr Hum Retrovirol*, 1995;9:172–175.
80. Gallo D, Georges JR, Fitchen JH, et al. Evaluation of a system using oral mucosal transudate for HIV-1 antibody screening and confirmatory testing. *JAMA*, 1997;277:254–258.

81. Urnovitz HB, Murphy WH, Gottfried TD, et al. Urine-based diagnostic technologies. *Trends Biotechnol*, 1996;14:361–364.
82. Phillips J, Qureshi N, Barr C, et al. Low level of cell-free virus detected at high frequency in saliva from HIV-1 infected individuals. *AIDS*, 1994;8:1011–1012.
83. Urnovitz HB, Clerici M, Shearer GM, et al. HIV-1 antibody serum negativity with urine positivity. *Lancet*, 1993;342:1458–1459.
84. Ohya H, Tsukano K, Ichkawa K, et al. ABC-Western blot method to confirm the antibody against HIV-1 in urine samples. In: Program and abstracts of the Int Conf AIDS; July 7–12, 1996;11:294; Abstract Tu.B.2170.
85. Cassol SA, Read S, Weniger BG, et al. Dried blood spots collected on filter paper: An international resource for diagnosis and genetic characterization of human immunodeficiency virus type-1. *Mem Inst Oswaldo Cruz*, 1996;91:351–358.
86. Branson BM. Home sample collection tests for HIV infection. *JAMA*, 1998;280:1699–1701.
87. Brodie S, Sax P, et al. Novel approaches to HIV antibody testing. *AIDS Clin Care*, 1997;9:1–5.
88. Bayer R, Stryker J, Smith MD. Testing for HIV at home. *N Engl J Med*, 1995;332:1296–1299.
89. Kassler WB. Advances in HIV testing technology and their potential impact on prevention. *AIDS Educ Prev*, 1997;9(suppl B):27–40.
90. Guèye-Ndiaye A, Clark R, Samuel K, et al. Cost-effective diagnosis of HIV-1 and HIV-2 by recombinant-expressed env peptide (566/996) dot-blot analysis. *AIDS*, 1993;7:1411–1417.
91. Thomas C, Quinn MD. Acute primary HIV infection. *JAMA*, 1997;278:58–62.
92. Constantine NT, Callahan J, Watts DM, eds. *Retroviral testing: Essentials for quality control and laboratory diagnosis*. Boca Raton: CRC Press, 1992.

8

Molecular Diagnosis of HIV Infection

Boris Renjifo

Department of Immunology and Infectious Diseases, Harvard School of Public Health and Harvard AIDS Institute Research Laboratories, Boston, Massachusetts, USA.

The genome of the human immunodeficiency viruses is found as two copies of single-stranded RNA within the virion or as double-stranded DNA within the infected cell. After infection, the RNA genome is used as template by the viral reverse transcriptase (RT) to generate a provirus, which is randomly integrated into the host chromosomes. Upon stimulation, the provirus transcribes mRNAs for protein synthesis and full-length RNA molecules that are assembled into virus particles (1,2). The minute amount of proviral DNA compared to cellular DNA within the infected cell and the small number of blood cells harboring a provirus (one in 10^4 to 10^5) had previously limited the use of standard molecular techniques to study HIV (3).

The ability of the polymerase chain reaction (PCR) to exponentially replicate one copy of the viral genome and to distinguish genetically related organisms such as HIV-1 from HIV-2 has greatly enhanced our ability to study HIV infection (4,5). However, the extraordinary sensitivity of PCR makes this assay prone to false positive results when laboratory setups and techniques are less than optimal. Prior to the development of PCR, laboratory diagnosis of HIV infection was achieved mostly by detecting antibodies against HIV viral proteins, or by virus isolation in cell-culture systems. Today, PCR and the reverse transcriptase polymerase chain reaction (RT PCR) are used to diagnose HIV infection, to monitor patients' responses to antiretroviral treatments, and to manipulate parts of the viral genome for experimental HIV research.

The extensive sequence diversity of HIV has been a constant challenge for diagnostic PCR tests, especially in African settings where all HIV genetic types (HIV-1 and HIV-2), groups (M, N, O for HIV-1), subtypes (A-D, F, H, J, K for HIV-1 and A-F for HIV-2), and circulating recombinant forms (CRFs) (CRF01 to CRF10 for HIV-1), have been found in the population (6–10).

PCR TECHNOLOGY

The principle behind PCR technology is the amplification of a nucleic acid fragment through repeated cycles of replication in vitro (11,12). The minimum reagents needed to perform a PCR are primers, a pH buffer, deoxynucleotide triphosphates (dNTPs), mono and divalent cations, and a thermostable and thermoactive polymerase enzyme (13,14). The amplified fragments can be detected and quantified by gel electrophoresis, by hybridization with radiolabeled probes, or by immunoassay-like colorimetric assays. Detailed information regarding specific PCR techniques and applications, access to PCR-related software, and direct links to providers of thermal cyclers and PCR equipment and supplies can be obtained through the PCR Jump Station (PJS) web page (Table 1).

PCR Components

Sample

It is important to follow appropriate protocols to reduce degradation of target sequences during collection, transport, and storage of samples because there may be very few HIV-infected cells in the peripheral blood (3,15). Almost any tissue can be used as a source of DNA and RNA, but peripheral blood mononuclear cells (PBMCs) or plasma are recommended for use in HIV diagnosis. Blood should be collected in ethylenediaminetetraacetic acid (EDTA) or acid citrate dextrose tubes (not heparin tubes, since heparin inhibits DNA polymerases) (16,18). Ideally, samples should be kept at room temperature and processed within 6 hours. This timing is particularly critical if the samples are to be used for RNA load quantification, due to degradation of the RNA. Technicians should observe universal blood precautions while processing samples inside laminar flow hoods. If the samples cannot be processed immediately, cell and plasma components should be separated and stored at –70°C (15,18).

Dried blood spots may be tested as an alternative; this type of sample is easier to collect, transport, and test for HIV infection in newborns. Likewise, cervical swabs may be used to collect and test cervicovaginal samples (19,20–22). There are a large number of protocols and commercial kits for the isolation of DNA and RNA suitable for PCR amplification (23,24) (Table 1). Technicians following manual protocols without an automated system for sample and PCR preparation should process a small number of samples

TABLE 1. Internet Resources

Name	Web address	Description
The PCR Jump Station	http://www.highveld.com/pcr.html	Provides information on all aspects of PCR. A comprehensive directory for PCR protocols, vendors, software, and literature. Links to other related web sites.
The National Center for Biotechnology Information, National Institutes of Heath, USA.	http://www.ncbi.nlm.nih.gov	Resource for molecular biology information, public databases including GenBank, literature searches, retrovirus resources, and software tools for analyzing genome data.
HIV Sequence Database, Theoretical Biology and Biophysics Group, Los Alamos National Laboratory, NM, USA.	http://hiv-web.lanl.gov/	Provides access to HIV sequence databases, alignments, tools and interfaces for the analysis of HIV sequences. Links to the HIV molecular immunology database, and the HIV drug resistance database.
Phylogeny Programs, J, Felsenstein, University of Washington, Seattle, USA.	http://evolution.genetics.washington.edu/phylip/software.html	Complete list of available phylogeny programs with contact information of developer site. Links to other specialized phylogeny sites.
The National Institutes of Health AIDS Research and Reference Reagent Program, USA.	http://www.aidsreagent.org/	State of the art reagents for AIDS research: cell lines, hybridomas, virus isolates, clones, sera, kits, literature for HMA and virus culture. Links to other web sites.
Virology Manual for HIV Laboratories, Laboratories, National Institute of Allergy and Infectious Diseases, USA.	http://www.niaid.nih.gov/daids/vir_manual/	Detailed laboratory protocols for virus isolation, drug resistance tests, PCR, RT PCR, neutralization assays, p24 quantification, titrations and other protocols.
All the Virology on the WWW, DM, Sander, East Sacramento, CA, USA.	http://www.virology.net/	Extensive collection of virology related web sites for all virologists, course material, organizations. Links to many other web sites including HIV and AIDS.

simultaneously. Processing fewer samples at a time ensures that incubation times and steps in the protocols can be followed accurately, and minimizes labeling errors and cross-contamination between samples.

Primers

Primers are synthetic oligonucleotides that correspond to sequences flanking the genomic region to be amplified. Primers are typically 18 to 30 bases long with 50% to 60% G+C content, and 100 to 500 nmol/liter of each primer should be used in the PCR. To avoid preferential amplification of one DNA strand, mispriming, or primer-dimer formation, the two primers used in the PCR should have similar melting temperatures and lack sequence homology between and within strands (14). Highly conserved regions across the HIV genome should be used when designing primers to detect HIV variants from all genotypes. A selection of primer pairs that have been used for detection and distinction of HIV-1 and HIV-2 and for full-length amplifications are shown in Table 2. For diagnostic PCR, short fragments are easier to amplify, thereby increasing sensitivity of the assay. In contrast, the entire viral genome can be amplified as a single molecule for research purposes. The National Center for Biotechnology Information and the Los Alamos National Laboratory HIV Database are extremely useful resources that should be consulted when designing new primers and analyzing HIV sequences (Table1). These databases are continuously updated and provide public access to sequence databases, a variety of software tools, interactive programs to analyze HIV sequences, and reviews.

Buffers and Ions

A buffer system of 10 to 50 mM Tris-HCl, pH 8.3 at 20°C is commonly used in PCR buffer preparations. The apparent alkalinity of the buffer is lowered by the dissociation of the Tris-HCl at the high temperatures used for polymerization. Other reagents, such as dimethyl sulfoxide, glycerol, sodium dodecyl sulfate, formamide, or urea have been added to some buffer preparations to increase annealing of primers to target sequences and to decrease the number of non-specific products (25). Monovalent cations provided by KCl in the buffer preparation facilitate annealing of primers to the target DNA by neutralizing the negative charge. The amount of $MgCl_2$ necessary for maximum polymerase activity is dependent on both the primer sequences and the concentration of dNTPs, because dNTPs also bind $MgCl_2$. Therefore when using new primer pairs titration of $MgCl_2$ concentrations should be performed to achieve optimal primer binding and DNA polymerization (26).

Deoxynucleotide Triphosphates

It is recommended to use the lowest possible amounts of dNTPs during PCR to ensure specificity, fidelity, and efficient amplification. Deoxyadenosine triphosphate (dATP), deoxyguanosine triphosphate (dGTP), deoxycytidine triphosphate (dCTP), and deoxythymidine triphosphate (dTTP) should be present in equivalent amounts (13). A concentration of 20 to 200 μmol/liter of each dNTP is sufficient to synthesize between 2 and 20 μg of DNA in a 100 μl reaction. When using uracil-N-glycosylase (UNG) to prevent carryover contamination, deoxyuridine triphosphate (dUTP) is substituted for dTTP (27–29). Adjustments of the dUTP concentration may be necessary, according to the DNA polymerase used or the presence of target sequences rich in A/T residues. Commercial dATP, dGTP, dCTP, and dTTP are available as individual preparations or as mix solutions (dATP/dGTP/dCTP/dTTP) in sodium or lithium salt preparations.

Enzyme

DNA polymerases used for PCR amplification are thermoactive and thermostable.

TABLE 2. Primers for HIV-1 and HIV-2 PCR Amplification

Name	Position[a]	5′-3′ Sequence	Region	Virus[b]	Ref.[c]
SK38	1551-1578 (SF2)	ATAATCCACCTATCCCAGTAGGAGAAAT	*gag*	(HIV-1)	41,42
SK19[d]	1595-1635 (SF2)	ATCCTGGGATTAAATAAAATAGTAAGAATGTATAGCCCTAC	*gag*	(HIV-1)	41,42
SK39	1665-1638 (SF2)	TTTGGTCCTTGTCTTATGTCCAGAATGC	*gag*	(HIV-1)	41,42
SK145	1366-1395 (SF2)	AGTGGGGGGACATCAAGCAGCCATGCAAAT	*gag*	(HIV-1/HIV-2)	42
SK102	1403-1435 (SF2)	CAGACCATCAATGAGGAAGCTGCAGAATGGGAT	*gag*	(HIV-1/HIV-2)	42
SK101	1506-1482 (SF2)	GCTATGTCAGTYCCCCTTGGTTCTC	*gag*	(HIV-1/HIV-2)	42
SK462[e]	1366-1395 (SF2)	AGTTGGAGGACATCAAGCAGCCATGCAAAT	*gag*	(HIV-1/HIV-2)	104
SK431[e]	1507-1481 (SF2)	TGCTATGTCAGTTCCCCTTGGTTCTCT	*gag*	(HIV-1/HIV-2)	104
OG53[f]	539-561 (ROD)	GTGGGAGATGGGCGCGAGAAACT	*gag*	(HIV-2)	5,105,103
OG63	637-660 (ROD)	TAAAACATATTGTGTGGGCAGCGA	*gag*	(HIV-2)	5,103
OG81	810-833 (ROD)	CACGCAGAAGAGAAAGTGAAAGAT	*gag*	(HIV-2)	5,103
OG106[f]	1062-1085 (ROD)	GGATTTCAGGCACTCTCAGAAGGC	*gag*	(HIV-2)	5,105,103
401	6539-6559 (HxB2)	GAGGATATAATCAGTTTATGG	*env*	(HIV-1)	5,103
404	6976-6953(HxB2)	AATTCCATGTGTACATTGTACTG	*env*	(HIV-1)	5,103
402	6560-6579 (HxB2)	GATCAAAGCCTAAAGCCATG	*env*	(HIV-1)	5,103
403	6876-6857 (HxB2)	CAATAATGTATGGGAATTGG	*env*	(HIV-1)	5,103
OG778	7782-7805 (ROD)	GGAATAGTGCAGCAACAGCAACAG	*env*	(HIV-2)	5,103
OG783	7837-7861 (ROD)	TGTTGCGACTGACCGTCTGGGGAAC	*env*	(HIV-2)	5,103
OG795	7950-7973 (ROD)	GTCTGCCACACTACTGTACCATGG	*env*	(HIV-2)	5,103
OG825	8259-8281 (ROD)	AAGGGCTATAGGCCTGTTTTCTC	*env*	(HIV-2)	5,103
626(+)[g]	626-652 (HxB2)	AGGGGGCCAAGTCGGCCTCTCTAGCAGTGGCGCCCGAACAGGG	*gag*	(HIV-1)	9,132
9690(−)	9690-9661 (HxB2)	AGTCGCGGCCGCGGTCTGAGGGATCTCTAGTTACCAGAGTC	LTR	(HIV-1)	9,132
9624(−)	9624-9603 (HxB2)	TAAGGCGGCCGCGGCAAGCTTTATTGAGGCTTA	LTR	(HIV-1)	9,132

[a]Nucleotide position of the primer according to the reference clone is shown in parentheses. The GenBank accession numbers for HxB2, SF2, and ROD molecular clones are K03455, K02007, and M15390, respectively.

[b]Indicates primer ability to anneal to HIV-1 and/or HIV-2 sequences.

[c]Reference.

[d]SK19 is the internal probe for SK38/SK39 and SK431/SK462 primer-pairs.

[e]SK431 and SK462 are 5′-biotinylated SK145 and SK101. SK431/SK462 are the primers and SK102 is the probe used in a commercial test (20,73,81,121–123).

[f]OG53 and OG106 primers were used to measure HIV-2 RNA viral load in plasma.

[g]The primer set 626/9690/9624 is used in a heminested PCR for the amplification of virtually full-length genome as a single amplicon that includes sequences from the primer binding site to the U5 region in the LTR.

The isolation and characterization of the *Thermus aquaticus* (Taq) DNA polymerase was essential for the development of PCR. Taq processivity at temperatures near 75°C ensures specific and stringent amplification, while its stability at 95°C guarantees complete DNA strand separation (11,30,31). However, it was soon recognized that Taq lacked the 3′-5′ exonuclease activity necessary to minimize detachment from the DNA template and early termination of polymerization. The resulting effects include the amplification of fragments with errors (1×10^4), the addition of one non-template nucleotide to the 3′ end of the DNA, and the inability to amplify pieces of DNA larger than a few kilobases (kb) (32). After the discovery of thermostable DNA polymerases with proofreading and exonuclease activities it was found that the mixing of nonproofreading enzymes with small amounts of proofreading enzymes allowed the amplification of fragments up to 22 kb from human genomic DNA or 44 kb from Lambda DNA (33–35). This provided the tools for the amplification of the entire HIV genome, which contributed significantly to our understanding of HIV classification, diversity, and recombination in samples of African origin (6,9,36–40).

PCR Amplification

Steps and Cycles

PCR amplification is the incubation of target DNA with PCR components at three different temperatures in repetitive cycles to achieve DNA denaturation, primer annealing, and DNA polymerization (Figure 1). The specific temperature and length of each step are dependent on the primer sequence and the size of the amplified fragments. The number of cycles required for detectable amplification is dependent on the initial number of target DNA copies and the method used to detect the amplified products. Incubation at 94°C for 10 to 60 seconds is sufficient to completely denature amplified DNA, but many protocols include an initial step of 3 to 10 minutes to ensure complete denaturation of the input genomic DNA (13,26,41,42). The input of total DNA and the number of target DNA copies are limiting factors for amplification during the initial PCR cycles. The consumption of dNTP and primers, the accumulation of amplicons and pyrophosphate molecules, and the decrease of the polymerase integrity are factors that limit amplification in the later cycles of PCR. Poorly standardized protocols may favor the generation and amplification of short or nonspecific sequences that drastically compromise the ability to detect and quantify HIV sequences in a sample. When the input of target DNA is very low, a nested PCR amplification is preferentially done instead of using more than 40 cycles of amplification. In theory, a fully optimized PCR protocol should be able to amplify a single copy of target DNA within a complex mixture of sequences.

Detection of PCR Amplification

Several methods that differ in sensitivity, specificity, and requirement for reagents and equipment can be used to detect amplified product (Table 3). Detection methods that rely on size separation and visualization of PCR products include agarose and polyacrylamide gel electrophoresis, solid phase assays, high-pressure liquid chromatography, and nonspecific capture of products in solid phase assays (43–45). These methods allow the assessment of the presence and the size of the amplified products (Figure 2A). Agarose gels are used to separate a wide range of DNA fragment sizes, are easy to run, and are convenient for most laboratories. Visualization is achieved by staining the gels with ethidium bromide, a chromogen dye that binds to nucleic acids and fluoresces under ultraviolet light. Polyacrylamide gels are preferably used to separate small size fragments or to separate fragments according to their

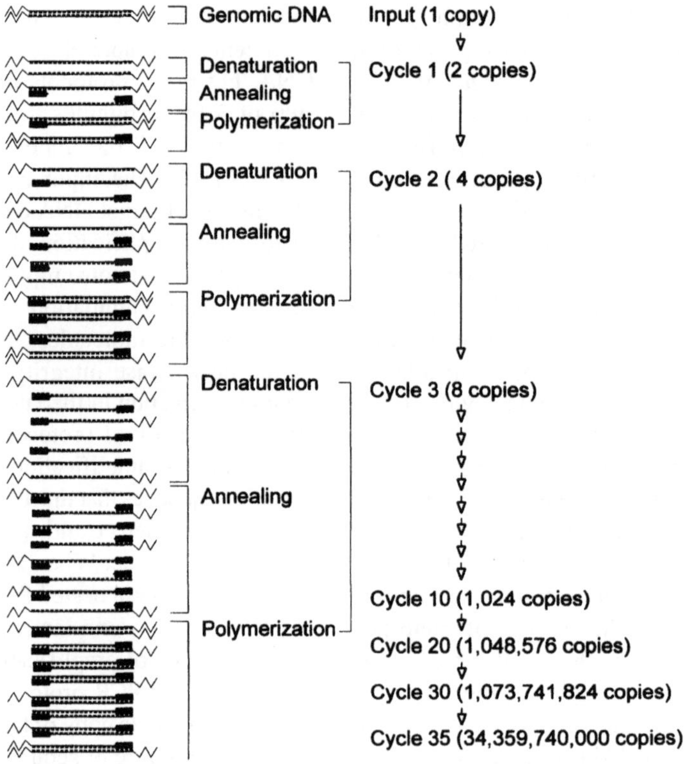

FIGURE 1. PCR amplification. Schematic representation of the molecular processes (left column), individual steps (middle column), and number of copies generated during PCR (right column). Primers are designed according to the sequence of the chosen target HIV sequence. Proviral DNA (dotted lines) integrated in the host genome (wavy lines) is first heated to ≥93°C to separate both DNA strands (denaturation). The primers (black boxes) are allowed to anneal to their complementary HIV sequences by briefly cooling the reaction to a temperature near the estimated melting temperature for the primers (annealing). One primer is complementary to the sense strand while the other is complementary to the anti-sense strand. Incubation at 70°C to 75°C allows the thermostable DNA polymerase to catalyze the synthesis of new DNA strands (polymerization). These three steps form a cycle that is repeated 20 to 40 times to generate 2^n number of DNA copies, where n is the number of cycles.

molecular conformation. To increase the sensitivity of the PCR, the amplification can be done in the presence of ^{32}P-radiolabeled dNTPs, ^{32}P-radiolabeled primers, or digoxigenin-dUTP (Figure 2B) (46). Other detection methods are based on the hybridization of labeled oligonucleotide to sequences within the amplified fragment. The denatured PCR products are exposed to the probe followed by autoradiographic, colorimetric, or chemiluminescent detection. Because the level of hybridization is greatly affected by sequence variation, these methods increase the sensitivity and specificity of the assay (Figure 2C). Southern blots are most commonly used, but dot blots, oligomer restriction, gel retardation, and specific capture of products in a solid phase are among other methods that involve a hybridization intermediate step (Table 3) (42,47–50).

Procedures to Minimize PCR Carryover

Clinical and research facilities wishing to use PCR-based protocols to test clinical samples must carefully plan the use of physical space, be equipped with appropriate laboratory equipment, and be staffed with trained personnel. Any investment toward containment and standardization will be

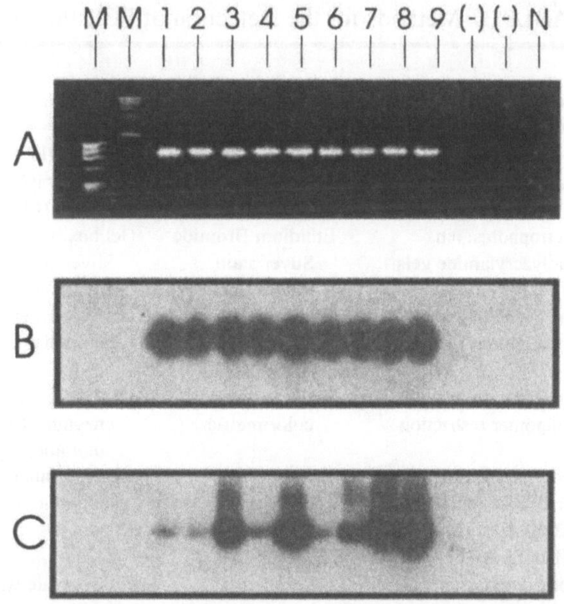

FIGURE 2. Sequence variation, sensitivity, and specificity in PCR amplification and detection. Nine HIV-1 infected samples (lines 1 to 9) from Tanzania were subjected to PCR amplification using envelope primers in a 100 μl PCR. Two HIV-1 negative samples (−) and one reaction without DNA (N) were amplified simultaneously as negative controls to detect carryover. Molecular weight markers (M); X174 DNA digested with Hae III and a 1 kb ladder.
A. PCR products (15 μl) were separated by agarose gel electrophoresis and visualized by ethidium bromide staining. This method relies only on size for identification of specific amplification and requires substantial amplification for visualization. All samples except the negative controls showed equivalent amounts of amplification product.
B. The same samples were amplified in the presence of ^{32}P-dATP. One μl of labeled PCR product was separated by agarose gel electrophoresis, transferred to a nylon membrane, and visualized by autoradiography. Although this method is more sensitive, it still relies only on the size of the PCR product to identify specific amplification.
C. The PCR products from panel 2A were transferred to a nylon membrane and hybridized under stringent conditions to a ^{32}P-labeled internal oligonucleotide probe. The use of a labeled internal probe makes this method both sensitive and specific. This experiment also illustrates how nucleic acid hybridization (probe to amplicons during detection or primer to target DNA during PCR) can be highly susceptible to sequence variation. All infected samples (lines 1 to 9) score positive using this test (diagnosis), and the signal obtained from each sample varied greatly (quantification) even though they have the same amount of PCR product. This suggests that sequence variation may have a larger effect on quantitative assays (viral RNA load) than qualitative assays (diagnosis of infection).

repaid by the generation of accurate and uniform results. The capacity of PCR to generate large numbers of molecules and to detect one copy of DNA as starting material for amplification makes contamination the most common problem in diagnostic PCR (14,28,29,51,52). False positives may arise by contamination with genomic DNA from positive samples or more commonly by previously PCR-amplified products known as carryover. Pipetting or opening PCR tubes can easily aerosolize small volumes of PCR product that may contain large numbers of DNA copies (6×10^{11} molecules in 100 μl), which can cause serious contamination of stock reagents, equipment, and personnel (51). Following strict laboratory guidelines and using enzymatic and chemical modifications have proven successful in keeping carryover problems to a minimum. The frequent changing of gloves, the use of clean, disposable laboratory coats, and wearing face masks at all times are additional precautions recommended to avoid carryover. Several known negative samples in addition to a control reaction without DNA should be included

TABLE 3. Methods for the Detection of PCR Products

Principle	System	Detection[a]	Equipment	Sensitivity[b]/ Specificity[c]
Size separation and direct visualization	Electrophoresis in agarose gels	Ethidium Bromide	Gel box, UV light, Photography recording system (PRS)	+/+
	Electrophoresis in polyacrylamide gels	Ethidium Bromide	Gel box, UV light, PRS	+/++
		Silver stain	Silver stain reagents	+/++
		Fluorescent dyes	Automated sequencer	+++/++ [d]
Liquid phase hybridization and size separation	Hybridization and gel retardation	Radioactive, colorimetric	Gel box, label probe, autoradiography, PRS	+++/+++
	Hybridization and oligomer restriction	Radioactive, colorimetric	Gel box, restriction enzymes, label probe, autoradiography, PRS	+++/++ [e]
Size separation and solid phase hybridization	Electrophoresis and hybridization (Southern Blot), hybridization only (Dot blot)[f]	Radioactive, colorimetric or chemiluminescent	Gel box, label probe, autoradiography, PRS	+++/+++
Solid phase hybridization	Biotinylated primers and plates coated with the internal probe[g]	Colorimetric	ELISA plate washer and reader	+++/+++

[a]Many reagents are toxic, carcinogenic, or radioactive. They require special handling and should be disposed of accordingly to minimize health hazards.
[b]+ indicates low sensitivity; +++, high sensitivity.
[c]+ indicates low specificity; +++, high specificity.
[d]It is possible to determine differences as small as one base pair by using internal size standards.
[e]A single nucleotide change can disrupt the restriction site despite specific HIV amplification.
[f]Dot blots do not involve size separation.
[g]The qualitative HIV-1 detection commercial assays use this system and principle.

with every PCR to monitor PCR carryover. Ideally, a diagnostic PCR laboratory should have at least three contained and physically separated spaces: a sample processing area, a PCR setup area, and a PCR analysis and detection area (51,52). No plasmid or amplified DNA should ever be brought into the sample processing and PCR setup areas. Each area should have its own set of laboratory equipment and reagents. Material should not be shared between the areas, particularly between the PCR analysis room and the PCR setup and sample processing rooms. Positive displacement pipets or aerosol barrier tips should be used to avoid contamination between samples. A major effort should be made to have unidirectional movement of personnel from the clean areas to the PCR analysis area, or to have separate personnel working in each PCR area. Additional strategies have been developed to decrease carryover of PCR products in the diagnostic laboratory such as the use of dUTP with UNG, UV irradiation, DNase treatment, and the incorporation of psoralen (14,27,53,54). UNG recognizes and modifies dUTP-containing DNA by opening the deoxyribose ring. This modified DNA breaks when exposed to elevated temperatures in an alkaline environment, while the UNG is inactivated during the initial denaturation step.

Thermal Cyclers

Today there are a large number of commercial thermal cyclers designed for repeated cycling between 0°C to 100°C. The cyclers come with blocks to hold 0.5 ml and 0.2 ml tubes, 48-well, 96-well, 192-well, and 384-well plates, and microscope slides for in situ reactions. Several models allow interchanging of the blocks in order to choose the optimum sample block for a given application. Most machines come with heated covers for reliable oil-free cycling, and the temperature is controlled directly in the block using in-sample probe control or by a calculated-temperature control. The machines offer a variety of default programs in addition to a memory space to store several hundred different programs. Standard functions include extension or decrement at each cycle of the temperature and cycling times in addition to variation of the ramping rates between 1.0°C/sec to 3.0°C/sec. They usually come with several connection ports to allow communication with a variety of computerized systems. The principal makers of thermal cyclers include Biometra, Bio-Rad, Eppendorf, Hybaid, MJ Research, Perkin Elmer, Stratagene, and Techne. The companies' web site addresses can be accessed through the PJS (Table 1).

PCR APPLICATIONS

PCR-based detection systems are some of the most sensitive tools developed for clinical and research applications. In addition to diagnosis and clinical assessment of HIV-infected individuals, PCR-based technologies have been fundamental to a large number of discoveries that have expanded our understanding of HIV biology, pathogenesis, variation, evolution, and epidemiology.

PCR Application in Clinical Settings

Detection of HIV Infection before Seroconversion

PCR studies of samples from initially HIV-seronegative commercial sex workers, men who have sex with men, and hemophiliacs have shown that the interval between infection and seroconversion ranges from a few weeks to 4 months (55–57). The length of this window has been taken into consideration in the definition of the time required to test an individual with a possible exposure to HIV. Because high plasma RNA load after seroconversion has been correlated with an increased risk of clinical progression of HIV disease, PCR-based assays can be used to study virologic and host interactions that determine HIV plasma RNA loads after seroconversion (58–62).

Solving Cases with Indeterminate Western Blot Results

In blood donor centers and laboratories that routinely screen large numbers of low-risk individuals, it is not uncommon to detect samples that are reactive by HIV-1 enzyme immunoassays (EIA) but have indeterminate Western blot profiles (63,64). PCR testing can be used as an additional tool to determine the HIV status of these samples. Long-term follow-up using serologic and repeated PCR testing has shown that individuals at low risk for HIV infection whose Western blot results are indeterminate are rarely infected with HIV (65,66).

Diagnosis of Perinatal Infection

The most common application of DNA PCR in clinical settings is the diagnosis of HIV infection in infants born to HIV-infected mothers (19,20,67–73). HIV-1–infected pregnant women transfer antibodies against HIV to their newborns regardless of the HIV-1 status of the infant. During the first 18 months of life, routine serologic assays such as EIA and Western blots are not valuable diagnostic tools because of the presence of maternal IgG antibodies in the infant (74–76). Because more than one-third of infants born to untreated infected mothers acquire HIV-1 infection, early diagnosis is critical to the evaluation of new treatment protocols and the identification of infants who could benefit from early treatment. The detection of p24 antigen, anti-HIV IgM and IgA antibodies, or in vitro antibody production shows low specificity and sensitivity for detecting HIV infection in newborns (76–78). Virus isolation requires special laboratory facilities and trained personnel and cannot be used as a routine rapid diagnostic test. In contrast, PCR diagnosis requires a smaller amount of sample than virus culture, and many samples can be tested simultaneously in a short period of time (79). Since infants are infected with one or a few infectious viruses, viral sequence diversity can be very limited during the first weeks of life and special attention should be given to the selection of primers and PCR conditions to avoid false negatives (73,80–83).

Monitoring HIV Resistance to Antiretrovirals

HIV isolates resistant to nucleoside analogs, nonnucleoside inhibitors, and protease inhibitors have been isolated from patients undergoing therapy (84–87). Nucleotide sequencing of field isolates and genetic manipulations of HIV-1 have been used to map RT mutations associated with resistance to antiretrovirals. Several PCR protocols and commercial kits have been developed that can be used to monitor the appearance of mutations in RT during antiretroviral treatment. The point mutation assay (PMA) has been developed to quantify ZDV resistance-associated mutations, while the line probe assay (LiPA) is able to screen for several mutations conferring resistance to a variety of antiretrovirals using a single PCR amplification product (88,89). These PCR protocols are less time consuming, less hazardous, and less expensive, and also allow processing of higher sample throughput than phenotypic assays that use cell culture systems.

Quantification of Viral Load by RT PCR

Because amplification is an exponential process, small differences in any component can dramatically affect the total amount of generated PCR product. RNA PCR uses the reverse transcription of the viral RNA to generate a DNA molecule, followed by standard PCR amplification. The use of competitive internal standards minimizes tube-to-tube and sample-to-sample variation, thus transforming PCR into a quantitative assay (5,90,91). This method is based on the co-amplification of a competitive template that uses the same primers as the target DNA but is distinguishable from the target DNA after amplification. As with DNA PCR, quantitative viral RNA load tests were developed using HIV-1 subtype B sequences for primer selection and test validation. Their performance on HIV-1 non-B subtypes showed differences in the ability of each test to quantify samples belonging to HIV-1 non-B subtypes in addition to differences in the total viral load detected by different methods on the same sample (92–97). These assays were re-evaluated and improved versions are currently being tested in African samples. In the United States and Europe, where HIV-1 subtype B is the predominant subtype circulating in the population, the RNA plasma load is routinely used to predict disease progression, to determine when to start antiretroviral therapy, and to assess viral response to therapy.

Differentiation between HIV-1 and HIV-2 Infection

In West African countries where both HIV-1 and HIV-2 are circulating in the population, it is not uncommon to find individuals dually infected with both HIV-1 and HIV-2 (2,98,99). The observation that antibodies against envelope proteins could be more stringent in discriminating between HIV-1 and HIV-2 motivated the development of serologic assays utilizing synthetic envelope peptides and recombinant envelope antigens (99–102). Since HIV-1 and HIV-2 share about 40% of their nucleotide sequence homology, primers and probes generic for HIV-1 and HIV-2 or specific for HIV-1 or HIV-2 have been designed (Table 2) (41,42,

103–105). PCR has proven to be 100% sensitive and specific for monotypic HIV-1 or HIV-2 infections, but only HIV-1 was detected in dually infected individuals with low $CD4^+$ cell counts (5). Accurate HIV typing is required for the counseling, prognosis, and treatment of patients because HIV-2 is less pathogenic, less transmissible, and shown to be protective against subsequent infection by HIV-1. In addition, HIV typing would aid in research studies to establish whether dually infected individuals follow the same disease course as individuals infected with only HIV-1 or HIV-2.

PCR Application in Research Settings

HIV Subtype Classification

In addition to serologic or phenotypic properties, HIV can be classified into groups, subtypes, and CRFs on the basis of its phylogenetic relationships (6). Nucleotide sequencing and the heteroduplex mobility assays (HMAs) rely on PCR to generate large amounts of template and are the most common methods for HIV subtyping (6,106, 107). Nucleotide sequencing is the most accurate method while HMA is less expensive, less time consuming, and may be performed in locations with limited resources (Figure 3). In African populations that have several circulating HIV subtypes and recombinants, at least two separate genomic regions should be used for genetic subtyping (Table 4) (83,107–109). The ability to use primer pairs targeted to any region of the HIV genome and the development of long range PCR for amplification of virtually full-length genome have been key factors in the rapid generation of nucleotide sequences from HIVs around the globe (6). Kits for *env* and *gag* HMA subtype classification are available for laboratories registered with the National Institutes of Health (NIH) Research and Reference Reagent Program (Table 1). The *gag* and *env* HMA kits provide reference plasmids for subtypes A–H, and J, positive controls, and primers for amplification of selected regions of the gp120 and *gag*. An extensive number of programs for genetic analysis of any organism including HIV can be accessed at the Phylogeny Program web site (Table 1).

In-Situ PCR

The sensitivity of PCR technology, combined with the ability to preserve the anatomical structure of tissues using in situ hybridization techniques, facilitates the identification and quantification of rare transcripts or single copy genes at the cellular and subcellular level. The tissue sample has to be fixed and permeabilized to preserve the cell architecture and the integrity of the nucleic acids while permitting the influx of PCR, RT PCR, and detection reagents (110). In-situ PCR has been used to determine the number of cells in the peripheral blood harboring HIV provirus, to describe the active replication of HIV in lymphoid tissues, and to identify the phenotype of HIV-infected cells from different organs (3,111–113).

Real-Time PCR

This new PCR innovation incorporates fluorescent technology with ultra rapid thermal cycling. This allows amplification and detection within the same tube, as well as analysis of the sample in real time while the amplification is in progress. Unlike a quantitative PCR, in which the detection methods only measure the final amount of the amplified product, real-time PCR detects per cycle the increment of fluorescent signal as it is incorporated into newly generated amplicons. The high cost of the equipment needed for this technique has limited its current use. However, this technology has been useful in studying several aspects of HIV biology, including viral entry, monitoring viral replication under antiretroviral therapy, and quantifying HIV-2 plasma RNA load (114–117).

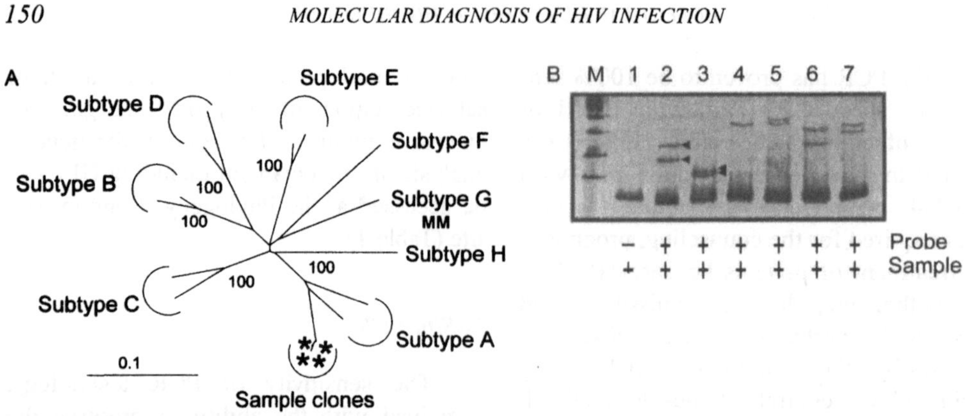

FIGURE 3. Subtype classification of HIV-1 samples. The same PCR product was classified using two methods: nucleotide sequencing and heteroduplex mobility assay (HMA).
A. For nucleotide classification the sample was gel purified, cloned into a plasmid, and used to transform prokaryotic cells. Individual bacterial colonies were screened for the presence of inserts by restriction enzyme analysis of plasmid DNA. Four clones with an insert of the appropriate size were sequenced in both directions by automated cycle sequencing with dye terminators. Nucleotide sequences were aligned to control sequences belonging to various HIV-1 subtypes and subjected to phylogenetic analysis. The four sample clones grouped together with subtype A controls. The sequences can also be used to study a variety of viral genetic questions, including the presence and extension of viral quasispecies, the location of mutations associated with specific biologic phenotypes, or to locate mutations conferring resistance to drugs.
B. HMA classification is based on slower migration of heteroduplex molecules formed between divergent DNA molecules in polyacrylamide gels. Aliquots of the PCR product were individually combined with *env* DNA from known subtypes A, C, and D. After a cycle of denaturation and annealing, the newly formed double-stranded DNA were separated in a polyacrylamide gel and visualized by silver staining. This sample has a low genetic diversity as indicated by the presence of one species of DNA heteroduplex molecules (lane 1). Heteroduplex molecules formed between sample plus subtype C controls (lanes 4 and 5) and sample plus subtype D controls (lanes 6 and 7) showed slower migration than the heteroduplex molecules formed between the sample plus subtype A controls (lanes 2 and 3, back arrows). This indicates that sequences in the sample are more related to subtype A sequences than subtype C or subtype D sequences.

TABLE 4. Importance of Using More than One Genomic Region for HIV-1 Subtype Classification[a]

Genotype	*gag*	*env*	*gag* and *env*[b]
A	25	41	22
C	26	28	22
D	42	19	19[c]
Recombinant	7	12	37[d]

[a]Nucleotide sequences of *gag* and *env* were obtained from one hundred perinatally infected infants (83).
[b]Both genes have the same subtype classification in A, C, and D genotypes but discordant *gag* and *env* subtypes in the recombinant group.
[c]Subtype D genotypes (19 samples) were overestimated when nucleotide sequences from only *gag* (42 samples) but not when only *env* (19 samples) genotypes were used for classification.
[d]Recombinants in Tanzania (37 samples) were significantly underestimated when nucleotide sequences from only *gag* (7 samples, $p < 0.0001$) or only *env* (12 samples, $p < 0.011$) were used for classification.

Genetic Manipulation and Other PCR Applications

The ability to design primers that contain internal restriction sites or selected nucleotide changes facilitated the manipulation of nucleic acids in the HIV research laboratory. Variations of PCR protocols have been used to clone individual genes, to clone the entire HIV genome, to construct infectious chimeric HIV genomes, to study virus quasispecies in distinct tissues, and to introduce specific mutations to observe the correlation between the role of viral genotypes and biologic phenotypes (21,22,40,118–120). Other applications include the generation of labeled probes, inverse PCR, multiplex PCR, DNase I footprinting, differential display, single-cell cDNA libraries, CHIP technology, and others (Table 1).

A PCR-Based Commercial Assay

The diagnosis of HIV infection by DNA PCR is particularly useful in neonates whose HIV status cannot be accurately established by serologic assays (73–77). Several PCR assays were developed that eliminated the use of radioisotopes and that allowed the analysis of numerous samples in a short period of time. One of them is commercially available and has been used as the diagnostic test in several clinical trials designed to decrease rates of mother-to-infant transmission in African settings (20,73,81,121–123). The kit consists of three components: a whole blood specimen preparation component, an amplification component, and a detection component. The system is set up in a 96-microwell format, comes with ready to use premixed reagents, positive and negative controls, and uses dUTP-UNG to avoid carryover. One-half milliliter of whole blood is treated with the specimen wash solution to selectively lyse red blood cells and to obtain a leukocyte pellet. A cell lysate ready for PCR is prepared by adding extraction reagent to cell pellets followed by two incubations, the first one to lyse the cell pellet and the second to inactivate the proteases present in the extraction reagent. An aliquot of this cell extract is added to a master mix containing the SK431 and SK462 biotinylated primers (Table 2), dATP, dCTP, dGTP, dUTP, buffer, mono and divalent cations, the polymerase, and UNG. The PCR reaction is subjected to 35 cycles of amplification, with the first five amplification cycles at a lower annealing temperature to amplify HIV-1 sequences that have few nucleotide mismatches. Once the amplification cycles are completed, the samples are immediately mixed with a denaturing solution to inactivate the UNG and to denature and stabilize the new amplicons. An aliquot of the denatured amplicons is transferred to individual wells coated with the HIV-1 SK102 probe of the detection plate (Table 2). Unhybridized DNA is washed away and avidin-horseradish peroxidase (HRP) is added to the wells. The avidin-HRP binds to biotin present in the primers of the PCR products that are bound to the plate through the SK102 probe. Color is developed after incubation with 3,3′,5,5′-tetramethylbenzidine (TMB), H_2O_2 substrate and a chromogen. The absorbance at 450 nm in positive and negative controls should fall between a predetermined value range for the test to be considered valid. No commercial kits have been developed to detect or to quantify HIV-2 DNA or RNA.

HIV CULTURE

Although the isolation of HIV is the most convincing evidence of the presence of infectious virus in a patient's blood, virus isolation per se is not a requirement for diagnosis of HIV infection. Virus isolation from clinical samples has been used as the standard by which new diagnostic methods, including PCR, have been evaluated (79). Due to the lengthy time required to isolate HIV, the high cost of running and maintaining cell-culture facilities in addition to its technical difficulties, virus isolation is not routinely used as a diagnostic method but rather as a unique research tool. Although HIV-1 has been isolated from saliva, spinal fluid, brain, semen, breast milk, urine, lymphoid tissue, and plasma, PBMCs are the preferred starting material for HIV isolation (124–128). The success rate of HIV isolation in cell cultures can be as high as 100%, but lower success rates are expected in the majority of laboratories (129,130). The isolation rate is dependent on the quality and quantity of the sample, the number of infected cells in each specific sample, and the technical skills of the person performing the isolation (3,128,131). Detailed protocols for HIV assays using cell culture can be obtained from the Virology Manual for HIV Laboratories (Table 1). Blood samples should be collected in the presence of an anticoagulant, kept at room temperature, and processed for co-cultivation within 24 hours after collection. When long delays are expected in the co-cultivation, it is recommended to separate and freeze the PBMCs under liquid nitrogen (128). HIV isolation is done by co-cultivating the patient cells with phytohemagglutinin-stimulated PBMC from an HIV-negative donor. The cells are maintained in media supplemented with glutamine, heat inactivated fetal calf serum, and Interleukin 2. Fresh culture media and supplements are added at regular intervals while aliquots of culture supernatants are used to detect HIV virus. The most common methods used to detect virus replication are the quantification of HIV viral gag antigen (HIV-1 p24 gag or HIV-2 p27 gag) or virus reverse transcriptase activity (RT assays) in culture supernatants. Additional methods include Western blot, radioimmunoprecipitation, appearance of cytopathic effects, electron microscopy, and the detection of HIV provirus DNA or genomic RNA by PCR and RT PCR. The isolation and growth of HIV in cell-culture systems offers the unique opportunity to determine phenotypic properties of HIV isolates that cannot be delineated by any other available laboratory technique. The phenotypic properties of transmitting viruses, the correlation of HIV in vivo cell tropism and pathogenesis, and the detection of virus resistance to antiretroviral drugs were found through cell-culture assays. In addition, culture systems are required to generate large quantities of viral antigens used in ELISA and Western blot diagnostic tests.

CONCLUSION

Although in specific instances PCR may offer some advantages over serologic techniques, efforts to capacitate more laboratories to perform PCR techniques should not replace efforts to maintain laboratories that are able to perform reliable serologic diagnosis of HIV. Even though numerous laboratories in major African cities are currently executing highly sophisticated laboratory protocols, including PCR-based assays, they are too few to keep pace with the scale of the HIV epidemic on the African continent. Several physical, human, and supply requirements must be fulfilled by any laboratory setting to consistently and accurately perform PCR-based tests. If laboratory personnel have a clear understanding of the detection power of PCR, guidelines designed to avoid cross-contamination and false negatives are more likely to be closely followed. It is difficult, time consuming, and extremely expensive to solve problems caused by inappropriate handling of samples, plasmid, or amplified products.

PCR diagnosis should be used when standard serologic tests have failed to provide a definitive result of infection in at-risk neonates or in patients with illnesses that make serologic testing of any kind unreliable. Paradoxically, the extreme sensitivity that characterizes PCR has been one of the main reasons for the lack of its widespread use in clinical laboratories. The development of PCR and RT PCR user-friendly kits with improved PCR primers, the understanding of the importance of containment spaces in addition to molecular aids to minimize carryover are allowing PCR assays to continuously gain acceptance as an important tool in clinical virology laboratories. The combination of information collected using PCR technology with virologic and immunologic assays will help broaden our understanding of HIV genetic variation and its role in transmission, pathogenesis, disease progression, drug resistance, and vaccine development.

REFERENCES

1. Luciw, PA. Human immunodeficiency viruses and their replication. In: Fields BN, Knipe DM, Howley PM, eds. *Fields Virology*. Philadelphia: Lippincott-Raven Publishers, 1996;1881–1882.
2. Kanki, PJ. Virologic and biologic features of HIV-2. In: Wormser GP, ed. *AIDS and other manifestations of HIV infection*. Philadelphia: Lippincott-Raven Publishers, 1988;161–173.

3. Harper ME, Marselle LM, Gallo RC, et al. Detection of lymphocytes expressing human T-lymphotropic virus type III in lymph nodes and peripheral blood from infected individuals by in situ hybridization. *Proc Natl Acad Sci U S A*. 1986;83:772–776.
4. Nakamura S, Katamine S, Yamamoto T, et al. Amplification and detection of a single molecule of human immunodeficiency virus RNA. *Virus Genes*. 1993;7:325–338.
5. Sarr AD, Hamel DJ, Thior I, et al. HIV-1 and HIV-2 dual infection: lack of HIV-2 provirus correlates with low CD4+ lymphocyte counts. *AIDS*. 1998; 12:131–137.
6. Robertson DL, Anderson AP, Bradac JA, et al: HIV-1 nomenclature proposal. A reference guide to HIV-1 classification. In: *Human Retroviruses and AIDS: A compilation and analysis of nucleic acid and amino acid sequences*. Kuiken C FB, Hahn BH, Korber B, McCutchan F, Marx PA, Mellors JW, Mullins JL, Sodroski J, Wolinsky S, eds. Los Alamos, NM: Theoretical biology and biophysics group, 1999; 492–505.
7. McCutchan, FE. Understanding the genetic diversity of HIV-1. *AIDS*. 2000;14(suppl):S31:S44.
8. Gao F, Yue L, Robertson DL, et al. Genetic diversity of human immunodeficiency virus type 2: evidence for distinct sequence subtypes with differences in virus biology. *J Virol*. 1994;68:7433–7447.
9. Koulinska IN, Ndung'u T, Mwakagile D, et al. A New Human Immunodeficiency Virus Type 1 Circulating Recombinant Form from Tanzania. *AIDS Res Hum Retroviruses*. 2000;17(5):423–431.
10. Essex M. Human immunodeficiency viruses of the developing world. *Adv Virus Res*. 1999;53:71–88.
11. Saiki RK, Scharf S, Faloona F, et al. Enzymatic amplification of beta-globin genomic sequences and restriction site analysis for diagnosis of sickle cell anemia. *Science*. 1985;230:1350–1354.
12. Saiki RK, Gelfand DH, Stoffel S, et al. Primer-directed enzymatic amplification of DNA with a thermostable DNA polymerase. *Science*. 1988; 239:487–491.
13. Innis MA, Gelfand DH. Optimization of PCRs. In Innis MA, Gelfand DH, Sninsky JJ, White T, eds. PCR protocols: *A guide to methods and applications*. San Diego: Academic Press, 1990;3–20.
14. Sirko DA, Ehrlich GD. Laboratory facilities, protocols and operations. In Ehrlich GD, Greenberg AJ, eds. *PCR-based diagnostic in infectious diseases*. Boston: Backwell Scientific Publications, 1994; 19–44.
15. Holodniy M. Effects of collection, processing and storage on RNA detection and quantification. In: Kochanowsli B, Reischl U, eds. *Quantitative PCR protocols*. New Jersey: Humana Press, 1999;43–59.
16. Gustafson S, Proper JA, Bowie EJ, et al. Parameters affecting the yield of DNA from human blood. *Anal Biochem*. 1987;165:294–299.
17. Holodniy M, Kim S, Katzenstein D, et al. Inhibition of human immunodeficiency virus gene amplification by heparin. *J Clin Microbiol*. 1991;29:676–679.
18. Holodniy M, Mole L, Yen-Lieberman B, et al. Comparative stability of quantitative human immunodeficiency virus RNA in plasma from samples collected in VACUTAINER CPT, VACUTAINER PPT, and standard VACUTAINER tubes. *J Clin Microbiol*. 1995;33:1562–1566.
19. Comeau AM, Pitt J, Hillyer GV, et al. Early detection of human immunodeficiency virus on dried blood spot specimens: sensitivity across serial specimens. Women and Infants Transmission Study Group. *J Pediatr*. 1996;129:111–118.
20. Biggar RJ, Miley W, Miotti P, et al. Blood collection on filter paper: a practical approach to sample collection for studies of perinatal HIV transmission. *J Acquir Immune Defic Syndr Hum Retrovirol*. 1997;14:368–373.
21. Clemetson DBA, Moss GB, Willerford DM et al. Detection of HIV DNA in cervical and vaginal secretions-prevalence and correlates among women in Nairobi, Kenya. *JAMA*. 1993;269:2860–2864.
22. Sankale JL, Mboup S, Essex ME, et al. Genetic characterization of viral quasispecies in blood and cervical secretions of HIV-1 and HIV-2-infected women. *AIDS Res Hum Retroviruses*. 1998;14:1473–1481.
23. Higuchi R. Simple and rapid preparation of samples for PCR. In: Erlich HA ed. *PCR technology: principles and applications for DNA amplification*. New York: Stockton Press, 1989;31–38.
24. Kawasaki ES. Sample preparation from blood, cells, and other fluids. In: Innis MA, Gelfand DH, Sninsky JJ, White T, eds. *PCR protocols: A guide to methods and applications*. San Diego: Academic Press, 1990;146–152.
25. Gelfand DH. Taq DNA polymerase. In: Erlich HA ed. *PCR technology: principles and applications for DNA amplification*. New York: Stockton Press, 1989;17–22.
26. Saiki RK. The design and optimization of the PCR. In: Erlich HA ed. *PCR technology: principles and applications for DNA amplification*. New York: Stockton Press, 1989;7–16.
27. Longon MC, Berninger MS, Hartley JL. Use of uracil DNA glycosylase to control carry-over contamination in polymerase chain reactions. *Gene*. 1990;93:125–128.
28. Kwok S, Higuchi R. Avoiding false positives with PCR. *Nature*. 1989;339:237–238.
29. Kwok S. Procedures to minimize PCR-product carry-over. In: Innis MA, Gelfand DH, Sninsky JJ, White T, eds. *PCR protocols: A guide to methods and applications*. San Diego: Academic Press, 1990;142–146.
30. Brock TD, Freeze H. Thermus aquaticus gen. n. and sp. n., a nonsporulating extreme thermophile. *J Bacteriol*. 1969;98:289–297.

31. Lawyer FC, Stoffel S, Saiki RK, et al. Isolation, characterization, and expression in Escherichia coli of the DNA polymerase gene from Thermus aquaticus. *J Biol Chem.* 1989;264:6427–6437.
32. Tindall KR, Kunkel TA. Fidelity of DNA synthesis by the Thermus aquaticus DNA polymerase. *Biochemistry.* 1988;27:6008–6013.
33. Abramson RD. Thermostable DNA polymerases: An update. In: Innis MA, Gelfand DH, Sninsky JJ, eds. *PCR applications. Protocols for functional genomics.* San Diego: Academic Press, 1999; 33–47.
34. Cheng S, Fockler C, Barnes WM, et al. Effective amplification of long targets from cloned inserts and human genomic DNA. *Proc Natl Acad Sci USA.* 1994;91:5695–5699.
35. Barnes WM. PCR amplification of up to 35-kb DNA with high fidelity and high yield from lambda bacteriophage templates. *Proc Natl Acad Sci USA.* 1994;91:2216–2220.
36. Carr JK, Salminen MO, Koch C, et al. Full-length sequence and mosaic structure of a human immunodeficiency virus type 1 isolate from Thailand. *J Virol.* 1996;70:5935–5943.
37. Carr JK, Salminen MO, Albert J, et al. Full genome sequences of human immunodeficiency virus type 1 subtypes G and A/G intersubtype recombinants. *Virology.* 1998;247:22–31.
38. Gao F, Robertson DL, Carruthers CD, et al. A comprehensive panel of near-full-length clones and reference sequences for non-subtype B isolates of human immunodeficiency virus type 1. *J Virol.* 1998;72:5680–5698.
39. Novitsky VA, Montano MA, McLane MF, et al. Molecular cloning and phylogenetic analysis of human immunodeficiency virus type 1 subtype C: a set of 23 full-length clones from Botswana. *J Virol.* 1999;73:4427–4432.
40. Ndung'u T, Renjifo B, Novitsky VA, et al. Molecular cloning and biological characterization of full-length HIV-1 subtype C from Botswana. *Virology.* 2000;278:390–399.
41. Ou CY, Kwok S, Mitchell SW, et al. DNA amplification for direct detection of HIV-1 in DNA of peripheral blood mononuclear cells. *Science.* 1988;239:295–297.
42. Kellogg DE, Kwok S. 1990. Detection of human immunodeficiency virus. In: Innis MA, Gelfand DH, Sninsky JJ, White T, eds. *PCR protocols: A guide to methods and applications.* San Diego: Academic Press, 1990:337–347.
43. Abbott M, Poiesz B, Sninsky J, et al. A comparison of methods for the detection and quantification of the polymerase chain reaction. *J Infect Dis.* 1988:158:1158–1169.
44. Katz ED, Bloch W, Wages J. HPLC quantification and identification of DNA amplified by the polymerase chain reaction. *Amplifications.* 1992;8:10–13.
45. Reischl U, Kocchanowski B. Quantitative PCR. In Kochanowsli B, Reischl U, eds. *Quantitative PCR protocols.* New Jersey: Humana Press, 1999;3–31.
46. King JA, Ball JK. Detection of HIV-1 by digoxigenin-labelled PCR and microtitre plate solution hybridization assay and prevention of PCR carry-over by uracil-n-glycosylase. *J Virol Methods.* 1993;44:67–76.
47. Saiki RK, Walsh DS, Erlich HA. Generic analysis of amplified DNA with immobilized sequence-specific oligonucleotide probes. *Proc Natl Acad Sci* USA. 1989;86:6230–6234.
48. Keller GH, Huang DP, Manak MM. Detection of human immunodeficiency virus type 1 DNA by polymerase chain reaction and capture hybridization in microtiter wells. *J Clin Microbiol.* 1991; 29:638–641.
49. Schmidt BL. A rapid chemiluminescence detection method for PCR-amplified HIV-1 DNA. *J Virol Meth.* 1991;32;233–244.
50. Kohsaka H, Taniguchi A, Richman DD, et al. Microtiter format gene amplification by covalent capture of competitive PCR products: Application to HIV-1 detection. *Nucleic Acids Res.* 1993;21:3469–3472.
51. Findlay JB. A containment system for PCR amplification and detection. In: Ehrlich GD and Greenberg SJ, eds. *PCR-based diagnostic in infectious diseases.* Boston: Backwell Scientific Publications, 1994 pp. 97–113.
52. Dennis Lo YM. Setting up a PCR laboratory. In: Dennis Lo YM, ed. *Clinical applications of PCR.* New Jersey: Humana Press, 1998;11–20.
53. Sarkar G, Sommer SS. Removal of DNA contamination in polymerase chain reaction reagents by ultraviolet irradiation. *Methods Enzylmol.* 1993; 218:381–388.
54. Cimino GD, Metchette KC, Tessman JW, et al. Post-PCR sterilization: a method to control carryover contamination by the polymerase chain reaction. *Nucleic Acid Res.* 1991;19:99–107.
55. Horsburgh CR, Jr, Ou CY, Jason J, Holmberg SD, et al. Duration of the human immunodeficiency virus infection before detection of antibody. *Lancet.* 1989;2:637–640.
56. Imagawa DT, Lee MH, Wolinsky SM, et al. Human immunodeficiency virus type 1 infection on homosexual men who remain seronegative for prolonged periods. *N Engl J Med.* 1989;320:1458–1462.
57. Farzadegan H, Vlahov D, Solomon L, et al. Detection of human immunodeficiency virus type 1 infection by polymerase chain reaction in a cohort of seronegative intravenous drug users. *J Infect Dis.* 1993;168:327–331.
58. Moore JP, Cao Y, Ho DD, et al. Development of the antigp120 antibody response during seroconversion to human immunodeficiency virus type 1. *J Virol.* 1994;68:5142–5155.

59. Koup RA, Safrit JT, Cao Y, et al. Temporal association of cellular immune response with the initial control of viremia in primary human immunodeficiency virus type 1 syndrome. *J Virol.* 1994;68:4650–4655.
60. Mellors JW, Rinaldo CR, Gupta P, et al. Prognosis in HIV-1 infection predicted by the quantity of virus in plasma. *Science.* 1996;272:1167–1170.
61. Stein DS, Lyles RH, Graham NM, et al. Predicting clinical progression or death in subjects with early-stage of human immunodeficiency virus (HIV) infection: a comparative analysis of quantification of HIV RNA, soluble tumor necrosis factor II receptors, neopterin, and beta2-microglobulin. Multicenter AIDS Cohort Study. *J Inectf Dis.* 1997;176:1161–1167.
62. Lefrere JR, Roudotthoraval F, Mariotti M, et al. The risk of disease progression is determined during the first year of human immunodeficiency virus type 1 infection. *J Infect Dis.* 1998;177:1541–1548.
63. Sethoe SY, Ling AE, Sng EH, et al. PCR as confirmatory test for human immunodeficiency virus type 1 infection in individuals with indeterminate Western blot (Immunoblot) profiles. *J Clin Microbiol.* 1995;33:3034–3036.
64. Schochetman G, Sninsky JJ. Direct detection of HIV infection using nucleic amplification techniques. In: Schochetman G, Geroge JR, eds. *AIDS testing.* New York; Springer-Verlag, 1994;141–169.
65. Jackson JB, Hanson MR, Johnson GM, et al. Long-term follow-up of blood donors with indeterminate human immunodeficiency virus type 1 results on Western blot. *Transfusion.* 1995;35:98–102.
66. Jackson JB, MacDonald KL, Cadwell J, et al. Absence of HIV infection in blood donors with indeterminate Western blot test for antibody to HIV-1. *N Engl J Med.* 1990;322:217–222.
67. Connors EM, Sperling RS, Gelber R, et al. Reduction of maternal-infant transmission of human immunodeficiency virus type 1 with zidovudine treatment. Pediatric AIDS Clinical Trials Group Protocol 076 Study Group. *N Engl J Med.* 1994;331:1173–1180.
68. Owens DK, Holodniy M, Mcdonald TW, et al. A meta-analytic evaluation of the polymerase chain reaction for the diagnosis of HIV infection in infants. *JAMA.* 1996;275:1342–1348.
69. Kuhn L, Abrams EJ, Matheson PB, et al. Timing of maternal-infant HIV transmission. Association between intrapartum factors and early polymerase chain reaction results. *AIDS.* 1997;11:429–435.
70. Shaffer N, Chuachoowong R, Mock PA, et al. Short-course zidovudine for perinatal HIV-1 transmission in Bangkok, Thailand: a randomized controlled trial. *Lancet.* 1999;353:773–780.
71. Cattaneo E, Zavattoni M, Baldanti F, et al. Diagnostic value of viral culture, polymerase chain reaction and western blot for HIV-1 infection in 218 infants born to HIV-infected mothers and examined at different ages. *Microbiologica.* 1999;22: 281–291.
72. Wiktor SZ, Ekpini E, Karon JM, et al. Short-course oral zidovudine for prevention of mother-to-child transmission of HIV-1 in Abidjan, Cote d'Ivoire: a randomized trial. *Lancet.* 1999;353:781–785.
73. Fawzi W, Msamanga G, Hunter D, et al. A randomized trial of vitamin supplements in relation to vertical transmission of HIV-1 in Tanzania. *J Acquir Immune Defic Syndr.* 2000;23:246–254.
74. Johnson JP, Nair P, Hines SE, et al. Natural history and serologic diagnosis of infants born to human immunodeficiency virus-infected women. *Am J Dis Chil.* 1989;143:1147–1153.
75. European Collaborative Study. Children born to women with HIV infection: natural history and risk of transmission. *Lancet.* 1991;337:253–269.
76. Rogers MF, Schochetman G. HIV infection in children. In: Schochetman G, Geroge JR, eds. *AIDS testing.* New York; Springer-Verlag, 1994;266–283.
77. Palomba E, Gay V, de Martino M, et al. Early diagnosis of human immunodeficiency virus infection in infants by the detection of free and complexed p24 antigen. *J Infect Dis.* 1992;165:394–395.
78. Quinn TC, Kline RL, Halsey N, et al. Early diagnosis of perinatal HIV infection by detection of viral-specific IgA antibodies. *JAMA.* 1991;266:3439–3442.
79. Krivine A, Yakudima A, Le May M, et al. A comparative study of virus isolation, polymerase chain reaction, and antigen detection in children of mothers infected with human immunodeficiency virus. *J Pediatr.* 1990;116:372–376.
80. Wolinsky SM, Wike CM, Korber BT, et al. Selective transmission of human immunodeficiency virus type-1 variants from mothers to infants. *Science.* 1992;255:1134–1137.
81. Lyamuya, E, Olausson-Hansson, E, Albert, J, et al. Evaluation of a prototype Amplicor PCR assay for detection of human immunodeficiency virus type 1 DNA in blood samples from Tanzanian adults infected with HIV-1 subtypes A, C and D. *Journal of Clinical Virology.* 2000;17:57–63.
82. Blackard JT, Renjifo B, Chaplin B, et al. Diversity of the HIV-1 long terminal repeat following mother-to-child transmission. *Virology.* 2000;274:402–411.
83. Renjifo B, Gilbert P, Chaplin B, et al. Emerging recombinant human immunodeficiency virus: Uneven representation of the envelope V3 region. *AIDS.* 1999;13:1613–1621.
84. Larder BA, Kemp, SD. Multiple mutations in HIV-1 reverse transcriptase confer high-level resistance to zidovudine (AZT). *Science.* 1988;246:1155–1158.
85. St Clair MH, Martin JL, Tudor-Williams G, et al. Resistance to ddI and sensitivity to AZT induced by a mutation in HIV-1 reverse transcriptase. *Science.* 1991;235:1557–1559.

86. Fitzgibbon JE, Howell RM, Haberzettl CA, et al. Human immunodeficiency virus type 1 pol gene mutations which cause decreased susceptibility to 2′,3′-dideoxycytidine. *Antimicrobial Agents Chemother*. 1992;36:153–157.
87. Hertogs K, Bloor S, Kemp SD, et al. Phenotypic and genotypic analysis of clinical HIV-1 isolates reveals extensive protease inhibitor cross-resistance: a survey of over 6000 samples. *AIDS*. 2000;14:1203–1210.
88. Kaye S. Viral genotyping by a quantitative point mutation assay: Application to HIV-1 drug resistance. In: Innis MA, Gelfand DH, Sninsky JJ, eds. *PCR applications. Protocols for functional genomics*. San Diego: Academic Press. 1999;153–169.
89. Rusconi S, Catamancio SL, Sheridan F, et al. A genotypic analysis of patients receiving Zidovudine with either Lamivudine, Didanosine or Zalcitabine dual therapy using the LiPA point mutation assay to detect genotypic variation at codons 41, 69, 70, 74, 184 and 215. *J Clin Virol*. 2000;19:135–142.
90. Ferre F. Quantitative or semi-quantitative PCR: reality versus myth. *PCR Meth and Appl.* 1992;2:1–9.
91. Gilliand G, Perrin S, Bunn HF. Competitive PCR for quantification of mRNA. In: Innis MA, Gelfand DH, Sninsky JJ, White T, eds. *PCR protocols: A guide to methods and applications*. San Diego: Academic Press, 1990;60–69.
92. Alaeus A, Lidman K, Sonnenborg A, et al. Subtype-specific problems with quantification of plasma HIV-1 RNA. *AIDS*. 1997;11:859–865.
93. Chew CB, Herring BL, Zheng F, et al. Comparison of three commercial assays for the quantification of HIV-1 RNA in plasma from individuals infected with different HIV-1 subtypes. *J Clin Virol*. 1999; 14:87–94.
94. Parekh B, Phillips S, Granade TC, et al. Impact of HIV type 1 subtype variation on viral RNA quantification. *AIDS Res Hum Retroviruses*. 1999; 81:123–129.
95. Mani I, Coa H, Johnson J, et al. Plasma RNA viral load as measured by the branched DNA and nucleic acid sequence-based amplification assays of HIV-1 subtype A and D in Uganda. *J Acquir Immune Defic Syndr Hum Retrovirol.* 1999;22:208–212.
96. Michael NL, Herman SA, Kwok S, et al. Development of calibrated viral load standard for group M subtypes of human immunodeficiency virus type 1 and performance of an improved AMPLICOR HIV-1 MONITOR test with isolates of diverse subtypes. *J Clin Microbiol.* 1999;37: 2557–2563.
97. Burgisser P, Vernazza P, Flepp M, et al. Performance of five different assays for the quantification of viral load in persons infected with various subtypes of HIV-1. *J Acquir Immune Defic Syndr.* 2000;23:138–144.
98. George JR, Ou CY, Parekh B, et al. Prevalence of HIV-1 and HIV-2 mixed infections in Cote d'Ivore. *Lancet.* 1992;340:337–339.
99. Kanki PJ. Epidemiology and natural history of HIV-2. *AIDS.* 1994;8:S1-S9.
100. Gnann JW Jr, McCormick JB, Mitchell S, et al. Synthetic peptides immunoassays distinguishes HIV type 1 and HIV type 2 infections. *Science.* 1987;137:1346–1349.
101. Zuber M, Samuel KP, Lautenberger JA, et al. Bacterially-produced HIV-2 Env polypeptides specific for distinguishing HIV-1 from HIV-1 infections. *AIDS Res Hum Retroviruses.* 1990; 6:525–534.
102. Gueye-Ndiaye A, Clark R, Samuel KP, et al. Cost-effective diagnosis of HIV-1 and HIV-2 by recombinant-expressed env peptide (566/996) dot-blot analysis. *AIDS.* 1993;7:475–481.
103. Grankvist O, Bredberg-Raden U, Gustafsson A, et al. Improved detection of HIV-2 DNA in clinical samples using a nested primer-based polymerase chain reaction. *J Acquir Immune Defic Syndr.* 1992;5:286–293.
104. Erlich GD. PCR-based laboratory methods for the detection of the human retroviridae and hepadnaviridae. In: Ehrlich GD, Greenberg SJ, eds. *PCR-based diagnostic in infectious diseases.* Boston: Backwell Scientific Publications, 1994;414–446.
105. Popper SJ, Sarr AD, Travers KU, et al. Lower human immunodeficiency virus (HIV) type 2 viral load reflects the difference in pathogenicity of HIV-1 and HIV-2. *J Infect Dis.* 1999;180:1116–1121.
106. Delwart EL, Shpaer EG, Louwagie J, et al. Genetic relationships determined by a DNA heteroduplex mobility assay: analysis of HIV-1 env genes. *Science.* 1993;262:1257–1261.
107. Heyndrickx L, Janssens W, Zekeng L, et al. Simplified strategy for detection of recombinant human immunodeficiency virus type 1 group M isolates by gag/env heteroduplex mobility assay. Study Group on Heterogeneity of HIV Epidemics in African Cities. *J Virol.* 2000;74:363–370.
108. Renjifo B, Chaplin B, Mwakagile D, et al. Epidemic expansion of HIV type 1 subtype C and recombinant genotypes in Tanzania. *AIDS Res Hum Retroviruses.* 1998;14:635–638.
109. Renjifo B, Fawzi W, Mwakagile D, et al. Differences in perinatal transmission between HIV-1 genotypes. *J Hum Virol.* 2001;4(1):16–25.
110. Hully JR. In situ PCR. In: Innis MA, Gelfand DH, Sninsky JJ, eds. *PCR applications. Protocols for functional genomics.* San Diego: Academic Press, 1999;169–194.
111. Bagasra O, Hauptman SP, Lischner HW, et al Detection of human immunodeficiency virus type 1 provirus in mononuclear cells by in situ polymerase chain reaction. *N Eng J Med.* 1992;326: 1385–1391.

112. Pantaleo G, Graziosi C, Demarest JF, et al. HIV infection is active and progressive in lymphoid tissue during the clinically latent stage of disease. *Nature.* 1993;362:355–358.
113. Embretson J. Analysis of human immunodeficiency virus-infected tissues by amplification and in situ hybridization reveals latent and permissive infections at single-cell resolution. *Proc Natl Acad Sci USA.* 1993;90:357–361.
114. Lewin SR, Vesanen M, Kostrikis L, et al. Use of real-time PCR and molecular beacons to detect virus replication in human immunodeficiency virus type 1-infected individuals on prolonged effective antiretroviral therapy. *J Virol.* 1999;73:6099–6103.
115. O'Doherty U, Swiggard WJ, Malim MH. (2000). Human immunodeficiency virus type 1 spinoculation enhances infection through virus binding. *J Virol.* 2000;74:10074–10080.
116. Valentin A, Trivedi H, Lu W, et al. CXCR4 mediates entry and productive infection of syncytia-inducing (X4) HIV-1 strains in primary macrophages. *Virology.* 2000;269:294–304.
117. Schutten M, van den Hoogen B, van der Ende ME, et al. Development of a real-time quantitative RT-PCR for the detection of HIV-2 RNA in plasma. *J Virol Meth.* 2000;88:81–87.
118. Wang WK, Lee CN, Dudek T, et al. Interaction between HIV type 1 glycoprotein 120 and CXCR4 coreceptor involves a highly conserved arginine residue in hypervariable region 3. *AIDS Res Hum Retroviruses.* 2000;16:1821–1829.
119. Wang WK, Dudek T, Zhao YJ, et al. CCR5 coreceptor utilization involves a highly conserved arginine residue of HIV type 1 gp120. *Proc Natl Acad Sci USA.* 1998;95:5740–5745.
120. Sankale JL, Hamel D, Woolsey A, et al. Molecular evolution of human immunodeficiency virus type 1 subtype A in Senegal: 1988–1997. *J Hum Virol.* 2000;3:157–164.
121. Lallemant M, Jourdain G, Le Coeur S, et al. A trial of shortened zidovudine regimens to prevent mother-to-child transmission of human immunodeficiency virus. *N Eng J Med.* 2000;343:982–991.
122. Shaffer N, Chuachoowong R, Mock PA, et al. Short-course zidovudine for perinatal HIV-1 transmission in Bangkok, Thailand: a randomised controlled trial. *Lancet.* 1999;353:773–780.
123. Cassol S, Butcher A, Kinard S, et al. Rapid screening for early detection of mother-to-child transmission of human immunodeficiency virus type 1. *J Clin Microbiol.* 1994;32:2641–2645.
124. Ho D, Rota R, Schooley R, et al. Isolation of HTLV-III from cerebrospinal fluid and neural tissues of patients with neurologic syndromes related to the acquired immunodeficiency syndrome. *N Engl J Med.* 1985;313;1493–1497.
125. Ho D, Byington R, Schooley R, et al. Isolation of HTLA-III from 83 saliva and 50 blood samples from 71 seropositive homosexual men. *N Engl J Med.* 1985;313;1606.
126. Gaines H, Albert J, Von Sydow M, et al. HIV antigenemia and virus isolation from plasma during primary HIV infection. *Lancet.* 1987;1:1317–1318.
127. Gendelman HE, Baca LM, Husayni H, et al. Macrophage-HIV interaction: virus isolation and target cell tropism. *AIDS.* 1990;4:221–228.
128. Rayfield MA. HIV culture. In: Schochetman G, Geroge JR, eds. *AIDS testing.* New York; Springer-Verlag, 1994:129–140.
129. Jackson JB, Kwok SY, Sninsky JJ, et al. Human immunodeficiency virus type 1 detected in all seropositive symptomatic and asymptomatic individuals. *J Clin Microbiol.* 1988;28:16–19.
130. Jackson JB. Human immunodeficiency virus type 1 antigen and culture assays. *Arch Pathol Lab Med.* 1990;114:249–254.
131. Ulrich PP, Busch MP, El-Beik T, et al. Assessment of human immunodeficiency virus expression in co-cultures of peripheral blood mononuclear cells from healthy seropositive subjects. *J Med Virol.* 1988;25:1–10.
132. Dittmar MT, Simmons G, Donaldson Y, et al. Biological characterization of human immunodeficiency virus type 1 clones derived from different organs of an AIDS patient by Long-Range PCR. *J Virol.* 1997;71:5140–5147.

9

Monitoring HIV-1 Subtype Distribution

*Francis R. Barin, †§Coumba Toure-Kane,
*‡Jean-Christophe Plantier, and †Martine Peeters

*Département de Microbiologie Médicale et Moléculaire, Université François Rabelais, Tours, France.
†Laboratoire Retrovirus, IRD, Montpellier, France. ‡Laboratoire de Virologie,
CHU Charles Nicolle, Rouen, France. §Hôpital Le Dantec, Dakar, Sénégal.

Assays for monitoring the HIV pandemic are absolutely necessary for any part of the world but particularly so for sub–Saharan Africa, a region where approximately two-thirds of global HIV infections have occurred and infection prevalence is among the highest worldwide. The HIV pandemic must be monitored both quantitatively—by measuring the prevalence and the incidence of HIV infection—and qualitatively, by tracking the various types and subtypes of the virus. Because the tools necessary to monitor the prevalence of HIV infection are based on assays for HIV antibodies that are already broadly used in many countries, but not necessarily applicable in Africa, we will focus on particular aspects of a practical approach that can be applied in Africa by countries seeking to monitor infection prevalence. In addition, because the incidence of HIV infection can be more difficult to document, we will review different technologic approaches for its determination. However, the need to monitor the prevalence and incidence of this infectious disease can pale when compared with the need to carefully, and precisely, monitor the extensive variability of its causative agent: HIV. Such data have the potential to significantly affect techniques for diagnosis, therapy, and prevention. Because all of the known groups, types, and subtypes of HIV circulate in the populations of sub–Saharan Africa, and because intersubtype recombinations occur frequently, we will devote the majority of this chapter to a discussion of the assays for monitoring HIV diversity.

MONITORING HIV PREVALENCE

In most countries, the prevalence of HIV infection has been determined using conventional assays that measure for HIV antibody. Indeed, diagnosis of HIV infection is usually made based on the results of serum testing for HIV antibody. However, this assay presents several difficulties when implemented in Africa. At times, the technical environment is very restricted. At other times, candidates for testing, particularly babies and children, may be reluctant to accept an invasive act such as a venous puncture. Although conventional antibody assays on serum samples, enzyme immunoassays for HIV antibody, and Western blot assays must remain the classic reference methods for attaining the highest specificity, several alternative approaches that have been tried and validated make surveillance studies more convenient, practical, and cost effective. Alternative algorithms using rapid tests only, have been shown to be perfectly acceptable for both population-based surveillance studies and diagnostic procedures (1–4).

To avoid the need for separating serum or plasma from cell components, a few, rapid, instrument-free assays have been developed and adapted as techniques for screening whole blood (5,6). Some of these assays have proved to be reliable and easy to perform and interpret, and, therefore, suitable for use in situations where laboratory support and personnel are scarce.

Another alternative approach is the use of dried blood spots (DBS) rather than blood and sera drawn and stored as liquid in a tube. The advantages of using DBS include the ability to collect only small volumes of blood, the opportunity to collect samples without invasive puncture, and the latitude to delay serologic assays because the DBS can be stored for long periods of time without decreasing the efficacy of the antibody screening tests. DBS have been used in a number of large field studies, especially in studies carried out in remote areas but also in those conducted in developed countries (7–9). In addition to antibody screening, DBS can be used also for detection or quantification of HIV genome, either viral RNA or proviral DNA (7,10,11).

The use of body fluids other than blood (such as saliva and urine) as alternative media for tests has also been evaluated. Several studies have shown that using urine to test for HIV antibodies produces results that show less sensitivity and specificity, eliminating this as an alternative technical approach to diagnostic testing (12,13). By contrast, many studies found that results from HIV antibody testing of saliva or other oral fluid produced sensitivities and specificities that were comparable to those achieved using serum specimens (12–17). However, if it is necessary to transport and/or store such samples before testing, it is important to use adapted collection devices and vials containing a preservative solution (18).

The use of HIV antibody testing with saliva has been evaluated in Africa and has been shown to yield results that are accurate and acceptable (6,19–23). In situations where HIV antibody testing using oral fluids is recommended for prevalence studies, those in charge of these studies must know the exact performance of the test system that they will use and apply the exact conditions validated to get accurate results.

MONITORING HIV INCIDENCE

Serologic monitoring of the HIV epidemic is generally limited to monitoring seroprevalence, the proportion of the population with antibodies to HIV, comprising both people with recent infection and people with infection of several years' duration. However, the best data for understanding recent changes in the HIV epidemic are obtained from determinations of the number of new infections occurring within a defined time period (incidence). HIV incidence can be determined by longitudinal studies of large cohorts. However, these longitudinal studies are logistically complex, costly, and require a long follow-up period, and their results can be skewed by the selective participation and loss to follow-up of participants.

Data collected from methods to detect primary infection can be used to estimate incidence. Because the symptomatology of primary infection can be atypical or even absent, it is important to define virologic markers or profiles that are specific to this early phase of infection. The detection of p24 antigen in the absence of HIV antibody during the period before seroconversion has been proposed as a means of identifying persons with primary infection, and, therefore, a method for estimating incidence (24,25). However, because the period of antigenemia before antibody detection is brief (14 to 22 days), the utility of this methodology is limited to large populations with high incidence (26,27). Although detection of plasma HIV

RNA during the period before seroconversion might be a more sensitive measure for estimating incidence than p24 antigenemia, the high cost and technologic requirements associated with nucleic acid technology are major obstacles to its use for this purpose.

In most viral infections, the diagnosis of recent infection is based on detection of IgM to viral antigens. This marker is used in the diagnosis of many viral infections such as rubella, hepatitis A, and hepatitis B (HBc IgM), as well as those associated with parvovirus B19, Epstein–Barr virus (VCA IgM or EA IgM), and human cytomegalovirus (28). However, for reasons that may be technical but more likely are linked to HIV's pathogenesis, there is no technique that consistently detects IgM to HIV. Therefore, this test is of no practical use for identifying recent HIV infections. Recently, a new strategy based on a sensitive/less-sensitive assay testing algorithm has been proposed as a method of identifying early HIV infection during the period when the antibody titer is increasing but before peak and persistently high antibody response (27). In this strategy, using both a sensitive and a less-sensitive enzyme immunoassay, also called a detuned assay, on a blood specimen from a person in the early phase of infection, the blood specimen is reactive on an enzyme immunoassay sensitive to HIV antibodies but is nonreactive on a less-sensitive enzyme immunoassay. In the detuned assay, the estimated mean time to being reactive to the sensitive assay and nonreactive to the less-sensitive assay was 129 days. In study populations from North America and Trinidad, where the subtype B variants predominate, this testing strategy accurately diagnosed 95% of individuals with early infection but incorrectly indicated early HIV-1 infection in 0.4% of men with established infection and in 2% of individuals with late-stage AIDS. The strategy was applied to various situations and produced, for example, an estimate of HIV incidence of 1.1% per year (1996–1998) in individuals seeking anonymous testing in San Francisco (29) and of 2.8% in a population of prison inmates in Sao Paulo, Brazil (30).

A sensitive/less-sensitive enzyme immuno-assay testing strategy would be a useful method for monitoring the HIV epidemic in Africa. However, because of the high diversity of HIV strains circulating in Africa and the low efficacy of commercial assays to detect early HIV-1 infections (31), it would be necessary to validate this strategy on well-documented blood specimens from different cohorts in Africa before applying it throughout the continent.

MONITORING HIV DIVERSITY

In the mid-1980s, serologic and genetic analyses of HIV began to show that the viruses circulating in Africa were highly diverse (Figure 1). This diversity was first demonstrated in 1985 with the discovery of HIV-2 based on serologic evidence of an SIV-related virus infecting West-African residents (32–34) and by the discovery that envelope proteins among HIV-1 isolates from Africa and the United States could differ in more than 35% of their amino-acid residues (35,36). This was followed by the identification of the highly divergent groups O and N within the HIV-1 type (37–40) and, within the group M of HIV-1, of at least five subtypes (41). The total number of HIV-1 group M viruses in Africa continues to expand, in part as a result of recombinations of subtypes that produce epidemiologically distinct circulating recombinant forms (CRFs) (42).

Distinguishing HIV-1 and HIV-2 from each other is relatively easy and does not require the use of sophisticated molecular technologies. In most of the cases, serologically based methods that are easy to perform give accurate results (43). Similarly, serologic subtyping, although usually restricted to specialized laboratories, has been shown to be an efficient method for discriminating between viral isolates of each of the three groups of HIV-1: M, O, and N (40,44,45).

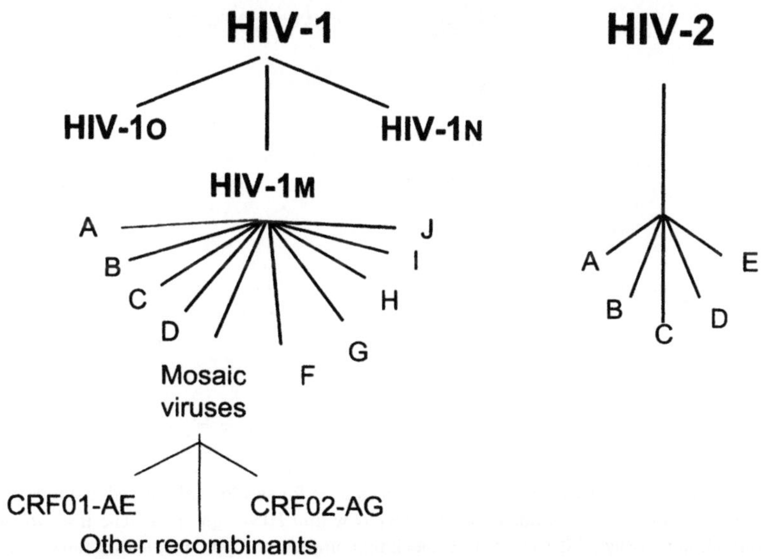

FIGURE 1. Types, groups, and subtypes of HIV identified in Africa.

This story changes, however, when it becomes necessary to identify and track subtypes within group M, a circumstance encountered throughout Africa. Full-length viral sequences are needed to optimally characterize the phylogenetic relationships between a new isolate and pre-existing HIV sequences, particularly in light of the potential for recombination (42,46–48). Generating complete sequences is a critical component of surveillance studies of global variation but is not feasible for large-scale molecular epidemiology surveys. Alternative approaches, including serologic methods as well as technologies based on polymerase chain reaction (PCR), have been commonly used and are continuously being refined (49). Because each of these methods has some advantages but also some real limitations, there is a clear need for continued development of inexpensive alternatives for tracking the genetic variation of the virus.

Serologically Based Methods of Subtyping

Serologic assays are highly desirable because of their ease of execution, their cost-effectiveness, and their capacity to be performed using stored serum. These assays detect host antibodies to immunogenic epitopes that are specific to type, group, or subtype. Two major epitopes are involved in serologic subtyping assays. Both epitopes are located within the envelope protein, and, because each corresponds to a linear epitope, each can be produced easily in large amounts by chemical synthesis (Figure 2).

The immunodominant epitope (IDE) of the transmembrane protein portion of the virus envelope is highly conserved within each type of HIV and therefore facilitates their differentiation. The IDE, however, is less useful for differentiating groups M, O, or N of HIV-1. Different enzyme immunoassay methodologies, either using a classic micro-plate support or a rapid immunoassay, as well as commercially available confirmatory assays such as immunoblots, rely on the use of synthetic peptides that represent sequences of the IDE. These formats are widely used and validated to discriminate between antibodies to HIV-1 and those to HIV-2 (43,50–52). Synthetic peptides representing consensus sequences of the IDE of the transmembrane protein have been also used to discriminate between

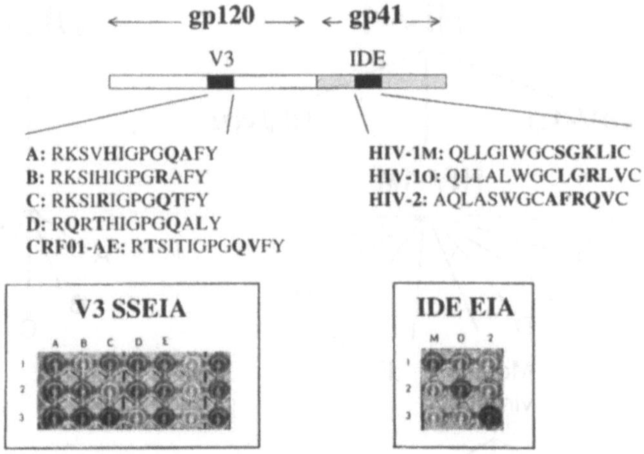

FIGURE 2. Locations and sequences of envelope epitopes used for serologically based methods of subtyping. The V3 region of gp120 is used for discrimination of subtypes within HIV-1 group M. The inset for the V3 subtype-specific enzyme immunoassay (SSEIA), using a blocking-competition approach, shows three samples reactive to peptides B, C, and D in lines 1, 2, and 3, respectively (no colored signal). The immunodominant epitope (IDE) of gp41 is used for discrimination of types and groups. The IDE enzyme immunoassay (EIA) inset shows three samples positive for antibodies to HIV-1 group M, HIV-1 group O, and HIV-2 in lines 1, 2, and 3, respectively (strongest colored signal). The amino acids upon which the determinations are based are indicated in bold for each epitope.

antibodies to either group M or group O viruses. This method allowed large serologic surveys of HIV-1 group O infections to be carried out. However, the sensitivity of these determinations can be improved by including V3 peptides (45) and by using a blocking-competition approach (44).

Like the IDE, the V3 loop, located within the surface glycoprotein of the virus is highly immunogenic during infection. At least 90% of infected individuals develop antibodies to V3 peptides (44,53) that become detectable a few months after exposure (54). Although the V3 region is highly variable, it is hypothesized that it is sufficiently conserved within the different subtypes to be useful in serologic analyses to discriminate between the subtypes of the group M virus. Following this hypothesis, consensus sequences of each subtype were defined with the intention of using them in tests to determine which HIV-1 subtypes had infected individuals. It was thought that sera from individuals infected by a virus of a given subtype of HIV-1 would react preferentially with peptides of the appropriate subtype. Different enzyme immunoassays, including indirect assays and assays using a blocking-competition approach were developed and gave similar results (55–57). The correlation between serotyping and genotyping was analyzed, and the data showed that V3 serotyping was closely related to the V3 loop amino-acid sequence of the analyzed sample (58,59).

However, several studies have shown V3 serotyping has a major limitation (58,60). Owing to high cross-reactivity between several subtypes, V3 serology is accurate only for differentiation of serotypes B/D versus serotypes A/C/E/F/G. Therefore, only in locations where a few serologically distinguishable serotypes are prevalent can large, population-based epidemiology studies using V3 serotyping be performed with a high degree of confidence. This is, for instance, the case in Europe for studies to distinguish between B and non-B serotypes (61,62); in Thailand, for studies of B and E serotypes (63), and in South Africa, for studies of B and C serotypes (64). However, in most of the African countries where different subtypes have been cocirculating for a long time, the use of V3 serologic subtyping results in a substantial percentage of mismatches between serologic result and actual genetic subtype (58,60). In addition, V3 serotyping assays focus on less than 1% of the total genome, the V3 loop, and, thus, cannot be used for conclusions regarding the other regions of the viral genome.

Polymerase Chain Reaction-Based Methods of Subtyping

Heteroduplex Mobility Assay

The heteroduplex mobility assay (HMA) is a PCR-based method that allows rapid subtyping using a set of reference reagents representing different subtypes. Less sophisticated equipment is required for this technique than is required for sequencing (65–67). The structural deformities in double-stranded DNA caused by nucleotide insertions or deletions are thought to result in "bubbles" in the heteroduplex that retard its mobility through the polyacrylamide matrix of electrophoretic analysis (Figure 3). This biochemistry is the basis of HMA.

Heteroduplexes are formed by denaturing and reannealing (usually by heating and cooling) partially complementary strands of DNA. HMA begins with PCR-amplified fragments of DNA. Substrates for PCR can include purified DNA or detergent-lysed cells from whole blood or from fresh or frozen white blood cells. Nested PCR reactions are used to generate sufficient quantities for the assay.

Nested PCR of highly conserved primers is used to generate 1.2-, 0.7-, or 0.5-kilobase (kb) fragments of envelope (*env*) gene from uncharacterized strains of HIV-1. For reference, the same size fragments are amplified from a series of plasmids containing *env* from different, known HIV-1 subtypes. Heteroduplexes that form between an unknown sample and its most closely

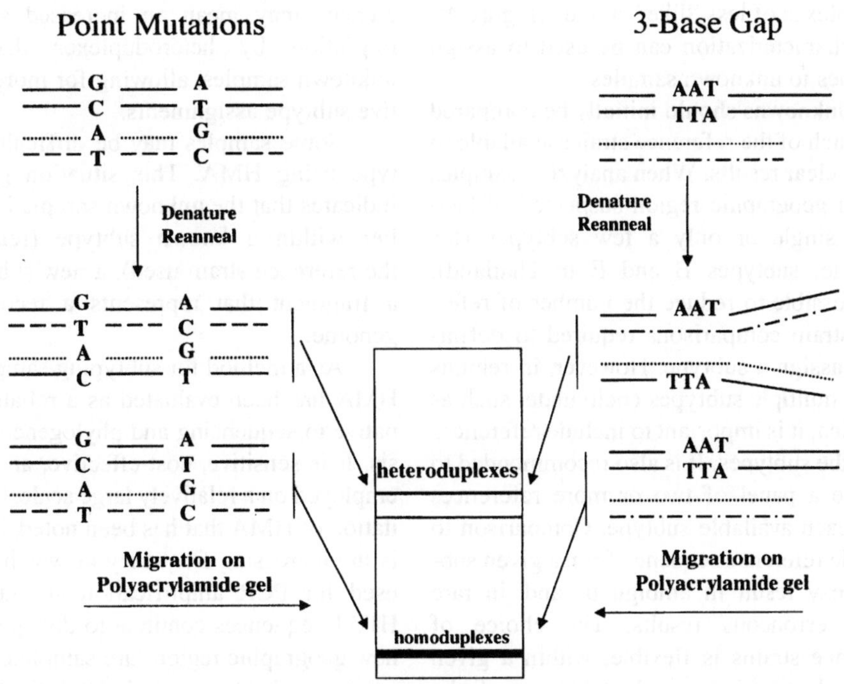

FIGURE 3. Schematic representation of heteroduplex mobility assay showing the potential results that point mutations (left) or a 3-base deletion (right) can yield.

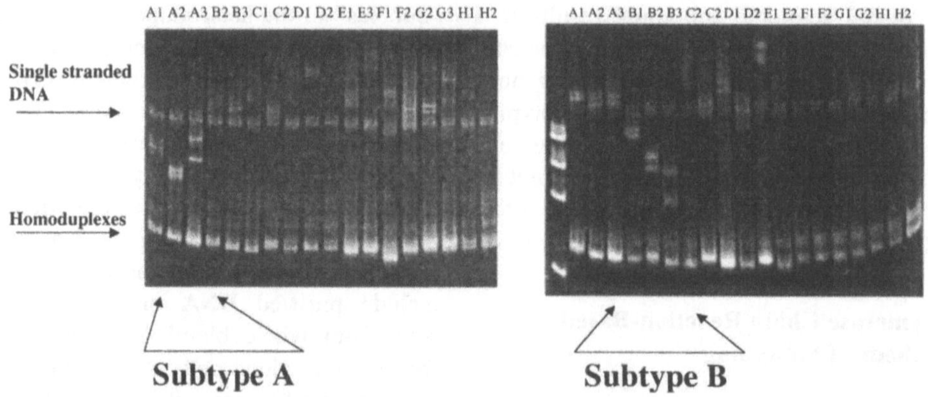

FIGURE 4. Heteroduplexes formed between pairs of PCR-amplified DNA fragments from subtype references with samples from individuals infected with HIV-1. A 700-bp fragment, covering the V3-V5 region of the envelope, was amplified from the unknown samples and from the plasmids representing the different HIV-1 group M subtypes. The amplified products from the unknown samples were mixed with each of the different references, and, after denaturation and reannealing, the fragments were separated on a polyacrylamide gel. Subtype reference fragments are noted above each lane. The subtype of the unknown sample was determined by identifying the reference subtype associated with the fastest migrating heteroduplexes. The unknown samples were identified as subtype A (left) and subtype B (right).

related reference sequence exhibit mobilities that are markedly faster than those of heteroduplexes of less "like" strands (Figure 4). This characterization can be used to assign subtypes to unknown samples.

Unknowns should initially be compared with each of the reference strains available to obtain clear results. When analyzing samples from a geographic region suspected of having a single or only a few subtypes (for example, subtypes B and E in Thailand), it is possible to reduce the number of reference strain comparisons required to definitively assign a subtype. However, in regions where multiple subtypes cocirculate, such as in Africa, it is important to include references of all the subtypes. It is also recommended to include a panel of two or more references from each available subtype. Comparison to a single reference sequence from a given subtype may result in ambiguous and, in rare cases, erroneous results. The choice of reference strains is flexible; within a given geographic region, resident strains of the same HIV-1 subtype are more likely to be closely related to each other than to other geographically more distant strains of the same subtype. The use of locally derived references may mean an increased speed of migration by heteroduplexes that form unknown samples, allowing for more definitive subtype assignments.

Some samples may be difficult to subtype using HMA. This situation generally indicates that the unknown sample is an outlier within a known subtype (relative to the reference strain used), a new subtype, or a fragment that represents a recombinant genome.

As a method for subtyping samples, *env* HMA has been evaluated as a reliable alternative to sequencing and phylogenetic analysis. It is sensitive, cost-effective, and can be employed on a relatively large scale. One limitation of HMA that has been noted, however, is the increasing frequency at which primers used for PCR amplification are failing as HIV-1 sequences continue to diverge, and as new geographic regions are sampled, causing more samples to remain indeterminate.

Another limitation is that *env* HMA can-not discriminate between subtype A and recombinant CRF02-AG, which remains genetically subtype A in the *env* region analyzed. This is particularly a problem in geographic regions were CRF02-AG and subtype A strains cocirculate, which is the case in West and West-Central Africa.

In an effort to extend HMA subtyping to another region of the HIV genome, and perhaps overcome the limitation introduced by intersubtype recombination, another HMA has been developed. This version characterizes *gag* genotypes. In contrast to *env* HMA, *gag* HMA can distinguish between subtype A and CRF02-AG. Simultaneous use of *gag* and *env* HMA can give a preliminary estimate of the frequency of recombinant viruses (68).

Subtype-Specific PCR Methodologies

This type of subtyping uses DNA that has been extracted from blood cells and subjected to nested PCR using universal first-round primers. The products are amplified with primer sets specific for the *env* subtypes to identify (Table 1). The PCR amplification products are detected by electrophoresis on agarose gel with ethidium bromide (EtB) staining or by Southern blot analysis (69–71). Subtype-specific PCR was initially described to distinguish North American/European variants from African variants (72). Since that application, it has been used successfully in molecular epidemiology studies to differentiate subtype B and CRF01-AE (former subtype E) in Southeast Asia (69,70,73,74). It provided evidence of dual infection with subtype B and CRF01-AE in Thai subjects (69). This methodology was adapted and applied in Africa for distinguishing subtype A from non-A subtypes in a study involving more than 400 samples. In this application, the method gave 98.7% specificity and an overall sensitivity of 72.8% (ranging from 87.5% in West Africa to 50% in Central Africa) (71). The major limitations of the methodology were found to be the capacity to distinguish only a limited number of subtypes and the fact that subtype A-specific PCR is an inefficient means for distinguishing CRF02-AG, a strain highly prevalent in West Africa.

PCR and Subtype-Specific Probe Hybridization

Several methodologies of this sort have been developed. They each consist of first amplifying a selected region by a

TABLE 1. Main Characteristics of the Different PCR-based Techniques[a]

Subtyping method	Analytic method	Target region of the genome	Type of probe	Discriminated subtypes
Subtype-specific PCR	Electrophoresis and EtB or Southern-blot	gp41 or C3-V4	N/A	B and CRF01-AE or A and non-A
PCR and probe hybridization	Dot-blot/microplate using digoxigenin labeling	C2-V3 or C2-V4	Consensus oligonucleotide	B and CRF01-AE or A and D
PCR and probe hybridization	DEIA	5′ end *env* – mid-C1	Consensus oligonucleotide	A to G, CRF01-AE, and CRF02-AG
PCR and probe hybridization	COMA	C2-V4	Reference single-stranded DNA	A to H
PCR and RFLP	Electrophoretic migration pattern	p17, p24 protease	Restriction enzymes	A to D and F

[a]PCR indicates polymerase chain reaction; EtB, ethidium bromide; DEIA, DNA enzyme immunoassay; COMA, combinatorial DNA melting assay; RFLP, restriction fragment-length polymorphism.

subtype-nonspecific nested PCR, followed by subtype detection using single-stranded subtype-specific probe hybridization. The formats differ by the nature of the probes and the method of revelation.

Oligonucleotide probe hybridization. In this approach, consensus sequences specific for different subtypes are defined and probes are obtained by chemical synthesis. Two dot-blot assays have been developed. One has been used to differentiate subtype B and CRF01-AE in Thailand (63) and another has been used to differentiate subtypes A and D in Uganda (75). The hybridization was done with digoxigenin-labeled consensus oligonucleotide probes, and the detection steps included the addition of alkaline phosphatase-conjugated anti-digoxigenin antibody followed by substrate. The hybridization and detection steps can also be adapted to a microplate format. Good sensitivity and specificity have been obtained.

These techniques were applied in large-scale molecular epidemiology studies in Thailand ($n>200$) and Uganda ($n>700$). They provided an effective screening of the respective two predominant subtypes. However, 20% of Ugandan samples could not be classified (76,77). The main limitation of these techniques is that they allow the discrimination of only two subtypes.

We recently developed a similar assay in a microplate format for discriminating subtypes A to G, and strains CRF01-AE and CRF02-AG using a set of nine probes. The PCR products (part of the *env* gene) are captured with consensus oligonucleotide probes, and the analysis is performed using an anti-double-stranded DNA mouse monoclonal antibody. This assay was evaluated on 128 samples from three different countries (France, Senegal, and Cameroon) and showed a global concordance of 83.5% with HMA (78). This assay is limited by the regional variability of the strains, however. The probes represent consensus sequences of the different subtypes. Too great a difference between regional sample sequences and consensus probes impair hybridization. Designing location-specific consensus probes and regularly re-evaluating the probes is necessary. This methodology can identify CRF01-AE and CRF02-AG but not other mosaic genomes.

Combinatorial DNA Melting Assay (COMA). The major difference between COMA and the assays previously described is the use of single-stranded DNA molecules as probes (79). These probes, corresponding to reference subtype and/or regional strains, are generated by asymmetrical PCR using primers that are conjugated to biotin to allow for capture on streptavidin-coated microplates. Complementary sense-stranded molecules from unknown samples are produced by asymmetrical PCR using digoxigenin-labeled primers. The analysis is performed using alkaline phosphatase-conjugated anti-digoxigenin antibody and its substrate. Development testing of this assay was performed on samples of subtypes A through H collected in 15 different countries. Complete agreement was found between results obtained from the COMA test and results obtained using the subtyping reference method (nucleotide sequencing and phylogenetic analysis of *env* sequences or HMA) (79). COMA was performed on 24 samples from Kenyan individuals and subtypes A and D were detected with 100% concordance (80). COMA, a variation of HMA on microplate, is based on representative strains, not consensus probes. It would, therefore, be necessary to select reference or regional strains appropriate to defining a pool specific to each geographic location in which it would be used and to also regularly re-evaluate these reference strains. It would also be necessary to prepare numerous reference capture single-stranded DNA molecules from genomic DNA or plasmids.

PCR and Subtype-Specific Restriction Fragment Length Polymorphism (RFLP)

This assay also uses a nested PCR to amplify the selected region of the viral genome for subtype discrimination. The PCR product is digested with a set of restriction enzymes and analyzed by agarose or polyacrylamide gel electrophoresis and EtB staining. The restriction site's polymorphism yields digested products having different electrophoretic mobility (81). This methodology was developed for distinguishing subtypes A, B, C, D, and F through an analysis of the protease and *gag*/protease regions using different enzymes (82). Molecular epidemiology studies using RFLP have shown high specificity in studies in Brazil, Puerto Rico, and Côte d'Ivoire but have shown lower specificity in the African study (83–85). This methodology was used to identify dual infections involving subtypes B, C, D, and F in individuals in Brazil and Puerto Rico (85,86). A sequential RFLP algorithm based on *gag* and using a different set of restriction enzymes was recently developed and used to efficiently detect subtypes A to D in studies in South Africa (87). As with other PCR-based assays, this methodology is limited by the fact that primer mismatches result in the non-amplification of divergent strains and the fact that a single nucleotide mutation in the endonuclease site can disrupt the recognition pattern or produce false positives. Technical limitations to the use of this approach are the requirement for sequential analysis and large amounts of viral DNA, and the occurrence of multiple distinct patterns for a single subtype as a result of sequence variability.

Sequencing and Sequence Analyses

Despite the limitations of the various PCR-based assays, sequencing remains the most accurate way to identify variants of HIV-1. Even only partial *gag* and/or *env* sequences give more precise information on subclades or recombinant viruses than do serotyping or PCR-based methods. Also, partial genome characterization allows for preliminary selection of important strains for full sequencing. Full-length genome sequencing is needed to determine whether a new isolate is a recombinant or whether the pattern of mosaicism within an isolate is that of a recombinant. Full-length genome sequencing is vital to efforts to maintain surveillance of HIV-1's global variation.

Sequencing

Genome fragments can be amplified and directly sequenced (without cloning) using a cycle-sequencing protocol adapted for the ABI automatic sequencer (Applied Biosystems). The direct-sequencing approach has the advantage that the average sequence of the clinical isolate is seen. It is also much faster than cloning a PCR product and sequencing several clones, a process that can produce PCR artifacts that cannot be discriminated from patient-derived variants. Recent advances in long-PCR technologies have made it possible to generate full-length sequences of HIV genomes on a routine basis.

Subtype Identification by Phylogenetic Tree Analysis

In order to determine the subtype of genome fragments or entire HIV-1 genomes, the sequences in question are aligned with reference strains of different known subtypes and, eventually, sub-subtypes. Reference alignments can be obtained from the Los Alamos HIV Sequence Database (http://hiv-web.lanl.gov). Nucleotide and protein sequences can be aligned using various software programs, such as Clustal W (88), and manually adjusted. Sites with gaps in sequences as well as areas of uncertain alignment must be excluded from all sequence comparisons. Once alignments have been made, pair-specific evolutionary distances can be estimated using the two-parameter method to correct for superimposed substitutions (89). Phylogenetic trees can be constructed using the neighbor-joining method (90), and the reliability of topologies can be estimated by performing bootstrap analyses with 100 or 1,000 replicates (91). Phylogenetic relationships can also be determined using maximum-likelihood approaches, used in certain software programs such as DNAPARS and DNAML from the PHYLIP package (92). The subtype of a newly derived sequence will correspond to the subtype of the reference strains with which it forms a separate cluster, a determination that also should be supported by high bootstrap values (>80%).

Analysis of Recombinant HIV-1 Genomes

Hybrid viruses can be detected because their phylogenetic affinities will vary with the region of the genome that is analyzed. Various complementary approaches have been developed to identify sequences that are recombinants and to map the breakpoint positions within mosaic sequences. Recombinant sequences are generally identified by determining whether relative distances between

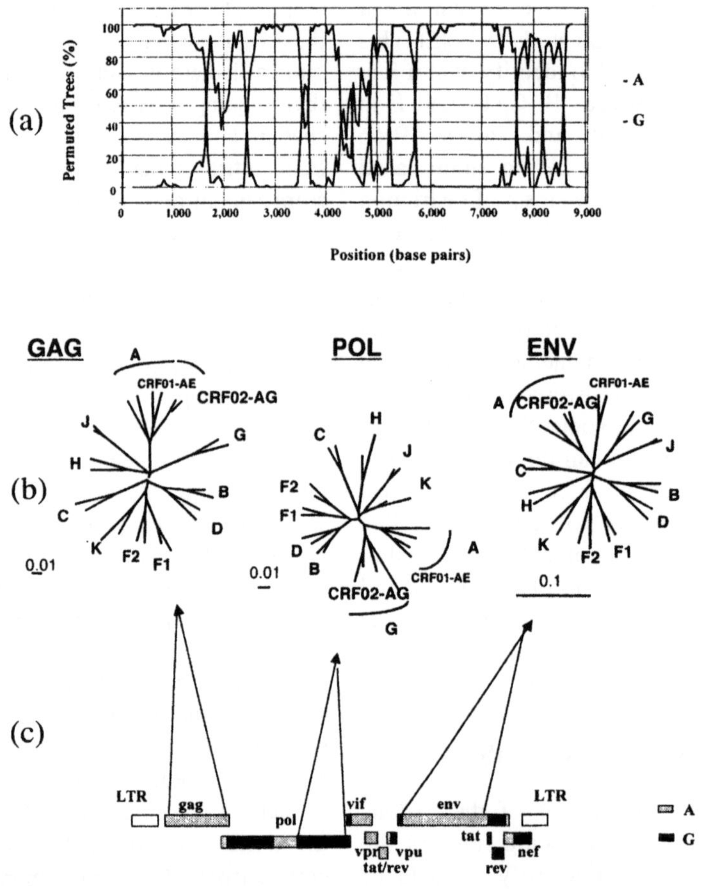

FIGURE 5. Structure of the CRF02-AG prototype recombinant: AG_{IBNG} from Nigeria. Bootscan analysis (a) evaluates systematically the bootstrap values supporting independent monophyletic phylogeny in different parts of the genome. For the bootscan plots, the Simplot software performed bootscanning on parsimony trees by using SEQBOOT, DNAPARS, and CONSENSUS from the PHYLIP package for a 500-bp (base pair) window moving along the alignment at 50-bp increments. The bootstrap values for the studied sequences were plotted at the midpoint of each window. Successive subtype A and G fragments were observed. Phylogenetic tree analysis from different genomic regions (b), confirmed the alternate subtype A and subtype G fragments. A schematic representation (c) of the mosaic structure of CRF02-AG.

sequences vary at different windows along a sequence alignment (93–95). Because the different subtypes of the M group of HIV-1 have been well defined, potential intersubtype recombinants can be analyzed in a more-or-less automated fashion. Moving-window analysis (96,97) can plot the diversity or similarity of a new sequence to representatives of other subtypes. Software such as a recombinant identification program (98) uses distance measures to assign subtypes to regions within the new sequence, and the strength of bootstrap support for the phylogenetic placement of the new sequence with any subtype representative can be assessed using software such as a bootscan program (99). Fine-scale mapping of recombination breakpoints has been performed using informative site analysis (48,96). Most of the software used to perform these analyses is freely available from their developers or can be accessed online. An example of the data that can be assembled from these computer analyses can be found in Figure 5, which shows the structure of the CRF02-AG strain, determined through bootscan analysis and phylogenetic tree analysis.

CONCLUSION

The global HIV epidemic is extremely heterogeneous and dynamic in nature, embracing several epidemics specific to different geographic locations and populations, as evidenced in Africa. Although the degree of surveillance for HIV-1 strains has increased in recent years, more information is needed. Both the current incidence and the current distribution of HIV subtypes need to be better established. Only with these data, will it be possible to track changes in subtype distribution over time and detect the introduction of novel subtypes or CRFs into populations. This information is vital to delineating the historical and dynamic details of the epidemic. Subtype and strain surveillance is necessary to monitor the emergence of new subtypes and strains that may be naturally resistant to antiretroviral drugs. Finally, knowing the distribution of HIV-1 strains will likely be relevant for vaccine development.

REFERENCES

1. Meda A, Gautier-Charpentier L, Soudré RB, et al. Serological diagnosis of human immunodeficiency virus in Burkina-Faso: reliable, practical strategies using less expensive commercial test kits. *Bull World Health Organ*, 1999;77:731–739.
2. Stetler HC, Granade TC, Nunez CA, et al. Field evaluation of rapid HIV serologic tests for screening and confirming HIV-1 infection in Honduras. *AIDS*, 1997;11:369–375.
3. UNAIDS/WHO. Revised recommendations for the selection and use of HIV antibody tests. *Wkly Epidemiol Rec*, 1997;72:81–87.
4. Wilkinson D, Wilkinson N, Lombard C, et al. On-site HIV testing in resource-poor settings: is one rapid test enough? *AIDS*, 1997;11:377–381.
5. Kemp E, Rylatt DB, Bundesen PG, et al. Autologous red cell agglutination assay for HIV-1 antibodies: simplified test with whole blood. *Science*, 1988;241:1352–1354.
6. Webber LM, Swanevelder C, Grabow WO, et al. Evaluation of a rapid test for HIV antibodies in saliva and blood. *S Afr Med J*, 2000;90: 1004–1007.
7. Biggar RJ, Miley W, Miotti P, et al. Blood collection on filter paper: a practical approach to sample collection for studies of perinatal HIV transmission. *J Acquir Immune Defic Syndr Hum Retrovirol*, 1997;14:368–373.
8. Boillot F, Peeters M, Kosia A, et al. Prevalence of the human immunodeficiency virus among patients with tuberculosis in Sierra Leone, established from dried blood spots on filter paper. *Int J Tuberc Lung Dis*, 1997;1:493–497.
9. Johnstone F, Goldberg D, Tappin D, et al. The incidence and prevalence of HIV infection among childbearing women living in Edinburgh city, 1985–1995. *AIDS*, 1998;12:911–918.
10. Cassol S, Gill MJ, Pilon R, et al. Quantification of human immunodeficiency virus type 1 RNA from dried plasma spots collected on filter paper. *J Clin Microbiol*, 1997;35:2795–2801.
11. Lallemant M, Jourdain G, Lallemant-Lecoeur S, et al. A trial of shortened zidovudine regimens to prevent mother-to-child transmission of human immunodeficiency virus type 1. *New England Journal of Medicine*, 2000;343:982–991.

12. Martinez PM, Torres AR, Ortiz de Lejarazu R, et al. Human immunodeficiency virus antibody testing by enzyme-linked fluorescent and western blot assays using serum, gingival-crevicular transudate, and urine samples. *J Clin Microbiol*, 1999;37:1100–1106.
13. Tribble DR, Rodier GR, Saad MD, et al. Comparative field evaluation of HIV rapid diagnostic assays using serum, urine, and oral mucosal transudate specimens. *Clin Diagn Virol*, 1997;7:127–132.
14. Granade TC, Phillips SK, Parekh B, et al. Detection of antibodies to human immunodeficiency virus type 1 in oral fluids: a large-scale evaluation of immunoassay performance. *Clin Diagn Lab Immunol*, 1998;5:171–175.
15. King SD, Wynter SH, Bain BC, et al. Comparison of testing saliva and serum for detection of antibody to human immunodeficiency virus in Jamaica, West-Indies. *J Clin Virol*, 2000;19:157–161.
16. Pasquier C, Bello PY, Gourney P, et al. A new generation of serum anti-HIV antibody immunocapture assay for saliva testing. *Clinical Diagnostic Virology*, 1997;8:195–197.
17. Schramm W, Angulo GB, Torres PC, et al. A simple saliva-based test for detecting antibodies to human immunodeficiency virus. *Clin Diagn Lab Immunol*, 1999;6:577–580.
18. Malamud D. Oral diagnostic testing for detecting human immunodeficiency virus-1 antibodies: a technology whose time has come. *Am J Med*, 1997;102:9–14.
19. Ettiegne-Traore V, Ghys PD, Maurice C, et al. Evaluation of an HIV saliva test for the detection of HIV-1 and HIV-2 antibodies in high-risk populations in Abidjan, Côte d'Ivoire. *Int J STD AIDS*, 1998;9:173–174.
20. Fylkesnes K, Kasumba K. The first Zambian population-based HIV survey: saliva-based testing is accurate and acceptable. *AIDS*, 1998;12:540–541.
21. Fylkesnes K, Ndhlovu Z, Kasumba K, et al. Studying dynamics of the HIV epidemic: population-based data compared with sentinel surveillance in Zambia. *AIDS*, 1998;12:1227–1234.
22. Grant RM, Piwowar EM, Katongole-Mbidde E, et al. Comparison of saliva and serum for human immunodeficiency virus type 1 antibody testing in Uganda using a rapid recombinant assay. *Clin Diagn Lab Immunol*, 1996;3:640–644.
23. Matee MI, Lyamuya EF, Simon E, et al. Detection of anti-HIV-1 IgG antibodies in whole saliva by GACELISA and western blot assays. *East Afr Med J*, 1996;73:292–294.
24. Brookmeyer R, Quinn TC. Estimation of current human immunodeficiency virus incidence rates from a cross-sectional survey using early diagnostic tests. *Am J Epidemiol*, 1995;141:166–172.
25. Beyrer C, Brookmeyer R, Natpratan C. Measuring HIV-1 incidence rates in Northern Thailand: prospective cohort results and estimates based on early diagnostic tests. *J Acquir Immune Defic Syndr Hum Retrovirol*, 1996;12:495–499.
26. Busch MP, Lee LLL, Satten DR, et al. Time course of detection of viral and serologic markers preceding human immunodeficiency virus type 1 seroconversion: implications for screening of blood and tissue donors. *Transfusion*, 1995;35:91–97.
27. Janssen RS, Satten GA, Stramer SL, et al. New testing strategy to detect early HIV-1 infection for use in incidence estimates and for clinical and prevention purposes. *JAMA*, 1998;280:42–48.
28. McIntosch K. Diagnostic virology. In: BN Fields, DM Knipe, PM Howley, eds. *Fields Virology*. Philadelphia: Lippincott-Raven, 1996;401–430.
29. McFarland W, Busch MP, Kellogg TA, et al. Detection of early HIV infection and estimation of incidence using a sensitive/less-sensitive enzyme immunoassay testing strategy at anonymous counseling and testing sites in San Francisco. *J Acquir Immune Defic Syndr Hum Retrovirol*, 1999;22: 484–489.
30. Diaz RS, Kallas EG, Castelo A, et al. Use of a less-sensitive enzyme immunoassay testing strategy to identify recently infected persons in a Brazilian prison: estimation of incidence and epidemiological tracing. *AIDS*, 1999;13:1417–1418.
31. Apetrei C, Lousset-Ajaka I, Descamps D, et al. Lack of screening test sensitivity during HIV-1 non-B subtype seroconversions. *AIDS*, 1996;10: F57–F60.
32. Barin F, M'Boup S, Denis F, et al. Serological evidence for virus related to simian T-lymphotic retrovirus III in residents of west-Africa. *Lancet*, 1985;II:1387–1389.
33. Clavel F, Guetard D, Brun-Vezinet F, et al. Isolation of a new human retrovirus from West African patients with AIDS. *Science*, 1986;233:343–346.
34. Kanki PJ, Barin F, M' Boup S, et al. New human T-lymphotropic retrovirus related to simian T-lymphotropic virus type III (STLV-III_{AGM}). *Science*, 1986;232:238–243.
35. Alizon M, Wain-Hobson S, Montagnier L, et al. Genetic variability of the AIDS virus: nucleotide sequence analysis of two isolates from African patients. *Cell*, 1986;46:63–74.
36. Benn S, Rutledge R, Folks T, et al. Genomic heterogeneity of AIDS retroviral isolates from North-America and Zaire. *Science*, 1985;230:949–951.
37. Charneau P, Borman AM, Quillent C, et al. Isolation and envelope sequence of a highly divergent HIV-1 isolate: definition of a new HIV-1 group. *Virology*, 1994;205:247–253.
38. De Leys R, Vanderborght B, Van den Haesevelde M, et al. Isolation and characterization of an unusual human immuodeficiency retrovirus from two persons of west-central African origin. *J Virol*, 1990;64:1207–1216.

39. Gurtler LG, Hauser PH, Eberle J, et al. A new subtype of human immunodeficiency virus type 1 (MVP–5180) from Cameroon. *J Virol*, 1994; 68:1581–1585.
40. Simon F, Mauclère P, Roques P, et al. Identification of a new human immunodeficiency virus type 1 distinct from group M and group O. *Nat Med*, 1998;4:1032–1037.
41. Myers G, Korber B, Wain-Hobson S, et al. Los Alamos, NM: a compilation and analysis of nucleic acid and amino acid sequences. Los Alamos National Laboratory, Los Alamos, NM, 1992.
42. Robertson DL, Anderson JP, Bradac JA, et al. HIV-1 nomenclature proposal. *Science*, 2000; 288:55–56.
43. Barin F, Mulanga-Kabeya C. Diagnostic tools for HIVs. In: M Essex, SM'Boup, PJ Kanki, MR Kalengayi, eds. *AIDS in Africa*. New York: Raven Press, 1994:109–131.
44. Mauclere P, Damond F, Apetrei C, et al. Synthetic peptide ELISAs for detection of and discrimination between group M and group O HIV-1 infection. *AIDS Res Hum Retroviruses*, 1997;13:987–993.
45. Peeters M, Gueye A, M'Boup S, et al. Geographical distribution of HIV-1 group O viruses in Africa. *AIDS*, 1997;11:493–498.
46. Carr JK, Laukkanen T, Salminen M, et al. Characterization of subtype A HIV-1 from Africa by full genome sequencing. *AIDS*, 1999;13:1819–1824.
47. Laukkanen T, Carr JK, Janssens W, et al. Virtually full-length subtype F and F/D recombinant HIV-1 from Africa and South America. *Virology*, 2000; 269:95–104.
48. Robertson DL, Sharp PM, McCutchan FE, et al. Recombination in HIV-1. *Nature*, 1995;374: 124–126.
49. Workshop report from the European Commission (DG XII, INCO-DC) and the joint United Nations program on HIV/AIDS. HIV-1 subtypes: implications for epidemiology, pathogenicity, vaccines and diagnostics. *AIDS*, 1997;11:UNAIDS17-UNAIDS36.
50. Baillou A, Janvier B, Leonard G, et al. Fine sero-typing of human immunodeficiency virus serotype 1 (HIV-1) and HIV-2 infections by using synthetic oligopeptides representing an immunodominant domain of HIV-1 and HIV-2/simian immunodeficiency virus. *J Clin Microbiol*, 1991;29: 1387–1391.
51. Gnann JW Jr, McCormick J, Mitchell S, et al. Synthetic peptide immunoassay distinguishes HIV type 1 and HIV type 2 infections. *Science*, 1987; 1346–1349.
52. Norrby E, Biberfeld G, Chiodi F, et al. Discrimination between antibodies to HIV and to related retroviruses using site-directed serology. *Nature*, 1987;339:248–250.
53. Baillou A, Brand D, Denis F, et al. High antigenic cross-reactivity of the V3 consensus sequences of HIV-1 gp120. *AIDS Res Hum Retroviruses*, 1994;9:1203–1209.
54. Turbica I, Simon F, Besnier JM, et al. Temporal development and prognostic value of the antibody response to the major neutralizing epitopes of gp120 during HIV-1 infection. *J Med Virol*, 1997;52:309–315.
55. Barin F, Lahbabi Y, Buzelay L, et al. Diversity of antibody binding to V3 peptides representing consensus sequences of HIV-1 genotypes A to E: an approach for HIV-1 serological subtyping. *AIDS Res Hum Retroviruses*, 1996;12:1279–1289.
56. Cheingsong-Popov R, Osmanov S, Pau CP, et al. Serotyping of HIV-1 infections: definition, classification, relationship to viral genetic subtypes and assay evaluation. *AIDS Res Hum Retroviruses*, 1998;14:311–318.
57. Sherefa K, Sönnenborg A, Steinbergs J, et al. Rapid grouping of HIV-1 infection in subtypes A to E by V3 peptide serotyping and its relation to sequence analysis. *Biochem Biophys Res Commun*, 1994; 205:1658–1664.
58. Hoelscher M, Hanker S, Barin F, et al. HIV-1 V3 serotyping in Tanzanian samples; probable reasons for mismatching with genetic subtyping. *AIDS Res Hum Retroviruses*, 1998;14:139–149.
59. Plantier JC, Damond F, Lasky M, et al. V3 serotyping of human immunodeficiency virus type 1 infection: correlation with genotyping, limitations and identification of signature sequences. *J Acquir Immune Defic Syndr*, 1999;20:432–441.
60. Candotti D, Tareau C, Barin F, et al. Genetic subtyping and V3 serotyping of HIV type 1 isolates in Congo. *AIDS Res Hum Retroviruses*, 1999;15: 309–314.
61. Barin F, Courouсé AM, Pillonel J, et al. Increasing diversity of HIV-1M serotypes in French blood donors over a 10-year period (1985–1995). *AIDS*, 1997;11:1503–1508.
62. Couturier E, Damond F, Roques P, et al. HIV-1 diversity in France, 1996–1998. *AIDS*, 2000;14: 289–296.
63. Subbarao S, Luo CC, Limpakarnjanarat K, et al. Evaluation of oligonucleotide probes for the determination of the two major HIV-l *env* subtypes in Thailand. *AIDS*, 1996;10:350–351.
64. Van Harmelen J, Wood R, Lambrick M, et al. An association beween HIV-1 subtypes and mode of transmission in Cape Town, South Africa. *AIDS*, 1997;11:81–87.
65. Bachmann MH, Delwar EL,, Shpaer EG, et al. Rapid genetic characterization of HIV type 1 strains from four World Health Organization sponsored vaccine evaluation sites using a heteroduplex mobility assay. WHO network for HIV isolation and characterization. *AIDS Res Hum Retroviruses*, 1994; 10:1345–1353.

66. Delwart E, Shpaer E, Louwagie J, et al. Genetic relationships determined by a DNA heteroduplex mobility assay: analysis of HIV-1 env genes. *Science*, 1993;262:1257–1261.
67. Delwart E, Herring B, Rodrigo AG, et al. Genetic subtyping of human immunodeficiency virus using a heteroduplex mobility assay. *PCR Methods Appl*, 1995;4:S202–S216.
68. Heyndrickx L, Janssens W, Zekeng L, et al. Simplified strategy for detection of recombinant human immunodeficiency virus type 1 group M isolates by gag/env heteroduplex mobility assay. *J Virol*, 2000;74:363–370.
69. Artenstein, AW, VanCott TC, Mascola JR, et al. Dual infection with human immunodeficiency virus type 1 of distinct envelope subtypes in humans. *J Infect Dis*, 1995;171:805–810.
70. McCutchan FE, Hegerich PA, Brennan TP, et al. Genetic variants of HIV-1 in Thailand. *AIDS Res Hum Retroviruses*, 1992;8:1887–1895.
71. Peeters M, Liegeois F, Bibollet-Ruche F, et al. Subtype-specific polymerase chain reaction for the identification of HIV-1 genetic subtypes circulating in Africa. *AIDS*, 1998;12:671–673.
72. McCutchan FE, Sanders-Buell E, Oster CW, et al. Genetic comparison of human immunodeficiency virus HIV-1 isolates by polymerase chain reaction. *J Acquir Immune Defic Syndr*, 1991;4:1241–1250.
73. Gaywee J, Artenstein AW, VanCott, TC, et al. Correlation of genetic and serologic approaches to HIV-1 subtyping in Thailand. *J Acquir Immune Defic Syndr*, 1996;13:392–396.
74. Porter KR, Mascola JR, Hupudio H, et al. Genetic, antigenic and serologic characterization of human immunodeficiency virus type 1 from Indonesia. *J Acquir Immune Defic Syndr*, 1997;14:1–6.
75. Luo CC, Downing, RG, Dela Torre N, et al. The development and evaluation of a probe hybridization method for subtyping HIV type 1 infection in Uganda. *AIDS Res Hum Retroviruses*, 1998;14:691–694.
76. Rayfield, MA, Downing RG, Baggs J, et al. A molecular epidemiologic survey of HIV in Uganda. *AIDS*, 1998;12:521–527.
77. Subbarao S, Limpakarnjanarat K, Mastro TD, et al. HIV type 1 in Thailand, 1994–1995: persistence of two subtypes with low genetic diversity. *AIDS Res Hum Retroviruses*, 1998;14:319–327.
78. Plantier JC, Vergne L, Damond F, et al. Feasibility of a molecular method using oligonucleotidic probe hybridization, for *env* genotyping of subtypes A through G of HIV-1 group M infection, with discrimination of the Circulating Recombinant Forms CRF01-AE and CRF02-AG. *J Clin Microbiol*, 2002;40:in press.
79. Kostrikis LG, Shin S, Ho DD, et al. Genotyping HIV-1 and HCV strains by a Combinatorial DNA Melting Assay (COMA). *Mol Med*, 1998; 4:443–453.
80. Robbins KE, Kostrikis LG, Brown TM, et al. Genetic analysis of human immunodeficiency virus type 1 strains in Kenya: a comparison using phylogenetic analysis and a combinatorial melting assay. *AIDS Res Hum Retroviruses*, 1999;15;329–335.
81. Janini LM, Pieniazek D, Peralta JM, et al. Identification of single and dual infections with distinct subtypes of human immunodeficiency virus type 1 by using restriction fragment length polymorphism analysis. *Virus Gene*, 1996;13: 69–81.
82. Pieniazek D, Janini LM, Ramos A, et al. HIV-1 patients may harbor viruses of different phylogenetic subtypes: implications for the evolution of the HIV/AIDS pandemic. *Emerg Infect Dis*, 1995; 1:86–88.
83. Ellenberger DL, Pieniazek D, Nkengasong, J, et al. Genetic analysis of human immunodeficiency virus in Abidjan, Ivory Coast reveals predominance of HIV type 1 subtype A and introduction of subtype G. *AIDS Res Hum Retroviruses*, 1999;15:3–9.
84. Nkengasong J, Luo CC, Abouya L, et al. Distribution of HIV type 1 subtypes among HIV-seropositive patients in the interior of Côte d'Ivoire. *J Acquir Immune Defic Syndr*, 2000;20; 430–436.
85. Pinto ME, Tanuri A, Schechter M. Molecular and epidemiologic evidence for the discontinuous introduction of subtypes B and F into Rio de Janeiro, Brazil. *J Acquir Immune Defic Syndr*, 1998;19: 310–312.
86. Flores I, Pieniazek D, Moran N, et al. HIV-1 subtype F in single and dual infections in Puerto-Rico: a potential sentinel site for monitoring novel genetic HIV variants in North America. *Emerg Infect Dis*, 1999;5:481–483.
87. Van Harmelen J, van der Ryst E, Wood R, et al. Restriction fragment length polymorphism analysis for rapid *gag* subtype determination of human immunodeficiency virus type 1 in South Africa. *J Virol Methods*, 1999;78:51–59.
88. Thompson JD, Higgins D, Gibson TJ. CLUSTAL W improving the sensitivity of progressive multiple sequence alignment through sequence weighting, position-specific gap penalties and weight matrix choice. *Nucleic Acids Res*, 1994;22:4673–4680.
89. Kimura, M. A simple method for estimating evolutionary rates of base substitutions through comparative studies of nucleotide sequences. *J Mol Evol*, 1980;16:111–120.
90. Saitou N, Nei M. The neighbor-joining method: a new method for reconstructing phylogenetic trees. *Mol Biol Evol*, 1987;4:406–425.
91. Felsenstein J. Confidence limits on phylogenies: an approach using the bootstrap. *Evolution*, 1985; 39:783–791.
92. Felsenstein J. *PHYLIP (Phylogeny Inference Package), Version 3.5c* [computer program]: Seattle,

WA: Department of Genetics, University of Washington; 1989.
93. Grassly NC, Holmes EC. A likelihood method for the detection of selection and recombination using nucleotide sequences. *Mol Biol Evol*, 1997; 14;239–247.
94. McGuire G, Wright F, Prentice MJ. A graphical method for detecting recombination in phylogenetic data sets. *Mol Biol Evol*, 1997;14:1125–1131.
95. Weiller GF. Phylogenetic profiles: a graphical method for detecting genetic recombinations in homologous sequences. *Mol Biol Evol*, 1998;15: 326–335
96. Gao F, Robertson DL, Carruthers CD, et al. A comprehensive panel of near-full-length clones and reference sequences for non-subtype B isolates of human immunodeficiency virus type 1. *J Virol*, 1998;7:5680–5698.
97. Lole K, Bollinger R, Paranjape R, et al. Full-length human immunodeficiency virus type 1 genomes from subtype C infected seroconverters in India, with evidence of intersubtype recombination. *J Virol*, 1999;73:142–160.
98. Siepel AC, Halpern AL, Macken C, et al. A computer program designed to screen rapidly for HIV type 1 intersubtype recombinant sequences. *AIDS Res Hum Retroviruses*, 1995;11:1413–1416.
99. Salminen MO, Carr J, Burke DS, et al. Identification of breakpoints in intergenotypic recombinants of HIV type 1 by bootscanning. *AIDS Res Hum Retroviruses*, 1995;11:1423–1425.

10

Monitoring Viral Load

Phyllis J. Kanki and Indu Mani

Department of Immunology and Infectious Diseases, Harvard School of Public Health, Boston, Massachusetts 02115, USA.

Human immunodeficiency virus (HIV) infection results in progressive loss of immune function marked by the depletion of CD4$^+$ T-lymphocytes, leading to the opportunistic infections and malignancies characteristic of acquired immune deficiency syndrome or AIDS. A number of host and viral factors influence the rate of disease progression. Studies conducted in developed countries prior to the implementation of antiretroviral therapy suggested a median time to AIDS ranging from 8 to 10 years.

Historically, CD4$^+$ T-lymphocyte counts provided the most reliable prognostic marker of HIV disease progression (1). Other prognostic markers have included immunologic markers of immune dysfunction such as cutaneous anergy (2,3), serum β_2 microglobulin, and neopterin levels (1). Quantitation of viral infection in the past was performed with imperfect and/or laborious methods. For example, the serologic quantitation of the viral core antigen p24 was frequently considered as a surrogate marker of high viral burdens (4,5). Quantitative viral culture was difficult to perform and not cost-effective for clinical monitoring on a regular basis (6,7). HIV viral expression measured by mRNA levels was also considered an important marker that preceded immunologic compromise (8,9). Qualitative characteristics of HIV infection that were often associated with viral burden included the syncytium-inducing properties of the virus; syncytium-inducing viruses were associated with high viral loads and rapid progression to disease, while nonsyncytium-inducing viruses were associated with lower viral loads and slower disease progression (10–12).

The development of sensitive PCR-based technology to reliably quantitate viral RNA levels, or viral load, in plasma has revolutionized our abilities to track HIV infection (13). Mellors and colleagues provided important new evidence that such measurements of plasma RNA levels were important predictors of disease progression (14,15). Based on data from large U.S. cohort studies of homosexual men, the risk of AIDS or AIDS-related death was significantly associated with baseline plasma viral loads, independent of $CD4^+$ T-lymphocyte counts (14,16). It is worth noting that these studies and many of the ensuing viral load studies were conducted in the United States and Europe, where infection with HIV-1 subtype B is predominant.

VIRAL LOAD AND THE NATURAL HISTORY OF HIV

Many studies that have followed the natural history of HIV infection have reported the utility of viral load determinations in tracking and predicting disease progression. A variety of other markers, most notably lymphocyte subset data, were frequently collected in many of these studies. Thus, the relationship of viral load with $CD4^+$ lymphocyte counts has also been frequently evaluated. It has been important to evaluate the predictive value of viral load measurements over the full course of HIV infection. This has required longitudinal analyses of data from large cohorts, where time of infection has been known and where observation times predated the use of antiretroviral therapy.

Data from the large U.S. Multicenter AIDS Cohort Study (MACS) have demonstrated a strong correlation between early viral load measurements and declines in $CD4^+$ T-lymphocyte counts (17). Both initial HIV RNA levels and slopes were associated with AIDS-free times. HIV RNA load measured at the first seropositive visit, and at 3 months after seroconversion, was highly predictive of AIDS; subsequent HIV RNA measurements showed even better prognostic discrimination. However, HIV RNA slopes in the 3 years preceding AIDS and HIV RNA levels at the time of AIDS diagnosis showed little variation according to total AIDS-free time (17). Because the MACS study population is largely a Caucasian, homosexual male cohort infected with HIV-1B, it may not be possible to generalize these findings to other population groups with different modes of transmission or different viral subtypes.

Sabin and colleagues' results from their study of large European hemophilia cohorts confirm the importance of HIV RNA levels in assessing the long-term prognosis of HIV-infected individuals (18). The risk of developing AIDS and death remained low when the HIV-1 RNA level was below 4 $\log_{10}$ copies/ml, but increased rapidly thereafter, supporting current guidelines for the initiation of antiretroviral therapy after the viral load has exceeded this level (19). In the French SEROCO study of HIV seroconverters ($n = 330$), patients who remained AIDS-free had lower early viral loads and, on average, a longer period of viral-load decline after infection (36 versus 18 months), followed by a slower viral load increase compared with those who progressed to AIDS (20). A true plateau-phase, lasting approximately 4 years after the seroconversion period, was observed only in patients who remained AIDS-free for at least 90 months. In multivariate analysis, both early viral load and later changes in load levels were significant predictors of progression to AIDS (20).

PRIMARY HIV INFECTION AND VIRAL SETPOINT

In recent years, through the study of primary HIV infection, we have learned that some degree of viral containment occurs during the very early phases of HIV infection in vivo. During this critical period, a complex dynamic of infecting virus and responding host and immune factors leads to the establishment of a "steady-state" level of viremia, or viral setpoint, that appears predictive of subsequent disease progression rates and survival (14,16). The period from initial infection to onset of symptoms is an average of 21.4 days (SD = 9.6 days, range: 10–55 days) and the self-limited illness usually resolves within 1–3 weeks. Current data suggests that HIV viral load in the blood reaches a peak in the first 15–30 days after infection, concurrent with a precipitous drop in $CD4^+$ T-cell count and an increase in absolute number of $CD8^+$ T-lymphocytes (21–23). Subsequent to this early acute response and associated with its resolution is the decline of viral load and the rebound of $CD4^+$ T-lymphocyte levels. Corey and colleagues have reported considerable variability in viral burdens during these early phases of HIV infection, 120 days after acquisition, plasma HIV RNAs rapidly decrease to an inflection point, after which they gradually increase (24). The early infection phase continues over the next 6–12 months, with seeding and establishment of viral load in blood and lymphoreticular tissues (25–27). The viral setpoint is established during this phase of infection and remains relatively invariant throughout much of the long incubation period that follows.

It is now well established that the level of HIV-1 plasma RNA early in infection is highly predictive of future clinical course (14,16,28). Cross-sectional studies have demonstrated that long-term nonprogressors have significantly lower cell and plasma viral burdens than do rapid progressors (29–31). Increases in plasma RNA load are correlated with increases in proviral burden, quantitative virus isolation, and quantity of virus in lymphoreticular tissue (26). The stability of virion-associated HIV-1 RNA levels suggests that an equilibrium between HIV-1 replication rate and the efficacy of immunologic response is established shortly after infection and persists throughout the asymptomatic period. Thus, host immunologic control of HIV-1 infection may be as important as viral replication rate in determining AIDS-free survival.

HIV THERAPY AND VIRAL LOAD

Treatment of HIV-1 infection with highly active antiretroviral therapy (HAART) has been shown to drastically lower plasma RNA load, a measurement now used as an indicator of the effectiveness of treatment (32,33). After discontinuing HAART, HIV-infected individuals have rebounds in their viral burdens approximating pre-HAART levels, even after a significant time on treatment (approximately 5 years) (34). In addition, viral load at baseline is predictive of the rate at which HIV-1 RNA levels decline during antiretroviral therapy (35). Multiple studies have shown that the current repertoire of antiretroviral drugs is insufficient to completely eradicate HIV-1 from infected individuals (36–38).

In the era of HIV treatment, the use of sequential HIV RNA measurements may be more meaningful than any single measurement. Putter et al. reported that pretreatment slopes of HIV-1 RNA decline in acutely infected individuals was significantly more dramatic ($p = 0.0001$) after initiation of antiretroviral therapy. However, post-treatment slopes were lower than those found in chronically infected individuals ($p = 0.012$). Slopes were inversely correlated ($p = 0.012$) with baseline HIV-1 RNA (39).

The multiple, adverse side-effects associated with HAART and the stringent demands of regimen adherence have prompted the design of new treatment strategies. Several studies have examined the longitudinal effects of multiple, scheduled treatment interruptions—the long term safety of which is largely unknown, particularly with respect to the development of resistant viruses. However, such a treatment strategy would likely improve long-term adherence. Individual viral load plateaus will serve as an important guide in selecting the aggressiveness and timing of such treatment interruptions (34).

VIRAL LOAD BY GENDER, RACE, AGE, AND MODE OF TRANSMISSION

A number of studies have demonstrated that viral loads may vary by gender, race, age, and perhaps mode of HIV transmission. In an Italian study of known seroconverters, the median viral load for women was roughly half that for men ($p = 0.002$). The association between viral load and gender remained significant after fitting a two-way analysis of variance ($p = 0.03$) and after adjusting for $CD4^+$ count, mode of HIV transmission, and age at enrollment in a regression model. Viral load was 0.27 $\log_{10}$ copies/ml lower in women (95% CI, 0.05–0.40; $p = 0.01$), that is, 50% lower in the raw scale (40). Similarly, Sterling et al. reported lower median plasma viral load in women, with viral load increasing more rapidly over time in women than in men (41). It is possible that women should be given highly aggressive antiretroviral therapy at lower HIV-RNA levels than those used to indicate therapy for men.

Data from the MACS study and the Women's Interagency HIV study (WIHS) showed that HIV RNA levels were 41% lower in individuals of color compared to whites and 21% lower in persons reporting a history of intravenous drug use compared to those reporting other HIV risk factors (42). In that study, 1,256 women and 1,603 men were studied at multiple time points, where viral loads in women were 32% to 50% lower than those in men after adjusting for baseline $CD4^+$ cell count, age and clinical symptoms (42).

Despite the clinical and prognostic utility of measuring the plasma viral loads of HIV-infected adults, viral loads remain relatively high and fluctuate over time in both symptomatic and long-term asymptomatic children (43). This makes viral load determinations less useful in children than in adults for predicting disease progression and for making therapeutic decisions (44). In a study of 106 perinatally infected infants, Shearer and coworkers confirmed high levels of HIV RNA that were slow to decline during the first two years of life. Infants with high peak HIV-1 RNA loads during their first two months of life were associated with more rapid disease progression than infants with lower peak loads (45,46). These findings suggest that early treatment with antiretroviral agents may be indicated for these infants.

HIV TYPES AND SUBTYPES AND VIRAL LOAD

Kanki et al. have developed an internally controlled quantitative reverse transcriptase polymerase chain reaction (RT PCR) to measure HIV-2 plasma RNA levels (47,48). The assay has a lower detection limit of 100 copies/ml, and is linear over 4 logs. We found that HIV-2 viral RNA was detectable in 56% of all samples tested from a cohort of registered commercial sex workers in Dakar, Senegal; the median load was 141 copies/ml. Levels of viral RNA in plasma were inversely related to $CD4^+$ cell counts. HIV-2 and HIV-1

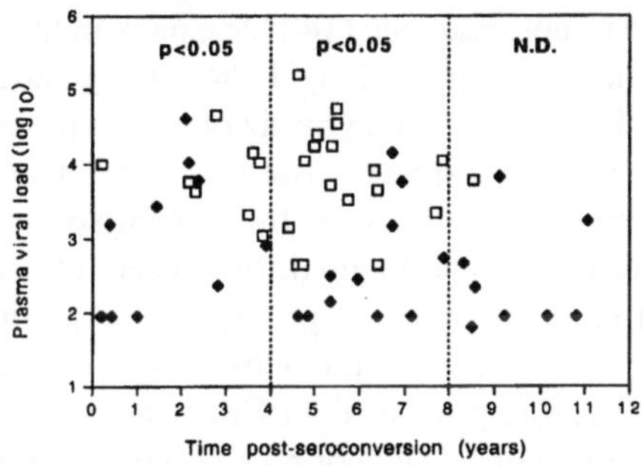

FIGURE 1. Time since seroconversion versus plasma viral load. HIV-1-infected subjects are represented by open squares (□); HIV-2 infected subjects by filled diamonds (♦). The *p* values correspond to the probability that HIV-1 and HIV-2 viral loads differ within the time interval defined by the dotted lines. N.D. indicates no statistical comparison was done (47).

viral loads were compared among the seroincident women in the cohort (Figure 1). The median viral load was 30 times lower in the HIV-2–infected women ($p < 0.001$, Wilcoxon rank sum test), irrespective of the length of time infected. We did not observe any association between length of time infected and either HIV-1 or HIV-2 viral load ($p > 0.05$, Spearman rank correlation) (47,48). The apparent stability of HIV-2 viral load, even many years after infection, is consistent with observations of lack of disease progression among HIV-2–infected individuals (49). Such comparative studies of HIV-1 and HIV-2 viral loads suggest that differences in plasma viremia are linked to the differences in the pathogenicity of the two viruses (47,48).

Few studies have rigorously evaluated viral load in individuals infected with non-B subtypes of HIV-1 in Africa. This has been partially due to the nature of commercial assays, which are expensive, have particular sample handling and storage requirements, and are time consuming. Furthermore, during the early development of commercial viral load assays, there were significant problems with reliable detection of the genetically divergent subtypes (as discussed later), which exist in Africa (50). The continuing identification of distinct and varied recombinant viruses in certain populations still begs the question of whether current assays will be capable of reliably measuring viral load in the future in settings with potentially new and divergent viruses.

METHODS FOR VIRAL LOAD QUANTITATION

Many factors can affect a viral load assay and its performance, including the following: the genotype of the target viral gene or virus, the sample compartment [plasma, semen, breast milk, cerebrospinal fluid (CSF), cervicovaginal fluid, or saliva], and the assay methodology. Since the assays are based on nucleic acid detection, and HIV viruses demonstrate significant genetic variability, consideration of the HIV subtypes to be evaluated is of critical importance. In Africa, where multiple HIV-1 subtypes are endemic, the selection of the appropriate RNA load assay is critical. It is also crucial to ensure appropriate sampling conditions and plasma storage for highly sensitive assays.

The three types of commercial assays currently in widespread use include the RT PCR assays, Amplicor Monitor versions 1.0 and 1.5 (Roche Diagnostic Systems, Branchburg, New Jersey); the branched DNA or bDNA assays, Quantiplex versions 2.0 and 3.0 (Bayer Diagnostics, Tarrytown, New York); and the nucleic acid sequence-based amplification assays, NASBA HIV-1 QT and NucliSens HIV-1 QT (Organon Teknika, Durham, North Carolina). Currently, these assays are for research use only, with the exception of the U.S. FDA-approved Amplicor Monitor 1.0.

These commercial assays apply two main technologies: signal amplification, in which a target nucleic acid is quantified in a sandwich hybridization assay and subsequently has its signal amplified through sequential steps; and target amplification, in which the target nucleic acid is amplified enzymatically and quantified.

The Quantiplex bDNA assay utilizes signal amplification through sequential hybridization of multiple probes to the *pol* of HIV-1. The probes are derived from nucleotide analyses of HIV-1 subtypes A, B and D. The virus is pelleted and lysed to release its RNA, and captured on a microtiter plate by hybridizing to 10 oligonucleotide target and capture probes which are chemically linked to the plate. Multiple bDNA amplifier molecules and 35 additional alkaline phosphatase (ALP)-labeled probes hybridize with the viral RNA such that each HIV-1 RNA molecule may display several thousand "branches," or ALP-conjugated probes. Finally, dioxetane is added, and the chemiluminescent signal is detected and quantitated by interpolation from a standard curve of single-strand DNA phage containing the HIV-1 *pol* sequence. In this assay, the HIV-1 RNA is quantified directly; amplification ensues by multiplication of the signal, not of the target RNA itself. The newest generation of the bDNA assay is the Quantiplex version 3.0, which requires a specimen volume of 1 ml of EDTA-preserved plasma. It yields a lower limit of detection of 50 copies/ml and a dynamic range of 50–500,000 copies/ml. The version 2.0 assay had a lower limit of detection of 500 copies/ml, a dynamic range of 500–800,000 copies/ml and required a larger specimen volume of 2 ml. The increased sensitivity of the newer version was attained by increasing the number of capture and target probe binding sites and by including non-natural oligonucleotides in the target probe binding regions, thereby reducing cross-hybridization of probes with non–HIV-1 genetic material and "background noise" (51,52).

In Roche's Amplicor Monitor assay, HIV-1 RNA is extracted from plasma by a salt guanidinium thiocyanate protocol, precipitated, and solubilized. RT PCR is then performed using the RT activity of recombinant *Thermus thermolyticus* DNA polymerase and two HIV-1 *gag* primers. After the reverse transcription of the RNA to cDNA, the target sequence (142 base pairs in the *gag* gene) is amplified by PCR and quantified and calculated by hybridization to a probe in a microwell-plate using a biotin-avidin enzyme immunoassay by comparison to an internal standard signal. In a recent ultrasensitive variation to the protocol, viral particles were first concentrated by high-speed centrifugation prior to RT PCR, with a resultant lower limit of detection of 50 copies/ml and a dynamic range of 50–75,000 copies/ml (51,52). The standard Amplicor Monitor 1.0 and 1.5 assays require a specimen volume of 200 μl of EDTA-preserved plasma, have a lower limit of detection of 400 copies/ml, and a dynamic range of 400–750,000 copies/ml. The version 1.5 utilizes a new *gag* primer set designed for use with non-B subtypes, improving on the version 1.0 which did not quantify all non-B subtypes equally well (53,54).

The NucliSens HIV-1 QT assay (NASBA) is also a target amplification protocol with isothermal amplification of RNA and quantification in comparison to three internal standard RNA calibrators. RNA is extracted from plasma using the salt guanidinium thiocyanate protocol, purified by adherence to acidified silica, and amplified with RT, RnaseH, T7 polymerase, and two HIV-1 *gag* primers. This results in numerous RNA target sequence copies, and the original target is indirectly measured by quantifying amplified product. The calibrators, which are very similar to the target RNA, act as controls for extraction and amplification errors and are included with the target in a chemiluminescent detection assay. The second generation NucliSens HIV-1 QT assay has a lower limit of detection of 40 copies/ml given a specimen volume of 2 ml, and a lower limit of detection of 1,600 copies/ml given a specimen volume of 50 μl. The dynamic range is 40–10,000,000 copies/ml. Both the sensitivity and dynamic range have been improved from the original NASBA HIV-1 QT assay. The specimen can be drawn using EDTA, heparin, or whole blood. According to the manufacturer, sample preservative and use of anticoagulants do not compromise the quality of results.

ASSAY PERFORMANCE ISSUES AND SUBTYPE PROBLEMS

Important characteristics with respect to assay performance include assay linearity, precision, accuracy, sensitivity, specificity, and problems with subtype variation. Linearity is the degree to which the given assay results are proportional to the concentration of virus in the sample. Accuracy is the degree that an assay measures in accordance with an accepted "gold standard," and is very difficult to characterize with the multiple assays in use today. Precision, or reproducibility, is the measure of agreement of repeat assays on the same sample. The bDNA assay appears less affected by the presence of heterogenous biologic molecules in plasma samples (55,56) (Table 1). Quantiplex versions 2.0 and 3.0 have yielded results with excellent reproducibility and a broad linear range (57–63). Sensitivity, or the lower limit of detection, is the lowest limit of virus that the assay can detect but not necessarily quantify with accuracy or precision. Initially, the NASBA HIV-1 QT assay was the methodology with superior sensitivity (64–67) and a second generation, NucliSens HIV-1 QT, has displayed even greater sensitivity (68). Currently, newer generations of both the Roche Amplicor and Bayer Quantiplex assays exhibit enhanced sensitivity compared with their earlier versions. The Quantiplex 3.0 has ten times greater sensitivity than its former version (51,69,70), as does the Amplicor 1.5. Quantiplex 2.0 appears to underquantify by 2- to 3-fold compared with Quantiplex 3.0 or Amplicor 1.5 (51,52) and it has a lower sensitivity (66,70), displaying greater differences at lower viral loads and smaller differences at higher viral loads (50,71,72).

The Quantiplex 3.0 and Amplicor 1.5 ultrasensitive results are highly correlated in multiple studies (51,52,73), although a few studies have found that Amplicor 1.5 quantified at consistently higher levels than Quantiplex 3.0 (63,74).

The bDNA assay has been the historical "gold standard" within the scientific community with respect to the effects of subtype genetic variation on viral load quantification. This assay's use of multiple probes is designed to detect and quantify multiple

TABLE 1. Comparison of Viral RNA Quantitative Assays

	NASBA	RT PCR	Branched DNA
Commercial assay	Nuclisens HIV-1 QT (Organon Technika)	Amplicor Monitor versions 1.0 and 1.5 (Roche)	Quantiplex versions 2.0 and 3.0 (Bayer)
Method of amplification	Target Amplification	Target Amplification	Signal Amplification
Sample volume required	50 µl to 2 ml	*Standard*: 200 µl *Ultrasensitive*: 500 µl	1 ml
Lower limit of detection	40 copies/ml to 1600 copies/ml	*Standard*: 400 copies/ml *Ultrasensitive*: 50 copies/ml	50 copies/ml
HIV-1 subtype problems (refs.)	Detects subtypes A–F Problems: G (81) and A (63,82)	*Version 1.0*: Problems with A, E, G and H (50,53,75,78,82,84) *Version 1.5*: Detects and quantifies all HIV-1 group M subtypes (54)	Detects and quantifies all HIV-1 group M subtypes (50,53,65,75–77)

subtypes (53,65). Signal amplification technology has led to its consistent detection of multiple subtypes (50,53,65,75–77). The initial design and validation of the Amplicor and NucliSens assays were carried out using subtype B samples (72,78), unlike the bDNA assays (65). The NASBA HIV-1 QT assay is not optimal for the detection of multiple subtypes, and has had difficulty detecting and quantifying non-B subtypes, particularly subtype G (50,53,72,75,76,78–80). The newer NucliSens HIV-1 QT appears to detect subtypes A through F, but not subtype G (81), and may still underestimate subtype A samples (63,82). However, another NASBA assay in development that uses long terminal repeat (LTR) primers appears to equally detect and quantify the major HIV-1 group M subtypes (83). The Amplicor 1.0 has also had difficulty in consistent quantification of multiple subtypes, although the Amplicor 1.5, with redesigned primers, is much improved and has demonstrated high sensitivity in the detection of multiple subtypes (50,53,54,71, 75–79,82,84). Few comparative studies have suggested that Amplicor 1.5 may overestimate subtypes A and E viral loads in certain African samples as compared with Quantiplex 3.0 (63,74,85).

In selecting the optimal viral load assay for use in regions with multiple non-B subtypes, one must consider genotypic shifts in virus populations, high inter- and intra-subtype variation, selective pressure on circulating viruses, and emerging viral diversification. It is therefore important to select a viral load assay that will accommodate "emerging diversity." The bDNA assay appears to be the most reliable for the detection of all subtypes; most likely due to its use of multiple probes which can more readily accommodate target sequence variation. In target amplification methods, primer mismatches and poor hybridization with a single probe may lead to poor detection of multiple diverse subtypes, requiring the need for continual "re-design" of primers in the face of diversifying virus populations. Furthermore, cost analysis based on labor, disposable materials, kit costs, and disposal and generation of biohazardous waste has shown the Quantiplex 3.0 assay to bring more significant savings than the Amplicor 1.5 or the NucliSens HIV-1 QT (52,63). At this writing, the bDNA assay still appears to be superior for viral load measurement in regions with multiple non-B subtypes, such as Africa.

HIV VIRAL LOADS IN NONBLOOD SPECIMENS

Few studies have evaluated the comparative efficacy of commercial viral load assays for detecting and quantifying virus in samples such as semen, seminal plasma, cervicovaginal fluid, saliva, breast milk, and cerebrospinal fluid (CSF). Quantification of viral load in these compartments could provide useful information about HIV-1 transmission and disease pathogenesis.

Of the three commercial assays, the NucliSens HIV-1 QT is advertised for use in a variety of tissue and fluid compartments. The types of assays commonly used for HIV-1 RNA quantification in nonblood specimens are RT PCRs, by both the commercial assay (Amplicor Monitor) or individually-designed noncommercial assays; and nucleic acid sequence-based amplification assays (NASBA HIV-1 QT and NucliSens HIV-1 QT). Studies comparing the utility of Amplicor Monitor, NASBA, and NucliSens have been performed in subtype B semen, seminal plasma, and cervicovaginal fluid samples. Viral RNA has been detected by all methods (86–88). The results were fairly concordant between NASBA and Amplicor Monitor assays in the quantification of HIV-1 RNA in semen and seminal plasma (86,87) and in female genital tract samples (88). However, the Amplicor Monitor RT PCR was prone to PCR inhibition, which could be eliminated by pretreatment with silica (87,89,90). Another study evaluated NASBA HIV-1 QT, NucliSens

HIV-1 QT, and Amplicor Monitor 1.0 for detection of HIV-1 viral RNA in saliva, CSF, breast milk, seminal plasma and cervicovaginal lavage (CVL) fluid (90). They concluded that Amplicor Monitor 1.0 had greater sensitivity in CSF and CVL, but was limited in the other fluids due to PCR inhibition. They also concluded that the NASBA HIV-1 QT and NucliSens HIV-1 QT were similar in their ability to detect HIV-1 RNA from all fluids without apparent inhibition, although at lower sensitivity in CSF and CVL. RT PCR (Amplicor Monitor 1.0) has also been used to quantitate non-B subtype HIV-1 RNA in cervicovaginal samples with a detection rate of 64% (91) and in cell-free breast milk specimens with a detection rate of 39%–63% (92,93). Further, multiple studies have quantified HIV-1 viral RNA by NASBA and RT PCR in CSF specimens with varying rates of detection (94–97). However, more detailed comparative studies must be performed to determine the optimal viral load assays for different compartments. This will provide a much greater understanding of transmission prevention as well as disease pathogenesis.

CONCLUSION

The ability to measure HIV-1 viral load has revolutionized our ability to track HIV infection and viral replication. The advent of viral load assays has been both a technologic and pragmatic feat, supplying a sturdy clinical measure to guide clinical AIDS management. Formerly, clinicians and scientists relied on difficult and cumbersome plasma and peripheral blood mononuclear cell cultures for virus isolation, or p24 antigen quantitation to monitor infection in the individual patient. The development of PCR-based methods to measure viral RNA levels has been particularly useful in following patients and managing therapy. Importantly, the measurement of viral load has provided new insights into the mechanisms of HIV transmission and pathogenesis.

REFERENCES

1. Fahey JL, Taylor JM, Detels R, et al. The prognostic value of cellular and serologic markers in infection with human immunodeficiency virus type 1. *N Engl J Med.* 1990;322:166–172.
2. Redfield R, Wright D, Tramont E. The Walter Reed staging classification for HTLV-III/LAV infection. *N Engl J Med.* 1986;314:131–132.
3. Blatt S, Hendrix C, Butzin C, et al. Delayed-type hypersensitivity skin testing predicts progression to AIDS in HIV-infected patients. *Ann Intern Med.* 1993;119:177–184.
4. Allain J, Laurian Y, Paul D, et al. Long-term evaluation of HIV antigen and antibodies to p24 and gp41 in patients with hemophilia: Potential clinical importance. *N Engl J Med.* 1987;317:1114–1121.
5. Dewolf F, Spijkerman I, Schellekens PT, et al. Aids prognosis based on HIV-1 RNA, CD4+ T-cell count and function-markers with reciprocal predictive value over time after seroconversion. *AIDS.* 1997;11(15):1799–1806.
6. Coombs RW, Collier AC, Allain J, et al. Plasma viremia in human immunodeficiency virus infection. *N Engl J Med.* 1989;321:1621–1631.
7. Ho DD, Moudgil T, Alam M. Quantitation of human immunodeficiency virus in the blood of infected persons. *N Engl J Med.* 1989;321:1621–1625.
8. Gupta P, Kingsley L, Armstrong J, et al. Enhanced expression of human immunodeficiency type 1 correlates with development of AIDS. *Virology.* 1993;196:586–595.
9. Saksela K, Steven C, Ribinstein P, et al. Human immunodeficiency virus type 1 mRNA expression in peripheral blood cells predicts disease progression independently of the numbers of CD4+ lymphocytes. *Proc Natl Acad Sci USA.* 1994;91:1104–1108.
10. Fenyo E, Albert J, Asjo B. Replicative capacity, cytopathic effect and cell tropism of HIV. *AIDS.* 1989;3(suppl 1):S5–S12.
11. Tersmette M, De Goede R, Al B, et al. Differential syncytium-inducing capacity of human immunodeficiency virus isolates: frequent detection of syncytium-inducing isolates in patients with acquired immunodeficiency syndrome (AIDS) and AIDS-related complex. *J Virol.* 1988;62:2026–2032.
12. Koot M, Keet, I, Vos A, et al. Prognostic value of HIV-1 syncytium-inducing phenotype for rate of CD4+ cell depletion and progression to AIDS. *Ann Intern Med.* 1993;118:681–688.
13. Pachl C, Todd JA, Kern DG, et al. Rapid and precise quantification of HIV-1 RNA in plasma using a branched DNA signal amplification assay. *J Acquir Immune Defic Syndr.* 1995;8(5):446–454.

14. Mellors J, Kingsley L, Rinaldo C, et al. Quantitation of HIV-1 RNA in plasma predicts outcome after seroconversion. *Ann Intern Med.* 1995;122:573–579.
15. Vergis EN, Mellors JW. Natural history of HIV-1 infection. *Infect Dis Clin North Am.* 2000; 14(4):809-+.
16. Mellors JW, Rinaldo CR, Gupta P, et al. Prognosis in HIV-1 Infection Predicted by the Quantity of Virus in Plasma. *Science.* 1996;272:1167–1170.
17. Lyles RH, Munoz A, Yamashita TE, et al. Natural history of human immunodeficiency virus type 1 viremia after seroconversion and proximal to AIDS in a large cohort of homosexual men. *J Infect Dis.* 2000;181(3):872–880.
18. Sabin CA, Devereux H, Phillips AN, et al. Immune markers and viral load after HIV-1 seroconversion as predictors of disease progression in a cohort of haemophilic men. *AIDS.* 1998;12(11):1347–1352.
19. Sabin CA, Devereux H, Phillips AN, et al. Course of viral load throughout HIV-1 infection. *J Acquir Immune Defic Syndr.* 2000;23(2):172–177.
20. Hubert JB, Burgard M, Dussaix E, et al. Natural history of serum HIV-1 RNA levels in 330 patients with a known date of infection. *AIDS.* 2000; 14(2):123–131.
21. Clark DR, Wolthers KC. T-cell dynamics and renewal in HIV-1 infection. In: Schuitemaker H and Miedema F, eds. *AIDS Pathogenesis.* Dordrecht: Kluwer Academic, 2000;28:55–64.
22. Clark S, Saag M, Decker W, et al. High titers of cytopathic virus in plasma of patients with symptomatic primary HIV-1 infection. *N Engl J Med.* 1991;324:954–960.
23. Clark SJ, Shaw GM. The Acute Retroviral Syndrome and the Pathogenesis of HIV-1 Infection. *Immunology.* 1993;5:149–155.
24. Schacker TW, Hughes JP, Shea T, et al. Biological and virologic characteristics of primary HIV infection. *Ann Intern Med.* 1998;128(8).
25. Fauci AS. Host factors and the pathogenesis of HIV-induced disease. *Nature.* 1996;384(6609):529–534.
26. Haynes BF, Pantaleo G, Fauci AS. Toward an understanding of the correlates of protective immunity to HIV infection [see comments]. *Science.* 1996; 271(5247):324–328.
27. Fauci AS. Immunopathogenesis of HIV Infection. *J Acquir Immune Defic Syndr.* 1993;6:655–662.
28. Stein D, Lyles R, Graham N, et al. Predicting Clinical Progression or Death in Subjects with Early-Stage Human Immunodeficiency Virus (HIV) Infection – a Comparative Analysis of Quantification of HIV RNA, Soluble Tumor Necrosis Factor Type I Receptors, Neopterin, and Beta(2)-Microglobulin. *J Infect Dis.* 1997;176(5): 1161–1167.
29. Cao Y, Qin L, Zhang L, et al. Virologic and immunologic characterization of long-term survivors of human immunodeficiency virus type 1 infection [see comments]. *N Engl J Med.* 1995;332(4):201–208.
30. Rinaldo C, Huang X-L, Fan Z, et al. High Levels of Anti-Human Immunodeficiency Virus Type 1 (HIV-1) Memory Cytotoxic T-Lymphocyte Activity and Low Viral Load are Associated with Lack of Disease in HIV-1-Infected Long-Term Nonprogressors. *J Virol.* 1995;69(9):5838–5842.
31. Pantaleo G, Menzo S, Vaccarezza M, et al. Studies in subjects with long-term nonprogressive human immunodeficiency virus infection [see comments]. *N Engl J Med.* 1995;332(4):209–216.
32. Saag MS, Holodniy M, Kuritzkes DR, et al. HIV viral load markers in clinical practice. *Nat Med.* 1996;2(6):625–629.
33. Obrien TR, Rosenberg PS, Yellin F, et al. Longitudinal HIV-1 RNA levels in a cohort of homosexual men. *J Acquir Immune Defic Syndr.* 1998; 18(2):155–161.
34. Hatano H, Vogel S, Yoder C, et al. Pre-HAART HIV burden approximates post-HAART viral levels following interruption of therapy in patients with sustained viral suppression. *AIDS.* 2000;14(10): 1357–1363.
35. Notermans DW, Goudsmit J, Danner SA, et al. Rate of HIV-1 decline following antiretroviral therapy is related to viral load at baseline and drug regimen. *AIDS.* 1998;12(12):1483–1490.
36. Wong JK, Ignacio CC, Torriani F, et al. In vivo compartmentalization of human immunodeficiency virus: evidence from the examination of pol sequences from autopsy tissues. *J Virol.* 1997; 71:2059–2071.
37. Finzi D, Hermankova M, Pierson T, et al. Identification of a reservoir for HIV-1 in patients on highly active antiretroviral therapy. *Science.* 1997; 278(5341):1295–1300.
38. Dornadula G, Zhang H, VanUitert B, et al. Residual HIV-1 RNA in blood plasma of patients taking suppressive highly active antiretroviral therapy. *JAMA.* 1999;282(17):1627–1632.
39. Putter H, Prins JM, Jurriaans S, et al. Slower decline of plasma HIV-1 RNA following highly suppressive antiretroviral therapy in primary compared with chronic infection. *AIDS.* 2000; 14(18):2831–2839.
40. Rezza G, Lepri AC, Monforte AD, et al. Plasma viral load concentrations in women and men from different exposure categories and with known duration of HIV infection. *J Acquir Immune Defic Syndr.* 2000;25(1):56–62.
41. Sterling TR, Lyles CM, Vlahov D, et al. Sex differences in longitudinal human immunodeficiency virus type 1 RNA levels among seroconverters. *J Infect Dis.* 1999;180(3):666–672.
42. Anastos K, Gange SJ, Lau B, et al. Association of race and gender with HIV-1 RNA levels and

immunologic progression. *J Acquir Immune Defic Syndr*. 2000;24(3):218–226.

43. Mofenson LM, Korelitz J, Meyer WA, et al. The relationship between serum human immunodeficiency virus type 1 (HIV-1) RNA level, CD4 lymphocyte percent, and long-term mortality risk in HIV-1-infected children. *J Infect Dis*. 1997; 175(5):1029–1038.
44. Naver L, Ehrnst A, Belfrage E, et al. Long-term pattern of HIV-1 RNA load in perinatally infected children. *Scand J Infect Dis*. 1999;31(4):337–343.
45. Shearer WT, Quinn TC, Larussa P, et al. Viral load and disease progression in infants infected with human immunodeficiency virus type 1. *N Engl J Med*. 1997;336(19):1337–1342.
46. Dickover RE, Dillon M, Leung KM, et al. Early prognostic indicators in primary perinatal human immunodeficiency virus type 1 infection: Importance of viral RNA and the timing of transmission on long-term outcome. *J Infect Dis*. 1998; 178(2):375–387.
47. Popper SJ, Dieng-Sarr A, Travers KU, et al. Lower HIV-2 viral load reflects the difference in pathogenicity of HIV-1 and HIV-2. *J Infect Dis*. 1999;180:1116–1121.
48. Popper SJ, Dieng-Sarr A, Guèye-NDiaye A, et al. Low Plasma HIV-2 viral load is independent of proviral load: low virus production in vivo. *J Virol*. 2000;74(3):1554–1557.
49. Berry N, Ariyoshi D, Jaffar S, et al. Low peripheral blood viral HIV-2 RNA in individuals with high CD4 percentage differentiates HIV-2 from HIV-1 infection. *J Hum Virol*. 1998;1:457–468.
50. Coste J, Montes B, Reynes J, et al. Comparative Evaluation of Three Assays for the Quantitation of Human Immunodeficiency Virus Type 1 RNA in Plasma. *J Med Virol*. 1996;50:293–302.
51. Anastassopoulou CG, Touloumi G, Katsoulidou A, et al. Comparative evaluation of the quantiplex HIV-1 RNA 2.0 and 3.0 (bDNA) assays and the amplicor HIV-1 monitor v1.5 test for the quantitation of human immunodeficiency virus type 1 RNA in plasma. *J Virol Methods*. 2001;91(1):67–74.
52. Elbeik T, Charlebois E, Nassos P, et al. Quantitative and cost comparison of ultrasensitive human immunodeficiency virus type 1 RNA viral load assays: Bayer bDNA Quantiplex versions 3.0 and 2.0 and Roche PCR Amplicor Monitor version 1.5. *J Clin Microbiol*. 2000;38(3):1113–1120.
53. Parekh B, Phillips S, Granade TC, et al. Impact of HIV type 1 subtype variation on viral RNA quantitation. *AIDS Res Hum Retroviruses*. 1999; 15(2):133–142.
54. Michael NL, Herman SA, Kwok S, et al. Development of calibrated viral load standards for group M subtypes of human immunodeficiency virus type 1 and performance of an improved amplicor HIV-1 monitor test with isolates of diverse subtypes. *J Clin Microbiol*. 1999;37(8): 2557–2563.
55. Todd J, Pachl C, White R, et al. Performance characteristics for the quantitation of plasma HIV-1 RNA using branched DNA signal amplification technology. *J Acquir Immune Defic Syndr*. 1995; 10(Suppl 2):44.
56. Alonso R, de Viedma DG, Rodriguez-Creixems M, et al. Effect of potentially interfering substances on the measurement of HIV-1 viral load by the bDNA assay. *J Virol Methods*. 1999;78(1–2):149–152.
57. Yeghiazarian T, Zhao WQ, Read SE, et al. Quantification of human immunodeficiency virus type 1 RNA levels in plasma by using small-volume-format branched-DNA assays. *J Clin Microbiol*. 1998;36(7):2096–2098.
58. Erice A, Brambilla D, Bremer J, et al. Performance characteristics of the quantiplex HIV-1 RNA 3.0 assay for detection and quantitation of human immunodeficiency virus type 1 RNA in plasma. *J Clin Microbiol*. 2000;38(8):2837–2845.
59. Murphy DG, Gonin P, Fauvel M. Reproducibility and performance of the second-generation branched-DNA assay in routine quantification of human immunodeficiency virus type 1 RNA in plasma. *J Clin Microbiol*. 1999;37(3):812–814.
60. Skidmore SJ, Zuckerman M, Parry JV. Accuracy of plasma HIV RNA quantification: A multicentre study of variability. *J Med Virol*. 2000;61(4): 417–422.
61. Gale H. Evaluation of the Quantiplex human immunodeficiency virus type 1 RNA 3.0 Assay in a tertiary-care center. *Clin Diagn Lab Immunol*. 2000;7(1):122–124.
62. Schuurman R, Descamps D, Weverling GJ, et al. Multicenter Comparison of Three Commercial Methods for Quantification of Human Immunodeficiency Virus Type 1 RNA in Plasma. *J Clin Microbiol*. 1996;34(12):3016–3022.
63. Murphy DG, Cote L, Fauvel M, et al. Multicenter Comparison of Roche COBAS amplicor monitor Version 1.5, Organon Teknika NucliSens QT with Extractor, and Bayer Quantiplex Version 3.0 for Quantification of Human Immunodeficiency Virus Type 1 RNA in Plasma. *J Clin Microbiol*. 2000;38(11):4034–4041.
64. Vandamme AM, Schmit JC, Vandooren S, et al. Quantification of HIV-1 RNA in plasma: Comparable results with the NASBA HIV-1 RNA QT and the Amplicor HIV Monitor test. *J Acquir Immune Defic Syndr*. 1996;13(2):127–139.
65. Mani I, Cao HY, Hom D, et al. Plasma RNA viral load as measured by the branched DNA and nucleic acid sequence-based amplification assays of HIV-1 subtypes A and D in Uganda. *J Acquir Immune Defic Syndr*. 1999;22(2):208–209.

66. Ginocchio CC, Tetali S, Washburn D, et al. Comparison of levels of human immunodeficiency virus type 1 RNA in plasma as measured by the NucliSens nucleic acid sequence-based amplification and quantiplex branched-DNA assays. *J Clin Microbiol.* 1999;37(4):1210–1212.
67. Bettini P, Boeri E, Lillo F, et al. HIV-1 RNA Quantification by one-tube quantitative NASBA in HIV-1 infected patients. *AIDS.* 1996;10:1735–1751.
68. Notermans DW, De Wolf F, Oudshoorn P, et al. Evaluation of a second-generation nucleic acid sequence-based amplification assay for quantification of HIV type 1 RNA and the use of ultrasensitive protocol adaptations. *AIDS Res Hum Retroviruses.* 2000;16(15):1507–1517.
69. O'Shea S, Chrystie I, Cranston R, et al. Problems in the interpretation of HIV-1 viral load assays using commercial reagents. *J Med Virol.* 2000; 61(2): 187–194.
70. Manegold C, Krempe C, Jablonowski H, et al. Comparative evaluation of two branched-DNA human immunodeficiency virus type 1 RNA quantification assays with lower detection limits of 50 and 500 copies per milliliter. *J Clin Microbiol.* 2000;38(2):914–917.
71. Nolte FS, Boysza J, Thurmond C, et al. Clinical Comparison of an Enhanced-Sensitivity Branched-DNA Assay and Reverse Transcription-PCR for Quantitation of Human Immunodeficiency Virus Type 1 RNA in Plasma. *J Clin Microbiol.* 1998; 36(3):716–720.
72. Emery S, Bodrug S, Richardson BA, et al. Evaluation of performance of the Gen-Probe human immunodeficiency virus type 1 viral load assay using primary subtype A, C, and D isolates from Kenya. *J Clin Microbiol.* 2000;38(7): 2688–2695.
73. Highbarger HC, Alvord WG, Jiang MK, et al. Comparison of the Quantiplex Version 3.0 Assay and a Sensitized Amplicor Monitor Assay for Measurement of Human Immunodeficiency Virus Type 1 RNA Levels in Plasma Samples. *J Clin Microbiol.* 1999;37(11):3612–3614.
74. Clarke JR, Galpin S, Braganza R, et al. Comparative quantification of diverse serotypes of HIV-1 in plasma from a diverse population of patients. *J Med Virol.* 2000;62(4):445–449.
75. Coste J, Montes B, Reynes J, et al. Effect of HIV-1 Genetic Diversity of HIV-1 RNA Quantification in Plasma: Comparative Evaluation of Three Commercial Assays. *J Acquir Immune Defic Syndr.* 1997;15(2):174–175.
76. Debyser Z, Vanwijngaerden E, Vanlaethem K, et al. Failure to quantify viral load with two of the three commercial methods in a pregnant woman harboring an HIV type 1 subtype G strain. *AIDS Res Hum Retroviruses.* 1998;14(5):453–459.
77. Dunne AL, Crowe SM. Comparison of Branched DNA and Reverse Transcriptase Polymerase Chain Reaction for Quantifying Six Different HIV-1 Subtypes in Plasma. *AIDS.* 1997;11(1):126–127.
78. Alaeus A, Lidman K, Sonnerborg A, et al. Subtype-specific problems with quantification of plasma HIV-1 RNA. *AIDS.* 1997;11(7):859–865.
79. Gobbers E, Fransen K, Oosterlaken T, et al. Reactivity and amplification efficiency of the NASBA HIV-1 RNA Amplification System with Regard to Different HIV-1 Subtypes. *J Virol Methods.* 1997;66:293–301.
80. Burgisser P, Vernazza P, Flepp M, et al. Performance of five different assays for the quantification of viral load in persons infected with various subtypes of HIV-1. *J Acquir Immune Defic Syndr.* 2000;23(2):138–144.
81. Segondy M, Ly T, Lapeyre M, et al. Evaluation of the Nuclisens HIV-1 QT Assay for Quantitation of Human Immunodeficiency Virus Type 1 RNA Levels in Plasma. *J Clin Microbiol.* 1998;36(11): 3372–3374.
82. Nkengasong JN, Bile C, Kalou M, et al. Quantification of RNA in HIV type 1 subtypes D and G by NucliSens and Amplicor assays in Abidjan, Ivory Coast. *AIDS Res Hum Retroviruses.* 1999; 15(6):495–498.
83. De Baar MP, van der Schoot AM, Goudsmit J, et al. Design and evaluation of a human immunodeficiency virus type 1 RNA assay using nucleic acid sequence-based amplification technology able to quantify both group M and O viruses by using the long terminal repeat as target. *J Clin Microbiol.* 1999;37(6):1813–1818.
84. Alaeus A, Lilja E, Herman S, et al. Assay of plasma samples representing different HIV-1 genetic subtypes: An evaluation of new versions of the Amplicor HIV-1 monitor assay. *AIDS Res Hum Retroviruses.* 1999;15(10):889–894.
85. Triques K, Coste J, Perret JL, et al. Efficiencies of four versions of the amplicor HIV-1 monitor test for quantification of different subtypes of human immunodeficiency virus type 1. *J Clin Microbiol.* 1999;37(1):110–116.
86. Fiscus SA, Brambilla D, Coombs RW, et al. Multicenter evaluation of methods to quantitate human immunodeficiency virus type 1 RNA in seminal plasma. *J Clin Microbiol.* 2000; 38(6):2348–2353.
87. Dyer JR, Gilliam BL, Eron JJ, et al. Quantitation of human immunodeficiency virus type 1 RNA in cell free seminal plasma - comparison of NASBA™ with Amplicor™ reverse transcription-PCR amplification and correlation with quantitative culture. *J Virol Methods.* 1996;60(2):161–170.
88. Bremer J, Nowicki M, Beckner S, et al. Comparison of two amplification technologies for detection and quantitation of human immunodeficiency virus type 1 RNA in the female genital tract. *J Clin Microbiol.* 2000;38(7):2665–2669.

89. Coombs RW, Speck CE, Hughes JP, et al. Association between culturable Human Immunodeficiency Virus Type 1 (HIV-1) in Semen and HIV-1 RNA Levels in Semen and Blood: Evidence for Compartmentalization of HIV-1 between Semen and Blood. *J Infect Dis*. 1998;177:320–330.
90. Shepard RN, Schock J, Robertson K, et al. Quantitation of human immunodeficiency virus type 1 RNA in different biological compartments. *J Clin Microbiol*. 2000;38(4):1414–1418.
91. Iversen AKN, Larsen AR, Jensen T, et al. Distinct determinants of human immunodeficiency virus type 1 RNA and DNA loads in vaginal and cervical secretions. *J Infect Dis*. 1998;177(5):1214–1220.
92. Lewis P, Nduati R, Kreiss JK, et al. Cell-free human immunodeficiency virus type 1 in breast milk. *J Infect Dis*. 1998;177(1):34–39.
93. Pillay K, Coutsoudis A, York D, et al Cell-free virus in breast milk of HIV-1-seropositive women. *J Acquir Immune Defic Syndr*. 2000;24(4):330–336.
94. Distefano M, Monno L, Fiore JR, et al. Neurological disorders during HIV-1 infection correlate with viral load in cerebrospinal fluid but not with virus phenotype. *AIDS*. 1998;12(7):737–743.
95. Kravcik S, Gallicano K, Roth V, et al. Cerebrospinal fluid HIV RNA and drug levels with combination ritonavir and saquinavir. *JAIDS: J Acquir Immune Defic Syndr*. 1999;21(5):371–375.
96. Gisolf EH, van Praag RM, Jurriaans S, et al. Increasing chemokine concentrations despite undetectable cerebrospinal fluid HIV RNA in HIV-1 infected patients receiving antiretroviral therapy. *J Acquir Immune Defic Syndr.* 2000;25(5):426–433.
97. Gisslen M, Hagberg L, Fuchs D, et al. Cerebrospinal fluid viral load in HIV-1-infected patients without antiretroviral treatment - a longitudinal study. *J Acquir Immune Defic Syndr*. 1998;17(4):291–295.

11

Monitoring Immune Function

***Gunnel Biberfeld and †Eligius Lyamuya**

**Swedish Institute for Infectious Disease Control and Microbiology and Tumorbiology Center, Karolinska Institute, Stockholm, Sweden.*
†Department of Microbiology and Immunology, Muhimbili University College of Health Sciences, University of Dar es Salaam, Dar es Salaam, Tanzania.

HIV infection, especially its advanced stages, is associated with profound immunologic abnormalities (1,2). The most characteristic immunologic perturbation is the progressive loss of $CD4^+$ T-lymphocytes, which are the primary target cells for HIV infection. Other immunologic abnormalities include an increase in the number of $CD8^+$ T-lymphocytes, a depression in delayed-type hypersensitivity (DTH) to various recall antigens, an in-vitro decrease in T-helper cell response to various recall antigens and mitogens, a decrease in cytotoxic T-lymphocyte (CTL) function, an elevation in the serum levels of immune activation markers and immunoglobulins, a poor antibody response to new antigens, and a decrease in the function of natural killer cells and monocyte macrophages. Many of these immunologic alterations are useful for monitoring the immune status of HIV-infected subjects.

In spite of the immunologic aberrations induced by HIV infection, virus-specific humoral and cellular immune responses occur in most HIV-infected individuals. HIV-specific antibodies are produced against multiple HIV antigens, including antibodies active in virus neutralization (3,4), antibody-dependent cell-mediated cytotoxicity (ADCC) (3,4), and HIV antigen binding. HIV-specific CD8$^+$ CTL activity is detectable early after infection and usually persists during the chronic, asymptomatic phase of infection (5–7). Some of these immune responses help control HIV replication during the clinical latency phase but none eradicate the virus. Over time, CD4$^+$ T-lymphocytes are destroyed leading ultimately to severe immunosuppression, the hallmark of AIDS.

Most diagnostic tests for HIV infection are based on detection of antibodies to various HIV proteins. In contrast, immune status monitoring, important in clinical management of patients, is based on quantification of CD4$^+$ and CD8$^+$ T-lymphocytes, assessment of T-lymphocyte function, and detection of immune activation markers. This chapter reviews the various aspects of immune status monitoring in HIV infection and looks at its utility in the African setting.

LYMPHOCYTIC AND SEROLOGIC MARKERS FOR MONITORING IMMUNE STATUS

CD4$^+$ T-Lymphocyte Levels

Dysfunction and destruction of CD4$^+$ T-lymphocytes lead to the severe immunodepression seen in patients with HIV or AIDS. The most commonly used and important marker for the monitoring of immune status of HIV-infected individuals is the CD4$^+$ T-lymphocyte level. Monitoring HIV progression is essential for it helps a clinician define a person's stage of infection, determine when to initiate prophylaxis against opportunistic infections such as *Pneumocystis carinii* pneumonia (PCP), or determine when to start antiretroviral (ARV) therapy, and monitor response to ARV treatment. According to the U.S. Centers for Disease Control and Prevention (CDC), an HIV-infected person with CD4$^+$ T-lymphocyte counts less than 200 cells/μl or a CD4$^+$ T-lymphocyte percentage less than 14%, is defined as having AIDS (8) and PCP prophylaxis is recommended (9). The level of HIV RNA in plasma is an important marker for monitoring HIV disease progression and viral response to ARV therapy (10). However, the quantification of CD4$^+$ T-cells provides additional essential information for the clinical management of HIV-infected patients and can be an alternative to the expensive viral load measurement in settings with limited resources. UNAIDS and the World Health Organization (WHO) have recommended monitoring CD4$^+$ T-lymphocyte counts when initiating ARV therapy and when monitoring patients on ARV treatment in countries where viral load assays are not easily available (11).

Natural history studies and clinical trials have demonstrated that a decreased CD4$^+$ T-lymphocyte percentage or count increases the risk of developing complications and is a strong predictor for progression to AIDS and death (12,13). There is considerable variation in the rate of CD4$^+$ T-cell decline among HIV-1–infected subjects; some individuals maintain stable counts for long periods while others show a rapid decline in their CD4$^+$ T-lymphocyte counts. In HIV-2 infection, the rate at which individuals develop abnormal CD4$^+$ T-lymphocyte counts and progress to clinical AIDS is lower than that found among individuals infected with HIV-1 (14). Among

HIV-1–infected individuals who were followed from the time of seroconversion, the decline in $CD4^+$ T-cell counts correlated with their progression to AIDS (12). It has also been shown that the higher the plasma viral load, the more rapid the rate of decline of $CD4^+$ T-lymphocytes (10). A study reported from Uganda has confirmed a correlation between plasma HIV-1 RNA and absolute $CD4^+$ T-lymphocyte counts but found no correlation between increasing plasma viral load and $CD4^+$ T-lymphocyte decline (15). However, further evidence from other studies strongly suggests that measuring both plasma HIV-1 RNA and $CD4^+$ cells provides a powerful tool for defining the prognosis of HIV-infected patients (10,16). In the late stages of HIV infection, $CD4^+$ T-lymphocyte counts have been shown to be better measures for predicting progression to AIDS than have viral load levels (17,18). The utility of $CD4^+$ T-lymphocyte counts for predicting mortality has been reported in studies conducted among HIV-1 infected children and adults in Africa (19,20). Low $CD4^+$ T-lymphocyte levels are also predictive of mother-to-infant transmission of HIV-1 (21,22).

It has been debated whether to use absolute $CD4^+$ T-cell counts or $CD4^+$ T-cell percentages in immune status monitoring. It has been shown that the $CD4^+$ T-cell percentages show less variability than absolute $CD4^+$ T-cell counts, a finding that possibly gives percentages greater prognostic significance (23).

With the use of ARV regimens that effectively suppress HIV replication, such as highly active antiretroviral therapy (HAART), significant immune recovery can be achieved, leading to an increase in $CD4^+$ T-lymphocyte counts (24–26). Such an increase has been shown to occur in two phases. The first phase is thought to reflect the re-circulation of memory $CD4^+$ T-lymphocytes that had been trapped in lymphoid tissues. The second phase is thought to result from the production of new naïve ($CD45^{RA+}CD45^{RO-}$) $CD4^+$ cells (26). The increase in $CD4^+$ T-lymphocyte counts appears to persist as long as the viral load remains below the levels measured before ARV therapy (27).

The reference method for quantification of $CD4^+$ and $CD8^+$ T-lymphocytes is flow cytometry. This technique is expensive, requires highly trained personnel, and has high maintenance costs. Consequently, it is unavailable for routine use in most laboratories with limited facilities, a situation found in most African countries. Determination of $CD4^+$ T-lymphocyte counts usually requires use of a separate hematologic analyzer that measures the total leukocyte count. This count is then combined with the proportions of $CD4^+$ and $CD8^+$ cells within the T-lymphocyte population, determined using flow cytometric immunophenotyping, and final counts of $CD4^+$ and $CD8^+$ T-lymphocytes are then calculated. Use of two separate instruments inevitably introduces an additional instrumental error to the final counts. Recently, single platform methods for flow cytometry have been developed. These methods do not require the use of a separate hematologic analyzer (28).

Because of the limited availability of flow cytometry in most developing countries, alternative methods for determination of $CD4^+$ and $CD8^+$ T-lymphocyte counts have been developed. These methods are simple, affordable, and "user friendly," and they can be adapted for use in resource-scarce settings. These alternative methods have been evaluated in various settings, and several have been shown to give reliable counts that are comparable to those achieved using flow cytometry (Table 1) (29–34). Accordingly, the WHO has recommended that these alternative methods be used to monitor ARV therapy in laboratories where flow cytometry is not available or affordable (35). Because only a few of these methods are being used, it is felt that their manufacturers need to promote the use of the alternative methods that have been shown to give reliable results by making them available at a reasonable cost for potential users. In addition to these alternatives, a

TABLE 1. Available Alternative Methods for the Determination of $CD4^+$ and $CD8^+$ T-Lymphocyte Counts

Method	Manufacturer	Detection system	References
FACSCount™	Becton Dickinson	Fluorochrome-labeled anti-CD3, -CD4, and -CD8 MAb[a]	(30–32)
Coulter manual $CD4^+$ count kit	Coulter Corp.	Beads conjugated to anti-CD4 MAb	(29)
Zymmune kit	Zynaxis Inc.	anti-CD4 and -CD8 MAb	(30,31)
Dynabeads™	Dynal A/S	Magnetic beads coated with anti-CD4 and -CD8 MAb	(32)
Capcellia	Sanofi Diagnostics Pasteur	anti-CD4 and -CD8 MAb	(34)
Immunoalkaline Phosphatase assay	Reagents available commercially	Slide-based staining with anti-CD3, -CD4, and -CD8 MAb	(33)

[a]MAb indicates monoclonal antibodies.

study in South Africa has shown that quantification of $CD4^+$ T-lymphocytes by flow cytometry can be made more affordable by use of a single tube, single color staining method in lieu of the conventional multicolor, multiple tube staining method (36).

In any given laboratory, accurate interpretation of $CD4^+$ and $CD8^+$ T-lymphocyte counts requires the use of reference values determined from analysis of blood samples taken from healthy individuals in the respective locality. Few studies have reported reference values for $CD4^+$ and $CD8^+$ T-lymphocytes in Africa (37–41), and several laboratories in Africa still use $CD4^+$ and $CD8^+$ T-lymphocyte reference values derived from European and North American populations. There is concern that hematologic parameters among African populations differ from those reported for Caucasians (42). For example, HIV-infected individuals in Abidjan, Côte d'Ivoire, had higher values for their total number of lymphocytes and for absolute number of $CD4^+$ T-lymphocytes for a given percentage of $CD4^+$ T-cells than did HIV-1–infected individuals in France (42). Total lymphocyte counts, $CD3^+$ T-cell counts, and $CD4^+$ and $CD8^+$ T-lymphocyte counts were higher among seronegative Cameroonians than among seronegative Caucasians (39). In addition, lymphocytosis is said to be a common occurrence within black African populations (43), but has not consistently been found in the results of other studies from Africa (40,41,44). Seronegative Ethiopians have been reported to have significantly lower leukocyte and $CD4^+$ T-lymphocyte counts and considerably higher $CD8^+$ T-lymphocyte counts when compared to corresponding values among seronegative Europeans and Israelis (40,41).

Factors other than race and geographic location that influence lymphocyte subset values in HIV-seronegative individuals include sex, age, diurnal changes, and physical exercise (37,39,45–48). In African and European populations, females have been shown to have higher $CD4^+$ T-lymphocyte levels than males (37,39,45). Higher $CD4^+$ levels in females have also been demonstrated in a cohort of HIV-1–infected individuals in France (49) and in a cohort of HIV-2–infected individuals in Guinea Bissau (50). $CD4^+$ and $CD8^+$ T-lymphocyte counts vary with age in childhood (46). In West Africa, it has been reported that healthy children under 2 years of age had lower levels of $CD4^+$ T-cells than did children in the same age group in developed countries (47). All these observations emphasize the importance both of establishing standard hematologic references for each local population in Africa and of exercising caution in making direct comparisons of T-lymphocyte values across different racial groups.

Immune Activation Markers

Immune activation changes during HIV infection include increased spontaneous lymphocyte proliferation, altered T-lymphocyte phenotypic expression, increased serum levels of several proteins, polyclonal hypergammaglobulinemia, and increased cytokine production in lymphoid tissues. This activation is associated with specific anti-HIV-1 responses, but may also induce responses that enhance disease pathogenesis. It has been argued that in the HIV epidemic in Africa, immune activation plays a key role in the pathogenesis of AIDS (51).

Cellular Markers

During immune activation, an increase of $CD8^+$ T-lymphocytes together with a decrease of $CD4^+$ T-lymphocytes results in a decrease of the ratio of $CD4^+$ to $CD8^+$ T-lymphocytes. This ratio, like the count and percentage of $CD4^+$ T-cells, is a useful marker for predicting progression to AIDS. The number of $CD8^+$ T-cells has little predictive value (13). The increase in $CD8^+$ T-cells includes an elevation of $CD8^+$ T-cells with such activation markers as CD38, HLA-DR, and CD71 (transferrin receptor). Some of these markers can be used to predict progression to AIDS (52–56). $CD8^+$ T-cells that are also positive for CD38 increase soon after seroconversion and become progressively more elevated throughout the infection period (52,55,56). A high level of $CD8^+CD38^+$ T-cells strongly correlates with HIV-1 disease progression, adding to the prognostic value of $CD4^+$ T-lymphocyte counts. Expression of CD38 is also correlated with high plasma HIV RNA (57). HIV-1–infected individuals have also been shown to have decreased CD25 (IL-2 receptor alpha chain) expression (58). Recently, HLA-DR and CD71 expression on $CD4^+$ T-cells has been shown to be a better marker for monitoring AIDS prognosis than the expression of the same markers on $CD8^+$ T-cells (59). The utility of these markers in efforts to monitor HIV infection and AIDS in Africa is scantly documented. For example, a gradual increase of activated $CD4^+$ and $CD8^+$ T-lymphocytes and a decrease of $CD8^+CD28^+$ T-lymphocytes was reported among HIV-1–infected Ethiopians as they progressed from the asymptomatic infection phase to AIDS (60).

It has been shown that immune activation, measured by the proportion of HLA-DR^+ cells in the total lymphocyte population and the serum concentrations of β_2 microglobulin and IgG, is reduced in HIV-2 compared with HIV-1 infection (61). Studies have documented that environmental factors may play a part in causing immune activation. One study reported that uninfected Ethiopians living in Africa had higher levels of activated $CD4^+$ and $CD8^+$ T-cells than did uninfected Dutch living in the Netherlands (60), while another study reported a higher immune activation among uninfected Ugandans and Italians living in Uganda than among uninfected Ugandans and Italians living in Italy (62). If one considers the multiple infectious diseases endemic to Africa that could cause immune activation and the documented immune activation associated with infections like helminthiasis among uninfected Ethiopians (63), it is not surprising that immune activation has been implicated in the pathogenesis of HIV in Africa (51). This is an area that could benefit from more research, despite the potentially limiting factor imposed on such research by the high cost of assays for cellular activation markers.

With introduction of ARV therapy, researchers have investigated its effect on some cellular activation markers. In general, most studies have reported a significant and rapid decrease in the proportions of activated T-lymphocytes, including $CD38^+$ and/or

$HLA\text{-}DR^+$ $CD8^+$ cells and $HLA\text{-}DR^+$ $CD4^+$ cells, following suppression of HIV replication by ARV treatment (24–26). A fall in the levels of $CD8^+$ cells with activation markers, including $CD38^+HLA\text{-}DR^+$, $CD38^+CD45^{RO+}$, $HLA\text{-}DR^+CD45^{RO+}$, and $CD38^+CD28^-$, has been strongly associated with the disappearance of HIV RNA following ARV therapy (64). Additionally, a decrease in memory $CD45^{RA-}CD45^{RO+}$ $CD8^+$ cells occurs during ARV treatment (24).

Soluble Markers

Immune activation in HIV infection is also associated with elevated serum levels of several markers, including neopterin, β_2 microglobulin, soluble TNFα-RII (tumor necrosis factor α-receptor II), sIL-2 (soluble interleukin 2) receptor, and sCD8 (soluble CD8) (13,18,65–67). Neopterin, a metabolite of guanosine triphosphate, is produced by macrophages following stimulation by IFN-γ (interferon γ). β_2 microglobulin is the light chain of the major histocompatibility class I molecule (MHC class I). IL-2 receptor is secreted by activated T-lymphocytes and monocytes, while sCD8 is shed from activated $CD8^+$ T-lymphocytes.

Some of these factors have been shown to be good surrogate markers for monitoring disease progression. In particular, β_2 microglobulin and neopterin levels have been reported to increase early in HIV infection, even before $CD4^+$ T-cell levels decline, and to remain high and increasing throughout the course of infection and disease (13,66). These markers have been shown useful in estimating an HIV-infected individual's risk of developing AIDS (13), and have therefore been recommended as additional or alternative markers for monitoring prognosis in HIV-infected persons. Additionally, β_2 microglobulin has been shown to be a predictive marker for mother-to-infant transmission of HIV-1 (22). Assays for some of these factors, especially β_2 microglobulin and neopterin, may be affordable in resource-scarce settings, thus making their use attractive for monitoring the disease in infected individuals in Africa. For markers like neopterin, urine samples, which can be obtained without the need for invasive procedures, can be used instead of blood.

Concomitant infection with agents other than HIV, however, can also cause immune activation, and a subsequent increase in serum levels of these markers (68,69). Furthermore, elevation of some immune activation markers has been documented among apparently healthy HIV-seronegative Africans (70). These observations may limit the usefulness of clinical application of these serologic markers in immune monitoring in Africa because of the prevalence of infections by agents other than HIV. Even with these potential limitations, data from African studies have shown serum levels of β_2 microglobulin and neopterin can be useful in monitoring the prognosis of HIV-infected individuals (44,71–73). The prognostic value of neopterin appears to remain useful even among HIV-infected patients who are under treatment for underlying opportunistic infections like tuberculosis (68). Documented data on the reference levels of the serum markers of immune activation in healthy HIV-seronegative African populations is scanty (44). It would therefore be desirable to establish such values to facilitate correct interpretation of these parameters when they are used in immune function monitoring for HIV-infected individuals.

Polyclonal activation of B-lymphocytes is a common immune disregulation following HIV infection. The resulting hypergammaglobulinemia involves all immunoglobulin isotypes. Studies of the levels of immunoglobulin isotypes in relation to disease progression have shown that high levels of IgA and IgG provide prognostic information for disease progression and monitoring that is independent of viral load (74). A previous study among HIV-infected Tanzanian adults also showed that serum levels of IgA, IgM, IgD, and IgG3 increased from the asymptomatic phase through the AIDS phase (75). An increase in the level of IgE has also been associated with disease progression among HIV-infected adults and children in Europe (76–78). In contrast, however, a study of immunoglobulin levels among HIV-infected children in Tanzania, showed an elevation of all classes, but no correlation between those levels and clinical disease staging by CDC criteria (79). The use of serum immunoglobulin levels to monitor individuals' disease progression could appeal to staff in laboratories with limited facilities because these levels can be easily determined through a single radial immunodiffusion assay using commercially available plates. This technique is simple and does not require highly trained personnel or sophisticated equipment. However, further work needs to be done among HIV-infected individuals in Africa to determine the value that measuring levels of serum immunoglobulin classes and subclasses holds for monitoring their disease progression.

T-LYMPHOCYTE FUNCTION

CD4⁺ T-Lymphocyte Function

CD4⁺ T-cell reactivity measurement in vivo and in vitro can complement CD4⁺ T-cell determinations used in the prognosis of HIV infection. DTH skin reactivity to recall antigens is an in-vivo measure that has been used as a marker to determine the immune status of HIV-infected individuals. The DTH reaction is mediated by CD4⁺ T-helper cells that produce IL-2 and IFN-γ. Although some correlation between DTH reactivity and CD4⁺ T-cell count has been observed in HIV-infected individuals, DTH anergy has been reported to be an independent predictor of HIV-1 progression (80–82). Studies in Africa of HIV-1– and HIV-2–infected individuals have also shown a correlation between DTH reactivity and clinical stage of infection (83–86). However, the rate of development of cutaneous anergy is slower in HIV-2 infection than it is in HIV-1 infection (14). DTH skin testing using one or more common recall antigens (such as tuberculin, tetanus toxoid, or candidin) is a fast and easy way to obtain information about the immunologic status of an HIV-infected individual.

CD4⁺ T-cell function can be analyzed in vitro by determining levels of lymphocyte proliferation, cytokine production, and helper activity for antibody production. A person must have been exposed to the antigen to show antigen-specific lymphocyte proliferation and cytokine production in in vitro tests. In the lymphocyte proliferation assay, peripheral blood mononuclear cells (PBMCs) are cultured with or without antigens or mitogens for up to 6 days and then measured for radioactive thymidine uptake. This methodology requires expensive equipment and reagents. Cytokine production in response to antigenic stimulation can be measured by the enzyme-linked immunospot assay (ELISPOT), by flow cytometry, or by quantification of cytokines in supernatants of PBMC cultures using an enzyme-linked immunosorbent assay (ELISA) or a bioassay for IL-2. In the ELISPOT assay, the number of cells producing a certain cytokine can be determined using a microscope.

Abnormalities in T-helper cell function have been shown to occur as early as the asymptomatic phase of HIV infection when CD4⁺ cell counts are still within the normal range (87,88). T-cell defects during the early infection phase include decreases in lymphocyte proliferation and in IL-2 production in response to various recall antigens or CD3 antibodies, and poor pokeweed mitogen-induced helper activity of immunoglobulin production.

The defects in T-cell function increase as HIV infection progresses. At advanced stages of HIV infection, T-cells also lose their capacity to respond to alloantigens and stimulation by mitogens (87). T-cell function, as measured by proliferation induced by CD3 antibodies or IL-2 production induced by recall antigens, has been shown to be useful for predictions of progression to AIDS and survival time independent of $CD4^+$ T-lymphocyte counts (89,90). In addition, a study of asymptomatic HIV-infected subjects showed direct correlation between decreased lymphocyte proliferation in response to CD3 antibodies and in vivo DTH anergy to recall antigens (91).

HIV-specific T-cell proliferative responses are usually poor or absent in HIV-1–infected individuals (92–94). However, strong HIV-specific $CD4^+$ T-cell proliferative responses associated with production of INF-γ and antiviral β-chemokines have been found among HIV-1–infected long-term nonprogressors whose viremia was controlled without ARV therapy (95). Strong HIV-1–specific lymphocyte proliferative responses have also been found in individuals treated with combination ARV therapy early during acute HIV-1 infection. In individuals with chronic HIV-1 infection, levels of virus-specific T-cell proliferative responses have been shown to be inversely correlated with plasma viral load (95). Studies among HIV-1–infected individuals treated effectively with ARV therapy have indicated that lymphocyte proliferation responses to common recall antigens such as cytomegalovirus (CMV), tuberculin, and candida improve (24). However, in ARV-treated individuals with chronic infection, lymphocyte proliferative responses to HIV-1 antigens do not improve (24). T-helper cell responses to HIV-1 have been demonstrated in a proportion of individuals who have repeatedly been exposed to HIV-1 without becoming infected (96). Enhanced HIV-1–specific $CD4^+$ T-helper cell function, measured by the ELISPOT assay, has been measured in ARV-treated HIV-1–infected individuals after they were immunized with inactivated gp120-depleted HIV-1 (97).

$CD8^+$ T-Lymphocyte Function

Cytotoxic T-Lymphocytes

CTLs play an important role in the control of many viral infections (7). Antigen-specific CTLs are generally HLA class I-restricted $CD8^+$ T-lymphocytes, but antigen-specific cytotoxicity mediated by $CD4^+$ T-lymphocytes also exists. Several methods can be used to measure virus-specific CTLs, including CTLs to HIV (98). In the standard CTL assay PBMCs are incubated with autologous ^{51}Cr-labeled virus-infected target cells followed by determining the degree of lysis by quantifying chromium release. Usually CTLs against HIV are measured after in-vitro culture of PBMCs with autologous cells that express HIV antigens so as to increase the number of HIV-specific CTLs. However, some HIV-infected individuals have HIV-specific CTLs that can be detected in freshly isolated PBMCs.

The CTL assay can be made more quantitative by measuring CTL-precursor frequency by limiting dilution analysis, but this is a difficult and cumbersome procedure. More recent quantitative methods to measure $CD8^+$ T-effector cells include the tetramer assay and the ELISPOT assay or flow cytometry for detection of T-cells that produce IFN-γ. $CD8^+$ CTLs recognize virus-infected target cells that display virus-derived antigenic peptides bound to HLA class I molecules at the cell surface. In the tetramer assay method, fluorescent HLA class I/peptide tetrameric complexes are allowed to bind to peptide- (epitope-) specific $CD8^+$ T-cells and flourescent cells are identified by flow cytometry. Although sensitive, use of the assay is limited by both the need to know the HLA class I type—and the corresponding epitope—of the individual being tested and the need to construct tetramers for each epitope and HLA class I type to be tested. Tetramer binding is not a functional assay, but the results it yields have been shown to correlate with functional activity as measured by uncultured peptide-specific cytolysis (99). However, it has been reported that in HIV-1–infected individuals with very low $CD4^+$ T-cell counts, HIV-1– and CMV-specific $CD8^+$ T-cells, as measured by tetramer assay, can persist but may lack direct effector activity (100). $CD8^+$ T-lymphocytes secrete IFN-γ and certain other cytokines following specific interaction between the T-cell receptor and the HLA class I/peptide complexes. The ELISPOT assay for quantification of antigen-specific $CD8^+$ T-lymphocytes that produce INF-γ is rapid and easy to perform. Using poxviruses that express HIV-1 genes as its source of antigens, the ELISPOT assay allows broad HIV-specific responses to be measured, responses that are not dependent upon using peptides restricted to one epitope and one HLA class I type (101).

It is of particular interest to monitor HIV-specific CTL activity since there is evidence that HIV-specific CTL responses are essential to the control of HIV-1 infection (6,7). The HIV-1–specific CTL response develops early during primary infection and is associated with the decrease in high viral load that occurs during acute infection (5). HIV-specific CTLs can usually be detected in individuals with untreated chronic HIV-1 infection. A number of studies have shown that levels of HIV-1–specific CTL activity decline with disease progression (6,7). By comparison, virus-specific CTL activity remains high in most HIV-1–infected long-term nonprogressors. A significant inverse correlation between the magnitude of HIV-1–specific CTL response, as measured by tetramer assay, and plasma RNA viral load has been documented (99). It has also been demonstrated that HIV-1–specific T-helper cell response, measured by p24 antigen-induced lymphocyte proliferation, correlates directly with the level of HIV-1 *gag*-specific CTL precursors (102). Studies of HIV-1–specific CTL levels after combination ARV therapy have reported a decay of HIV-specific CTL to low or undetectable levels in individuals with undetectable plasma HIV RNA (103). Among seronegative individuals who have been repeatedly exposed to HIV, a high proportion have virus-specific $CD8^+$ HLA class I-restricted CTLs which are believed to play an important role in the resistance to infection (7,104–106).

There are few reported studies of HIV-2–specific CTLs (7). Among asymptomatic HIV-2–infected individuals tested, a majority demonstrated virus-specific CTL activity in freshly isolated PBMCs (107). An inverse correlation between HIV-2–specific CTL activity and HIV-2 proviral load has been observed in HIV-2–infected individuals in Gambia (108). CTLs against HIV-2 as well as HIV-1 peptides have been detected in uninfected female prostitutes in Gambia (104). Some CTL epitopes show cross-reactivity between HIV-1 and HIV-2 (104,109).

Noncytolytic Antiviral Suppressor Activity

It is well documented that $CD8^+$ T-cells can suppress HIV-1 replication in the absence of cell killing (110,111). This antiviral suppressor activity does not require HLA compatibility and is mediated by various soluble proteins, including the β-chemokines, RANTES, MIP-1α and MIP-1β (112), as well as by other factors called T-cell antiviral factors (CAF) (111).

Determining $CD8^+$ T-cell anti-HIV suppressor activity is technically demanding. It requires culture of $CD8^+$ T-cells at various concentrations with HIV-infected $CD4^+$ T-cells or culture of HIV-infected PBMCs with or without the addition of supernatants from mitogen-stimulated $CD8^+$ T-cells (111). β-chemokines inhibit HIV infection in vitro by competing with HIV for binding to the β-chemokine receptor CCR5, which also serves as a coreceptor for macrophage-tropic HIV-1 strains (113). Both $CD8^+$ and $CD4^+$ T-cells can produce β-chemokines. In vitro, β-chemokine production can be induced by mitogen stimulation of purified $CD8^+$ T-cells or by antigen-specific stimulation of PBMCs (114–116).

It has been shown that $CD8^+$ T-cell anti-HIV suppressor activity correlates with the clinical state of the infected individual (111,117) and that $CD8^+$ T-cells from long-term nonprogressors are more effective at suppressing HIV-1 replication than the corresponding cells from progressors (118). Furthermore, noncytotoxic anti-HIV $CD8^+$ T-cell activity has been observed in a high proportion of HIV-exposed uninfected individuals (119).

The level of β-chemokine production by $CD8^+$ T-cells in vitro correlates with the clinical status in HIV-1 infection (114,115). Plasma levels of β-chemokines, however, do not show such a correlation (114). High levels of mitogen- or antigen-induced production of β-chemokines have been associated with asymptomatic HIV infection and a decreased risk of HIV disease progression (114–116). A significant inverse correlation between plasma HIV-1 RNA and antigen-specific production of the β-chemokines, RANTES, MIP-1α and MIP-1β, has been demonstrated in ARV-naïve individuals (120). Moreover, sustained suppression of plasma HIV RNA by ARV therapy has been associated with an increased production of mitogen-induced MIP-1α and MIP-1β (121).

There are several reports of increased production of β-chemokines in HIV-exposed uninfected individuals. An association between reduced HIV-1 infectibility of $CD4^+$ T-cells in vitro and high β-chemokine production in HIV-exposed uninfected individuals has been described (122). In hemophiliacs who had been repeatedly exposed to HIV-contaminated blood products, resistance to infection was associated with high β-chemokine production by mitogen-stimulated PBMCs (123). Increased production of MIP-1α by unstimulated PBMCs has been observed in seronegative individuals at risk for HIV infection (115). Furthermore, high levels of antigen-induced β-chemokine production by $CD4^+$ T-cells have been found in HIV-exposed uninfected individuals (124).

CONCLUSION

The growing HIV epidemic in Africa increases the need for immunologic assays that will provide data that can guide clinical decisions about disease management. Use of ARV drugs for the treatment of HIV and AIDS is currently beyond the economic reach of most Africans infected with HIV. However, there is growing interest among donor organizations and international agencies to initiate programs that would reduce or subsidize the cost of ARV drugs to individuals in African countries. In such programs, immune status monitoring will be required to provide the information for decisions on when to initiate ARV treatment, how to evaluate the clinical response of patients, and how to assess the effect of such therapy on disease progression. Methods for the quantification of $CD4^+$ T-lymphocyte counts will therefore be needed as a complement or alternative to viral load measurement, depending upon available resources. Determining the levels of immune activation markers may also be of value. However, the use of surrogate markers for immune status monitoring in Africa will have to address some challenges, including a paucity of baseline reference values for most of the markers, and the role of genetic factors, other tropical diseases, and environment in immune activation.

In view of the need for a safe, effective vaccine for HIV that will complement other prevention strategies, efficacy trials of candidate vaccines will require the participation of countries in Africa where the incidence of HIV is high. Monitoring immune system responses in vaccine trials will demand measuring HIV-specific $CD4^+$ and $CD8^+$ T-lymphocyte activity as well as viral neutralization activity.

REFERENCES

1. Rosenberg ZF, Fauci AS. The immunopathogenesis of HIV infection. *Adv Immunol*, 1989;47:377–431.
2. Seligmann M, Pinching AJ, Rosen FS, et al. Immunology of human immunodeficiency virus infection and the acquired immunodeficiency syndrome. An update. *Ann Intern Med*, 1987;107:234–242.

3. Fenyo EM, Albert J, McKeating J. The role of the humoral immune response in HIV infection. *AIDS*, 1996;10 Suppl A:S97–S106.
4. Haigwood NL, Zolla-Pazner S. Humoral immunity to HIV, SIV and SHIV. *AIDS*, 1998;12 Suppl A:S121–S132.
5. Koup RA, Safari JT, Cao Y, et al. Temporal association of cellular immune responses with the initial control of viremia in primary human immunodeficiency virus type 1 syndrome. *J Virol*, 1994;68:4650–4655.
6. Bollinger RC, Egan MA, Chun Tae-Wook, et al. Cellular immune responses to HIV-1 in progressive and non-progressive infections. *AIDS*, 1996;10 Suppl A:S85–S96.
7. Rowland-Jones S, Tan R, McMichael A. Role of cellular immunity in protection against HIV infection. *Adv. Immunol*, 1997;65:277–346.
8. CDC 1993. Revised classification system for HIV infection and expanded surveillance case definition for AIDS among adolescents and adults. *MMWR*, 1992;41:1–19.
9. CDC 1997. USPHS/IDSA Guidelines for prevention of opportunistic infections in persons infected with human immunodeficiency virus. *MMWR*, 1999;48:1–59.
10. Mellors JW, Munoz A, Giorgi JV, et al. Plasma viral load and CD4+ lymphocytes as prognostic markers of HIV-1 infection. *Ann Intern Med*, 1997; 126:946–954.
11. UNAIDS/WHO 1998. Guidance modules on antiretroviral treatments: Module 1–9 WHO/AIDS/98.1 UNAIDS/98.7.
12. Stein DS, Korvick JA, Vermund SH. CD4+ lymphocyte cell enumeration for prediction of clinical course of human immunodeficiency virus disease: A review. *J Infect Dis*, 1992;165:352–363.
13. Fahey JL, Taylor JM, Detels R, et al. The prognostic value of cellular and serologic markers in infection with human immunodeficiency virus type 1. *N Engl J Med*, 1990;322:166–172.
14. Marlink R, Kanki P, Thior I, et al. Reduced rate of disease development after HIV-2 infection as compared to HIV-1. *Science*, 1994;265:1587–1590.
15. Morgan D, Rutebemberwa A, Malamba S, et al. HIV-1 RNA levels in an African population-based cohort and their relation to CD4 lymphocyte counts and World Health Organization clinical staging. *J Acquir Immune Defic Syndr*, 1999;22:167–173.
16. Kim S, Hughes MD, Hammer SM, et al. Both serum HIV type 1 RNA levels and CD4+ lymphocyte counts predict clinical outcome in HIV type 1-infected subjects with 200 to 500 CD4+ cells per cubic millimeter. AIDS Clinical Trials Group Study 175 Virology Study Team. *AIDS Res Hum Retroviruses*, 2000;16:645–653.
17. de Wolf F, Spijkerman I, Schellekens PT, et al. AIDS prognosis based on HIV-1 RNA, CD4+ T-cell count and function: markers with reciprocal predictive value over time after seroconversion. *AIDS*, 1997;11:1799–1806.
18. Fahey JL, Taylor JMG, Manna B, et al. Prognostic significance of plasma markers of immune activation, HIV viral load and CD4 T-cell measurements. *AIDS*, 1998;12:1581–1590.
19. Taha TE, Kumwenda NI, Hoover DR, et al. Association of HIV-1 load and CD4 lymphocyte count with mortality among untreated African children over one year of age. *AIDS*, 2000;14:453–459.
20. French N, Mujugira A, Nakiyingi J, et al. Immunologic and clinical stages in HIV-1-infected Ugandan adults are comparable and provide no evidence of rapid progression but poor survival with advanced disease. *J Acquir Immune Defic Syndr*, 1999;22:509–516.
21. European Collaborative Study: Risk factors for mother-to-child transmission of HIV-1. *Lancet*, 1992;339:1007–1012.
22. Bredberg-Râdén U, Urassa W, Urassa E, et al. Predictive markers for mother-to-child transmission of HIV-1 in Dar es Salaam, Tanzania. *J Acquir Immune Defic Syndr Hum Retrovirol*, 1995;8: 182–187.
23. Taylor JM, Fahey JL, Detels R, et al. CD4 percentage, CD4 number, and CD4:CD8 ratio in HIV infection: which to choose and how to use. *J Acquir Immune Defic Syndr*, 1989;2:114–124.
24. Gea-Banacloche JC, Clifford Lane H. Immune reconstitution in HIV infection. *AIDS*, 1999;13 Suppl A:S25–S38.
25. Plana M, Garcia F, Gallart T, et al. Immunological benefits of antiretroviral therapy in very early stages of asymptomatic chronic HIV-1 infection. *AIDS*, 2000;14:1921–1933.
26. Autran B, Carcelain G, Li TS, et al. Positive effects of combined antiretroviral therapy on CD4+ T cell homeostasis and function in advanced HIV disease. *Science*, 1997;277:112–116.
27. Daniel Kuritzkes. Viral Pathogenesis: Update and Clinical Implications. [Medscape Web site]. May 31, 2000. Available at: http://www.medscape.com/medscape/HIV/AnnualUpdate/2000/mha.update05.02.kuritzes/mha05.kuritzkes-01.html. Accessed July 9, 2001.
28. CDC 1997. Revised guidelines for performing CD4+ T-cell determinations in persons with human immunodeficiency virus (HIV). *MMWR*, 1997; 46:1–29.
29. Landay A, Ho JL, Hom D, et al. A rapid manual method for CD4+ T-cell quantification for use in developing countries. *AIDS*, 1993;7:1565–1568.
30. Nicholson JK, Velleca WM,. Jubert S, et al. Evaluation of alternative CD4 technologies for the enumeration of CD4 lymphocytes. *J Immunol Methods*, 1994;177:43–54.

31. Johnson D, Hirschkorn D, Busch MP. Evaluation of four alternative methodologies for determination of absolute CD4+ lymphocyte counts. *J Acquir Immune Defic Syndr Hum Retrovirol,* 1995; 10: 522–530.
32. Lyamuya EF, Kagoma C, Mbena EC, et al. Evaluation of the FACScount, TRAx CD4 and Dynabeads methods for CD4 lymphocyte determination. *J Immunol Methods,* 1996;195:103–112.
33. Lisse IM, Bottiger B, Christensen LB, et al. Evaluation of T cell subsets by an immunocytochemical method compared to flow cytometry in four countries. *Scand J Immun,* 1997;45: 637–644.
34. Diagbouga S, Durand G, Sanou PT, et al. Evaluation of a quantitative determination of CD4 and CD8 molecules as an alternative to CD4+ and CD8+ T lymphocyte counts in Africans. *Trop Med Int Health,* 1999;4:79–84.
35. UNAIDS/WHO 1998. Guidance Modules on Antiretroviral treatments: Module 5, Laboratory requirements for the safe and effective use of antiretrovirals. WHO/AIDS/98.1 UNAIDS/98.7.
36. Sherman GG, Galpin JS, Patel JM, et al. CD4+ T cell enumeration in HIV infection with limited resources. *J Immunol Methods,* 1999;222:209–217.
37. Tugume SB, Piwowar EM, Lutalo T, et al. Hematological reference ranges among healthy Ugandans. *Clin Diagn Lab Immunol,* 1995; 2:233–235.
38. Levin A, Brubaker G, Shao JS, et al. Determination of T-lymphocyte subsets on site in rural Tanzania: results in HIV-1 infected and non-infected individuals. *Int J STD AIDS,* 1996;7:288–291.
39. Zekeng L, Sadjo A, Meli J, et al. T lymphocyte subset values among healthy Cameroonians. *J Acquir Immune Defic Syndr Hum Retrovirol,* 1997;14:82–83.
40. Kalinkovich A, Weisman Z, Burstein R, et al. Standard values of T-lymphocyte subsets in Africa. *J Acquir Immune Defic Syndr Hum Retrovirol,* 1998;17:183–185.
41. Tsegaye A, Messele T, Tilahun T, et al. Immunohematological reference ranges for adult Ethiopians. *Clin Diagn Lab Immunol,* 1999; 6:410–414.
42. Anglaret X, Diagbouga S, Mortier E, et al. $CD4^+$ T-lymphocyte counts in HIV infection: are European standards applicable to African patients? *J Acquir Immune Defic Syndr Hum Retrovirol,* 1997; 14: 361–367.
43. Gilles HM. Normal haematological values in tropical areas. *Clin Haematol,* 1981;10:697–706.
44. Urassa WK, Lyamuya EF, Mbena E, et al. Immunohaematological findings in healthy and HIV-1 infected adults in Dar es Salaam, Tanzania. *East Afr Med J,* 1996;73:670–674.
45. Maini MK, Gilson RJ, Chavda N, et al. Reference ranges and sources of variability of CD4 counts in HIV-seronegative women and men. *Genitourin Med,* 1996;72:27–31.
46. Denny T, Yogev R, Gelman R, et al. Lymphocyte subsets in healthy children during the first 5 years of life. *JAMA,* 1992;267:1484–1488.
47. Lisse IM, Aaby P, Whittle H, et al. T-lymphocyte subsets in West African children: impact of age, sex and season. *J Pediatr,* 1997;130:77–85.
48. Signore A, Lugini P, Lefizia C, et al. Study of the diurnal variation of human lymphocyte subsets. *J Clin Lab Immunol,* 1985;17:25–28.
49. Delmas M-C, Jadand C, De Vincenzi I, et al. Gender differences in CD4+ cell counts persist after HIV-1 infection. *AIDS,* 1997;11:1071–1073.
50. Norrgren H, Da Silva ZJ, Andersson S, et al. Clinical features, immunological changes and mortality in a cohort of HIV-2-infected individuals in Bissau, Guinea-Bissau. *Scand J Infect Dis,* 1998;30: 323–329.
51. Bentwich Z, Kalinkovich A, Weisman Z. Immune activation is a dominant factor in the pathogenesis of African AIDS. *Immunol Today,* 1995;16: 187–191.
52. Giorgi JV, Liu Z, Hultin LE, et al. Elevated levels of CD38+ CD8+ T cells in HIV infection add to the prognostic value of low CD4+ T cell levels: results of 6 years of follow-up. The Los Angeles Center, Multicenter AIDS Cohort Study. *J Acquir Immune Defic Syndr,* 1993;6:904–912.
53. Yagi MJ, Chu FN, Jiang JD, et al. Increases in soluble CD8 antigen in plasma, and CD8+ and CD8+CD38+ cells in human immunodeficiency virus type-1 infection. *Clin Immunol Immunopathol,* 1992;63:126–134.
54. Bass HZ, Nishanian P, Hardy WD, et al. Immune changes in HIV-1 infection: significant correlations and differences in serum markers and lymphoid phenotypic antigens. *Clin Immunol Immunopathol,* 1992;64:63–70.
55. Autran B, Giorgi JV. Activated CD8+ cells in HIV-related diseases. In: Janossy G, Autran B, Miedema F, eds. *Immunodeficiency in HIV infection and AIDS,* Basel, Switzerland: S. Karger AG. 1992: 171–184.
56. Mocroft A, Bofill M, Lipman M, et al. CD8+, CD38+ lymphocyte percent: a useful immunological marker for monitoring HIV-1-infected patients. *J Acquir Immune Defic Syndr Hum Retrovirol,* 1997;14:158–162.
57. Bouscarat F, Levacher-Clergeot M, Dazza MC, et al. Correlation of CD8 lymphocyte activation with cellular viremia and plasma HIV RNA levels in asymptomatic patients infected by human immunodeficiency virus type 1. *AIDS Res Hum Retroviruses,* 1996;12:17–24.
58. Zola H, Koh LY, Mantzioris BX, et al. Patients with HIV infection have a reduced proportion of

lymphocytes expressing the IL2 receptor p55 chain (TAC, CD25). *Clin Immunol Immunopathol*, 1991;59:16–25.

59. Plaeger S, Bass HZ, Nishanian P, et al. The prognostic significance in HIV infection of immune activation represented by cell surface antigen and plasma activation marker changes. *Clin Immunol*, 1999;90:238–246.
60. Messele T, Abdulkadir M, Fontanet AL, et al. Reduced naive and increased activated CD4 and CD8 cells in healthy adult Ethiopians compared with their Dutch counterparts. *Clin Exp Immunol*, 1999;115:443–450.
61. Michel P, Balde AT, Roussilhon C, et al. Reduced immune activation and T cell apoptosis in human immunodeficiency virus type 2 compared with type 1: correlation of T cell apoptosis with β_2 microglobulin concentration and disease evolution. *J Infect Dis*, 2000;181:64–75.
62. Clerici M, Butto S, Lukwiya M, et al. Immune activation in Africa is environmentally-driven and is associated with upregulation of CCR5. Italian-Ugandan AIDS Project. *AIDS*, 2000;14:2083–2092.
63. Kalinkovich A, Weisman Z, Greenberg Z, et al. Decreased CD4 and increased CD8 counts with T cell activation is associated with chronic helminth infection. *Clin Exp Immunol*, 1998;114:414–421.
64. Bouscarat F, Levacher M, Landman R, et al. Changes in blood CD8+ lymphocyte activation status and plasma HIV RNA levels during antiretroviral therapy. *AIDS*, 1998;12:1267–1273.
65. Fuchs D, Jager H, Popescu M, et al. Immune activation markers to predict AIDS and survival in HIV-1 seropositives. *Immunol Lett*, 1990;26:75–79.
66. Fuchs D, Kramer A, Reibnegger G, et al. Neopterin and beta 2-microglobulin as prognostic indices in human immunodeficiency virus type 1 infection. *Infection,* 1991;19 Suppl 2:S98–S102.
67. Hofmann B, Wang YX, Cumberland WG, et al. Serum beta 2-microglobulin level increases in HIV infection: relation to seroconversion, CD4 T-cell fall and prognosis. *AIDS*, 1990;4:207–214.
68. Hosp M, Elliott AM, Raynes JG, et al. Neopterin, beta 2-microglobulin, and acute phase proteins in HIV-1-seropositive and -seronegative Zambian patients with tuberculosis. *Lung,* 1997;175:265–275.
69. Bentwich Z, Weisman Z, Moroz C, et al. Immune dysregulation in Ethiopian immigrants in Israel: relevance to helminth infections? *Clin Exp Immunol*, 1996;103:239–243.
70. Rizzardini G, Piconi S, Ruzzante S, et al. Immunological activation markers in the serum of African and European HIV-seropositive and seronegative individuals. *AIDS*, 1996;10: 1535–1542.
71. Garden GA, Moss GB, Emonyi W, et al. Beta-2 microglobulin as a marker of HIV disease status in Nairobi, Kenya. *Int J STD AIDS*, 1993;4:49–51.
72. Dyer JR, Hoffman IF, Eron JJ Jr, et al. Immune activation and plasma viral load in HIV-infected African individuals. *AIDS*, 1999;13:1283–1285.
73. Hengster P, Schmutzhard E, Fuchs D, et al. Evaluation on HIV serology and immune-stimulation on patients in Tanzania. *Int J STD AIDS* 1991; 2:180–184.
74. Sabin CA, Devereux H, Phillips AN, et al. Immune markers and viral load after HIV-1 seroconversion as predictors of disease progression in a cohort of haemophilic men. *AIDS*, 1998;12:1347–1352.
75. Lyamuya EF, Maselle SY, Matre R. Serum immunoglobulin profiles in asymptomatic HIV-1 seropositive adults and in patients with AIDS in Dar es Salaam, Tanzania. *East Afr Med J*, 1994; 71:24–28.
76. Israel-Biet D, Labrousse F, Tourani JM, et al. Elevation of IgE in HIV-infected subjects: a marker of poor prognosis. *J Allergy Clin Immunol*, 1992; 89:68–75.
77. Vigano A, Principi N, Crupi L, et al. Elevation of IgE in HIV-infected children and its correlation with the progression of disease. *J Allergy Clin Immunol*, 1995;95:627–632.
78. de Martino M, Rossi ME, Azzari C, et al. Low IgG3 and high IgG4 subclass levels in children with advanced human immunodeficiency virus-type 1 infection and elevated IgE levels. *Ann Allergy Asthma Immunol*, 1999;83:160–164.
79. Lyamuya EF, Matee MI, Kasubi M, et al. Immunoglobulin profile in HIV-1 infected children in Dar es Salaam. *East Afr Med J*, 1999;76:370–375.
80. Birx DL, Brundage J, Larson K, et al. The prognostic utility of delayed-type hypersensitivity skin testing in the evaluation of HIV-infected patients. Military Medical Consortium for Applied Retroviral Research. *J Acquir Immune Defic Syndr*, 1993; 6:1248–1257.
81. Blatt SP, Hendrix CW, Butzin CA, et al. Delayed-type hypersensitivity skin testing predicts progression to AIDS in HIV-infected patients. *Ann Intern Med*, 1993;119:177–184.
82. Gordin FM, Hartigan PM, Klimas NG, et al. Delayed-type hypersensitivity skin tests are an independent predictor of human immunodeficiency virus disease progression. Department of Veterans Affairs Cooperative Study Group. *J Infect Dis*, 1994;169:893–897.
83. Miller WC, Thielman NM, Swai N, et al. Delayed-type hypersensitivity testing in Tanzanian adults with HIV infection. *J Acquir Immune Defic Syndr Hum Retrovirol*, 1996;12:303–308.
84. Colebunders RL, Lebughe I, Nzila N, et al. Cutaneous delayed-type hypersensitivity in patients with human immunodeficiency virus infection in Zaire. *J Acquir Immune Defic Syndr*, 1989; 2:576–578.

85. Nauclér A, Albino P, Andersson S, et al. Clinical and immunological follow-up of previously hospitalized HIV-2 seropositive patients in Bissau, Guinea-Bissau. *Scand J Inf Dis*, 1992;24:725–731.
86. Whittle H, Egboga A, Todd J, et al. Immunological responses of Gambians in relation to clinical stage of HIV-2 disease. *Clin Exp Immunol*, 1993; 93:45–50.
87. Shearer GM, Clerici M. Early T-helper cell defects in HIV infection. *AIDS* 1991;5:245–253.
88. Miedema F, Meyaard L, Koot M, et al. Changing virus-host interactions in the course of HIV-1 infection. *Immunol Rev*, 1994;140:35–72.
89. Roos MT, Miedema F, Koot M, et al. T cell function in vitro is an independent progression marker for AIDS in human immunodeficiency virus-infected asymptomatic subjects. *J Infect Dis*, 1995; 171: 531–536.
90. Dolan MJ, Clerici M, Blatt SP, et al. In vitro T cell function, delayed-type hypersensitivity skin testing, and CD4+ T cell subset phenotyping independently predict survival time in patients infected with human immunodeficiency virus. *J Infect Dis*, 1995;172:79–87.
91. Maas JJ, Roos MT, Keet IP, et al. In vivo delayed-type hypersensitivity skin test anergy in human immunodeficiency virus type 1 infection is associated with T cell nonresponsiveness in vitro. *J Infect Dis*, 1998;178:1024–1029.
92. Wahren B, Morfeldt-Mansson L, Biberfeld G, et al. Characteristics of the specific cell-mediated immune response in human immunodeficiency virus infection. *J Virol*, 1987;1:2017–2023.
93. Pontesilli O, Carlesimo M, Varani AR, et al. HIV-specific lymphoproliferative responses in asymptomatic HIV-infected individuals. *Clin Exp Immunol*, 1995;100:419–424.
94. Caruso A, Licenziati S, Canaris AD, et al. T cells from individuals in advanced stages of HIV-1 infection do not proliferate but express activation antigens in response to HIV-1-specific antigens. *J Acquir Immune Defic Syndr Hum Retrovirol*, 1997;15:61–69.
95. Rosenberg ES, Billingsley JM, Caliendo AM, et al. Vigorous HIV-1-specific CD4+ T cell responses associated with control of viremia. *Science*, 1997;278:1447–1450.
96. Shearer GM, Clerici M. Protective immunity against HIV infection: has nature done the experiment for us? *Immunol Today*, 1996;17:21–24.
97. Moss R, Webb E, Giermakowska WK, et al. HIV-1-specific CD4 helper function in persons with chronic HIV-1 infection on antiviral drug therapy as measured by ELISPOT after treatment with an inactivated, gp120-depleted HIV-1 in incomplete Freund's adjuvant. *J Acquir Immune Defic Syndr*, 2000;24:264–269.
98. Goulder PJR, Rowland-Jones SL, McMichael AJ, et al. Anti-HIV cellular immunity: recent advances towards vaccine design. *AIDS*, 1999; 13 Suppl A:S121–S136.
99. Ogg GS, Jin X, Bonhoeffer S, et al. Quantitation of HIV-1-specific cytotoxic T lymphocytes and plasma load of viral RNA. *Science*, 1998;279: 2103–2106.
100. Spiegel HML, Ogg GS, De Falcon E, et al. Human immunodeficiency virus type 1- and cytomegalovirus-specific cytotoxic T lymphocytes can persist at high frequency for prolonged periods in the absence of circulating peripheral CD4+ T cells. *J Virol*, 2000;74:1018–1022.
101. Larsson M, Jin X, Ramratnam B, et al. A recombinant vaccinia virus based ELISPOT assay detects high frequencies of Pol-specific CD8 T cells in HIV-1-positive individuals. *AIDS*, 1999;13: 767–777.
102. Kalams SA, Buchbinder SP, Rosenberg ES, et al. Association between virus-specific cytotoxic T-lymphocyte and helper responses in human immunodefiency virus type 1 infection. *J Virol*, 1999;73:6715–6720.
103. Ogg GS, Jin X, Bonhoeffer S, et al. Decay kinetics of human immunodeficiency virus-specific effector cytotoxic T lymphocytes after combination antiretroviral therapy. *J Virol*, 1999;73:797–800.
104. Rowland-Jones S, Sutton J, Ariyoshi K, et al. HIV-specific cytotoxic T-cells in HIV-exposed but uninfected Gambian women. *Nat Med*, 1995;1:59–64.
105. Rowland-Jones SL, Dong T, Fowke KR, et al. Cytotoxic T cell responses to multiple conserved HIV epitopes in HIV-resistant prostitutes in Nairobi. *J Clin Invest*, 1998;102:1758–1765.
106. Bernard NF, Yannakis CM, Lee JS, et al. Human immunodeficiency virus (HIV)-specific cytotoxic lymphocyte activity in HIV-exposed seronegative persons. *J Infect Dis*, 1999;179:538–547.
107. Gotch F, McAdam SN, Allsopp CE, et al. Cytotoxic T cells in HIV-2 seropositive Gambians. Identification of a virus specific MHC-restricted peptide epitope. *J Immunol*, 1993;151:3361–3369.
108. Ariyoshi K, Cham F, Berry N et al. HIV-2 specific cytotoxic T-lymphocyte activity is inversely related to proviral load. *AIDS*, 1995;9:555–559.
109. Nixon DF, Huet S, Rothbard J, et al. An HIV-1 and HIV-2 cross-reactive cytotoxic T-cell epitope. *AIDS*, 1990;4:841–845.
110. Walker CM, Moody DJ, Stites DP, et al. $CD8^{+}$ lymphocytes can control HIV infection in vitro by suppressing virus replication. *Science*, 1986;234: 1563–1566.
111. Levy JA, Mackewicz CE, Barker E. Controlling HIV pathogenesis: the role of the noncytotoxic anti-HIV response of $CD8^{+}$ T cells. *Immunol Today*, 1996;5:217–224.

112. Cocchi F, DeVico A, Garcino-Demo A, et al. Identification of RANTES, MIP-1α and MIP-1β as the major HIV-suppressive factors produced by CD8⁺ T cells. *Science,* 1995;270:1811–1815.
113. Berger EA, Murphy PM, Farber JM. Chemokine receptors as HIV-1 coreceptors: Roles in viral entry, tropism and disease. *Annu Rev Immunol,* 1999;17:657–700.
114. Cocchi F, DeVico AL, Yarchoan R, et al. Higher macrophage inflammatory protein MIP-1α and MIP-1β levels from CD8⁺ cells are associated with asymptomatic HIV-1 infection. *PNAS,* 2000; 97:13812–13817.
115. Garzino-Demo A, Moss RB, Margolick JB, et al. Spontaneous and antigen-induced production of HIV-inhibitory β-chemokines are associated with AIDS-free status. *PNAS,* 2000;96:11986–11991.
116. Ullum H, Cozzi Lepri A, Victor J, et al. Production of β-chemokines in human immunodeficiency virus (HIV) infection: Evidence that high levels of macrophage inflammatory protein-1β are associated with a decreased risk of HIV disease progression. *J Infect Dis* 1998;177:331–336.
117. Mackewicz CE, Ortega HW, Levy JA. CD8⁺ cell anti-HIV activity correlates with the clinical state of the infected individual. *J Clin Invest,* 1991;87: 1462–1466.
118. Cao Y, Qin L, Zhang L, et al. Virologic and immunologic characterization of long-term survivors of human immunodeficiency virus type 1 infection. *N Engl J Med,* 1995;332:201–208.
119. Stanford SA, Skurnick J, Louria D, et al. Lack of infection in HIV-exposed individuals is associated with a strong CD8⁺ cell noncytotoxic anti-HIV response. *Proc Natl Acad Sci USA,* 1999; 96: 1030–1035.
120. Ferbas J, Giorgi JV, Amini S, et al. Antigen-specific production of RANTES, macrophage inflammatory protein MIP-1α and MIP-1β in vitro is a correlate of reduced human immunodeficiency virus burden in vivo. *J. Infect Dis,* 2000;182:1247–1250.
121. Kumar D, Parato K, Kumar A, et al. Sustained suppression of plasma HIV RNA is associated with an increase in the production of mitogen-induced MIP-1α and MIP-1β. *AIDS Res Hum Retroviruses,* 1999;15:1073–1077.
122. Paxton WA, Liu R, Kang S, et al. Reduced HIV-1 infectability of CD4⁺ lymphocytes from exposed-uninfected individuals: association with low expression of CCR5 and high production of β-chemokines. *Virology,* 1998;244:66–73.
123. Zagury D, Lachgar A, Chams V, et al. C-C chemokines, pivotal in protection against HIV type 1 infection. *Proc Natl Acad Sci USA,* 1998;95:3857–3861.
124. Furci L, Scarlatti G, Burastero, et al. Antigen-driven C-C chemokine-mediated HIV-1 supression by CD4⁺ T cells from exposed uninfected individuals expressing the wild-type CCR-5 allele. *J Exp Med,* 1997;186:455–460.

12

The Epidemiology of HIV and AIDS

Peter Piot and Michael Bartos

Joint United Nations Programme on HIV/AIDS, Geneva, Switzerland.

Twenty years after the initial reports of AIDS and some 18 years since it was first observed in Africa, the HIV epidemic has spread throughout the continent to devastating effect. As of the end of 2001, there are an estimated 28.1 million adults and children living with HIV in sub–Saharan Africa and an additional 440,000 in North Africa and the Middle East (1). Over the course of 2001 an estimated 3.4 million Africans became infected with HIV, 700,000 of whom were children under the age of 15. In 2001 there were an estimated 2.3 million deaths due to AIDS in sub–Saharan Africa, and sub–Saharan Africans account for some three-quarters of the total global toll of 20 million AIDS deaths since the epidemic began (1,2). AIDS has become the leading cause of death in Africa. It is responsible for one in five deaths in sub–Saharan Africa, twice as many as for the second leading cause of death (3).

Across sub–Saharan Africa, the average prevalence of HIV in adults aged 15 to 49 is 8.8% (2). However, within sub–Saharan Africa, HIV prevalence is not uniformly distributed. East Africa once had the highest infection rates on the continent but has now been overtaken by the southern cone. Among some urban populations, for example in Francistown, Botswana, prevalence among pregnant women[a] has been found to be as high as 44% (4). In southern Africa, Botswana, Lesotho, Malawi, South Africa, Swaziland, Zambia, and Zimbabwe all have at least some regions where prevalence among pregnant women at antenatal surveillance sites is 25% or higher (5). But even in these countries, the situation is different in different areas. For example, the prevalence among antenatal clinic attendees in South Africa's KwaZulu Natal province in 2000 was 36.2%, while in the Western Cape it was only 8.7% (6).

Among specific population groups that are disproportionately affected by the epidemic, there are a number of locations where HIV prevalence has been found to exceed 70%. For example, this rate has been found among sex workers and people with sexually transmitted diseases (STDs) (5), and high rates of HIV prevalence have also been found among occupational groups such as mine workers and military personnel. High prevalence among certain occupational or other population groups can sit alongside much lower background prevalence. For example, Ghana, a country with a very extensive surveillance system, has found only one site

[a]Antenatal surveillance has become the standard instrument for estimating HIV prevalence globally. In most of Africa, antenatal surveillance data are the basis for population estimates of HIV prevalence. Other broad-based population samples of prevalence or incidence are not common in Africa.

of 23 where antenatal prevalence is above 5%, and national adult prevalence is estimated at 3.4%. However, prevalence among sex workers in Accra, Ghana, has been found to be 72.6% (7,8).

Over time, the size of the HIV epidemics across sub–Saharan Africa has become steadily larger (Figure 1). However, this trend has not been universal. In parts of sub–Saharan Africa prevalence has remained low. In Senegal, for example, national HIV prevalence is estimated at less than 2%, and antenatal surveillance sites find an average prevalence of only 1% (9). There are also national as well as more local examples of high prevalence rates that have been reduced as a result of large-scale and sustained changes in behavior, such as in urban Uganda, in Lusaka, Zambia, and in the Mbeya region of Tanzania. Even though the aggregate rate of growth of the HIV epidemic across Africa appears to be stable, it is not clear to what extent a natural epidemiologic equilibrium has been reached, even in the most heavily affected countries (1).

This chapter deals with the determinants of the spread of HIV, together with prevention interventions, the demographic and social impact of AIDS, and the future of responses to the epidemic.

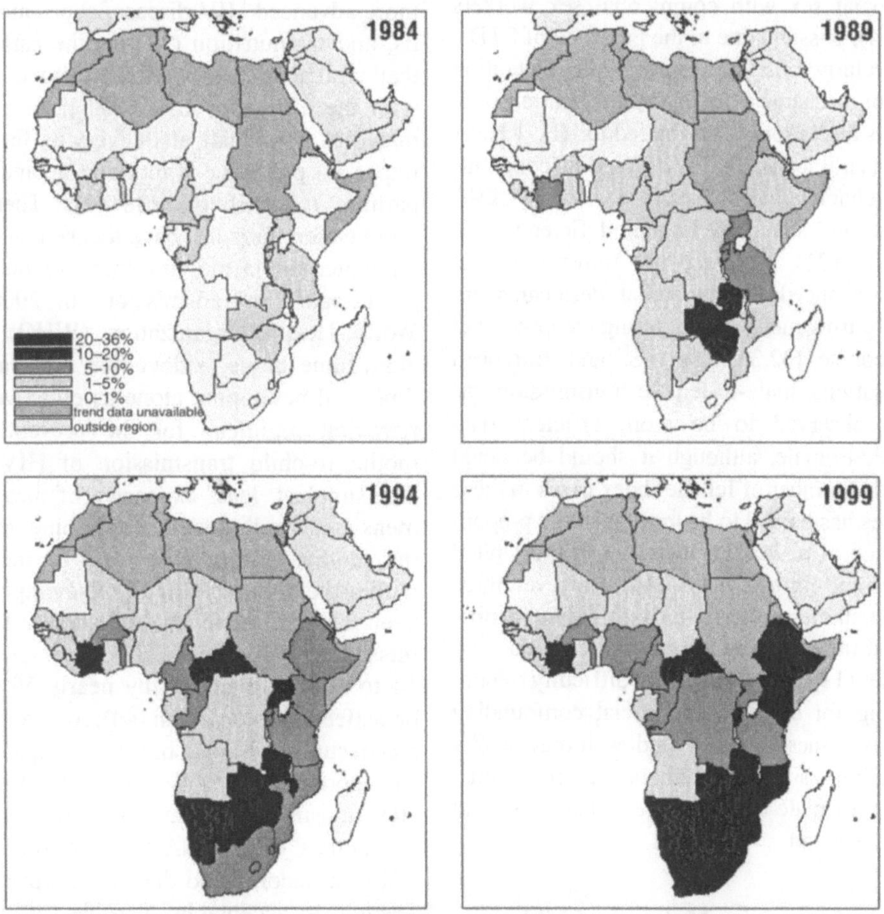

FIGURE 1. Spread of HIV in Africa, 1984–1999: Estimated HIV prevalence rates among 15- to 49-year-olds in sub–Saharan African countries in 1984, 1989, 1994 and 1999.

MODES OF TRANSMISSION

Heterosexual Transmission

In Africa, the predominant mode of HIV transmission is heterosexual contact. Nonetheless, heterosexual intercourse is a relatively inefficient mode of transmission. Studies conducted in Europe, the United States, Thailand, and Uganda have found transmission probabilities for heterosexual couples to be between .0001 and .0020 per episode of sexual intercourse, although such probability can be increased several-fold in the presence of genital inflammation and lesions due to STDs (10–22). Higher probabilities of transmission were reported in Thailand and Kenya for heterosexual sex with commercial sex workers (23,24), possibly due to the presence of STDs, particularly those that cause genital ulceration (11) or discharge (25). Probability of transmission is also strongly correlated to HIV-1 RNA level (viral load) (11,26–29), and its concomitant characteristics, such as lower $CD4^{+}$ counts and advanced immunodeficiency (13, 15–18,30,31). Heterosexual transmission is also enhanced when vaginal desiccants are used, during menses, and during receptive anal intercourse (32,33). In U.S. and European populations, male-to-female transmission has been observed to be more efficient than female-to-male, although it should be noted that the number of female index cases in these studies has tended to be low, given the preponderance of male HIV infection in the United States and Europe (12–17,34). However, three recent studies in Africa have found no significant differences in transmission efficiency by gender (11,18,25). Given the difficulty of controlling for biologic and social confounding factors in these types of studies, it may be that prevailing assumptions about the greater efficiency of male-to-female transmission should be questioned.

Transmission from Mother to Child

Over 90% of the 2.4 million children under the age of 15 who are living with HIV in sub–Saharan Africa acquired infection from their mothers (1,2). In the absence of drug intervention and with breastfeeding by HIV-1–infected mothers, there is a 30% to 35% cumulative HIV-1 transmission rate through intrauterine, intrapartum, and postpartum exposure (35). In contrast, in industrialized countries, where antiretroviral therapy is available, the rate of transmission is 4% to 6% (36), and has been reduced even further by frequent caesarian section. In sub–Saharan Africa the high rate of mother-to-child transmission is attributable to a lack of access for women to both HIV care and to ante- and postnatal care, together with the predominance of breastfeeding, and the higher proportion of women in Africa with more advanced HIV disease, chorioamnionitis, and malnutrition (37). In the same way that viral load has been found to correlate with the efficiency of sexual transmission, maternal viral load at delivery is the most important predictor of intrauterine and intrapartum transmission (38–42). Therefore, intervention therapies have focused on reducing maternal plasma viral load to reduce risk of intrapartum transmission. In 2000, the World Health Organization (WHO) listed zidovudine alone, zidovudine plus lamivudine, and nevirapine alone as effective antiretroviral regimens for the prevention of mother-to-child transmission of HIV (43). The simplest, least expensive of these regimens is a single dose of nevirapine given to the mother during labor and to the baby within the first days of life. Nevirapine has been found to reduce the risk of HIV-1 transmission from mother to child during the first 14 to 16 weeks of life by nearly 50% in a breastfeeding population (44). According to a recent study in Kenya, breastfeeding accounts for approximately 44% of the total rate of HIV transmission from mother to child over 24 months (45). UNAIDS, the WHO, and UNICEF recommend that when replacement feeding is acceptable, feasible, affordable, sustainable, and safe, HIV-infected mothers should avoid all breastfeeding, and otherwise, exclusive breastfeeding is recommended during the first months of life (35). Among the evidence that informed this recommendation was a study conducted in Durban, South Africa; the results of this study, which were first published in 1999, showed that exclusive breastfeeding is associated with a lower risk of HIV transmission than mixed feeding, possibly because of the damage to the bowel caused by contaminated formula, facilitating the entry of HIV in breast milk into infant tissues (46).

Transfusion

Blood transfusion is the third most important mode of HIV-1 transmission in Africa, although its proportional significance has declined in comparison to the massive increases in sexual transmission. Transfusion is the most efficient way to transmit HIV-1: 90% of recipients of seropositive blood become infected (47). African women and children in particular are exposed to HIV-1–contaminated blood because of the high rate of transfusion required for malaria-induced anemia, sickle cell disease, and obstetric complications (48–51). Data on HIV transmission by blood transfusion in Africa are scarce. AIDS surveillance data collated by UNAIDS and WHO for 20 countries in sub–Saharan Africa are categorized by mode of transmission: the proportion of total AIDS cases between 1996 and 1999 caused by contaminated blood ranges from 0.1% to 5.3% in the 10 countries for which some transmission via blood or blood products is reported (52).

In 1994, Kenya became the first sub–Saharan country to evaluate risk of transmission by transfusion. Collection and screening of blood in Kenya is done at the hospital level, which is the most cost-effective approach for a developing country (50). The National Blood Transfusion Service serves as an oversight agency, rather than a centralized blood bank. The study found that 2% of transfusions transmitted HIV infections (51). Though blood screening eliminated more than two-thirds of infected donations, poor laboratory practices were faulted as the major source of error. In response, the Ministry of Health introduced a quality assurance program and reforms to its training programs. In Cameroon, a five-year evaluation study found one transfusion-related HIV infection in over 40,000 blood donations, and 20% of blood donations were rejected following screening for HIV and Hepatitis B (53). Transmission of HIV by transfusion has been reduced to minimal numbers in industrialized countries (54, 55). Many developing countries mandate screening systems, but international support for such programs has waned (56). The basic components of a successful blood safety system are: the consistent and reliable use of HIV screening tests; donor deferral; the recruitment of safe donors; and the more conservative use of blood. The implementation of such precautionary measures will also certainly decrease the transmission of hepatitis B, C, and D, syphilis, and HTLV by transfusion (50). Blood-transfusion-acquired HIV infection is one of the more dismal consequences of poverty and the deterioration of health services in many African countries.

Injections

The risk of HIV infection among health care workers exposed to a needlestick injury is 0.3% (57–60). This figure may underestimate the risk of HIV infection associated with unsafe injections since the studies upon which this estimate was generated were conducted in industrialized countries where post-exposure prophylaxis is available. One study has estimated that unsafe injection accounts for around 100,000 or 2% of the new cases of HIV that occur globally each year (61).

Transmission through the other principal modes known globally, namely needle sharing by injecting drug users and male-to-male sex, are not well documented in Africa. As elsewhere in the world, there is no evidence of routes of transmission other than those mentioned in this section. In particular, arthropod-borne transmission has never been documented and the epidemiology of HIV does not support this mode of transmission.

FACTORS AFFECTING THE SPREAD OF HIV-1

The patterns of spread of HIV-1 in Africa are heterogeneous, even at village levels. Understanding this heterogeneity is important for adapting prevention strategies to specific populations and areas. No single factor, whether biologic or behavioral, determines the epidemiologic patterns of HIV-1 infection. Instead, it is the complex interaction between several factors, including a degree of historical accident, that determines how and where HIV-1 spreads in populations. The timeframe over which the spread of HIV should be gauged is measured in decades. In the absence of facilitating factors, HIV-1 can remain endemic for many years. However, in the presence of the compounding social and biologic factors that facilitate its spread, the growth of the epidemic can become explosive, with major shifts in prevalence apparent within periods of less than a year. In general, the HIV epidemic is characterized by a long incubation period of slow viral spread until a critical rate of prevalence is reached and spread accelerates.

Viral Parameters

There is a high degree of genetic variability in HIV, due to its high rate of recombination (62), the error-prone nature of its reverse transcriptase (63,64), and the speed of its replication in vivo (65,66). Thus, there is variation in the virus genome within each host, and even greater variation between hosts (67,68). Phylogenetic analysis of nucleotide sequences of the HIV-1 genome has made it possible to classify the various forms of HIV, which is helpful in tracking local and global transmission patterns. HIV-1 strains can be classified into three groups: M (major), N (non-M, non-O), and O (outlier). The latter two are limited to west central Africa (Cameroon and neighboring countries). Group O's highest prevalence in these areas is only 2% to 5% of HIV-1–positive samples (69,70), and group N has only been identified in two isolates from Cameroonian patients (71,72). Group M, the most common globally, is further divided into nine subtypes (A–D, F–H, J, K), and several circulating recombinant forms (CRFs). The highly variable *env* and *gag* genes of the HIV-1 genome were originally used to classify subtypes. With the increased efficiency of full-length genomic sequencing (73,74), it was proposed that at least three full-length genomes be required to identify novel forms of the virus (74–76). Amino acid sequences vary by as much as 20% within a subtype, and by 25% to 35% between subtypes (77). Subtypes E and I have been reclassified as recombinant. Recombination can occur when an individual is superinfected with two or more subtypes or groups of HIV-1. Coinfection with HIV-1 and HIV-2 can also occur, but recombinants of the two types have not been reported. Twenty percent to 25% of HIV-1 viruses are estimated to be recombinant in areas where multiple subtypes cocirculate (67,78).

The proportional distribution of HIV-1 subtypes may remain consistent over time in areas where the HIV epidemic is stable (for example, subtypes A and D in Uganda). Alternatively, the introduction of new subtypes may lead to an increased spread of HIV-1 in a short period of time (for example, in injecting drug users in Kaliningrad, Russia) (79,80). Subtype C is the most predominant globally, accounting for 48% of prevalent HIV-1 infections and a higher proportion of new infections (67) (Figure 2). It dominates southern and southeast Africa. The greatest genetic diversity is found in central Africa, where all HIV-1 groups and subtypes have been reported (69,72,81). The most common subtypes in East Africa are A

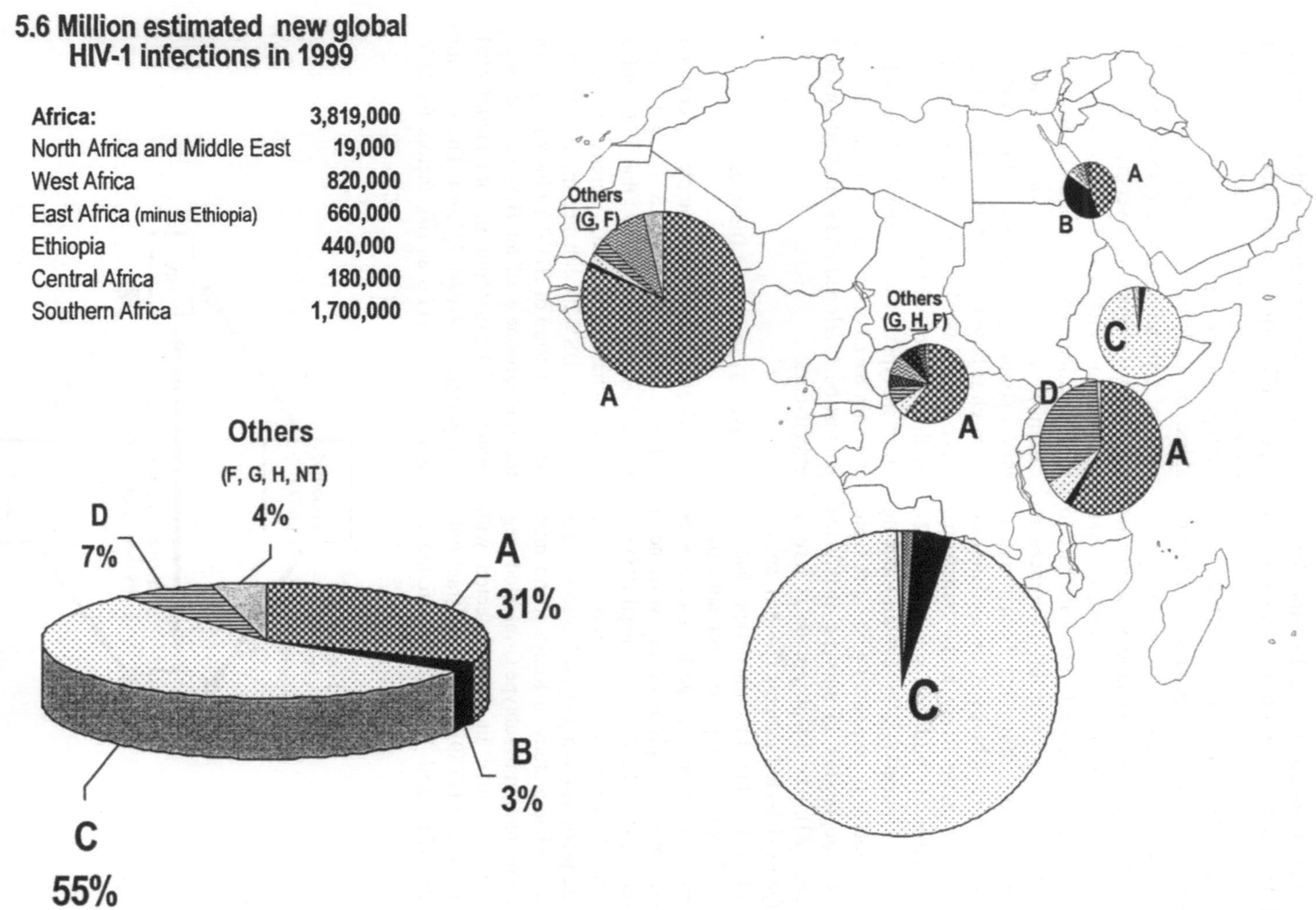

FIGURE 2. Estimated distribution of new HIV-1 infections in Africa in 1999 by *env* subtypes.

and D (67), and in West and central Africa, CRF02_AG. HIV-2 has been limited mainly to West Africa.

The relationship between HIV-1 subtype and the biologic properties that affect its transmissibility and disease progression is not well understood. Intersubtype studies are complicated by factors such as host, societal, and virologic characteristics that are hard to control. Recent evidence of differences in subtype transmissibility has been found in Tanzania where subtype A or recombinant forms were more likely to be transmitted from mother to child than subtype D (82). The fast-replicating, syncytium-inducing (SI) phenotype is associated with more rapid disease progression in subtype B-infected patients (83). The SI phenotype is rare in subtype C-infected patients (84–86), so it is not clear whether this phenotype has the same clinical consequences for subtype C infection. It has been suggested that subtype D is the most strongly associated with the SI phenotype (87). Studies in Senegal (88) and Uganda (80) have shown that there is slower disease progression in subtype A-infected individuals, while a study in Kenya found more rapid progression in subtype C-infected pregnant women than in those infected with subtypes A or D (89). Studies in Israel (90), Sweden (91), and Thailand (92) found no differences among patients with varying subtypes. It is hard to know whether these results are actually due to biologic factors relating to subtype, or are confounded by other variables. In addition to possible variation in rates of transmission and disease progression, HIV-1's genetic diversity has other implications. Viral load assays, an important tool in patient management and assessment, can have varying sensitivities to different HIV strains (67,93,94). Most vaccine research is based on subtype B antigens and it is not clear whether the vaccines developed by this research will offer protection against other subtypes as well. Therefore, candidate vaccines based on strains other than subtype B must be developed and evaluated for their effectiveness.

Sexually Transmitted Diseases

Figure 3 shows the complex interaction between HIV infection and STDs (95). There is substantial evidence that ulcerative STDs—chanchroid and, increasingly predominant, HSV-2—enhance the risk of sexual transmission of HIV-1 by increasing both the infectiousness of an HIV-infected individual and the susceptibility of an uninfected sex partner to HIV-1 (21,96). The case for nonulcerative STDs as risk factors for HIV

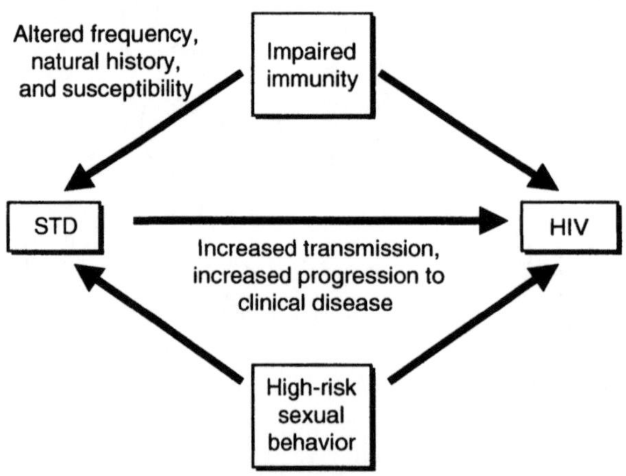

FIGURE 3. Interactions between sexually transmitted diseases and HIV.

transmission is less certain. In a prospective study among female sex workers in Kinshasa, infection with gonorrhea, chlamydia, or trichomoniasis during the presumed period of exposure to HIV were all significantly associated with HIV-1 seroconversion, even after controlling for the number of sexual contacts and frequency of condom use (33). A multicenter study of factors determining the differential spread of HIV in four African cities found trichomoniasis was more common in the two high-prevalence cities studied than in the two low-prevalence ones (97). Sexually transmitted disease prevalence rates are generally higher in urban populations, but vary between regions. The attributable risk of STDs in the transmission of HIV remains to be quantified, and the impact of STD control on the spread of HIV remains a complex issue. Apparently contradictory results were obtained from large-scale randomized trials: in Mwanza, Tanzania, STD management was significantly associated with reduced HIV incidence, while in Rakai, Uganda, STD treatment resulted in no such effect (98,99). Irrespective of the magnitude of the effects of STDs on HIV-1 transmission, sexual behavior change remains relatively powerful in reducing HIV-1 transmission compared to STD treatment at the levels achieved in the Mwanza and Rakai trials (100). Nevertheless, treatment of systemic and genital tract infections does have overall preventive benefits in reducing HIV infectivity and susceptibility (11,25,101). As well, there are service-provision synergies to be obtained from including STD management in the context of HIV control (102).

Recent meta-analyses have concluded that male circumcision is associated with a reduced risk of HIV infection, especially in high-risk populations where genital ulcerative diseases are more prevalent (103,104). However, it is not at all clear how a widescale program of prepubertal circumcision could be implemented, given religious, cultural, and service-provision considerations.

Sexual Behavior

Sexual behavior is undoubtedly the most important determinant of the spread of HIV. Patterns of sexual behavior are not uniform within or between countries, age groups, genders, or different social classes, and this diversity contributes to the epidemiologic heterogeneity of the HIV epidemic in Africa (105). High numbers of lifetime sexual partners have been consistently found to be associated with greater likelihood of HIV infection (106). In addition, higher rates of partner change, particularly in commercial sex, are associated with greater likelihood of HIV infection at the individual level. The rate of engagement in commercial sex may be increased in populations with large numbers of single migrant men, high male-to-female ratios (as is the case in many large cities in eastern and southern Africa) (107), and in situations where marriage for men tends to be delayed due to a lack of resources or higher education, or the ease of finding partners outside of marriage (108). There is major variation across Africa in age at first sexual intercourse and the extent of sex with non-regular partners, including commercial sex workers (109). At least during the initial phase of an epidemic, when HIV prevalence in the general population is still low, there may be slower spread of HIV where the predominant sexual mixing pattern is one of serial relationships involving roughly equal numbers of men and women, rather than patterns of multiple concurrent relationships (110). As the HIV epidemic progresses, an increasing number of people are infected who do not necessarily practice particularly elevated HIV risk behaviors. Thus, surveys in Rwanda, former Zaire, and Kenya found that an increasing proportion of women with HIV-1 infection reported regular partners or husbands as their sole sexual contact (111–113). Across sub–Saharan Africa, women now have higher HIV-1 infection rates than men, accounting for 55% of cumulative infections (114). This may be due to higher rates of transmission from men to women, but it may also be an effect of the younger age at which women tend to be infected (115). Also, in many societies throughout the world, men have sexual relationships with younger women.

Accounting for different rates of HIV spread resulting from demographic factors that affect sexual transmission is complex. In a major study comparing two high-prevalence cities in sub–Saharan Africa (Kisumu in Kenya and Ndola in Zambia), with two low-prevalence cities (Cotonou in Benin and Yaoundé in Cameroon), factors such as high rates of partner change, sex with sex workers, concurrent sexual partners, and condom use did not differ between the high- and low-prevalence cities. Young age at women's first sexual intercourse, young age at first marriage, age difference between spouses, prevalence of HSV-2 or trichomoniasis, and lack of male circumcision were the factors that were more common in the high-prevalence cities (116). This study suggests that variation in rates of HIV-1 prevalence can be explained in part by differences in transmissibility; that HIV and STD epidemics, especially HSV-2, reinforce one another; and that the degree of sexual behavior change required to alter the dynamics of the HIV epidemic is substantial.

Demographic Variables

The most sexually active age groups represent a much larger proportion of the population in sub–Saharan Africa than in the industrialized world. This circumstance alone leads to higher incidence rates of STDs and HIV infection in sub–Saharan Africa. In addition, because of high birth rates, the population of young adults will become even larger in the near future, although HIV is having an impact on population patterns. The gender balance of a population, affecting the supply and demand of sexual contact between men and women, is an important determinant of HIV-1 epidemiology (117). Cities with an imbalance in this supply and demand may experience a more rapid spread of HIV-1. The urban preponderance of men (usually due to migration of male laborers into cities), social constraints on sexuality (such as the tendency of men to marry later in life than women), and the social prohibition of premarital and extramarital sex for women, may lead to such imbalances. Urban demographic patterns may have a marked influence on sexual behavior by favoring sex work and high rates of STDs. The distribution of HIV-1 in urban and rural populations also changes over the course of the epidemic: while earlier in the epidemic, prevalence among rural populations was often lower than in urban populations, these differences have been reduced as the epidemic has matured (118). In some cases, response to the epidemic has been more marked in urban settings, resulting in reductions in incidence that have not been matched in rural settings (119)

Economic and Political Parameters

Poverty has always been a driving force of epidemics. This is true of HIV, with migration, separation of families, poor education, and prostitution catalyzing the spread of the virus. It is striking, however, that at least in Rwanda, Zaire, and Zambia, HIV-1 infection rates among men were initially highest among those with the highest income or education levels (120,121). These higher rates may reflect increased opportunities for travel and sexual encounters. However, the spread of HIV among the highly educated upper classes was more significant only at the beginning of the epidemic, and may have been specific to men.

AIDS exacerbates and prolongs poverty in every context, while poverty increases vulnerability to HIV and AIDS. In particular, this relationship between AIDS and poverty has had a tremendously negative impact on households. For example, in 1996 the proportion of people living in poverty in Botswana had fallen to 38% from 49% a decade earlier, but in another decade, AIDS will result in its returning to 45% (122). In poorer households, AIDS-related expenses require a greater proportion of the available expenditure, and limits access to everything from health care to food.

War in Uganda has likely contributed greatly to the country's AIDS epidemic, and social disturbance is often accompanied by an increased incidence of STDs. In addition, both preventive and curative health services are largely disrupted, if not interrupted, in such times. For example, all preventive efforts, including social marketing and interventions targeted to sex workers, were interrupted in Kinshasa in 1991 as a result of a major political crisis.

THE IMPACT ON MORBIDITY AND MORTALITY

AIDS has a uniquely devastating impact on mortality: the toll of AIDS deaths will continue to rise in the coming years as a result of infections that have already occurred, and HIV infection rates are highest among young women and men in their most productive years and when transmission from mother to child is a further risk. In twenty years time in a number of African countries the standard population pyramid will have turned upside down, with more adults in their 60s and 70s than those in their 40s and 50s. Based on the current incidence and mortality patterns, the lifetime risk of contracting HIV, and in all probability dying from AIDS, exceeds 50% for today's 15-year-olds in a number of African countries where HIV prevalence exceeds 20% (2) (Figure 4).

Drops in life expectancies are beginning to occur (Figure 5), and four countries—Botswana, Malawi, Mozambique, and Swaziland—now have a life expectancy of less than 40 years. Were it not for HIV/AIDS, average life expectancy in sub-Saharan Africa would be approximately 62 years; instead, it is currently about 47 years. In South Africa, the average life expectancy is only 47 years instead of 66, the number it would have been if AIDS were not a factor (1).

The number of African children who had lost their mother or both parents to the AIDS epidemic by the end of 2000—12.1 million—is forecast to more than double over the next decade (1). These orphans are

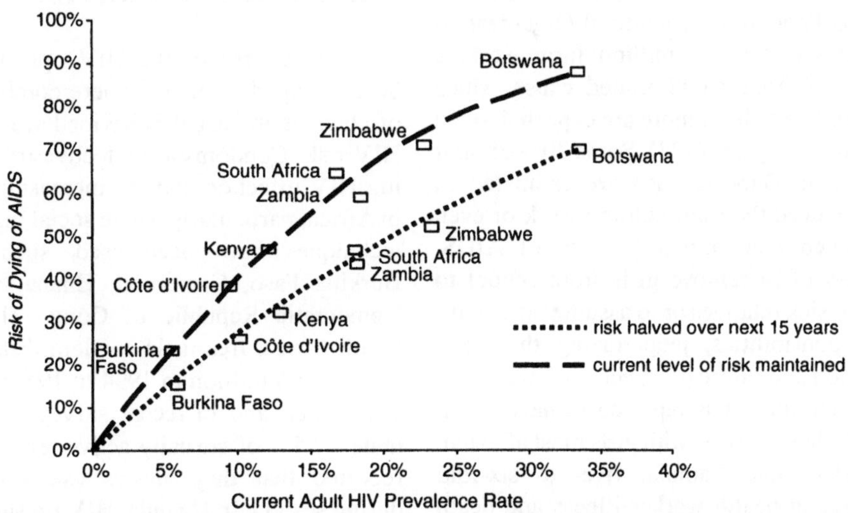

FIGURE 4. Lifetime risk of AIDS death for 15-year-old boys, assuming unchanged or halved risk of becoming infected with HIV, selected countries.

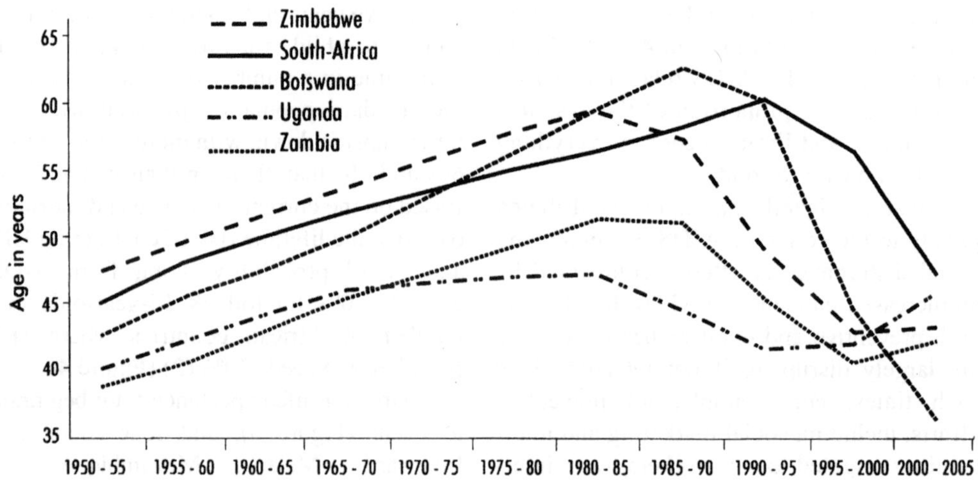

FIGURE 5. Changes in life expectancy in selected African countries with high HIV-1 prevalence.

especially vulnerable to the epidemic and the impoverishment and precariousness it brings.

AIDS has its most severe economic impact on those who are already economically or socially vulnerable. Studies in Rwanda have shown that households with an HIV or AIDS patient spend, on average, 20 times more on health care annually than households without an AIDS patient. Only a third of those households can manage to meet these extra costs (1). The United Nations Food and Agricultural Organization estimates that seven million farm workers have died from AIDS-related causes since 1985 and 16 million more are expected to die in the next 20 years (123). Some 20% of rural families in Burkina Faso are estimated to have reduced their agricultural work or even abandoned their farms because of AIDS. Families often remove girls from school to care for sick relatives or to assume other family responsibilities, jeopardizing the girls' education and future prospects. In Swaziland, school enrollment is reported to have fallen by 36% due to AIDS, with girls most affected. In Malawi and Zambia, five- to six-fold increases in health worker illness and death rates have reduced personnel, increasing stress levels and workload for the remaining employees. In 1999 alone, an estimated 860,000 children lost their teachers to AIDS in sub–Saharan Africa. In the Central African Republic, AIDS was the cause of 85% of the 300 teacher deaths that occurred in 2000. Already, by the late 1990s, the death toll had forced the closure of more than 100 educational establishments in that country (1).

THE IMPACT OF PREVENTION

The course of the HIV epidemic has been changed in places where combinations of changes in sexual behavior have reduced HIV risk. Condoms are effective in preventing HIV infection and are increasingly used in Africa, particularly where social marketing techniques have been used, such as in Burkina Faso, Cameroon, Ghana, and the Democratic Republic of Congo (124). In South Africa, free male condom distribution rose from 6 million in 1994 to 198 million 5 years later, and in recent surveys, approximately 55% of sexually active teenage girls reported that they always use a condom during sex (1). In Uganda, HIV prevalence in pregnant women in urban areas has fallen for 8 years in a row, from a high of 29.5% in

1992 to 11.25% in 2000. With comprehensive HIV prevention efforts that reach down to village levels, Uganda's response to AIDS has boosted condom use across the country. In the Masindi and Pallisa districts, for instance, condom use with casual partners rose from 42% and 31% respectively in 1997, to 51% and 53% respectively in 2000 (1). In the capital, Kampala, almost 98% of sex workers surveyed in 2000 said they had used a condom the last time they had sex (1). The impact of condom use on the incidence of HIV-1 infection in prostitutes has been well documented in Kinshasa and Nairobi (125, 126), and condom promotion, where successful, has slowed the spread of HIV.

The effects of behavioral change on HIV prevalence are clearest in younger populations. In Zambia, for example, HIV prevalence for women under 20 attending antenatal clinics in Lusaka declined from 27% in 1993 to 17% by 1998 and outside major urban areas the rate has declined from 14% in 1994 to 6% in 1998 (9). In the Mbeya region of Tanzania prevalence in antenatal clinic attendees aged 15 to 24 has dropped from its 1994 peak of 20% to 15% in 1999 (127). In Uganda the peak of prevalence across the population of close to 14% in the early 1990s has since declined to around 8%, and the declining prevalence observed in pregnant women attending sentinel antenatal clinics has been confirmed by rural cohort data (128).

TUBERCULOSIS AND HIV

At least one disease of major public health significance has been greatly affected by HIV infection: the incidence of tuberculosis (TB) has risen drastically wherever HIV has become endemic in Africa (129–132). Surveillance data from Burundi, the Central African Republic, Tanzania, and Zambia show that the incidence of TB has at least doubled in recent years, suggesting that the increased incidence is attributable to HIV infection. HIV-induced immunodeficiency is thought to lead to reactivation of latent infection with *Mycobacterium tuberculosis* and may be the driving force behind the resurgence of TB. Reported HIV seroprevalence rates among TB patients in Africa now range from between 12% and 55%, with most studies finding rates between 30% and 50% (129). The incidence of TB among people with HIV has been estimated at 4% per year, which is 30 to 40 times higher than that in HIV-uninfected people (133–135).

One problem hampering TB control programs is the high mortality rate among TB patients with HIV infection, which is primarily due to HIV-related diseases (136). A 5- to 10-fold increase in skin rashes, including the fatal Stevens-Johnson syndrome, has been described during anti-TB therapy in HIV-positive patients (137). The relapse rate of TB is markedly increased in people with HIV (138).

CONCLUSION

The impact of HIV-1 on Africa has been devastating, and the number of people already infected with HIV means that its impact will inevitably worsen in coming decades. However, the lessons learned from the successful responses to this problem, which have resulted in sustained reductions in HIV prevalence in some areas, demonstrate that it is possible to reduce the spread of the epidemic and to mitigate its impact. To do so requires comprehensive responses that take account not only of the heterogeneity of the epidemic but the complex social, population, and biologic dynamics that determine the course of the epidemic.

There can be no shortcut substitute for broad social mobilization in responding to HIV. The two-decade-long history of responses to AIDS is already littered with failed attempts to devise one-time, universally applicable, technically driven solutions. Massive rollout of antiretroviral therapy, STD treatment, and male circumcision are merely the latest of these. Despite the intrinsic merits, at least of antiretroviral therapy and STD treatment, these interventions alone will not provide plausible solutions to the crises caused by the spread and impact of HIV in Africa. Even an effective HIV vaccine is unlikely to be universally available and acceptable, or to confer complete sterilizing immunity. For the foreseeable future, the solutions to AIDS will be developed in the complex territory formed at the intersection of politics, science, and mass mobilization. The principal determinant of the future course of the HIV epidemic in Africa will remain African leadership, from village levels and up.

ACKNOWLEDGMENTS

We thank Mark Krakauer for his contributions to this chapter while an intern with UNAIDS. We also thank Johan Goeman and Marie Laga, Institute of Tropical Medicine, Antwerp, Belgium who with Peter Piot authored the version of this chapter in the first edition of *AIDS in Africa*.

REFERENCES

1. UNAIDS and WHO. AIDS Epidemic Update December 2001. Geneva, Switzerland: UNAIDS and WHO, 2001.
2. Piot P, Bartos M, Ghys PD, et al. The global impact of HIV/AIDS. *Nature*, 2001;410:968–973.
3. World Health Organization. The World Health Report 2000. Health systems: improving performance. Geneva: World Health Organization, 2000.
4. Mogae F, Phumaphi HJ, Khan AB, et al. Botswana 2000 HIV Sero-Prevalence Sentinel Survey amongst Pregnant Women and Men with Sexually Transmitted Diseases. Technical Report. National AIDS Coordinating Agency, AIDS/STD Unit, District Health Teams, WHO, CDC, December 2000. Cited in: US Census Bureau HIV/AIDS Surveillance Data Base Summary Tables. Table 3: Detailed Listing of Estimates of HIV-1 & HIV-2 Seroprevalence, by Residence and Risk Factor, for Developing Countries: Circa 2000. Available at: http://www.census.gov/ipc/www/hivtable.html. Accessed 5 February 2002.
5. HIV/AIDS surveillance data base, June 2000. United States Bureau of the Census, Population Division, International Programs Center. Available at: http://www.census.gov.
6. Department of Health, Republic of South Africa. *National HIV and Syphilis Sero-Prevalence Survey of Women Attending Public Antenatal Clinics in South Africa*. Pretoria: Department of Health, 2001.
7. Ghana Ministry of Health. HIV Sentinel Surveillance 1998. Report. Accra, Ghana: Disease Control Unit, Ministry of Health, July 1999. Cited in US Census Bureau HIV/AIDS Surveillance Data Base Summary Tables. Table 3: Detailed Listing of Estimates of HIV-1 & HIV-2 Seroprevalence, by Residence and Risk Factor, for Developing Countries: Circa 2000. Available at: http://www.census.gov/ipc/www/hivtable.html. Accessed 5 February 2002.
8. Mingle JA, Asamoah-Adu A, Bekoe V. Trends in Human Immunodeficiency Virus (HIV) Infection in Sexually Active Ghanaian Women. Poster at: 12th World AIDS Conference; June 28–July 3, 1998; Geneva, Switzerland. Poster 23593. Cited in US Census Bureau HIV/AIDS Surveillance Data Base Summary Tables. Table 3: Detailed Listing of Estimates of HIV-1 & HIV-2 Seroprevalence, by Residence and Risk Factor, for Developing Countries: Circa 2000. Available at: http://www.census.gov/ipc/www/hivtable.html. Accessed 5 February 2002.
9. UNAIDS. AIDS in Africa, Country by Country. UNAIDS/00.30E. Geneva, Switzerland: UNAIDS, 2000.
10. de Vincenzi I. A longitudinal study of human immunodeficiency virus transmission by heterosexual partners. European Study Group on Heterosexual Transmission of HIV. *N Engl J Med*, 1994;331:341–346.
11. Gray RH, Wawer MJ, Brookmeyer R, et al. Probability of HIV-1 transmission per coital act in monogamous, heterosexual, HIV-1-discordant couples in Rakai, Uganda. *Lancet*, 2001;357:1149–1153.
12. Mastro TD, Kitayaporn D. HIV type 1 transmission probabilities: estimates from epidemiological studies. *AIDS Res Hum Retroviruses*, 1998; 14(Suppl 3):S223–S227.
13. Nicolosi A, Correa Leite ML, Musicco M, et al. The efficiency of male-to-female and female-to-male sexual transmission of the human immunodeficiency virus: a study of 730 stable couples. Italian Study Group on HIV Heterosexual Transmission. *Epidemiology*, 1994;5:570–575.
14. Padian NS, Shiboski SC, Jewell NP. Female-to-male transmission of human immunodeficiency virus. *JAMA*, 1991;266:1664–1667.

15. Royce RA, Sena A, Cates W, Jr., et al. Sexual transmission of HIV. *N Engl J Med*, 1997;336: 1072–1078.
16. Mayer KH, Anderson DJ. Heterosexual HIV transmission. *Infect Agents Dis*, 1995;4:273–284.
17. O'Brien TR, Busch MP, Donegan E, et al. Heterosexual transmission of human immunodeficiency virus type 1 from transfusion recipients to their sex partners. *J Acquir Immune Defic Syndr*, 1994;7:705–710.
18. Fideli US, Allen SA, Musonda R, et al. Virologic and immunologic determinants of heterosexual transmission of human immunodeficiency virus type 1 in Africa. *AIDS Res Hum Retroviruses*, 2001;17:901–910.
19. Auvert B, Buonamico G, Lagarde E, et al. Sexual behavior, heterosexual transmission, and the spread of HIV in sub–Saharan Africa: a simulation study. *Comput Biomed Res*, 2000;33:84–96.
20. Cohen MS. Sexually transmitted diseases enhance HIV transmission: no longer a hypothesis. *Lancet*, 1998;351(Suppl 3):5–7.
21. Fleming DT, Wasserheit JN. From epidemiological synergy to public health policy and practice: the contribution of other sexually transmitted diseases to sexual transmission of HIV infection. *Sex Transm Infect*, 1999;75:3–17.
22. Cameron DW, Simonsen JN, D'Costa LJ, et al. Female to male transmission of human immunodeficiency virus type 1: risk factors for seroconversion in men. *Lancet*, 1989; 2:403–407.
23. Laga M, Nziia N, Goeman J. The interrelationship of sexually transmitted diseases and HIV infection: implications for the control of both epidemics in Africa. *AIDS*, 1991:5:555–563.
24. Mastro TD, Satten GA, Nopkesorn T, et al. Probability of female-to-male transmission of HIV-1 in Thailand. *Lancet*, 1994;343:204–207.
25. Quinn TC, Wawer MJ, Sewankambo N, et al. Viral load and heterosexual transmission of human immunodeficiency virus type 1. Rakai Project Study Group. *N Engl J Med*, 2000;342:921–929.
26. Lee TH, Sakahara N, Fiebig E, et al. Correlation of HIV-1 RNA levels in plasma and heterosexual transmission of HIV-1 from infected transfusion recipients. *J Acquir Immune Defic Syndr Hum Retrovirol*, 1996;12:427–428.
27. Operskalski EA, Stram DO, Busch MP, et al. Role of viral load in heterosexual transmission of human immunodeficiency virus type 1 by blood transfusion recipients. Transfusion Safety Study Group. *Am J Epidemiol*, 1997;146:655–661.
28. Pedraza MA, del Romero J, Roldan F, et al. Heterosexual transmission of HIV-1 is associated with high plasma viral load levels and a positive viral isolation in the infected partner. *J Acquir Immune Defic Syndr*, 1999;21:120–125.
29. Ragni MV, Faruki H, Kingsley LA. Heterosexual HIV-1 transmission and viral load in hemophiliac patients. *J Acquir Immune Defic Syndr Hum Retrovirol*, 1998;17:42–45.
30. Laga M, Taelman H, Van der Stuyft P, et al. Advanced immunodeficiency as a risk factor for heterosexual transmission of HIV. *AIDS*, 1989;3: 361–366.
31. Nelson KE, Rungruengthanakit K, Margolick J, et al. High rates of transmission of subtype E human immunodeficiency virus type 1 among heterosexual couples in Northern Thailand: role of sexually transmitted diseases and immune compromise. *J Infect Dis*, 1999;180:337–343.
32. Cameron DW, Simonsen JN, D'Costa W, et al. Female to male transmission of human immunodeficiency virus type I: risk factors for seroconversion in men. *Lancet*, 1989;2:403–407.
33. Laga M, Manoka A, Kivuvu M, et al. Non-ulcerative sexually transmitted diseases as risk factors for HIV-I transmission in women: results from a cohort study. *AIDS*, 1993;7:95–102.
34. Padian N, Marquis L, Francis DP, et al. Male-to-female transmission of human immunodeficiency virus. *JAMA*, 1987;258:788–790.
35. UNAIDS. New Data on the Prevention of Mother-to-Child Transmission of HIV and their Policy Implications. WHO Technical Consultation on Behalf of the UNFPA/UNICEF/WHO/UNAIDS Inter-Agency Task Team on Mother-to-Child Transmission of HIV; October 11–13, 2000; Geneva, Switzerland.
36. Luo C. Strategies for prevention of mother-to-child transmission of HIV. *Reprod Health Matters*, 2000; 8:144–155.
37. Wiktor SZ, Ekpini E, Nduati RW. Prevention of mother-to-child transmission of HIV-1 in Africa. *AIDS*, 1997;11(Suppl B):S79–S87.
38. Garcia PM, Kalish LA, Pitt J, et al. Maternal levels of plasma human immunodeficiency virus type 1 RNA and the risk of perinatal transmission. Women and Infants Transmission Study Group. *N Engl J Med*, 1999;341:394–402.
39. McGowan JP, Shah SS. Prevention of perinatal HIV transmission during pregnancy. *J Antimicrob Chemother*, 2000;46:657–668.
40. Mock PA, Shaffer N, Bhadrakom C, et al. Maternal viral load and timing of mother-to-child HIV transmission, Bangkok, Thailand. Bangkok Collaborative Perinatal HIV Transmission Study Group. *AIDS*, 1999;13:407–414.
41. Mofenson LM, Lambert JS, Stiehm ER, et al. Risk factors for perinatal transmission of human immunodeficiency virus type 1 in women treated with zidovudine. Pediatric AIDS Clinical Trials Group Study 185 Team. *N Engl J Med*, 1999;341: 385–393.

42. Shaffer N, Roongpisuthipong A, Siriwasin W, et al. Maternal virus load and perinatal human immunodeficiency virus type 1 subtype E transmission, Thailand. Bangkok Collaborative Perinatal HIV Transmission Study Group. *J Infect Dis*, 1999;179: 590–599.
43. World Health Organization. New Data on the Prevention of Mother-to-Child Transmission of HIV and their Policy Implications. Geneva: World Health Organization, 2000.
44. Guay LA, Musoke P, Fleming T, et al. Intrapartum and neonatal single-dose nevirapine compared with zidovudine for prevention of mother-to-child transmission of HIV-1 in Kampala, Uganda: HIVNET 012 randomised trial. *Lancet*, 1999;354:795–802.
45. Nduati R, John G, Mbori-Ngacha D, et al. Effect of breastfeeding and formula feeding on transmission of HIV-1: a randomized clinical trial. *JAMA*, 2000;283:1167–1174.
46. Coutsoudis A, Pillay K, Kuhn L, et al. Method of feeding and transmission of HIV-1 from mothers to children by 15 months of age: prospective cohort study from Durban, South Africa. *AIDS*, 2001;15: 379–387.
47. Donegan E, Lee H, Operskalski EA, et al. Transfusion transmission of retroviruses: human T-lymphotropic virus types I and II compared with human immunodeficiency virus type 1. *Transfusion*, 1994;34:478–483.
48. Greenberg AE, Nguyen-Dinh P, Mann JM, et al. The association between malaria, blood transfusions, and HIV seropositivity in a pediatric population in Kinshasa, Zaire. *JAMA*, 1988;259:545–549.
49. Izzia KW, Lepira B, Kayembe K, et al. Acquired immunodeficiency syndrome and homozygote sickle cell anemia. Apropos of a Zairian case. *Ann Soc Belg Med Trop*, 1984;64:391–396.
50. Jacobs B, Mercer A. Feasibility of hospital-based blood banking: a Tanzanian case study. *Health Policy Plan*, 1999;14:354–362.
51. Moore A, Herrera G, etc. Estimated risk of HIV transmission by blood transfusion in Kenya. *Lancet*, 2001;358:657–660.
52. UNAIDS and WHO 2000 Global HIV/AIDS and STD Surveillance Epidemiological Factsheets by Country. Available at: http://www.unaids.org/hivaidsinfo/statistics/fact_sheets/index_en.htm. Accessed: January 17, 2002.
53. Mbanya D, Binam F, Kaptue L. Transfusion outcome in a resource-limited setting of Cameroon: a five-year evaluation. *Int J Infect Dis*, 2001;5: 70–73.
54. Lackritz EM, Satten GA, Aberle-Grasse J, et al. Estimated risk of transmission of the human immunodeficiency virus by screened blood in the United States. *N Engl J Med*, 1995;333:1721–1725.
55. Schreiber GB, Busch MP, Kleinman SH, et al. The risk of transfusion-transmitted viral infections. The Retrovirus Epidemiology Donor Study. *N Engl J Med*, 1996;334:1685–1690.
56. Lackritz EM. Prevention of HIV transmission by blood transfusion in the developing world: achievements and continuing challenges. *AIDS*, 1998; 12(Suppl A):S81–S86.
57. Gerberding JL. Incidence and prevalence of human immunodeficiency virus, hepatitis B virus, hepatitis C virus, and cytomegalovirus among health care personnel at risk for blood exposure: final report from a longitudinal study. *J Infect Dis*, 1994;170: 1410–1417.
58. Henderson DK, Fahey BJ, Willy M, et al. Risk for occupational transmission of human immunodeficiency virus type 1 (HIV-1) associated with clinical exposures. A prospective evaluation. *Ann Intern Med*, 1990;113:740–746.
59. Ippolito G, Puro V, De Carli G. The risk of occupational human immunodeficiency virus infection in health care workers. Italian Multicenter Study. The Italian Study Group on Occupational Risk of HIV infection. *Arch Intern Med*, 1993;153:1451–1458.
60. Tokars JI, Marcus R, Culver DH, et al. Surveillance of HIV infection and zidovudine use among health care workers after occupational exposure to HIV-infected blood. The CDC Cooperative Needlestick Surveillance Group. *Ann Intern Med*, 1993;118: 913–919.
61. Hauri AM, Armstrong G, Hutin Y. Estimation of the global burden of disease attributable to contaminated injections given in health-care settings. Unpublished paper. World Health Organization, 2001.
62. Hu WS, Temin HM. Retroviral recombination and reverse transcription. *Science*, 1990;250:1227–1233.
63. Preston BD, Poiesz BJ, Loeb LA. Fidelity of HIV-1 reverse transcriptase. *Science*, 1988;242:1168–1171.
64. Roberts JD, Bebenek K, Kunkel TA. The accuracy of reverse transcriptase from HIV-1. *Science*, 1988;242:1171–1173.
65. Ho DD, Neumann AU, Perelson AS, et al. Rapid turnover of plasma virions and CD4 lymphocytes in HIV-1 infection. *Nature*, 1995;373:123–126.
66. Wei X, Ghosh SK, Taylor ME, et al. Viral dynamics in human immunodeficiency virus type 1 infection. *Nature*, 1995;373:117–122.
67. Alaeus A. Significance of HIV-1 genetic subtypes. *Scand J Infect Dis*, 2000;32:455–463.
68. Nowak MA. Variability of HIV infections. *J Theor Biol*, 1992;155:1–20.
69. Peeters M, Gueye A, MBoup S, et al. Geographical distribution of HIV-1 group O viruses in Africa. AIDS, 1997;11:493–498.
70. Zekeng L, Gurtler L, Afane ZE, et al. Prevalence of HIV-1 subtype O infection in Cameroon: preliminary results. *AIDS*, 1994;8:1626–1628.
71. Peeters M, Sharp PM. Genetic diversity of HIV-1: the moving target. *AIDS*, 2000;14(Suppl 3):S129–S140.

72. Simon F, Mauclere P, Roques P, et al. Identification of a new human immunodeficiency virus type 1 distinct from group M and group O. *Nat Med*, 1998;4:1032–1037.
73. Gao F, Robertson DL, Morrison SG, et al. The heterosexual human immunodeficiency virus type 1 epidemic in Thailand is caused by an intersubtype (A/E) recombinant of African origin. *J Virol*, 1996;70:7013–7029.
74. Salminen MO, Koch C, Sanders-Buell E, et al. Recovery of virtually full-length HIV-1 provirus of diverse subtypes from primary virus cultures using the polymerase chain reaction. *Virology*, 1995;213: 80–86.
75. McCutchan FE. Understanding the genetic diversity of HIV-1. *AIDS*, 2000;14(Suppl 3):S31–S44.
76. Robertson DL, Anderson JP, Bradac JA, et al. HIV-1 nomenclature proposal. *Science*, 2000; 288:55–56.
77. Heeney JL, Hahn BH. Vaccines and immunology: elucidating immunity to HIV-1 and current prospects for AIDS vaccine development. AIDS, 2000; 14(Suppl 3):S125–S127.
78. Robertson DL, Sharp PM, McCutchan FE, et al. Recombination in HIV-1. *Nature*, 1995;374: 124–126.
79. Liitsola K, Tashkinova I, Laukkanen T, et al. HIV-1 genetic subtype A/B recombinant strain causing an explosive epidemic in injecting drug users in Kaliningrad. *AIDS*, 1998;12:1907–1919.
80. Kaleebu P, Ross A, Morgan D, et al. Relationship between HIV-1 Env subtypes A and D and disease progression in a rural Ugandan cohort. *AIDS*, 2001;15:293–299.
81. Janssens W, Buve A, Nkengasong JN. The puzzle of HIV-1 subtypes in Africa. *AIDS*, 1997;11:705–712.
82. Blackard JT, Renjifo B, Fawzi W, et al. HIV-1 LTR subtype and perinatal transmission. *Virology*, 2001;287:261–265.
83. Tersmette M, Lange JM, de Goede RE, et al. Association between biological properties of human immunodeficiency virus variants and risk for AIDS and AIDS mortality. *Lancet*, 1989;1: 983–985.
84. Abebe A, Demissie D, Goudsmit J, et al. HIV-1 subtype C syncytium- and non-syncytium-inducing phenotypes and coreceptor usage among Ethiopian patients with AIDS. *AIDS*, 1999;13:1305–1311.
85. Peeters M, Vincent R, Perret JL, et al. Evidence for differences in MT2 cell tropism according to genetic subtypes of HIV-1: syncytium-inducing variants seem rare among subtype C HIV-1 viruses. *J Acquir Immune Defic Syndr Hum Retrovirol*, 1999;20:115–121.
86. Tscherning C, Alaeus A, Fredriksson R, et al. Differences in chemokine coreceptor usage between genetic subtypes of HIV-1. *Virology*, 1998; 241:181–188.
87. de Wolf F, Hogervorst E, Goudsmit J, et al. Syncytium-inducing and non-syncytium-inducing capacity of human immunodeficiency virus type 1 subtypes other than B: phenotypic and genotypic characteristics. WHO Network for HIV Isolation and Characterization. *AIDS Res Hum Retroviruses*, 1994;10:1387–1400.
88. Kanki PJ, Hamel DJ, Sankale JL, et al. Human immunodeficiency virus type 1 subtypes differ in disease progression. *J Infect Dis*, 1999;179:68–73.
89. Neilson JR, John GC, Carr JK, et al. Subtypes of human immunodeficiency virus type 1 and disease stage among women in Nairobi, Kenya. *J Virol*, 1999;73:4393–4403.
90. Weisman Z, Kalinkovich A, Borkow G, et al. Infection by different HIV-1 subtypes (B and C) results in a similar immune activation profile despite distinct immune backgrounds. *J Acquir Immune Defic Syndr*, 1999;21:157–163.
91. Alaèus A, Lidman K, Bjorkman A, et al. Similar rate of disease progression among individuals infected with HIV- 1 genetic subtypes A–D. *AIDS*, 1999;13:901–907.
92. Amornkul PN, Tansuphasawadikul S, Limpakarnjanarat K, et al. Clinical disease associated with HIV-1 subtype B′ and E infection among 2104 patients in Thailand. *AIDS*, 1999;13: 1963–1969.
93. Alaeus A, Lidman K, Sonnerborg A, et al. Subtype-specific problems with quantification of plasma HIV-1 RNA. *AIDS*, 1997;11:859–865.
94. Debyser Z, Van Wijngaerden E, Van Laethem K, et al. Failure to quantify viral load with two of the three commercial methods in a pregnant woman harboring an HIV type 1 subtype G strain. *AIDS Res Hum Retroviruses*, 1998;14:453–459.
95. Laga M, Nziia N, Goeman J. The interrelationship of sexually transmitted diseases and HIV infection: implications for the control of both epidemics in Africa. *AIDS*, 1991:5:555–563.
96. Johnson AM, Laga M. Heterosexual transmission of HIV. *AIDS*, 1988:2:549–556.
97. Buve A, Weiss HA, Laga M, et al. Study Group on Heterogeneity of HIV Epidemics in African Cities. The epidemiology of trichomoniasis in women in four African cities. *AIDS*, 2001;15(Suppl 4):S89–S96.
98. Grosskurth H, Mosha F, Todd J, et al. Impact of improved treatment of sexually transmitted diseases on HIV infection in rural Tanzania: randomized control trial. *Lancet*, 1995;346:530–536.
99. Wawer MJ, Gray RH, Sewankambo NK, et al. A randomized, community-based trial of intense sexually transmitted disease control for AIDS prevention, Rakai, Uganda. *AIDS*, 1998;12:1211–1225.
100. Korenromp E. *Treatment of sexually transmitted diseases as an HIV prevention strategy?*

[Unpublished MD thesis]. 264p. Rotterdam: Erasmus University, 2001.
101. Cohen MS. Preventing sexual transmission of HIV—new ideas from sub-Saharan Africa. *N Engl J Med*, 2000;342:970–972.
102. UNAIDS & WHO Consultation on STD interventions for preventing HIV: what is the evidence? Geneva, Switzerland: UNAIDS, 2001.
103. O'Farrell N, Egger M. Circumcision in men and the prevention of HIV infection: a 'meta-analysis' revisited. *Int J STD AIDS*, 2000;11:137–142.
104. Weiss HA, Quigley MA, Hayes RJ. Male circumcision and risk of HIV infection in sub-Saharan Africa: a systematic review and meta-analysis. *AIDS*, 2000;14:2361–2370.
105. Caraël M, Cleland I, Adeokun L. Overview and selected findings of sexual behavior survevs. *AIDS*, 1991;5(suppl 1):565–574.
106. Auvert B, Buve A, Ferry B, et al. Study Group on the Heterogeneity of HIV Epidemics in African Cities. Ecological and individual level analysis of risk factors for HIV infection in four urban populations in sub-Saharan Africa with different levels of HIV infection. *AIDS*, 2001;15(Suppl 4):S15–S30.
107. Larson A. Social context of human immunodeficiency virus transmission in Africa: historical and cultural bases of east and central African sexual relations. *Rev Infect Dis*, 1989;ll:716–731.
108. Caraël M., Van de Perre P, Allen S, et al. Sexually active young adults in Central Africa. In: Schinazi RF, Nahmias AJ, eds. *AIDS in Children, Adolescents and Heterosexual Adults*. New York: Elsevier Science Publishing Co., Inc., 1988:346–349.
109. Caraël M, Buvé A, Awusabo-Asare K. The Making of HIV epidemics: what are the driving forces? *AIDS*, 1997;11(B):S23–S31.
110. Morris M, Kretzschmar M. Concurrent partnerships and the spread of HIV. *AIDS*, 1997;11: 641–648.
111. Temmerman M, All FM, Ndinya-Achola J, et al. Rapid increase of both HIV-1 and syphilis among pregnant women in Nairobi, Kenya. *AIDS*, 1992;6:1181–1185.
112. Allen S, Lindan C, Serufllira A, et al. Human immunodeficiency virus infection in urban Rwanda. Demographic and behavioral correlates in a representative sample of childbearing women. *JAMA*, 1991;266:1657–1663.
113. Kamenga M, Ryder RW, Jingu M, et al. Evidence of marked sexual behavior change associated with low HIV-1 seroconversion in 149 married couples with discordant HIV-1 serostatus: experiences at an HIV counselling center in Zaire. *AIDS*, 1991;5:6167.
114. UNAIDS. Report on the global HIV/AIDS epidemic, June 2000. Geneva, Switzerland: UNAIDS, 2000.
115. Berkley S, Naamara W, Okware S, et al. AIDS and HIV infection in Uganda: are more women infected than men? *AIDS*, 1990;4:1237–1242.
116. Buve A, Carael M, Hayes RJ, et al. Study Group on Heterogeneity of HIV Epidemics in African Cities. The multicentre study on factors determining the differential spread of HIV in four African cities: summary and conclusions. *AIDS*, 2001;15(Suppl 4):S127–S131.
117. Piot P, Laga M, Ryder R, et al. The global epidemiology of HIV infection: continuity, heterogeneity, and change. *J Acquir Immune Defic Syndr*, 1990;3:403–412.
118. Glynn JR, Ponnighaus J, Crampin AC, et al. The development of the HIV epidemic in Karonga District, Malawi. *AIDS*, 2001;15:2025–2029.
119. Fylkesnes K, Musonda RM, Sichone M, et al. Declining HIV prevalence and risk behaviours in Zambia: evidence from surveillance and population-based surveys. *AIDS*, 2001;15:907–916.
120. Ryder RW, Ndilu M, Hassig SE, et al. Heterosexual transmission of HIV-1 among employees and their spouses at two large businesses in Zaire. *AIDS*, 1990;4:725–732.
121. Melbye M, Njelesani EK, Bayley A, et al. Evidence for heterosexual transmission and clinical manifestations of human immunodeficiency virus infection and related conditions in Lusaka, Zambia. *Lancet*, 1986;3:1113–1115.
122. BIDPA. Macroeconomic Impacts of the HIV/AIDS Epidemic in Botswana. Gaborone: Botswana Institute for Development Policy Analysis, 2000.
123. Food and Agriculture Organisation Web site. Focus: AIDS, A Threat to Africa. Available at: http://www.fao.org/FOCUS/E/aids/aids1-e.htm. Accessed: January 18, 2002.
124. Lamptey P, Goodridge GAW. Condom issues in AIDS prevention in Africa. *AIDS*, 1991;5(suppl 1):S183–S191.
125. Tuliza M, Manoka AT, Nzila N, et al. The impact of STD control and condom promotion on the incidence of HIV in Kinshasa prostitutes. In: Abstracts of the VII International Conference on AIDS; June 1991; Florence, Italy. Abstract MC2.
126. Moses S, Plummer FA, Ngugi EN, et al. Controlling HIV in Africa: effectiveness and cost of an intervention in a high-frequency STD transmitter core group. *AIDS*, 1991;5:407–411.
127. Jordan-Harder B, Koshuma YA, Pervilhac C, et al. Hope for Tanzania: Lessons Learned from a Decade of Comprehensive AIDS Control in Mbeya Region. Eschborn, Germany: GTZ and Dar-es-Salaam: Ministry of Health, United Republic of Tanzania, 2000.
128. Kamali A, Carpenter L, Whitworth J, et al. Seven-year trends in HIV-1 infection rates, and changes in sexual behaviour, among adults in rural Uganda. *AIDS*, 2000;14:427–434.
129. Perriens SH, Mukadi Y, Nunn P. Tuberculosis and HIV infection: implications for Africa. *AIDS*, 1991;5(suppl I):5127–5133.

130. Styblo K. Overview and epidemiological assessment of the current global tuberculosis situation with an emphasis on control in developing countries. *Rev Infect Dis*, 1989;11(suppl 2):S339–S346.
131. Standaert B, Niragira F, Kadende P, et al. The association of tuberculosis and HIV infection in Burundi. *AIDS Res Hum Retroviruses*, 1989;5:247–251.
132. Lesbordes IL, Baqillon G, Georges MC, et al. La tuberculose au cours de l'infection par le virus de l'immunodéficience humaine à Bangui (République Centrafricaine). *Méd Trop*, 1988;48:21–25.
133. Badi N, Braun M, Ryder R, et al. A retrospective cohort study of the incidence of tuberculosis (TB) among child-bearing women with HIV infection in Kinshasa, Zaire. In: Abstracts of the VI International Conference on AIDS; June 1990; San Francisco, California, USA. Abstract ThB485.
134. Wadhawan D, Hira S, Mwanza N, et al. Isoniazid prophylaxis among patients with HIV-I infection. Abstracts of the VI International Conference on AIDS; June 1990; San Francisco, California, USA. Abstract ThB510.
135. Batungwanayo I, Allen S, Bogaerts J, et al. Etude prospective du risque de tuberculose dans une cohorte de femmes VIH seropositives ~ Kigali, Rwanda. In: Abstracts of the V International Conference on AIDS in Africa; October 1990; Kinshasa, Zaire. Abstract WOD4.
136. Perriens JH, Colebunders R, Karahunga C, et al. Increased mortality and tuberculosis treatment failure rate among human immunodeficiency virus (HIV) seropositive patients compared with HIV seronegative patients with pulmonary tuberculosis treated with "standard" chemotherapy in Kinshasa, Zaire. *Am Rev Respir Dis*, 1991;144:750–755.
137. Nunn P, Kibuga D, Elliott A, et al. Impact of human immunodeficiency virus on transmission and severity of tuberculosis. *Transact Roy Soc Trop Med Hyg*, 1990;84(suppl 1):9–13.
138. Girardi E, Goletti D, Antonucci G, et al. Tuberculosis and HIV: a deadly interaction. *J Biol Regul Homeost Agents*, 2001;15:218–223.

13

Transmission of HIV

*Sibylle Kristensen, †Moses Sinkala, and *‡Sten H. Vermund

**University of Alabama School of Medicine, Birmingham, Alabama, USA.*
†Lusaka District Health Management Board, Lusaka, Zambia.
‡University of Alabama School of Public Health, Birmingham, Alabama, USA.

Sub–Saharan Africa alone bears an estimated 70% of the current burden of HIV and AIDS; 25.3 of the 36.1 million persons living with HIV or AIDS live in sub–Saharan Africa (1). Of all HIV deaths since the start of the epidemic (17.5 million adults and 4.3 million children), over three-fourths have occurred in Africa (1). Sexual transmission of HIV causes 75% to 85% of HIV infections worldwide. In Europe, North America, and parts of

Asia, men who have sex contact with men, and injection drug users (IDUs) remain at the highest risk of contracting HIV. In contrast, the spread of HIV in Africa is primarily heterosexual (2–4). HIV infection has an immense negative impact on population growth, life expectancy, and infant mortality rates in sub–Saharan Africa (5). The magnitude of HIV spread in Africa is unlike anything seen on other continents: in many countries the epidemic is generalized, affecting the general population at rates seen only among high-risk populations elsewhere.

The early spread of HIV in Africa can be viewed as that of an emerging infectious disease, influenced by changes in equilibrium between the viral agent, the human host, and the sociocultural environment (6). The severe economic and political disruptions of the 1970s (e.g., civil wars in Nigeria, Sudan, Angola; civil unrest in Zaire, South Africa, Uganda) accompanied by large-scale migrations from rural to urban areas probably brought HIV to new locations. In urban areas, sexual behaviors are not as limited by traditional taboos and familial and tribal customs as in rural settings, potentially facilitating the spread of the emerging virus. As background HIV prevalence rises, the likelihood of encountering an HIV-infected person increases, thereby improving the efficiency of HIV transmission or acquisition, and as partner exchange rates rise, HIV incidence rises (7). High partner exchange rates are common in settings where men are away from their families, a circumstance often driven by civil strife or economic hardship. Such settings include mining communities, roadside bars serving truck drivers or soldiers, and other settings where transient men have access to women selling or offering sex often accompanied by alcohol use (4).

Economic and political factors that increase HIV transmission are numerous. Lack of access to voluntary counseling and testing in many areas reduces opportunities to identify and educate HIV-infected individuals (8). Poor primary health care diminishes the control of sexually transmitted diseases (STDs), boosting the efficiency of HIV transmission. Poverty can increase the number of women in sex work, as does the number of absentee, transient men working far from home. Political leaders often fail to include HIV in their action items, to implement programs targeting marginalized populations such as commercial sex workers and alcoholics, to finance HIV prevention activities, and to respond aggressively when opportunities arise to stem the epidemic.

Many countries have distinct epidemiologic profiles. Attempts to explain the severity and magnitude of the emergence of the HIV epidemic must take into consideration the extreme heterogeneity of the contributing factors in different regions. Such factors include: frequency of sexual contact (9,10); number of sexual partners (11); risk characteristics of sexual partners (4); alcohol use and occasional use of other drugs (12); condom use (13); use of vaginal drying agents (14); background immunologic status and coinfections (15); stage of the epidemic and likelihood of encountering an infectious individual (15); circumcision in men or women (16,17); frequency of sexually transmitted diseases and access to prompt treatment (11, 18,19); plasma HIV-1 RNA levels and access to antiretroviral chemotherapies (20–24); and frequency of selected chemokine receptors and mutations (25,26). Improved understanding of the way in which these factors influence the infectiousness of HIV, individuals' susceptibility to HIV, and individuals' risk behaviors has facilitated efforts to prevent transmission of the virus.

BIOLOGIC COFACTORS OF HIV SEXUAL TRANSMISSION

Viral Factors

A variety of biologic factors are associated with risk of HIV transmission. Viral characteristics may be associated with transmission and may vary in different parts of the world. Some of these risk factors are well confirmed while others are speculative. To date, all known HIV subtypes have been identified in Africa and several subtypes are cocirculating in multiple African countries. Whether subtype B, which is uncommon in Africa but prevalent in the Americas and Europe, is less infectious than the subtypes predominantly circulating in Africa, is the subject of considerable speculation and competing laboratory claims (27). Not in dispute, however, is the observation that HIV-1 is more infectious and more pathogenic than HIV-2 (28–31). Additionally some HIV-1s are far more virulent and infectious than others in tissue-culture assays, suggesting that viral factors may play an important role in the varying infectiousness of different individuals (32).

Risk of Sexual Transmission

It seems logical that HIV transmission might be more efficient from male-to-female than from female-to-male. The posterior vaginal fornix has evolved to help retain semen to assist in procreation. In contrast, the penis has no such function and sexually acquired secretions typically dry quickly or are rubbed off by friction with clothing or bedding. In uncircumcised males, however, subprepucal retention of infectious cervicovaginal secretions may be prolonged.

Two early European and North American studies reported that HIV-infected men were more likely than HIV-infected women to transmit HIV to their partners (33,34). These studies argued that women were more susceptible to HIV, a plausible hypothesis since women are exposed to a large inoculum of infected seminal fluid, deposited on a large surface area that may be abraded during sexual activity. In contrast, men are exposed to a relatively smaller volume of infected vaginal fluids on a different type of epithelial surface for relatively shorter periods of time (33, 34). However, these studies included small numbers of transmission events and few HIV-infected women. Another European study conducted in multiple centers did not see a difference in male-to-female or female-to-male transmission rates (13).

Two recent studies, one in Uganda (35), the other in Zambia (30), studied discordant couples with substantial numbers of male-to-female and female-to-male transmission events. The study conducted in Uganda showed a seroconversion rate of 11.8 per 100 person-years. Female-to-male transmission rates (11.6 per 100 person-years) were similar to male-to-female rates (12.0 per 100 person-years) (35). The study conducted in Zambia showed a seroconversion rate of 8.5 per 100 person-years with no notable difference between female-to-male (8.1 per 100 person-years) and male-to-female (8.8 per 100 person-years) transmission rates (30). These more recent African data on the equivalence of female-to-male and male-to-female transmission rates support other large studies conducted in Africa (36,37), Haiti (38), and Europe (13).

Viral Load

Both studies from Zambia and Uganda showed that levels of plasma viral load were consistently higher among transmitters than among nontransmitters (30,35). These strong associations between transmission risk and viral load suggest that reducing plasma RNA levels could significantly reduce transmission risk. Such reductions in transmission have been documented in studies of perinatal transmission (39–43), but not yet in studies of sexual transmission. One study showed no sexual transmission occurred among women treated with zidovudine (44), but studies of antiretroviral therapy and HIV levels in the genital tract have not yielded consistent results (45–48). A reasonably good correlation between viral load in peripheral blood and that in seminal plasma and cervical secretions has been reported (36,49,50). Viral loads in genital secretions decline along with viral load in peripheral blood as a result of combination antiretroviral therapy (23,37,49). Risk of transmission is substantially reduced along with the reductions in peripheral blood and seminal plasma viral load. Measuring the effects of antiretroviral drugs on sexual transmission will help quantify the potential impact of expanded drug therapies in Africa.

Sexually Transmitted Diseases

Numerous studies leave no doubt that the attributable risk of coinfection with other STDs both ulcerative and nonulcerative—in heterosexual HIV transmission is substantial (4). It is now well established that unprotected sexual contact in the presence of other STDs enhances the likelihood of HIV transmission (19,51–53). STDs damage the integrity of the epithelial lining of the cervix, vagina, urethra, vulva, and anus (51,54–56), thereby facilitating the efficiency of HIV transmission (55). Mucosal ulceration, inflammation, or exudation is likely to increase the frequency of viral contact with target cells through macroscopic or microscopic breaks in mucosal integrity and the recruitment of immune cells that are readily infected (dendritic cells, macrophages, $CD4^+$ lymphocytes) into the genitourinary tract (57). The most dramatic evidence of STDs as cofactors in HIV transmission in Africa comes from a study conducted in Mwanza, Uganda (58) in which immediate syndromic management of STDs at the village level reduced HIV transmission by approximately 42% over a two-year period; see chapter 14, *this volume*.

The interactions between STDs and HIV have contributed substantially to the AIDS epidemic, particularly where HIV prevalence is low (59). HIV spreads rapidly among high-risk populations such as STD patients, who commonly report high-risk activities and high-risk partners (59). In simulations of the first decade of the HIV epidemic (1981 to 1990), over 90% of HIV infections were attributed to STD coinfections worldwide (60). Even under more conservative assumptions about the prevalence of STDs and their role in HIV transmission, STDs can be demonstrated to play a critical role in the rapid and extensive spread of HIV infection in many diverse settings (61). The identification and treatment of STDs as risk factors for HIV transmission should therefore be a crucial element of HIV prevention efforts (59–61).

Bacterial Vaginosis

STD treatment and subsequent restoration of the integrity of mucosal barriers can reduce sexual transmission of HIV. It is postulated that treatment of bacterial vaginosis and the restoration of a normal vaginal ecology, dominated by hydrogen peroxide-producing lactobacilli, may also inhibit the sexual spread of HIV. Similarly, it is postulated that mother-to-child HIV transmission may be reduced by antibiotic treatment of mothers who have bacterial vaginosis (62). This concept is based on the association of lower genital tract bacterial vaginosis with risk of histologic chorioamnionitis and the additional increased risk of HIV transmission among mothers with chorioamnionitis. Bacterial vaginosis has been associated with HIV in Africa, suggesting this causal pathway to be plausible and worthy of investigation for both sexual and perinatal transmission reduction (63).

Host Factors

Host factors can augment the risk of HIV transmission or acquisition. For example, the homozygous Δ32 mutation of the CCR5 gene confers almost total protection against sexual HIV transmission (64,65). Because this gene mutation is more common among Caucasian populations than among black African populations, it has been speculated that it may have contributed to the relatively indolent epidemic seen in North

America, Europe, and Australia, compared to that seen in Africa (66).

Other genetic predispositions for HIV transmission or disease progression are topics of intense investigation (67–69). Results of studies of discordant couples and studies of commercial sex workers indicate that while some persons are infected by repetitive exposure to HIV, others may be immunized and remain uninfected. Meanwhile, others seem to be completely resistant to the virus, but show no immunologic responses that suggest immunization-like events. While we are in our infancy in understanding the complexities of the human genome to affect sexual transmission of HIV, research toward this end is critical to assist vaccine development, elucidate correlates of protective immunity, and explain the diversity of HIV in different populations.

Systemic Coinfections

Infection with systemic viruses or other microorganisms, many of which are transmitted sexually, may activate the immune system. An activated immune system with up-regulated primary and secondary target molecules presented to infectious particles is easier to infect with HIV than a quiescent one. In addition, systemic coinfections may stimulate HIV production, thus increasing infectiousness (57). These relationships are not very well documented, but some organisms have been studied for their effects on HIV transmission, including cytomegalovirus, Epstein-Barr virus, human T-cell lymphotropic virus (HTLV) types I and II, and human herpesviruses types 6, 7, and 8. In addition, malaria may be the most important such organism in the African setting (70). The immune activation associated with chronic malaria, for example, might increase risk of HIV infection due to the presence of a higher proportion of target lymphocytes (71). While in-vitro studies and case reports suggest an association between malaria and HIV infection, epidemiologic data are needed, as was the case with *Mycoplasma fermentans*, formal epidemiologic analysis of which did not support the speculations of case reports (72). Severe HIV disease was reportedly associated with HTLV-I coinfection compared to persons with mild disease (73); it is not known whether this suggests that HTLV-I is a coinfection that contributes to HIV disease progression, or whether coinfection may be related to duration of risk behavior and HIV infection.

Young Women

Young women are at a comparatively higher risk for HIV acquisition than older women because of both behavioral and biologic mechanisms (57). Adolescents with immature vaginal mucosa (large cervical ectopy zones) may be more susceptible to trauma during sexual activity, and may be especially prone to STD infection due to large transformation zones and exposed squamocolumnar epithelia (4). HIV transmission may be facilitated by sexual activity at times when blood exposure is likely, such as during menses, rape, or first coital experience (57). In addition, older men, who are more likely to be HIV-infected than younger men, often seek younger sexual partners (74). This accounts for the higher incidence of HIV seroconversion in Africa among young women compared to males of the same age (75).

Cervical Ectopy

Cervical ectopy is a normal developmental variation in cervical growth, causing the exocervical exposure of the columnar epithelium, which is typically located in the endocervix of a mature woman. Cervical ectopy exposes the transformation zone, where the columnar epithelium transitions to squamous epithelium. Pathogens accompanying semen can infect cells in this vulnerable tissue. The transformation zone is more susceptible to infection with HIV and other

STDs because it lacks both the physical protection of the squamous epithelium and the high vascularity of the columnar epithelium. Cervical ectopy may thereby increase HIV susceptibility among uninfected women (57). Bleeding during intercourse occurs more often among young women with cervical ectopy; hence, an HIV-infected woman with cervical ectopy may be more infectious than one without this condition. An association of cervical ectopy with HIV risk was reported in an African study (76), though it was not confirmed in a U.S. study (77). Because neither study reported prospective data on seroconversion, the conclusions remain unclear.

Oral or injectable contraceptive hormones may also increase HIV risk since they are thought to increase cervical ectopy (57). However, this is not yet known. Risk factors for cervical ectopy, other than adolescence, may include lack of exposure to semen (77). If exposure to semen accelerates squamous metaplastic changes in the cervix with the consequent involution of the transformation zone into the endocervix, the ectopy-related increased risk for HIV may be especially critical for youth just initiating their sexual debut (57,59,77).

BEHAVIORAL COFACTORS FACILITATING HIV TRANSMISSION

To better formulate effective HIV/AIDS prevention campaigns in sub–Saharan Africa, it is critical to understand the factors that have given rise to and sustained patterns of risky sexual behavior that permit the rapid and efficient transmission of HIV.

Female Circumcision

Female circumcision is a likely risk factor for HIV transmission, although it has not been described as such. The abnormal bleeding, anatomic distortion, coital trauma, scarring, and infection associated with female circumcision would be expected to increase susceptibility to HIV transmission (78,79). However, since Muslim families in the Sudan and other nations in the Sahel region have the highest rates of female circumcision, and low rates of HIV infection, it may be that these women are not often exposed to HIV.

Vaginal Drying Agents

Vaginal drying agents include a variety of herbs or other plant products, sometimes mixed with nonorganic, excoriative agents (Sinkala M, personal observation). These agents have been associated with HIV risk, presumably due to the resulting bleeding and epithelial trauma during intercourse (4,14).

Male Circumcision

Male circumcision is speculated to be a cofactor of HIV transmission in sub–Saharan Africa. Several studies have suggested a protective effect of male circumcision. In a study of serodiscordant couples, Quinn et al. found an HIV incidence of 16.7 per 100 person-years among 137 uncircumcised male partners, whereas there were no seroconversions among the 50 circumcised male partners ($p < 0.001$) (35). In a cross-sectional study conducted among men with genital ulcer disease, HIV-1 infection was independently associated with being uncircumcised (OR 4.8); this association could not be explained by measures of sexual exposure to HIV-1 among this population (80). No clinical trial or prospective data are available. Since men who practice Islam are most likely to be circumcised, there is potential confounding of circumcision with religious practice and social tradition that may explain much of the protective association now attributed to circumcision. However, if it were feasible in a given setting, male circumcision could be considered as an intervention strategy for HIV control.

Rates of Partner Exchange

The current economic and political situations in most African countries result in many men migrating for work and living away from their families for several months each year. Soldiers, refugees, miners, truck drivers, and migrant farm workers are all absent from home for long periods of time. Rates of partner exchange increase tremendously when men are living or traveling away from their families. Transient men may have sex with commercial sex workers or with multiple high-risk partners, bringing STDs, including HIV, home to their families.

Auvert et al. used a stochastic simulation model to show that, of the various risk factors related to sexual behavior, the most important determinant of the spread of HIV was the proportion of men engaging in sexual relationships with people other than their spouses (78). Interventions aimed at reducing extramarital sex with multiple high-risk partners may substantially limit the potential for the spread of HIV infection in Africa (81). It is thought that the single greatest behavior change in Uganda, where HIV infections have dropped considerably, has not been condom use, but rather, the decrease in casual sexual liaisons, which correlates with declining HIV and STD incidence rates (81).

Researchers in Tanzania reported that numbers of sexual partners were higher among men than women. Fifty-three percent of the men and 15% of the women reported having casual sex during the previous year. Only 2% of the men in this study reported having sexual contact with bar girls or commercial sex workers, indicating that the promiscuous men are having sex with women who are not themselves identified as "high risk" (82).

Very little attention has been paid to the practices of men who have sex with men in Africa. Most African societies are based upon extended families and clan structures and discourage male-to-male sexual contact. Estimates of African men who have experienced sexual contact with other men are lacking.

Interventions aimed at reducing numbers of sexual partners should not be limited to men. In some countries, marital dissolution and remarriage are common (82). Women may have multiple or inconsistent sexual partners for economic reasons. For example, more than one sexual partner may help support a woman and her children. Dissatisfaction with the infidelities, alcohol consumption, or appearance of a partner; fear of getting an STD from a partner; lack of leisure time with a partner; and influence of a partner's relatives and/or children with other women, have all been reported as motives for women to have other sexual partners (83).

Condom Use

Despite some recent increases, rates of condom use remain very low throughout Africa (84). The 1993–1994 Ghana Demographic Health Survey found that high levels of AIDS-related knowledge among Ghanaian women have yet to translate into increased condom use (85). A study of Ethiopian sailors reported a 14% rate of condom use, though even this low rate was reported as inconsistent (86). Munguti et al. reported that in Tanzania only 20% of the men and 3% of the women in their study had ever used a condom; again, the use was not reported as regular (82). Quinn et al. found that the highest reported rates of condom use among discordant couples in rural Uganda were 7.4% among women and 16.9% among men (35). In such settings, culturally-sensitive approaches that could help increase the use of all types of contraceptives, including barrier methods, are needed. Condom use seems to be markedly increased in settings where there are sustained programs of education, primary care, and condom distribution (51). Furthermore, when couples are counseled and trained together so that each knows his or her own HIV status, and that of his or her partner, subsequent condom use rates have been quite high (3,8,36). As contraceptive use increases, it is speculated that the use of condoms for both AIDS prevention and for family planning will increase in sub–Saharan Africa (85).

Alcohol Abuse

Alcohol use, although rare in many Muslim populations in Africa, may impact HIV transmission in a number of settings. Alcohol use in some areas is closely related to the highly mobile male population, the social norms affecting the use of substances that lower sexual inhibitions (11), and contact with commercial sex workers (12). In rural areas, problems with alcohol abuse reside mostly with men (87). Women are less likely to use alcohol then men, but due to gender inequity, may be unable to practice safe sex. The results of a study conducted in two rural areas of Zimbabwe suggested that male alcohol consumption obstructed effective female behavioral change regarding fertility control and HIV prevention methods (87). Alcohol use is more widespread, however, among women in urban areas than among women in rural areas. A study among married African women attending an STD clinic in Lusaka, Zambia, showed that female alcohol use before sex was associated with increased rates of female STDs (88).

Gender

In a survey of 1,117 adults aged 15 to 54 years in rural Tanzania, 50% of women and 46% of men reported having sexual intercourse for the first time before age 16 (82). On average, women married 2 years, and men 6 years, after their sexual debut. Men married later in life than did women, and men typically married women around 5 to 10 years younger than themselves (82). Notably, in the Rakai study of discordant couples, the incidence of seroconversion was highest among the partners who were 15 to 19 years of age (15.3 per 100 person-years) (35). In a cross-sectional study of 200 adolescents conducted in Kenyan truck stops, 93% of girls and 87% of boys reported having had sexual intercourse, and of these, 54% of girls and 38% of boys reported having used a condom (89). Fifty-two percent of the girls and 30% of the boys reported having had an STD. Seventy-eight percent of girls reported usually exchanging sex for gifts or money, while 59% of boys reported usually giving gifts or money for sex (89).

Women may have negligible negotiating power within the context of sex and reproduction in patriarchal societies (90); see chapter 43, *this volume*.

Awareness of AIDS

In a cross-sectional study of Ethiopian sailors, the prevalence of HIV-1 infection was observed to decrease with increasing levels of education (86). A cross-sectional survey carried out in western Kenya detected STDs (including HIV) in 36.2% of women at an urban clinic and 21.2% of women at a rural clinic (91). Knowledge of STDs and HIV was nearly universal in both rural and urban clinic populations; over 96% of the patients were aware of AIDS. There was a heightened consciousness among women at the urban clinic: 76.3% of them felt they could get HIV or another STD, compared to 48.8% of the women at the rural clinic ($p < 0.02$) (91).

HIV voluntary counseling and testing services have been shown to effectively reduce HIV transmission by raising levels of HIV/AIDS awareness and knowledge (8,92). Voluntary counseling and testing allows individuals to know their infection status and promotes behavior change to allow them to protect themselves and others from infection (92). It also allows people to cope with the anxiety associated with HIV status, and can improve medical and psychosocial support to those who are infected (92); see chapter 34, *this volume*.

BLOODBORNE TRANSMISSION

While sexual transmission of HIV is clearly the dominant route of transmission among adolescents and adults in Africa, use of contaminated needles is problematic, particularly in the formal and informal health care sectors.

Unsafe Injections

The probability of HIV seroconversion after injection with a needle that is contaminated with infected blood is 0.3%. This rate varies considerably according to the infectious stage and age of the HIV-infected individual whose blood is the source of contamination (93). Recent data show that the percentage of observed unsafe injections in sub–Saharan Africa ranges from 70% to over 90% (94). Not only are unsafe injections common in Africa, but many injections and transfusions are not medically indicated; shots are given when oral medicines would suffice and transfusions are given when more benign therapies should be preferred (93). An average 95% of all injections in developing countries are therapeutic, the majority of which have been judged unnecessary by WHO policy researchers (93). Most "injection doctors" have flourishing businesses based on the popular belief that injections are more efficient cures than oral medications. Two studies from Tanzania reported that 77% of all therapeutic injections given were unnecessary (95, 96). Overall, the most frequently injected medications include antibiotics, vitamins, analgesics, and quinine. The reasons cited for using injections typically include nonspecific symptoms such as mild diarrhea, fever, cold, and fatigue—symptoms for which injections are almost never indicated (97). There is evidence that childhood immunizations are safer than therapeutic injections. However, several recent national surveys estimated that 31% to 90% of childhood vaccinations were unsafe (94).

Risk to Medical Personnel

The transmission of HIV among medical personnel is facilitated by unsanitary working conditions, which, in many settings, are the result of a lack of resources; see chapter 37, *this volume*. We have observed midwives in Zambia deliver babies without gloves or with only one glove. With the current HIV prevalence rates among women of childbearing age in Lusaka, such practices put the midwives at an increased risk for HIV transmission. There is at least one well-documented case of a Zambian midwife with a reported HIV infection caused by handling unsafe blood during a delivery (Sinkala M, personal observation). However, the attributable risk of occupational exposure among African health workers is difficult to quantify due to the widespread prevalence of nonoccupational risk factors among African populations.

The frequency of skin exposure to HIV-infected blood was estimated in a serosurvey conducted among traditional birth attendants practicing in a rural, but densely populated area in southern Rwanda (98). Almost 2% of these traditional birth attendants tested positive for HIV-1 antibodies, but all had reported nonoccupational risk factors for HIV infection. No evidence of HIV infection caused by occupational blood contact was discovered (98). It is likely, however, that the poor conditions in most African health care settings facilitate health care worker exposure on a regular basis, even if it is not easily quantified. In 1994, Habimana et al. estimated that among 215 HIV-negative traditional birth attendants in Rwanda, 2,234 potentially infectious blood–skin contacts occurred out of a total of approximately 35,000 deliveries assisted in a 5-year period (98). This estimate of the number of potential exposures would be considerably higher in African countries with higher HIV prevalence rates than those of Rwanda; the Rwandan epidemic is one-half to one-third the size of that in more southern African countries (1,2).

Injection Drug Users

Drug injecting is increasing in a number of developing countries, often followed quickly by outbreaks of HIV infection as seen in Bangkok, Thailand; Manipur, India, and urban centers of eastern Europe (99). Rates of injection drug use in Africa are low and the spread of HIV due to injection drug use is nowhere near that due to heterosexual transmission. A 2% HIV antibody positivity rate was found among IDUs in Johannesburg, South Africa, a rate substantially lower than that among IDUs elsewhere in the world (100). Given the continued recruitment of new injectors where injection drug use is endemic, and the potential diffusion of drug injecting in countries where the practice was formerly rare, HIV prevention efforts must discourage drug injecting. Countries in drug-producing regions and along drug-transit routes in Africa are particularly at risk. Africans are used as couriers for drugs in Southeast and southwestern Asia and South America (99). Such persons are often paid in drugs, which creates demand for drugs in their home countries. In a cross-sectional study carried out in a population of Ethiopian sailors, the prevalence of HIV-1 infection was 9.6% and the risk of acquiring infection was found to increase with the use of hypodermic injections (OR 3.4) (86). Injection drug use could spread rapidly in Africa, outstripping HIV prevention activities. Public health systems need to target current injectors and high-risk youth for behaviorial change to discourage drug use and its diffusion to new populations.

CONCLUSION

Interventions are sorely needed to reduce the high rates of sexual partner exchange and casual sex, and to increase the low rates of condom use recorded in sub–Saharan Africa. Targeting interventions to traditional "core groups" may be of limited value in rural areas. Additional strategies that focus on teenagers and on male partners are needed. Biologic and behavioral interventions often have overlapping goals, such as to discourage use of vaginal drying agents, to encourage traditions of safe male circumcisions where practiced, to provide rapid access to STD treatment, to encourage condom use, to encourage a reduction in sexual partner number, to encourage counseling and testing for HIV, and to provide sustained antiretroviral therapy wherever feasible.

Interventions still in the research arena include microbicides and HIV vaccines, neither of which has yet demonstrated efficacy in human studies for HIV prevention. It is hard to estimate the proportion of infections in Africa that might be attributable to needle- or employment-related exposure compared to sexual exposure; this area requires further research.

ACKNOWLEDGMENTS

The authors wish to thank Ms. Adrienne Ellis for her help. Financial support was provided by the AIDS International Training and Research Program from the Fogarty International Center, NIH (1 D43 TW01035-03) at the University of Alabama.

REFERENCES

1. UNAIDS/WHO. *AIDS epidemic update: December 2000.* UNAIDS/00.44E-WHO/CDS/CSR/EDC/2000.9. Geneva: UNAIDS/WHO; 2000.
2. UNAIDS. *Report on the global HIV/AIDS epidemic.* UNAIDS/00.13E. Geneva: UNAIDS; June 2000.
3. Allen S, Serufilira A, Bogaerts J, et al. Confidential HIV testing and condom promotion in Africa. Impact on HIV and gonorrhea rates. *JAMA*, 1992; 268:3338–3343.
4. Vermund SH, Kristensen S, Bhatta MP. HIV as an STD. In: Mayer KH, ed. *The Emergence of AIDS: The Impact on Immunology, Microbiology, and Public Health.* Washington: American Public Health Association, 2000;1:121–138.

5. Coggins C, Segal S. AIDS and reproductive health. *J Reprod Immunol*, 1998;4:3–15.
6. De Cock KM. The emergence of HIV/AIDS in Africa. *Rev Epidemiol Sante Publique*, 1996;44: 511–580.
7. Gupta S, Anderson RM. Population structure of pathogens: the role of immune selection. *Parasitol Today*, 1999;15:497–501.
8. Allen SA, Karita E, N'Gandu N, et al. The evolution of voluntary testing and counseling as an HIV prevention strategy. In: Gibney L, DiClemente RJ, Vermund SH, eds. *Preventing HIV in Developing Countries: Biomedical and Behavioral Approaches*. New York: Kluwer Academic/Plenum Publishers, 1998.
9. Vittinghoff E, Douglas J, Judson F, et al. Per-contact risk of human immunodeficiency virus transmission between male sexual partners. *Am J Epidemiol*, 1999;150:306–311.
10. Shiboski SC, Padian NS. Epidemiologic evidence for time variation in HIV infectivity. *J Acquir Immune Defic Syndr Hum Retrovirol*, 1999;19:527–535.
11. Royce RA, Sena A, Cates WJ Jr., et al. Sexual transmission of HIV. *N Engl J Med*, 1997;336: 1072–1078 [Erratum, *N Engl J Med*, 1997; 337:799].
12. Boerma JT, Urassa M, Senkoro K, et al. Spread of HIV infection in a rural area of Tanzania. *AIDS*, 1999;13:1233–1240.
13. de Vincenzi I. A longitudinal study of human immunodeficiency virus transmission by heterosexual partners. *N Engl J Med*, 1994;331:341–346.
14. Dallabetta GA, Miotti PG, Chiphangwi JD, et al. Traditional vaginal agents: use and association with HIV infection in Malawian women. *AIDS*, 1995; 9:293–297.
15. Nelson KE, Rungruengthanakit K, Margolick J, et al. High rates of transmission of subtype E human immunodeficiency virus type 1 among heterosexual couples in northern Thailand: role of sexually transmitted diseases and immune compromise. *J Infect Dis*, 1999;180:337–343 [Erratum, *J Infect Dis*, 1999;180:1756].
16. Moses S, Bailey RC, Ronald AR. Male circumcision: assessment of health benefits and risks. *Sex Transm Infect*, 1998;74:368–373.
17. Halperin DT, Bailey RC. Male circumcision and HIV infection: 10 years and counting. *Lancet*, 1999;354:1813–1815.
18. Fleming DT, Wasserheit JN. From epidemiological synergy to public health policy and practice: the contribution of other sexually transmitted diseases to sexual transmission of HIV infection. *Sex Transm Infect*, 1999;75:3–17.
19. Cohen MS. Sexually transmitted diseases enhance HIV transmission: no longer a hypothesis. *Lancet*, 1998;351(Suppl 3):5–7.
20. Lee TH, Sakahara N, Fiebig E, et al. Correlation of HIV-1 RNA levels in plasma and heterosexual transmission of HIV-1 from infected transfusion recipients. *J Acquir Immune Defic Syndr Hum Retrovirol*, 1996;12:427–428.
21. Ragni MV, Faruki H, Kingsley LA. Heterosexual HIV-1 transmission and viral load in hemophilic patients. *J Acquir Immune Defic Syndr Hum Retrovirol*, 1998;17:42–45.
22. Operskalski EA, Stram DO, Busch MP, et al. Role of viral load in heterosexual transmission of human immunodeficiency virus type 1 by blood transfusion recipients. *Am J Epidemiol*, 1997;146:655–661.
23. Pedraza MA, del Romero J, Roldan F, et al. Heterosexual transmission of HIV-1 is associated with high plasma viral load levels and a positive viral isolation in the infected partner. *J Acquir Immune Defic Syndr Hum Retrovirol*, 1999;21:120–125.
24. Musicco M, Lazzarin A, Nicolosi A, et al. Antiretroviral treatment of men infected with human immunodeficiency virus type 1 reduces the incidence of heterosexual transmission. *Arch Intern Med*, 1994;154:1971–1976.
25. Moore JP. Co-receptors: implications for HIV pathogenesis and therapy. *Science*, 1997;276:51–52.
26. Hoffman TL, MacGregor RR, Burger H, et al. CCR5 genotypes in sexually active couples discordant for human immunodeficiency virus type 1 infection status. *J Infect Dis*, 1997;176:1093–1096.
27. Essex M. Human immunodeficiency viruses in the developing world. *Adv Virus Res*, 1999;53:71–88.
28. Kanki PJ, Travers KU, Mboup S, et al. Slower heterosexual spread of HIV-2 than HIV-1. *Lancet*. 1994;343:943–946.
29. Marlink R, Kanki P, Thior I, et al. Reduced rate of disease development after HIV-2 infection as compared to HIV-1. *Science*, 1994;265:1587–1590.
30. Fideli US, Allen SA, Musonda R, et al. Virologic and immunologic determinants of heterosexual transmission of human immunodeficiency virus type 1 in Africa. *AIDS Res Hum Retroviruses*, 2001; 17:901–910.
31. Li Q, Tsang B, Ding L, et al. Infection with the human immunodeficiency virus type 2: epidemiology and transmission. *Int J Mol Med*, 1998;2: 573–576.
32. Clumeck N, Hermans P, De Wit S. Some epidemiological and clinical characteristics of African AIDS. *Antibiot Chemother*, 1987;38:41–51.
33. Saracco A, Musicco M, Nicolosi A, et al. Man-to-woman sexual transmission of HIV: longitudinal study of 343 steady partners of infected men. *J Acquir Immune Defic Syndr*, 1993;6:497–502.
34. Padian NS, Shiboski SC, Glass SO, et al. Heterosexual transmission of human immunodeficiency virus (HIV) in northern California: results from a ten-year study. *Am J Epidemiol*, 1997;146: 350–357.

35. Quinn TC, Wawer MJ, Sewankambo N, et al. Viral load and heterosexual transmission of human immunodeficiency virus type 1. Rakai Project Study Group. *N Engl J Med*, 2000;342:921–929.
36. Allen S, Tice J, Van de Perre P, et al. Effect of serotesting with counseling on condom use and seroconversion among HIV discordant couples in Africa. *BMJ*, 1992;304:1605–1609.
37. Serwadda D, Gray RH, Wawer MJ, et al. The social dynamics of HIV transmission as reflected through discordant couples in rural Uganda. *AIDS*, 1995; 9:745–750.
38. Deschamps MM, Pape JW, Hafner A, et al. Heterosexual transmission of HIV in Haiti. *Ann Intern Med*, 1996;125:324–330.
39. Dickover RE, Garratty EM, Herman SA, et al. Identification of levels of maternal HIV-1 RNA associated with risk of perinatal transmission. Effect of maternal zidovudine treatment on viral load. *JAMA*, 1996;275:599–605.
40. Coll O, Hernandez M, Boucher CA, et al. Vertical HIV-1 transmission correlates with a high maternal viral load at delivery. *J Acquir Immune Defic Syndr Hum Retrovirol*, 1997;14:26–30.
41. Boyer PJ, Dillon M, Navaie M, et al. Factors predictive of maternal-fetal transmission of HIV-1. Preliminary analysis of zidovudine given during pregnancy and/or delivery. *JAMA*, 1994;271: 1925–1930.
42. Mofenson LM, Lambert JS, Stiehm ER, et al. Risk factors for perinatal transmission of human immunodeficiency virus type 1 in women treated with zidovudine. *N Engl J Med*, 1999;341:385–393.
43. Shaffer N, Chuachoowong R, Mock PA, et al. Short-course zidovudine for perinatal HIV-1 transmission in Bangkok, Thailand: a randomised controlled trial. *Lancet*, 1999;353:773–780.
44. Nicolosi A, Musicco M, Saracco A, et al. Risk factors for woman-to-man sexual transmission of the human immunodeficiency virus. Italian Study Group on HIV Heterosexual Transmission. *J Acquir Immune Defic Syndr*, 1994;7:296–300.
45. Liuzzi G, Chirianni A, Clementi M, et al. Analysis of HIV-1 load in blood, semen and saliva: evidence for different viral compartments in a cross-sectional and longitudinal study. *AIDS*, 1996;10:F51–F56.
46. Gupta P, Mellors J, Kingsley L, et al. High viral load in semen of human immunodeficiency virus type 1-infected men at all stages of disease and its reduction by therapy with protease and nonnucleoside reverse transcriptase inhibitors. *J Virol*, 1997; 71:6271–6275.
47. Mayer KH, Boswell S, Goldstein R, et al. Persistence of human immunodeficiency virus in semen after adding indinavir to combination antiretroviral therapy. *Clin Infect Dis*, 1999;28: 1252–1259.
48. Zhang H, Dornadula G, Beumont M, et al. Human immunodeficiency virus type 1 in the semen of men receiving highly active antiretroviral therapy. *N Engl J Med*, 1998;339:1803–1809.
49. Peterson B, George SL. Sample size requirements and length of study for testing interaction in a 2 x k factorial design when time-to-failure is the outcome. *Control Clin Trials*, 1993;14:511–522.
50. Trask S, Derdeyn C, Musonda R, et al. Sequencing algorithms to establish phylogenetic linkage between spouses in a prospective study of discordant heterosexual couples from Zambia. *AIDS Res Hum Retroviruses*, submitted.
51. Laga M, Alary M, Nzila N, et al. Condom promotion, STD treatment leading to a declining incidence of HIV-1 infection in female Zairean sex workers. *Lancet*, 1994;344:246–248.
52. Robinson NJ, Mulder DW, Auvert B, et al. Proportion of HIV infections attributable to other sexually transmitted diseases in a rural Ugandan population: simulation model estimates. *Int J Epidemiol*, 1997;26:180–189.
53. Klouman E, Masenga EJ, Klepp KI, et al. HIV and reproductive tract infections in a total village population in rural Kilimanjaro, Tanzania: women at increased risk. *J Acquir Immune Defic Syndr Hum Retrovirol*, 1997;14:163–168.
54. Rodrigues JJ, Mehendale SM, Shepherd ME, et al. Risk factors for HIV infection in people attending clinics for sexually transmitted diseases in India. *BMJ*, 1995;311:283–286.
55. Cleghorn FR, Jack N, Murphy JR, et al. HIV-1 prevalence and risk factors among sexually transmitted disease clinic attenders in Trinidad. *AIDS*, 1995;9:389–394.
56. Coplan PM, Gortmaker S, Hernandez-Avila M, et al. Human immunodeficiency virus infection in Mexico City. Rectal bleeding and anal warts as risk factors among men reporting sex with men. *Am J Epidemiol*, 1996;144:817–827.
57. Vermund SH. Transmission of HIV-1 among adolescents and adults. In: DeVita VT, Hellman S, Rosenberg SA, eds. *AIDS: Etiology, Diagnosis, Treatment and Prevention*, Fourth Edition. Philadelphia: Lippincott-Raven Publishers, 1996; 147–165.
58. Grosskurth H, Mosha F, Todd J, et al. Impact of improved treatment of sexually transmitted diseases on HIV infection in rural Tanzania: randomized controlled trial. *Lancet*, 1995;346:530–536.
59. Wasserheit JN. Epidemiological synergy: Interrelationships between human immunodeficiency virus infection and other sexually transmitted diseases. *Sex Transm Dis*, 1992;19:61–77.
60. The World Bank. Efficient and Equitable Strategies for Preventing HIV/AIDS. In: *Confronting AIDS: Public Priorities in a Global Epidemic*, First

Edition. New York: Oxford University Press, 1997;103–172.
61. Gertig DM, Kapiga SH, Shao JF, et al. Risk factors for sexually transmitted diseases among women attending family planning clinics in Dar-es-Salam, Tanzania. *Genitourin Med*, 1997;73:39–43.
62. Goldenberg RL, Vermund SH, Goepfert AR, et al. Choriodecidual inflammation: a potentially preventable cause of perinatal HIV-1 transmission? *Lancet*, 1998;352:1927–1930.
63. Taha TE, Hoover DR, Dallabetta GA, et al. Bacterial vaginosis and disturbances of vaginal flora: association with increased acquisition of HIV. *AIDS*, 1998;12:1699–1706.
64. Katzenstein TL, Eugen-Olsen J, Hofmann B, et al. HIV-infected individuals with the CCR delta32/CCR5 genotype have lower HIV RNA levels and higher CD4 cell counts in the early years of the infection than do patients with the wild type. Copenhagen AIDS Cohort Study Group. *J Aquir Immune Defic Syndr*, 1997;16:10–14.
65. D'Aquila RT, Sutton L, Savara A, et al. CCR5/delta(ccr5) heterozygosity: a selective pressure for the syncytium-inducing human immunodeficiency virus type 1 phenotype. NIAID AIDS Clinical Trials Group Protocol 241 Virology Team. *J Infect Dis*, 1998;177:1549–1553.
66. Martinson JJ, Chapman NH, Rees DC, et al. Global distribution of the CCR5 gene 32-basepair deletion. *Nat Gene*, 1997;16:100–103.
67. Philpott S, Burger H, Charbonneau T, et al. CCR5 genotype and resistance to vertical transmission of HIV-1. *J Acquir Immune Defic Syndr*, 1999;21: 189–193.
68. Kaslow RA, Carrington M, Apple R, et al. Influence of combinations of human major histocompatibility complex genes on the course of HIV-1 infection. *Nat Med*, 1996;2:405–411.
69. Tang J, Costello C, Keet IP, et al. HLA class I homozygosity accelerates disease progression in human immunodeficiency virus type 1 infection. *AIDS Res Hum Retroviruses*, 1999;15:317–324.
70. French N, Gilks CF. Fresh from the field: some controversies in tropical medicine and hygiene. HIV and malaria, do they interact? *Trans R Soc Trop Med Hyg*, 2000;94:233–237.
71. Parise ME, Ayisi JG, Nahlen BL, et al. Efficacy of sulfadoxine-pyrimethamine for prevention of placental malaria in an area of Kenya with a high prevalence of malaria and human immunodeficiency virus infection. *Am J Trop Med Hyg*, 1998;59:813–822.
72. Hawkins RE, Rickman LS, Vermund SH, et al. Association of mycoplasma and human immunodeficiency virus infection: detection of amplified *Mycoplasma fermentans* DNA in blood. *J Infec Dis*, 1992;165:581–585.
73. Schechter M, Harrison LH, Halsey NA, et al. Coinfection with human T-cell lymphotropic virus type I and HIV in Brazil: Impact on markers of HIV disease progression. *JAMA*, 1994;271:353–357.
74. Campbell T, Kelly M. Women and AIDS in Zambia: a review of the psychosocial factors implicated in the transmission of HIV. *AIDS Care*, 1995;7:365–373.
75. Wawer MJ, Serwadda D, Musgrave SD, et al. Dynamics of spread of HIV-1 infection in a rural district of Uganda. *BMJ*, 1991;303:1303–1306.
76. Moss GB, Clemetson D, D'Costa L, et al. Association of cervical ectopy with heterosexual transmission of human immunodeficiency virus: results of a study of couples in Nairobi, Kenya. *J Infec Dis*, 1991;164:588–591.
77. Moscicki AB, Ma Y, Holland C, et al. Cervical ectopy in adolescent girls with and without human immunodeficiency virus infection. *J Infect Dis*, 2001;183:865–870.
78. Auvert B, Buonamico G, Lagarde E, et al. Sexual behavior, heterosexual transmission, and the spread of HIV in sub–Saharan Africa: a simulation study. *Comput Biomed Res*, 2000;33:84–96.
79. Odoi A, Brody SP, Elkans TE. Female genital mutilation in rural Ghana, West Africa. *Int J Gynecol Obstet*, 1997;56:179–180.
80. Tyndall MW, Ronald AR, Agoki E, et al. Increased risk of infection with human immunodeficiency virus type 1 among uncircumcised men presenting with genital ulcer disease in Kenya. *Clin Infect Dis*, 1996;23:449–453.
81. Robinson NJ, Mulder D, Auvert B, et al. Type of partnership and heterosexual spread of HIV infection in rural Uganda: results from simulation modeling. *Int J STD AIDS*, 1999;10:718–725.
82. Munguti K, Grosskurth H, Newell J, et al. Patterns of sexual behavior in a rural population in north-western Tanzania. *Soc Sci Med*, 1997;44:1553–1561.
83. Twa-Twa J, Nakanaabi I, Sekimpi D. Underlying factors in female sexual partner instability in Kampala. *Health Transit Rev*, 1997;7 Suppl:83–88.
84. Statistics Department, Ministry of Finance and Economic Planning and Demographic Health Surveys. *Uganda demographic and health survey 1995.* Calverton, Md.: Macro International, 1996:48.
85. Takyi BK. AIDS-related knowledge and risks and contraceptive practices in Ghana: the early 1990s. *Afr J Reprod Health*, 2000;4:13–27.
86. Demissie K, Amre D, Tsega E. HIV-1 infection in relation to educational status, use of hypodermic injections and other risk behaviors in Ethiopian sailors. *East Afr Med J*, 1996;73:819–822.
87. Gregson S, Zhuwau T, Anderson RM, et al. Is there evidence for behavior change in response to AIDS in rural Zimbabwe? *Soc Sci Med*, 1998;46:321–330.
88. Morrison CS, Sunkutu MR, Musaba E, et al. Sexually transmitted disease among married

Zambian women: the role of male and female sexual behavior in prevention and management. *Genitourin Med*, 1997;73:555–557.
89. Nzyuko S, Lurie P, McFarland W, et al. Adolescent sexual behavior along the Trans-Africa Highway in Kenya. *AIDS*, 1997;11(Suppl 1):S21–S26.
90. Sibanda A. A nation in pain: why the HIV/AIDS epidemic is out of control in Zimbabwe. *Int J Health Serv*, 2000;30:717–738.
91. Wools KK, Menya D, Muli F, et al. Perception of risk, sexual behaviour and STD/HIV prevalence in western Kenya. *East Afr Med J*, 1998;75:679–683.
92. Sweat M, Gregorich S, Sangiwa G, et al. Cost-effectiveness of voluntary HIV-1 counseling and testing in reducing sexual transmission of HIV-1 in Kenya and Tanzania. *Lancet*, 2000;356:113–121.
93. Simonsen L, Kane A, Lloyd J, et al. Unsafe injections in the developing world and transmission of blood-borne pathogens: a review. *Bull Who*, 1999;77:789–800.
94. WHO Expanded program on immunization. Country reports including special studies of injection safety. Geneva: World Health Organization, 1998, unpublished documents.
95. Gumodoka B, Vos J, Berege ZA, et al. Injection practices in Mwanza Region, Tanzania: prescriptions, patient demand and sterility. *Trop Med Int Health*, 1996;1:874–880.
96. Vos J, Gumodoka B, vam Asten HA, et al. Improved injection practices after the introduction of treatment and sterility guidelines in Tanzania. *Trop Med Int Health*, 1998;3:291–296.
97. Lepage P, Van de Perre P. Nosocomial transmission of HIV in Africa: what tribute is paid to contaminated blood transfusions and medical injections. *Infect Control Hosp Epidemiol*, 1988;9:200–203.
98. Habimana P, Bulterys M, Usabuwera P, et al. A survey of occupational blood contact and HIV infection among traditional birth attendants in Rwanda. *AIDS*, 1994;8:701–704.
99. Stimson GV. The global diffusion of injecting drug use: implications for human immunodeficiency virus infection. *Bull Narc*, 1993;45:3–17.
100. Williams PG, Ansell SM, Milne FJ. Illicit intravenous drug use in Johannesburg—medical complications and prevalence of HIV infection. *S Afr Med J*, 1997;87:889–891.

14

Role of Sexually Transmitted Diseases in HIV-1 Transmission

*Saidi H. Kapiga and *†Iain W. Aitken

*Department of Population and International Health, Harvard School of Public Health, Boston, Massachusetts 02115, USA. †Department of Maternal and Child Health, Harvard School of Public Health, Boston, Massachusetts 02115, USA.

The emergence of the HIV-1 pandemic, and the recognition that bacterial and viral sexually transmitted diseases (STDs) and HIV-1 interact and reinforce each other, has dramatically increased research interest in STDs. Some of the initial evidence of possible associations between conventional STDs and HIV-1 infection came from studies conducted in the mid-1980s in both developed and developing countries (1,2). By the end of the 1980s, the accumulating evidence from additional studies led Pepin and colleagues to suggest that STD control could be used as an indirect strategy to reduce the transmission of HIV-1 (3). This hypothesis spurred researchers and public health officials to further examine the role of STDs in HIV-1 transmission in the 1990s. During this last decade, impressive progress has been made in understanding the determinants of heterosexual HIV-1 transmission, and the role of STDs in enhancing both the acquisition and infectiousness of HIV-1. The prevention and control of STDs has thus become a major public health priority and a critical component of HIV-1 intervention programs.

This chapter examines the results from epidemiologic, clinical, and laboratory studies of the role of the STDs that are prevalent in Africa in increasing the susceptibility to and the infectiousness of HIV-1. This chapter does not discuss how HIV-1 disease alters the natural history, diagnosis, or response to therapy of other STDs. Readers are advised to consult other sources that have reviewed this subject more extensively (4). Because of the difficulties in interpreting cross-sectional and case-control studies, the findings from prospective studies will be emphasized when available.

PUBLIC HEALTH IMPORTANCE OF STDs

Sexually transmitted diseases continue to cause significant morbidity and mortality among sexually active men and women throughout the world (5,6). Although the lack of case notification and national surveillance systems in most developing countries precludes making precise estimates of STD prevalence and incidence, results from numerous epidemiologic studies show that STDs are a major public health problem in these countries (7).

In 1995, following an extensive review of the published and unpublished prevalence data, the World Health Organization (WHO) estimated that more than 333 million new cases of syphilis, gonorrhea, chlamydia, and trichomoniasis occur globally each year (8). A disproportionate number of these curable infections occur in developing countries. When adjusted for population size, the estimated annual incidence rates are highest in sub–Saharan Africa, where they range from 12 to 120 per 1000 adults aged 15 to 49 years. Table 1 shows the estimated annual incidence rates of each of these infections based on their prevalence and estimated mean duration in different regions of the world.

The estimates shown in Table 1, although based on a comprehensive review of the available information, are affected by differences in the quality of data available from various regions, and differences in the geographic location, type, and size of the populations studied (8). Most STD estimates that are based on the number of cases reported in health facilities substantially underestimate the burden of STDs on the general population in developing countries. Many people with STDs, particularly women, tend to have asymptomatic infections and thus do not seek services from health facilities (9). Others do not seek treatment because of the social stigma associated with STDs, or because their access to health services is limited. Even when patients with STDs experience symptoms and go to health facilities, lack of appropriate diagnostic tests limits the ability of health workers in most developing countries to make precise etiologic diagnoses and provide appropriate treatments.

Sexually transmitted diseases are associated with serious social and economic consequences, and are a major cause of the loss of healthy years of life in developing countries. According to 1993 World Bank estimates, STDs were the second most important cause of healthy life lost in women aged 15 to 44 years after maternal morbidity and mortality (10). Most of the disease burden attributable to STDs is caused by the severe medical complications that arise when these infections are left untreated. These complications disproportionately affect women of reproductive age, and their offspring, causing cervical cancer, congenital and neonatal infections, low birth weight, miscarriage, stillbirth, and premature birth (11,12). Untreated STDs may also lead to upper reproductive tract infections, resulting in pelvic inflammatory disease, chronic pelvic pain, tubo-ovarian abscesses, and ectopic pregnancies (11,13). Inflammation of the uterus, fallopian tubes, and other pelvic structures is a major cause of infertility among women in developing countries. In Africa, genital

TABLE 1. Estimated Annual Incidence Rate of New STDs (per 1000) in Adults Aged 15 to 49 Years[a]

	Syphilis		Gonorrhea		Chlamydia		Trichomoniasis	
Regions of the world	Males	Females	Males	Females	Males	Females	Males	Females
North America	0.094	0.094	10.85	12.04	21.46	30.73	49.36	55.42
Western Europe	0.94	0.94	5.59	6.01	21.46	30.73	49.36	55.42
Australasia	0.94	0.94	10.85	12.04	21.46	30.73	49.36	55.42
Latin America and Caribbean	4.48	5.59	27.56	29.23	40.03	40.77	68.05	72.45
Sub–Saharan Africa	12.33	15.39	57.71	65.47	55.04	65.95	119.18	119.91
North Africa and Middle East	3.37	4.24	9.15	9.76	19.93	16.29	27.59	28.20
Eastern Europe and Central Asia	0.63	0.63	14.83	14.67	27.29	37.09	62.13	65.66
East Asia and Pacific	0.63	0.78	4.35	3.79	6.53	6.75	11.68	11.65
South and Southeast Asia	5.48	6.85	30.03	31.80	41.65	44.32	81.63	78.41

[a]Data from Gerbase AC, et al: Global prevalence and incidence estimates of selected curable STDs (8).

infections account for almost two-thirds of the cases of infertility in women. The prevalence of tubal occlusion in Africa is more than three times higher than that in any other region of the world (14,15). Infertility may also occur in males due to ascending infections of the urethra and epididymis (16).

ROLE OF STDs IN HIV-1 TRANSMISSION

Numerous studies have been conducted to examine the interactions between conventional STDs and HIV-1 infection (4,17–20). These studies have described how HIV-1 and other STDs may alter the rate of transmission and the natural history of each other, leading to increased prevalence and incidence of both infections. The complex reciprocal relationship between these infections has been described as "epidemiologic synergy" (4,19).

Results from cross-sectional and case-control studies provided initial evidence of the associations between HIV-1 infection and other STDs (4). However, these studies failed to determine whether STDs were independent risk factors for HIV-1 infection because the temporal sequence of events was not known and a cause-and-effect relationship could not be established. Prospective studies provide an opportunity to address issues of causality more adequately. Nonetheless, there are several other methodologic challenges that must be considered when analyzing data on the role of STDs in HIV-1 transmission. First, the observed associations between HIV-1 and other STDs might be a result of their shared mode of transmission and behavioral risk factors, rather than causal links. Hence, analyses that adjust for sexual behavior are important in assessing whether STDs are independent risk factors for HIV-1 transmission. Second, with increasing HIV-1–related immunosuppression, susceptibility to other infections, including bacterial and viral STDs, increases. Hence, STDs could be opportunistic complications of HIV-1 disease rather than risk factors for HIV-1 transmission. Third, the presence of multiple STDs in the same individual is relatively common. This might result in an observed, yet spurious association between one STD and HIV-1 that is actually due to an underlying association between another STD and HIV-1 (4).

Many factors determine the risk of HIV-1 transmission during sexual intercourse, including the mode of sexual contact, the infectiousness of the index case, and the susceptibility of the HIV-1–uninfected partner exposed to the virus. Increasing evidence suggests that infection with bacterial or viral STDs influences both the susceptibility to HIV-1 of uninfected individuals, and the infectiousness of individuals who are infected with HIV-1.

STDs and HIV-1 Susceptibility

Nonulcerative STDs and HIV-1 Susceptibility

Seven prospective studies have examined the risk of HIV-1 acquisition among women with nonulcerative STDs in Africa (Table 2). These studies were conducted among commercial sex workers (CSWs) (21–23), STD clinic attendees (24,25), pregnant women at antenatal clinics (26), or family planning clients (27). Appropriate laboratory tests, including culture, microscopy, and serology, were used to confirm etiologic diagnosis of STDs in each of these studies. As shown in Table 2, only three of these studies assessed the association between chlamydial infection and HIV-1 acquisition (21–23). Accurate detection of chlamydial infection requires expensive diagnostic facilities that are not routinely available in many African countries. The study conducted in Kinshasa reported a significantly increased risk of HIV-1 acquisition among women with chlamydial infection (adjusted RR 3.6; 95% CI, 1.4 to 9.1). Relatively modest HIV-1 risk increases were

TABLE 2. Studies on the Association between Nonulcerative STDs and HIV-1 Acquisition[a]

Study population, site (Year)	Author (Reference)	STDs studied	Adjusted RR (95% CI)
CSWs, Nairobi (1991)	Plummer et al. (21)	Chlamydia	2.7 (0.9–7.8)
CSWs, Kinshasa (1993)	Laga et al. (22)	Gonorrhea	4.8 (2.4–9.8)
		Chlamydia	3.6 (1.4–9.1)
		Trichomoniasis	1.9 (0.9–4.1)
STD patients, Yaounde (1994)	Weir et al. (24)	Gonorrhea	1.4 (0.4–4.9)
		Trichomoniasis	2.4 (0.7–8.0)*
STD patients, Nairobi (1994)	Plourde et al. (25)	Gonorrhea	1.3 (0.4–4.5)*
CSWs, Mombasa (1998)	Martin et al. (23)	Gonorrhea	1.8 (1.0–3.3)
		Chlamydia	1.3 (0.5–3.3)
		Trichomoniasis	1.2 (0.7–2.2)
Pregnant women, Blantyre (1998)	Taha et al. (26)	Gonorrhea	4.3 (1.2–15.7)
		Trichomoniasis	1.7 (0.7–3.8)*
FP clients, Dar es Salaam (1998)	Kapiga et al. (27)	Gonorrhea	3.8 (1.7–8.5)
		Trichomoniasis	1.5 (0.7–3.2)*

[a]STDs indicates sexually transmitted diseases; RR, relative risk; CI, confidence interval; CSWs, commercial sex workers; FP, family planning; *, relative risks that are not adjusted for other risk factors.

reported among women with trichomoniasis (22–24,26,27). Data from three of these studies showed gonorrhea to be a significant risk factor for sexual transmission of HIV-1 in women; the relative risk ranged from 3.8 to 4.8 (22,26,27).

Two other prospective studies conducted in Thailand assessed the association between nonulcerative STDs and HIV-1 acquisition. In the study conducted among CSWs in northern Thailand, the risk of HIV-1 acquisition was more than three times higher (RR 3.6; 95% CI, 1.4 to 9.7) among women who had chlamydia at one visit during the follow-up period, and about ten times higher (RR 10.4; 95% CI, 4.3 to 25.2) among those who had chlamydia at two or more visits (28). Similarly, the risk of HIV-1 acquisition was significantly increased among women with gonorrhea at one visit during follow-up (RR 3.5; 95% CI, 1.4 to 9.0), and among those with gonorrhea at two or more visits (RR 6.2; 95% CI, 2.0 to 19.3). However, only chlamydial infection remained significantly associated with HIV-1 acquisition after adjusting for other risk factors in multivariate analysis (RR 3.3; 95% CI, 1.4 to 7.9). The other study found that self-reported urethritis was associated with significantly increased risk of HIV-1 acquisition (RR 6.0; 95% CI, 1.8 to 20.9) among 1,115 young men conscripted in the Thai army (29). The results of this study provide evidence of the role of nonulcerative STDs in female-to-male transmission of HIV-1. However, there are no prospective studies that have examined the susceptibility to HIV-1 infection of African men with nonulcerative STDs.

There are no studies that have specifically examined whether the risk of HIV-1 acquisition among patients with symptomatic nonulcerative STDs is higher than that of patients with asymptomatic infections. Since most STD-related symptoms and signs are markers of the STDs themselves, it is difficult to make any firm conclusions about the role of symptomatic and asymptomatic nonulcerative STDs on HIV-1 acquisition. However, a few studies have reported a significantly increased risk of HIV-1 acquisition among patients with symptoms and signs related to STDs. For example, in a study of CSWs in Kinshasa (22), the presence of cervical pus was associated with a marginally significant increased risk of HIV-1 acquisition (adjusted RR 2.6; 95% CI, 1.0 to 6.7). In another study involving CSWs in Kenya (23), vulvitis and abnormal vaginal discharge were significantly associated with HIV-1 acquisition after adjusting for other predictors in multivariate analyses.

There are a number of plausible biologic mechanisms that could explain the increased susceptibility to HIV-1 of people with nonulcerative STDs. The microscopic disruption of mucosal barriers that occurs during these infections could contribute to substantial HIV-1 risk (18). Inflammation resulting from nonulcerative STDs is associated with the recruitment of lymphocytes, Langerhans cells, and macrophages in the genital tract mucosa (30–32). Thus, infection with nonulcerative STDs might enhance susceptibility to HIV-1 by increasing the number of HIV-1 target cells in the genital mucosa. In addition, factors released at sites of inflammation have been shown to greatly enhance HIV-1 subtype C viral replication (33). Results from in-vitro studies suggest that polymorphonuclear leukocytes (PMNs) from HIV-1–seronegative donors induce HIV-1 replication in mononuclear cells from HIV-1–infected patients (34). Hence, recruitment of PMNs into the genital tract may increase the risk of HIV-1 transmission. It is also possible that STDs interact with other cells at the molecular level to facilitate HIV-1 transmission. For example, *Chlamydia trachomatis* has been shown in vitro to enhance HIV-1 replication in the presence of PMNs (34), possibly through the generation of reactive oxygen products secreted by granulocytes (35). Chlamydial infection also causes secretion of cytokines that could affect the replication of HIV-1 and/or increase the number of receptive cells (36).

Ulcerative STDs and HIV-1 Susceptibility

The most common causes of genital ulcer disease (GUD) are *Treponema pallidum*, *Haemophilus ducreyi*, herpes simplex virus type 2 (HSV-2), lymphogranuloma venereum, and granuloma inguinale (37). Other less common causes of GUD are trauma, adverse drug reactions, other infections not transmitted by sexual contact, neoplasms, vesiculobullous skin diseases, and other nonspecific causes. The causes of GUD vary across geographic areas of the world, and sometimes within the same country. The frequency of different causes also changes over time. For instance, during the 1980s, chancroid and syphilis were reported to be the most common causes of GUD in most parts of Africa (38) while studies suggested that HSV-2 was not a major cause of GUD in this region (39–41). Findings from more recent studies, however, suggest that the relative importance of HSV-2 in Africa is increasing (42).

Researchers in Rwanda were among the first to report a relatively high prevalence of HSV-2 in Africa (43); 18% of the men and 20% of the women with GUD in their study had HSV-2 detected by culture. In a recent study of 558 men attending STD clinics in three major South African cities, about 36% of those with GUD had HSV-2, the most frequently identified etiologic agent (44). Other studies have reported the prevalence of HSV-2 antibodies to be higher than 60% among randomly selected men and women from rural populations in some African countries (45,46). Similar findings have been reported in other countries in Southeast Asia (47), and in Central and South America (48,49), although rates may be lower in most developed countries (50).

There are a number of potential explanations for the increasing prevalence of HSV-2 in developing countries. Most of the developing countries with relatively high HSV-2 prevalence tend to also have high prevalence of HIV-1 infection. Increasing HSV-2 prevalence in these countries could be a result of the changing spectrum and natural history of GUD caused by increasing HIV-1 disease in the general population. It is also possible that the increase in reports of genital herpes among patients with GUD is the result of increased detection of HSV-2. Recent advancements in type-specific serologic assays and nucleic acid amplification techniques have availed improved tools for the estimation of HSV-2 prevalence and incidence in many populations in developing countries (51,52).

Numerous studies have examined the association between GUD and HIV-1 transmission. Studies conducted among female CSWs and their male clients in Kenya were among the earliest prospective studies to support initial findings from cross-sectional and case-control studies. The first study, reported in 1989 by Cameron et al., involved 422 men who presented with STD-related symptoms at a clinic in Nairobi (53). These men had sexual contact with a group of CSWs during the 4 weeks preceding their clinic visit. The majority of them had been sexually exposed to HIV-1 as over 85% of the CSWs were known to be HIV-1–seropositive. During the follow-up period, 24 (8.2%) of the 293 initially HIV-1–seronegative men acquired a new HIV-1 infection. After adjusting for other risk factors, men with a genital ulcer at enrollment had about a five-fold increased risk of HIV-1 seroconversion (RR 4.7; 95% CI, 1.3 to 17.0) compared with men without a genital ulcer. About 50% of the ulcers were culture positive for *Haemophilus ducreyi*. This study provided the first evidence of the role of GUD in facilitating female-to-male transmission of HIV-1.

Of the 595 CSWs approached to participate in the second study, the 196 (32.9%) who were HIV-1–seronegative were enrolled in 1985 and followed up to the end of June 1987 (21). At the end of follow-up, 83 (67%) of the 124 women who participated until the end of the study, were found to have acquired a new HIV-1 infection. The annual incidence of HIV-1 infection in this population was estimated to be 47%. The presence of genital ulcers was associated with a more than three-fold increased risk of HIV-1 seroconversion (adjusted RR 3.3; 95% CI, 1.2 to 10.1). This study suggested a dose–response relationship; HIV-1 seroconversion rates increased from about 58% among those without an ulcer or with a single episode of an ulcer, to almost 100% among those with more than three episodes of an ulcer in a year. Results from this study provided the first evidence of the role of GUD in facilitating transmission of HIV-1 from men to women.

These and other studies that have examined the role of GUD in HIV-1 acquisition within and outside Africa are listed in Table 3 (21,22,29,47,53–57). Most of these studies used laboratory tests to determine the etiologic causes of GUD. These studies report a great range of risk estimates—possibly due to varying durations of the ulcers before they were diagnosed and treated, and differences in the rate of partner change and HIV-1 prevalence in the general population. Overall, these studies report high risk estimates, suggesting relatively strong associations between the various causes of GUD and the risk of HIV-1 acquisition among both men and women.

There are several biologic mechanisms to account for the increased risk of HIV-1 acquisition among individuals with GUD. Most infections that cause GUD induce an intense inflammatory response with subsequent development of microscopic and macroscopic ulcers in the genital tract. These processes are associated with disruption of the genital tract mucosal integrity and increased susceptibility to HIV-1 infection. Genital ulcers bleed easily and can come in contact with genital secretions during sex. The inflammatory response that follows these infections also increases the presence and activation of HIV-1–susceptible cells, such as PMNs, and $CD4^+$ lymphocytes and macrophages in the genital tract and on the ulcer surface (58–60). The increased presence of these cells in the genital tract increases the likelihood of GUD patients acquiring HIV-1 from infected sexual partners.

Furthermore, there is evidence to suggest that the interactions between acute or

TABLE 3. Studies on the Association between Ulcerative STDs and HIV-1 Acquisition[a]

Study population, site (Year)	Sex	Author (Reference)	Etiology of Genital Ulcer Disease (GUD)	Adjusted RR (95% CI)
STD patients, Nairobi (1989)	Male	Cameron et al. (53)	GUD by clinical exam at enrollment (50% *H. ducreyi* positive, 4% syphilis, 5% HSV-2)	4.7 (1.3–17.0)
CSWs, Nairobi (1991)	Female	Plummer et al. (21)	*H. ducreyi* and syphilis	3.3 (1.2–10.1)
CSWs, Kinshasa (1993)	Female	Laga et al. (22)	*H. ducreyi*	1.9 (0.0–69.5)*
			Syphilis	3.4 (0.7–17.6)*
STD patients, New York (1993)	Male	Telzak et al. (54)	*H. ducreyi*	3.3 (1.1–10.1)
			New STDs between visits	3.2 (1.0–10.1)
STD patients, Baltimore (1994)	Male and Female	Kassler et al. (55)	Syphilis	2.0 (0.1–32.0)*
			GUD by clinical exam	11.3 (1.6–80.2)
STD patients, Pune (1995)	Male and Female	Mehendale et al. (56)	GUD by clinical exam at previous visit	4.3 (2.2–8.4)
			GUD at recurrent visits	8.2 (3.8–17.9)
Factory workers, Harare (1996)	Male	Mbizvo et al. (57)	Self-reported GUD during follow-up	3.6 (1.5–8.3)
Military conscripts, Northern Thailand (1997)	Male	Nelson et al. (47)	*H. ducreyi*	2.2 (0.9–5.5)
			HSV-2	3.1 (1.2–7.9)
			Syphilis	1.5 (0.02–27.6)*
Military conscripts, Northern Thailand (1998)	Male	Nopkesorn et al. (29)	*H. ducreyi*	1.8 (0.2–8.0)*
			HSV-2	2.0 (0.6–6.1)
			Syphilis	2.2 (0.1–14.3)*
			Self-reported GUD during follow-up	13.5 (3.4–89.9)

[a]STDs indicates sexually transmitted diseases; RR, relative risk; CI, confidence interval; CSWs, commercial sex workers; *, relative risks that are not adjusted for other risk factors; HSV-2, herpes simplex virus type 2.

reactivated viral STDs and HIV-1 at the molecular level may induce HIV-1 expression and transactivation. For example, HSV genes have been shown to enhance HIV-1 replication by binding directly to the HIV-1 long terminal repeat (LTR) or by processes mediated through cellular transcription factors (61,62). More recently, *Treponema pallidum* lipoproteins were shown to increase HIV-1 replication (63). HIV-1 infects and multiplies in activated $CD4^+$ T-lymphocytes by using the $CD4^+$ molecule as a receptor for entry (64). In-vivo studies suggest that HIV-1 may also be capable of infecting cells that lack the $CD4^+$ molecule, such as keratinocytes, in tissues coinfected with herpesviruses (65). Hence, people with GUD caused by viral STDs may be at a relatively increased risk of acquiring HIV-1 infection because the virus is capable of infecting both cells that express $CD4^+$ receptors and other cells.

STDs and HIV-1 Infectiousness

In addition to the susceptibility of the HIV-1–uninfected partner, the infectiousness of the index case is an important determinant of the sexual transmission of HIV-1 (66,67). In general, the transmission of an infectious pathogen is determined by the inoculum size and the infectiousness of the pathogen itself (67). The viral concentration of HIV-1 in the blood and seminal plasma, and in the female genital secretions is a major determinant of the infectivity of HIV-1–infected individuals. High concentration of HIV-1 in the blood plasma is associated with HIV-1 disease progression in both adults and children (68–70), and with significantly increased risk of bloodborne (71), vertical (72), and sexual (73) transmission of HIV-1 infection. High concentrations of HIV-1 in the genital tract have also been shown to be associated with increased vertical (74) and sexual (75) transmission of HIV-1 infection.

The concentration of HIV-1 in seminal plasma and female genital secretions is weakly correlated with that in blood plasma (76–78), suggesting that factors other than the viral load in blood plasma determine the levels of HIV-1 RNA in the genital tract. Numerous clinical studies have assessed the association between ulcerative and nonulcerative STDs, and HIV-1 shedding in the genital tract (79). Cross-sectional studies have reported detection of HIV-1 in the exudates from the surfaces of genital ulcers. In 1989, Kreiss et al. reported that HIV-1 had been detected by culture from four (11%) of the 36 ulcers of 33 HIV-1–positive CSWs seen at an STD clinic in Nairobi (80). In another study conducted at the same clinic, Plummer et al. reported isolating HIV-1 by culture from two out of seven (30%) ulcers of HIV-1 seropositive men with GUD in 1990 (81).

Eight other studies have used nucleic acid amplification techniques to compare HIV-1 shedding in the genital tracts of individuals infected with STDs with that of individuals not infected with STDs (Table 4). Two of these studies assessed the association between HIV-1 shedding and ulcerative STDs (76,82); the others examined the role of nonulcerative STDs in genital HIV-1 shedding (83–88). Two of the three studies that assessed the presence of both gonorrheal and chlamydial infection reported significantly increased risk of genital HIV-1 shedding

TABLE 4. Studies on the Association between STDs and HIV-1 Genital Shedding among HIV-1 Seropositive Populations[a]

Study population, site (Year)	Sex	Author (Reference)	STDs studied	Adjusted OR (95% CI)
Nonulcerative STDs				
HIV-1–positive men, Boston and San Francisco (1992)	Male	Anderson et al. (83)	Seminal leukocytosis	7.0 (1.3–39.3)
STD patients, Nairobi (1993)	Female	Clemetson et al. (84)	Cervical mucopus	6.2 (0.9–41.4)
			N. gonorrhoeae	4.3 (0.7–25.3)*
CSWs, Nairobi (1994)	Female	Kreiss et al. (85)	Cervicitisx (Gram's stain microscopy and Pap smear cytology)	8.7 (2.0–37.2)
STD patients, Nairobi (1995)	Male	Moss et al. (86)	*N. gonorrhoeae*	3.2 (1.6–6.4)
CSWs, Abidjan (1997)	Female	Ghys et al. (76)	*N. gonorrhoeae*	1.9 (1.2–3.0)
			C. trachomatis	2.5 (1.1–5.8)
Pregnant women, Nairobi (1997)	Female	John et al. (87)	Mucopus	2.1 (1.1–3.9)*
			N. gonorrhoeae	2.2 (0.7–6.4)*
			C. trachomatis	1.2 (0.4–3.4)*
STD patients, Nairobi (1997)	Female	Mostad et al. (88)	*N. gonorrhoeae*	3.1 (1.1–9.8)*
			C. trachomatis	1.3 (0.4–4.6)*
Ulcerative STDs				
CSWs, Abidjan (1997)	Female	Ghys et al. (76)	Cervical or vaginal ulcer	3.9 (2.1–7.4)
STD patients, Seattle (1998)	Male	Schacker et al. (82)	HSV-2	4.6 (1.8–8.7)

[a]STDs indicate sexually transmitted diseases; RR, relative risk; CI, confidence interval; CSWs, commercial sex workers; *, relative risks that are not adjusted for other risk factors; HSV-2, herpes simplex virus type 2.

among subjects with gonorrhea compared to those without this type of infection. These results were supported by a pooled analysis of data from five other studies (79), in which 41% of patients with gonorrhea and 32% of those without gonorrhea had detectable HIV-1 in the genital tract ($p = 0.004$).

Other studies have compared viral load in the genital secretions of STD patients with that of HIV-infected individuals without STDs. Some of these studies have also examined the effect of STD therapy on the level of HIV-1 shedding in the genital tract. Researchers in North Carolina reported a 32-year-old white male with chlamydial urethritis whose seminal plasma HIV-1 RNA concentration was 375,000 copies/ml before treatment (89). Four weeks after the patient completed therapy for chlamydial infection, his seminal plasma HIV-1 RNA concentration was reduced to 7,500 copies/ml. This patient did not receive any antiretroviral therapy during this interval. Another study involving four homosexual men with urethritis (three with gonorrhea and one with nongonococcal urethritis) was conducted in London between October 1994 and June 1995 (90). The mean HIV-1 proviral concentration in the semen of these men declined from about 550 copies/ml to 120 copies/ml ($p < 0.05$) following successful STD treatment. The large difference between the patients' seminal plasma viral loads in these two studies might be due to several factors, including differences in their clinical stages of HIV-1 disease and the different laboratory techniques used to measure their viral loads.

The largest study to examine the impact of STD treatment on HIV-1 shedding was conducted between January and March 1996 in Malawi (91). In this study, HIV-1 RNA concentration was measured in the seminal plasma of 86 HIV-1–seropositive men with urethritis and 49 HIV-1–seropositive men without urethritis who served as controls. Although both groups of men had similar $CD4^+$ lymphocyte counts and blood plasma viral loads, the median seminal plasma HIV-1 RNA concentration at baseline was eight times higher in men with urethritis than in the controls (12.4 vs. 1.51×10^4 copies/ml; $p = 0.035$). Among men with urethritis, those with gonorrhea had higher concentrations of HIV-1 RNA in semen than those with nongonococcal urethritis (median 15.8 vs. 2.52×10^4 copies/ml; $p = 0.003$). Two weeks after completion of antibiotic treatment for their urethritis, the median seminal plasma HIV-1 RNA concentration in these men had declined from 12.4 to 4.12×10^4 copies/ml ($p = 0.0001$). At that point, the concentration of seminal plasma HIV-1 RNA among these patients was no longer significantly different from that of the controls. The blood plasma HIV-1 RNA concentration did not change significantly during the study in any group, including the group that received antibiotic STD treatment.

In summary, the findings from the studies presented in this section confirm that both ulcerative and nonulcerative STDs are associated with increased HIV-1 shedding in seminal plasma and other genital tract secretions. Because increased concentration of HIV-1 in the genital tract is associated with increased infectiousness in the index case, these findings also provide plausible biologic explanations for the increased rate of sexual HIV-1 transmission from individuals with both HIV-1 and other STDs to their HIV-1–uninfected partners. Furthermore, these studies show that antibiotic treatment of patients with conventional STDs reduces their infectiousness by decreasing the shedding of HIV-1 in the genital tract. However, treatment of STDs does not eradicate HIV-1 shedding in the genital tract and transmission can still occur following completion of STD therapy.

CONTROL OF STDs FOR HIV-1 PREVENTION

STDs can be controlled by preventing new infections (primary prevention), and providing treatment for existing infections (secondary prevention). Most STD control programs seek to change sexual behavior through risk-reduction education and condom promotion. Secondary prevention includes provision of prompt and effective STD therapy to patients and their sexual partners, and screening for asymptomatic cases. Optimal STD case management and case finding shorten the duration of infections, thereby interrupting the chain of transmission and helping to reduce STD prevalence.

A number of investigators have used observational study designs and community-based, randomized, controlled trials to evaluate the effectiveness of STD control as a strategy for HIV-1 prevention. Most observational studies have evaluated a range of service delivery strategies, including raising awareness about STD symptoms, promoting condoms, providing periodic STD screening followed by treatment, treating STDs presumptively, and increasing access to STD diagnosis and treatment services.

One of the earliest observational studies of the effects of STD control on HIV-1 incidence was conducted between 1988 and 1991 among female CSWs in Kinshasa (92). During this period, 531 initially HIV-1–negative CSWs received monthly STD screening and treatment, individual health education, and condoms. A decline of HIV-1 incidence was observed over a 3-year period, from 11.7 per 100 person-years during the first 6 months, to 4.4 per 100 person-years during the last 6 months ($p = 0.003$). Over the same time period, the incidence of gonorrhea, trichomoniasis, and GUD declined significantly. The results of this study were the first to suggest that provision of effective STD treatment and condoms for CSWs could lead to significant reductions of both STD and HIV-1 incidence. Another study conducted in a mining company in South Africa showed that monthly presumptive STD treatment of CSWs reduced STD prevalence not only in this high-risk group, but also in the surrounding population of miners (93). However, the effect on HIV-1 transmission was not directly measured in this study.

Observational studies conducted in selected populations cannot directly measure the effect of STD control on HIV-1 incidence in the general population. Hence, they are less useful in assessing the overall impact of STD interventions on HIV-1 transmission. Well-designed, randomized, controlled trials with clearly defined endpoints have become the gold standard for evaluating public health interventions. Such studies provide stronger evidence of a causal association, since random allocation of the interventions helps to minimize confounding by enhancing the comparability of intervention and comparison groups (94). STD interventions can be applied at both the individual and the community level. At the individual level, persons can be randomized into the intervention and control arm and then followed to find out the impact of the intervention on HIV-1 incidence. However, randomizing communities rather than individuals is likely to have a greater impact on HIV-1 incidence since the intervention operates both on HIV-1 acquisition (susceptibility) and HIV-1 transmission (infectiousness) (95). Community randomization also helps to minimize "contamination," and allows evaluation of interventions delivered at the population level.

Two major community-based, randomized, controlled, intervention trials have been conducted to assess the impact of STD control on HIV-1 incidence at the population level. The first trial, conducted between 1991 and 1994 in the Mwanza region of Tanzania, tested the impact of improved STD treatment within the existing primary health care system on HIV-1 transmission in the general population (96). This trial was implemented in six pairs of large rural communities. In each pair, one community was randomly allocated to receive the intervention while the other community served as a comparison area and received the existing unimproved services. The intervention comprised of three main coordinated activities: (*i*) a community educational campaign to raise STD awareness and improve treatment-seeking behavior, (*ii*) regular supervision and training for health workers on the syndromic approach to STD management, and (*iii*) provision of inexpensive and effective STD drugs. In these communities, the prevalence of HIV-1 was 4% and the incidence was about 1 per 100 person-years.

After 24 months of follow-up, the Mwanza trial demonstrated a statistically significant 38% reduction in HIV-1 incidence in the intervention communities (97). Furthermore, the interventions reduced the prevalence of active syphilis by 29%, the incidence of active syphilis by 38%, and the prevalence of symptomatic male urethritis by 49% (98). However, the interventions were not successful in reducing the prevalence of reproductive tract infections among pregnant women in the study communities. No significant differences in reported sexual behavior or condom use were noted between the intervention and comparison communities at baseline or during the implementation of the study.

The second trial was conducted between 1994 and 1998 in 56 rural communities in the Rakai district of Uganda (99). These communities were aggregated into 10 clusters of four to seven contiguous villages. Five of these clusters were randomly assigned to receive the intervention, which comprised of intermittent mass treatment of STDs in the general population, administered every 10 months. During the treatment rounds, all residents of the intervention communities between the ages of 15 and 59 were administered highly effective single-dose oral antibiotics in their homes. All residents of the comparison communities received a single-dose of vitamins, iron, folic acid, and antihelminths. At the time this study was initiated, the HIV-1 epidemic in Rakai was generalized with HIV-1 incidence estimated at 1.5–2.0 per 100 person-years and prevalence at approximately 16%. Unlike the trial conducted in Mwanza, the Rakai trial found no difference in the incidence of HIV-1 infection between the intervention and the comparison communities after three rounds of mass treatment (adjusted RR 0.97; 95% CI, 0.81 to 1.16) (100). However, the Rakai trial reported significant reductions in the number of serologically-diagnosed active syphilis and culture-confirmed trichomoniasis cases in the intervention communities at the end of the second follow-up period. The incidence of trichomoniasis was also significantly reduced (adjusted RR 0.52; 95% CI, 0.35 to 0.79), but the incidence of syphilis was not significantly changed. The prevalence rates of trichomoniasis, bacterial vaginosis, gonorrhea, and chlamydia were significantly reduced by 30% to 70% among pregnant women in the intervention areas. These changes were not influenced by differential sexual behavior changes in the two study groups.

The findings from the Mwanza trial provided the first evidence that simple and inexpensive STD control activities integrated into the existing primary health care services in a typical developing country setting could significantly reduce HIV-1 transmission. The estimated cost-effectiveness of this intervention, US$218 per HIV-1 infection averted and US$10 per disability-adjusted life year (DALY) saved, compared favorably with other highly effective public health interventions (101). As expected, these findings generated a great deal of interest among public health workers, donor agencies and policy-makers. The unexpected results of the Rakai trial, however, have generated considerable uncertainty about the effectiveness of STD control in HIV-1 prevention programs.

Several factors may have contributed to the discrepancy between the results of the Mwanza and Rakai trials. First, because of the more severe inflammatory response that accompanies symptomatic STDs, such infections may be more important in the transmission of HIV-1 than asymptomatic STDs (19). In Rakai, the clinical infrastructure to treat symptomatic STDs between treatment rounds was not well developed. The continuous services for the treatment of symptomatic STDs that were provided in Mwanza, might be more effective in reducing HIV-1 transmission than intermittent mass STD treatment of the general population. Second, the two trials were conducted in populations at different stages of the HIV-1 epidemic. The HIV-1 epidemic in Rakai was mature and generalized, with a 16% prevalence rate. In Mwanza, the prevalence of HIV-1 was about 4%, indicating that the epidemic was in its early stages. The divergent results of these trials suggest that STDs may have a greater cofactor effect on HIV-1 transmission in early rather than late stages of the HIV-1 epidemic (102). Results from mathematical models (103,104), and empirical data from both of the trials support this hypothesis. Third, the proportion of new HIV-1 infections attributable to treatable or untreatable STDs might have been different in the two areas. In Mwanza, 43% of the new HIV-1 infections among men in the comparison group could be attributed to treatable symptomatic STDs or new episodes of syphilis (105); in Rakai, only 10% of new HIV-1 infections were attributable to STD symptoms or treatable STDs in both the intervention and the comparison communities (106). In Rakai, HSV-2 was detected in 45% of genital ulcers, while the prevalence of bacterial vaginosis among women was about 50%. Although these infections were not directly investigated in Mwanza, their prevalence is likely to be less than what was found in Rakai (107). Hence, the lack of impact of STD control on HIV-1 incidence in the Rakai trial may be due to high incidence and prevalence of incurable STDs and difficult-to-treat genital tract infections.

BACTERIAL VAGINOSIS

Bacterial vaginosis (BV) is the most common cause of vaginitis in women of childbearing age. This condition was first described as "nonspecific vaginitis," partly because no single causative microorganism could be identified (108). In more recent years, the name of this infection was changed from "nonspecific vaginitis" to "bacterial vaginosis." The term "vaginosis" was adopted because inflammatory response is not a common characteristic of this condition. It is now recognized that BV is associated with complex pathophysiologic changes in the vaginal flora that are characterized by a reduction in the concentration of hydrogen peroxide-producing lactobacilli (109). These changes are associated with overgrowth of certain bacterial species, including *Gardnerella vaginalis*, *Mobiluncus* spp., *Mycoplasma hominis*, *Bacteroides* spp., and anaerobic bacteria belonging to the genera *Prevotella*, *Porphyromonas*, and *Peptostreptococcus* spp. (110). The precise determinants and mechanisms by which these changes occur are not known, although overgrowth of bacterial species is associated with biochemical changes, including elevated pH, increased concentrations of diamines, polyamines, and organic acids, and enzymes such as mucinases, sialidase, and collagenases in vaginal fluid (111,112). Women with BV present with an unpleasant, "fishy smelling" discharge that is more noticeable after unprotected intercourse. The discharge is off-white, thin, and homogeneous. Because of lack of inflammatory response, most women with BV tend to be asymptomatic.

Although precise estimates of the prevalence of BV in Africa have not been determined, studies conducted in African countries suggest that BV might be more common than most other causes of genital infections. About 51% of the women who participated in a community-based, STD control trial in Rakai, had BV at baseline (113). Studies conducted in other sub–Saharan African countries have reported prevalence rates ranging from 20% to 50% (114–116). Bacterial vaginosis has been associated with a number of gynecologic complications, including increased rate of abnormal Pap smears (117). A few studies have reported increased risk of pelvic inflammatory disease (PID) among women with BV (118), although others have not shown any association (119). The microorganisms associated with BV have been isolated from the upper genital tract and some studies have associated BV with postcesarean delivery endometritis, and salpingitis (120,121). Several obstetric complications have been associated with BV including chorioamnionitis, premature rupture of membranes, and late miscarriages (122). The associations between BV and increased risk of preterm birth and low birthweight have been demonstrated by multiple case-control and prospective cohort studies (112).

Role of Bacterial Vaginosis in HIV-1 Transmission

Data from recent studies have associated presence of abnormal vaginal flora and lack of lactobacilli with increased risk of HIV-1 infection (123). Most of the early studies that investigated the associations between STDs and HIV-1 did not examine the role of BV in HIV-1 transmission, partly because BV is not traditionally regarded as an STD. In addition, the lack of mucosal disruption and inflammation in women with BV might have led most investigators to assume that this condition was unlikely to be associated with a significantly increased risk of HIV-1 transmission.

Initial evidence of the association between BV and HIV-1 transmission came from cross-sectional studies conducted among members of both high-risk populations and the general population. The first study, involving 144 CSWs in Thailand, was reported in 1995 by Cohen et al. (124). In this study, women with clinical BV had a significantly increased risk of HIV-1 infection (adjusted OR 4.0; 95% CI, 1.7 to 9.4). In a community-based study in a rural district of Uganda, the prevalence of HIV-1 increased from 14.2% among women with normal vaginal flora to 26.7% among women with severely abnormal vaginal flora or BV ($p < 0.0001$) (113). After adjusting for other risk factors, the risk of HIV-1 was significantly increased among women with moderate abnormalities (adjusted OR 1.50; 95% CI, 1.18 to 1.89), and among those with severe abnormalities or BV (adjusted OR 2.08; 95% CI, 1.48 to 2.94). The third study was conducted among pregnant women who participated in cross-sectional surveys in Blantyre, southern Malawi (116). This study demonstrated a "dose–response" relationship between the risk of HIV-1 infection and the severity of the vaginal flora disturbances. The adjusted HIV-1 risk estimate increased from 1.65 (95% CI, 1.32 to 2.07) among women with mild disturbances to 3.04 (95% CI, 2.43 to 3.84) among women with severe disturbances or BV. In a similar study involving 724 pregnant women in the United States, the prevalence of HIV-1 infection increased with increasing severity of abnormal flora ($p = 0.03$) (125).

Two prospective studies have reported increased risk of HIV-1 acquisition among women with disturbances of the vaginal flora and BV. In a cohort study involving 657 CSWs in Mombasa, Kenya (126), women with abnormal vaginal flora had an almost two-fold increased risk of HIV-1 acquisition (adjusted RR 1.9; 95% CI, 1.1 to 3.1). The largest cohort study was conducted in Blantyre, Malawi, in which 1,196 women were followed during pregnancy and after delivery (26). In this cohort, women with BV had an increased risk of HIV-1 seroconversion during pregnancy (adjusted OR 3.68) and the postnatal period (adjusted OR 1.84). As observed in the cross-sectional study previously conducted in this population (116), the risk of HIV-1 acquisition increased with increasing severity of the vaginal flora disturbances ($p = 0.04$).

There are a number of mechanisms by which BV might enhance susceptibility to HIV-1 infection. First, hydrogen peroxide produced by lactobacilli plays an important role as a natural microbicide within the vaginal ecosystem, and is toxic to a number of organisms, including HIV-1 (127,128). Hence, reduced concentration of the hydrogen peroxide-producing lactobacilli could facilitate HIV-1 transmission. Second, low vaginal pH has been postulated to inhibit $CD4^+$ lymphocyte activation, resulting in reduced numbers of HIV-1 target cells in the vagina (129). Reduced production of lactic acid among women with BV increases the vaginal pH, making it more conducive to HIV-1 survival (130,26). Third, BV and several nonulcerative STDs have been shown to increase the levels of endocervical interleukin-10, which increases the susceptibility of macrophages to HIV-1 (131).

Although there are no clinical studies that have shown increased HIV-1 shedding in the genital tracts of women with BV, there is evidence to suggest that BV may increase HIV-1 infectiousness. BV is associated with increased levels of proinflammatory cytokines, such as TNF-α and IL-1β, in the cervical secretions (132). These cytokines could up-regulate local HIV-1 replication through activation of the LTR promoter region, leading to increased HIV-1 transmission (132). Membrane components of BV-related microorganisms have been shown to activate in-vitro transcription of HIV-1. For example, *Gardnerella vaginalis* has been found to significantly stimulate HIV-1 expression in monocytoid cells and certain T-cell lines (133). In addition, *G. vaginalis* activates LTR transcription in HIV-1 infected cells and increases NF-κB binding activity (133). Investigators have observed that other BV-associated anaerobic bacteria, such as *Peptostreptococcus asaccharolyticus* and *Prevotella bivia*, stimulate HIV-1 expression in monocytoid cells (134). Others have found that several bacterial and fungal species, especially diphtheroid-like bacteria and *Mycoplasma* spp., induce HIV-1 expression (135). These investigators identified *M. hominis* as a potential source of the heat stable soluble HIV-1 inducing factor (HIF) activity in the female genital tract.

Treatment and Prevention of Bacterial Vaginosis

Prevention and treatment of BV could help to restore normal vaginal flora and reduce the susceptibility of women to HIV-1 infection. A number of clinical trials have been conducted to assess the effectiveness of antimicrobial compounds for the treatment of BV and two reviews on this subject have been published (136,137). Metronidazole has been shown to be highly efficacious and has been widely used in the treatment of BV since the early 1980s. In general, the cure rates are much higher for a 7-day oral course (500 mg twice a day for 7 days), ranging from 86% 5 to 10 days following therapy to 78% 4 weeks after treatment completion. However, the most commonly used antimicrobial regimen for BV is a single 2 g dose of metronidazole. This regimen has a cure rate of about 84% at 1 week and 62% at 3 to 4 weeks after completion of treatment (136). This single oral dose regimen may be the most cost-effective regimen in Africa because it is inexpensive and does not require extended patient compliance. Clindamycin cream 2% (5 g at bedtime for 7 consecutive days) or metronidazole gel 0.75% (5 g twice a day for 5 days) are considered as effective as oral metronidazole therapy (137).

There are no studies that have directly assessed the impact of BV treatment on HIV-1 transmission. The impact of a single oral dose of metronidazole (2 g metronidazole given at 10 monthly intervals) on BV prevalence was assessed in Rakai, Uganda as part of the STD mass treatment community trial (100). In this study, the prevalence of BV at baseline in the intervention and control communities (50.4% vs. 51.2%) was not significantly different from that reported after the second round of treatment (46.6% vs. 53.8%). A substudy of pregnant women in this population showed a 26% reduction in BV prevalence after delivery (adjusted RR 0.74; 95% CI, 0.67 to 0.81), but no concomitant reduction in incidence of HIV-1 infection either during pregnancy or after delivery.

CONCLUSION

The scientific evidence of the role of STDs in facilitating sexual transmission of HIV-1 strongly justifies STD control as a strategy to reduce further expansion of the HIV-1 epidemic in Africa. However, it remains to be determined how best to achieve this goal. Results from intervention studies suggest that treating symptomatic rather than asymptomatic STDs may be more effective in reducing the transmission of HIV-1. Findings from intervention studies also suggest that continuous access to improved STD services, as was provided in Mwanza, may have a greater impact on HIV-1 transmission than periodic STD treatment in the general population. Operations research is required to determine cost-effective strategies to deliver improved STD services within existing health facilities in Africa, and to validate effective treatment algorithms. Results from mathematical models suggest that the contribution of STDs to the spread of HIV-1 may decline as HIV-1 prevalence in the general population increases. Hence, STD control for HIV-1 prevention should be targeted to populations with substantial rates of curable STDs in the early or intermediate phases of the HIV-1 epidemic. Additional studies are required to determine the effects of incurable infections, such as HSV-2, on the transmission of HIV-1, and to identify strategies that may be used to prevent and reduce the recurrence rate of these infections.

Existing evidence suggests that the risk of HIV-1 acquisition is increased in women with BV. The risk ratios reported in most studies are comparable to those reported in other studies that have examined the role of nonulcerative STDs in HIV-1 transmission. Since BV is more prevalent than many other genital infections in Africa, the proportion of HIV-1 infections that could be attributable to BV is likely to be higher than that of most STDs. Prevention efforts directed at BV are hampered by limited knowledge of the microbiologic and host risk factors for BV acquisition. Hence, studies to describe the natural history of this infection and to determine the risk factors are urgently needed. Genital hygienic practices in women and their male partners may be important risk factors; further research is required to define their contribution. Although the role of sexual transmission in BV is not well established, promotion of safer sexual practices might help to reduce the burden of this condition. In addition, clinical trials to determine the impact of BV treatment and prevention on HIV-1 transmission should be given the highest priority.

REFERENCES

1. Carael M, Van de Perre PH, Lepage PH, et al. Human immunodeficiency virus transmission among heterosexual couples in Central Africa. *AIDS*, 1988;2:201–205.
2. Chmiel JS, Detels R, Kaslow RA, et al. Factors associated with prevalent human immunodeficiency virus (HIV-1) infection in multicenter AIDS cohort study. *Am J Epidemiol*, 1987;128:568–575.
3. Pepin J, Plummer FA, Brunham RD, et al. The interaction of HIV-1 and other sexually transmitted diseases: an opportunity for intervention. *AIDS*, 1989;3:3–9.
4. Wasserheit JN. Epidemiological synergy: interrelationships between human immunodeficiency virus infection and other sexually transmitted diseases. *Sex Transm Dis*, 1992;5(suppl I):S55–S63.
5. Yankauer A. Sexually transmitted diseases: a neglected public health priority. *Am J Public Health*, 1994;84:1894–1897.
6. Over M, Piot P. Human immunodeficiency virus infection and other sexually transmitted diseases in developing countries: public health importance and priorities for resource allocation. *J Infect Dis*, 1996;174(Suppl 2):S162–S175.
7. Piot P, Islam MQ. Sexually transmitted diseases in the 1990s: Global epidemiology and challenges for control. *Sex Transm Dis*, 1994;21(Suppl 2):S7–S13.
8. Gerbase AC, Rowley JT, Mertens TE. Global epidemiology of sexually transmitted diseases. *Lancet*, 1998;351(suppl III):2–4.

9. Dallabetta G, Gerbase AC, Holmes KK. Problems, solutions, and challenges in syndromic management of sexually transmitted diseases. *Sex Transm Infect*, 1998;74(Suppl 1):S1-S11.
10. The World Bank. *World Development Report 1993.* Investing in Health. New York: Oxford University Press; 1993.
11. Temmerman M. Sexually transmitted diseases and reproductive health. *Sex Transm Dis*, 1994; 21(Suppl 2):S55–S58.
12. Wasserheit JN, Holmes KK. Reproductive tract infections: challenges for international health policy, programs and research. In: Germaine A, Holmes KK, Piot P, Wasserheit JN, eds. *Reproductive Tract Infections: Global Impact and Priorities for Women's Reproductive Health.* New York: Plenum Press, 1992:7–33.
13. Muir DG, Belsey MA. Pelvic inflammatory disease and its consequences in the developing world. *Am J Obstet Gynecol*, 1980;138:913–928.
14. Cates W, Farley TM, Rowe PJ. Worldwide patterns of infertility: is Africa different? *Lancet*, 1985; 2:596–598.
15. World Health Organization. Infections, pregnancies, and infertility: perspectives on prevention. *Fertil Steril*, 1987;47:964–968.
16. Drotman DP. Epidemiology and treatment of epididymitis. *Rev Infect Dis*, 1982;4:S788–S792.
17. Laga M. Epidemiology and control of sexually transmitted diseases in developing countries. *Sex Transm Dis*, 1994;21(Suppl 2):S45–S50.
18. Plummer FA. Heterosexual transmission of human immunodeficiency virus type 1 (HIV-1): Interactions of conventional sexually transmitted diseases, hormonal contraception and HIV-1. *AIDS Res Hum Retroviruses*, 1998;14(Suppl 1):S5–S10.
19. Fleming DT, Wasserheit JN. From epidemiological synergy to public health policy and practice: the contribution of other sexually transmitted diseases to sexual transmission of HIV-1 infection. *Sex Transm Infect*, 1999;75:3–17.
20. Mabey D. Interactions between HIV-1 infection and other sexually transmitted diseases. *Trop Med Int Health*, 2000;5:A32–A36.
21. Plummer FA, Simonsen JN, Cameron DW, et al. Cofactors in male-female sexual transmission of human immunodeficiency virus type 1. *J Infect Dis*, 1991;163:233–239.
22. Laga M, Manoka A, Kivuvu M, et al. Non-ulcerative sexually transmitted diseases as risk factors for HIV-1 transmission in women: results from a cohort study. *AIDS*, 1993;7:95–102.
23. Martin Jr. HL, Nyange PM, Richardson BA, et al. Hormonal contraception, sexually transmitted diseases, and risk of heterosexual transmission of human immunodeficiency virus type 1. *J Infect Dis*, 1998;178:1053–1059.
24. Weir SS, Feldblum PJ, Roddy RE, et al. Gonorrhea as a risk factor for HIV acquisition. *AIDS*, 1994; 8:1605–1608.
25. Plourde PJ, Pepin J, Agoki E, et al. Human immunodeficiency virus type 1 seroconversion in women with genital ulcers. *J Infect Dis*, 1994;170:313–317.
26. Taha TE, Hoover DR, Dallabetta GA, et al. Bacterial vaginosis and disturbances of vaginal flora: association with increased acquisition of HIV. *AIDS*, 1998;12:1699–1706.
27. Kapiga SH, Lyamuya EF, Lwihula GK, et al. The incidence of HIV infection among women using family planning methods in Dar es Salaam, Tanzania. *AIDS*, 1998;12:75–84.
28. Kilmarx PH, Limpakarnjanarat K, Mastro TD, et al. HIV-1 seroconversion in a prospective study of female sex workers in northern Thailand: continued high incidence among brothel-based women. *AIDS*, 1998;12:1889–1898.
29. Nopkesorn T, Mock PA, Mastro TD, et al. HIV-1 subtype E incidence and sexually transmitted diseases in a cohort of military conscripts in northern Thailand. *J Acquir Immune Defic Syndr Hum Retrovirol*, 1998;18:372–379.
30. Kiviat NB, Paavonen JA, Wolner-Hanssen P, et al. Histopathology of endocervical infection caused by *Chlamydia trachomatis*, herpes simplex virus, *Trichomonas vaginalis*, and *Neisseria gonorrhea*. *Human Pathol*, 1990;21:831–837.
31. Levine WC, Pope V, Bhoomkar A, et al. Increase in endocervical CD4 lymphocytes among women with nonulcerative sexually transmitted diseases. *J Infect Dis*, 1998;177:167–174.
32. Edwards JNT, Morris HB. Langerhans' cells and lymphocyte subsets in the female genital tract. *Br J Obstet Gynecol*, 1985;92:974–982.
33. Montano MA, Nixon CP, Ndung'u T, et al. Elevated tumor necrosis factor-α activation of human immunodeficiency virus type 1 subtype C in Southern Africa is associated with an NF-KB enhancer gain-of-function. *J Infect Dis*, 2000;181:76–81.
34. Ho JL, He S, Hu A, et al. Neutrophils from human immunodeficiency virus (HIV)-seronegative donors induce HIV replication from HIV-infected patients' mononuclear cells and cell lines: An in vitro model of HIV transmission facilitated by chlamydia trachomatis. *J Exp Med*, 1995;181: 1493–1505.
35. Cohen MS. Sexually transmitted diseases enhance HIV-1 transmission: no longer a hypothesis. *Lancet*, 1998;351(Suppl III):5–7.
36. Rasmussen SJ, Eckmann L, Quayle AJ, et al. Secretion of proinflammatory cytokines by epithelial cells in response to chlamydia infection suggests a central role for epithelial cells in chlamydial pathogenesis. *J Clin Invest*, 1997;99:77–87.
37. Engelkens HJH, Stolz E. Genital ulcer disease. *Int J Dematol*, 1993;32:169–181.

38. Buve A. Genital ulcer disease in Africa: many pieces are still missing from the puzzle. *Sex Transm Infect*, 1999;75:85–86.
39. Dangor Y, Fehler G, Exposto F, et al. Causes and treatment of sexually acquired genital ulceration in southern Africa. *South Afr Med J*, 1989;76:339–341.
40. Nsanze H, Fast MV, D'Costa LJ, et al. Genital ulcers in Kenya: Clinical and laboratory study. *Br J Vener Dis*, 1981;57:378–381.
41. Mabey DC, Wall RA, Bello CS. Aetiology of genital ulceration in the Gambia. *Genitourin Med*, 1987;63:312–315.
42. O'Farrell N. Increasing prevalence of genital herpes in developing countries: implications for heterosexual HIV transmission and STI control programs. *Sex Transm Infect*, 1999;75:377–384.
43. Bogaerts J, Ricart CA, Van Dyck E, et al. The etiology of genital ulceration in Rwanda. *Sex Transm Dis*, 1989;16:123–126.
44. Chen CY, Ballard RC, Beck-Sague CM, et al. Human immunodeficiency virus infection and genital ulcer disease in South Africa: the herpetic connection. *Sex Transm Dis*, 2000;27:21–29.
45. Obasi A, Mosha F, Quigley M, et al. Antibody to herpes simplex virus type 2 as a marker of sexual risk behavior in rural Tanzania. *J Infect Dis*, 1999; 179:16–24.
46. Kamali A, Nunn AJ, Mulder DW, et al. Seroprevalence and incidence of genital ulcer disease in a rural Ugandan population. *Sex Transm Infect*, 1999;75:98–102.
47. Nelson K, Eiumtrakul S, Celantano D, et al. The association of herpes simplex virus type 2 (HSV-2), Hemophilus ducreyi, and syphilis with HIV infection in young men in northern Thailand. *J Acquir Immune Defic Syndr Hum Retrovirol*, 1997;16: 293–300.
48. Conde-Glez CJ, Juarez-Figueroa L, Uribe-Salas F, et al. Analysis of herpes simplex virus 1 and 2 infection in women with high risk sexual behavior in Mexico. *Int J Epidemiol*, 1999;28:571–576.
49. Carvalho M, de Carvalho S, Pannuti CS, et al. Prevalence of herpes simplex type 2 antibodies and a clinical history of herpes in three different populations in Campinas City, Brazil. *Int J Infect Dis*, 1999;3:94–98.
50. Fleming DT, McQuillan GM, Johnson RE, et al. Herpes simplex virus type 2 in the United States, 1976–1994. *New Engl J Med*, 1997;337:1105–1111.
51. Orle KA, Gates CA, Martin DH, et al. Simultaneous PCR detection of Haemophilus ducreyi, Treponema pallidum, and herpes simplex viruses types-1 and -2 from genital ulcers. *J Clin Microbiol*, 1996;34:49–54.
52. Sanchez-Martinez D, Schmid DS, Whittington W, et al. Evaluation of a test based on baculovirus-expressed glycoprotein G for detection of herpes simplex virus type-specific antibodies. *J Infect Dis*, 1991;164:1196–1199.
53. Cameron DW, Simonsen JN, D'Costa LJ, et al. Female to male transmission of human immunodeficiency virus type 1: risk factors for seroconversion in men. *Lancet*, 1989;2:403–407.
54. Telzak EE, Chiasson MA, Bevier PJ, et al. HIV-1 seroconversion in patients with and without genital ulcer disease: a prospective study. *Ann Intern Med*, 1993;119:1181–1186.
55. Kassler WJ, Zenilman JM, Erickson B, et al. Seroconversion in patients attending sexually transmitted disease clinics. *AIDS*, 1994;8:351–355.
56. Mehendale SM, Rodrigues JJ, Brookmeyer RS, et al. Incidence and predictors of human immunodeficiency virus type 1 seroconversion in patients attending sexually transmitted disease clinics in India. *J Infect Dis*, 1995;172:1486–1491.
57. Mbizvo MT, Machekano R, McFarland W, et al. HIV seroincidence and correlates of seroconversion in a cohort of male factory workers in Harare, Zimbabwe. *AIDS*, 1996;10:895–901.
58. King R, Gough J, Ronald A, et al. An immunohistochemical analysis of naturally occurring chancroid. *J Infect Dis*, 1996;174:427–430.
59. Spinola SM, Orazi A, Aruo JN, et al. *Haemophilus ducreyi* elicits a cutaneous infiltrate of CD4 cells during experimental human infection. *J Infect Dis*, 1996;173:394–402.
60. van Laer L, Vingerhoets J, Vanham G, et al. In vitro stimulation of peripheral blood mononuclear cells (PBMC) from HIV− and HIV+ chanroid patients by *Haemophilus ducreyi* antigen. *Clin Exp Immunol*, 1995;102:243–250.
61. Laurence J. Molecular interactions among herpesviruses and human immunodeficiency viruses. *J Infect Dis*, 1990;162:338–346.
62. Rando RF, Pelett PE, Luciw PA, Bohan CA, Srinivasan A. Transactivation of human immunodeficiency virus by herpesviruses. *Oncogene*, 1987;1:13–18.
63. Theus SA, Harrich DA, Gaynor R, Radolf D, Norgard MV. Treponema pallidum lipoproteins analogues induce human immunodeficiency virus type 1 gene expression in monocytes via NF-kB activation. *J Infect Dis*, 1998;177:941–950.
64. Fauci AS. The human immunodeficiency virus: infectivity and mechanisms of pathogenesis. *Science*, 1988;239:617–622.
65. Heng MCY, Heng SY, Allen SG. Co-infection and synergy of human immunodeficiency virus-1 and herpes simplex virus-1. *Lancet*, 1994;343: 255–258.
66. Royce RA, Sena A, Cates W, Cohen MS. Sexual transmission of HIV. *N Eng J Med*, 1997;336: 1072–1078.
67. Vernazza PL, Eron JJ, Fiscus SA, et al. Sexual transmission of HIV: infectiousness and prevention. *AIDS*, 1999;13:155–166.

68. Mellors JW, Rinaldo CR Jr, Gupta P, et al. Prognosis in HIV-1 infection predicted by the quantity of virus in plasma. *Science*, 1996;272:1167–1170.
69. Shearer WT, Quinn TC, LaRussa P, et al. Viral load and disease progression in infants infected with human immunodeficiency virus type 1. *N Engl J Med*, 1997;336:1337–1342.
70. Semple M, Loveday C, Weller I, et al. Direct measurement of viraemia in patients infected with HIV-1 and its relationship to disease progression and zidovudine therapy. *J Med Virol*, 1991;35:38–45.
71. Gerberding JL. Incidence and prevalence of human immunodeficiency virus, hepatitis B virus, and cytomegalovirus among health care personnel at risk for blood exposure: final report from a longitudinal study. *J Infect Dis*, 1994;170:1410–1417.
72. Garcia PM, Kalish LA, Pitt J, et al. Maternal levels of plasma human immunodeficiency virus type 1 RNA and the risk of perinatal transmission. *N Engl J Med*, 1999;341:394–402.
73. Quinn TC, Wawer MJ, Sewankambo N, et al. Viral load and heterosexual transmission of human immunodeficiency virus type 1. *N Engl J Med*, 2000;342:921–929.
74. Panther LA, Tucker L, Xu C, et al. Genital tract human immunodeficiency virus type 1 (HIV-1) shedding and inflammation and HIV-1 env diversity in perinatal HIV-1 transmission. *J Infect Dis*, 2000;181:555–563.
75. Mostad SB, Kreiss JK. Shedding of HIV-1 in the genital tract. *AIDS*, 1996;10:1305–1315.
76. Ghys PD, Fransen K, Diallo MO, et al. The association between cervicovaginal HIV shedding, sexually transmitted diseases and immunosuppression in female sex workers in Abidjan, Cote d'Ivore. *AIDS*, 1997;11:F85–F93.
77. Coombs RW, Speck CE, Hughes JP, et al. Association between culturable human immunodeficiency virus type 1 (HIV-1) in semen and HIV-1 RNA levels in semen and blood: evidence for compartmentalization of HIV-1 between semen and blood. *J infect Dis*, 1998;177:320–330.
78. Dyer JR, Kazembe P, Vernazza PL, et al. High levels of HIV-1 in blood and semen of seropositive men in sub-Saharan Africa. *J Infect Dis*, 1998;177: 1742–1746.
79. Rotchford K, Strum AW, Wilkinson D. Effect of coinfection with STDs and of STD treatment on HIV shedding in genital-tract secretions: systematic review and data synthesis. *Sex Transm Dis*, 2000;27:243–248.
80. Kreiss JK, Coombs R, Plummer F, et al. Isolation of human immunodeficiency virus from genital ulcers in Nairobi, Kenya. *J Infect Dis*, 1989; 160:380–384.
81. Plummer FA, Wainberg MA, Plourde P, et al. Detection of human immunodeficiency virus type 1 (HIV-1) in genital ulcer exudate of HIV-1-infected men by culture and gene amplification. *J Infect Dis*, 1990;161:810.
82. Schacker T, Ryncarz AJ, Goddard J, et al. Frequent recovery of HIV-1 from genital herpes simplex virus lesions in HIV-1-infected men. *JAMA*, 1998;280: 61–66.
83. Anderson DJ, O'Brien TR, Politch JA, et al. Effects of disease stage and zidovudine therapy on the detection of human immunodeficiency virus type 1 in semen. *JAMA*, 1992;267:2769–2774.
84. Clemetson DBA, Moss GB, Willerford DM, et al. Detection of HIV DNA in cervical and vaginal secretions: prevalence and correlates among women in Nairobi, Kenya. *JAMA*, 1993;269: 2860–2864.
85. Kreiss J, Willerford DM, Hensel M, et al. Association between cervical inflammation and cervical shedding of human immunodeficiency virus DNA. *J Infect Dis*, 1994;170:15597–15601.
86. Moss GB, Overbaugh J, Welch M, et al. Human immunodeficiency virus DNA in urethral secretions in men: association with gonococcal urethritis and CD4 cell depletion. *J Infect Dis*, 1995; 172:1469–1474.
87. John GC, Nduati RW, Mbori-Ngacha D, et al. Genital shedding of human immunodeficiency virus type 1 DNA during pregnancy: association with immunosuppression, abnormal cervical or vaginal discharge, and severe vitamin A deficiency. *J Infect Dis*, 1997;175:57–62.
88. Mostad SB, Overbaugh J, DeVange DM, et al. Hormonal contraception, vitamin A deficiency, and other risk factors for shedding of HIV-1 infected cells from the cervix and vagina. *Lancet*, 1997;350:922–927.
89. Eron JJ, Gilliam B, Fiscus S, et al. HIV-1 shedding and chlamydial urethritis. *JAMA*, 1996;275:36.
90. Atkins MC, Carlin EM, Emery VC, et al. Fluctuations of HIV load in semen of HIV positive patients with newly acquired sexually transmitted diseases. *BMJ*, 1996;313:341–342.
91. Cohen MS, Hoffman IF, Royce RA, et al. Reduction of concentration of HIV-1 in semen after treatment of urethritis: implications for prevention of sexual transmission of HIV-1. *Lancet*, 1997;349:1868–1873.
92. Laga M, Alary M, Nzila N, et al. Condom promotion, sexually transmitted diseases treatment, and declining incidence of HIV-1 infection in female Zairian sex workers. *Lancet*, 1994;344:246–248.
93. Steen R, Vuylsteke B, De Coito T, et al. Evidence of declining STDs prevalence in a South African mining community following a core-group intervention. *Sex Transm Dis*, 2000;27:1–8.
94. Mertens T, Hayes RJ, Smith PG. Epidemiologic methods to study the interaction between HIV infection and other sexually transmitted diseases. *AIDS*, 1990;4:57–65.

95. Hayes R, Wawer M, Gray R, et al. Randomised trials of STD treatment for HIV prevention: report of an international workshop. *Genitourin Med*, 1997;73:432–443.
96. Hayes R, Mosha F, Nicoll A, et al. A community trial of the impact of improved STD treatment on the HIV epidemic in rural Tanzania: 1. Design. *AIDS*, 1995;9:916–926.
97. Grosskurth H, Mosha F, Todd J, et al. Impact of improved treatment of sexually transmitted diseases on HIV infection in rural Tanzania: randomized controlled trial. *Lancet*, 1995;346:530–536.
98. Mayaud P, Mosha F, Todd J, et al. Improved treatment services significantly reduce the prevalence of sexually transmitted diseases in rural Tanzania: results of a randomized controlled trial. *AIDS*, 1997;11:1873–1880.
99. Wawer MJ, Gray RH, Sewankambo NK, et al. A randomized, community-based trial of intense sexually transmitted disease control for AIDS prevention, Rakai, Uganda. *AIDS*, 1998;12:1211–1225.
100. Wawer M, Sewankambo N, Serwadda D, et al. Control of sexually transmitted diseases for AIDS prevention in Uganda: a randomized community trial. *Lancet*, 1999;353:525–535.
101. Gilson L, Mkanje R, Grosskurth H, et al. Cost-effectiveness of improved treatment services for sexually transmitted diseases in preventing HIV-1 infection in Mwanza region, Tanzania. *Lancet*, 1997;350:1805–1809.
102. Hitchcock P, Fransen L. Preventing HIV infection: lessons from Mwanza and Rakai. *Lancet*, 1999; 353:513–514.
103. Anderson RM, May RM. Epidemiological parameters of HIV transmission. *Nature*, 1988;333: 514–519.
104. Robinson NJ, Mulder DW, Auvert B, et al. Proportion of HIV infection attributable to other sexually transmitted diseases in a rural Ugandan population: simulation model estimates. *Int J Epidemiol*, 1997;26:180–189.
105. Orroth KK, Gavyole A, Todd J, et al. Syndromic treatment of sexually transmitted diseases reduces the proportion of incident HIV infections attributable to these diseases in rural Tanzania. *AIDS*, 2000;14:1429–1437.
106. Gray RH, Wawer MJ, Sewankambo NK, et al. Relative risks and population attributable fraction of incident HIV associated with symptoms of sexually transmitted diseases and treatable symptomatic sexually transmitted diseases in Rakai District, Uganda. *AIDS*, 1999;13:2113–2123.
107. Grosskurth H, Gray R, Hayes R, Mabey D, Wawer M. Control of sexually transmitted diseases for HIV-1 prevention: understanding the implications of the Mwanza and Rakai trials. *Lancet*, 2000; 355:1981–1987.
108. Thomason JL, Gelbart SM, Broekhuizen FF. Advances in the understanding of bacterial vaginosis. *J Reprod Med*, 1989;34:581–587.
109. Eschenbach DA, Davick PR, Williams BL, et al. Prevalence of hydrogen peroxide-producing *Lactobacillus* species in normal women and women with bacterial vaginosis. *J Clin Microbiol*, 1989;27: 251–256.
110. Hill GB. The microbiology of bacterial vaginosis. *Am J Obstet Gynecol*, 1993;169:450–454.
111. Chen KCS, Amsel R, Eschenbach DA, et al. Biochemical diagnosis of vaginitis: Determination of diamines in vaginal fluid. *J Infect Dis*, 1982;145:337–347.
112. McGregor JA, French JI. Bacterial vaginosis in pregnancy. *Obstet Gynecol Survey*, 2000;55 (Suppl 1): S1–S19.
113. Sewankambo N, Gray RH, Wawer MJ, et al. HIV-1 infection associated with abnormal vaginal flora morphology and bacterial vaginosis. *Lancet*, 1997;350:546–550.
114. Govender L, Hoosen AA, Moodley P, et al. Bacterial vaginosis and associated infections in pregnancy. *Int J Gynaecol Obstet*, 1996;55:23–28.
115. Ledru S, Nicolas M, Mohamed F, et al. Etiologic study of genitourinary infections in women of childbearing age in Bobo-Dioulasso, Burkina Faso, 1992. *Sex Transm Dis*, 1996;23:151–156.
116. Taha ET, Gray RH, Kumwenda NI, et al. HIV infection and disturbances of vaginal flora during pregnancy. *J Acquir Immune Defic Syndr Hum Retrovirol*, 1999;20:52–59.
117. Byrne MA, Turner MJ, Griffiths M, et al. Evidence that patients presenting with dyskaryotic cervical smears should be screened for genital-tract infections other than human papillomavirus infection. *Eur J Obstet Gynecol Reprod Biol*, 1991; 41:129–133.
118. Paavonen J, Teisala K, Heinonen PK, et al. Microbiological and histopathological findings in acute pelvic inflammatory disease. *Br J Obstet Gynecol*, 1987;94:454–460.
119. Faro S, Martens M, Maccato M, et al. Vaginal flora and pelvic inflammatory disease. *Am J Obstet Gynecol*, 1993;169:470–474.
120. Hillier SL, Kiviat NB, Hawes SE, et al. Role of bacterial vaginosis-associated microorganisms in endometritis. *Am J Obstet Gynecol*, 1996;175: 435–441.
121. Soper DE. Gynecologic sequelae of bacterial vaginosis. *Int J Gynecol Obstet*, 1999;67(Suppl 1): S25–S28.
122. Sweet RL. New approaches for the treatment of bacterial vaginosis. *Am J Obstet Gynecol*, 1993; 169:479–482.
123. Schmid G, Markowitz L, Joesoef R et al. Bacterial vaginosis and HIV infection. *Sex Transm Infect*, 2000;76:3–4.

124. Cohen CR, Duerr A, Pruithithada N, et al. Bacterial vaginosis and HIV seroprevalence among female commercial sex workers in Chiang Mai, Thailand. *AIDS*, 1995;9:1093–1097.
125. Royce RA, Thorp J, Granados JL, et al. Bacterial vaginosis associated with HIV infection in pregnant women from North Carolina. *J Acquir Immune Defic Syndr Hum Retrovirol*, 1999;20:382–386.
126. Martin HL, Richardson BA, Nyange PM, et al. Vaginal lactobacilli, microbial flora, and risk of human immunodeficiency virus type 1 and sexually transmitted disease acquisition. *J Infect Dis*, 1999;180:1863–1868.
127. Klebanoff SL, Coombs RW. Virucidal effect of Lactobacillus acidophilus on human immunodeficiency virus type-1; possible role in heterosexual transmission. *J Exp Med*, 1991;174:289–292.
128. Hillier SL. The vaginal microbial ecosystem and resistance to HIV. *AIDS Res Hum Retroviruses*, 1998;14(Suppl 1):S17–S21.
129. Hill JA, Anderson DJ. Human vaginal leukocytes and the effects of vaginal fluid on lymphocyte and macrophage defense functions. *Am J Obstet Gynecol*, 1992;166:720–726.
130. Mardh P-A. The vaginal ecosystem. *Am J Obstet Gynecol*, 1991;165:1163–1168.
131. Cohen CR, Plummer FA, Mugo N, et al. Increased interleukin-10 in the endocervical secretions of women with non-ulcerative sexually transmitted diseases: a mechanism for enhanced HIV-1 transmission? *AIDS*, 1999;13:327–332.
132. Sturm-Ramirez K, Gaye-Diallo A, Eisen G, et al. High levels of tumor necrosis factor-α and interleukin–1β in bacterial vaginosis may increase susceptibility to human immunodeficiency virus. *J Infect Dis*, 2000;182:467–473.
133. Hashemi FB, Ghassemi M, Roebuck KA, et al. Activation of human immunodeficiency virus type 1 expression by Gardnerella vaginalis. *J Infect Dis*, 1999;179:924–930.
134. Hashemi FB, Ghassemi M, Faro S, et al. Induction of human immunodeficiency virus type 1 expression by anaerobes associated with bacterial vaginosis. *J Infect Dis*, 2000;181:1574–1580.
135. Al-Harthi L, Roebuck KA, Olinger GG, et al. Bacterial vaginosis – associated microflora isolated from the female genital tract activates HIV-1 expression. *JAIDS*, 1999;21:194–202.
136. Joesoef MR, Schmid GP. Bacterial vaginosis: review of treatment options and potential clinical indications for therapy. *Clin Infect Dis*, 1995; 20(Suppl 1):S72–S79.
137. Joesoef MR, Schmid GP, Hillier SL. Bacterial vaginosis: review of treatment options and potential clinical indications for therapy. *Clin Infec Dis*, 1999;28(Suppl 1):S57–S65.

15

Mother-to-Child Transmission of HIV

Anne Willoughby

Center for Research for Mothers and Children, National Institute of Child Health and Human Development, Rockville, Maryland, USA.

EXTENT OF THE HIV EPIDEMIC IN AFRICA AND ITS IMPACT ON WOMEN AND CHILDREN

In December 2000, UNAIDS and the World Health Organization (WHO) shared their most recent grim statistics on HIV with the world health community. They estimated that there are 36.1 million adults and children living with HIV infection worldwide (1). Seventy percent of these infected individuals live in sub–Saharan Africa, where more than half of the HIV-infected adults are women. The percentages of female cases of HIV are estimated to range from 53% in Botswana and Nigeria to 58% in Rwanda and Niger (2). Furthermore, high HIV seroprevalence rates have been documented among African women of childbearing age (3). Some investigators have suggested and reported evidence that HIV-infected women have lower fertility rates than their uninfected counterparts (4). However, high rates of infection, especially among adolescent African women (5), assure the continuation of the pediatric HIV epidemic in Africa until Afro-centric strategies to prevent mother-to-child transmission (MTCT) of HIV are developed and effectively implemented.

Of all HIV-infected children worldwide, 87% are estimated to live in Africa (1). A decade ago, mathematical modeling projections supported the conclusion that, "the recent gains made in ensuring child survival [were] likely to be increasingly reversed in regions where HIV-1 infection is being transmitted in a substantial proportion of pregnancies and births" (6). More recent analyses of trends in all-cause child mortality in Africa argue convincingly that HIV may be responsible for worsening trends in child death (among children less than five years of age) in Zimbabwe and Zambia, and for the slowing of the decline in child mortality rates in other African nations (7). A study conducted in rural Uganda documented that HIV-uninfected children less than five years of age have a death rate of 12.3 per 1,000 person-years, while their HIV-infected counterparts have a death rate of 397 per 1,000 person-years (8).

TIMING OF TRANSMISSION

In order to target safe, rational, and effective interventions to reduce MTCT of HIV, it is essential to understand the timing of transmission from pregnant, HIV-infected women to their offspring (Table 1). The timing of HIV transmission may also affect the viral and immune status of the young child (9).

TABLE 1. Evidence Supporting Mother-to-Child Transmission of HIV During Different Maternal–Child Stages

Gestation	Late gestation through labor/delivery	Postnatal
Identification of HIV in placental and fetal tissues	Twin studies	HIV-positive wet nurse infects children of HIV-negative mother
Rapidly progressive disease in ill infants	Presence of virus in birth canal fluids	Postpartum transfusion of infected blood to breastfeeding HIV-negative mother who seroconverts and infects child
Comparison of mother and child viruses	Partially effective prophylaxis given in late pregnancy and during labor/delivery	Higher infection rates in breastfed vs. formula-fed infants of HIV-positive mothers
Experimental infectability of placental tissues	Neonates culture/PCR-negative shortly after birth but later proven infected	
Immunoreactivity to HIV by neonates who are not infected	Some efficacy of C-Section in preventing transmission	
	Higher rates of infection after prolonged rupture of membrances	

Very early studies in fetuses and infants have provided evidence that HIV can be transplacentally transmitted (10–12). However, Brossard and colleagues studied 100 fetuses (mean fetal age 22.4 ± 4.6 weeks) of HIV-infected mothers. They took extraordinary care to prepare tissue samples and to standardize and validate polymerase chain reaction (PCR) procedures. Their study revealed only two fetal thymic samples to be HIV-positive (13). Based on data from this relatively large cohort, it appears that early in-utero transmission contributes only modestly to perinatally transmitted infection in children.

Investigations of the clinical status of infants born to HIV-infected women reveal two distinct patterns. According to a large French cohort study of 1,386 children born to HIV-infected mothers, a small percentage of these infants (10% to 15%) are severely immunocompromised, have signs of gravely impaired central nervous system (CNS) function, suffer from opportunistic infections early in life, and may die of rapidly progressive disease (9). A much larger percentage of infected children have a slower, indolent, and varied course of disease. The existence of these two apparently distinct clinical courses suggests that a minority of HIV-infected children suffer from a chronic intrauterine infection that was well established during gestation, while the vast majority of children are infected late in pregnancy or during the process of labor and delivery. The higher rate of infection among first-born twins documented in Goedert's twin studies (14); the presence of virus in the cervicovaginal secretions of pregnant women (15); the observations that prolonged rupture of membranes increases the risk of transmission (16); and the results from Bryson's studies of infants who test culture- and PCR-negative in the first days or weeks of life, but positive during the first few months of life (17), suggest that infants can be infected during late gestation and the delivery process (17).

Using a sophisticated and complex statistical modeling of time of transmission and data from a French cohort study, analysts estimated that in nonbreastfeeding, pregnant,

HIV-infected women, the risk of early intrauterine, late in-utero, and intrapartum transmission was 25.2%, 39.0 %, and 35.8%, respectively (18). When these analysts applied the methods used by Bryson et al. (17) to their data, rates were 20.4%, 39.2%, and 40.4%, respectively (18). These and other studies suggest that the majority of mother-to-child transmission occurs late in pregnancy and during delivery.

It is clear from anecdotal case reports of transmission from HIV-infected wet nurses to the infants of HIV-uninfected mothers, from the detection of virus in breast milk, and from the results of a carefully constructed trial comparing breastfeeding with formula-feeding among the children of HIV-infected women, that HIV infection is transmitted via breastfeeding. Kreiss and Nduati made a landmark contribution to our understanding of this all-important issue in Africa (see chapter 36, *this volume*). They randomized 425 Kenyan HIV-infected pregnant women to breastfeeding vs. formula-feeding for their infants. The rate of infection at 24 months was 36.7% in the breastfed infants and 20.6% in the formula-fed group with the implication that 16.2% of infants are infected via breastfeeding. In fact, this figure may be an underestimate because a sizeable minority of women whose infants were randomized to the formula-fed group in fact breastfed their infants to some degree, while 96% of the breastfeeding group complied with the randomization. It appears that 75% of the infections among breastfed children in this group occurred before 6 months of age (19).

Other earlier observational studies had estimated similar rates. Several of these studies raised the question of the risk of infection per unit time of exposure to the milk of HIV-infected mothers. An international pooled analysis of late postnatal transmission clearly illustrated that the risk of infection continues to climb with longer duration of breastfeeding (20,21). Another study showed data that suggested that early termination of breastfeeding might form a viable strategy for reducing mother-to-infant HIV transmission in developing countries (22,23). An even more intriguing study by Coutsoudis suggested that while the exclusively breastfed infants of HIV-infected mothers have a higher rate of infection than never breastfed infants (25% vs. 18% at 15 months), the highest rate of infection is seen in children who receive both breast milk and supplemental foods (36%) (24). Future research will be directed toward efforts to understand whether manipulation of the duration of breastfeeding and type of feeding (exclusive breastfeeding vs. formula only vs. mixed feeding) might define an optimal strategy for minimizing the risk of HIV transmission while allowing the beneficial effects of breastfeeding to occur. Other research will examine whether the use of antiretroviral agents in nursing mothers or very young infants during all or part of breastfeeding may permit nursing to continue while offering infants some additional protection against infection.

RISK FACTORS

Epidemiologic, natural history, and observational studies (especially those with carefully devised laboratory analyses of biologic materials) have provided many insights into the etiology and pathogenesis of perinatal HIV transmission. A substantial and occasionally contradictory body of literature outlines factors that are generally believed to be associated with increased risk of MTCT of HIV.

Maternal factors which likely contribute to increased risk of MTCT include cigarette smoking (25), illicit drug use (26–28), frequency of intercourse during pregnancy (29), multiple sexual partners (30), increased viral load (31–36), anemia (37), low maternal $CD4^+$ lymphocyte count (28,29,38–41), and presence of sexually transmitted disease (42). Obstetric factors that may increase perinatal transmission are prolonged rupture of amniotic membranes (16,29,43–45), mode of

TABLE 2. Factors Postulated to Increase the Risk of Mother-to-Child Transmission of HIV-1

Maternal factors	Obstetric factors
Smoking	Prolonged rupture of amniotic membranes
Illicit drug use	Mode of delivery
Frequency of intercourse during pregnancy	Birth order
Multiple sexual partners	Placental disruption, inflammation
Increased viral load	Obstetric complications
Low maternal $CD4^+$ lymphocyte count	
Presence of sexually transmitted disease	
Low maternal vitamin A	
Anemia	

delivery (with elective C-section thought to be protective) (34,46–50), birth order in twin gestations (51), placental disruption or inflammation (52–54), and obstetric complications. Table 2 enumerates these factors.

It is interesting to note that some factors are "discovered" to be important (for example, advanced maternal age) and then fade from prominence. Other factors are intuitively appealing because a causal explanation is both simple and apparent (instrumentation during parturition, episiotomy, and fetal skin tears), but despite their logical appeal, they are apparently not important determinants of transmission (55). Many studies are methodologically flawed or attempt to draw conclusions from very small numbers of mother–child pairs. St. Louis emphasized early on that the same risk factor may vary in impact over the course of HIV infection and that factors that each predict increased risk do not necessarily act synergistically or additively (56). He also cautioned that while certain factors may be important across studies from different geographic locations, the use of absolute values or cut-offs to determine risk is not appropriate (56). Other authors emphasize that the determination of risk is multifactorial and that risk factors vary widely in their magnitude or importance (57). Some risk factors are interrelated and independent effects may be difficult or impossible to discern. Future research of risk factors may focus on the genetic make-up of transmitter and host as MacDonald has shown that when mothers and their offspring manifest major histocompatibility discordance, the risk of transmission appears low (58). This result remains to be confirmed, refuted, or examined across a number of studies.

Estimates of transmission rates from a variety of geographic locations show that infants born to HIV-infected mothers in Africa are at a higher risk of HIV transmission than those in the northern hemisphere. The Working Group on Mother-to-Child Transmission of HIV examined methodologic variation among studies from the United States, Europe, the Caribbean, and Africa (59). In African studies direct methods estimated transmission rates from 24.2% to 42.1% while direct estimates from U.S. and European data revealed rates that ranged from 14.1% to 24.9% (59). The authors of this report speculated that transmission rates may vary among women from different geographic locations due to differences in intrapartum and peripartum interventions, prevalence of chorioamnionitis, maternal viral load, viral subtype, or the prevalence of sexually transmitted or other diseases, such as malaria. In an earlier paper, Ryder had compared rates of transmission from various studies and acknowledged some of the same methodologic problems as well as selection bias in recruiting for MTCT studies in developing countries. He also pointed out that the "case mix"—the number of maternal cases of primary HIV infection during pregnancy and the number of severely immunocompromised pregnant women with advanced HIV disease—will affect study rates, as may other systematic differences (for example, nutritional status or the maturity of the epidemic among women) between and among cohorts from different geographic locations (60). Lallemant and LeCoeur have underscored some of the same points and emphasized that breastfeeding, especially prolonged breastfeeding, may contribute to the higher rates seen in African cohorts (61).

Some researchers have generated data that raise intriguing questions about, "... the hypothesis that genetically distinct subtypes of HIV-1 might also differ in their biologic properties" and "...whether the distribution of subtypes reflects the dynamics of different subtype-specific transmission potentials" (62). Murray and colleagues tried to determine whether the maternal infecting HIV-1 subtype had an impact on the rate of MTCT in a Kenyan cohort. They found no relationship between rate of transmission and viral subtype (63). In contrast, Renjifo and associates recently presented evidence from an analysis of HIV perinatal transmission in African mothers that HIV-1 subtypes A, C, and inter-subtype recombinants are more transmissible than subtype D (64). Others have documented an abnormal immune hyperactivation in some Africans and question whether this phenomenon increases susceptibility to HIV (65). Further study is needed to determine definitively whether certain subtypes of HIV are more transmissible than others and whether hyperactivation of the immune systems of Africans living in Africa plays a role in heightened transmissibility (66).

ANTIRETROVIRAL CLINICAL TRIALS

The U.S. and French ACTG 076 trial demonstrated that zidovudine (ZDV) administered to mothers during gestation and parturition, and to neonates early in life, results in a two-thirds reduction of HIV transmission to nonbreastfeeding infants (67). Since then, increasing attention has been directed toward studying antiretroviral use to reduce MTCT in developing countries. In fact, after the 076 trial, prominent researchers and public health policy experts from both developed and developing countries strongly advocated for similarly diligent and rigorous studies of the safety, efficacy, tolerability, and sustainability of modified ZDV regimens (68,69).

In an expeditiously mounted trial in Thailand, researchers from the Thai and U.S. Centers for Disease Control and Prevention demonstrated that oral ZDV administered twice a day during the last 4 weeks of pregnancy followed by oral dosing of ZDV every 3 hours from the onset of labor through delivery resulted in a reduction of HIV transmission by 51% in a nonbreastfeeding group of HIV-infected Thai women (69). These results were achieved even though the regimen differed markedly from the 076 regimen, which started much earlier in pregnancy, involved five-times daily dosing to the mother, used intravenous ZDV during labor and delivery, and gave oral ZDV to the infant in a syrup during the first 6 weeks of life. This bold yet essential Thai study conducted by Shaffer et al. accelerated the pace of clinical therapeutic research in developing countries.

A second Thai study performed in collaboration with Harvard researchers compared four different ZDV regimens. All HIV-infected pregnant women in this study were given oral ZDV from the onset of labor through delivery, but the duration of antenatal ZDV dosing was systematically varied. ZDV was given twice daily to mothers during gestation for a long (L) period of 12 weeks, or a short (S) period of 4 weeks. Zidovudine syrup was administered four times daily to infants for a long (l) period of 6 weeks, or a short (s) period of 3 days. The groups of differently treated pregnant women and children (termed here Ll, Ls, Sl, and Ss, noting that the upper case letter represents the mother's treatment and the lower case letter the infant's) had rates of transmission of 6.5% (Ll), 4.7% (Ls), 8.6% (Sl), and 10.5% (Ss). The Ss regimen was deemed inferior during the interim monitoring of the trial and was discontinued early. Although the three other arms were judged statistically equivalent, the apparent excess of gestational transmission in the Sl arm suggests that, where feasible, the longer gestational treatment should be implemented. The Thai women who participated in this study did not breastfeed (70).

A study in Cote d'Ivoire that mirrored the Thai-Shaffer study in a breastfeeding population noted a 37% reduction in HIV transmission in the children of the treated women at 3 months and an efficacy of 24% when the cohort was followed for 24 months (71).

A similar study in Cote d'Ivoire and Burkina Faso used yet another ZDV regimen—ZDV for HIV-infected pregnant women for the last 2 to 4 weeks of pregnancy, one oral 600 mg dose of ZDV during labor and delivery, and twice daily oral ZDV to the breastfeeding mother for one week postpartum. All infants in this study were breastfed. Researchers noted a 38% reduction in MTCT at 6 months of infant age in the treated group and a 30% reduction at 15 months of infant age in the control group (72,73).

The PETRA study of ZDV and 3TC in Uganda, Tanzania, and South Africa systematically varied antepartum, intrapartum and postpartum antiretroviral treatment of mothers and newborns. Group 1 received antenatal ZDV and 3TC for the last week of gestation, oral intrapartum dual therapy, and dual therapy to the mother and newborn for one week postpartum. Group 2 did not receive the antenatal treatment. Group 3 received only the intrapartum ZDV/3TC. Group 4 was placebo-controlled in all three phases. Group 1 showed an efficacy of 57% and Group 2 had an efficacy of 36%, while there was no reduction of transmission in Group 3 at 6 weeks of infant age. Efficacy of 21% and 7% was noted in Groups 1 and 2 respectively at 18 months, a difference that is no longer statistically significant (74).

The HIVNET 012 trial compared the use of oral ZDV for mothers during parturition followed by ZDV syrup for newborns for 1 week, with the use of oral nevirapine (NVP) during labor and delivery followed by one oral dose to the newborn within 72 hours. The efficacy of NVP over ZDV was 47% at age 14–16 weeks (75).

The SAINT study sponsored by Boehringer-Ingelheim found no advantage to intrapartum and postpartum NVP over intrapartum and postpartum combination ZDV/3TC in South African women (40% of whom breastfed their infants) (76).

A four-arm study sponsored by Bristol-Myers Squibb compared the effects of didanosine (ddI), d4T, ddI plus d4T, and ZDV on MTCT among the formula-fed children of HIV-infected South African women. An interim analysis that was performed when about half of the children were 6 weeks of age showed no significant differences in HIV transmission between the four groups (77). A number of other studies are planned or under way in Africa and India that will attempt to find more optimal ways to reduce HIV transmission from mother to child in breastfeeding populations.

OTHER MODES OF PREVENTION OF MTCT IN AFRICA

Clearly the most effective way to prevent MTCT of HIV globally would be to prevent HIV infection in women who bear children. Effective and proposed methods to reduce heterosexual transmission include male and female condom use, vaginal microbicides, rectal microbicides, reduction in number of sexual partners, treatment and prevention of sexually transmitted diseases, and reduction of other practices that promote and enhance transmission. Behavioral change presents a multifold challenge because many practices are fostered by cultural norms, economics, and gender roles. Economic considerations and low per capita health care expenditures encumber both the research process that guides development of health policy, and the implementation of improved public health practices.

Researchers have explored a number of preventive strategies, including some potentially suited to address some of the economic and other constraints of health care systems in Africa. These strategies have included the use of vitamin A and other micronutrients to reduce MTCT in Malawi, Tanzania, and South Africa (24,78,79). Unfortunately, vitamin A does not reduce HIV perinatal transmission rate (79). Passive immunization with various preparations of hyperimmune, anti-HIV–specific immunoglobulins did not prove effective in ACTG 185, possibly due to the efficacy of the ZDV prophylaxis even in this group of women with relatively advanced HIV disease (80). A number of strategies for vaginal cleansing or lavage before delivery with or without washing of the babies of HIV-infected mothers after delivery have been examined and are still under evaluation in some places. Biggar's study of vaginal washing with 0.25% chlorhexidine in Malawi showed no effect on HIV transmission from mother to child (81). Antibiotic prophylaxis to prevent chorioamnionitis in combination with multivitamin and NVP prophylaxis will be evaluated. It is gratifying that some MTCT interventions have resulted in decreased neonatal sepsis, improved pregnancy outcome, and reduced maternal and infant morbidity and mortality (82). Evaluation of some of these strategies in HIV-uninfected maternal and infant populations are under way.

COST-EFFECTIVENESS EVALUATION OF ANTIRETROVIRAL REGIMENS

Although research is planned and under way to optimize HIV chemoprophylaxis for HIV-infected mothers and their offspring, the financial implications of implementing known efficacious regimens to reduce MTCT must be considered. UNAIDS has stated that efficacious preventive interventions must move out of the realm of pilot and research projects and into regular practice (83). In this context, it is important to note that the cost of basic medical care for an HIV-infected child, excluding therapeutic antiretrovirals exceeds the cost of care for an uninfected child by 74% (84).

Marseille and colleagues examined the cost-effectiveness of the HIVNET 012 regimen using both a targeted strategy (counseling, testing, and giving NVP to infected pregnant women and their newborns) and a universal strategy (mass treatment of all pregnant women). They modeled cost-effectiveness assuming a 20,000-woman cohort with a 30% HIV seroprevalence rate. The universal treatment would cost US$138 per case of perinatal HIV prevented with more than 600 cases averted. Targeted treatment in a 30% seroprevalence area would cost US$298 per case avoided with 302 cases prevented. For either the universal or the targeted strategy in a 30% seroprevalence area, the cost of the 012 regimen was more favorable than the PETRA or Thai regimens (85). Other analyses have looked at cost-effectiveness using different strategies in both developed (86) and developing (87) countries.

Some investigators have reviewed Marseille's cost-effectiveness model and noted that a number of issues were not taken into account. One major issue was whether universally treated women, unsure of their HIV serostatus, would keep the NVP pill and then use it as instructed (potentially enduring social censure if they could not take the pill secretly). They noted that some women might give their pills to ill friends or family members. These investigators have comparatively evaluated universal and targeted strategies with the limitations of the Marseille analysis in mind (88). Commendably, Stringer and colleagues caution that, "Such issues as ethics, equity, legality, and compassion quite rightly deserve their place beside cost-effectiveness information as decision makers work together to address the many important societal challenges presented by the HIV epidemic" (88).

ECONOMIC AND SOCIOCULTURAL CONSIDERATIONS IN THE PREVENTION OF HIV MTCT

Marseille reported that the cost of a mother/child 012 dose of NVP would be US$4, excluding shipping and the cost of potentially lost or expired drugs (85). This is the cheapest regimen to date that shows promising efficacy in rigorous, controlled trials. Although the issue of cost of antiretroviral drugs to prevent MTCT in developing countries is important, it is by no means the only factor that will affect feasibility of implementation. Serologic testing where mass treatment strategies are not feasible or proposed, adequate and responsive counseling of women both pre-test and post-test, adequate and timely antenatal care for women, adequate intrapartum and postpartum care, and structured medical care regimens for women identified as HIV-infected in order to limit morbidity and prolong and improve their lives, are also needed. A woman's HIV status is not only important in relationship to childbearing; basic health care packages for women that recognize this must be created. Fortunately, voluntary counseling and testing programs appear to be acceptable in the antenatal setting to many African women (89). Rapid HIV testing procedures may improve the follow-up of women who have consented to testing. However, these procedures must be formally evaluated and compared to more standard programs where there is a delay between counseling and testing and the woman making herself available to hear results.

There are subtler and yet very real obstacles to implementation of prevention programs that are less easy to calculate than the cost of a pill or a counseling and testing session. Although Africa is a large and varied continent with hundreds of important tribal groups with their own rules and cultural expectations, one common concern is the relegation of women to a low sociocultural status (90). As Harrison points out, a number of conditions, directly or indirectly related to health, may result from low female status, including early assumption of the role of wife and mother, lack of methods or even the right to limit family size, short interpregnancy intervals, inadequate availability of food, and very burdensome physical labor. Maternal morbidity and mortality is high in some areas and the economically and socially disadvantaged position of women makes it difficult to improve their health, regardless of their HIV status.

Another sociocultural reality that must be better defined and explored is that an HIV-infected person often may suffer social stigma and even social isolation, the latter a life threatening condition in some settings of communal inter-dependence. It is heartening that a number of African nations are confronting the problem of reducing social stigma and actively fostering better societal knowledge and understanding concerning HIV. A national response is essential because in many African nations all classes of society are affected and it is clear that interventions must address all groups, from women who are the main workers in agricultural production in Africa to more affluent groups who are critical to the economic and intellectual life of the nations (91).

One of the evolving consequences of the AIDS epidemic is the rapidly increasing number of AIDS orphans (see chapter 44, *this volume*). Although Ryder's early report in 1994 suggested at least a short-term capacity for extended family and guardians to care for these children, the burden is likely to continue to grow (92). Although there are some very encouraging signs of decline of HIV infection among young pregnant women in Uganda (93) and downward trends among young women in Tanzania (94), there is still cause for concern. There is a very high risk of HIV infection in some African women (95), relatively high rates of childbearing in some groups of infected women, and large numbers of women who are progressing to more advanced stages of disease, a condition thought to greatly increase risk of perinatal transmission.

AFROCENTRIC STRATEGIES FOR THE PREVENTION OF MTCT OF HIV

The development and evaluation of appropriate and effective strategies to prevent MTCT of HIV in Africa will require an understanding of both African-specific and global data on the timing of transmission and the risk factors involved. It will also require the further development and long-term support of a vigorous, active, and sustainable research infrastructure that focuses on African health issues. The world health community has made an admirable beginning in this regard. After the conclusion of the ACTG 076 protocol, experts quickly assessed the applicability of its findings to developing nations. Trials aimed at validating this antiretroviral approach to preventing MTCT and evaluating the safety of its use in developing countries were mounted. The Thai-CDC study, the Cote d'Ivoire study supported by CDC, the Thai-Harvard study, and the HIVNET 012 study underscored the necessity of using antiretrovirals to prevent MTCT effectively in the developing world. Furthermore, in a press release issued after a technical consultation with experts in Geneva from October 11–13, 2000 (95), UNAIDS officials stated, "... the prevention of mother-to-child transmission of HIV—the virus that causes AIDS—should be included in the minimum standard package of care for HIV-positive women and their children" and "there is no justification to restrict use of any of these [antiretroviral] regimens to pilot project or research settings." Dr. Winnie Mpanju-Shumbusho, director of the HIV/AIDS/STI Initiative of the WHO, stated in the same press release, "a number of available regimens are known to be effective and safe. The choice should be determined according to local circumstances on the grounds of costs and practicality, particularly as related to the availability and quality of antenatal care." The press release also addressed the issue of breastfeeding: "There is continued concern that up to 20% of infants born to HIV-positive mothers may acquire HIV through breastfeeding. The meeting concluded that the guidelines issued in 1998 remain valid (see chapter 36, *this volume*) (95).

These and other antiretroviral studies are attempting to maximally reduce the risk of MTCT of HIV in primarily breastfeeding populations while trying to use simplified, potentially sustainable, cost-effective regimens with minimal toxicity and minimal development and spread of drug-resistant virus.

ACKNOWLEDGMENTS

The author is grateful for the substantial assistance of Drs. Lynne Mofenson and John Moye, Ms. Sandra Ott, and Dana and Jonathan Gordin. The opinions expressed in this chapter are solely those of the author and do not represent any official position of the U.S. Public Health Service.

REFERENCES

1. UNAIDS/WHO. AIDS epidemic update: December 2000. UNAIDS/00.44E-WHO/CDS/CSR/EDC/2000.9. UNAIDS: Geneva, 2000.
2. UNAIDS. Global trends in HIV/AIDS. June, 2000. Printed from the UNAIDS website 11/27/00.
3. Fylkesnes K, Musonda R, Kasumba K, et al. The HIV epidemic in Zambia: sociodemographic prevalence patterns and indications of trends among childbearing women. *AIDS*, 1997;11:339–345.

4. Zaba B, Gregson S. Measuring the impact of HIV on fertility in Africa. *AIDS*, 1998;12 (suppl 1):S41–S50.
5. Bulterys M, Chao A, Habimana P, et al. Incident HIV-1 infection in a cohort of young women in Butare, Rwanda. *AIDS*, 1994;8:1585–1591.
6. Valleroy L, Harris J, Way P. The impact of HIV-1 infection on child survival in the developing world. *AIDS*, 1990;4:667–672.
7. Timaeus I. Impact of the HIV epidemic on mortality in sub-Saharan Africa: evidence from national surveys and censuses. *AIDS*, 1998;12(suppl 1): S15–S27.
8. Nunn A, Mulder D, Kamali A, et al. Mortality associated with HIV-1 infection over five years in a rural Ugandan population: cohort study. *BMJ*, 1997;315:767–771.
9. Mayaux M, Burgard M, Teglas J, et al. Neonatal characteristics in rapidly progressive perinatally acquired HIV-1 disease. *JAMA*, 1996;275:606–610.
10. Lapointe N, Michaud J, Pekovic D, et al. Transplacental transmission of HTLV-III virus (letter). *N Engl J Med*, 1985;312:1325–1326.
11. Lyman W, Kress Y, Kure K, et al. Detection of HIV in fetal central nervous system tissue. *AIDS*, 1990;4: 917–920.
12. Langston C, Lewis D, Hammill H, et al. Excess intrauterine fetal demise associated with maternal human immunodeficiency virus infection. *J Infect Dis*, 1995;172:1451–1460.
13. Brossard Y, Aubin J, Mandelbrot L, et al. Frequency of early in utero HIV-1 infection: a blind DNA polymerase chain reaction study on 100 fetal thymuses. *AIDS*, 1995;9:359–366.
14. Goedert J, Duliege A, Amos C, et al. High risk of HIV-1 infection for first-born twins. *Lancet*, 1991; 338:1471–1475.
15. Nielsen K, Boyer P, Dillon M, et al. Presence of human immunodeficiency virus (HIV) type 1 and HIV-1-specific antibodies in cervicovaginal secretions of infected mothers and in the gastric aspirates of their infants. *J Infect Dis*, 1996;173:1001–1004.
16. Minkoff H, Burns D, Landesman S, et al. The relationship of the duration of ruptured membranes to vertical transmission of human immunodeficiency virus. *Am J Obstet Gynecol*, 1995;173: 585–589.
17. Bryson Y, Luzuriaga K, Wara D. Proposed definitions for in utero versus intrapartum transmission of HIV-1. *N Engl J Med*, 1992;327:1246–1247.
18. Chouquet C, Richardson S, Burgard M, et al. Timing of human immunodeficiency virus type 1 (HIV-1) transmission from mother to child: Bayesian estimation using a mixture. *Statist Med*, 1999;82:815–833.
19. Nduati R, John G, Mbori-Ngacha D, et al. Effect of breastfeeding and formula feeding on transmission of HIV-1: a randomized trial. *JAMA*, 2000;283: 1167–1174.
20. Leroy V, Newell M, Dabis F, et al. International multicentre pooled analysis of late postnatal mother-to-child transmission of HIV-1 infection. *Lancet*, 1998;352:597–600.
21. Leroy V, Newell M, Davis F, et al. Late postnatal mother-to-child transmission of HIV-1 (letter). *Lancet*, 1998;352:1630.
22. Ekpini E, Wiktor S, Satten, et al. Late postnatal mother-to-child transmission of HIV-1 in Abidjan, Cote d'Ivoire. *Lancet*, 1997;345:1054–1059.
23. Nagelkerke N, Moses S, Embree J, et al. The duration of breastfeeding by HIV-1-infected mothers in developing countries; balancing benefits and risks. *J Acquir Immune Defic Syndr*, 1995;8:176–181.
24. Coutsoudis A, Pillay K, Spooner E, et al. Randomized trial of the effect of vitamin A supplementation on pregnancy outcomes and early mother-to-child HIV transmission in Durban, South Africa. *AIDS*, 1999;13:1517–1524.
25. Turner B, Hauck W, Fanning T, et al. Cigarette smoking and maternal-child HIV transmission. *J Acquir Immune Defic Syndr*, 1997;14: 327–337.
26. Bulterys M, Landesman S, Burns D, et al. Sexual behavior and injection drug use during pregnancy and vertical transmission of HIV-1. *J Acquir Immune Defic Syndr*, 1997;15:76–82.
27. Rodriguez E, Mofenson L, Chang B, et al. Association of maternal drug use during pregnancy with maternal HIV culture positivity and perinatal HIV transmission. *AIDS*, 1996;10:273–282.
28. Bulterys M, Chao A, Dushimimana A, et al. Multiple sexual partners and mother-to-child transmission of HIV-1. *AIDS*, 1993;7:1639–1645.
29. Burns D, Landesman S, Wright D, et al. Influence of other maternal variables on the relationship between maternal virus load and mother-to-infant transmission of human immunodeficiency virus type 1. *J Infect Dis*, 1997;175:1206–1210.
30. Landesman S, Kalish L, Burns D, et al. Obstetrical factors and the transmission of human immunodeficiency virus type 1 from mother to child. *N Engl J Med*, 1996;34:1617–1623.
31. O'Shea S, Newell M, Dunn D, et al. Maternal viral load, CD4 cell count and vertical transmission of HIV-1. *J Med Virol*, 1998;54:113–117.
32. Thea D, Steketee R, Pliner V, et al. The effect of maternal viral load on the risk of perinatal transmission of HIV-1. AIDS, 1997;11:437–444.
33. St. Louis M, Kamenga M, Brown C, et al. Risk for perinatal HIV-1 transmission according to maternal immunologic, virologic, and placental factors. *JAMA*, 1993;269:2853–2859.
34. The European Collaborative Study. Maternal viral load and vertical transmission of HIV-1: an important factor but not the only one. *AIDS*, 1997;13: 1377–1385.

35. Coll O, Hernandez M, Boucher C, et al. Vertical HIV-1 transmission correlates with a high maternal viral load at delivery. *J Acquir Immune Defic Syndr*, 1997;14:26–30.
36. Dickover R, Garratty E, Herman S, et al. Identification of levels of maternal HIV-1 RNA associated with risk of perinatal transmission. *JAMA*, 1996;275:599–605.
37. Bobat R, Coovadia H, Coutsoudis A, et al. Determinants of mother-to-child transmission of human immunodeficiency virus type 1 infection in a cohort from Durban, South Africa. *Pediatr Infect Dis J*, 1996;15:604–610.
38. Pitt J, Brambilla D, Reichelderfer P, et al. Maternal immunologic and virologic risk factors for infant human immunodeficiency virus type 1 infection: findings from the Women and Infants Transmission Study. *J Infect Dis*, 1997;175:567–575.
39. Mazza C, Ravaggi A, Rodella A, et al. Influence of maternal CD4 levels on the predictive value of virus load over mother-to-child transmission of human immunodeficiency virus type 1 (HIV-1). *J Med Virol*, 1999;58:59–62.
40. Bredberg-Raden U, Urassa W, Urassa E, et al. Predictive markers for mother-to-child transmission of HIV-1 in Dar es Salaam, Tanzania. *J Acquir Immune Defic Syndr*, 1995;8:182–187.
41. The European Collaborative Study. Vertical transmission of HIV-1: maternal immune status and obstetric factors. *AIDS*,1996;10:1675–1681.
42. Tovo P, Gabiano C, Tulisso S. Maternal and clinical factors influencing HIV-1 transmission. *Acta Paediatr Suppl*, 1997;421:52–55.
43. Umans-Eckenhausen M. Prolonged rupture of membranes and transmission of the human immunodeficiency virus (letter). *N Engl J Med*, 1996;335: 1533–1534.
44. The International Perinatal HIV Group. Duration of ruptured membranes and vertical transmission of HIV-1: a meta-analysis from fifteen prospective cohort studies. *AIDS*, 2001;15:357–368.
45. McCarthy M. Timing of fetal membrane rupture predicts HIV risk. *Lancet*, 1996;347:1821.
46. Minkoff H, Mofenson L. The role of obstetric interventions in the prevention of pediatric human immunodeficiency virus infection. *Am J Obstet Gynecol*, 1994;171:1167–1175.
47. Mofenson L. A critical review of studies evaluating the relationship of mode of delivery to perinatal transmission of human immunodeficiency virus. *Pediatr Infect Dis J*, 1995;14: 169–176.
48. Dunn D, Newell M, Mayaux J, et al. Mode of delivery and vertical transmission of HIV-1: a review of prospective studies. *J Acquir Immune Defic Syndr*, 1994;7:1064–1066.
49. The European Collaborative Study. Caesarean section and the risk of vertical transmission of HIV-1. *Lancet*, 1994;343:1464–1467.
50. Kuhn L, Stein Z, Thomas P, et al. Maternal-infant HIV transmission and circumstances of delivery. *Am J Public Health*, 1994;84:1110–1115.
51. Duliege A, Amos C, Felton S, et al. Birth order, delivery route, and concordance in the transmission of human immunodeficiency virus type 1 from mothers to twins. *J Pediatr*, 1995;126:625–632.
52. Bloland P, Wirima J, Steketee RW, et al. Maternal HIV infection and infant mortality in Malawi: evidence for increased mortality due to placental malarial infection. *AIDS*, 1995;9:721–726.
53. Wabwire-Mangen F, Gray R, Mmiro F, et al. Placental membrane inflammation and risks of maternal-to-child transmission of HIV-1 in Uganda. *J Acquir Immune Defic Syndr*, 1999;22: 379–385.
54. Temmerman M, Nyong'o A, Bwayo J, et al. Risk factors for mother-to-child transmission of human immunodeficiency virus infection. *Am J Obstet Gynecol*, 1995;172:700–705.
55. Mandelbrot L, Mayaux M, Bongain A, et al. Obstetric factors and mother-to-child transmission of human immunodeficiency virus type 1: the French perinatal cohorts. *Am J Obstet Gynecol*, 1996;175:661–667.
56. St. Louis M, Kamenga M, Brown C, et al. Risk for perinatal HIV-1 transmission according to maternal immunologic, virologic, and placental factors. *JAMA*, 1993;269:2853–2859.
57. Zorrilla C. Obstetric factors and mother-to-infant transmission of HIV-1. *Infectious Disease Clinics of North America*. 1997;11:109–118.
58. MacDonald K, Embree J, Njenga S, et al. Mother-child class 1 HLA concordance increases perinatal human immunodeficiency virus type 1 transmission. *J Infect Dis*, 1998;177:551–556.
59. The Working Group on Mother-to-Child Transmission of HIV. Rates of mother-to-child transmission of HIV-1 in Africa, America, and Europe: results from 13 perinatal studies. *J Acquir Immune Defic Syndr*, 1995;8:506–510.
60. Ryder R, Behets F. Reasons for the wide variation in reported rates of mother-to-child transmission of HIV-1. *AIDS*, 1994;8:1495–1497.
61. Lallemant M, Le Coeur S, Samba L, et al. Mother-to-child transmission of HIV-1 in Congo, central Africa. *AIDS*, 1994;8:1451–1456.
62. Kanki P, Hamel D, Sankale J, et al. Human immunodeficiency virus type 1 subtypes differ in disease progression. *J Infect Dis*, 1999;179:68–73.
63. Murray M, Embree J, Ramdahin S, et al. Effect of human immunodeficiency virus (HIV) type 1 viral genotype on mother-to-child transmission of HIV-1. *J Infect Dis*, 2000;181:746–749.

64. Renjifo B, Fawzi W, Mwakagile D, et al. Differences in perinatal transmission between HIV-1 genotypes. *J Hum Virol*, 2001;4:16–25.
65. Rizzardini G, Trabattoni D, Saresella M, et al. Immune activation in HIV-infected African individuals. *AIDS*, 1998;12:2387–2396.
66. Cohen J. Is AIDS in Africa a distinct disease? *Science*, 2000;288:2153–2155.
67. Connor E, Sperling R, Gelber R, et al. Reduction of maternal-infant transmission of human immunodeficiency virus type 1 with zidovudine treatment. *N Engl J Med*, 1994;331:1173–1180.
68. Dabis F, Msellati P, Newell M, et al. Methodology of intervention trials to reduce mother to children transmission of HIV with special reference to developing countries. *AIDS*, 1995;9(suppl A): S67–S74.
69. Shaffer N, Chuachoowong R, Mock P, et al. Short-course zidovudine for perinatal HIV-1 transmission in Bangkok, Thailand: a randomized controlled trial. *Lancet*, 1999;353:773–780.
70. Lallemant M, Jourdain G, Le Coeur S, et al. A trial of shortened zidovudine regimens to prevent mother-to-child transmission of human immunodeficiency virus type 1. *N Engl J Med*, 2000; 343: 982–991.
71. Wiktor S, Ekpini E, Karon J, et al. Short-course oral zidovudine for prevention of mother-to-child transmission of HIV-1 in Abidjan, Cote d'Ivoire: a randomized trial. *Lancet*, 1999;353:781–785.
72. Dabis F, Msellati P, Meda N, et al. 6-month efficacy, tolerance, and acceptability of a short regimen of oral zidovudine to reduce vertical transmission of HIV in breastfed children in Cote d'Ivoire and Burkina Faso: a double-blind placebo-controlled multicentre trial. *Lancet*, 1999;353:786–792.
73. DITRAME ANRS 049 Study Group. 15-month efficacy of maternal oral zidovudine to decrease vertical transmission of HIV-1 in breastfed African children. *Lancet*, 1999;354:2050–2051.
74. Gray G. The PETRA study: early and late efficacy of three short ZDV/3TC combination regimens to prevent mother-to-child transmission of HIV-1. In: Program and abstracts of the XIII International AIDS Conference: July 2000; Durban, South Africa. Abstract LbOr5.
75. Guay L, Musoke P, Fleming T, et al. Intrapartum and neonatal single-dose nevirapine compared with zidovudine for prevention of mother-to-child transmission of HIV-1 in Kampala, Uganda: HIVNET 012 randomized trial. *Lancet*, 1999;354:795–802.
76. Moodley D. The SAINT trial: Nevirapine (NVP) versus zidovudine (ZDV)=lamivudine (3TC) in prevention of peripartum HIV transmission. In: Program and abstracts of the XIII International AIDS Conference. July 2000; Durban, South Africa. Abstract LbOr2.
77. Gray G, McIntyre J, Jivkvov B, et al. Preliminary efficacy, safety, tolerability, and pharmacokinetics of short course regimens of nucleoside analogues for the prevention of mother-to-child transmission (MTCT) of HIV. In: Program and abstracts of the XIII International AIDS Conference. July 2000; Durban, South Africa. Abstract TuOrB355.
78. Semba R. Overview of the potential role of vitamin A in mother-to-child transmission of HIV-1. *Acta Paediatr*, 1997;421(Suppl):107–112.
79. Fawzi W, Msamanga G, Hunter D, et al. Randomized trial of vitamin supplements in relation to vertical transmission of HIV-1 in Tanzania. *J Acquir Immune Defic Syndr*, 2000;23: 246–254.
80. Mofenson LM, Lambert JS, Stiehm ER, et al. Risk factors for perinatal HIV transmission in HIV-infected women and infants receiving zidovudine prophylaxis. *N Engl J Med* 1999;341:385–393.
81. Biggar RJ, Miotti PG, Taha TE, et al. Perinatal intervention trial in Africa: effect of a birth canal cleansing intervention to prevent HIV transmission. *Lancet*, 1996;347:1647–1650.
82. Fawzi W, Msamanga G, Spiegelman D, et al. Randomized trial of effects of vitamin supplements on pregnancy outcomes and T cell counts in HIV-1 infected women in Tanzania. *Lancet*, 1998;351: 1477–1482.
83. Joint UNAIDS/WHO Press Release. Preventing mother-to-child HIV transmission-technical experts recommend use of antiretroviral regimens beyond pilot projects. October 25, 2000. Available at: http://www.unaids.org/whatsnew/press/eng/pressarc00/geneva251000.html. Accessed November 22, 2001.
84. Leroy V, Giraudon I, Viho I, et al. Medical care costs of children born to HIV-infected mothers in Abidjan, Cote d'Ivoire 1996–1997. *AIDS*, 2000;14:1976–1077.
85. Marseille E, Kahn J, Mmiro F, et al. Cost effectiveness of single-dose nevirapine regimen for mothers and babies to decrease vertical HIV-1 transmission in sub-Saharan Africa. *Lancet*, 1999;354:803–809.
86. Ratcliffe J, Ades A, Gibb D, et al. Prevention of mother-to-child transmission of HIV-1 infection: alternative strategies and their cost-effectiveness. *AIDS*, 1998;12:1381–1388.
87. Mansergh G, Haddix A, Steketee R, et al. Cost-effectiveness of short-course zidovudine to prevent perinatal HIV type 1 infection in a sub-Saharan African developing country setting. *JAMA*, 1996;276:139–145.
88. Stringer J, Rouse D, Vermund S, et al. Cost-effective use of nevirapine to prevent vertical HIV transmission in sub-Saharan Africa. *J Acquir Immune Defic Syndr*, 2000;24:369–377.
89. Cartoux M, Meda N, Van de Perre, et al. Acceptability of voluntary HIV testing by pregnant

women in developing countries: an international survey. *AIDS*, 1998;12:2489–2493.
90. Harrison K. The importance of the educated healthy woman in Africa. *Lancet*, 1997;349: 644–647.
91. Berkley S. HIV in Africa: what is the future? *Ann Intern Med*, 1991;116:339–341.
92. Ryder R, Kamenga M, Nkusu M, et al. AIDS orphans in Kinshasa, Zaire. Incidence and socioeconomic consequences. *AIDS*, 1994;8:673–679.
93. Asiimwe-Okiror G, Opio A, Musinguzi J, et al. Change in sexual behaviour and decline in HIV infection among young pregnant women in urban Uganda. *AIDS*, 1997;11:1757–1763.
94. Kwesigabo G, Killewo J, Godoy C, et al. Decline in the prevalence of HIV-1 infection in young women in the Kagera region of Tanzania. *J Acquir Immune Defic Syndr*, 1998;17:262–268.
95. Konde-Lule J, Wawer M, Sewankambo N, et al. Adolescents, sexual behavior, and HIV-1 in rural Rakai district, Uganda. *AIDS*, 1997;11:791–799.

16

HIV-1 Subtypes and Recombinants

Boris Renjifo and Max Essex

Department of Immunology and Infectious Diseases,
Harvard School of Public Health, Boston, Massachusetts, USA.

Regardless of their host tropism or associated illnesses, retroviruses share similarities in structure, genome organization, and steps in the replication cycle. Behavioral, social and biologic factors, including evolutionary versatility have allowed HIV-1 to cause one of the most devastating epidemics of our times. The genomic diversity of HIV-1 has been a continuous challenge for the development of diagnostic tests, antiretroviral therapies, and the development of a preventive vaccine.

THE HIV COMPONENTS AND REPLICATION CYCLE

The HIV-1 particle has a diameter of approximately 100 nm and is made up of proteins encoded by the *gag*, *pol*, and *env* genes. The outer component is the envelope membrane containing the viral envelope proteins gp41 and gp120 in addition to a variety of host-derived proteins (1). The internal nucleocapsid is assembled by complex nucleic acid-protein and protein-protein interactions to guarantee stability of the particle. A matrix protein p17 is located between the envelope membrane and the capsid formed by the p24 protein. The genomic RNA is single-stranded, of positive polarity, about 9–10 kilobases long, and composed of two usually identical copies wrapped by p7 nucleoprotein molecules. The viral reverse transcriptase (RT), protease (PR), and integrase (IN) are required for various replication steps and provirus integration. Accessory genes (*tat, rev, vif, vpr, vpu*, and *nef*) with regulatory and accessory functions are encoded within the middle and 3′ end of the genome. These accessory genes allow novel ways for interaction with the host cell machinery as well as evasion of immune recognition (2).

HIV GENETIC VARIATION

A hallmark of HIV is the large genomic diversity of viruses within and between infected individuals. Factors determining the overall rate of HIV genetic variation include the number of mutations per replication cycle, the time required to complete each replication cycle, the propensity of the viruses for recombination, and the overall effect of sequence changes on the fitness of the generated viruses for subsequent replications. It has been widely assumed that reverse transcription is responsible for generating the majority of mutations in HIV. Reverse transcriptase does not have the exonuclease activity necessary for correcting misincorporations during synthesis. Without proofreading activity, insertions, deletions, and point mutations are incorporated into the new genome and passed to the progeny. The amount of mutations incorporated by RT has been estimated at between 1/1,700 and 1/4,000 per nucleotide per replication cycle (3). Once integrated, the proviral DNA is only replicated when the infected cell goes through cell division. Cellular DNA polymerases introduce only a negligible number of mutations because a proofreading activity detects and corrects misincorporations. The last source of mutations is during synthesis of full-length RNA by cellular RNA polymerases. The number of mutations introduced by cellular RNA polymerases while transcribing full-length HIV RNA genomes from proviral DNA has not been characterized, but it may be as significant as that of viral RT.

In theory, mutations introduced by viral RT, and cellular DNA and RNA polymerases can be located in any position within the HIV genome. Whether a mutation is retained in the genome depends on the effect of the mutation on the ability of the progeny virus to replicate as successfully as the progenitor virus and evade immune responses. The high genetic variation of HIV appears to be due to high replication rates and to a lesser extent to a higher rate of misincorporation by the HIV RT (4,5).

When dual infections with different viruses occur in the same cell, different nucleotide sequences can be incorporated as genomes of progeny virus particles. This can result in recombination between different parental genomes in the next replication cycle, causing rapid diversification in viral gene sequences. This has been easiest to identify when sequences from different viral subtypes appear in the same genomes. Such viruses are designated intersubtype recombinants. Presumably recombinants for which both parental viruses come from the same subtype, intrasubtype recombinants, emerge much more frequently, but are extremely difficult to identify.

Because mutant viruses are constantly emerging, analysis of multiple viruses in a single blood sample usually reveals minor genotypic variants that may be described as quasispecies (6). The sequences of dominant clones may change by as much as 1% per year in an infected individual (7).

Mutations or recombinatorial events that result in phenotypic changes of the progeny virus may result in rapid positive selection. A dramatic example is the selection of drug-resistant mutants of HIV-1 that occurs in individuals treated with reverse transcriptase inhibitors. For drug resistance, antibody neutralization, cytolytic T-cell attack, and cell tropism mediated by coreceptors, only one or a few mutations can rapidly change the viral phenotype (8). Some regions of the viral genome, such as envelope, appear to vary more rapidly, presumably because of immunoselection. While changes in envelope and polymerase have been most extensively analyzed, selection for variants appears to happen in all regions of the genome, including noncoding areas involved in transcriptional regulation (9).

METHODS FOR HIV GENOTYPE CLASSIFICATION

At the beginning of the HIV-1 epidemic, viral strains were grouped according to the geographic origin of the sample. With the use of a gag-anchored polymerase chain reaction (PCR) and nucleotide sequence analysis it became evident that African strains showed more extensive genetic variation than European and U.S. viruses (10). This genetic variation stimulated the development of molecular and immune-based techniques for the categorization of HIV viruses. Methods that utilize PCR include nucleotide sequencing, heteroduplex mobility assays (HMA), subtype-specific PCR, oligonucleotide probe hybridization, and restriction fragment polymorphism (11–13). Serology-based techniques such as V3 peptide enzyme-linked immunosorbent assays have also been used for subtype determination (14–17). Even though nucleotide sequencing is the most accurate method of HIV genotyping, other methods are widely used because of their lower cost and their utility in large-scale population studies and in locations with limited resources. In addition, the existence of intersubtype recombinants makes it more expensive and time consuming to characterize and compare pure nonrecombinant subtypes.

Entries in the Los Alamos HIV sequence databases generally reflect the way our knowledge of the HIV epidemic has evolved with continuous improvement and development of newer methods for cloning and sequencing HIV genomes. Initially, the majority of sequences originated from subtype B samples from the United States and Europe, but later studies have focused on samples from African populations. Today, while numbers of full-length sequences in the database are increasing, the majority of new entries are still fragments or complete individual genes such as p24, RT, gp120, V3 region, and gp41 and various accessory genes. However, the largest numbers of full-length sequences are now from non-B subtypes and most are from African samples.

Since there has not been a consistent and systematic program for the surveillance of HIV-1 subtypes in Africa, our knowledge of the subtype prevalence in some African countries is fragmented. The HIV-1C virus predominates in southern Africa and in Ethiopia and the horn of Africa. The HIV-1A and HIV-1D subtypes are most common in East Africa, and the A/G recombinant virus, HIV-1 CRF02_AG, is most common in West Africa (18) (Figure 1). While some countries and regions have epidemics that are dominated by a single subtype, countries such as Cameroon and Tanzania have multiple subtypes and recombinants circulating concurrently at significant levels (19–21).

Nucleotide Sequencing

Early efforts to sequence HIV genomes used manual sequencing techniques. As automated sequencing became widely available, it has become feasible for many laboratories to sequence full-length genomes. Once the nucleotide sequence is obtained, a variety of phylogenetic algorithms are used for subtype classification. Software packages and interactive programs to generate alignments for building phylogenetic trees are available through the internet (see Table 1 in Chapter 8, *this volume*). Reference sequences spanning the same genetic region as the sample are used to create sequence alignments.

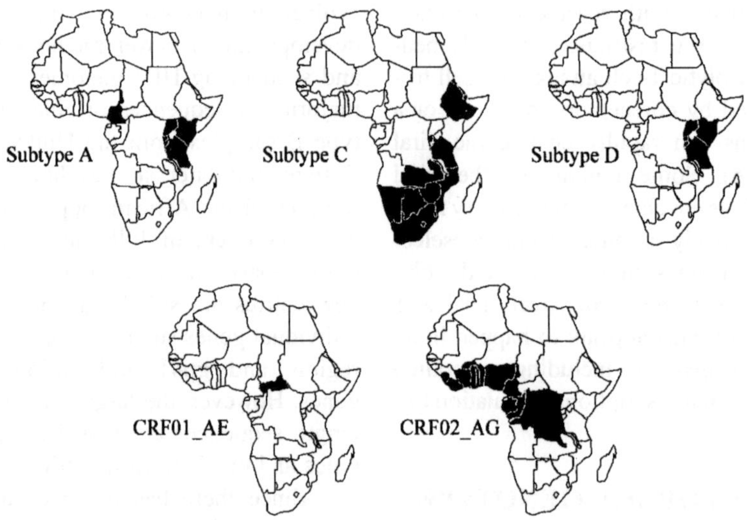

FIGURE 1. Geographical representation of HIV-1 subtypes and circulating recombinant forms estimated to occur at a total prevalence of at least 2% in particular African countries.

Phylogenetic trees can be created using character- or distance-based methods. Distance-based methods, such as the Neighbor Joining method, are frequently used because they generate trees very rapidly that are accurate enough for use in subtype classification. Character-based methods, such as Maximum Parsimony and Maximum Likelihood, may yield trees from which genetic distance can be calculated. However, the amount of computer time required for the analysis restricts their use to selected samples, and for answering more detailed questions.

The diversity of HIV-1 sequences seen in the late 1980s also stimulated the creation of the HIV Sequence Database at the Los Alamos National Laboratory (http://hiv-web.lanl.gov), as well as the development of phylogenetic algorithms for the analysis of viral sequences. The categorization of HIV-1 subtypes originated as a result of phylogenetic comparison of nucleotide sequences from *gag* and envelope sequences from isolates collected in countries around the globe (22,23). Nucleotide sequencing of subgenomic fragments is still the most common method used for HIV subtyping, for monitoring HIV-1 genetic diversity, and for studying the origin and molecular evolution of HIV within the human population.

Full-length genome PCR amplification will be a key factor in the identification of new recombinants and the surveillance of known subtypes and circulating recombinant forms (CRFs) in the global HIV pandemic (24). A list of HIV-1 clones used as representatives of individual subtypes and CRFs known to exist in Africa is shown in Table 1A and B respectively.

Heteroduplex Mobility Assays

The heteroduplex mobility assay (HMA) relies on the principle that dsDNA molecules that are formed by two DNA molecules with dissimilar sequences run more slowly in polyacrylamide gels than the homoduplex dsDNA molecules from which they originated. Distortions in the DNA structure created by nucleotide mismatches, gaps, and insertions retard their mobility through polyacrylamide gels. Standard dsDNA molecules representing each HIV-1 subtype are combined individually with DNA aliquots from the sample being tested. The more sequence similarity between the standard and the sample DNA, the lower the number of mismatches that will occur and the faster the molecule will migrate in a gel. The subtype designation is obtained by comparing the mobility of the duplexes formed by the sample with a set of references from any given subtype. The env V3–V5 region was the first genomic fragment used to show the use of HMA for HIV-1 genetic classification but other regions of the HIV genome, including gp41 and gag, have been used for HMA assays (11,25). In geographic locations known to contain a limited number of HIV-1 subtypes, the number of references required for each run can be restricted (see Figure 3 in Chapter 8, *this volume*). However, a periodic surveillance with all subtype references to detect new incoming subtypes is recommended.

Since its description, HMA has been used as the primary subtyping technique or as a screening technique for subsequent sequencing in many locations, including several African countries (26–31). The HIV-1 group M *env* Heteroduplex Mobility Analysis Subtyping Kit, available to registered laboratories in the AIDS Reagent Program of the U.S. National Institutes of Health, improves on previous versions by the inclusion of new subtype standards and the ability to analyze *env* fragments of different sizes (see Table 1 in Chapter 8, *this volume*) (11). A new HMA based on *gag* sequences has been developed as a tool for the detection of intersubtype recombinants when used in conjunction with *env* HMA (32). This HIV-1 group M *gag* Heteroduplex Mobility Analysis Subtyping Kit is also available through the AIDS Reagent Program.

Other Methods Based on PCR Amplification

The need for fast, cheap, and reliable methods to use in large-scale population studies within specific geographic regions stimulated the development of alternative protocols for HIV genotype classification. These methods still require a PCR step to generate a dsDNA molecule for molecular manipulation and they commonly analyze a single fragment in the HIV genome, which decreases their ability to detect recombinant genomes. Individual methods vary in the specificity of their PCR primers, hybridization probes, and methodologies for detection. Oligonucleotide probes with V3 nucleotide sequences corresponding to circulating subtypes B and CRF01_AE, or A and D, were used in Thailand and Uganda respectively (12,33). A restriction fragment length polymorphism (RFLP) analysis generated by digesting *gag* PCR products with distinct restriction enzymes was used for determination of subtype A, B, C, and D infections in South Africa (13). The combinatorial melting assay (COMA) is a PCR-capture technique in which a combination of oligonucleotides corresponding to specific subtypes was used for subtype A, C, and D determination in Kenyan samples (34). COMA relies on the dissimilar melting temperatures of each individual oligonucleotide to the target sequences. A subtype A-specific PCR was developed to be used in regions where subtype A predominates compared to other circulating subtypes. This system was tested in samples from West and central Africa and showed sensitivity ranging from 50% to 87%, depending on the geographic origin of the samples (35).

V3 Serotyping

The presence of antibodies against viral antigens has also been used for the development of serologic assays for HIV-1 subtype classification. The V3 loop of the HIV-1 envelope protein gp120 is involved in early viral-host interactions, including chemokine coreceptor utilization and cell tropism, in addition to eliciting neutralizing antibodies. It was hypothesized that the amino acid differences in the V3 region would be sufficient to accurately discriminate serologically between distinct HIV-1 subtypes.

Variations of a V3-loop peptide enzyme-linked immunosorbent assay (PEIA) were developed and tested on serum samples from people known to be infected with specific subtypes of HIV-1 (15–17,36). A comparison by several laboratories on the same set of samples showed poor correlation with genetic subtype in addition to considerable variation in their accuracy to predict HIV-1 subtypes A, B, C, D, F, G, and H (14). In another study, a panel of samples of known HIV-1 genotype and diverse geographic origin were tested by V3 serotyping and it was found that the predictive value of PEIA was good for subtypes B, D, and CRF01_AE; inadequate to differentiate between subtypes A and C; and insensitive for detection of subtypes G or H (36). Despite these limitations, serologic assays have been valuable in locations where only two subtypes appear to circulate in the population, such as subtypes B and CRF01-AE in Thailand or subtypes B and C in South Africa, Russia, or Israel (13,37).

Based on our current knowledge that circulation of several subtypes and their recombinants characterizes the HIV-1 epidemics in most African countries, the use of PEIA may not be the most appropriate method for use in this region.

HIV-1 NOMENCLATURE

Phylogenetic analyses have become an important tool in the genetic analysis and classification of HIV. The clustering patterns formed when nucleotide sequences are structured through phylogenetic analysis into related lineages have been the fundamental method for HIV classification. Phylogenetic assessment has also been used to track linkage among samples and to follow epidemiologic trends.

The phylogenetic classification of HIV-1 subtypes into groups, subtypes, subsubtypes and CRFs has been the result of a continuous compilation from fragments, complete gene sequences, and more recently, full-length genomic sequences from samples around the globe (24,38). Currently, full-length HIV sequences obtained from three epidemiologically unlinked individuals are required for the description of a new HIV-1 group, subtype, or CRF. Due to the large number of recombinant genomes circulating in many African regions, the use of a single gene for subtyping would erroneously misclassify intersubtype recombinants, making it difficult to establish phenotypes associated with particular subtypes.

HIV-1 Groups

Currently, HIV-1 viruses fall into three separate groups, the main group (M), the outlier group (O), and the non-M/non-O group (N) (24,38,39). Viruses in the M group cause the vast majority of HIV-1 infections in the world. Infections by viruses belonging to the O group have been confined to West and central African countries, and their prevalence compared to viruses belonging to the M group is low (40–42). The description of HIV-1 viruses from group N has also been confined to a limited number of samples from Cameroon (43,44).

HIV-1 Subtypes

In 1992, a classification based on genetic subtypes, rather than geographic origin, began to be used to better reflect the diversity of nucleotide sequences from isolates collected around the globe (23,45,46). Within the M group, subtypes form phylogenetically equidistant clusters, independent of the genomic region used for the analysis. Currently, nine different subtypes, designated A, B, C, D, F, G, H, J, and K, have been identified (24,45,47). Two viruses originally designated as subtypes, HIV-1E and HIV-1I, were subsequently recognized to be recombinants. They are mentioned in the next section under "HIV-1 Circulating Recombinant Forms." The distribution and prevalence of individual subtypes varies extensively within the African continent. Prevalence rates of HIV-1 infections in women attending antenatal care clinics have varied from 0.5% to 43%, with the highest rates in the southern African countries (48).

While in some central African countries (Democratic Republic of Congo, Cameroon, Congo, Central African Republic) it is possible to find most of the known subtypes and many different recombinants, in other regions (Namibia, Botswana, Zimbabwe, Zambia and Mozambique), subtype C is the most common or the only prevalent circulating subtype (Figure 1).

HIV-1 Subtype A

Subtype A is responsible for a large number of HIV-1 infections in Africa (Figure 1). It has been described as the most common subtype detected in countries such as Côte d'Ivoire (49, 50), Mali (27), Rwanda (51–53), Central African Republic (28), Democratic Republic of Congo (26), Ghana (54–56), Uganda (57–60), Congo (61), and Kenya (34,62,63). However, the analysis of samples from west African locations such as Senegal (31,64,65), Equatorial Guinea (66), Cameroon (19,20,67), Nigeria (68,69), Benin (32,70), and Gabon (71–73) showed that many samples thought to be subtype A were found to be CRF02_AG (Figure 1).

In the Democratic Republic of Congo, which is sometimes suggested as the location where the HIV-1 epidemic originated, subtype A sequences have been described to account for 43% to 68% of all detected genotypes (26). The extensive diversity of subtype A genotypes has been established by several lines of evidence. Phylogenetic trees of full-length sequences showed that two subclusters, designated A1 and A2, are formed when new samples from Cyprus and the Democratic Republic of Congo are included in the analysis (74) (Table 1A). Three distinct subclusters of HIV-1A *gag* sequences were detected among African samples. The gag region of nonrecombinant genomes from East Africa formed a subcluster separate from CRF01_AE from Central African Republic or the CRF02_AG genomes from West and central Africa (75).

The ability of subtype A genomes to generate recombinants with a capacity for epidemic spread (for example, CRF01_AE in Thailand and CRF02_AG in West Africa) has been well established. In addition, six of the 12 CRFs reported in the Los Alamos National Laboratory HIV Sequence Database include subtype A sequences (24,47).

HIV-1 Subtype B

Since the beginning of the HIV-1 epidemic, subtype B viruses have been responsible for the majority of infections detected in the United States and Europe. Consequently a large number of subtype B sequences have been characterized and reported in the databases. However, except for North Africa and selected high-risk subpopulations in the cities of the Republic of South Africa, HIV-1B viruses are rarely found in Africa (76–78). Because HIV-1B has not been linked to any major epidemics in Africa, it seems plausible that most of the isolated infections observed may have been related to direct or indirect contact with the United States or western Europe (19,20,22,26,28, 31,50,66,73,77,79).

Sequence comparisons showed that overall diversity between subtype B and D genomes is not greater than the diversity observed within other subtypes. However, the *env* of subtype B was found to be more similar to subtype F than to subtype D *env*. It was suggested that the subtype B epidemic in the United States and Europe may have originated with a subtype D virus that was arbitrarily named subtype B.

HIV-1 Subtype C

HIV-1 subtype C has become the most prevalent subtype in the HIV-1 pandemic, accounting for the majority of all circulating subtypes in the world (18,80). Subtype C infections account for the intense epidemics observed in southern Africa (29,30,32,46,76, 81–86) and Ethiopia (87,88) (Figure 1).

HIV-1C has also been described in various other countries in East and central Africa (21,26,28,34,51,52,59,63,66,89–93). Outside Africa, subtype C and its recombinants account for the majority of infections in India and China (45,82,94–97).

Phylogenetic analysis has shown that subtype Cs from India and different regions of Africa form distinct subclusters, and that viruses from India show considerably less diversity than African strains. In addition, a C′ sub-subtype in Ethiopia has been reported (87, 88). Efforts to characterize subtype C viruses show that the majority of subtype C sequences from southern Africa have three NF-κB binding sites in the long terminal repeat (LTR) and a five amino acid insertion in the Vpu (86).

The prevalence rates of HIV-1 infection in African countries where subtype C predominates are the highest in the world. HIV-1 subtype C infections in Botswana, Lesotho, Swaziland, Namibia, Zimbabwe, Zambia, and South Africa often represent 20% to 40% of the infections in women attending antenatal care clinics (48). In East Africa, where other subtypes were predominant, subtype C infections appear to be expanding and generating large numbers of de-novo recombinants (21,90).

HIV-1 Subtype D

The first comparison between African and U.S. full-length clones was done in the mid 1980s, when the ELI strain from the Democratic Republic of Congo, which subsequently became the first HIV-1D, was fully sequenced (98). Further studies showed that some African strains were phylogenetically closer to European or U.S. sequences (99,100).

Subtype D is among the most prevalent subtypes in Uganda (57–59), Tanzania (21,53, 90,101–104) and Kenya (62,63) (Figure 1). Subtype D has also been detected in various other sites, especially in central and West Africa (20,26,28,49,50,56,66,67,72, 76,105).

A characteristic of subtype D genomes is that they appear to have the most divergent V3 sequences. The number of amino acid changes within the V3 regions compared to changes outside the V3 region in subtype D genomes is larger than in other subtypes (106). Within subtype D, full-length genomes from central Africa group separately from genomes from East Africa (45). The cocirculation of subtype D genomes and other subtypes in many African regions has favored the generation of a large number of recombinants with subtype D sequences.

HIV-1 Subtype F

Infections by HIV-1 subtype F viruses have been described in South America, Europe, and Africa. This subtype was first classified, based on *gag* and *env* sequences, into three phylogenetic sub-subtypes designated F1, F2, and F3 (107). Full-length analysis showed that F3 genomes correspond to the new subtype K (108). Sequences within the F1 have been reported from several countries in West and central Africa (26,31,67,107, 109), as well as Europe (110,111) and South America (112–114). Sequences clustering within the sub-subtype F2 have been reported from Cameroon, Nigeria, Gabon, and the Democratic Republic of Congo (26,19, 20,115). Subtype F sequences have also been found in recombinants such as CRF05_DF and CRF12_BF (47,116). Reference sequences 93BR020.1, VI850, FIN9363, and MP411 belong to sub-subtype F1 while sequences 95CMMP255 and P5CMMP257 from Cameroon belong to sub-subtype F2 (Table 1A).

HIV-1 Subtype G

The first full-length genomes of HIV-1G completely sequenced were strains SE6165 and HH8793, obtained from a Congolese patient living in Sweden and an individual with close contact to an infected individual from Kenya (Table 1A) (117). It was found that the LTR of subtype G genomes have two AP1, two NF-κB, and three SP1 binding sites

TABLE 1. HIV-1 Clones Frequently Used as Reference Sequences for Subtypes (A) and Circulating Recombinant Forms (B) Present in Africa

A. Subtypes			B. Circulating Recombinant Forms		
Subtype	Clone	GenBank Accession #	CRF	Clone	GenBank Accession #
A1	U455	M62320	CRF01_AE	CM240	U54771
A1	92UG037.1	U51190	CRF01_AE	93TH253.3	U51189
A1	Q2317	AF004885	CRF01_AE	90CF402.1	U51188
A1	SE7253	AF069670	CRF01_AE	CM235	L03698
A2	94CY017.41	AF286237	CRF01_AE	90CF11697	AF197340
A2	97CDKTB48	AF286238	CRF01_AE	90CF4071	AF197341
A2	97CDKS10	AF286241	CRF02_AG	IbNG	L39106
B	HXB2	K03455, M38432	CRF02_AG	DJ264	AF063224
B	JRFL	U63632	CRF02_AG	DJ263	AF063223
B	RF	M17451, M12508	CRF02_AG	98SE-MP1211	AJ251056
B	WEAU160	U21135	CRF02_AG	98SE-MP1213	AJ251057
C	ETH2220	U46016	CRF05_DF	VI1310	AF193253
C	92BR025.8	U52953	CRF05_DF	VI961	AF076998
C	IN21068	AF067155	CRF06_cpx	BFP90	AF064699
C	96BW05.02	AF110967	CRF06_cpx	95ML84	AJ245481
D	NDK	M27323	CRF06_cpx	95ML127	AJ288982
D	ELI	K03454	CRF06_cpx	97SE1078	AJ288981
D	94UG114.1	U88824	CRF09_cpx	p2911	NA
D	84ZR085	U88822	CRF10_CD	TZBFL061	AF289548
F1	93BR020.1	AF005494	CRF10_CD	TZBFL071	AF289549
F1	VI850	AF077336	CRF10_CD	TZBFL110	AF289550
F1	FIN9363	AF075703	CRF11_cpx	GR17	AF179368
F1	MP411	AJ249238	CRF11-cpx	97CM-MP818	AJ291718
F2	95CMMP255	AJ249236	CRF11-cpx	99FR-MP129	AJ291719
F2	P5CMMP257	AJ249237	CRF11-cpx	99FR-MP1307	AJ291720
G	SE6165	AF061642			
G	HH8793	AF061640			
G	DRCBL	AF084936			
G	92NG0083	U88826			
H	90CF056.1	AF005496			
H	VI991	AF190127			
H	VI997	AF190128			
H	VI557	U09666			
J	SE9280.9	AF082394			
J	SE9173.3	AF082395			
K	97ZR-EQTB11	AJ249235			
K	96CM-MP535	AJ249239			

upstream from a normal TATAA box. The TAR loop has a three-nucleotide bulge similar to subtypes B, C, and D. In addition, an insertion of 20 nucleotides was detected downstream of the primer binding site.

Subtype G infections have been described in diverse locations from East to West Africa, though rarely as a major proportion of the infections (22,26,27,31,32,34,46, 49,50,54–56,59,61,63,66,67,69,70,72,89, 109,115,118–123). In some locations such as Mali, Benin, and Nigeria, subtype G may account for more than 20% of all HIV-1 infections (27,32,124). The wide distribution of this subtype in the African continent and the existence of several recombinants with subtype G sequences suggest that subtype G viruses have been circulating for a long period of time. However, except for the recombinant CRF02_AG, HIV-1G viruses have not shown fitness for the same high prevalence rates observed with HIV-1A, HIV-1C, or HIV-1D in Africa.

HIV-1 Subtype H

The first full-length sequence of a subtype H genome, clone 90CR056.1, was obtained from an asymptomatic patient from the Central African Republic (60). The V3 region from this sample was initially unclassified, but then found to belong to a new subtype once the full-length clone was sequenced (89). Additionally, two full-length sequences have been obtained from individuals in Belgium with links to the Democratic Republic of Congo (125). These clones, V1991 and V1997, contain LTRs with two NF-κB and three SP1 binding sites in addition to a truncated *tat* (125).

In the African continent, subtype H infections have been described in central and West Africa (26,31,60,67,89,109,120,121), but the number of subtype H infections tends to be small as compared to other circulating subtypes. Subtype H has also been reported in Africans residing in Europe and in individuals from Europe who visited Africa (110,126–128).

HIV-1 Subtype J

HIV-1 J viruses are rare, but have been identified in Zambia (129), the Democratic Republic of Congo (26), and Cameroon (130). HIV-1J viruses have also been identified in individuals in Europe who had an association with central Africa (131–133). Recombinants that contain J sequences have also been identified in one individual from Botswana (134) and another who was presumed to be exposed in Sierra Leone (135).

HIV-1 Subtype K

Based on *gag* and *env* sequences, genomes belonging to this subtype were initially classified as the sub-cluster F3 within subtype F genomes (107). Using several sequencing analysis tests, it was decided that subtype F3 genomes corresponded to nonrecombinant viruses from a new subtype designated K (108). Reference sequences of subtype K include 96CM-MP535 and 97ZR-EQTB11, recovered from two epidemiologically unlinked samples from the Democratic Republic of Congo and Cameroon (Table 1A). It has been suggested that subtype K may be present in several central African countries, since the env region of a sample from Gabon (VI354) and the env region from a recombinant sample from the Democratic Republic of Congo (Z36) cluster within subtype K prototype sequences (72,107,108). The fact that subtype K genomes are equidistant to the subtypes A through J suggests that subtype K has been circulating in the African continent as long as other subtypes. The longevity of subtype K is also suggested by the presence of subtype K-like sequences in CRF04_cpx and CRF06_cpx, as well as in other intersubtype recombinants.

HIV-1 Circulating Recombinant Forms

A CRF is defined as a recombinant HIV-1 genome showing evidence of expansion in a population, as suggested by its isolation from at least three epidemiologically unlinked individuals (24,38,47). These recombinants must have an identical mosaic configuration over the entire viral genome that indicates a common ancestor from the same recombination event. The denomination used for CRF includes a number followed by letters indicating the subtypes involved in the recombination. When more than two subtypes are present in the CRF, the letters "cpx" are used to indicate the "complex" composition of the recombinant. Currently there are twelve CRFs described in the Los Alamos National Laboratory HIV Sequence Database, but the impact of each CRF on the global AIDS pandemic is vastly uneven. Some, such as CRF01_AE and CRF02_AG, have been responsible for regional epidemics, while others have only been described in a few individuals. Several CRFs, particularly CRF03_AB (136), CRF04_cpx (137, 138), CRF07_BC (94), CRF08_BC (95), and CRF12_cpx (47) have only been described from sites outside Africa. CRF04_cpx was originally described as subtype HIV-1I (139). A schematic representation of the genomic organization of CRFs known to occur in Africa is shown in Figure 2. The distribution of two CRFs that occur at a prevalence of 2% or higher in African populations is shown in Figure 1.

CRF01_AE

The introduction of CRF01_AE in Thailand resulted in the first known and well-characterized epidemic caused by a recombinant virus (140–142). Since the early 1990s, CRF01_AE has caused a large number of infections in Thailand where it is now the most prevalent virus (142,143). Recent reports have described the introduction of CRF01_AE in other areas of Southeast Asia (144–147). Although CRF01_AE appears to have originated in central Africa (19,26,47), it does not appear to have spread as successfully as HIV-1A, HIV-1C, HIV-1D, or CRF02_AG. Prototype viruses belonging to CRF01_AE were first designated as subtype E based on *env* nucleotide sequences, but were found to be recombinant when the *gag* gene was sequenced (140,141,148). Full-length sequencing of samples from Thailand and the Central African Republic showed that these viruses possess the gag and pol regions derived from subtype A, while most of the envelope regions, *vpu*, and LTR are derived from subtype E (140, 141). The fact that no full-length subtype E parental strain has been identified has raised questions about the true recombinant origin of

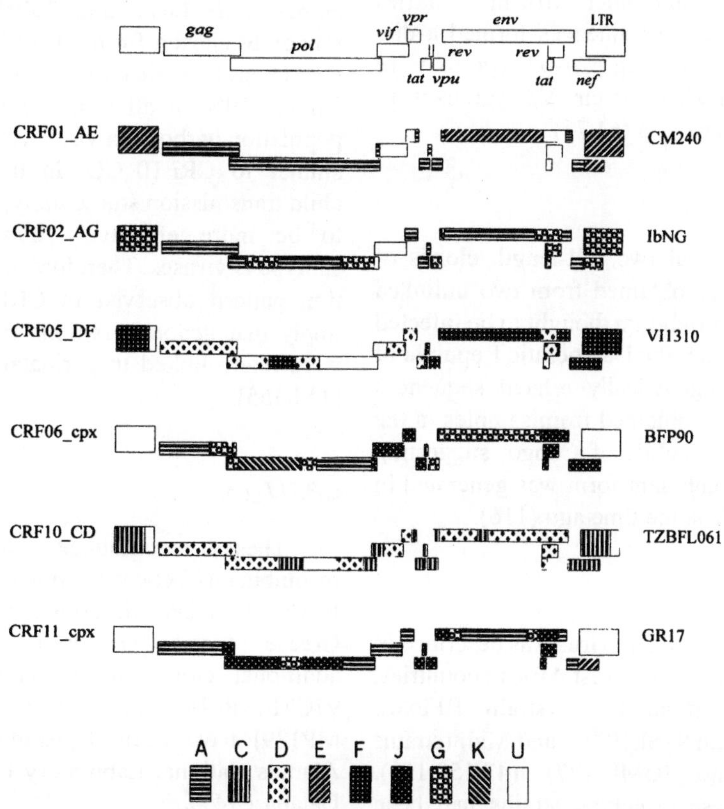

FIGURE 2. Genomic organization scheme of circulating recombinant forms known to be present in Africa.

CRF01-AE viruses. It has been suggested that CRF01-AE may not be a de-novo recombinant but a sub-subtype A genome according to a recent analysis of samples from Thailand and the Central African Republic (149) (Figure 1).

CRF02_AG

This CRF is often designated as "IbNG," the name given to the first sample described, from Ibadin, Nigeria (68). This is the most widely spread recombinant virus on the African continent and among the predominant HIV-1 in Côte d'Ivoire (49,50), Guinea Bissau (66), Senegal (31,64), Nigeria (68, 69), and Cameroon (20,32,109) (Figure 1). CRF02_AG genomes had also been described in Congo (61), Uganda (59), Kenya (34,63), and Djibouti (75). Many genomes within the "IbNG" CRF cluster may have erroneously been classified as subtype A. Phylogenetic analysis of samples from Senegal and other African countries showed that IbNG sequences formed a distinct cluster when gag p24-p7 regions were used, but not when the env V3 regions were used for the analysis (64,75).

CRF05_DF

The original two full-length clones of this CRF were obtained from two unlinked individuals in Belgium thought to be infected by partners from the Democratic Republic of Congo. Phylogenetically related sequences have also been obtained from samples in the Democratic Republic of Congo, suggesting that this recombinant form was generated in central Africa some time ago (116).

CRF06_cpx

This recombinant virus was described in samples from several West African countries, including Burkina Faso (strain BFP90), Senegal (strain 97SE1078), and Mali (strains 95ML84 and 95ML-127) (47,150,151). Some of these prototype strains had been given several different names until the origin of a complex recombinant between subtypes A, G, J, and K was recognized.

CRF09_cpx

Information about this recombinant is very limited. CRF09_cpx was mentioned in a review article but the sequences and the genomic structure have not been made available to the scientific community. Samples were collected in Senegal and also in a seroconvertor from the United States Army (45).

CRF10_CD

Full-length clones were obtained shortly after infection from three newborn infants enrolled in a large mother-to-child transmission cohort in Dar es Salaam, Tanzania (152, 153). The prototype strain TZBFL061, and clones TZBFL071 and TZBFL110, were randomly chosen from 13 different D(gag)-D/C/D(env) perinatally infected infants. Almost 10% of all infants infected in this population harbored a virus with an envelope similar to CRF10_CD. In this mother-to-child transmission study, subtype C appeared to be more effectively transmitted than subtype D viruses. Therefore, the recombination pattern observed in CRF10_CD may imply that genomic regions representing C were likely linked to perinatal transmission (154,155).

CRF11_cpx

These recombinants are complex recombinants between subtypes A, G, J, and E. They have been described in samples from Greece (prototype strain GR17), but additional clones from Cameroon (strain 97CM-MP818) and France (strain 99FR-MP129) have been deposited in the Los Alamos National Laboratory HIV Sequence Database (47).

CONCLUSION

HIV-1 undergoes rapid genetic diversification due to high mutation rates as well as frequent genomic recombination. Some regions of the genome such as the envelope gene show particularly high rates of evolution due to selection pressure exerted by the host. While only one or a few point mutations are enough to show major phenotypic changes for properties such as drug resistance or immune evasion, HIV-1s are phylogenetically classified into subtypes on the basis of 20%–35% differences in their amino acid sequences.

The main group of HIV-1 has 9 subtypes, all of which have been found in Africa. However, only three (A, C, and D) have spread to cause large numbers of infections at the present time. A growing number of CRFs—at least 6—have been described in Africa. Only CRF02_AG, which is the dominant virus in West Africa, has already accounted for a large number of infections. However, CRF01_AE, which is present in the Central African Republic, is also the dominant virus in the heterosexual epidemic of Thailand. HIV-1 subtypes can be most reliably classified using nucleotide sequencing or HMA. To be sure that a given virus is not a recombinant, it is necessary to check the sequences of multiple regions of the viral genome.

REFERENCES

1. Arthur LO, Bess JW Jr, Sowder RC 2nd, et al. Cellular proteins bound to immunodeficiency viruses: implications for pathogenesis and vaccines. *Science*, 1992;258:1935–1938.
2. Emerman M, Malim MH. HIV-1 regulatory/accessory genes: keys to unraveling viral and host cell biology. *Science*, 1998;280:1880–1884.
3. Lukashov VV, Goudsmit J. HIV heterogeneity and disease progression in AIDS: a model of continuous virus adaptation. *AIDS*, 1998;12(Suppl): S43–S52.
4. Coffin JM. Genetic diversity and evolution of retroviruses. *Curr Top Microbiol Immunol*, 1992;176: 143–164.
5. Preston BD, Poiesz BJ, Loeb LA. Fidelity of HIV-1 reverse transcriptase. *Science*, 1988;242:1168–1171.
6. Goodenow M, Huet T, Saurin W, et al. HIV-1 isolates are rapidly evolving quasispecies: evidence for viral mixtures and preferred nucleotide substitutions. *J Acquir Immune Defic Syndr*, 1989;2:344.
7. Myers G, Pavlakis GN. Evolutionary potential of complex retroviruses. In: Levy J, ed. *The Retroviridae* (volume 1). New York: Plenum Press, 1992:51.
8. Shioda T, Levy J, Chang-Mayer C. Small amino acid changes in the V3 hypervariable region of gp120 can affect T-cell line and macrophage tropism of human immunodeficiency virus type 1. *Proc Natl Acad Sci USA*, 1992;89:9434.
9. Montano M, Nixon C, Ndung'u T, et al. Elevated TNFα Activation of Human Immunodeficiency Virus Type 1 Subtype C in Southern Africa Associated with a NFκB Enhancer Gain-of-Function. *J Infect Dis*, 2000;181:76–81.
10. Louwagie J, McCutchan F, Van der Groen G, et al. Genetic comparison of HIV-1 isolates from Africa, Europe, and North America. *AIDS Res Hum Retroviruses*, 1992;8:1467–1469.
11. Delwart EL, Shpaer EG, Louwagie J, et al. Genetic relationships determined by a DNA heteroduplex mobility assay: analysis of HIV-1 env genes. *Science*, 1993;262:1257–1261.
12. Luo CC, Downing RG, Dela Torre N. The development and evaluation of a probe hybridization method for subtyping HIV type 1 infection in Uganda. *AIDS Res Hum Retroviruses*, 1998;14: 691–694.
13. van Harmelen J, van der Ryst E, Wood R, et al. Restriction fragment length polymorphism analysis for rapid gag subtype determination of human immunodeficiency virus type 1 in South Africa. *J Virol Methods*, 1999;78:51–59.
14. Nkengasong JN, Willems B, Janssens W, et al. Lack of correlation between V3-loop peptide enzyme immunoassay serologic subtyping and genetic sequencing. *AIDS*, 1998;12:1405–1412.
15. Barin F, Lahbabi Y, Buzelay L, et al. Diversity of antibody binding to V3 peptides representing consensus sequences of HIV type 1 genotypes A to E: an approach for HIV type 1 serological subtyping. *AIDS Res Hum Retroviruses*, 1996;12:1279–1289.
16. Moore JP, Cao Y, Leu J, et al. Inter- and intraclade neutralization of human immunodeficiency virus type 1: genetic clades do not correspond to neutralization serotypes but partially correspond to gp120 antigenic serotypes. *J Virol*, 1995;70:427–444.
17. Hoelscher M, Hanker S, Barin F, et al. HIV type 1 V3 serotyping of Tanzanian samples: probable reasons for mismatching with genetic subtyping. *AIDS Res Hum Retroviruses*, 1998;14:139–149.
18. Essex, M. Human Immunodeficiency Viruses of the Developing World. *Advan Virus Res*, 1999;53:71–88.
19. Nkengasong JN, Janssens W, Heyndrickx L, et al. Genotypic subtypes of HIV-1 in Cameroon. *AIDS*, 1994;8:1405–1412.

20. Tkehisa J, Zekeng L, Miura T, et al. Various types of HIV mixed-infections in Cameroon. *Virology*, 1998;245:1–10.
21. Renjifo B, Chaplin B, Mwakagile D, et al. Epidemic expansion of HIV type 1 subtype C and recombinant genotypes in Tanzania. *AIDS Res Hum Retroviruses*, 1998;14:635–638.
22. Louwagie J, McCutchan FE, Peeters M, et al. Phylogenetic analysis of gag genes from 70 international HIV-1 isolates provides evidence for multiple genotypes. *AIDS*, 1993;7:769–780.
23. Myers G, Korber B, Berzofky JA, Smith TF, Pavlakis GN, eds. *Human Retroviruses and AIDS*. Los Alamos: Los Alamos National laboratory, 1992.
24. Robertson DL, Anderson AP, Bradac JA, et al. HIV-1 nomenclature proposal. A reference guide to HIV-1 classification. In: *Human Retroviruses and AIDS: A compilation and analysis of nucleic acid and amino acid sequences*. Kuiken CFB, Hahn BH, Korber B, McCutchan F, Marx PA, Mellors JW, Mullins JL, Sodroski J, Wolinsky S, eds. Los Alamos, NM: Theoretical Biology and Biophysics Group, 1999:492–505.
25. Agwale SM, Robbins KE, Odama L, et al. Development of an env gp41-based heteroduplex mobility assay for rapid human immunodeficiency virus type 1 subtyping. *J Clin Microbiol*, 2001;39: 2110–2114.
26. Vidal N, Peeters M, Mulanga-Kabeya C, et al. Unprecedented degree of human immunodeficiency virus type 1 (HIV-1) group M genetic diversity in the Democratic Republic of Congo suggests that the HIV-1 pandemic originated in Central Africa. *J Virol*, 2001;74:10498–10507.
27. Peeters M, Koumare B, Mulanga C, et al. Genetic subtypes of HIV type 1 and HIV type 2 strains in commercial sex workers from Bamako, Mali. *AIDS Res Hum Retroviruses*, 1998;14:51–58.
28. Muller-Trutwin MC, Chaix ML, Letourneur F, et al. Increase of HIV-1 subtype A in Central African Republic. *J Acquir Immune Defic Syndr*, 1999;21: 164–171.
29. Tien PC, Chiu T, Latif A, et al. Primary subtype C HIV-1 infection in Harare, Zimbabwe. *J Acquir Immune Defic Syndr Hum Retrovirol*, 1999;20: 147–153.
30. Bredell H, Williamson C, Sonnenberg P, et al. Genetic characterization of HIV type 1 from migrant workers in three South African gold mines. *AIDS Res Hum Retroviruses*, 1998;14:677–684.
31. Toure-Kane C, Montavon C, Faye MA, et al. Identification of all HIV type 1 group M subtypes in Senegal, a country with low and stable seroprevalence. *AIDS Res Hum Retroviruses*, 2000;16: 603–609.
32. Heyndrickx L, Janssens W, Zekeng L, et al. Simplified strategy for detection of recombinant human immunodeficiency virus type 1 group M isolates by gag/env heteroduplex mobility assay. Study Group on Heterogeneity of HIV Epidemics in African Cities. *J Virol*, 2000;74:363–370.
33. Subbarao S, Luo CC, Limpakarnjanarat K, et al. Evaluation of oligonucleotide probes for the determination of the two major HIV-1 env subtypes in Thailand. *AIDS*, 1996;10:350–351.
34. Robbins KE, Kostrikis LG, Brown TM, et al. Genetic analysis of human immunodeficiency virus type 1 strains in Kenya: a comparison using phylogenetic analysis and a combinatorial melting assay. *AIDS Res Hum Retroviruses*, 1999;15:329–335.
35. Peeters M, Liegeois F, Bibollet-Ruche F, et al. Subtype-specific polymerase chain reaction for the identification of HIV-1 genetic subtypes circulating in Africa. *AIDS*, 1998;12:671–673.
36. Plantier JC, Damond F, Lasky M, et al. V3 serotyping of HIV-1 infection: correlation with genotyping and limitations. *J Acquir Immune Defic Syndr Hum Retrovirol*, 1999;20:432–441.
37. Gaywee J, Artenstein AW, VanCott TC, et al. Correlation of genetic and serologic approaches to HIV-1 subtyping in Thailand. *J Acquir Immune Defic Syndr Hum Retrovirol*, 1996;13:392–396.
38. Robertson DL, Anderson JP, Bradac JA, et al. HIV-1 nomenclature proposal. *Science*, 2000;288:55–56.
39. Bibollet-Ruche F, Peeters M, Montavon C, et al. Molecular characterization of the envelope transmembrane glycoprotein of 13 new human immunodeficiency virus type 1 group O strains from six different African countries. *AIDS Res Hum Retroviruses*, 1998;14:1281–1285.
40. Mauclere P, Loussert-Ajaka I, Damond F, et al. Serological and virological characterization of HIV-1 group O infection in Cameroon. *AIDS*, 1997;11:445–453.
41. Peeters M, Gueye A, Mboup S, et al. Geographical distribution of HIV-1 group O viruses in Africa. *AIDS*, 1997;11:493–498.
42. Gurtler LG, Hauser PH, Eberle J, et al. A new subtype of human immunodeficiency virus type 1 (MVP-5180) from Cameroon. *J Virol*, 1994;68:1581–1585.
43. Ayouba A, Souquieres S, Njinku B, et al. HIV-1 group N among HIV-1-seropositive individuals in Cameroon. *AIDS*, 2000;14:2623–2625.
44. Simon F, Mauclere P, Roques P, et al. Identification of a new human immunodeficiency virus type 1 distinct from group M and group O. *Nat Med*, 1998;4:1032–1037.
45. McCutchan FE. Understanding the genetic diversity of HIV-1. *AIDS*, 2000;14:S31–S44.
46. Louwagie J, Janssens W, Mascola J, et al. Genetic diversity of the envelope glycoprotein from human immunodeficiency virus type 1 isolates of African origin. *J Virol*, 1995;69:263–271.

47. Peeters M. Recombinant HIV sequences: their role in the global epidemic. In: *Human Retroviruses and AIDS: A compilation and analysis of nucleic acid and amino acid sequences*. Kuiken C FB, Hahn BH, Korber B, McCutchan F, Marx PA, Mellors JW, Mullins JL, Sodroski J, Wolinsky S, eds. Los Alamos, NM: Theoretical Biology and Biophysics Group, 2000:I39–I54.
48. UNAIDS/WHO. Report on the global HIV/AIDS epidemic. UNAIDS/00.13E. Geneva: UNAIDS/WHO, 2000.
49. Ellenberger DL, Pieniazek D, Nkengasong J, et al. Genetic analysis of human immunodeficiency virus in Abidjan, Ivory Coast reveals predominance of HIV type 1 subtype A and introduction of subtype G. *AIDS Res Hum Retroviruses*, 1999;15:3–9.
50. Janssens W, Heyndrickx L, Van de Peer Y, et al. Molecular phylogeny of part of the env gene of HIV-1 strains isolated in Cote d'Ivoire. *AIDS*, 1994;8:21–26.
51. Mulder-Kampinga GA, Simonon A, Kuiken CL, et al. Similarity in env and gag genes between genomic RNAs of human immunodeficiency virus type 1 (HIV-1) from mother and infant is unrelated to time of HIV-1 RNA positivity in the child. *J Virol*, 1995;69:2285–2296.
52. Kampinga GA, Simonon A, Van de Perre P, et al. Primary infections with HIV-1 of women and their offspring in Rwanda: findings of heterogeneity at seroconversion, coinfection, and recombinants of HIV-1 subtypes A and C. *Virology*, 1997;227: 63–76.
53. Cornelissen M, Kampinga G, Zorgdrager F, et al. Human immunodeficiency virus type 1 subtypes defined by env show high frequency of recombinant gag genes. The UNAIDS Network for HIV Isolation and Characterization. *J Virol*, 1996;70:8209–8012.
54. Takehisa J, Osei-Kwasi M, Ayisi NK, et al. Phylogenetic analysis of human immunodeficiency virus 1 in Ghana. *Acta Virol*, 1997;41:51–54.
55. Brandful JA, Ampofo WK, Janssens W, et al. Genetic and phylogenetic analysis of HIV type 1 strains from southern Ghana. *AIDS Res Hum Retroviruses*, 1998;14:815–819.
56. Ishikawa K, Janssens W, Brandful J, et al. Genetic and phylogenetic analysis of HIV type 1 env subtypes in Ghana, West Africa. *AIDS Res Hum Retroviruses*, 1996;12:1575–1578.
57. Buonaguro L, Del Guadio E, Monaco M, et al. Heteroduplex mobility assay and phylogenetic analysis of V3 region sequences of human immunodeficiency virus type 1 isolates from Gulu, northern Uganda. The Italian-Ugandan Cooperation AIDS Program. *J Virol*, 1995;69:7971–7981.
58. Rayfield MA, Downing RG, Baggs J, et al. A molecular epidemiologic survey of HIV in Uganda. HIV Variant Working Group. *AIDS*, 1998;12: 521–527.
59. Becker-Pergola G, Mellquist JL, Guay L, et al. Identification of diverse HIV type 1 subtypes and dual HIV type 1 infection in pregnant Ugandan women. *AIDS Res Hum Retroviruses*, 2000;16: 1099–1104.
60. Gao F, Robertson DL, Carruthers CD, et al. A comprehensive panel of near-full-length clones and reference sequences for non-subtype B isolates of human immunodeficiency virus type 1. *J Virol*, 1998;72:5680–5698.
61. Candotti, D, Tareau C, Barin F, et al. Genetic subtyping and V3 serotyping of HIV-1 isolates from Congo. *AIDS Res Hum Retroviruses*, 1999;15: 309–314.
62. Janssens W, Heyndrickx L, Fransen K, et al. Genetic variability of HIV type 1 in Kenya. *AIDS Res Hum Retroviruses*, 1994;10:1577–1579.
63. Neilson JR, John GC, Carr JK, et al. Subtypes of human immunodeficiency virus type 1 and disease stage among women in Nairobi, Kenya. *J Virol*, 1999;73:4393–4403.
64. Sankale JL, Hamel D, Woolsey A, et al. Molecular evolution of human immunodeficiency virus type 1 subtype A in Senegal: 1988–1997. *J Hum Virol*, 2000;3:157–164.
65. Sarr AD, Sankale JL, Hamel DJ, et al. Interaction with human immunodeficiency virus (HIV) type 2 predicts HIV type 1 genotype. *Virology*, 2000;268: 402–410.
66. Ortiz M, Sanchez I, Gonzalez MP, et al. Molecular epidemiology of HIV type 1 subtypes in Equatorial Guinea. *AIDS Res Hum Retroviruses*, 2001;17: 851–885.
67. M'Vouenze R, Zekeng L, Tkehisa J, et al. HIV type 1 genetic variability in the northern part of Cameroon. *AIDS Res Hum Retroviruses*, 1999;15: 951–956.
68. Howard TM, Olaylele DO, Rasheed S. Sequence analysis of the glycoprotein 120 coding region of a new HIV type 1 subtype A strain (HIV-1IbNg) from Nigeria. *AIDS Res Hum Retroviruses*, 1994;10: 1755–1757.
69. McCutchan FE, Carr JK, Bajani M, et al. Subtype G and multiple forms of A/G intersubtype recombinant human immunodeficiency virus type 1 in Nigeria. *Virology*, 1999;254:226–234.
70. Heyndrickx L, Janssens W, Alary M, et al. Genetic variability of HIV type 1 in Benin. *AIDS Res Hum Retroviruses*, 1996;12:1495–1497.
71. Montavon C, Toure-Kane C, Liegeois F, et al. Most env and gag subtype A HIV-1 viruses circulating in West and West Central Africa are similar to the prototype AG recombinant virus IBNG. *J Acquir Immune Defic Syndr*, 2000;23:363–374.
72. Delaporte E, Janssens W, Peeters M, et al. Epidemiological and molecular characteristics of HIV infection in Gabon, 1986–1994. *AIDS*, 2000;10:903–910.

73. Huet T, Dazza MC, Brun-Vezinet F, et al. A highly defective HIV-1 strain isolated from a healthy Gabonese individual presenting an atypical Western blot. *AIDS*, 1989;3:707–715.
74. Gao F, Vidal N, Li Y, et al. Evidence of two distinct subsubtypes within the HIV-1 subtype A radiation. *AIDS Res Hum Retroviruses*, 2001;17:675–88.
75. Carr JK, Laukkanen T, Salminen MO, et al. Characterization of subtype A HIV-1 from Africa by full genome sequencing. *AIDS*, 1999;13: 1819–1826.
76. Engelbrecht S, Laten JD, Smith TL, et al. Identification of env subtypes in fourteen HIV type 1 isolates from South Africa. *AIDS Res Hum Retroviruses*, 1995;11:1269–1271.
77. De Baar MP, De Ronde A, Berkhout B, et al. Subtype-specific sequence variation of the HIV type 1 LTR and primer-binding site. *AIDS Res Hum Retroviruses*, 2000;16:499–504.
78. El Sayed NM, Gomatos PJ, Beck-Sague CM, et al. Epidemic transmission of human immunodeficiency virus in renal dialysis centers in Egypt. *J Infect Dis*, 1995;81:91–97.
79. Kiwelu IE, Nakkestad HL, Shao J, et al. Evidence of subtype B-like sequences in the V3 loop region of human immunodeficiency virus type 1 in Kilimanjaro, Tanzania. *AIDS Res Hum Retroviruses*, 2000;16:1191–1195.
80. Esparza J, Bhamarapravati N. Accelerating the development and future availability of HIV-1 vaccines: why, when, where, and how?. *Lancet*, 2000;355:2061–2066.
81. Engelbrecht S, Koulinska I, Smith TL, et al. Variation in HIV type 1 V3 region env sequences from Mozambique. *AIDS Res Hum Retroviruses*, 1998;14:803–805.
82. Rodenburg CM, Li Y, Trask SA, et al. Near full-length clones and reference sequences for subtype C isolates of HIV type 1 from three different continents. *AIDS Res Hum Retroviruses*, 2001;17:161–168.
83. Ping LH, Nelson JA, Hoffman IF, et al. Characterization of V3 sequence heterogeneity in subtype C human immunodeficiency virus type 1 isolates from Malawi: underrepresentation of X4 variants. *J Virol*, 1999;73:6271–6281.
84. Gao F, Morrison SG, Robertson DL, et al. Molecular cloning and analysis of functional envelope genes from human immunodeficiency virus type 1 sequence subtypes A through G. The WHO and NIAID Networks for HIV Isolation and Characterization. *J Virol*, 1996;70:1651–1667.
85. Orloff GM, Kalish ML, Chiphangwi J, et al. V3 loops of HIV-1 specimens from pregnant women in Malawi uniformly lack a potential N-linked glycosylation site. *AIDS Res Hum Retroviruses*, 1993;9:705–706.
86. Novitsky VA, Montano MA, McLane MF, et al. Molecular cloning and phylogenetic analysis of human immunodeficiency virus type 1 subtype C: a set of 23 full-length clones from Botswana. *J Virol*, 1999;73:4427–4432.
87. Abebe A, Lukashov VV, Pollakis G, et al. Timing of the HIV-1 subtype C epidemic in Ethiopia based on early virus strains and subsequent virus diversification. *AIDS*, 2001;15:1555–1561.
88. Abebe A, Lukashov VV, Rinke De Wit TF, et al. Timing of the introduction into Ethiopia of subcluster C' of HIV type 1 subtype C. *AIDS Res Hum Retroviruses*, 2001;17:657–661.
89. Murphy E, Korber BT, Georges-Courbot MC, et al. Diversity of V3 region sequences of human immunodeficiency viruses type 1 from the Central African Republic. *AIDS Res Hum Retroviruses*, 1993;9:997–1006.
90. Renjifo B, Gilbert P, Chaplin B, et al. Emerging recombinant human immunodeficiency viruses: uneven representation of the envelope V3 region. *AIDS*, 1999;13:1613–1621.
91. Salminen MO, Johansson B, Soennerborg A, et al. Full-length sequence of an Ethiopian human immunodeficiency virus type 1 (HIV-1) isolate of genetic subtype C. *AIDS Res Hum Retroviruses*, 1996;12:1329–1339.
92. Hoelscher M, Kim B, Maboko L, et al. High proportion of unrelated HIV-1 intersubtype recombinants in the Mbeya region of southwest Tanzania. *AIDS*, 2001;15:1461–1470.
93. Keys B, Karis J, Fadeel B, et al. V3 sequences of paired HIV-1 isolates from blood and cerebrospinal fluid cluster according to host and show variation related to the clinical stage of disease. *Virology*, 1993;196:475–483.
94. Su L, Graf M, Zhang Y, et al. Characterization of a Virtually Full-Length Human Immunodeficiency Virus Type 1 Genome of a Prevalent Intersubtype (C/B') Recombinant Strain in China. *J Virol*, 2000;74:11367–11376.
95. Piyasirisilp S, McCutchan FE, Carr JK, et al. A recent outbreak of human immunodeficiency virus type 1 infection in southern China was initiated by two highly homogeneous, geographically separated strains, circulating recombinant form AE and a novel BC recombinant. *J Virol*, 2000;74:11286–11295.
96. Tripathy S, Renjifo B, Wang WK, et al. Envelope glycoprotein 120 sequences of primary HIV type 1 isolates from Pune and New Delhi, India. *AIDS Res Hum Retroviruses*, 1996;12:1199–1202.
97. Lole KS, Bollinger RC, Paranjape RS, et al. Full-length human immunodeficiency virus type 1 genomes from subtype C-infected seroconverters in India, with evidence of intersubtype recombination. *J Virol*, 1999;73:152–160.
98. Alizon M, Wain-Hobson S, Montagnier L, et al. Genetic variability of the AIDS virus: nucleotide sequence analysis of two isolates from African patients. *Cell*, 1986;46:63–74.

99. Albert J, Franzen L, Jansson M, et al. Ugandan HIV-1 V3 loop sequences closely related to the U.S./European consensus. *Virology*, 1992;190: 674–681.
100. Potts KE, Kalish ML, Bandea CI, et al. Genetic diversity of human immunodeficiency virus type 1 strains in Kinshasa, Zaire. *AIDS Res Hum Retroviruses*, 1993;9:613–618.
101. Zwarf G, Wolfs TFW, Bookelman R, et al. Greater diversity of the HIV-1 V3 neutralization domain in Tanzania compared with The Netherlands: serological and genetic analysis. *AIDS*, 1993;7:467–474.
102. Siwka W, Schwinn A, Baczko K, et al. Vpu and env sequence variability of HIV-1 isolates from Tanzania. *AIDS Res Hum Retroviruses*, 1994;12: 1753–1754.
103. Holm-Hansen C, Ayehunie S, Johansson B, et al. HIV-1 proviral DNA sequences of env gp41 PCR amplificates from Tanzania. *APMIS*, 1996;104: 459–464.
104. Robbins KE, Bandea CI, Levin A, et al. Genetic variability of human immunodeficiency virus type 1 in rural northwest Tanzania. *AIDS Res Hum Retroviruses*, 1996;12:1389–1391.
105. Spire B, Sire J, Zachar V, et al. Nucleotide sequence of HIV1-NDK: a highly cytopathic strain of the human immunodeficiency virus. *Gene*, 1989;81:275–284.
106. Korber BT, MacInnes K, Smith RF, et al. Mutational trends in V3 loop protein sequences observed in different genetic lineages of human immunodeficiency virus type 1. *J Virol*, 1994;68:6730–6744.
107. Triques K, Bourgeois A, Saragosti S, et al. High diversity of HIV-1 subtype F strains in Central Africa. *Virology*, 1999;259:99–109.
108. Triques K, Bourgeois A, Vidal N, et al. Near-full-length genome sequencing of divergent African HIV type 1 subtype F viruses leads to the identification of a new HIV type 1 subtype designated K. *AIDS Res Hum Retroviruses*, 2000;16:139–151.
109. Tkehisa J, Harada Y, Bikandou B, et al. Genetic diversity of HIV-1 group M from Cameroon and Republic of Congo. *Arch Virol*, 1999;144:2291–2311.
110. Simon F, Loussert-Ajaka I, Damond F, et al. HIV type 1 diversity in northern Paris, France. *AIDS Res Hum Retroviruses*, 1996;12:1427–1433.
111. Dumitrescu O, Kalish ML, Kliks SC, et al. Characterization of human immunodeficiency virus type 1 isolates from children in Romania: identification of a new envelope subtype. *J Infect Dis*, 1994;169:281–288.
112. Campodonico M, Janssens W, Heyndrickx L, et al. HIV type 1 subtypes in Argentina and genetic heterogeneity of the V3 region. *AIDS Res Hum Retroviruses*, 1996;12:79–81
113. Morgado MG, Sabino EC, Shpaer EG, et al. V3 region polymorphisms in HIV-1 from Brazil: prevalence of subtype B strains divergent from North American/European prototype and detection of subtype F. *AIDS Res Hum Retroviruses*, 1994;10:569–576.
114. Potts KE, Kalish ML, Lott T, et al. Genetic heterogeneity of the V3 region of the HIV-1 envelope glycoprotein in Brazil. Brazilian Collaborative AIDS Research Group. *AIDS*, 1993;7:1191–1197.
115. Myers G, Korber B, Berzofksy JA, Smith RF, and Pavlakis GN, eds. *Human Retroviruses and AIDS: A Compilation and Analysis of Nucleic Acid and Amino Acid Sequences*. Los Alamos: Theoretical Biology and Biophysics Group, Los Alamos National Laboratory, 1992.
116. Laukkanen T, Carr JK, Janssens W, et al. Virtually full-length subtype F and F/D recombinant HIV-1 from Africa and South America. *Virology*, 2000;269:95–104.
117. Carr JK, Salminen MO, Albert J, et al. Full genome sequences of human immunodeficiency virus type 1 subtypes G and A/G intersubtype recombinants. *Virology*, 1998;247:22–31.
118. Kaleebu P, Bobkov A, Cheingsong-Popov R, et al. Identification of HIV-1 subtype G from Uganda. *AIDS Res Hum Retroviruses*, 1995;11:657–659.
119. Abimiku AG, Stern TL, Zwandor A, et al. Subgroup G HIV type 1 isolates from Nigeria. *AIDS Res Hum Retroviruses*, 1995;10:1581–1583
120. Janssens W, Heyndrickx L, Fransen K, et al. Genetic and phylogenetic analysis of env subtypes G and H in central Africa. *AIDS Res Hum Retroviruses*, 1994;10:877–879.
121. Murphy E, Korber B, Georges-Courbot MC, et al. Diversity of V3 region sequences of human immunodeficiency viruses type 1 from the Central African Republic. *AIDS Res Hum Retroviruses*, 1993;9:997–1006.
122. Debyser Z, Van Wijngaerden E, Van Laethem K, et al. Failure to quantify viral load with two of the three commercial methods in a pregnant woman harboring an HIV type 1 subtype G strain. *AIDS Res Hum Retroviruses*, 1998;14:453–459.
123. Oelrichs RB, Vandamme AM, Van Laethem K, et al. Full-length genomic sequence of an HIV type 1 subtype G from Kinshasa. *AIDS Res Hum Retroviruses*, 1999;15:585–589.
124. Peeters M, Mboup S, Ndoyi-Mbiguino A, et al. Genetic diversity of HIV-1 in West and West Central Africa. In: Program and Abstracts of the XIII International Conference on AIDS; July 9–14, 2000; Durban, South Africa. Abstract TuOrA411.
125. Janssens W, Laukkanen T, Salminen MO, et al. HIV-1 subtype H near-full length genome reference

strains and analysis of subtype-H-containing inter-subtype recombinants. *AIDS*, 2000;14: 1533–1543.

126. Bobkov A, Cheingsong-Popov R, Selimova L, et al. Genetic heterogeneity of HIV type 1 in Russia: identification of H variants and relationship with epidemiological data. *AIDS Res Hum Retroviruses*, 1996;12:1687–1690.
127. Heyndrickx L, Janssens W, Coppens S, et al. HIV type 1 C2V3 env diversity among Belgian individuals. *AIDS Res Hum Retroviruses*, 1998;14: 1291–1296.
128. Alaeus A, Leitner T, Lidman K, et al. Most HIV-1 genetic subtypes have entered Sweden. *AIDS*, 1997;11:199–202.
129. Trask SA, Derdeyn CA, Fideli U, et al. Molecular Epidemiology of Human Immunodeficiency Virus Type 1 Transmission in a Heterosexual Cohort of Discordant Couples in Zambia. *J Virol*, 2002;76: 397–405.
130. Fonjungo PN, Mpoudi EN, Torimiro JN, et al. Presence of diverse human immunodeficiency virus type 1 viral variants in Cameroon. *AIDS Res Hum Retroviruses*, 2000;16:1319–1324.
131. Machuca R, Bogh M, Salminen M, et al. HIV-1 subtypes in Denmark. *Scand J Infect Dis*, 2001;33: 697–701.
132. Boni J, Pyra H, Gebhardt M, et al. High frequency of non-B subtypes in newly diagnosed HIV-1 infections in Switzerland. *J Acquir Immune Defic Syndr*, 1999;22:174–179.
133. Laukkanen T, Albert J, Liitsola K, et al. Virtually full-length sequences of HIV type 1 subtype J reference strains. *AIDS Res Hum Retroviruses*, 1999;15:293–297.
134. Novitsky VA, Gaolekwe S, McLane MF, et al. HIV type 1 A/J recombinant with a pronounced pol gene mosaicism. *AIDS Res Hum Retroviruses*, 2000;16:1015–1020.
135. Paraskevis D, Magiorkinis E, Magiorkinis G, et al. Molecular characterization of a complex, recombinant human immunodeficiency virus type 1 (HIV-1) isolate (A/G/J/K/?): evidence to support the existence of a novel HIV-1 subtype. *J Gen Virol*, 2001;82(Pt10):2509–2514.
136. Liitsola K, Tashkinova I, Laukkanen T, et al. HIV-1 genetic subtype A/B recombinant strain causing an explosive epidemic in injecting drug users in Kaliningrad. *AIDS*, 1998;12:1907–1919.
137. Kostrikis LG, Bagdades E, Cao Y, et al. Genetic analysis of human immunodeficiency virus type 1 strains from patients in Cyprus: identification of a new subtype designated subtype I. *J Virol*, 1995;69:6122–6230.
138. Nasioulas G, Paraskevis D, Magiorkinis E, et al. Molecular analysis of the full-length genome of HIV type 1 subtype I: evidence of A/G/I recombination. *AIDS Res Hum Retroviruses*, 1999;15:745–758.
139. Salminen M, Gao F, Janssens W, et al. The loss of HIV-1 subtype I. In: Program and Abstracts of the XIII International Conference on AIDS; July 9–14, 2000; Durban, South Africa. Abstract A2065.
140. Carr JK, Salminen MO, Koch C, et al. Full-length sequence and mosaic structure of a human immuno-deficiency virus type 1 isolate from Thailand. *J Virol*, 1996;70:5935–5943.
141. Gao F, Robertson DL, Morrison SG, et al. The heterosexual human immunodeficiency virus type 1 epidemic in Thailand is caused by an intersubtype (A/E) recombinant of African origin. *J Virol*, 1996;70:7013–7029.
142. Weginer B. Experience from incidence cohorts in Thailand: Implications for HIV vaccines efficacy trials. *AIDS*, 1998;8:1007–1010.
143. UNAIDS. UNAIDS/WHO Working group on global HIV/AIDS and STD surveillance report on the global HIV/AIDS epidemic. Geneva, Switzerland: World Health Organization, 1997.
144. Beyrer C, Razak MH, Lisam K, et al. Overland heroin trafficking routes and HIV-1 spread in south and south-east Asia. *AIDS*, 2000;14:75–83.
145. Yu XF, Chen J, Shao Y, et al. Emerging HIV infections with distinct subtypes of HIV-1 infection among injection drug users from geographically separate locations in Guangxi Province, China. *J Acquir Immune Defic Syndr*, 1999;22:180–188.
146. Kato K, Shiino T, Kusagawa S, et al. Genetic similarity of HIV type 1 subtype E in a recent outbreak among injecting drug users in northern Vietnam to strains in Guangxi Province of southern China. *AIDS Res Hum Retroviruses*, 1999;15:1157–1168.
147. Motomura K, Kusagawa S, Kato K, et al. Emergence of new forms of human immunodeficiency virus type 1 intersubtype recombinants in central Myanmar. *AIDS Res Hum Retroviruses*, 2000;16:1831–1843.
148. McCutchan FE, Salminen MO, Carr JK, et al. HIV-1 genetic diversity. *AIDS*, 1996;10:S13–S20.
149. Anderson JP, Rodrigo AG, Learn GH, et al. Testing the hypothesis of a recombinant origin of human immunodeficiency virus type 1 subtype E. *J Virol*, 2000;74:10752–10765.
150. Montavon C, Bibollet-Ruche F, Robertson D, et al. The identification of a complex A/G/I/J recombinant HIV type 1 virus in various West African countries. *AIDS Res Hum Retroviruses*, 1999;15: 1707–1712.
151. Oelrichs RB, Workman C, Laukkanen T, et al. A novel subtype A/G/J recombinant full-length HIV type 1 genome from Burkina Faso. *AIDS Res Hum Retroviruses*, 1998;14:1495–1500.
152. Koulinska IN, Ndung'u T, Mwakagile D, et al. A new human immunodeficiency virus type 1 circulating recombinant form from Tanzania. *AIDS Res Hum Retroviruses*, 2001;17:423–431.

153. Fawzi WW, Msamanga G, Hunter D, et al. Randomized trial of vitamin supplements in relation to vertical transmission of HIV-1 in Tanzania. *J Acquir Immune Defic Syndr*, 2000;23:246–254.
154. Renjifo B, Fawzi W, Mwakagile D, et al. Differences in perinatal transmission among human immunodeficiency virus type 1 genotypes. *J Hum Virol*, 2001;4:16–25.
155. Blackard JT, Renjifo B, Fawzi W, et al. HIV-1 LTR subtype and perinatal transmission. *Virology*, 2001;287:261–265.

17

Current Estimates and Projections for the Epidemic

Karen A. Stanecki and Neff Walker

United States Census Bureau, International Programs Center, Washington, DC, USA.
United Nations Joint Programme on HIV/AIDS, Geneva, Switzerland.

Although it may be easier to estimate HIV prevalence in parts of the world where superior surveillance techniques are available, it still remains a challenging effort throughout the world. Despite advancements in our understanding of the epidemiology of HIV and techniques for monitoring the epidemic, HIV incidence levels are still unknown in most parts of the world.

Projecting the future of the HIV epidemic presents an additional challenge. When the first edition of this book was published, the HIV epidemics in Africa appeared to be most severe in central and eastern Africa, with very little evidence of HIV in southern African countries such as Botswana, Lesotho, Swaziland, or South Africa. Today, these countries are among those with the highest levels of HIV prevalence in the world. All estimates and projections are based on what we know today. The future may hold an altogether different picture.

HIV/AIDS SURVEILLANCE

Epidemiologic surveillance has been defined as "the ongoing and systematic collection, analysis, and interpretation of health data in the process of describing and monitoring a health event" (1). The HIV epidemic represents a health event of unprecedented magnitude.

HIV and AIDS surveillance provides information that allows researchers to determine the extent of the epidemic and to track changes or trends in the epidemic over time. Given the long period of incubation between HIV infection and the development of full-blown AIDS, a surveillance system that relies solely on AIDS case reporting is not effective. In resource-poor countries with underdeveloped health infrastructures, reports of AIDS or HIV cases are usually not complete enough to be considered reliable measures of the scope of the epidemic. In richer countries, where fewer people are progressing to AIDS as a result of the provision of therapy, the reporting of AIDS cases is even less useful in estimating numbers of persons living with HIV.

In 1988, the World Health Organization (WHO) proposed the introduction of HIV sentinel surveillance systems to monitor the magnitude and trends of the HIV epidemic (2). More recently, UNAIDS and the WHO have put forth guidelines for second-generation surveillance of HIV (3). These guidelines make recommendations for strengthening and expanding surveillance systems to collect behavioral data and information on a set of HIV/AIDS indicators to increase their ability to track the course of the epidemic and to assess the impact of interventions.

Surveillance data can be used in many ways in addition to estimating the magnitude of the epidemic and monitoring its trends. The information provided by a functioning surveillance system is essential to developing strategies to respond to the HIV epidemic. For example, if used for advocacy, surveillance data enable decision makers to strengthen commitment to research and prevention, to ensure sufficient allocation of resources to national programs, and to target interventions to the highest risk groups or areas. Surveillance data are also essential in planning and evaluating prevention activities and monitoring their impact. Finally, estimates of current and expected HIV and AIDS caseloads can be useful in planning for and providing health and social services.

Targeting Appropriate Populations for Sentinel Surveillance

The guidelines put forth by UNAIDS and the WHO for second-generation surveillance are based on the state of the epidemic in a given country. HIV epidemics are classified in three states: low-level, concentrated, and generalized. Definitions of these states and their respective recommended surveillance systems follow (3).

Low-level: HIV prevalence has not consistently exceeded 5% in any defined subpopulation whose behavior places them at highest risk. These groups include injection drug users, commercial sex workers, and men who have sex with men, among others. At this level of the epidemic, HIV surveillance should be carried out in the groups at highest risk in the country.

Concentrated: HIV prevalence is consistently over 5% in at least one defined subpopulation at highest risk, but prevalence remains below 1% in the general adult population (ages 15–49) in urban areas. At this level of the epidemic, surveillance of high-risk groups should continue and surveillance of the general population in urban areas should begin.

Generalized: HIV prevalence reaches 1% in the general adult population (ages 15–49) in urban areas. At this level, surveillance of the general population in rural areas should begin in addition to the continued surveillance of the general population in urban settings and of at least one high-risk group.

Data that are representative of the general adult population in the most sexually active years (ages 15–49) are hard to gather. Women receiving clinical antenatal care are often used as a proxy for the general adult population (2,4; WHO Global Program on AIDS, unpublished field guidelines, 1989).

Antenatal clinics often provide the most accessible cross-section of healthy, sexually active women in the general population, and have therefore become the most frequently used sites for sentinel surveillance of the general population. In most developing countries, antenatal services are among the most utilized health services, provide the broadest levels of coverage, and do not have as many confounding problems as do other potential surveillance sites (such as voluntary blood donation centers or general health clinics). Women at antenatal clinics often give blood for syphilis screening, so the additional procedure of unlinked, anonymous HIV testing of surplus blood sample is a low-cost and ethically acceptable method of surveillance. Of course, data from pregnant women are not representative of both men and women, but population-based studies that compare HIV prevalence in samples from antenatal clinic attendees with samples from men and women in the general population can be used to calibrate data (5,6). Several studies comparing data from antenatal clinics with community-based data have shown that HIV prevalence among women attending antenatal clinics gives a reasonable overall estimate of HIV prevalence in the general adult population (7,8).

Assessing the Quality of Sentinel Surveillance Systems

UNAIDS recently assessed the quality of sentinel surveillance systems around the world (9). This assessment was based on four criteria: (i) the frequency and timeliness of data collection; (ii) the appropriateness of the populations under surveillance; (iii) the consistency of the sites/locations and groups selected for surveillance over time; and (iv) the coverage/representativeness of the proxy groups for the adult populations (either for high-risk groups or for the general adult population). An assessment of the systems in the regions of sub–Saharan and North Africa follows.

Sub–Saharan Africa

Sub–Saharan Africa is the most affected by HIV and AIDS. Most countries in this region have generalized epidemics, making surveillance coverage of the general adult population more important in both rural and urban areas. Surveillance systems in sub–Saharan Africa vary considerably in quality. For example, 13 countries have systems that are categorized by UNAIDS as fully implemented (Table 1). On the other hand, 18 countries do not have even the basic elements required for an HIV/AIDS surveillance system. The remaining 13 countries have some or most of the components of a fully implemented surveillance system, but have yet to build a system that is capable of providing the data required for accurate tracking of the epidemic. Fortunately, those countries that are most affected by the epidemic generally have systems that are fully or substantially implemented.

North Africa

The countries in North Africa all have low-level or concentrated epidemics, with the exception of Sudan, where the epidemic is generalized (Table 2). Overall, the countries in this region have less developed surveillance systems than other African countries. Fortunately, most of these countries have sufficient information in the form of blood screening data or reports from occasional studies to suggest that HIV has not spread significantly in the general population. However, few countries have developed a surveillance system that would be able to detect the beginning of an epidemic in groups at highest risk.

Strengths and Weaknesses of Sentinel Surveillance Systems

A weakness of many systems is poor coverage of rural populations. In some countries with generalized epidemics little is known about HIV prevalence outside of cities.

TABLE 1. Adult Prevalence of HIV/AIDS, State of the Epidemic, and Quality of Surveillance System Rating by Country in Sub–Saharan Africa

Country	Adults living with HIV/AIDS (ages 15–49)[a]	Adult rate (%)[a]	State of epidemic[b]	Quality rating[c]
Regional Total for sub–Saharan Africa	23,400,000	8.57	—	—
Angola	150,000	2.78	G	1
Benin	67,000	2.45	G	3
Botswana	280,000	35.80	G	3
Burkina Faso	330,000	6.44	G	3
Burundi	340,000	11.32	G	3
Cameroon	520,000	7.73	G	3
Central African Republic	230,000	13.84	G	2
Chad	88,000	2.69	G	1
Comoros	400	0.12	L	1
Congo	82,000	6.43	G	1
Cote d'Ivoire	730,000	10.76	G	3
Dem. Republic of Congo	1,100,000	5.07	G	2
Djibouti	35,000	11.75	G	1
Equatorial Guinea	1,000	0.51	C	1
Eritrea	49,000	2.87	G	1
Ethiopia	2,900,000	10.63	G	2
Gabon	22,000	4.16	G	1
Gambia	12,000	1.95	G	1
Ghana	330,000	3.60	G	3
Guinea	52,000	1.54	G	2
Guinea Bissau	13,000	2.50	G	1
Kenya	2,000,000	13.95	G	3
Lesotho	240,000	23.57	G	1
Liberia	37,000	2.80	G	1
Madagascar	10,000	0.15	L	3
Malawi	760,000	15.96	G	2
Mali	97,000	2.03	G	1
Mauritania	6,300	0.52	C	1
Mauritius	500	0.08	L	1
Mozambique	1,100,000	13.22	G	2
Namibia	150,000	19.54	G	2
Niger	61,000	1.35	G	1
Nigeria	2,600,000	5.06	G	2
Rwanda	370,000	11.21	G	2
Senegal	76,000	1.77	G	3
Sierra Leone	65,000	2.99	G	1
Somalia	—	—	G	1
South Africa	4,100,000	19.94	G	3
Swaziland	120,000	25.25	G	2
Togo	120,000	5.98	G	2
Uganda	770,000	8.30	G	3
United Republic of Tanzania	1,200,000	8.09	G	3
Zambia	830,000	19.95	G	2
Zimbabwe	1,400,000	25.06	G	2

[a]Data from UNAIDS (14).
[b]L indicates low-level; C, concentrated; G, generalized.
[c]1 indicates poorly or nonfunctioning system; 2, some or most aspects of a fully implemented system; 3 fully implemented system.

TABLE 2. Adult Prevalence of HIV/AIDS, State of the Epidemic, and Quality of Surveillance System Rating by Country in North Africa

Country	Adults living with HIV/AIDS (15–49)[a]	Adult rate (%)[a]	State of epidemic[b]	Quality rating[c]
Regional total for North Africa and the Middle East	210,000	0.12	—	—
Algeria	11,000	0.07	L	1
Egypt	8,100	0.02	L	2
Libyan Arab Jamahiriya	1,400	0.05	L	1
Morocco	5,000	0.03	L	1
Sudan	140,000	0.99	G	1
Tunisia	2,200	0.04	L	1

[a]Date from UNAIDS (14).
[b]L indicates low-level; G, generalized.
[c]1 indicates poorly or nonfunctioning system; 2, some or most aspects of a fully implemented system; 3, fully implemented system.

Inconsistent data collection over time is another major weakness of surveillance systems in many countries. For example, some countries have collected data most years, but have done so in differing populations and regions, making the analysis of trends difficult.

Congo and Liberia have revamped their surveillance programs and have resumed collection of seroprevalence data. Other countries, such as Madagascar and Lesotho, which had good systems in the recent past, have discontinued data collection due to financial or other restrictions. Some countries, such as Namibia and Zambia, have chosen to collect data only every two years. While this may free funds for use in prevention and care efforts, it does limit the ability to track changes in trends in the epidemic. Finally, some of the countries whose surveillance systems received a UNAIDS quality rating of 2 (having some or most aspects of a fully implemented system) may have sufficient data to track the status and trends in the epidemic if their HIV case reporting system is of sufficient quality.

Data generated by surveillance efforts alone cannot fully explain the dynamics of the epidemic. Seroprevalence data must be analyzed by age group, and calibrated with periodically collected information from groups not regularly included in the sentinel surveillance system. In addition, behavioral data and data on sexually transmitted diseases are needed in order to discern whether observed changes in prevalence might be attributed to a successful national response, or are simply the results of the natural course of the epidemic. In concentrated epidemics, these data can also act as an early warning, guiding surveillance managers in their choice of populations or sites for future surveillance activities.

Many of the African countries most affected by HIV and AIDS have sound and functioning surveillance systems that can be gradually expanded to meet the criteria of second-generation surveillance systems. However, more must be done to establish the basics of functional surveillance systems in many other countries. Fortunately, the UNAIDS analysis suggests that most sub–Saharan African countries' current surveillance systems do produce sufficient data for estimating current HIV/ AIDS prevalence and HIV-related burden of disease.

COUNTRY-SPECIFIC ESTIMATES AND MODELS OF HIV AND AIDS: METHODS AND LIMITATIONS

In June 2000, UNAIDS and the WHO published new, country-specific estimates of HIV infections. Working with national governments and research institutions, researchers compiled and analyzed the most recent data from a number of sources, which were then used to estimate the number of men, women, and children living with HIV and AIDS at the end of 1999, as well as the number of AIDS deaths and the number of children orphaned by AIDS in each country. Similar exercises were carried out in 1995, when the WHO's Global Programme on AIDS estimated end-1994 HIV prevalence for all countries (10,11), and in 1997 by UNAIDS and the WHO. In this section, the methods and types of data used to generate the UNAIDS/WHO end-1999 estimates are discussed.

The HIV and AIDS epidemics in the eastern parts of sub–Saharan Africa started to level off in the mid-1990s after having spread at a dramatic pace since the late 1970s. In some countries of western Africa, levels of HIV have stayed relatively low for more than a decade. In southern Africa, a massive and rapid spread of HIV started only in the late 1980s and early 1990s (12). Although the HIV epidemic in southern Africa started later than that in eastern Africa, it has been explosive. For example, in Botswana, HIV prevalence among antenatal women in Francistown increased from 7% in 1991 to 42% in 1996. In KwaZulu-Natal, South Africa, HIV prevalence among antenatal women increased from no evidence of infection in 1991 to 33% in 1998.

As mentioned earlier, in developing countries with generalized epidemics, prevalence estimates are based primarily on surveillance data collected from women attending antenatal clinics. These data are then used to estimate prevalence among men, based on an assumed female-to-male ratio. Although surveillance in antenatal clinics samples only women, in most developing countries it provides the best available estimates of HIV prevalence within the general population. This is especially true for developing countries where fertility is very high and the rate of contraceptive use is low.

The UNAIDS/WHO report on the global HIV/AIDS epidemic used data from two categories of antenatal clinics, based on their location. One category included clinics located in "major urban areas" (usually the capital city and other major urban agglomerations). The other category included clinics located "outside major urban areas," defined as all other clinics in periurban or rural settings. Although imperfect, this distinction represents an attempt to take into account indications that the HIV epidemic often varies widely between rural and urban areas within a single country. Of course, variation in prevalence also occurs within major urban areas and within rural areas. However, the data are not at a level of specificity to capture this variation.

Making Adjustments for Urban–Rural Differentials to Estimate Prevalence in Countries with Generalized Epidemics

Adjustments were made to arrive at rural adult prevalence figures for both the end-1997 and end-1999 UNAIDS/WHO reports. Median prevalence values from antenatal clinics formed the basis for estimating prevalence among pregnant women in rural areas. However, because these values are usually collected in regional trading centers or towns that may have higher rates of HIV infection than that of truly rural sites, it was assumed that figures for rural areas were overestimated. For the 1997 estimates, the sentinel sites were reviewed and the estimated prevalence among women was lowered from the median value if the sites seemed not to be representative of rural areas. The adjustment factor was most often between 30% and 50%. For the end of 1999 estimates, the location of the sentinel sites, population density, and major highways were overlaid on a map for consideration. This allowed researchers to make more informed decisions about the coverage and representativeness of the rural sentinel surveillance sites and to make adjustments to median HIV prevalence among pregnant women who lived outside of major urban areas.

Establishing Female-to-Male Ratio

HIV prevalence among women in the general population is higher than that among women attending antenatal clinics, most likely due to the effects of HIV and AIDS on fertility. Thus, women who are infected are less likely to be included in a sample drawn from an antenatal clinic. Furthermore, prevalence among women attending antenatal clinics was found to be slightly higher than that among men in the general population (based on comparison with data from community-based surveys). Consequently, data from antenatal clinics that were used to set overall adult prevalence had to be adjusted to reflect the female-to-male differential. Total number of adults living with HIV/AIDS was calculated by applying the prevalence rate (in major urban areas and outside major urban areas) to the adult population (ages 15–49). Then the number of women and men infected was calculated by multiplying the total times 55% for women and 45% for men. This produced a rough 1.2 to 1 ratio of women to men living with HIV/AIDS in sub–Saharan Africa. For the end of 1997 estimates this ratio had been assumed to be 1 to 1.

Reduction in Fertility Rates for HIV-Infected Pregnant Women

Adjustments must be made to estimates of the number of children who acquire HIV from their mothers at birth or through breast-feeding to reflect the effects of HIV infection on fertility. The number of children who acquire HIV via mother-to-child transmission (MTCT) was calculated for both the end of 1997 and end of 1999 estimates by first establishing the number of women of childbearing age (15–49) who were HIV-positive, and then using regional, age-specific, fertility rates to estimate the number of children born to these infected women. A 35% rate of MTCT was assumed in the countries of sub–Saharan Africa. The one exception was South Africa, where a 30% transmission rate was used based on national data.

For the end of 1999 estimates, the estimate of children with HIV/AIDS was adjusted by reducing the overall fertility rate by 20% (13). This reduction was done not only for births in 1999, but for all years. This means that the end of 1999 estimates have reduced the number of children acquiring HIV/AIDS via MTCT, by 20% from the previous estimates.

Curve Fitting and Additional Assumptions Required to Produce Estimates of Incidence and Mortality for Adults and Children over Time

To estimate mortality and incidence, one must produce estimates of prevalence over time. For the end of 1999 report, point prevalence estimates were made for each year for which data were available. With these data and an estimated start date of the spread of HIV/AIDS, a prevalence curve was produced. Once a prevalence curve has been established, adult prevalence rates can be analyzed to produce incidence estimates, or combined with assumptions about the survival time of adults with HIV/AIDS to produce mortality estimates.

Estimates of children infected with HIV/AIDS were also made, as described earlier, based on assumptions about age-specific fertility rates and MTCT rates for countries in the region. Child mortality was calculated by applying a survival schedule to the number of children born with HIV. For countries with an under-five mortality rate above 50 per 1,000, it was assumed that 80% of children infected via MTCT would die before their fifth birthday. For countries with an under-five mortality rate below 50 per 1,000, it was assumed that 43% would die by their fifth birthday.

PROJECTION INTO THE FUTURE

Making accurate projections of the HIV/AIDS epidemic has been very difficult. Projections made in the early 1990s accounted for only half the number of infections that have now been estimated for the year 2000. The number of deaths projected to have occurred due to AIDS in sub–Saharan Africa by the year 2000 was 5 to 6 million. We now estimate that 15 million deaths have occurred in sub–Saharan Africa since the beginning of the epidemic.

The types of models that have been developed to understand the dynamics of HIV spread and to estimate the eventual magnitude of the epidemic include simple extrapolation and curve-fitting models as well as complex models that use multivariate equations to simulate the process of infection and progression of disease. The data required to use these models vary enormously.

The demographic impacts that are presented in this chapter were estimated using the iwgAIDS model, developed under the sponsorship of the Interagency Working Group (iwg) on AIDS Models and Methods of the U.S. Department of State. This model is a complex, deterministic model of the spread of HIV and the development of AIDS in a population. Given a set of user inputs, the iwgAIDS model can project the future path of an AIDS epidemic in both urban and rural sectors. Among the model's many potential outputs are age- and sex-specific seroprevalence levels, AIDS cases, AIDS deaths, and AIDS-related mortality rates.

Long-Term Demographic Impact of HIV/AIDS

AIDS increases mortality rates many times over among people aged 20 to 45 years (Figure 1). New HIV infections among adults are concentrated among those in their late teens to about age 30 to 35—ages of peak sexual activity. Because of the 10-year average incubation period between HIV infection and the onset of AIDS, and about a 1-year survival period after acquiring AIDS, deaths from AIDS are shifted into older ages and tend to occur most often in the 20- to 45-year age range. Normally, non-AIDS mortality rates for this age group are among the lowest of all age groups.

Cohort studies in Uganda have reported high levels of mortality due to AIDS in those age groups that generally have low levels of mortality. In Masaka Uganda, where 8% of

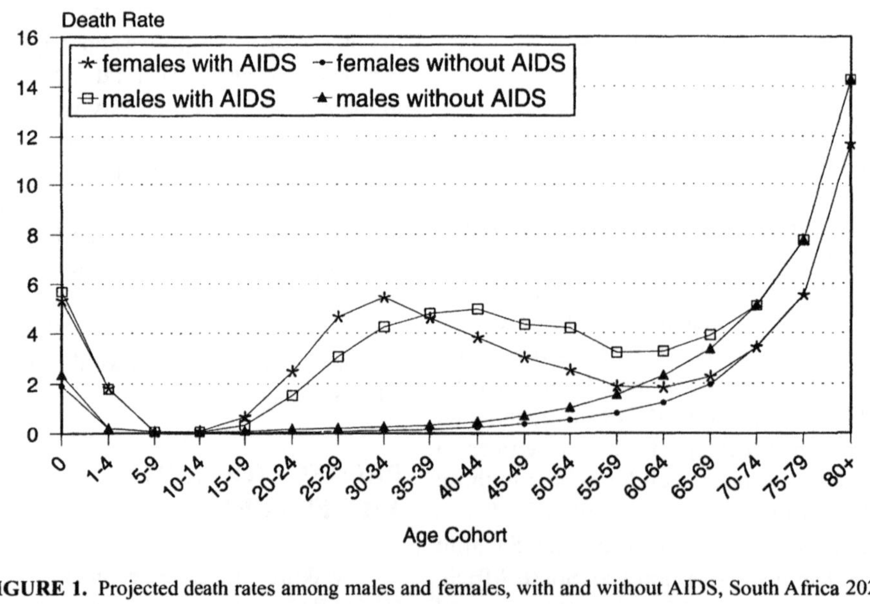

FIGURE 1. Projected death rates among males and females, with and without AIDS, South Africa 2020. Source: US Census Bureau, Global Population Profile 2000.

adults aged 13 years or older are HIV-positive, 89% of deaths of people between the ages of 25 and 34 were due to AIDS in 1989–90 (15). In Rakai District, where 21% of the adult population (15 years or older) was HIV-positive, 87% of deaths between the ages of 20 and 39 were due to AIDS in 1990–91 (16).

Mortality patterns are driven by HIV prevalence patterns. All demographic indicators will be affected by high HIV prevalence and increased mortality rates. Within the next decade, crude death rates will increase by more than 50% in some African countries and will more than double in others. Infant mortality rates and child mortality rates will be higher than they would have been without AIDS. And perhaps the most significant impact will be seen in the drop in projected life expectancies due to the increases in mortality rates among young adults. In South Africa, by 2020, mortality for adults aged 20 to 45 will be much higher than it would have been without AIDS. Mortality for women will peak between the ages of 30 and 34, earlier than the peak seen for men, which is between the ages of 40 and 44.

Population Growth Rates

As of the beginning of the 21st century, the population growth rate in Zimbabwe has been reduced to nearly zero due to AIDS mortality (Table 3A). Other southern African countries show sharply reduced growth rates: Botswana, Malawi, Namibia, South Africa, Swaziland, and Zambia.

By the year 2003, Botswana, South Africa and Zimbabwe will experience negative population growth. This negative population growth is due to high levels of HIV prevalence coupled with relatively low fertility rates in these countries. Population growth rates in these countries by 2003 will be −0.1% to −0.3% instead of 1.1% to 2.3%. By 2010, the growth rate for these countries will be approximately −1% (Table 3B). Without AIDS, growth rates in 2010 would have been between 1.0% and 2.0% in these countries. In 2010, other countries in southern Africa, including Lesotho, Malawi, Mozambique, Namibia, and Swaziland, will experience a growth rate of nearly 0, whereas without AIDS, these countries would have had a growth rate of 2% or higher.

This is the first time the U.S. Census Bureau estimates negative population growth due to AIDS in any country. Previously, HIV/AIDS experts did not expect HIV prevalence rates to reach such high national levels in any country, but by the end of 1999, adult HIV prevalence had reached an estimated 36% in Botswana, 20% in South Africa, and 25% in Zimbabwe (14).

With the exception of Botswana, South Africa, and Zimbabwe, populations in most sub–Saharan African countries will continue to increase despite the high levels of mortality. Although AIDS mortality has resulted in lower population growth rates in such countries, fertility rates remain high and population growth is still positive. The populations of Botswana, South Africa, and Zimbabwe will take a long time to rebound from the current levels of HIV prevalence and AIDS mortality, even if current AIDS control programs result in lower HIV incidence and prevalence in the future.

New Population Pyramids

AIDS mortality will produce population pyramids that have never been seen before. Particularly in those countries with projected negative population growth rates, population pyramids will have a new shape, known as "the population chimney" (Figure 2). The implications of this new population structure are not clear. By 2020, there will be more men than women between the ages of 15 and 44 in each of the 5-year age cohorts in Botswana. This phenomenon may push men to seek female partners in increasingly younger age cohorts, which may in turn increase HIV infection rates among younger women. Current evidence indicates that older

TABLE 3A. Demographic Indicators With and Without AIDS in Developing Countries: 2000

	Growth rate (%)			Life expectancy			Crude death rate (per 1,000 population)			Infant mortality rate			Child mortality (under age 5)			
Country	With AIDS	Without AIDS	Net decrease	With AIDS	Without AIDS	Net decrease	With AIDS	Without AIDS	Net increase	With AIDS	Without AIDS	Net increase	With AIDS	Without AIDS	Net increase	Total fertility
Benin	3.0	3.2	0.2	50.2	53.0	2.8	14.5	13.1	1.4	90.8	87.8	3.1	159.9	150.9	9.0	6.3
Botswana	0.8	2.5	1.8	39.3	70.5	31.2	22.8	5.4	17.4	61.7	27.6	34.1	136.0	38.9	97.1	3.8
Burkina Faso	2.7	3.2	0.5	46.7	55.5	8.8	17.0	12.8	4.3	108.5	100.4	8.2	178.3	155.7	22.6	6.4
Burundi	3.1	3.7	0.6	46.2	56.8	10.6	16.4	11.0	5.4	71.5	61.8	9.8	145.4	117.9	27.5	6.3
Cameroon	2.5	2.8	0.4	54.8	62.7	7.8	11.9	8.6	3.3	70.9	64.9	6.0	128.4	111.1	17.4	4.9
Central African Republic	1.8	2.5	0.8	44.0	58.3	14.3	18.4	11.0	7.4	106.7	94.2	12.5	168.4	133.2	35.3	5.0
Congo, Republic of the (Brazzaville)	2.2	2.8	0.5	47.4	57.3	9.9	16.4	11.2	5.2	101.6	93.1	8.4	165.5	141.5	24.0	5.1
Congo, Democratic Republic of the (Kinshasa)	3.2	3.5	0.3	48.8	54.4	5.6	15.4	12.6	2.8	101.7	96.7	5.1	153.9	139.2	14.7	6.9
Côte d'Ivoire	2.2	2.9	0.7	45.2	58.1	12.9	16.6	9.8	6.8	95.1	83.4	11.7	144.7	111.0	33.6	5.8
Ethiopia	2.8	3.4	0.6	45.2	56.1	10.9	17.6	11.8	5.9	101.3	90.8	10.5	155.6	125.8	29.8	7.1
Gabon	1.1	1.4	0.3	50.1	55.4	5.3	16.8	13.9	2.9	96.3	90.5	5.8	146.9	128.0	18.9	3.7
Ghana	1.9	2.1	0.2	57.4	61.3	3.9	10.2	8.5	1.7	57.4	53.9	3.5	103.6	91.8	11.8	4.0
Kenya	1.5	2.3	0.8	48.0	64.9	17.0	14.1	6.5	7.6	68.7	54.9	13.8	110.1	70.1	39.9	3.7
Lesotho	1.7	2.3	0.6	50.8	63.6	12.8	14.6	8.5	6.1	83.0	62.5	20.4	132.6	85.9	46.7	4.2
Malawi	1.6	2.6	1.0	37.6	53.3	15.7	22.4	12.9	9.5	122.3	105.2	17.1	219.6	175.4	44.2	5.3

Mozambique	1.5	2.4	0.9	37.5	50.3	12.7	23.3	14.4	8.9	139.9	123.1	16.8	225.5	174.9	50.5	4.9
Namibia	1.6	2.9	1.3	42.5	65.1	22.7	19.5	7.4	12.1	70.9	44.6	26.3	139.0	63.4	75.6	4.9
Nigeria	2.7	3.0	0.3	51.6	57.0	5.4	13.7	11.0	2.7	74.2	68.8	5.4	150.0	132.2	17.8	5.7
Rwanda	1.1	2.1	1.0	39.3	53.1	13.7	21.0	12.5	8.5	120.1	105.6	14.5	194.6	156.0	38.7	5.1
South Africa	0.5	1.2	0.7	51.1	65.7	14.6	14.7	7.4	7.3	58.9	41.1	17.8	119.6	65.6	54.0	2.5
Swaziland	2.0	3.1	1.1	40.4	57.7	17.2	20.4	10.3	10.1	109.0	86.1	22.9	183.2	118.4	64.9	5.9
Tanzania	2.6	3.1	0.5	52.3	64.0	11.8	12.9	7.9	5.0	81.0	71.6	9.4	127.5	101.2	26.3	5.5
Togo	2.7	3.0	0.3	54.7	62.3	7.6	11.2	8.0	3.2	71.6	65.5	6.0	128.8	110.3	18.5	5.5
Uganda	2.7	3.4	0.7	42.9	54.2	11.2	18.4	12.3	6.2	93.3	82.2	11.1	163.0	132.5	30.5	7.0
Zambia	1.9	3.2	1.2	37.2	58.9	21.7	22.1	9.7	12.4	92.4	69.6	22.8	168.8	106.5	62.3	5.6
Zimbabwe	0.3	2.2	1.9	37.8	69.9	32.1	22.4	4.9	17.5	62.3	30.0	32.3	132.8	41.3	91.6	3.3
Bahamas, The	1.0	1.3	0.3	71.1	79.7	8.7	6.8	3.8	3.0	17.0	11.8	5.2	32.5	12.5	20.0	2.3
Brazil	0.9	1.3	0.3	62.9	71.2	8.2	9.4	5.8	3.6	38.0	34.3	3.8	48.9	38.4	10.5	2.1
Guyana	−0.1	0.1	0.2	64.0	68.3	4.3	8.4	6.7	1.8	39.1	35.6	3.5	57.8	46.9	10.8	2.1
Haiti	1.4	1.8	0.4	49.2	56.5	7.3	15.1	11.6	3.5	97.1	90.8	6.3	155.0	137.8	17.1	4.5
Honduras	2.5	2.6	0.1	69.9	73.3	3.4	5.3	4.2	1.1	31.3	28.9	2.4	43.4	36.1	7.3	4.3
Burma	0.6	0.8	0.2	54.9	57.7	2.8	12.4	10.8	1.5	75.3	73.1	2.2	109.4	101.8	7.6	2.4
Cambodia	2.3	2.4	0.2	56.5	60.2	3.6	10.8	9.2	1.6	66.8	63.8	3.0	107.7	98.5	9.2	4.8
Thailand	0.9	1.0	0.1	68.6	71.2	2.6	7.5	6.4	1.1	31.5	30.2	1.2	41.9	36.8	5.1	1.9

Note: Life expectancy (e_0), infant mortality, and child mortality ($_5q_0$) are for both sexes combined.

Source: US Census Bureau, International Database 2001 and unpublished tables.

TABLE 3B. Demographic Indicators With and Without AIDS in Developing Countries: 2010

	Growth rate (%)			Life expectancy			Crude death rate (per 1,000 population)			Infant mortality rate			Child mortality (under age 5)			
Country	With AIDS	Without AIDS	Net decrease	With AIDS	Without AIDS	Net decrease	With AIDS	Without AIDS	Net increase	With AIDS	Without AIDS	Net increase	With AIDS	Without AIDS	Net increase	Total fertility
Benin	2.5	2.9	0.5	48.2	57.0	8.7	14.6	10.2	4.4	79.2	71.2	8.0	140.7	117.5	23.1	5.4
Botswana	−1.3	2.0	3.3	29.0	73.2	44.2	36.0	4.5	31.5	71.1	20.1	51.1	169.5	27.1	142.4	2.9
Burkina Faso	2.4	3.1	0.7	45.3	59.5	14.2	16.7	9.7	7.0	92.1	79.5	12.6	153.6	119.5.	34.1	5.5
Burundi	2.3	3.0	0.7	45.3	60.7	15.4	16.3	8.5	7.8	62.7	49.4	13.3	125.5	88.3	37.2	5.3
Cameroon	1.9	2.5	0.6	52.7	66.3	13.6	12.9	7.0	5.9	60.4	50.3	10.1	109.7	81.3	28.4	4.1
Central African Republic	1.4	2.3	0.9	42.8	62.2	19.4	19.0	9.0	10.0	91.5	74.8	16.6	149.8	103.5	46.3	4.1
Congo, Republic of the (Brazzaville)	1.9	2.5	0.6	48.4	61.2	12.8	15.3	8.8	6.5	83.1	72.8	10.3	135.6	107.1	28.6	4.4
Congo, Democratic Republic of the (Kinshasa)	2.9	3.2	0.3	50.7	58.4	7.7	13.4	9.8	3.6	83.2	76.7	6.5	126.3	107.8	18.6	6.1
Cote d'Ivoire	1.9	2.8	0.9	43.4	62.0	18.5	17.5	7.8	9.6	80.0	63.9	16.1	129.1	83.5	45.5	4.8
Ethiopia	2.3	3.3	1.0	42.1	60.1	17.9	18.7	9.2	9.4	87.8	70.8	16.9	142.6	96.0	46.6	6.4
Gabon	0.5	1.3	0.8	45.7	59.4	13.7	20.5	12.5	8.0	83.0	71.0	12.0	132.5	98.1	34.4	3.3
Ghana	1.1	1.6	0.4	55.5	65.0	9.5	11.5	7.1	4.4	48.9	42.1	6.8	88.0	67.6	20.4	2.8
Kenya	0.4	1.6	1.2	44.3	68.4	24.0	17.9	5.4	12.5	60.4	40.6	19.8	107.4	50.9	56.5	2.4
Lesotho	0.2	2.0	1.8	37.7	67.2	29.5	24.6	7.0	17.6	79.9	46.7	33.3	144.6	62.3	82.3	3.5
Malawi	0.8	2.1	1.4	35.8	57.3	21.5	24.1	10.2	14.0	110.0	85.3	24.7	202.6	137.3	65.3	3.9
Mozambique	0.1	2.0	1.9	31.4	54.2	22.9	29.9	11.7	18.2	131.8	100.5	31.3	225.3	140.4	85.0	3.9

Namibia	0.2	2.7	2.4	32.7	68.5	35.8	28.6	5.7	22.9	76.1	32.8	43.3	165.0	44.8	120.3	4.3
Nigeria	2.0	2.7	0.7	47.0	60.9	13.9	15.9	8.7	7.2	66.1	54.6	11.5	131.2	98.3	32.9	4.8
Rwanda	0.4	1.8	1.4	36.4	57.1	20.6	24.1	9.9	14.2	107.6	84.8	22.8	183.3	122.3	61.1	3.5
South Africa	−1.3	1.0	2.3	35.5	68.3	32.8	30.3	7.1	23.2	67.4	31.6	35.7	146.6	47.6	98.9	2.1
Swaziland	0.5	3.0	2.5	29.7	61.5	31.8	31.7	8.3	23.4	108.5	66.4	42.1	204.2	89.3	114.9	5.4
Tanzania	2.1	2.9	0.7	50.5	67.5	17.0	13.4	6.1	7.4	65.8	53.0	12.7	108.9	72.6	36.3	4.6
Togo	1.7	2.3	0.7	50.9	66.0	15.0	12.8	6.1	6.6	61.1	50.0	11.1	111.5	79.4	32.1	3.8
Uganda	3.0	3.5	0.5	46.6	58.2	11.6	15.1	9.5	5.6	75.4	65.5	9.9	129.7	101.6	28.1	6.1
Zambia	1.7	2.8	1.2	38.9	62.8	23.9	20.5	7.6	13.0	77.9	54.3	23.7	145.7	79.9	65.8	4.7
Zimbabwe	−0.9	1.9	2.7	32.5	72.8	40.3	31.6	4.4	27.1	65.9	21.8	44.1	153.0	28.8	124.2	2.6
Bahamas	0.4	0.9	0.6	66.3	81.0	14.6	10.2	4.5	5.7	17.4	9.1	8.4	34.2	9.6	24.6	2.1
Brazil	0.6	0.9	0.3	66.3	73.8	7.6	9.1	6.0	3.1	27.8	23.9	3.9	37.5	26.7	10.7	1.8
Guyana	0.4	1.1	0.7	57.0	71.4	14.4	13.5	6.4	7.1	35.9	25.7	10.3	63.3	32.9	30.5	2.0
Haiti	1.5	1.9	0.4	51.5	60.4	8.9	13.9	9.6	4.3	78.7	72.2	6.4	124.7	106.3	18.4	3.5
Honduras	1.6	2.0	0.4	63.6	75.7	12.1	8.0	3.8	4.2	27.8	20.4	7.4	47.2	25.0	22.2	3.2
Burma	0.3	0.5	0.2	57.7	61.6	4.0	12.0	9.8	2.2	59.7	56.4	3.3	86.6	76.6	10.0	1.9
Cambodia	2.1	2.3	0.2	59.8	64.0	4.2	9.5	7.7	1.8	53.0	49.4	3.5	88.5	73.2	10.4	4.0
Thailand	0.6	0.7	0.1	71.7	73.8	2.1	7.8	6.9	0.9	22.2	21.3	0.9	29.3	25.5	3.8	1.8

Note: Life expectancy (e_0), infant mortality, and child mortality (5q0) are for both sexes combined.

Source: US Census Bureau, International Database 2001 and unpublished tables.

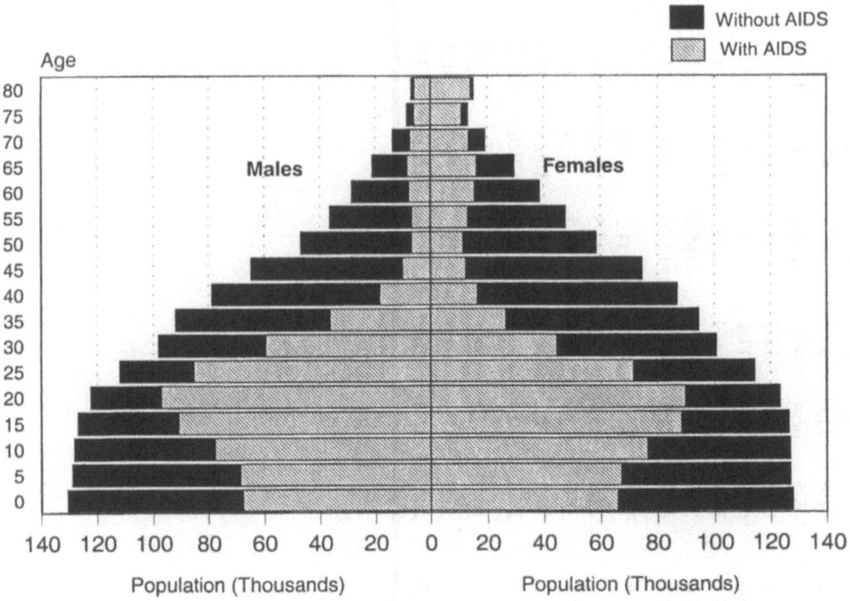

FIGURE 2. Population of Botswana: pyramid projections with and without AIDS by the year 2020. Source: US Census Bureau, Global Population Profile 2000.

men are infecting younger women, who then go on to infect their partners, particularly through marriage (8). This vicious cycle could result in even higher HIV infection levels.

In countries with moderate epidemics, AIDS mortality will have less of an effect on the population structure. For example, in Uganda, the greatest relative differences in future population size by cohort are evident in the youngest age groups and in those 30 to 50 years of age. However, the population pyramid continues to maintain its traditional shape.

Life Expectancy

AIDS mortality is resulting in falling life expectancies. Already, life expectancies in many countries in sub-Saharan Africa have dropped from the number of years they would have been without AIDS. For example, in Botswana, life expectancy is now 39 instead of 71 and in Zimbabwe, 38 instead of 70. In fact, six countries in sub-Saharan Africa—Botswana, Malawi, Mozambique, Rwanda, Zambia, and Zimbabwe—now have life expectancies below 40 years of age. Without AIDS, these figures would have been 50 years or greater.

By 2010, many countries in southern Africa will see life expectancies fall to approximately 30 years of age, a figure not seen since the beginning of the 20th century. By 2010, in this region that could have anticipated life expectancies to reach 70 years of age, many countries will see life expectancies reduced by about 40 years to the following rates: in Botswana, 29; in Namibia, 33; in Swaziland, 30; and in Zimbabwe, 33. Many other countries will see life expectancies drop from 50–60 years to 30–40 years of age.

Mortality

The most direct impact of AIDS is an increase in the number of deaths in the populations affected. Crude death rates, the number of people dying per 1,000 in the population, have already been affected by AIDS.

Seven countries in sub-Saharan Africa now have an estimated adult HIV prevalence of approximately 20% or greater: Botswana,

Lesotho, Namibia, South Africa, Swaziland, Zambia, and Zimbabwe (14). An additional nine countries have adult HIV prevalence levels higher than 10%. In many of these countries, reports indicate that HIV has been present since the early 1980s.

As a result of these long-term, high levels of HIV infection, estimated crude death rates including AIDS mortality rates in eastern and southern Africa are greater by 50% to 500% compared to what they would have been without AIDS. For example, in Kenya where adult HIV prevalence was estimated to be 14% at the end of 1999, crude death rates are estimated to be double (14.1) the level they would have been without AIDS (6.5). In South Africa, where adult HIV prevalence is estimated to be 20%, crude death rates are also doubled due to AIDS (14.7 compared to 7.4).

In many sub–Saharan African countries, crude death rates will be even higher in 2010 than in 2000, even though mortality due to non-AIDS causes will continue to decline. In Botswana, crude death rates will increase from 22.8 in 2000 to 36.0 in 2010. In South Africa, crude death rates will increase from 14.7 to 30.3, and in Zimbabwe from 22.4 to 31.6. In all three of these countries, crude death rates would have been between 5 and 7 without AIDS.

In some sub-Saharan African countries, infant mortality rates are now higher than they were in 1990 (U.S. Census Bureau, International Database and unpublished tables, 2001). AIDS mortality has reversed the direction of the declines that had been occurring in mortality rates during the 1980s and early 1990s. Over 30% of all children born to HIV-infected mothers in sub–Saharan Africa will become infected either through the birth process or due to breastfeeding. The relative impact of AIDS on infant mortality will depend on both the levels of HIV prevalence in the population and the infant mortality rates from other causes. In 1990, infant mortality in Zimbabwe was 54; in 2000 it was 62. In Kenya, infant mortality in 1990 was 67, while in 2000 it was 69. Without AIDS, infant mortality in Zimbabwe would have been 30 and in Kenya it would have been 55.

In countries with less severe epidemics, such as those in western and central Africa, infant mortality rates are still higher than they would have been without AIDS. The increase ranges from 3% in Benin to 12% in Côte d'Ivoire and 15% in Rwanda.

In four countries of sub–Saharan Africa (Botswana, Zimbabwe, South Africa, and Namibia), more infants will die from AIDS in 2010 than from all other causes. In Botswana and Zimbabwe, twice as many infants will die from AIDS than from all other causes. Although overall infant mortality rates are projected to decline between 2000 and 2010, infant mortality due to AIDS is projected to increase.

The impact on child mortality is highest among those countries which had significantly reduced child mortality due to other causes but have high levels of HIV prevalence. In 26 sub–Saharan African countries, child mortality rates have increased due to AIDS. Many HIV-infected children survive their first birthdays, only to die before the age of 5. In Zimbabwe, 70% of all deaths among children under the age of 5 are due to AIDS, and in South Africa, that percentage is 45.

In Zimbabwe and Botswana, where child mortality rates may have been below 30 without AIDS, over 150 children per 1,000 will die. Of that total, 80% will be due to AIDS. In many of the countries in southern Africa, over 50% of childhood deaths will be due to AIDS. In Malawi and Mozambique, where child mortality rates due to other causes are already high, AIDS mortality will increase those rates by 30%.

CONCLUSION

At the beginning of the 21st Century, AIDS is the number one cause of death in Africa and the 4th cause globally (17). Because the HIV epidemic emerged just 20 years ago, few would have predicted its current magnitude, particularly in sub–Saharan Africa. It was unthinkable that 25% of adults in any country would be living with HIV. Yet, this is the situation in four countries. Given the current rates, many more millions will die of AIDS over the next decade than have already died of AIDS in the past 2 decades. Many southern African countries are only beginning to see the impacts of their high levels of HIV prevalence.

Nevertheless, there have been success stories in countries such as Thailand, Senegal, and Uganda. In Thailand and Uganda, concerted efforts by members of all levels of society have turned around increasing HIV prevalence rates. In Senegal, programs put into place early in the epidemic have kept HIV prevalence rates low. These successes can and must be repeated. However, the current burden of disease, death, and orphanhood will be a significant problem in many countries of sub–Saharan Africa in the near future.

ACKNOWLEDGEMENTS. We would like to express our appreciation for the national HIV/AIDS programs in countries that have made their data available. We would also like to acknowledge the work of the regional and national program offices of the WHO, and the UNAIDS country program advisors for their work in compiling HIV and AIDS surveillance data.

REFERENCES

1. World Health Organization. *Protocol for the evaluation of epidemiological surveillance systems.* WHO/EMC/DIS/97.2. Geneva: World Health Organization; 1997.
2. World Health Organization. *Sentinel surveillance for HIV infection.* WHO/GPA/DIR/88.8. Geneva: World Health Organization; 1988.
3. WHO/UNAIDS. *Guidelines for Second Generation HIV Surveillance.* Geneva: World Health Organization and the Joint United Nations Programme on HIV/AIDS; 2000.
4. Chin J. Public health surveillance of AIDS and HIV infections. *Bulletin of the World Health Organization*, 1990;68:529–536.
5. Schwartländer B, Stanecki KA, Brown T, et al. Country-specific estimates and models of HIV and AIDS: methods and limitations. *AIDS*, 1999;13:2445–2458.
6. United States Bureau of the Census, Population Division, International Programs Center. HIV/AIDS surveillance data base. Washington, DC: June 2000.
7. Fylkesnes K, Ndhlovu Z, Kasumba K, et al. Studying dynamics of the HIV epidemic: population-based data compared with sentinel surveillance in Zambia. *AIDS*, 1998;12:1227–1234.
8. Buve A, Musonda RM, Carael M, et al. Multicentre Study on Factors Determining the Differential Spread of HIV in 4 African Towns. Paper presented at: Late Breaker Session of the XI International Conference on AIDS and STDs in Africa; September 12–16, 1999; Lusaka, Zambia.
9. Walker N, Garcia-Calleja JM, Heaton L, et al. Epidemiological analysis of the quality of HIV sero-surveillance in the world: how well do we track the epidemic? *AIDS*, 2001;15:1545–1554.
10. Burton AH, Mertens TE. Provisional country estimates of prevalent adult human immunodeficiency virus infections as of the end of 1994: a description of the methods. *International Journal of Epidemiology*, 1998;27:101–107.
11. World Health Organization. Provisional working estimates of adult HIV prevalence as of the end of 1994, by country. *Weekly Epidemiological Record*, 1995;70:355–357.
12. Tarantola D, Schwartländer B. HIV/AIDS epidemics in sub-Saharan Africa: dynamism, diversity and discrete declines? *AIDS*, 1997;11(suppl B): S5–S21.
13. Gray RH, Wawer MJ, Serwadda D, et al. Population-based study of fertility in women with HIV-1 infection in Uganda. *The Lancet*, 1998;351:98–103.
14. UNAIDS. *Report on the global HIV/AIDS epidemic, June 2000.* UNAIDS/00.13E, Geneva: United Nations Joint Programme on HIV/AIDS; 2000.
15. Mulder DW, Nunn AJ, Wagner HU, et al. HIV-1 Incidence and HIV-1 Associated Mortality in Rural Ugandan Population Cohort. *AIDS*, 1994;8:87–92.
16. Sewankambo NK, Wawer MJ, Gray RH, et al. Demographic Impact of HIV Infection in Rural Rakai District, Uganda: Results of a Population-Based Cohort Study. *AIDS*, 1994;8:1707–1713.
17. The World Health Organization. *The World Health Report 1999, Making a Difference.* 99/12368-SADAG-2000. France: The World Health Organization; 1999.

18

Clinical Diagnosis of AIDS and HIV-Related Diseases

Churchill Lukwiya Onen

Department of Medicine, Princess Marina Hospital, Gaborone, Botswana.

Nowhere in the world is the problem of HIV/AIDS worse than it is in sub–Saharan Africa. Virtually every practicing doctor on the continent will be required to become familiar with the diagnosis of HIV and AIDS as well as the work-up, management, and specific treatment of HIV-related disorders. HIV-infected individuals are presenting in increasing numbers to all cadres of health care professionals with clinical problems that may be directly or indirectly related to their HIV infection. UNAIDS and the World Health Organization's (WHO) recent estimates of people living with HIV or AIDS in 1999 and the first quarter of 2000 indicate that HIV prevalence has reached a plateau among some sentinel populations such as blood donors, pregnant women, and sexually transmitted disease (STD) clinic attendees (1), but this plateau does not signal the beginning of the end of the pandemic. Rather, it may indicate that a state of equilibrium has been attained between the number of new infections and the number of infected individuals who are dropping out of sentinel pools because of severe illness, infertility, or death (2).

This chapter discusses the clinical diagnosis of AIDS and HIV-related diseases in Africa. Weaknesses and strengths of current case definitions for AIDS and proposed modifications of certain criteria are highlighted. The chapter is by no means exhaustive, but rather attempts to emphasize problems likely to confront the clinician working in Africa.

PRIMARY HIV INFECTION

Little is known about the prevalence of acute primary HIV infection in different African population groups. Among patients, this may be in part due to delayed health-seeking behavior, and among physicians, due to underdiagnosis. Underdiagnosis may result from lack of clinical suspicion and lack of facilities, underreporting, and failure to differentiate the symptoms of acute HIV syndrome from a myriad of other conditions commonly seen in tropical and subtropical Africa. Individuals who experience acute HIV syndrome following primary infection manifest acute mononucleosis-like illness characterized by lethargy, anorexia, sweating, fever, malaise, headache, myalgia, arthralgia, sore throat, diarrhea, generalized lymphadenopathy, macular eruption involving the trunk and arms, and thrombocytopenia. Occasionally patients develop hepatomegaly, splenomegaly, oral candidiasis, pruritus, transitory asceptic meningoencephalitis, mononeuritis, or polyneuritis. The acute illness occurs within 3 months (usually within 10 to 30 days after exposure to

HIV) and resolves within 3 to 21 days (3). These symptoms are well correlated with the presence of viremia, which contributes to virus dissemination. Some individuals remain asymptomatic at this stage or, during later stages of their illness, do not recall experiencing acute symptoms.

DISEASE PROGRESSION

Acute HIV syndrome is followed by a stage of clinical latency. This does not mean disease latency; HIV infection generally progresses steadily during this asymptomatic period, except in very few persons with primary or acquired resistance to HIV infection or in those given postexposure prophylaxis. Several mechanisms of HIV's immune evasion have been proposed. These include its high rate of mutation, direct damage of HIV-specific T-cells resulting in early loss and functional defects of $CD4^+$ lymphocytes, inhibition of antigen presentation by HIV-infected cells, and qualitative abnormalities in anti-HIV $CD8^+$ T-cell response. However, in some individuals, the virus may be either less virulent or it may mutate to less aggressive forms. In such individuals, quantitative and qualitative aspects of their HIV-specific immune response, in addition to unrecognized genetic factors, may also contribute to their long-term nonprogression or acquired immunity to HIV (4). In general, HIV-resistant individuals and long-term nonprogressors manifest robust HIV-specific humoral (neutralizing antibodies) and cell-mediated (HIV-specific cytolytic T-lymphocytes) immune responses (5,6).

The diagnosis of early infection depends on the demonstration of antibodies to HIV, which generally appear in the circulation 4 to 8 weeks after infection. The standard screening test for HIV-1 and HIV-2 is the enzyme-linked immunosorbent assay (ELISA) (see Chapter 7, *this volume*). The natural history of HIV infection in sub–Saharan Africa is not well understood, partly because it is not always possible to establish the exact timing of infection.

The clinical consequences of HIV infection progress in stages from the acute syndrome associated with primary infection, to an asymptomatic period, to advanced disease. Much of the understanding of HIV-1 disease progression is derived from studies in the developed world where HIV-1 infection is almost exclusively due to subtype B. It is questionable whether the properties and consequences of HIV-1 infection observed in such studies can be generalized across the multiple subtypes that cocirculate in sub–Saharan Africa. A prospective study by Kanki et al. (7) that tracked the introduction and spread of HIV-1 subtypes A, C, D, and G among female sex workers from 1985 to 1997, showed that women infected with non-A subtypes were eight times more likely to develop AIDS than those who were infected with subtype A. These data suggested that infection with different HIV-1 subtypes results in different rates of progression to AIDS. People infected with HIV-2, as well as those with dual HIV-1 and HIV-2 infections, manifest a spectrum of AIDS-associated symptoms and signs that are not appreciably dissimilar to those in HIV-1–infected patients (8,9). However, HIV-2 appears to have reduced pathogenicity.

Some experts believe that in Africa, time from seroconversion to the development of AIDS may be shorter than that among HIV-infected individuals in industrialized countries (10,11). Furthermore, a decade ago, one study in Kinshasa, Zaire (now Democratic Republic of Congo), showed that the rate of progression to CDC-defined AIDS among recipients of HIV-contaminated blood transfusions was 6% after 1 year of follow-up (12). An earlier study by N'Galy et al. in the same country showed that within 2 years of seroconversion, 16% of 101 asymptomatic HIV-infected persons had developed symptomatic HIV disease, 3% had AIDS, and 12% had died (13). A more definitive study of a cohort of prostitutes in Nairobi revealed that the median time from seroconversion to the occurrence of symptomatic HIV disease and AIDS was 34.2 months, and 44.6 months, respectively (14).

CLASSIFICATION SYSTEMS FOR SURVEILLANCE AND CLINICAL STAGING

The Centers for Disease Control and Prevention's Surveillance Case Definition of AIDS

AIDS was originally defined by the Centers for Disease Control and Prevention (CDC) for the purpose of surveillance as follows: the presence of a reliably diagnosed "opportunistic" disease that is at least moderately predictive of an underlying defect in cell-mediated immunity in the absence of known causes of immune defects such as immunosuppressive therapy or malignancies (15). This definition, created prior to the identification of HIV as the etiologic agent of AIDS, has undergone several revisions based on the identification of HIV as the causative agent and also due to the advent of sensitive and specific diagnostic tests.

The latest revision took place in 1993 when the CDC put forth its revised HIV classification system and expanded its surveillance case definition for AIDS (Table 1). The revised HIV classification system for adolescents

TABLE 1. The Centers for Disease Control and Prevention's Revised HIV Classification System for Adolescents (aged at least 13 years) and Adults

	Clinical categories		
$CD4^+$ T-cell categories	A[a]	B[b]	C[c]
	Asymptomatic HIV infection, acute HIV infection with accompanying illness or history of acute HIV infection, or PGL	Symptomatic, not A or C conditions	AIDS-indicator conditions
1 >500/mm³	A1	B1	C1
2 200–499/mm³	A2	B2	C2
3[d] <200/mm³	A3	B3	C3

[a]Patients with documented HIV infection and one or more of the conditions listed in this column. The conditions listed for categories B and C must not have occurred. PGL indicates persistent generalized lymphadenopathy.

[b]HIV-infected patients presenting with symptomatic conditions that are not those listed for category C, and that meet at least one of the following criteria: (1) the conditions are attributed to HIV infection or are indicative of a defect in cell-mediated immunity; or (2) the conditions are considered by physicians to have a clinical course or require management that is complicated by HIV infection. Examples include, but are not limited to, the following: Bacillary angiomatosis; Candidiasis, oropharyngeal (thrush); Candidiasis, vulvovaginal, persistent, frequent or poorly responsive to therapy; Cervical dysplasia (moderate to severe)/cervical carcinoma in-situ; Constitutional symptoms, such as fever (38.5°C) or diarrhea lasting longer than 1 month; Hairy leukoplakia, oral; Herpes zoster (shingles), involving at least two distinct episodes or more than one dermatome; Idiopathic thrombocytopenic purpura; Listeriosis; Pelvic inflammatory disease, particularly complicated by tubo-ovarian abscess; Peripheral neuropathy.

[c]HIV-infected patients presenting with conditions listed in the AIDS surveillance case definition, including: Candidiasis of bronchi, trachea, or lungs; Candidiasis, esophageal; Cervical cancer, invasive; Coccidioidomycosis, disseminated or extrapulmonary; Cryptococcosis, extrapulmonary; Cryptosporidiosis, chronic intestinal (>1 month); Cytomegalovirus retinitis (with loss of vision); Encephalopathy, HIV-related; Herpes simplex: chronic ulcers, (>1 month), or bronchitis, pneumonia, or esophagitis; Histoplasmosis, disseminated or extrapulmonary; Isosporiasis, chronic intestinal (>1 month); Kaposi's sarcoma; Lymphoma, Burkitt or equivalent term; Lymphoma, primary, of brain; *Mycobacterium avium* complex, or *M. kansasii*, disseminated or extrapulmonary; *M. tuberculosis*, any site (pulmonary or extrapulmonary); *Mycobacterium*, other species or unidentified species, disseminated or extrapulmonary; *Pneumocystis carinii* pneumonia (PCP); Pneumonia (recurrent); Progressive multifocal leukoencephalopathy (PML); Salmonella septicemia, recurrent; Toxoplasmosis of brain; Wasting Syndrome.

[d]In the revised HIV classification system, individuals with $CD4^+$ T-cell counts <200/mm³ have AIDS by definition, regardless of the presence of symptoms or opportunistic diseases.

(aged at least 13 years) and adults identifies nine mutually exclusive subcategories of clinical conditions associated with HIV infection and $CD4^+$ T-lymphocyte counts. According to this classification system, any HIV-infected individual with a $CD4^+$ T-cell count $<200/mm^3$ has AIDS by definition, regardless of the presence of symptoms or opportunistic diseases. Individuals in subcategories A3, B3, and C3 thus meet the immunologic criteria of the surveillance AIDS case definition, and those in subcategories C1, C2, and C3 meet the clinical criteria for surveillance purposes. The clinical AIDS-indicator conditions in category C now include pulmonary tuberculosis (TB), recurrent bacterial pneumonia, and, in women, invasive cervical cancer (16). Once individuals have a clinical condition in category B or C, their disease cannot again be reclassified from category B to A or from C to B even if the condition resolves.

The CDC case definition for AIDS is complex, comprehensive, and universally standardized. Because this AIDS case definition was established for surveillance purposes, and not for the practical care of patients, some of the conditions listed in the CDC case definition (category C) are very rare or virtually impossible to diagnose in many parts of sub–Saharan Africa. The clinician working in Africa, faced with gross limitations to the application of this elaborate case definition, should view the spectrum of HIV disease to range from primary infection with or without the acute syndrome, to the asymptomatic stage, to advanced disease associated with protean manifestations and conditions, some of which cannot be reliably diagnosed in many settings in sub–Saharan Africa.

The WHO AIDS Case Definitions

Because of the inherent limitations of AIDS case definitions that rely on advanced diagnostic facilities for application in developing countries, the WHO held a workshop in Bangui, Central African Republic in October 1985 to create an African AIDS case definition for surveillance purposes. This case definition relies on clinical criteria without the need for serologic verification (17) (Table 2). In the absence of known causes of immunosuppression such as cancer, severe malnutrition, or other recognized etiologies, the WHO/Bangui case definition requires the existence of two major signs and one minor of AIDS, or the existence of generalized Kaposi's sarcoma (KS) or cryptococcal meningitis (two conditions considered AIDS-defining in themselves).

TABLE 2. The World Health Organization/Bangui AIDS Case Definition

Two or more major signs:	AND	One or more minor signs	OR	Sufficient for an AIDS diagnosis in themselves
• Weight loss of >10% of body weight • Chronic diarrhea lasting longer than 1 month • Prolonged fever (constant or intermittent) lasting longer than 1 month		• Persistent cough lasting longer than 1 month • Generalized pruritic dermatitis • Recurrent herpes zoster • Oropharyngeal candidiasis • Chronic progressive and disseminated herpes simplex infection • Generalized lymphadenopathy		• Disseminated Kaposi's sarcoma • Cryptococcal meningitis

The WHO/Bangui clinical case definition has been widely used in many African countries. Certain countries modified the case definition to suit local circumstances, and many now accept or encourage a positive HIV test as supportive evidence. Some researchers have criticized the WHO/Bangui case definition because of its low sensitivity (52% to 59%) and positive predictive value (50% to 74%), despite its high specificity (78% to 90%) (18–23). Its performance is poor in low seroprevalence groups (below 20%), such as among pediatric patients. Sensitivity in such groups ranges from 35% to 41% and positive predictive values from 25% to 48% (24–26). However, there appears to be a good concordance between the WHO/Bangui case definition and the CDC system (27).

Capabilities for monitoring HIV and AIDS in Africa have progressed tremendously since the WHO/Bangui case definition was first proposed. High quality serologic testing is now available to an extent that was not anticipated fifteen years ago. Much more is now known about the pandemic and its clinical consequences. Some experts have rightly questioned the logic in persisting with a provisional surveillance definition for AIDS that is imprecise and outdated (18,21,28). Authorities like De Cock and others (18) suggested modifying the WHO/Bangui case definition of AIDS in individuals aged 12 years and older to classify AIDS cases if the following conditions were met: (i) the CDC surveillance case definition for AIDS was fulfilled, or (ii) a test for HIV was positive, and (iii) one or more of the following were present: >10% body-weight loss or cachexia, with diarrhea or fever or both (intermittent or constant) for at least one month, not known to be due to a condition unrelated to HIV infection; TB with symptoms listed above or disseminated TB (involving at least two different organs), or miliary or extrapulmonary TB (which may be presumptively diagnosed); KS; neurologic impairment sufficient to prevent independent daily activities, not known to be due to a condition unrelated to HIV infection (for example trauma or hypertension). These proposed changes were widely incorporated into the WHO/Bangui case definition and gained extensive clinical application in many centers in Africa.

In 1994, the expanded WHO AIDS case definition for AIDS surveillance was developed. Greenberg et al. compared the 1985 WHO/Bangui clinical case definition with the 1994 expanded WHO case definition (29). Their study, which took place from March 1994 to December 1996, involved 8,648 patients in three university hospitals in Abidjan and 18,661 patients with TB in eight TB centers in Côte d'Ivoire. The following points emerged: (i) the inclusion of multiple, severe HIV-related illnesses in the expanded definition increased the number of reportable AIDS cases in HIV-seropositive patients by 31.3% in the university hospitals and 217% in the TB centers; (ii) the inclusion of HIV seropositivity as a criterion for the expanded definition enhanced the specificity of AIDS case reporting, eliminating 14.7% of cases in the university hospitals and 14.0% of cases in the TB centers in which HIV-seronegative patients had clinical signs consistent with AIDS; and (iii) based on these observations, the investigators recommended the use of the 1994 expanded definition for surveillance purposes in areas of the developing world where HIV serologic testing is available.

In the absence of diagnostic facilities, some doctors use the WHO/Bangui AIDS case definition for clinical diagnosis without relying on HIV antibody testing. Some investigators have found this approach disturbing, as the probability that a patient who fulfills the WHO clinical case definition criteria tests positive for HIV may fall well below 50% in populations with low seroprevalence (28).

It is important to distinguish between the symptoms that define AIDS and those that are not AIDS-defining in patients who are positive for HIV antibody. For instance, a middle-aged person with hypertension could present with a literalizing neurologic deficit and positive test for HIV antibody. In this case, the diagnoses could include thrombotic stroke, cerebral hemorrhage, toxoplasmosis, tuberculoma, meningovascular syphilis, brain abscess, or primary lymphoma of the central nervous system (CNS). Persistent diarrhea with weight loss can be associated with opportunistic as well as endemic parasitic or bacterial infections. Such difficulties are clearly amplified in settings where morbidity not associated with AIDS—caused by nonopportunistic conditions such as gastroenteritis, bacterial pneumonia, TB, or endemic KS—is common in HIV-uninfected individuals.

Tuberculosis may be the most important opportunistic infection related to HIV infection in Africa. Many patients with pulmonary or extrapulmonary TB, irrespective of their HIV status, have weight loss, fever, and lymphadenopathy and might therefore fulfill the WHO/Bangui clinical case definition for AIDS. Unless the results of an HIV test are known, such patients with TB might be reported as AIDS cases even if they are not HIV-infected. Abandoning the clinical case definition may reduce the undue emphasis currently being placed on opportunistic infections that can lead to the exclusion of other HIV-associated problems. Also, without recourse to HIV serology, it can be difficult to determine whether chronic diseases like diabetes mellitus, chronic renal failure, or underlying non-HIV-associated malignancies are AIDS-defining.

Staging HIV Disease

In developed countries, two classification systems for staging HIV disease are the CDC classification system (Table 3) and the Walter Reed Medical Center system (30); the latter is not used very often presently. The WHO clinical staging system is better suited for use in developing countries than the CDC or Walter Reed systems. Clinical staging systems, established to improve the clinical care and management of patients, are to be distinguished from the case definitions for AIDS, which are used for surveillance purposes. Each classification system has its advantages and disadvantages.

TABLE 3. CDC Classification System

Group	Clinical stage
I	Acute HIV syndrome
II	Asymptomatic infection
III	Persistent generalized lymphadenopathy
IV	Other diseases
-Subgroup A	Constitutional symptoms
-Subgroup B	Neurologic disease
-Subgroup C	Secondary infectious diseases
-Subgroup D	Secondary neoplasms
-Subgroup E	Other conditions

Source: Modified from the Centers for Disease Control and Prevention, USPHS, 1986, and 1987.

The CDC classification system relies heavily on clinical conditions, and is quite comprehensive. However, many of the conditions included in the CDC classification system cannot be reliably diagnosed in most health facilities in sub–Saharan Africa. For instance, the use of any complex criteria requiring brain imaging or brain biopsy, such as those used for the diagnosis of CNS toxoplasmosis or primary lymphoma, is impractical in this setting. Also, in most African countries, facilities to diagnose extrapulmonary TB are often limited; extrapulmonary TB is often diagnosed solely on clinical grounds without laboratory confirmation.

The main disadvantage of the Walter Reed system for use in developing countries is its inclusion of markers of immunologic status, such as $CD4^+$ T-cell counts and the presence or absence of delayed-type cutaneous hypersensitivity.

The WHO clinical staging system for HIV infection and disease (Table 4) closely mirrors the CDC classification system in terms of its spectrum. However, it is better

TABLE 4. WHO Clinical Staging System for HIV Infection and Disease

Clinical stage I: Asymptomatic
1. Asymptomatic/acute HIV infection
2. Persistent generalized lymphadenopathy (PGL)
3. History of acute HIV infection

And/or performance scale 1: asymptomatic, normal activity

Clinical stage II: Early (mild) disease
4. Weight loss, <10% of body weight
5. Minor mucocutaneous manifestations (seborrheic dermatitis, prurigo, fungal nail infections, recurrent oral ulcerations, angular cheilitis)
6. Herpes zoster within the last 5 years
7. Recurrent respiratory tract infections (e.g. bacterial sinusitis)

And/or performance scale 2: symptomatic, normal activity

Clinical stage III: Intermediate (moderate) disease
8. Weight loss, >10% of body weight
9. Unexplained chronic diarrhea, >1 month
10. Unexplained prolonged fever (intermittent or constant), >1 month
11. Oral candidiasis (thrush)
12. Oral hairy leukoplakia
13. Pulmonary tuberculosis within the past year
14. Severe bacterial infections (e.g. pneumonia, pyomyositis)

And/or performance scale 3: bedridden <50% of the daytime during the last month

Clinical stage IV: Late (severe) disease, AIDS
15. HIV wasting syndrome, as defined by CDC[a]
16. *Pneumocystis carinii* pneumonia
17. Toxoplasmosis of the brain
18. Cryptosporidiosis with diarrhea, >1 month
19. Isosporiasis with diarrhea, >1 month
20. Cryptococcosis, extrapulmonary
21. Cytomegalovirus (CMV) disease of an organ other than the liver, spleen, or lymph nodes
22. Herpes simplex virus (HSV) infection; mucocutaneous, >1 month, or visceral, any duration
23. Progressive multifocal leukoencephalopathy (PML)
24. Any disseminated endemic mycosis (e.g. histoplasmosis, coccidioidomycosis)
25. Candidiasis of the esophagus, trachea, bronchi, or lungs
26. Atypical mycobacteriosis, disseminated
27. Nontyphoidal salmonella septicaemia
28. Extrapulmonary tuberculosis
29. Lymphoma
30. Kaposi's sarcoma (KS)
31. HIV encephalopathy, as defined by CDC[b]

And/or performance scale 4: bedridden >50% of the daytime during the last month

Note: Both definitive and presumptive diagnoses are acceptable.

[a]HIV wasting syndrome: weight loss of >10% of body weight, plus either unexplained chronic diarrhea (>1 month) or chronic weakness and unexplained prolonged fever (>1 month).

[b]HIV encephalopathy: clinical findings of disabling cognitive and/or motor dysfunction interfering with activities of daily living, progressive over weeks to months, in the absence of a concurrent illness or condition other than HIV infection that could explain the findings.

tailored to the needs of developing countries because of its provision of both definitive and presumptive diagnoses of HIV-associated opportunistic diseases and conditions. Additionally, its use of a performance scoring system facilitates the assessment of AIDS patients who require home-based care. Certain cadres of health care providers might, however, experience difficulties with the Karnofsky Performance scoring system.

A further refinement of the WHO staging system introduced, in addition to the clinical component, a laboratory component that uses total lymphocyte counts where $CD4^+$ cell counts cannot be performed (Table 5). There appears to be a good correlation between total lymphocyte counts and $CD4^+$ T-lymphocyte counts, although leukocyte counts in general, and $CD4^+$ counts in particular, are lower in black Africans.

EARLY SYMPTOMATIC DISEASE

Early symptomatic disease is characterized by persistent generalized lymphadenopathy (PGL), oral lesions, reactivation of herpes zoster, thrombocytopenia, miscellaneous clinical conditions that include prurigo, seborrheic dermatitis, molluscum contagiosum, condyloma acuminatum, recurrent oral or genital herpes simplex, weight loss, unexplained fever, and diarrhea (31).

Persistent generalized lymphadenopathy is defined as the presence of enlarged lymph nodes greater than 1 cm in two or more extrainguinal sites for more than 3 months without an obvious cause (32). The nodes are generally discrete and freely mobile. Later in the course of HIV disease, the differential diagnosis of generalized lymphadenopathy expands to include mycobacterial infection, lymphadenopathic KS, lymphoma, toxoplasmosis, nocardiosis, and rarely, bacillary angiomatosis. Lymph node biopsy or fine needle aspiration helps to establish the diagnosis. The most common oral lesions at this stage include oral candidiasis, hairy leukoplakia, and recurrent aphthous ulcers.

OPPORTUNISTIC INFECTIONS

Fungal Infections

Candidiasis is the most frequent opportunistic fungal infection in HIV-infected patients in Africa (33–36). Oral candidiasis is most commonly associated with *Candida albicans* (37), although other species such as *C. tropicalis* and *C. glabrata* form the normal flora of the oral cavity. *Candida* is readily diagnosed by symptoms such as oropharyngeal pseudomembranous exudates, but recognition of erythematous, atrophic, hypertrophic, or angular cheilitis is more difficult and requires detection of organisms in smears

TABLE 5. WHO Staging System for HIV Infection and Disease: Clinical/Laboratory Classification

	Laboratory axis[a]		Clinical axis[b]			
	Total lymphocyte count	$CD4^+$ count	(1) Asymptomatic/PGL	(2) Early	(3) Intermediate	(4) Late
(A)	>2,000	>500	1A	2A	3A	4A
(B)	1,000–2,000	200–500	1B	2B	3B	4B
(C)	<1,000	<200	1C	2C	3C	4C

[a]Strata by laboratory values: A, B, and C.
[b]Strata by clinical status: 1, 2, 3, and 4.

or scrapings taken from the lesions. Specimens should be examined using potassium hydroxide (KOH), periodic acid-Schiff (PAS), or Gram stain. Smears are taken by gently drawing a wooden spatula across the suspect lesion. The specimen is then transferred into a drop of KOH on a glass slide and protected by a cover slip. Under the light microscope, *Candida* organisms appear as hyphae or blastospores. Cultures are grown on specific media, such as Sabouraud's agar. However, culture capabilities are limited in sub–Saharan Africa.

Cryptococcus neoformans is an encapsulated round to oval yeast measuring 4 to 6 μm with a surrounding polysaccharide capsule ranging in size from 1 to more than 30 μm in laboratory media. The early manifestations of cryptococcal infections in HIV-infected patients in Africa are rarely seen, partly because the majority of patients present late with cryptococcal meningitis as their index AIDS-defining diagnosis (38,39). In industrialized nations, cryptococcal pneumonia is reportedly the most frequent fungal pneumonia encountered in persons with AIDS (40). Because it is often asymptomatic or minimally symptomatic with or without evidence of dissemination, cryptococcal pneumonia is undiagnosed or not recognized until infection has disseminated. Patients with cryptococcal pneumonia present with nonspecific symptoms such as cough, fever, malaise, shortness of breath, and pleuritic chest pain. Physical examination may reveal lymphadenopathy, tachypnea, and crepitations. Chest x-rays are variable but generally abnormal, frequently showing focal or diffuse interstitial infiltrates, focal or widespread alveolar consolidation, or ground glass shadowing (41,42). These lesions may simulate those caused by other opportunistic pathogens such as bacterial pneumonia or *Pneumocystis carinii* pneumonia (PCP). Less common findings include solitary subpleural nodules, mass lesions, consolidation, hilar and mediastinal lymphadenopathy, or pleural effusion; rarely does cavitation or empyema occur (43,44). Sputum examination for cryptococci is usually negative but the isolation yield of bronchoalveolar lavage may be higher (45). Serology for cryptococcal antigen may be positive, suggesting disseminated disease. Very few facilities in sub–Saharan Africa provide bronchoscopy and/or cryptococcal antigen testing.

Cryptococcal meningitis is the most common opportunistic fungal meningitis and is the most life-threatening fungal meningitis in AIDS patients, especially where antifungal therapy is unavailable (39,46–48). In a study by Heyderman et al. (48) from Zimbabwe, cryptococcal meningitis was the index AIDS-defining illness in 88% of patients. Infection typically occurs subacutely within 2 weeks with headache, fever, photophobia, neck pain, and vomiting. The most common signs include pyrexia, neck stiffness, and a positive Kernig's sign. Mental status is normal in one-third of patients, confused in 40%, drowsy in 12%, stuporous in 12%, and comatose in about 1.5%. Cranial nerve palsies occur as part of the ocular manifestations of cryptococcal invasion of the CNS. Complications of CNS infection include obstructive hydrocephalus, motor or sensory deficits, cerebellar dysfunction, seizures, and dementia. Cerebrospinal fluid (CSF) examination reveals a high opening pressure in the majority, but the leukocyte count, glucose, and protein concentrations in CSF tend to be nonspecific (49). In general, a lymphocytic pleocytosis, hypoglycorrhachia, and high protein concentrations predominate the CSF characteristics. Moosa and Coovadiah in Durban, South Africa, found 17% of AIDS patients with cryptococcal meningitis had normal CSF (39). Therefore, the finding of apparently normal CSF should not preclude the diagnosis of cryptococcal meningitis.

Other sites affected by disseminated cryptococcosis include skin, adrenal glands, endocardium, joints, bones, and gastrointestinal tract. Cutaneous lesions may appear as papules, tumors, vesicles, plaques, abscesses, cellulitis, purpura, sinuses, ulcers, or subcutaneous swellings, thereby mimicking other skin lesions.

The diagnosis of cryptococcosis is confirmed by isolation of organisms from a body site, by histopathologic examination of tissues, or by detection of cryptococcal capsular antigen. The India ink stain that outlines the polysaccharide capsule of the fungus is positive on direct examination of the CSF in more than 80% of patients with AIDS. Encapsulated yeasts seen on Alcian blue or Gomori methenamine-silver stain are also diagnostic of cryptococcosis. Stains such as PAS reveal yeast cells but are not specific for cryptococcosis. Cryptococcal antigen in serum is usually indicative of disseminated systemic disease. Detection of cryptococcal antigen in CSF has greater than 95% sensitivity and specificity in the diagnosis of truly invasive CNS cryptococcosis. False positive tests can occur due to infection with *Trichosporon beigelii* or from residual contamination on laboratory slides. A wider availability of cryptococcal antigen tests, especially for CSF analysis, should be strongly advocated in Africa.

Other fungi seem to rarely infect patients with HIV or AIDS in Africa. *Histoplasma capsulatum*, which has become a significant opportunistic fungal pathogen in AIDS patients in North America, is limited to a few case reports, mainly from tropical central and West Africa, in both HIV-negative and HIV-positive individuals (50–53). The diagnosis of disseminated histoplasmosis is easily confused with TB. Examination of specimens such as sputum, purulent materials from skin lesions, lymph node aspirates, or biopsies will usually reveal numerous fungal elements that are readily interpreted as *Candida*. The definitive diagnosis of African histoplasmosis is established by staining the smears with PAS or by culture on Sabouraud's medium where cream-colored molds grow within 3 weeks.

Viral Infections

Infections by some members of Herpesviridae are the most common opportunistic viral infections in HIV-infected individuals in Africa (54–57). Primary infection by herpes simplex virus type 1 (HSV-1) and herpes simplex virus type 2 (HSV-2) typically results in painful, ulcerative mucosal and cutaneous lesions, which may not be distinguishable from lesions in HIV-negative individuals. Recurrences are, however, more frequent in HIV-infected persons, ranging from recurrent fever blisters on the lips, tongue, or buccal mucosa, to severe mucocutaneous infections, gingivostomatitis, intranasal ulcerations, esophagitis, prostatitis, keratitis, visceral infections, and herpetic encephalitis. The severity of illness depends on several factors including the site of infection, the degree of HIV-induced immunosuppression and whether it is caused by primary infection, infection by a new strain of HSV, or a recurrent infection. Recurrent genital herpes is particularly common in HIV-infected patients (58). Although both HSV-1 and HSV-2 can cause infection at any anatomic site, HSV-1 more often infects orolabial sites, and HSV-2 more commonly affects the genital and anorectal sites. In advanced HIV disease, mucocutaneous lesions may enlarge steadily with progressive ulceration, which may show no signs of spontaneous healing (59) due to the severe immunosuppression, lack of antiviral therapy, or possibly, as in industrialized countries, due to acyclovir-resistant HSV strains (60).

The severity of illness depends on the clinical diagnosis of typical mucocutaneous herpetic lesions can be made with confidence based on patient history and the characteristic appearance of crops of fragile vesicles or pustules. Patients with herpetic esophagitis present with dysphagia and/or odynophagia that must be differentiated from other causes of these symptoms, such as esophageal candidiasis or cytomegalovirus (CMV) esophagitis. An abnormal barium esophagram showing cobblestone appearance is nonspecific for herpetic esophagitis. Specific diagnosis requires esophagoscopy with biopsy and submission of specimens for histology and viral cultures. Lack of these diagnostic facilities in many African countries limits efforts to provisional diagnoses only. Likewise, the diagnosis of HSV encephalitis in patients with advanced HIV disease by clinical features alone is extremely difficult. Furthermore, attempts to confirm the diagnosis seem unwarranted in resource-poor settings, as specific antiviral therapy may be either locally unavailable or unaffordable. Cerebrospinal fluid examination is nonspecific, often revealing a lymphocytic pleocytosis, occasional red blood cells, and elevated protein content. Viral cultures of CSF are usually negative. Computerized tomography (CT), magnetic resonance imaging (MRI), and electroencephalography may be useful in localizing areas of severe brain involvement, but definitive diagnosis rests on the examination of brain biopsy materials.

Varicella-zoster virus (VZV) causes both varicella (chickenpox) and zoster (shingles) with increased frequency in HIV-infected individuals. Herpes zoster infection may occur at any stage of HIV infection; in some African patients it is the presenting AIDS-defining diagnosis (61–63). In high HIV-seroprevalence areas, herpes zoster has a positive predictive value for the diagnosis of HIV/AIDS of 90% to 100% (64,65); this value drops to about 40% in low-seroprevalence regions (66).

Typical herpes zoster lesions are clinically recognizable, with pain and vesicles limited to easily identifiable dermatomes. The presentation is subtle when few lesions occur, sparse lesions are covered with hair, vesicles have not erupted, existing lesions are grouped close to the midline or limited to the distribution of a division of the trigeminal nerve. Occasionally, herpes zoster affects the facial nerve, resulting in Ramsay Hunt syndrome (67). In western literature, there have been patients with HIV infection, presenting with prolonged lesion formation, progressive local extension, and dissemination of VZV (68,69). Herpes zoster usually appears in HIV-infected patients as multidermatomal erythematous maculopapular eruption that evolves within a few days to form true vesicles, pustules, and crusts. Painful bullae with hemorrhages and necrosis may occur in those with advanced HIV disease. Blisters and crusts usually last 2 to 3 weeks while necrotic lesions may take up to 6 weeks, healing with severe scarring or keloid formation. Recurrences are frequent but there is no evidence to suggest that postherpetic neuralgia is more common in HIV-infected patients than in HIV-uninfected individuals.

Progressive primary varicella, a syndrome characterized by persistent new lesion formation and visceral dissemination, may be life threatening. The rash of chickenpox typically appears 10 to 21 days after infection. Prodromal symptoms like malaise, low-grade fever, and myalgia in adults occur a day or two before the eruption of skin lesions that begin as small erythematous macules and progress over 12 to 36 hours to become papules and true vesicles. Lesions appear first and are most concentrated on the trunk, neck, and face while fewer lesions appear on the proximal aspects of the limbs. The vesicles, which are filled with straw-colored fluid, are variable in size and shape and rest on erythematous bases. They may ulcerate, dry up, and form scabs in the healing process, resulting in pruritus in some patients. Lesions in all stages of development (macules, papules, vesicles, ulcers, crusts) are characteristic of varicella. HIV-infected patients are at risk of secondary bacterial infection of the lesions. Also, all adults, especially pregnant women with chickenpox, with or without HIV infection, are at increased risk of varicella pneumonia. Many patients have only mild respiratory symptoms. Severe lung involvement with hypoxemia, cyanosis, and death may occur in severely immunocompromised individuals. Chest radiographic abnormalities in patients with VZV pneumonia are usually more pronounced than the clinical symptoms and signs. Differential diagnoses of varicella include other viral infections (measles, coxsackie, rubella, disseminated herpes simplex viral infection), typhus, secondary syphilis, scabies, and allergic drug reactions.

The diagnosis of VZV should be based on clinical symptoms because sensitive diagnostic tests are generally not available. Staining scrapings obtained directly from the base of either varicella or zoster skin ulcers to demonstrate multinucleated giant cells (Tzanck preparation) is not sensitive and cannot differentiate VZV from other herpesvirus infections such as HSV or CMV. The diagnostic procedure of choice is the detection of virus antigens expressed on the surface of infected cells obtained from scrapings and stained with specific fluorescein-conjugated monoclonal antibodies. Viral culture is less sensitive and requires about 2 weeks to demonstrate the cytopathic effects.

Hairy Leukoplakia

Immunodeficiency-associated hairy leukoplakia appears in early HIV disease as nonremovable, corrugated white lesions usually on the lateral margins of the tongue. There is now overwhelming evidence that hairy leukoplakia is caused by Epstein-Barr virus (EBV) infection in both latent forms and stages of active viral replication (70–73). Experienced clinicians can readily make presumptive diagnosis of hairy leukoplakia, but definitive diagnosis requires a biopsy of the lesion. The typical histologic appearance includes acanthosis, marked parakeratosis with formation of ridges and keratin projections, areas of ballooning cells, and usually no inflammatory reaction in the connective tissue. Demonstration of EBV by various techniques clinches the definitive diagnosis but is generally unavailable and lacks any additional value in the management of the patient. Differential diagnoses include lichen plannus, idiopathic leukoplakia, pseudomembranous candidiasis, dysplasia, white sponge nevus, and squamous cell carcinoma.

Cytomegalovirus Infection

There are very few reports of infection by CMV of African patients with HIV/AIDS. This may be partly because of underdiagnosis, but some authorities have suggested that the early death of AIDS patients in Africa stifles manifestations of CMV infection. In North America, autopsy studies showed that more than 90% of AIDS cases had evidence of disseminated CMV infection (74). Chorioretinitis most commonly occurs in patients with $CD4^+$ lymphocyte counts below 50/mm^3 and accounts for 80% to 90% of CMV disease in AIDS patients in the developed world. The reported prevalence of CMV retinitis in African AIDS patients varies from 0% to 8% (75). In a cross-sectional survey of 120 patients with HIV-1 (56 cases), HIV-2 (52 cases), or dual infection (12 cases), in Gambia, Jaffar and colleagues (76) found no cases of CMV retinitis, even among the 47.5% whose $CD4^+$ counts were below 14 cells/mm^3. A prospective study of patients in Burundi with higher $CD4^+$ counts ($>$100 cells/mm^3 in three-quarters of the cases), almost all of whom (99%) had serologic evidence of CMV exposure, showed only five cases of retinal perivasculitis and two cases of viral retinitis (77). Ophthalmoscopic examination of patients with CMV retinitis typically reveals large creamy to yellowish-white granular areas with perivascular exudates, either at the periphery or at the center of the fundus. The disease may be unilateral but progression to bilateral disease is common, becoming sight-threatening within 2 to 3 weeks if untreated.

Cytomegalovirus enterocolitis, though rare in immunocompetent hosts, is common in patients with AIDS and can occur in patients on immunosuppressive therapy for autoimmune or inflammatory diseases and in allograft recipients. It is characterized by diarrhea, weight loss, abdominal pain, anorexia, and fever (78). In sub–Saharan Africa, the diagnosis of CMV enterocolitis is usually tentative and must be differentiated from other HIV-associated gastrointestinal pathogens, lymphoma, or KS. Patients with CMV esophagitis present with dysphagia and odynophagia due to large distal ulcerations that are easily observed using barium esophagrams (79,80). Esophagoscopy usually reveals diffuse submucosal hemorrhages and mucosal ulceration; rarely is the mucosa normal. Biopsy reveals vasculitis, neutrophilic infiltration, and nonspecific inflammation. The presence of characteristic CMV inclusions and the absence of other pathogens confirm the diagnosis. Most cases of CMV pneumonia in severely immunocompromised HIV-infected adults are believed to be due to reactivation of latent CMV infections. Pneumonitis caused by CMV presents with fever, cough, hypoxemia, and diffuse radiographic opacities (81). There are minimal findings on chest auscultation. Chest x-ray shows diffuse interstitial pneumonitis. These clinicoradiographic features are indistinguishable from other causes of interstitial pneumonitis in AIDS patients. The most frequent neurologic syndrome caused by CMV is radiculopathy, a spinal cord syndrome characterized by pain in the lower extremities, weakness, spasticity, areflexia, urinary retention, and hypoesthesia. The CSF findings of polymorphonuclear pleocytosis and moderately low glucose concentrations are nondiagnostic. Viral culture from the CSF is usually negative, but, where available, CMV antigen or DNA assays may be positive. Subacute encephalitis caused by CMV resembles that caused by other pathogens and also requires brain biopsy for confirmation of diagnosis. The limitations of such diagnostic approaches in sub–Saharan Africa have already been emphasized.

Bacterial Infections

The clinical diagnosis of bacterial infections in HIV-infected patients follows the same standard approach in general medicine as in HIV-uninfected individuals. Although a good patient history, physical examination, and ancillary investigations such as radiography or ultrasound examinations may facilitate the localization or possible source of infection, definitive diagnosis rests on isolation of the organism. The most frequent organisms include *Streptococcus pneumoniae, Haemophilus influenzae, Staphylococcus aureus, Escherichia coli*, nontyphoidal *Salmonella* species, *Shigella* species, *Pseudomonas aeruginosa*, and *Klebsiella* species. Quite often there is bacteremia or septicemia. Therefore definitive diagnosis can easily be made on timely blood cultures. Culture of other specimens like sputum, pus, stool, urine, CSF, pleural effusions, pericardial effusion, or ascites may be of additional diagnostic value. Nocardiosis involving the lungs or lymph nodes affects less than 5% of HIV-infected African patients (82,83). Pulmonary nocardiosis is easily confused with TB. Patients with clinically suspected pulmonary TB who are smear negative for acid-fast bacilli should be considered for bronchoscopy and bronchoalveolar lavage.

Tuberculosis

The diagnosis of pulmonary TB in patients with HIV coinfection poses little problem when the sputum examination is positive for acid-fast bacilli. However, the diagnostic yield depends on the number of smears examined and the method of sputum examination (84,85). The sensitivity of sputum smears increases from about 80% with the first specimen, to 92% with the second, to nearly 100% with the third (86). Economic analysis shows that the incremental cost of performing a third test increases rapidly with only a small gain in additional cases of TB identified; a policy of examining only two samples in resource-poor settings has been suggested. Polymerase chain reaction (PCR) assay of sputum specimens gives a sensitivity and specificity of 91% and 90%, respectively, thereby adding little value to the diagnostic workup. Sputum induction is a useful technique for improving the case detection rate of smear-positive TB in patients who are unable to raise sputum (87). Sputum culture for mycobacteria should be performed for those whose smears are negative.

Patients who are sputum smear-negative or who have extrapulmonary TB pose greater diagnostic challenges. Less than 2% of those with extrapulmonary intrathoracic TB, such as pleural effusion, have positive sputum smears even after multiple sputum examinations; the proportion hardly exceeds 3% for patients with lymphadenopathy, miliary TB, and TB meningitis (88). Chest radiography is a weak tool because there is a wide overlap of radiologic features in HIV-infected patients with TB and those with other pulmonary conditions (89). The tuberculin skin test is of little diagnostic value in HIV-infected patients due to high rates of cutaneous anergy and also instability of tuberculin skin test reactivity (90,91).

Extrapulmonary TB is nearly twice as common in HIV-infected patients as in HIV-seronegative individuals, with extrathoracic manifestations in nearly two-thirds of the cases. Frequently involved sites include lymph nodes, CNS especially meninges, liver, spleen, genitourinary tract, spine, joints, and adrenals (92). The diagnosis of tuberculous lymphadenitis requires lymph node biopsy or needle aspiration. Given the relative ease with which the latter procedure is performed, it is recommended that patients with asymmetrical lymphadenopathy, or rapidly enlarging or tender nodes, should undergo needle aspiration of readily accessible glands before biopsy is contemplated.

Difficulties encountered in the diagnostic confirmation of tuberculous serositis (pleural effusion, pericardial effusion, ascites) are due to limitations in the identification of mycobacteria in the fluid, given that the bacillary population is small and immune mechanisms are largely responsible for the effusion. Pleural biopsy gives a diagnosis in 50% to 90% of cases of exudative pleural effusion. However, it is invasive and technically demanding. Biochemical examination of effusions is useful but not diagnostic. Tuberculous pleural effusion, for example, is characteristically exudative, with elevated protein content, lactic dehydrogenase, adenosine deaminase, and a lymphocytic predominance. The mononuclear cellularity might help to distinguish TB from parapneumonic effusion or empyema. Sometimes the pleural fluid may be hemorrhagic, thereby raising consideration of differential diagnoses like pulmonary embolism, malignancies including pleural involvement by KS, and amoebic liver abscess with rupture into the pleural cavity.

Tuberculous pericarditis results from bloodborne infection, rupture of adjacent lymph node or parenchymal lung lesion. Large pericardial effusion or rapidly accumulating fluid results in a raised jugular venous pressure with a sharp ‘xy’ descent. Ascites tends to be out of proportion with leg edema. The biochemical characteristics of the fluid are similar to those of pleural effusion, but are more often hemorrhagic. Cardiomegaly on chest x-ray is readily confirmed on two-dimensional echocardiography, which typically demonstrates serofibrinous pericardial effusion with or without features of cardiac tamponade. Clinical misdiagnosis arises in cases involving congestive cardiac failure especially due to idiopathic dilated cardiomyopathy, hepatocellular carcinoma, liver abscess, or liver cirrhosis. Constrictive pericarditis is rare, but some patients have features of effusive-constrictive pericarditis resulting from organized fibrinous pericarditis.

Tuberculous peritonitis results from mesenteric, intestinal, or hematogenous spread. The ascites is also usually exudative. Tuberculous meningitis occurs because of bloodborne infection or rupture of a tuberculoma within the brain. The CSF tends to be under high pressure; it may be clear or cloudy with web clot if the protein content is very high. There is a lymphocytic pleocytosis, although polymorphonuclear reaction may occur in early infection. The level of adenosine deaminase is also elevated. Tuberculous meningitis must be distinguished from cryptococcal, viral, and partially treated bacterial meningitis, as well as from toxoplasmosis and meningovascular syphilis. In a few patients, dual infections occur, thus complicating their diagnostic evaluation.

Miliary TB always follows hematogenous spread of infection and is characterized by miliary mottling of chest x-rays, elevated liver enzymes, and positive bone marrow culture for acid-fast bacilli. Sputum examination is of very little diagnostic value in cases of miliary TB. Bone and joint TB often affects the spine and less commonly the hips, the knees, and other peripheral joints (93).

Tuberculosis of peripheral joints tends to be monoarticular, mainly involving weight-bearing joints. Involvement of the spine begins with the disc before spreading to affect vertebral bodies. The thoracolumbar region is most frequently affected, followed by the upper thoracic spine and the lumbar region. Progressive destruction of the spine results in gibbus formation or kyphoscoliosis. Cold paravertebral abscesses may form. The diagnosis of TB of the gastrointestinal tract requires imaging such as barium series and endoscopy with biopsy. Isolated reports indicate that TB due to *Mycobacterium* other than tuberculosis (MOTT) occurs in both HIV-uninfected and HIV-infected individuals, especially miners (94,95). Diagnosis of MOTT requires a high index of suspicion and involves culture of sputum, aspirate, or biopsy specimen.

Parasitic Diseases

Toxoplasmosis

Toxoplasma gondii is a zoonotic obligate intracellular protozoan, which is recognized as a major cause of neurologic morbidity and mortality among patients with advanced HIV disease. Many seroepidemiologic studies involving the general population, children, young adults, and pregnant women have demonstrated a high rate of primary infection with seroprevalence rates ranging from 34% to 80% (96–99). Antitoxoplasma IgG antibody seroprevalence rates in HIV-infected individuals using the Sabin-Feldman dye test and immunosorbent agglutination assay are not significantly different from rates in HIV-uninfected persons (96). There are marked geographic differences in seroprevalence rates in HIV-infected patients, ranging from as low as 4% among HIV-infected patients in Zambia to 34% among those in Uganda (100).

Acute reactivation of toxoplasmosis is characterized by symptomatic dissemination of the once dormant parasite. Between 5% and 17% of HIV-infected persons from one African study developed toxoplasmosis (101). Disseminated toxoplasmosis occurs in severely immunocompromised patients, manifesting with fever, encephalitis, or brain abscesses, and occasionally pneumonia, myocarditis, hepatosplenomegaly, or skin rash. Toxoplasmosis of the CNS with features of encephalitis or focal neurologic deficits may be the first AIDS-defining diagnosis in some patients. This late presentation has led some authorities to regard the condition as relatively rare in African AIDS patients, although toxoplasmosis was a major underlying pathology in an autopsy study of HIV-positive adults with advanced disease in Côte d'Ivoire (102).

Symptoms of neurologic toxoplasmosis are vague and nonspecific. They include headache, fever, confusion, lethargy, meningism, and seizures. The clinicoradiologic features of toxoplasma pneumonia are indistinguishable from those of PCP (103). Ocular involvement is uncommon (104). The differential diagnosis of toxoplasmosis in HIV-infected patients is broad and includes neurologic deficits caused by TB, pyogenic brain abscess, fungal abscesses (*Cryptococcus, Aspergillus, Candida*), primary CNS lymphoma, progressive multifocal leukoencephalopathy, HSV encephalitis, HIV meningoencephalitis, and non–HIV-related conditions such as cerebrovascular accidents and vasculitides. Computerized tomography and, where available, MRI scan of the head, are sensitive but nonspecific methods of identifying the ring-enhancing lesions that are suggestive of cerebral toxoplasmosis (105). Multiple lesions may be seen in the frontal lobes, basal ganglia, and parietal lobes as well as within the cerebral white matter or subcortical grey matter. Calcification rarely occurs. Lumbar puncture is valuable in excluding other opportunistic infections. In toxoplasmosis, the CSF glucose tends to be normal, protein slightly elevated, and a significant number of patients exhibit a mononuclear pleocytosis. Diagnosis of pulmonary toxoplasmosis requires demonstration of the protozoan in the bronchoalveolar lavage fluid. HIV-infected patients with active toxoplasmosis tend to have higher titres of antitoxoplasma IgG antibodies than those with asymptomatic latent infection. Positive IgM titres are unusual. Positive antitoxoplasma IgG in CSF is an indication of CNS involvement (106). Although a positive antitoxoplasma IgG in blood cannot prove or disprove the diagnosis of toxoplasmosis, a negative test should prompt the clinician to consider alternative diagnoses. A good response to antitoxoplasma therapy may serve as a retrospective diagnosis.

Pneumocystis carinii Pneumonia

Pneumocystis carinii pneumonia is generally considered to be rare in adult patients with HIV/AIDS in Africa (107,108). Certain clinical and radiologic features, including tachypnea, hypoxemia, and reticulonodular infiltrates on chest x-rays, have been found to be strongly predictive of PCP (109). However, confirmation of diagnosis of PCP requires examination of bronchoalveolar lavage or an appropriately sampled large volume of sputum, specifically stained with methenamine silver or Grocott-Gomori staining technique.

Coccidiosis (Cryptosporidiosis, Cyclosporiasis, Isosporiasis, Microsporidiosis)

Coccidia are protozoa with subcellular organelles and a life cycle similar to that of *Toxoplasma gondii*. Intestinal coccidia (cryptosporidiosis, cyclosporiasis, isosporiasis and microsporidiosis) account for about one-half of cases of etiologically diagnosed persistent diarrhea in HIV-infected persons in the developed world (110). In central Africa, approximately 30% of persons with advanced HIV disease and persistent diarrhea had cryptosporidiosis in a study by Colebunders et al. in the Democratic Republic of Congo and in a study by Conlon et al. in Zambia (111,112). Sewankambo and his colleagues found a much higher prevalence (61%) of cryptosporidiosis and isosporiasis in a smaller but very similar study involving 23 Ugandan patients with enteropathic AIDS (113). Nausea, vomiting, abdominal cramps, flatulence, anorexia, and marked wasting commonly accompany the diarrhea associated with these coccidia. Stool oocyst excretion rates reportedly correlate with the intensity of infection. However, routine fecal examination for ova, parasites, and cysts is not sufficient to detect *Cryptosporidium* oocysts. There are numerous sedimentation, flotation, and staining techniques to identify oocysts in feces, including modified Ziehl-Neelsen carbolfuchsin, Giemsa, auramine, and rhodamine stains. Reports from some countries in sub–Saharan Africa cite rates of infection caused by *Isospora belli* that range from 8% to 24% (112,114–116).

The clinical features of isosporiasis are indistinguishable from those of cryptosporidiosis. However, for diagnosis of isosporiasis, stool samples should be stained with a modified Kinyoun stain (a modified acid-fast stain using carbol fuchsin and a bright green counter stain that colors cryptosporidia and *I. belli* bright red). Isospora cysts tend to be larger and elliptical in shape. Oocysts may be difficult to find in stool, in which case duodenal aspirates may be useful. Biopsy of small intestinal villous epithelium may be diagnostic but is considered overly invasive with little management value. Microsporidia are small spore-forming obligate intracellular protozoa that are found in the intestine, liver, kidney, cornea, brain, nerves, and muscles of animals. Unfortunately, the parasites have not been extensively studied in sub–Saharan Africa because diagnosis requires electron microscopy, which is of very limited availability within the continent (117).

Spirochetal Infections

The interaction of syphilis and HIV infection is complex. Most HIV-infected patients with *Treponema pallidum* infection present with typical clinical stages of disease (primary, secondary, latent, and tertiary syphilis). However, they are more likely to exhibit accelerated manifestations of disease with overlap of these stages, such that a patient with primary chancre may show symptoms and signs of secondary syphilis before the chancres heal. There have been reports in western literature of atypical lesions including multiple chancres, chancres appearing as fissures or abrasions, gummatous penile ulcerations, unusual rashes, severe necrotic ulcerations, and keratoderma (118–120). Early forms of neurosyphilis include syphilitic meningitis, meningovascular syphilis with thrombotic strokes, syphilitic meningomyelitis, and polyradiculopathy. Tabes dorsalis is rare. Paretic neurosyphilis would be very difficult to differentiate from AIDS-dementia complex. Ocular and otologic involvements may result in chorioretinitis, retrobulbar neuritis, vitreitis, scleritis, papillitis, optic neuritis, and sensorineural deafness with tinnitus, imbalance, and a sensation of ear fullness (121–126). These lesions are either uncommon or poorly documented in HIV-infected Africans (127). Other organs such as the liver, bones, lungs, stomach, skin, and mucous membranes may be affected by gummatous syphilis.

The serodiagnosis of syphilis in HIV-infected patients is complicated by low positive predictive values and a significant rate of biologic false positive (128) and false negative tests (129). Negative nontreponemal serologic tests such as rapid plasma reagent (RPR) and venereal disease reference laboratory (VDRL), which detect antibodies directed against cardiolipin-lecithin, do not rule out the diagnosis of syphilis in patients with HIV infection. Specific treponemal tests (fluorescent treponemal antibody-absorption [FTA-ABS], *Treponema pallidum* hemagglutination [TPHA], and *Treponema pallidum* immobilization [TPI] tests) are of sufficiently high sensitivity in untreated HIV-infected patients who are beyond the primary stage of infection. Beware of the prozone phenomenon—a nontreponemal serologic test read as negative simply because the specimen was not sufficiently diluted, thereby obviating detection of antigen-antibody complexes due to high antigen concentrations. Dark field examination or direct fluorescent antibody staining of exudates from suspicious primary or secondary lesions are of diagnostic value in patients with negative serology. The diagnosis of neurosyphilis is based on the CSF findings of a leukocytic pleocytosis, raised proteins, and a positive CSF VDRL or TPHA result. Neuroimaging such as CT and MRI scans may identify sites of cerebral infarction but do not surpass CSF serology.

HIV-Associated Malignancies

Kaposi's sarcoma is the most common AIDS-related malignancy (130). The risk of developing HIV-associated KS is almost three times greater among males than among females (131–132). Both endemic and epidemic forms of African KS are histologically similar and include a spindle cell component, slit-like vascular spaces containing erythrocytes, and a variable inflammatory cell infiltrate (133). There is a wide range in the distribution and clinical manifestations of HIV-associated KS. The disease usually causes violaceous skin lesions, but oral, visceral, or nodal KS may precede cutaneous involvement. In blacks, KS lesions may appear dark brown or black. Using chemotherapy, lesions may fade to grey but pigmentation may persist even in the absence of active disease. Biopsy is recommended to distinguish KS lesions from other pigmented skin conditions such as dermatophyte or bacterial infections, leprosy, non-Hodgkin lymphoma, neurofibromatosis, and bacillary angiomatosis. Oral lesions are particularly common on the palate, appearing as focal, flat, red or purple plaques, which may be completely asymptomatic and therefore easily overlooked. In time, lesions become larger, diffuse, or nodular and have a propensity to ulcerate and bleed easily. Kaposi lesions in the gingiva, tongue, uvula, tonsils, oropharynx, and lips may interfere with mastication, deglutition, speech, and breathing. Gastrointestinal KS is usually asymptomatic and only diagnosed at autopsy. The formal evaluation of the gastrointestinal tract through, for example, endoscopy, is only recommended in those patients with symptoms referable to the gastrointestinal tract, such as pain, bleeding, or obstruction. Kaposi's sarcoma that involves the lung parenchyma, tracheobronchial tree, and pleural spaces are late manifestations of HIV disease and portend a poor prognosis. Patient symptoms may include shortness of breath, cough, wheezing, hemoptysis, respiratory failure, and recurrent pleural effusions. Chest x-rays may show ill-defined nodules, interstitial infiltrates, or pleural effusion. The pleural fluid tends to be hemorrhagic exudates with nondiagnostic cytology. Lymphadenopathic KS also tends to be asymptomatic, and routine lymph node biopsies are therefore not recommended. Patients with massive lymphadenopathy will, however, benefit from biopsy as a means of differentiating KS from TB, nocardiosis, suppurative lymphadenitis, or lymphoma. Other visceral sites for KS include the liver, spleen, heart, pericardium, bone marrow, eyelids, conjunctivae, ears, and nose. Occasionally, KS may cause edema, usually affecting the feet and legs, but may involve other sites such as the groin, external genitalia, periorbital region, and rarely, the upper limbs, trunk, and abdomen.

HIV-associated lymphomas occur in patients with advanced AIDS and tend to cause widespread disease with extranodal involvement (134). The majority of these tumors are diffuse large cell lymphomas (DLCL), while a small proportion are small noncleaved cell lymphomas such as Burkitt lymphoma. Virtually all HIV-associated lymphomas are of B-cell origin. The occurrence of AIDS-related DLCL is preceded by decreasing EBV cytotoxic T-lymphocyte precursors and increasing EBV load. Failing EBV control might therefore be an important step in the pathogenesis of AIDS-related DLCL (135). However, while transplantation-associated lymphomas are uniformly associated with the EBV, this association is not seen in all systemic AIDS-related lymphomas (136). Body-cavity-based HIV-1–associated lymphomas are associated with human herpesvirus type 8 (HHV-8), which was initially described in association with KS.

HIV-infected patients with primary CNS lymphoma commonly experience confusion, lethargy, and memory loss. They may also have headaches, hemiparesis, aphasia, seizures, and cranial nerve palsies. It is difficult to distinguish lesions of primary CNS lymphomas from granulomatous mass lesions, such as intracranial toxoplasmosis, on CT or MRI. Brain biopsy, the standard diagnostic procedure, is impractical in most African settings. Primary effusion lymphomas are probably underdiagnosed in Africa, because it is very difficult to distinguish them from tuberculous serositis and effusions due to KS. HIV-infected individuals with Hodgkin disease show a shift in histologic subtype from nodular sclerosis to mixed cellularity and lymphocyte-depleted disease. The majority present in stage III or IV and involve extranodal sites, especially the bone marrow.

Anogenital neoplasia, which includes both cervical and anal cancer as well as their precursor lesions, are more common in HIV-infected individuals. Infection by human papilloma virus (HPV) is one of the most important risk factors associated with these neoplasms. Although studies in the United States have shown that the prevalence of HPV-associated anal squamous intraepithelial lesions (ASIL) and squamous neoplasia are high among HIV-positive homosexual and bisexual men (137,138), there are reports of these lesions in heterosexual men and women, and sometimes in women who have sex with women (139–141). Some of the risk factors for anogenital HPV infection in heterosexual individuals, especially women, include a younger age group, frequent sexual activities, anal sex, multiple sexual partners in their lifetime, and alcohol consumption. Direct visualization and biopsy of lesions in the anogenital region is the recommended diagnostic approach since cytology is unreliable. HIV may alter the clinical course of other malignancies including lung cancers and germ-cell malignancies, but the diagnostic evaluation of such patients follows the standard procedures for HIV-uninfected individuals.

Some HIV-Specific Disorders

Wasting syndrome, originally described as "slim disease" in Uganda (142), is currently defined by weight loss of at least 10% of body weight in the presence of diarrhea or chronic weakness and documented fever for at least 30 days, none of which are attributable to a concurrent condition other than HIV infection. The recently suggested use of body mass index (calculated by dividing weight in kilograms by the square of height in meters) instead of >10% weight loss is realistic because the majority of patients do not routinely know their weights. A cut-off value of <20 kg/m^2 is an indicator of wasting. Also severe cachexia as judged by the clinician can be taken as a feature of the wasting syndrome. Because of the large burden of comorbidity in AIDS patients in Africa and difficulties related to establishing the diagnoses of certain diseases in Africa, it is reasonable to expand the definition of wasting syndrome, even when other HIV-associated conditions, such as TB, are present. In practice, any involuntary weight loss resulting in clinically obvious depletion of body cell mass is considered wasting. The determinants of wasting in sub–Saharan African AIDS patients include poverty, malnutrition, concurrent infections like TB, recurrent bacterial pneumonias, recurrent diarrheas with or without vomiting, and malignancies such as KS. Factors contributing to weight loss include metabolic alterations, anorexia, malabsorption, hypogonadism, excessive cytokine production (interferon-α, tumor necrosis factor-α, interleukin-1) and rapid bowel transit due to diarrhea. Ideally, weight should be recorded on the same scale each time, without heavy clothing or jewelry, and after the patient has voided urine. Anthropometric measurements such as mid-arm circumference and tricep skin-fold thickness are impractical in most settings.

Neurologic Manifestations of HIV Infection

Neurologic manifestations of AIDS in Africa have received relatively little attention, and their prevalence is probably underestimated. A study of 200 patients with AIDS from Tanzania showed that 72% had some abnormal neurologic problems; 11% had focal abnormalities; and 54% had AIDS dementia complex (ADC) (143). Scarcity of diagnostic facilities as well as lack of human resources and severely constrained doctor-patient contact time preclude adequate evaluation of patients. Therefore, the inclusion of complex criteria in the case definition is bound to meet with restricted application of the surveillance tool.

AIDS dementia complex is a neurologic condition characterized by impaired concentration and memory, slowness of hand movements, ataxia, incontinence, apathy, and gait difficulties associated with HIV-1 viral infection of the CNS. Pathologic examination of the brain reveals white matter rarefaction, perivascular infiltrates of lymphocytes, foamy macrophages, and multinucleated giant cells (144). A major feature of this entity is the development of dementia, which is defined as a decline in cognitive ability to concentrate, increased forgetfulness, difficulty in reading, or increased difficulty performing complex tasks. Initially, the symptoms of ADC may be indistinguishable from reactive depression (145). However, patients with ADC also manifest motor and behavioral abnormalities such as psychomotor slowing, generalized myoclonus, unsteadiness of gait, poor balance, tremors, dysdiadochokinesia, brisk deep tendon jerks, apathy, loss of volition, and eventual progression to coma and vegetative state (146,147). Methods of staging ADC, as well as Mini-Mental Status examination (a simple screening test of cognitive impairment) need to be adapted to local circumstances. Interestingly, a study of 93 AIDS patients in Bangui, Central African Republic, by Belec et al. (148) appeared to suggest a lower prevalence of neuropsychiatric manifestations than rates reported in Europe and North America.

Spinal cord diseases in AIDS patients are of three types: vacuolar myelopathy, pure sensory ataxia, and sensory impairment. Their symptoms need to be differentiated from those of subacute combined degeneration of the cord due to avitaminosis B12, spinal cord compression, acute inflammatory polyneuropathy, or drug-induced peripheral neuropathies. Seizures in HIV-infected patients may result from opportunistic infections, neoplasms, HIV-encephalopathy, and progressive multifocal leukoencephalopathy due to Creutzfeldt Jakob disease. It may also be due to electrolyte abnormalities resulting from diarrhea and vomiting.

CONCLUSION

This chapter reviewed the development, refinement, and expansion of AIDS case definitions. Their limitations have been discussed, and the need to develop more accurate, regularly updated second-generation surveillance case definitions was emphasized. While many clinicians might apply these surveillance case definitions and HIV/AIDS clinical staging classifications interchangeably, it is important to make a clear distinction between surveillance tools and clinical staging systems. The diagnostic approach to any patient follows a distinctly different clinical algorithm to the principles of epidemiologic surveillance.

A cross-section of HIV-related disorders was selected to highlight the magnitude of diagnostic problems facing most clinicians working in sub–Saharan Africa. The list is by no means exhaustive. Given the meager resources in many African countries, our zeal to clinch difficult diagnoses in HIV-infected patients must be carefully balanced by efforts to give patients the best palliative care possible.

REFERENCES

1. Epidemiological fact sheet on HIV/AIDS and Sexually Transmitted Infections: UNAIDS/WHO 2000 Update. UNAIDS web site. Available at: http://www.unaids.org/hivaidsinfo/statistics/june00/fact_sheets/index.html. Accessed September 25, 2001.
2. Bigger RJ. Preventing AIDS now. *BMJ*, 1991;303:1150–1151.
3. Piot P, Colebunders R. Clinical manifestations and the natural history of HIV infection in adults. *West J Med*, 1987;147(6):709–712.
4. Fowke KR, Nagelkerke NJ, Kimani J, et al. Resistance to HIV-1 infection among persistently seronegative prostitutes in Nairobi, Kenya. *Lancet*, 1996;348:1347–1351.
5. Kaul R, Plummer FA, Kimani J, et al. HIV-1-specific mucosal CD8+ lymphocyte responses in the cervix of HIV-1-resistant prostitutes in Nairobi. *J Immunol*, 2000;164:1602–1611.
6. Willerford DM, Bwayo JJ, Hensel M, et al. Human immunodeficiency virus infection among high-risk seronegative prostitutes in Nairobi. *J Infect Dis*, 1993;167:1414–1417.
7. Kanki PJ, Hamel DJ, Sankale JL, et al. Human immunodeficiency virus type 1 subtypes differ in disease progression. *J Infect Dis*, 1999;179: 68–73.

8. De Cock KM, Odehouri K, Colebunders RL, et al. A comparison of HIV-1 and HIV-2 infections in hospitalized patients in Abidjan, Cote d'Ivoire. *AIDS*, 1990;4:443–448.
9. Ndour M, Sow P, Coll-Seck AM, et al. AIDS caused by HIV-1 and HIV-2 infection: are there clinical differences? Results of AIDS surveillance 1986–97 at Fann Hospital in Dakar, Senegal. *Trop Med Int Health*, 2000;5:687–691.
10. Grant AD, Djomand G, De Cock KM. Natural history and spectrum of disease in adults with HIV/AIDS in Africa. *AIDS*, 1997;11(Suppl B):S43–S54.
11. Lifson AR, Rutherford GW, Jaffe HW. The natural history of human immunodeficiency virus infection. *J Infect Dis*, 1988;158:1360–1367.
12. Colebunders R, Ryder RW, Francis H, et al. Seroconversion rate, mortality and clinical manifestations associated with the receipt of a human immunodeficiency virus-infected blood transfusion in Kinshasa, Zaire. *J Infect Dis*, 1991;164:450–456.
13. N'Galy B, Ryder RW, Bila K, et al. Human immunodeficiency virus infection among employees in an African hospital. *N Engl J Med*, 1988;319: 1123–1127.
14. Anzala A, Wambugu P, Plummer F, et al. Incubation time to symptomatic disease and AIDS in women with known duration of infection. In: Program and abstracts of the VII International Conference on AIDS; June 16–21, 1991; Florence, Italy. Abstract TU 103.
15. Centers for Disease Control. Mortality attributable to HIV infection/AIDS-United States, 1981–90. MMWR, 1991;40:41–44.
16. Centers for Disease Control and Prevention. 1993 revised classification system for HIV infection and expanded surveillance case definition for AIDS among adolescents and adults. *JAMA*, 1993;269:729–730.
17. World Health Organization. Workshop on AIDS in Central Africa. Bangui, Central African Republic, WHO/CDS/SIDA/85-1; October 22–24, 1985.
18. De Cock KM, Selik RM, Soro B, et al. AIDS surveillance in Africa: a reappraisal of the case definitions. *BMJ*, 1991;303:1185–1188.
19. Colebunders R, Mann JM, Francis H, et al. Evaluation of a clinical case-definition of acquired immunodeficiency syndrome in Africa. *Lancet*, 1987;1:492–494.
20. De Cock KM, Colebunders R, Francis H, et al. Evaluation of the WHO clinical case definition for AIDS in rural Zaire. *AIDS*, 1988;2:219–221.
21. Gilks CF. What use is a clinical case definition for AIDS in Africa? *BMJ*, 1991;303:1189–1190.
22. Keou FX, Belec L, Esunge PM, et al. World Health Organization clinical case definition for AIDS in Africa: an analysis of evaluations. *East Afr Med J*, 1992;69:550–553.
23. Miller WC, Thielman NM, Swai N, et al. Diagnosis and screening of HIV/AIDS using clinical criteria in Tanzanian adults. *J Acquir Immune Defic Syndr Hum Retrovirol*, 1995;9:408–414.
24. Colebunders RI, Greenberg A, Nguyen-Dinh P, et al. Evaluation of a clinical case definition of AIDS in African children. *AIDS*, 1987;1:151–153.
25. Lepage P, van de Perre P, Dabis F, et al. Evaluation and simplification of the World Health Organization clinical case definition for paediatric AIDS. *AIDS*, 1989;3:221–225.
26. Chintu C, Malek A, Nyumbu M, et al. Case definitions for paediatric AIDS: the Zambian experience. *Int J STD AIDS*, 1993;4:83–85.
27. Nelson AM, Perriens JH, Kapita B, et al. A clinical and pathological comparison of the WHO and CDC case definitions for AIDS in Kinshasa, Zaire: is passive surveillance valid? *AIDS*, 1993;7:1241–1245.
28. Nicoll A, Killewo J. AIDS surveillance in Africa. *BMJ*, 1991;303:1151–1152.
29. Greenberg AE, Coulibaly IM, Kadio A, et al. Impact of the 1994 expanded World Health Organization AIDS case definition on AIDS surveillance in university hospitals and tuberculosis centers in Cote d'Ivoire. *AIDS*, 1997;11:1867–1872.
30. Redfield RR, Wright DC, Tramont EC. The Walter Reed staging classification for HTLV-III/LAV infection. *N Engl J Med*, 1986;314:131–132.
31. Colebunders RL, Latif AS. Natural history and clinical presentation of HIV-1 infection in adults. *AIDS*, 1991;5:S103–S112.
32. Centers for Disease Control. Current trends: classification system for human T-cell lymphotropic virus type III/lymphadenopathy associated virus infections. *MMWR*, 1986;35:334–339.
33. Mayanja B, Morgan D, Ross A, et al. The burden of mucocutaneous conditions and the association with HIV-1 infection in a rural community in Uganda. *Trop Med Int Health*, 1999;4:349–354.
34. Jonsson N, Zimmerman M, Chidzonga MM, et al. Oral manifestations in 100 Zimbabwean HIV/AIDS patients referred to a specialist centre. *Cent Afr J Med*, 1998;44:31–34.
35. Arendorf TM, Bredekamp B, Cloete CA, et al. Oral manifestations of HIV infection in 600 South African patients. *J Oral Pathol Med*, 1998;27:176–179.
36. Hodgson TA. HIV-associated oral lesions: prevalence in Zambia. *Oral Dis*, 1997;3:(Suppl) 1:S46–S50.
37. Hauman CH, Thompson IO, Theunissen F, et al. Oral carriage of Candida in healthy and HIV-seropositive persons. *Oral Surg Oral Med Oral Pathol*, 1993;76:570–572.
38. Heyderman RS, Gangaidzo IT, Hakim JG, et al. Cryptococcal meningitis in human immunodeficiency

virus-infected patients in Harare, Zimbabwe. *Clin Infect Dis*, 1998;26:284–289.

39. Moosa MY, Coovadia YM. Cryptococcal meningitis in Durban, South Africa: a comparison of clinical features, laboratory findings, and outcome for human immunodeficiency virus (HIV)-positive and HIV-negative patients. *Clin Infect Dis*, 1997; 24:131–134.
40. Grant IH, Armstrong D. Fungal infections in AIDS. Cryptococcosis. *Infect Dis Clin North Am*, 1988;2:457–464.
41. Cameron ML, Bartlett JA, Gallis HA, et al. Manifestations of pulmonary cryptococcosis in patients with acquired immunodeficiency syndrome. *Rev Infect Dis*, 1991;13:64–67.
42. Miller WT Jr, Edelman JM, Miller WT. Cryptococcal pulmonary infection in patients with AIDS: radiographic appearance. *Radiology*, 1990;175:725–728.
43. Friedman EP, Miller RF, Severn A, et al. Cryptococcal pneumonia in patients with the acquired immunodeficiency syndrome. *Clin Radiol*, 1995;50:756–760.
44. Flickinger FW, Sathyanarayana, White JE, et al. Cryptococcal pneumonia occurring as an infiltrative mass simulating carcinoma in an immunocompetent host: plain film, CT, and MRI findings. *South Med J*, 1993;86:450–452.
45. Malabonga VM, Basti J, Kamholz SL. Utility of bronchoscopic sampling techniques for cryptococcal disease in AIDS. *Chest*, 1991;99:370–372.
46. Bogaerts J, Rouvroy D, Taelman H, et al. AIDS-associated cryptococcal meningitis in Rwanda (1983–1992): epidemiologic and diagnostic features. *J Infect*, 1999;39:32–37.
47. Mayanja-Kizza H, Oishi K, Mitarai S, et al. Combination therapy with fluconazole and flucytosine for cryptococcal meningitis in Ugandan patients with AIDS. *Clin Infect Dis*, 1998;26:1362–1366.
48. Heyderman RS, Gangaidzo IT, Hakim JG, et al. Cryptococcal meningitis in human immunodeficiency virus-infected patients in Harare, Zimbabwe. *Clin Infect Dis*, 1998;26:284–289.
49. Maher D, Mwandumba H. Cryptococcal meningitis in Lilongwe and Blantyre, Malawi: *J Infect*, 1994;28:59–64.
50. Koffi N, Boka JB, Anzouan-Kacou JB, et al. African histoplasmosis with ganglionic localization. Apropos of 1 case in an HIV negative patient. *Bull Soc Pathol Exot*, 1997;90:182–183.
51. Chandenier J, Goma D, Moyen G, et al. African histoplasmosis due to Histoplasma capsulatum var. duboisii: relationship with AIDS in recent Congolese cases. *Sante*, 1995;5:227–234.
52. Colebunders R, van den Abbeele K, Hauben E, et al. Histoplasma capsulatum infection in three AIDS patients living in Africa. *Scand J Infect Dis*, 1995;27:89–91.
53. Carme B, Ngaporo AI, Ngolet A, et al. Disseminated African histoplasmosis in a Congolese patient with AIDS. *J Med Vet Mycol*, 1992;30:245–248.
54. Gwanzura L, McFarland W, Alexander D, et al. Association between human immunodeficiency virus and herpes simplex virus type 2 seropositivity among male factory workers in Zimbabwe. *J Infect Dis*, 1998;177:481–484.
55. Chen CY, Ballard RC, Beck-Sague CM, et al. Human immunodeficiency virus infection and genital ulcer disease in South Africa: the herpetic connection. *Sex Transm Dis*, 2000;27: 21–29.
56. Kamali A, Nunn AJ, Mulder DW, et al. Seroprevalence and incidence of genital ulcer infections in a rural Ugandan population. *Sex Transm Infect*, 1999;75:98–102.
57. Ghebrekidan H, Ruden U, Cox S, et al. Prevalence of herpes simplex virus types 1 and 2, cytomegalovirus, and varicella-zoster virus infections in Eritrea. *J Clin Virol*, 1999;12:53–64.
58. Kạmya MR, Nsubuga P, Grant RM, et al. The high prevalence of genital herpes among patients with genital ulcer disease in Uganda. *Sex Transm Dis*, 1995;22:351–354.
59. Bagdades EK, Pillay D, Squire SB, et al. Relationship between herpes simplex virus ulceration and CD4 cell counts in patients with HIV infection. *AIDS*, 1992;6:1317–1320.
60. Tyring SK, Carlton SS, Evans T. Herpes. Atypical clinical manifestations. *Dermatol Clin*, 1998;16:783–788.
61. Van de Perre P, Bakkers E, Batungwanayo J, et al. Herpes zoster in African patients: an early manifestation of HIV infection. *Scand J Infect Dis*, 1988;20:277–282.
62. Karstaedt AS. AIDS-the Baragwanath experience. Part III. HIV infection in adults at Baragwanath Hospital. *S Afr Med J*, 1992;82:95–97.
63. Tyndall MW, Nasio J, Agoki E, et al. Herpes zoster as the initial presentation of human immunodeficiency virus type 1 infection in Kenya. *Clin Infect Dis*, 1995;21:1035–1037.
64. Naburi AE, Leppard B. Herpes zoster and HIV infection in Tanzania. *Int J STD AIDS*, 2000;11:254–256.
65. Edhonu-Elyetu Y. Significance of herpes zoster in HIV/AIDS in Kweneng district, Botswana. *East Afr Med J*, 1998;75:379–381.
66. Yedomon HG, Doango-Padonou F, Adjibi A, et al. Herpes Zoster, predictive element of human immunodeficiency virus infection (HIV). Epidemio-clinical study in Cotonou. *Bull Soc Pathol Exot*, 1993;86:87–89.

67. Belec L, Gherardi R, Georges AJ, et al. Peripheral facial paralysis and HIV infection: report of four African cases and review of the literature. *J Neurol*, 1989;236(7):411–414.
68. Cohen PR, Grossman ME. Clinical features of human immunodeficiency virus-associated disseminated herpes zoster virus infection-a review of the literature. *Clin Exp Dermatol*, 1989;14: 273–276.
69. Cohen PR, Beltrani VP, Grossman ME. Disseminated herpes zoster in patients with human immunodeficiency virus infection. *Am J Med*, 1988;84:1076–1080.
70. Mabruk MJ, Antonio M, Flint SR, et al. A simple and rapid technique for the detection of Epstein-Barr virus DNA in HIV-associated oral hairy leukoplakia biopsies. *J Oral Pathol Med*, 2000;29:118–122.
71. Triantos D, Leao JC, Porter SR, et al. Tissue distribution of Epstein-Barr virus genotypes in hosts coinfected by HIV. *AIDS*, 1998;12:2141–2146.
72. Webster-Cyriaque J, Raab-Traub N. Transcription of Epstein-Barr virus latent cycle genes in oral hairy leukoplakia. *Virology*, 1998;248: 53–65.
73. Raab-Traub N, Webster-Cyriaque J. Epstein-Barr virus infection and expression in oral lesions. *Oral Dis*, 1997;3(Suppl 1):S164–S170.
74. Reichert CM, O'Leary TJ, Levens DL, et al. Autopsy pathology in the acquired immunodeficiency syndrome. *Am J Pathol*, 1993;112: 357–382.
75. Kestelyn P. The epidemiology of CMV retinitis in Africa. *Ocul Immunol Inflamm*, 1999;7: 173–177.
76. Jaffar S, Ariyoshi K, Frith P, et al. Retinal manifestations of HIV-1 and HIV-2 infections among hospital patients in The Gambia, West Africa. *Trop Med Int Health*, 1999;4:487–492.
77. Cochereau I, Mlika-Cabanne N, Godinaud P, et al. AIDS related eye disease in Burundi, Africa. *Br J Ophthalmol*, 1999;83:339–342.
78. Soderlund C, Bratt GA, Engstrom L, et al. Surgical treatment of cytomegalovirus enterocolitis in severe human immunodeficiency virus infection. Report of eight cases. *Dis Colon Rectum*, 1994;37: 63–72.
79. Levine MS, Woldenberg R, Herlinger H, et al. Opportunistic esophagitistis in AIDS: radiographic diagnosis. *Radiology*, 1987;165:815–820.
80. Balthazar EJ, Megibow AJ, Hulnick D, et al. Cytomegalovirus esophagitistis in AIDS: radiographic features in 16 patients. *AJR Am J Roentgenol*, 1987;149: 919–923.
81. Salomon N, Perlman DC. Cytomegalovirus pneumonia. *Semin Respir Infect*, 1999;14:353–358.
82. Koffi N, Aka-Danguy E, Ngom A, et al. Prevalence of nocardiosis in an area of endemic tuberculosis. *Rev Mal Respir*, 1998;15:643–647.
83. Lucas SB, Hounnou A, Peacock C, et al. Nocardiosis in HIV-positive patients: an autopsy study in West Africa. *Tuber Lung Dis*, 1994;75:301–307.
84. Kinyanjui MG, Githui WA, Kamunyi RG, et al. Quality control in the laboratory diagnosis of tuberculosis. *East Afr Med J*, 1991;68:3–9.
85. Githui W, Kitui F, Juma ES, et al. A comparative study on the reliability of the fluorescence microscopy and Ziehl-Neelsen method in the diagnosis of pulmonary tuberculosis. *East Afr Med J*, 1993;70:263–266.
86. Walker D, McNerney R, Mwembo MK, et al. An incremental cost-effectiveness analysis of the first, second and third sputum examination in the diagnosis of pulmonary tuberculosis. *Int J Tuberc Lung Dis*, 2000;4:246–251.
87. Parry CM, Kamoto O, Harries AD, et al. The use of sputum induction for establishing a diagnosis in patients with suspected pulmonary tuberculosis in Malawi. *Tuber Lung Dis*, 1995;76:72–76.
88. Kwanjana IH, Harries AD, Hargreaves NJ, et al. Sputum-smear examination in patients with extrapulmonary tuberculosis in Malawi. *Trans R Soc Trop Med Hyg*, 2000;94:395–398.
89. Noronha D, Pallangyo KJ, Ndosi BN, et al. Radiological features of pulmonary tuberculosis in patients infected with human immunodeficiency virus. *East Afr Med J*, 1991;68:210–215.
90. Johnson JL, Nyole S, Okwera A, et al. Instability of tuberculin and Candida skin test reactivity in HIV-infected Ugandans. The Uganda-Case Western Reserve University Research Collaboration. *Am J Respir Crit Care Med*, 1998;158:1790–1796.
91. Duncan LE, Elliott AM, Hayes RJ, et al. Tuberculin sensitivity and HIV-1 status of patients attending a sexually transmitted diseases clinic in Lusaka, Zambia: a cross-sectional study. *Trans R Soc Trop Med Hyg*, 1995;89:37–40.
92. Richter C, Perenboom R, Mtoni I, et al. Clinical features of HIV-seropositive and HIV-seronegative patients with tuberculous pleural effusion in Dar es Salaam, Tanzania. *Chest*, 1994;106:1471–1475.
93. Jellis JE. Orthopaedic surgery and HIV disease in Africa. *Int Orthop*, 1996;20:253–256.
94. Corbett EL, Hay M, Churchyard GJ, et al. Mycobacterium kansasii and M. scrofulaceum isolates from HIV-negative South African gold miners: incidence, clinical significance and radiology. *Int J Tuberc Lung Dis*, 1999;3:501–507.
95. Corbett EL, Churchyard GJ, Hay M, et al. The impact of HIV infection on Mycobacterium kansasii disease in South African gold miners. *Am J Respir Crit Care Med*, 1999;160:10–14.

96. Doehring E, Reiter-Owona I, Bauer O, et al. *Toxoplasma gondii* antibodies in pregnant women and their newborns in Dar es Salaam, Tanzania. *Am J Trop Med Hyg*, 1995;52:546–548.
97. Morvan JM, Mambely R, Selekon B, et al. Toxoplasmosis at the Pasteur Institute of Bangui, Central African Republic (1996–1998): serological data. *Bull Soc Pathol Exot*, 1999;92:157–160.
98. Woldemichael T, Fontanet AL, Sahlu T, et al. Evaluation of the Eiken latex agglutination test for anti-Toxoplasma antibodies and seroprevalence of Toxoplasma infection among factory workers in Addis Ababa, Ethiopia. *Trans R Soc Trop Med Hyg*, 1998;92:401–403.
99. Guebre-Xabier M, Nurilign A, Gebre-Hiwot A, et al. Sero-epidemiological survey of *Toxoplasma gondii* infection in Ethiopia. *Ethiop Med J*, 1993;31:201–208.
100. Zumla A, Savva D, Wheeler RB, et al. Toxoplasma serology in Zambian and Ugandan patients infected with the human immunodeficiency virus. *Trans R Soc Trop Med Hyg*, 1991;85:227–229.
101. Kapita B, Colebunders R, Lusakumunu K, et al. Opportunistic parasitic diseases in Africa. Clinical aspects and diagnosis. *Ann Parasitol Hum Comp*, 1990;65(Suppl 1):45–47.
102. Lucas SB, Hounnou A, Peacock C, et al. The mortality and pathology of HIV infection in a West African city. *AIDS*, 1993;7:1569–1579.
103. Mariuz P, Bosler EM, Luft BJ. Toxoplasma pneumonia. *Semin Respir Infect*, 1997;12: 40–43.
104. Mwanza JC, Kayembe DL. Uveitis in patients with HIV infection. *Sante*, 2000;10:311–313.
105. Ramsey RG, Gean AD. Neuroimaging of AIDS. I. Central nervous system toxoplasmosis. *Neuroimaging Clin N Am*, 1997;7:171–186.
106. Makuwa M, Loemba H, Beuzit Y, et al. Intrathecal synthesis of anti-*Toxoplasma gondii* antibodies during cerebral toxoplasmosis associated with African AIDS. *Bull Soc Pathol Exot*, 1999;92:95–98.
107. Lucas SB, Hounnou A, Peacock C, et al. The mortality and pathology of HIV infection in a West African city. *AIDS*, 1993;7:1569–1579.
108. Batungwanayo J, Taelman H, Lucas S, et al. Pulmonary disease associated with the human immunodeficiency virus in Kigali, Rwanda. A fiberoptic bronchoscopic study of 111 cases of undetermined etiology. *Am J Respir Crit Care Med*, 1994;149:1591–1596.
109. Malin AS, Gwanzura LK, Klein S, et al. Pneumocystis carinii pneumonia in Zimbabwe. *Lancet*, 1995;346:1258–1261.
110. Goodgame RW. Understanding intestinal spore-forming protozoa: Cryptosporidia, Microsporidia, Isospora and Cyclospora. *Ann Intern Med*, 1996;124:429.
111. Colebunders R, Lusakumuni K, Nelson AM, et al. Persistent diarrhoea in Zairian AIDS patients: an endoscopic and histologic study. *Gut*, 1988;29:1687–1691.
112. Conlon CP, Pinching AJ, Perera CU, et al. HIV-related enteropathy in Zambia: a clinical, microbiological, and histological study. *Am J Trop Med Hyg*, 1990;42:83–88.
113. Sewankambo N, Mugerwa RD, Goodgame R, et al. Enteropathic AIDS in Uganda. An endoscopic, histological and microbiological study. *AIDS*, 1987;1:9–13.
114. Kelly P, Davies SE, Mandanda B, et al. Enteropathy in Zambians with HIV related diarrhoea: regression modeling of potential determinants of mucosal damage. *Gut*, 1997;41: 811–816.
115. Dieng T, Ndir O, Diallo S, et al. Prevalence of Cryptosporidium sp. and Isospora belli in patients with acquired immunodeficiency syndrome (AIDS) in Dakar (Senegal). *Dakar Med*, 1994;39:121–124.
116. Henry MC, De Clercq D, Lokombe B, et al. Parasitological observations of chronic diarrhoea in suspected AIDS adult patients in Kinshasa (Zaire). *Trans R Soc Trop Med Hyg*, 1986;80:309–310.
117. Drobniewski F, Kelly P, Carew A, et al. Human microsporidiosis in African AIDS patients with chronic diarrhea. *J Infect Dis*, 1995;171:515–516.
118. Garcia-Silva J, Velasco-Benito JA, Pena-Penabad C. Primary syphilis with multiple chancres and porphyria cutanea tarda in an HIV-infected patient. *Dermatology*, 1994;188:163–165.
119. Don PC, Rubinstein R, Christie S. Malignant syphilis (lues maligna) and concurrent infection with HIV. *Int J Dermatol*, 1995;34:403–407.
120. Fiumara NJ. Unusual location of condyloma lata. A case report. *Br J Vener Dis*, 1977;53:391–393.
121. Kuo IC, Kapusta MA, Rao NA. Vitritis as the primary manifestation of ocular syphilis in patients with HIV infection. *Am J Ophthalmol*, 1998;125:306–311.
122. Shalaby IA, Dunn JP, Semba RD, et al. Syphilitic uveitis in human immunodeficiency virus-infected patients. *Arch Ophthalmol*, 1997;115:469–473.
123. Becerra LI, Ksiazek SM, Savino PJ, et al. Syphilitic uveitis in human immunodeficiency virus-infected and noninfected patients. *Ophthalmology*, 1989;96: 1727–1730.
124. Passo MS, Rosenbaum JT. Ocular syphilis in patients with human immunodeficiency virus infection. *Am J Ophthalmol*, 1988;106:1–6.
125. Grimaldi LM, Luzi L, Martino GV, et al. Bilateral eighth cranial nerve neuropathy in human immunodeficiency virus infection. *J Neurol*, 1993;240:363–366.
126. Linstrom CJ, Gleich LL. Otosyphilis: diagnostic and therapeutic update. *J Otolaryngol*, 1993;22: 401–408.

127. Ronday MJ, Stilma JS, Barbe RF, et al. Aetiology of uveitis in Sierra Leone, West Africa. *Br J Ophthalmol*, 1996;80:956–961.
128. Gwanzura L, Latif A, Bassett M, et al. Syphilis serology and HIV infection in Harare, Zimbabwe. *Sex Transm Infect*, 1999;75:426–430.
129. Johnson PD, Graves SR, Stewart L, et al. Specific syphilis serological tests may become negative in HIV infection. *AIDS*, 1991;5:419–423.
130. Sitas F, Pacella-Norman R, Carrara H, et al. The spectrum of HIV-1 related cancers in South Africa. *Int J Cancer*, 2000;88:489–492.
131. Petruckevitch A, Del Amo J, Phillips AN, et al. Risk of cancer in patients with HIV disease. London African HIV/AIDS Study Group. *Int J STD AIDS*, 1999;10:38–42.
132. Amir H, Shibata HR, Kitinya JN, et al. HIV-1 associated KS in an African population. *Can J Oncol*, 1994; 4:302–306.
133. Kaaya EE, Parravicini C, Sundelin B, et al. Spindle cell ploidy and proliferation in endemic and epidemic African Kaposi's sarcoma. *Eur J Cancer*, 1992;28A:1890–1894.
134. Ng VL, McGrath MS. HIV-associated lymphomas. In: Cohen PT, Sande MA, Volbering PA, eds. *The AIDS Knowledge Base*, 3rd ed. Philadelphia: Lippincott Williams & Wilkins, 1999:831–835.
135. Kersten MJ, Klein MR, Holwerda AM, et al. Epstein-Barr virus-specific cytotoxic T cell responses in HIV-1 infection: different kinetics in patients progressing to opportunistic infection or non-Hodgkin's lymphoma. *J Clin Invest*, 1997; 99:1525–1533.
136. Levine AM. Lymphoma complicating immunodeficiency disorders. *Ann Oncol*, 1994;5(Suppl 2): 29–35.
137. Palefsky JM, Holly EA, Ralston ML, et al. Anal squamous intraepithelial lesions in HIV-positive and HIV-negative homosexual and bisexual men: prevalence and risk factors. *J Acquir Immune Defic Syndr Hum Retrovirol*, 1998;17:320–326.
138. Friedman HB, Saah AJ, Sherman ME, et al. Human papillomavirus, anal squamous intraepithelial lesions, and human immunodeficiency virus in a cohort of gay men. *J Infect Dis*, 1998;178:45–52.
139. Baken LA, Koutsky LA, Kuypers J, et al. Genital human papillomavirus infection among male and female sex partners: prevalence and type-specific concordance. *J Infect Dis*, 1995;171:429–432.
140. Palefsky J. Human papillomavirus-associated malignancies in HIV-positive men and women. *Curr Opin Oncol*, 1995;7:437–441.
141. Marrazzo JM, Koutsky LA, Stine KL, et al. Genital human papillomavirus infection in women who have sex with women. *J Infect Dis*, 1998; 178:1604–1609.
142. Serwadda D, Mugerwa RD, Sewankambo NK, et al. Slim disease: a new disease in Uganda and its association with HTLV-III infection. *Lancet*, 1985; 2:849–852.
143. Howlett WP, Njkya WM, Mmuni KA, et al. Neurological disorders in AIDS and HIV disease in the northern zone of Tanzania. *AIDS*, 1989;3:286–296.
144. Lipton SA, Gendelman HE. Seminars in medicine of the Beth Israel Hospital, Boston. Dementia associated with the acquired immunodeficiency syndrome. *N Engl J Med*, 1995;332:934–940.
145. Atkinson JH, Grant I. Natural history of neuropsychiatric manifestations of HIV disease. *Psychiatr Clin North Am*, 1994;17:17–33.
146. Sacktor NC, Bacellar H, Hoover DR, et al. Psychomotor slowing in HIV infection: a predictor of dementia, AIDS and death. *J Neurovirol*, 1996;2:404–410.
147. Maher J, Choudhri S, Halliday W, et al. AIDS dementia complex with generalized myoclonus. *Mov Disord*, 1997;12:593–597.
148. Belec L, Martin PM, Vohito MD, et al. Low prevalence of neuro-psychiatric clinical manifestations in central African patients with acquired immune deficiency syndrome. *Trans R Soc Trop Med Hyg*, 1989;83:844–866.

19

Antiretroviral Therapy in Resource-Limited Settings

Anthony Amoroso, Charles E. Davis, and Robert R. Redfield

Institute of Human Virology, University of Maryland, Baltimore, MD USA.

Over the past 15 years, clinicians in the United States and Europe have learned hard lessons about the limitations of antiretroviral chemotherapy. Prior to the use of AZT, physicians targeted intervention efforts to prevent opportunistic infection and expand access to mental health and palliative health care services. With the 1986 *Lancet* publication of the initial study of AZT monotherapy, a euphoria crept across the United States and Europe (1). In patients with advanced disease, AZT monotherapy prolonged disease-free survival. With the development and approval of zalcitabine (ddC) and didanosine (ddI), mono- and dual therapy rapidly became the standard of care. At the time few physicians or patients asked at what cost. Today, we recognize that a precious price was paid by many of these early patients. Monotherapy and dual combinations of the available nucleoside reverse transcriptase inhibitors (NRTIs)—zidovudine (ZDV), ddC, ddI, lamivudine (3TC)—resulted in drug resistance which impacted the efficacy of future treatment strategies (three-drug regimens) in these patients, as well as in others infected with these drug-resistant isolates. As a consequence, the therapeutic durability of the remarkable advancement of the 1990s may be limited to a single generation. Between 1998 and 2000, major U.S. cities had detected a significant rise, from 3.5% to 14%, in the spread of drug-resistant virus to newly HIV-infected individuals (2). Today the suboptimal use of antiretroviral drugs by both physicians and patients has set the stage for a public health crisis—an epidemic of multidrug-resistant HIV infection. For the United States and Europe, the race is on. Hindered by the occurrence of cross-class drug resistance, the future success of antiretroviral therapeutics is dependent on research, development, and approval of newer antiretroviral drugs with unique resistance mutation patterns.

The use of antiretroviral therapy (ART) continues to evolve: beginning with ZDV monotherapy and dual NRTI therapy; moving through combination triple-drug regimens such as two NRTIs and one PI (protease inhibitor), one NRTI plus one NNRTI (nonnucleoside reverse transcriptase inhibitor) plus one PI, combination PIs with an NRTI or NNRTI, two NRTIs and one NNRTI, or three NRTIs; and now using four-drug regimens, five-drug regimens, and salvage therapy. This scenario of rapid development of treatment failure is at the heart of the future use of antiretroviral drugs in Africa.

In addition, although ART causes profound suppression of HIV replication and results in improved immune function, the chance of achieving long-term control of HIV infection with ART alone seems very unlikely. Multiple studies have indicated that current antiretroviral treatments are insufficient to completely eradicate HIV from infected individuals (3–8). The data provides no evidence that amounts of residual virus decrease with time on typical ART (two NRTIs and one PI). After stopping ART, viral load can rebound to higher levels than pretreatment viral loads (9,10). Rebound rates seen after 1 to 5 years of ART are similar to those seen after short courses of therapy (9–13). Furthermore it is now clear that suppression of viral load (total plasma HIV-1 RNA) to levels below the detectable limit after 1 year of ART may be attainable in only approximately half of patients (14). Antiretroviral therapy demands stringent adherence to complex dosing regimens. The rate of virologic failure over a 6-month period has been demonstrated to be as high as 60% in patients who do not achieve greater than 95% adherence (15). Another unexpected consequence of prolonged viral suppression induced by ART is the loss of HIV-specific cell-mediated immunity. Although the clinical relevance of this observation is not completely understood, studies continue to support an association between preserved cellular immune function and improved disease outcome (16–20).

The combination of multiple adverse side effects associated with ART (21), the emergence of drug resistance, and the requirement of strict adherence for therapeutic benefit has prompted reconsideration of the current strategies for achieving the goals of HIV therapy. A rational approach to therapeutic interactions will be needed to successfully curb the HIV epidemic in Africa.

PRINCIPLES OF ANTIRETROVIRAL THERAPY

Like any new form of treatment, ART has created many clinical challenges. The best overall strategic approach to the use and management of these complicated, potent regimens is still being elucidated and will likely continue to change as more information is gained about HIV pathogenesis and host immune interactions. See Table 1 for principles of HIV therapy and Table 2 for important terminology related to ART.

The current goal of antiretroviral chemotherapy is to reduce viral load to the lowest level possible (undetectable) for as long as possible. This principle is based on the clear relationships between viral burden and disease progression, and between rate of viral replication and the development of drug resistance (22). A tremendous amount of viral replication occurs throughout the entire course of HIV infection (23,24). Detailed kinetic studies demonstrate that the viral life cycle is 1.6 days, that HIV plasma half-life is 5.6 hours, and that the half-life of an infected T-cell is 1.1 days. These kinetics indicate that 50% of an HIV-infected individual's measurable plasma viral load at any given time was produced during the previous 24 hours and that 99% of the

TABLE 1. Principles of HIV Therapy

1. Preservation of immune function
2. Reduction of HIV-related morbidity and mortality
3. Maximal and durable suppression of viral load
   a. Identify and minimize adherence barriers
   b. Use clinically proven triple combinations
   c. Avoid mono- or dual drug therapy
   d. Reduce viral load to the lowest levels possible (< 50 copies/ml)
4. Preservation of future treatment options
   a. Pre-plan sequencing of drugs
   b. Use resistance testing in selected clinical settings
   c. Avoid adding a single drug to a "failing" regimen
5. Minimization of toxicity
6. Reduction of HIV transmission

Source: Report of the NIH Panel to Define Principles of Therapy of HIV Infection. *MMWR*, 1989;47:1–41.

TABLE 2. Important Terminology Related to Antiretroviral Therapy

Latent Reservoir: Because of early establishment of infection in long-lived memory T-cells, cure of HIV has been deemed implausible with current therapy.

Undetectable virus: The threshold at which measurements of plasma HIV RNA levels (viral load) are not detectable depends on the assay used. Common thresholds are <400 copies/ml or <50 copies/ml.

Quantifying viral load: The Roche version 1.0 only detects subtype B virus, whereas version 1.5 detects subtypes A–G. The Bayer bDNA version 3.0 has been shown to detect HIV-2 and a wide diversity of the non-B subtype virus genome. All tests require freezing to −20°C prior to shipment. Obtaining a test with reliable performance for the subtypes in the region of intended use will be important. Viral loads will increase with other active infections or recent vaccinations. The standard deviation within these assays is 0.3–0.5 logs or 2–3-fold.

Virologic failure: Detectable virus after 24 weeks from initiating therapy or changing therapy indicates virologic failure. HIV RNA level greater 500 copies/ml at 12 to 16 weeks is a good predictor of failure.

Strategic treatment interruption (STI): STI is the discontinuation of ART in order to potentially boost immune response, decrease toxicities, improve adherence, or capitalize on more susceptible (wild-type) virus to overcome drug resistance. In chronically infected patients, virtually all studies have shown a rebound in viral load to pretreatment levels within 3 to 30 days regardless of how long viral suppression had occurred prior to STI, and in some cases a rapid decrease in $CD4^+$ cells has been observed. Clinical trials are ongoing.

Cyclic treatment interruptions, also referred to as "structured intermittent therapy:" These very short periods of treatment interruption, lasting 7 days, are showing promise in ongoing clinical studies. Such studies will have obvious implications on drug costs in developing countries. However, cyclic treatment interruptions are not recommended for routine clinical practice.

Immune-based therapies: Treatments involving IL-2 or therapeutic vaccines which are designed to either increase $CD4^+$ cell counts or decrease viral load.

Therapeutic vaccines: Therapeutic vaccines may be given to stimulate HIV-specific immunity. Second generation vaccines are beginning clinical trials in 2001 and have obvious immense implications in developing countries. However, none are likely to be ready for routine use in the next 3 to 4 years.

Immune Reconstitution: Immune reconstitution is the regeneration of memory and naïve T-cells in response to ART. At 6 months the impact of immune reconstitution has been demonstrated by the safety of discontinuation of prophylaxis for certain opportunistic infections (OIs), and the resolution of chronic, untreatable OIs. An associated immune reconstitution syndrome has been observed with several OIs, including tuberculosis.

Salvage therapy: Salvage therapy is used after primary treatment has failed. With the accumulation of drug resistance, the use of multiple drug regimens has had moderate success, but difficult adherence and toxicities are concerns.

Viral fitness: As HIV obtains certain genetic mutations, its ability to replicate can be diminished compared to that of wild type strain.

Resistance testing: Genotype testing measures mutations on reverse transcriptase and protease genes that are known to confer resistance to available drugs. Phenotype testing provides inhibitory concentrations. The inhibitory thresholds that define *in vivo* resistance have not yet been established. Both tests are expensive. Virtual phenotypes are also available.

viral load was produced by cells that were infected during the previous 48 to 72 hours (24,25). Successful ART typically leads to a decrease in viral load to <400 copies/ml in 12 weeks and <50 copies/ml at 16 to 24 weeks, and an increase in $CD4^+$ cell counts of about 100–200 cells/mm^3 in a year. It has been shown that $CD4^+$ cell increases are related to the degree of viral load suppression (26).

With the realization that the current antiretroviral drugs do not "cure" HIV (5–8), the clinician must view the treatment of HIV as a chronic illness (27). This approach places emphasis on the overall goal of preventing the clinical progression of disease for as long as possible, which, in turn, highlights the other primary goal of ART: durable suppression of viral load. One of the primary challenges in the treatment of HIV infection is the development of drug resistance, which is associated with clinical and immunologic relapse. It has been established that maximal viral suppression is the key to preventing the emergence of resistance (28). Continuing ART despite ongoing viral replication will allow for the accumulation of drug resistance mutations, leading to an eventual clinical decline.

CURRENT ANTIRETROVIRAL DRUGS

HIV has three viral enzymes: reverse transcriptase (RT), protease, and integrase. The currently available anti-HIV drugs have targeted the RT and protease enzymes. However, integrase inhibitors, fusion inhibitors, and coreceptor antagonists are under development. Fusion inhibitors are showing some early promise (29).

There are 15 available anti-HIV medications comprising the three classes (NRTIs, NNRTIs, and PIs), and more in the developmental pipeline. Initial monotherapy with AZT achieved a 10-fold decrease in viral load, maintainable for several weeks. Monotherapy with NNRTIs also produced similar reductions in viral load but resistance emerged within 4 to 6 weeks. Protease inhibitors have been shown to be the most potent agents as a class, reducing viral load 100-fold or more. Impressive clinical results from daily treatment with combinations of one PI and two NRTIs were evident as early as January 1996 (30). Since then, over 50 large clinical trials have shown multiple combinations of drugs to be able to suppress viral replication, improve immune function, and delay clinical deterioration (30). New clinical studies have shown such combinations can rapidly achieve viral suppression in about 90% to 95% of patients (31). Yet in general clinical practice, these combinations have an overall success rate of only about 50%, underscoring the complexity of effective ART.

Nucleoside Reverse Transcriptase Inhibitors (NRTIs)

The first five anti-HIV drugs developed were NRTIs and this class has remained the backbone of ART since 1986. There are now six available NRTIs. Each drug is an analog of a cellular nucleoside. ZDV and stavudine (d4T) are thymidine analogs. 3TC, emtricitibine (FTC) and ddC are cytosine analogs. DDI is an adenosine analog, and abacavir is a guanosine analog. The NRTIs require intracellular kinase phosphorylation to become active. Once phosphorylated, they become incorporated into proviral DNA by RT, which results in chain termination. NRTIs can also inhibit cellular DNA polymerases, particularly mitochondrial polymerase γ. It is felt that mitochondrial toxicity may explain some of the long-term side effects caused by drugs in this class (32–34). In addition, lactic acidosis with hepatic steatosis, although uncommon, is increasingly being observed, and has been linked to mitochondrial toxicity (35,36).

Two NRTIs are typically used in combination with the more potent NNRTIs or PIs for "highly active antiretroviral therapy" or HAART. However, the newest NRTI, abacavir, has outstanding potency and in combination with 3TC and ZDV had antiviral effects that were comparable to a PI-containing regimen in patients with viral loads less than 100,000 copies/ml (37). Abacavir, 3TC, and ZDV are now available combined in a single pill, Trizivir, which is dosed as 1 pill twice a day (bid), but Trizivir is not currently available at a discounted price in developing nations. Abacavir has low selectivity for mitochondrial polymerase γ, low potential for drug interaction because it is metabolized by alcohol dehydrogenase, and a low side-effect profile (38). The most clinically significant adverse effect of abacavir is a hypersensitivity reaction that occurs in about 3% to 5% of patients. The reaction has been characterized as a flu-like illness with fever, rash, and gastrointestinal side effects that usually occur within the first 6 weeks of initiation. The nonspecific nature of these symptoms can complicate the diagnosis. An accurate diagnosis is critical since hypersensitivity requires that the drug be stopped. Re-initiation of abacavir after a hypersensitivity reaction has resolved, can result in anaphylaxis and death (38,39).

Nucleotide Analogs

The newest type of reverse transcriptase inhibitors are the nucleotide analogs. The only approved nucleotide for clinical use is tenofovir (Viread). Tenofovir is a nucleoside diphosphate (nucleotide) analog of adenosine. It is a potent inhibitor of HIV replication, decreasing viral load by 1.6 log in antiretroviral naïve patients. It is a weak inhibitor of DNA polymerase gamma. Cross-resistance among other NRTIs has been recognized, and AZT- and ddI-associated mutations may confer reduction in efficacy.

Tenofovir is renally metabolized and has no known interactions with the cytochrome P-450 system. Its dosing in renal insufficiency has not yet been established. The most common reported adverse reactions have been mild gastrointestinal events such as nausea, diarrhea, and vomiting, although less than 1% of patients discontinued medication secondary to gastrointestinal intolerance. Animal toxicity data point to the potential of osteomalcia and phosphaturia. Tenofovir has been listed in pregnancy class B. Its most significant drug interaction is its ability to increase ddI levels by 44%.

At the time of writing there are no study results demonstrating tenofovir's effect on clinical progression of HIV disease. Its FDA approval was gained from strong results in salvage therapy trials (Viread Full Prescribing Information Guide. Gilead Sciences, Inc; October 2001).

Protease Inhibitors (PIs)

There are currently 6 PIs available in the United States. They all have the same mechanism of action. HIV requires active viral protease to cleave a precursor polyprotein to form mature, infectious, viral particles. Protease inhibitors act by blocking the viral protease, resulting in the production of noninfectious viral particles. PIs are the most potent inhibitors of HIV replication (40–45). The use of this class of drugs is largely responsible for reduced HIV mortality rates.

Protease inhibitors are typically combined with two NRTIs, and their success in combination therapy has led to the current focus on maximal suppression of viral load. A study of monotherapy with indinavir showed potent dose-response effects: viral load decreased by 1.5–3.1 log copies/ml in 12 to 24 weeks, showing indinavir to be one of the most potent PIs (46). Nelfinavir has dose effect up to a dose of 1000 mg three times a day (tid). Monotherapy with nelfinavir, at a dose of 750 mg tid, has been shown to reduce viral load by 1.5 log at 28 days (47). Clinical trials of amprenavir monotherapy have achieved a 2.0 log decrease in viral load at 28 days. When used in combination with 2 NRTIs, all PIs have similar 48-week response rates of about 60% in clinical trials (48,49).

Poor bioavailability remains the major limitation of the currently available PIs: oral bioavailability ranges from 4% for hard gel saquinavir to more than 70% for nelfinavir and ritonavir (40). Poor bioavailability results in short half-lives, food requirements, high pill burdens, large pills, and increased toxicities. Because of a favorable pharmacokinetic interaction between PIs, combining them is a strategy used to potentially overcome these limitations. For example, ritonavir is the most potent cytochrome P-450 inhibitor. Low-dose ritonavir (100 mg or 200 mg bid) added to a PI-containing regimen appears to have the best pharmacokinetic interaction because it inhibits cytochrome P-450 and thus allows for decreased pill burden, decreased frequency of dosing, and decreased drug costs, without significantly increasing toxicities. The newest PI, Kaletra, is lopinavir combined with 100 mg of ritonavir, given once a day. Clinical studies have demonstrated outstanding antiviral effects: more than 85% of those treated with Kaletra had their viral load reduced to less than 50 copies/ml after 36 weeks (50).

All PIs have distinct side effects. Dosed at 600 mg bid, ritonavir is the least-well tolerated PI: 50% of patients discontinue this medication due to gastrointestinal side effects (51). Attempts to manage PI's adverse side effects should not include decreasing drug dosage. Recently class-wide toxicities have been observed. PI therapy may be associated with hypertriglyceridemia, hypercholesterolemia, insulin resistance leading to diabetes, and fat redistribution syndrome (21).

Nonnucleoside Reverse Transcriptase Inhibitors (NNRTIs)

The U.S. Food and Drug Administration (FDA) approved the first NNRTI in 1996. NNRTIs have since proven to have impressive results in clinical trials and are playing an increasing role in the treatment of HIV infection. As a class, NNRTIs have excellent oral absorption, long half-lives, and are well tolerated.

NNRTIs noncompetitively inhibit RT. It is presumed that NNRTIs cause an inactivating conformational change in the RT enzyme. Because of their high selectivity for HIV-1 RT, they are not active against HIV-2, which is endemic in West Africa (52). They are highly active in vivo, but their durability is limited by the rapid emergence of resistance through single amino acid point mutations. One such mutation is the K103N substitution, which confers cross-class resistance. Thus the failure of one NNRTI typically precludes the successful use of another NNRTI. Because nevirapine monotherapy is increasingly being used or considered for perinatal prophylaxis throughout the developing world, public health authorities have raised concerns about increased NNRTI resistance. In the HIVNET 012 study of single-dose nevirapine to prevent perinatal transmission, 19% (21/111) of patients showed evidence of NNRTI resistance postpartum. K103N was the predominant mutation (53). Also of concern was the finding of transmission of a nevirapine-resistant isolate from mother to child through breastfeeding.

Although NNRTIs are all metabolized by the cytochrome P-450 enzyme system, they have different potential drug interactions due to P-450 induction (nevirapine), inhibition (delavirdine), or both (efavirenz). P-450 inhibition gives delavirdine a pharmacokinetic advantage, enhancing other PI levels when used in combination. P-450 induction by nevirapine and efavirenz may require increased dosing of PIs in some cases. Since efavirenz is both an inducer and inhibitor of the cytochrome P-450 system, it is often difficult to predict potential drug interactions. Efavirenz has been shown to decrease the indinavir area under the curve (AUC) by 31%, saquinavir AUC by 62%, amprenavir AUC by 36%, and rifabutin AUC by 38%, and can precipitate opioid withdrawal (54).

NNRTIs share common toxicities; the most frequent side effects are skin rashes and hepatotoxicity. Efavirenz, however, is commonly associated with unusual central nervous system (CNS) side effects. Toxicities are usually self-limited and occur early in the course of treatment. Unless the rash is associated with fever, vomiting, elevated liver enzymes, oral ulceration, or myalgias, it can typically be relieved with antihistamines and use of the drug can be continued. Severe cutaneous reactions, including Stevens-Johnson syndrome and toxic epidermal necrolysis, occur rarely with NNRTIs, estimated in about 0.3% of patients taking nevirapine (55).

Asymptomatic hepatitis has been known to occur in 8% to 20% of patients receiving nevirapine (56). However, awareness of the increasing potential for nevirapine hepatotoxicity is emerging. A recent South African study evaluating the NRTI, FTC, in combination with nevirapine reported a surprisingly high rate of hepatotoxicity. Seventeen percent of patients in the nevirapine group developed grade 3–4 hepatotoxicity, a condition that resulted in the deaths of

2 of the 351 patients. No clear risk factors contributing to the liver toxicities, such as hepatitis B or C coinfection, were identified (57). Two-thirds of NNRTI-related side effects occur shortly after the initiation of treatment, indicating the need to monitor liver function during the patient's first 1–3 months of therapy. Screening for liver abnormalities prior to the prescription of nevirapine is probably warranted.

Efavirenz was first approved in 1998, and in combination with ZDV and 3TC, it has been shown to be equal to, or slightly superior to the combination of ZDV, 3TC, and indinavir (58). Its excellent pharmacokinetic profile allows for once-daily dosing. The CNS side effects occur in about 50% of patients, but fewer than 3% of them have to discontinue treatment as a result of these side effects. Symptoms include disorientation, dizziness, irritability, vivid dreams, nightmares, and hallucinations. CNS side effects usually occur soon after the initiation of therapy and generally resolve after 2–4 weeks. Efavirenz is a preferred agent for initial treatment of HIV because of its excellent clinical data, limited side-effect profile, and ease of dosing.

CELL CYCLE AGENTS

Cell cycle agents, such as hydroxyurea (HU), deplete intracellular nucleotide pools. Hydroxyurea is an inhibitor of the enzyme ribonucleoside diphosphate reductase. This enzyme catalyzes the conversion of ribonucleotides to deoxyribonucleotides, an essential step in DNA synthesis. Hydroxyurea has been used for more than 30 years in the treatment of several neoplastic conditions and more recently with sickle cell anemia (59). By inhibition of ribonucleoside reductase, HU reduces the intracellular pool of deoxynucleotide triphosphates (dATP, dCTP, and dTTP), depriving cells of the triphosphate nucleotides that are needed by RT for DNA synthesis and HIV replication. DATP is depleted more extensively than any of the other nucleotides. DDI competes with dATP, thus the combination of ddI and HU has been shown to decrease the dATP pool-size by 84%. Hydroxyurea has also been shown to cause an increase in both the uptake and intracellular phosphorylation of the NRTIs to their active form (60,61).

The combination of ddI and HU *in vitro* has been shown to have a synergistic effect in resting cells as well as actively replicating lymphocytes and macrophages. *In vitro*, ddI combined with HU results in total suppression of viral production and protects lymphocytes from the cytopathic effects of viral replication, while ddI alone does not. Several clinical studies have also noted consistent and sustained viral suppression for as long as 40 weeks in HIV-infected patients receiving only HU and ddI. The combination of HU (500 mg bid) and ddI (200 mg bid) in treatment-naïve patients showed a 1.7 log reduction in viral load and a $CD4^+$ count increase of 120 cells/mm^3 (62–66).

Most of the published studies to date have linked the use of HU with ddI for obvious reasons based on *in-vitro* data. No controlled data is available using HU with more potent regimens, such as those containing NNRTIs or protease inhibitors. The clinical benefit of HU therapy remains an important research question. There are, however, concerns that HU may increase the side effects associated with ddI. There are reports of cases of fatal pancreatitis when used in combination with ddI and d4T. Additional toxicities include increased risk of persistent cytopenias, hepatotoxicity, and neuropathy. Hydroxyurea also has teratogenic properties. However, the many unique features of HU—ease of administration, rapid absorption, extensive tissue distribution, activity in different cell types, limited drug interaction, favorable resistance profile, and low cost—may create a role for HU in the design of durable treatment regimes for use in resource-limited countries.

CURRENT DRUG TREATMENT STRATEGIES

Two of the most important questions influencing HIV treatment are centered around the timing of initiating ART, and the selection of the initial regimen. These are important questions in any patient's care, but are also crucial public health questions in resource-limited countries.

When to Start: Issues to Consider

The fundamental question regarding the initiation of therapy is: at what point is the benefit of preventing immunologic damage offset by the realities of drug toxicities, development of resistance, and costs? The optimal threshold at which to initiate therapy has not yet been established. The most recent studies demonstrate a clear increase in mortality if therapy is initiated at or below a $CD4^+$ count of 200/mm^3 (67–69). The viral load at the time of initiation of therapy does not appear to predict mortality (67–69). Additional data suggests the difference in mortality between starting therapy at $CD4^+$ cell counts of 201–350/mm^3 or >350 cell/mm^3 is not significant. Complicating the matter is data showing that higher $CD4^+$ counts and lower viral loads prior to initiating therapy are associated with an increased ability to obtain and sustain virologic and immunologic response to therapy (70). To date, it is unclear how far above 200 cells/mm^3 therapy should be initiated. The decision of when to start ART may be more straightforward in resource-limited countries, because priority will have to be given to symptomatic patients with obvious immunologic damage.

The U.S. Department of Health and Human Services (DHHS) revised their guidelines on when to start ART in February 2001. Although there is no clear benefit in short-term mortality between starting therapy when a patient's $CD4^+$ cell count is between 200 and 350 cells/mm^3, the threshold of 350/mm^3 was set by the DHHS. This threshold is based on an analysis of the Multicenter AIDS Cohort Study (MACS). MACS data showed that patients with a $CD4^+$ cell count of 350/mm^3 had a 15% probability of developing an AIDS-defining illness within 1 year in the absence of treatment, unless their viral load was <20,000 copies/ml (22). Wherever possible, national guidelines should be established by individual countries with consideration of costs and the feasibility of acquiring, delivering, and monitoring ART in their respective regions (71).

The logic behind initiating therapy later, rather than earlier, in the course of illness is based on the following assumptions: (*i*) there is strong evidence that the currently available antiretroviral drugs cannot cure HIV infection; (*ii*) immune reconstitution appears to be consistent even with late initiation of treatment; (*iii*) to date, treatment trials have not demonstrated a clear short-term benefit of initiating therapy at a $CD4^+$ threshold of greater then 200/mm^3; (*iv*) there is increasing recognition of serious long-term toxicities associated with ART; and (*v*) long-term durability of treatment is dependent on extremely tight adherence in order to avoid drug resistance.

The patient must be ready for long-term daily administration of multiple drugs. Poor compliance, leading to treatment failure, may preclude further successful therapy, particularly in settings with limited availability of antiretroviral drugs.

What to Start: Issues to Consider

The first treatment intervention will likely be the most successful in achieving the maximal and most durable virologic response, as emergence of resistance may limit the success of future treatment. When choosing combinations, physicians must consider practical issues such as drug interactions, adverse effects, cross-resistance, previous drug exposures, pharmacokinetic enhancement, pill burden, food requirements, dosing complexity, likelihood of adherence, costs, and future availability of antiretroviral drugs.

The starting regimen should be a highly potent combination of three to four drugs. Certain starting regimens are strongly recommended based on demonstrated suppression of viral load and increases in $CD4^+$ cell counts for up to 48 weeks in controlled clinical trials (Tables 3, 4). Selection of the starting regimen will be heavily dependent on the cost and availability of drugs, although baseline viral load and degree of immunosuppression should also be considered. Most patients in resource-limited countries will begin treatment in advanced stages of disease because of lack of testing and available treatment. Patients in advanced stages of disease are likely to require more aggressive therapy and are at increased risk for drug toxicities.

TABLE 3. What to Start: DHHS Guidelines

Choose an NRTI combination from Column 1 PLUS one regimen from Column 2

Column 1[a]	Column 2[b]
Two NRTIs:	Efavirenz, 600 mg qhs
ZDV + 3TC,	Indinavir, 800 mg tid
ZDV + DDI,	Nelfinavir, 1250 mg bid or 750 mg tid
DDI + D4T,	Saquinavir, 400 mg bid + Ritonavir, 400 mg bid
D4T + 3TC, or	Indinavir, 800 mg bid + Ritonavir, 200 mg bid
DDI + 3TC	Lopinavir/Ritonavir, 400 mg/100 mg bid
OR	
Three NRTIs: ZDV + 3TC + ABC (Trizivir)	

[a]Combining ZDV with d4T should be avoided due to antagonism.
[b]qhs indicates at bedtime; tid, three times a day; bid, twice a day.

TABLE 4. Unacceptable Therapies (94)

- Monotherapy
- Dual therapy
- DDC + DDI
- DDC + D4T
- DDC + 3TC
- ZDV + D4T
- Saquinavir (Invirase) as the only PI
- Initial regimen involving a drug from all three classes
- D4T + DDI + HU in pregnant females
- D4T + DDI in pregnant females

Given the clinical data that shows the durable viral suppression achieved by PIs, PI-containing regimens have been the first choice for initiating ART since 1997. However, high occurrences of side effects related to PI use has increased interest in identifying effective antiretroviral drug combinations that do not contain PIs. The NNRTI, efavirenz, has once-daily dosing and side effects that can usually be tolerated. A PI-sparing regimen using efavirenz with ZDV and 3TC has been shown to be superior: 75% of patients on this regimen reached undetectable viremia compared with 60% of those receiving standard ART (1 PI and 2 NRTIs) (57). The NRTI, abacavir, has greater antiviral activity than other members of its class. The combination of abacavir, 3TC, and ZDV was shown to suppress viremia below detectable limits in 66% of patients, similar to PI-containing regimens (37). In a recent trial, efavirenz + abacavir + 3TC + ZDV suppressed viremia to undetectable levels in 96% of patients, far exceeding the results of previous PI-containing regimens. This combination was well tolerated and suppression of viremia was sustained for over 48 weeks (31). These trials suggest that regimens without PIs can be as effective as, or more effective than standard HAART using PIs.

The development of long-term treatment strategies is essential to sustain therapeutic benefit over time. It is critical to anticipate failure at the time of initiation of therapy. In a resource-poor setting, treatment choices after initial failure may be very limited. Since most antiretrovirals within a class have some degree of cross-resistance, the initial regimen should be designed in such a way that preserves the successful use of the alternative antiretrovirals available. Future treatment options may be compromised if the initial regimen is not chosen wisely. Thus, a contingency plan for an alternative regimen should be defined when selecting the initial regimen.

When to Switch: Issues to Consider

Although in various clinical trials 60% to 95% of patients may obtain viral suppression below the levels of detection, such suppression of virus in clinical practice in developed countries is actually around 50% (72). Inability to suppress viral load to an undetectable level is heavily related to the degree of compliance. Other important factors such as previous drug exposure, quality of follow-up, high baseline viral loads, low $CD4^+$ cell counts, decreased absorption, and increased drug metabolism also play a role (73–75). Thus, it is important to identify the reason for treatment failure prior to switching ART.

It should be expected that between 50% and 70% of patients receiving ART will achieve viral suppression (<50 copies/ml) by 12 to 16 weeks. A detectable viral load beyond 16 weeks or a persistent rebound in viral load after viral suppression had been achieved can be considered a virologic treatment failure. For patients on a stable regimen with viral suppression, periodic monitoring of viral load is recommended, and should be followed on the average of every 3 to 4 months in order to evaluate the effectiveness of therapy. A persistent rise in viral load that is greater than 3-fold the achieved nadir is a reasonable indication of the need to change therapy. Frequent monitoring of viral loads allows for early detection of failure and can be used to initiate an early change in therapy. This strategy is used to avoid development of multidrug resistance and to improve response to a new regimen.

Frequent monitoring of viral load may be a luxury in clinical practice in developing countries. However, consistent decreases in $CD4^+$ counts of $>30\%$ can also indicate a failing regimen. In addition, $CD4^+$ cell counts are useful in deciding when to start or stop prophylactic therapy for opportunistic infections.

In the absence of monitoring viral loads and $CD4^+$ cell counts, clinical deterioration may be the first sign of a failing regimen. Clinical deterioration will lag behind virologic failure since reduction of viral load without complete viral suppression appears to have some clinical benefit. (76–78). Most importantly, evidence from a large cohort study indicated that most new cases of AIDS-defining illnesses strike patients who are off treatment (79,80). Therefore, in resource-limited countries, the urgency of changing therapy as a result of detectable viremia in order to prevent the accumulation of resistance must be weighed against obtaining some degree of clinical benefit. Nonetheless, the sustainability of such clinical benefit in the face of viral replication is unclear. Because the effectiveness of ART is closely tied to adherence, creating a structure of tight adherence may decrease the need for close monitoring of virologic control.

What to Switch To: Issues to Consider

Along with poor adherence, drug resistance is one of the major causes of treatment failure (Table 5). If treatment failure is due to drug resistance, it is detrimental to add one additional drug to the failing regimen. A detailed history of current and past antiretroviral use is of vital importance. Patients frequently do not know which medications they have received, thus good record keeping in this regard will be important.

The 2001 U.S. DHHS guidelines recommend resistance testing when selecting new treatment regimens after virologic failure. Data support the use of resistance testing in clinical practice. The VIRADAPT (81) and GART (82) studies demonstrated an improved virologic response among patients whose therapy was changed using resistance testing compared to those whose therapy changes were based on treatment history

TABLE 5. Therapy Options after Drug Failure Considering Likelihood of Cross-Class Resistance

Drug class	Potential for drug sequencing within the class	Assumptions in the absence of genotypic data
NRTIs	Low likelihood of cross-class resistance, high chance of successful sequencing	Cross-class resistance may be due to unique multidrug-resistant mutations.
NNRTIs	High cross-class resistance, poor chance of successful sequencing	Consider failure of one drug to confer resistance to entire class.
PIs	Moderate cross-class resistance, high chance of successful sequencing	Resistance to other PIs cannot be reliably predicted by drug history alone.

alone. Although drug resistance is discussed in greater detail in chapter 20 (*this volume*), a few simple principles for the clinician are outlined here as follows: (*i*) there is no antiretroviral drug available which is free from the development of resistance; (*ii*) resistance to each drug is associated with specific genetic mutations; (*iii*) once resistance develops, it is long-lasting; (*iv*) cross-resistance within drug classes is frequent; (*v*) resistance can be evaluated by genotypic and phenotypic testing, although the sensitivity and specificity of each method remains to be established; (*vi*) if drug-resistant virus constitutes less than 10% to 20% of the circulating virus population, it may not be detected by the current resistance assays; (*vii*) resistance testing should be conducted while patients are taking antiretrovirals; (*viii*) resistance that developed to a drug that was subsequently discontinued may not be detected by resistance assays; (*ix*) the benefits of resistance testing have been demonstrated to be significant in the short term; (*x*) when testing, the presence of resistance is more useful as a guide for treatment changes than the absence of detectable resistance; and (*xi*) transmission of drug-resistant strains of HIV is well documented and is increasing (2,83).

While conducting resistance tests in a resource-poor country may be seen only as an "ideal," it may play an important role where new treatment options are limited. Early virologic failure in many cases is associated with resistance to only one drug out of the regimen (84). With the capability of doing genotypic or phenotypic testing, it may be possible to switch only the failing drugs. Without resistance data, the clinician will be obligated to change the entire regimen, an obvious challenge in a setting of limited drug options.

The widespread use of ART in settings where monitoring of viral response is limited, adherence education is poor, and the supply of medication may be interrupted, has the potential to quickly result in widescale resistance. The WHO recommends the establishment of reliable regulatory mechanisms to prevent misuse and misappropriation of antiretroviral drugs and to maximize the long-term effects of ART (71).

LIMITATIONS OF ANTIRETROVIRAL THERAPY

The widespread, publicized success and the increasing availability of ART has led to the generation of unrealistic expectations. There are many limitations to ART, particularly the development of drug resistance and failure, toxicities and drug interactions, the need for frequent monitoring of side effects and response, and most restrictive, costs and availability. Patients must be informed that ART is not a cure and that drugs will need to be taken for an indefinite period of time.

Impact of Antiretroviral Therapy on Established Infection

Antiretroviral therapy improves several immunologic parameters in chronically infected patients, irrespective of the stage of disease in which it was started. There is an increase in $CD4^+$ cells which usually follows a biphasic pattern: during the first 8 to 12 weeks of therapy, $CD4^+/CD45^{RO}$ cells (memory phenotype) increase rapidly, followed by a slower, steady regeneration of $CD4^+/CD45^{RA}$ cells (naïve phenotype) with significant peripheral expansion in almost all patients. The effect of successful ART on immune reconstitution is limited, with few exceptions, to non-HIV antigens (pathogens). The clinical importance of these events is that previously intractable opportunistic infections are controlled and prophylactic antimicrobial therapy can be suspended (85). In contrast, the impact of ART on HIV-specific immunity has been strikingly different. HIV-specific T-cell proliferative (memory) and CTL effector responses, which gradually diminish with progressive disease, are not maintained or restored with ART (19), except perhaps in very early infection. The use of ART in established infection is associated with the disappearance of HIV-specific CTL response, demonstrated by both functional assays and direct staining with HLA/peptide tetrameric complexes (86). A decrease in the HIV-specific CTL response has been observed after 3 to 6 months of successful ART (20). A decline in HIV-specific immunity might contribute to the rapid resumption of viral replication after ART is discontinued, and certainly does not facilitate efforts to promote immunologic responses that might allow for the eventual discontinuation of ART.

Toxicities

Adverse effects and toxicities are frequently encountered as a result of

TABLE 6. Major Toxicities and Side Effects Caused by Antiretroviral Drugs

Major toxicities	Antiretroviral drug(s)
Metabolic disorders: lipodystrophy, hyperlipidemia, diabetes	PIs
Anemia	ZDV
Peripheral neuropathy	DDI, D4T, DDC
Hypersensitivity reaction (life threatening)	Abacavir
Lactic acidosis (life threatening)	NRTIs
Stevens-Johnson syndrome (life threatening)	NNRTIs
Hepatic toxicity (life threatening)	Nevirapine, ritonavir, others
Pancreatitis (life threatening)	DDI
Kidney stones	Indinavir
Major side effects	**Antiretroviral drug(s)**
Nausea/diarrhea	PIs
CNS changes	Efavirenz[a]
Headache, nausea, fatigue	NRTIs
Other considerations	
Teratogenicity (in animal models), avoid during pregnancy	Efavirenz[a]

[a]Also known as Stocrin.

TABLE 7. HIV-Related Drugs with Overlapping Toxicities

Toxicity						
Bone marrow suppression	Peripheral neuropathy	Pancreatitis	Hepatoxicity	Rash	Diarrhea	Ocular effects
Cotrimoxazole	DDI	Cotrimoxazole	Delavirdine	Abacavir	DDI	DDI
Dapsone	Isoniazid	DDI	Efavirenz	Amprenavir	Nelfinavir	Ethambutol
Hydroxyurea	D4T	3TC (children)	Fluconazole	Cotrimoxazole	Ritonavir	Rifabutin
Primaquine	DDC	Pentamidine	Isoniazid	Dapsone	Lopinavir	
Pyrimethamine		D4T	Itraconazole	NNRTIs		
Rifabutin			Ketoconazole	Sulfadiazine		
Sulfadiazine			Nevirapine			
Trimetrexate			NRTIs			
ZDV			PIs			
			Rifabutin			
			Rifampin			

TABLE 8. Strategies to Improve Adherence

- Have patient commit to a negotiated treatment plan, focusing on need for life-long treatment
- Educate patient, linking poor adherence to the development of resistance
- Inform patient of potential side effects and educate on recognition/initial management of these toxicities
- Capitalize on strengths of family and community by involving family members or other social supports as adherence "partners"
- Provide culturally sensitive and appropriate educational materials (pictorials) on ART, dosing/food requirements, and toxicity recognition/management
- Provide pill boxes or similar labeled containers for storage and arrangement of medications
- Consider a home evaluation before or shortly after initiating ART to identify any potential adherence barriers
- Involve other clinic-based personnel in adherence counseling education (i.e. medication adherence counselors, HIV-clinical pharmacists, etc.)
- Avoid drug interactions with tuberculosis medications
- Postpone or interrupt ART in patients with proven difficulties with adherence
- Directly observed therapy

antiretroviral treatment, and pose significant roadblocks to the initiation and maintenance of successful ART (Tables 6, 7). Certain toxicities are common to an entire class, such as rash with NNRTI use, but there are important, distinctive, adverse effects to each individual drug that may cause serious safety concerns. Clinicians must be aware of these potential complications and have a sense of when to monitor for them. In addition, certain preexisting medical conditions may make some toxicities intolerable, as is the case with preexisting diabetes mellitus and PI-induced glucose intolerance. Complete lists of side effects can be found in package inserts.

Adherence

Poor adherence leads to the development of resistance, virologic failure, and increased morbidity and mortality (87,88) (Table 8). Paterson et al. showed that virologic failure occurred in up to 55% of patients whose adherence was as good as 90% to 95%, while failure occurred in only 22% of those whose adherence was greater than 95% (15).

The consequence of intermittent or suboptimal dosing to minimize drug costs or maximize drug supplies should be discussed at both the patient and the care provider levels. The psychosocial impact of high drug cost should also be considered. Patients may have spouses and children who also require treatment but cannot afford it. Family resources may be diverted to buy medications instead of other items needed for the well-being of the family.

SELECTION OF ANTIRETROVIRAL THERAPIES FOR USE IN AFRICA

Key factors that will influence the selection of antiretroviral agents for use in Africa include: cost, resistance threshold, drug half-life (pharmacokinetic profile), pill burden, dietary restrictions or requirements, side effects, toxicity monitoring requirements, tuberculosis drug interactions, and the ability to maintain a reliable, uninterrupted supply of drug (Table 9). Pill burden, toxicity profile, cold storage and clinical monitoring requirements are particular limitations to the use of PIs. Table 10 outlines several NRTI-, and NNRTI-based regimens that we believe should be considered as ART regimens of choice for in African settings.

Limitations of ART for Implementation in Africa

In the year 2000, most of the focus related to the use of ART in Africa has centered on the cost of the drugs themselves. Drug costs were assumed by many to be an insurmountable barrier. Yet just a year later, most of the major pharmaceutical companies agreed to reduce the cost of antiretroviral drugs for distribution in Africa by 90% or more. However, additional barriers remain. Most notable is the status of health care infrastructure in both urban and rural Africa. This includes the lack of infrastructure required to monitor for drug toxicity (complete blood count, liver function test, lipid profiles), the need to monitor therapeutic response ($CD4^+$ values) and responses to treatment (viral loads). In addition, a strong education effort will be required to attain general cultural acceptance of the regular use of daily pills. It is of critical importance that the implementation of ART in new settings be conducted in a prudent and step-wise fashion. Obstacles must be identified and corrective measures implemented and evaluated for effectiveness.

The high cost of medications may also continue to limit the ability to maintain long-term adherence, depending on the stability of the funding mechanisms in place to purchase medications. Evaluating the ability to create a successful long-term regimen will be dependent on drug cost and supply.

The following will be crucial to the introduction of ART: (*i*) long-term assurance of an adequate supply of quality manufactured drugs; (*ii*) sufficient resources to pay for treatment on a long-term basis; (*iii*) funding to train caregivers in the appropriate use of antiretrovirals and the care of patients who are taking antiretroviral medications; (*iv*) funding to establish reference labs for the monitoring of drug toxicities and viral response; and (*v*) funding to establish an infrastructure for early diagnosis, contact tracing, and prevention education.

Preventing the emergence of multidrug-resistant HIV variants must be a cornerstone of any implementation policy to provide antiretroviral drugs in resource-limited countries. If multidrug-resistant virus emerges to any significant degree, the impact of antiretroviral drugs on the course of HIV disease in Africa will be limited. It is unlikely that newer drugs with novel resistant patterns and the necessary toxicity and pharmacokinetic profiles will become available in a timely fashion for widescale use in Africa. The United States

TABLE 9.[a] Current Available Antiretrovirals

Drug	Annual costs (USD) per patient[b]		1/2-Life (hours)	Pill burden	Key side effects	Potential toxicities requiring monitoring[c]	Laboratory requirements	Resistance threshold	TB Drug interaction	Food/ storage restrictions
NRTIs	**U.S. price**	**Discounted price**								
ZDV	$3,540	$730	3.0	1 bid or 3 bid	Headache, nausea	Anemia, leukopenia, neutropenia, myopathy	Full hematology	Moderate	No	None
DDC	$2,532	NA	3.0	1 bid	Peripheral neuropathy	Pancreatitis	Amylase	Moderate	No	None
DDI	$2,316	$310	25–40	2 bid; 4qd; 1 EC qd	Peripheral neuropathy, nausea	Pancreatitis	Amylase	Low-Moderate	No	Empty stomach
3TC	$2,760	$219	12.0	1 bid	Limited	Minimal	None	High	No	None
D4T	$3,120	$55	3.5	1 bid	Peripheral neuropathy	Pancreatitis, neuropathy	Amylase	Moderate-High	No	None
Abacavir	$4,679	ND	3.3	1 bid	Hypersensitivity reaction	Hypersensitivity reaction	LFT, CPK, CBC	High	No	None
Combivir (ZDV+3TC)	$6,384	$720	3.0	1 bid	Headache	Anemia, leukopenia, neutropenia, myopathy	Full hematology	Moderate	No	None
Trizivir (ZDV+ 3TC + Abacavir)	$12,194	ND	3.0	1 bid	Hypersensitivity reaction, headache	Hypersensitivity reaction, anemia, leukopenia, neutropenia, myopathy	LFT, CPK, CBC	Moderate	No	None
Tenofovir	$3,054	ND	12–18	1 qd	GI intolerance	Osteomalacia	BSL	High	No	With food
NNRTIs						Phosphaturia				
Nevirapine	$2,976	$437	25–30	1 bid	Rash	Hepatotoxicity Hypersensitivity reaction	LFT	Low	Yes	None

Efavirenz	$2,796	$500	40–55	3 qhs	Rash, CNS	Hepatotoxicity Contraindicated during pregnancy	LFT	Low	Yes- dose at 600–800 mgs qhs	None
Delavirdine	$3960	$500	5.8	2 tid	Rash	Hepatotoxicity	LFT	Low	Yes	None
PIs										
Saquinavir (Fortovase)	$6864	$2,482	1–2	6 tid	GI intolerance	Hepatotoxicity, hyperglycemia, hyperlipidemia	LFT, BSL, lipids	Moderate	Yes- use only in combination with ritonavir	W/ large meal levels ↑ 6-fold, Cold storage.
Ritonavir	$8,016	At cost	3–5	6 bid	GI intolerance	Hepatotoxicity, hyperglycemia, hyperlipidemia	LFT, BSL, lipids, CPK, uric acid	Moderate	Yes	W/ food, Refrigerate
Indinavir	$5,400	$600	1.5	2 tid	Renal calculi	Nephrotoxicity, hepatotoxicity, hyperbilirubinemia, hyperglycemia, hyperlipidemia	Urinalysis, creatinine, LFT, BSL, lipids	Moderate	Yes-rifampin is contraindicated	On a full stomach levels ↓ 77%
Nelfinavir	$6,684	$3,467	3–5	5 bid or 3 tid	Diarrhea	Hepatotoxicity, hyperglycemia, hyperlipidemia	LFT, BSL, lipids	Moderate	Yes	W/ meal levels ↑ 2–3-fold
Amprenavir	$8,080	ND	7.1–10.6	8 bid	GI intolerance	Hepatotoxicity, hyperglycemia, hyperlipidemia	LFT, BSL, lipids	High	Yes	Avoid high fat meal, Cold storage
Lopinavir/ ritonavir	$6,500	At cost	5–6	3 bid	GI intolerance	Hepatotoxicity, hyperglycemia, hyperlipidemia	LFT, BSL, lipids	High	Yes	High fat meal ↑ AUC 48%, Cold storage

[a]NA indicates not available; ND, not discounted; bid, twice a day; qd, once a day; EC, enteric-coated; qhs, at bedtime; tid, three times a day; GI, gastrointestinal; LFT, liver function test; CPK, creatine phosphokinase; CBC, complete blood count; BSL, basic serum lytes; AUC, area under the curve.

[b]2001 estimates

[c]NRTIs can cause lactic acidosis with hepatic steatosis; rare, but life-threatening.

TABLE 10. Suggested Regimens for Use in Africa

Regimen	Advantages	Possible disadvantages
Trizivir (ZDV + 3TC + ABC)	• Simple 1 pill bid dosing • Saves Nevirapine for use in perinatal transmission programs	• Hypersensitivity reaction • Not yet discounted • Less activity if viral load > 100,000
Trizivir + Efavirenz (Stocrin)	• Simple dosing • Highly active	• CNS toxicity
Trizivir + Nevirapine	• Simple dosing • Nevirapine can be dosed 400 mg qd	• Concern of hepatic toxicity • Impact on perinatal transmission programs
Abacavir + 3TC + Efavirenz/Nevirapine	• 3-drug anti-RT regimen independent of cell cycle • Potential for once-a-day dosing	• Hypersensitivity reaction
DDI + 3TC + Efavirenz (Stocrin)/Nevirapine	• Once-a-day regimen • Saves ZDV for use in perinatal transmission programs	• Concern of hepatic toxicity/ Nevirapine
Combivir (ZDV + 3TC) + Efavirenz (Stocrin) Combivir + Nevirapine	• Simple dosing • Excellent clinical data • Simple dosing	• Expense • CNS toxicity • Concern of hepatic toxicity • Impact on perinatal transmission programs
DDI + D4T + Efavirenz (Stocrin)/Nevirapine	• Has the potential to be a qd-dosed regimen when sustained released formulation is approved • Inexpensive	• Concern of hepatic toxicity • Increased potential for drug toxicity, i.e., peripheral neuropathy, pancreatitis, and severe skin rash secondary to Nevirapine
3TC + D4T + Efavirenz (Stocrin)/Nevirapine	• Inexpensive • Potential for qd dosing	• CNS toxicity/Efavirenz • Concern of hepatic toxicity/ Nevirapine need for monitoring
Tenofovir + 3TC + Efavirenz (Stocrin)/Nevirapine	• qd dosing	• No clinical data
Tenofovir + Trizivir	• Class sparing	• No clinical data

and Europe bought into a treatment paradigm of sequential combination chemotherapy, where treatment failure was anticipated not once but several times (i.e., first failure, second failure, salvage, deep salvage). It is of critical importance that this scenario be anticipated and hopefully prevented in Africa.

Directly Observed Antiretroviral Therapy

Data in the United States continue to document the poor durability of combination ART in real-life treatment settings. Adherence appears to be the key factor. The experience in the United States and Europe confirms the limitations of self-administered antiretroviral drugs for the treatment of HIV infection. Treatment failure within the first year of ART has been reported in clinical cohort studies in Baltimore, Cleveland, and San Francisco at failure rates of 63%, 53%, and 50%, respectively (14,89,90). Similar studies in Europe reported 40% treatment failure in Amsterdam (91). Switzerland cohort studies reported 2-year treatment failure rates of 38% for patients who were antiretroviral-experienced and 20% for patients who were initially treatment-naïve (76). Results from these studies underscore the severe limitations of the currently available antiretroviral drugs to sustain viral control and provide long-term clinical benefit.

Similar problems of adherence to complex regimens have lead to the resurgence of multidrug-resistant *Mycobacterium tuberculosis* in the United States and worldwide. Multidrug resistance prevalence rates have reached as high as 36% in some eastern European countries (92). Alternative health care delivery systems were developed to provide medications under some form of supervision and to combat multidrug resistance. The most notable of these systems is directly observed therapy (DOT). This strategy, first developed in Tanzania in the 1980s, maximizes use of community health workers and volunteers to provide support and to ensure that patients take their medications. The key principle of DOT is the provision of effective, standardized treatment regimens in a supportive and patient-friendly environment, with direct observation of the treatment to maximize adherence and reduce drug resistance. Currently, over 300,000 people in Africa are being treated for tuberculosis using the DOT strategy. In the United States, widespread use of DOT has been successful in containing the multidrug-resistant tuberculosis epidemic. The WHO currently recommends DOT as the standard of care in the treatment of tuberculosis. Recently, pilot studies to evaluate DOT for the treatment of HIV reinforce the potential of this approach. After 24 weeks using DOT, Fischl et al. obtained sustained viral loads of <400 copies/ml, and <50 copies/ml in 100%, and 94% of patients, respectively (93). These rates were unmatched by intensively educated controls who self-administered ART, despite having on average lower baseline viral loads and higher $CD4^+$ cell counts at the time of therapy initiation. Unfortunately these rates have not been shown to hold up when DOT was used in treatment-experienced patients. Nonetheless, DOT appears to be the most effective way to increase adherence and sustain virologic suppression. Recent availability of once-daily dosed ART regimens will make DOT a more feasible option (Table 11).

Increasing the availability of DOT in Africa is considered key not only to curing tuberculosis cases but also to organizing community health infrastructure for the future provision of antiretroviral drugs. African countries, spending tremendous resources on HIV drugs, yet forced to deliver ART without the ability to measure virologic response, without trained adherence educators, and with a limited choice of second-line treatment options, may find DOT a highly effective and cost-efficient method of administering sustainable ART. DOT eliminates the impact of adherence on the maintenance of long-term viral suppression. Such an approach would maximize proper use of antiretroviral drugs, minimize the emergence of drug resistance,

TABLE 11. Clinically Proven Once-Daily Dosed Regimens

Clinically proven once-daily dosed ART regimens[a]	
Regimen, Dosage (reference)	% HIV RNA <400
Efavirenz,[b] 600 mg qhs DDI, 400 mg qd 3TC, 300 mg qd (85)	78
DDI, 400 mg qd FTC, 200 mg qd Efavirenz,[b] 600 mg qd (86)	>90 at 64 weeks

[a]qhs indicates at bedtime; qd, once a day.
[b]Also known as Stocrin.

maximize the ability to manage drug-related side effects, and maximize patient-specific education. If such an approach could be developed and validated to sustain viral control and provide long-term clinical benefits in a majority of patients, it might minimize the necessity to monitor $CD4^+$ cell counts and viral loads, allowing for further expansion of treatment access to more rural areas throughout Africa.

If DOT is implemented and evaluated to be a successful health care delivery model by African physicians and public health departments, its success will provide important insights for the redesign of ART delivery in the United States and Europe.

Future Directions

Clinical research efforts continue to focus on the search for new anti-HIV treatment approaches that will enhance the feasibility of sustainable ART for worldwide application. Several alternative strategies are under development. These include the use of inhibitors of cellular enzymes to potentiate nucleoside analogs (such as HU and mycophenolate mofetil); the use of cell cycle agents to maximize potency of specific antiretroviral drugs; and the development of HIV-specific therapeutic vaccines to be used in conjunction with antiretroviral medication. Each of these approaches holds potential to enhance the long-term feasibility of sustainable ART. For example, the development of an efficacious therapeutic vaccine would provide an inexpensive, easy to deliver, adherence-friendly therapy, which would also have minimal requirements for toxicity or therapeutic monitoring. Most importantly, the use of an efficacious therapeutic vaccine would not require sophisticated medical training or facilities for use, thus it would be rapidly available for broader worldwide use.

These approaches, coupled with the new development of antiretroviral agents that have a profile for worldwide use (similar to that described above for therapeutic vaccines) hold promise to enable the implementation of broader use of ART in resource-limited and resource-poor areas of the world over the next decade.

In the meantime, however, it is important to recognize and embrace antiretroviral treatment of HIV-infected people as a critical prevention strategy, which needs to be successfully implemented in Africa if the social, economic, and political consequences of the raging epidemic are to be confronted and impacted by the tools available to our common humanity. Even if an efficacious, preventive HIV vaccine were available today, the immediately catastrophic effect of the AIDS epidemic in Africa would still be unavoidable without the successful implementation of antiretroviral treatment. It is thus crucial to begin now in a measured, stepwise fashion to successfully develop and implement African strategies for the use of ART.

REFERENCES

1. Yarchoan R, Klecker RW, Weinhold KJ, et al. Administration of 3′-azido-3′-deoxythymidine, an inhibitor of HTLV-III/LAV replication, to patients with AIDS or AIDS-related complex. *Lancet*, 1986;1:575–580.
2. Simon V, Vanderhoeven J, Hurley A, et al. Prevalence of drug-resistant HIV-1 variants in newly infected individuals during 1999–2000. In: Program and abstracts of the 8th Conference on Retrovirus and Opportunistic Infections; February 4–8, 2001; Chicago, Illinois, USA. Abstract 423.
3. Cochrane J. Narrowing the gap; access to HIV treatment in developing countries. A pharmaceutical company's perspective. *J of Med Ethics*, 2000; 26:47–50.
4. Chun TW, Carruth L, Finzi D, et al. Quantification of latent tissue reservoirs and total body viral load in HIV-1 infection. *Nature*, 1997;387:183–187.
5. Chun TW, Stuyver L, Mizell SB, et al. Presence of an inducible HIV-1 latent reservoir during highly active antiretroviral therapy. *Proc Natl Acad Sci USA*, 1997;94:13193–13197.
6. Finzi D, Siliciano RF, et al. Identification of a Reservoir for HIV-1 in Patients on Highly Active Antiretroviral Therapy. *Science*, 1997;278: 1295–1300.
7. Wong JK, Richman DD, et al. Recovery of Replication-Competent HIV Despite Prolonged

Suppression of Plasma Viremia. *Science*, 1997;278: 1291–1294.

8. Chun TW, Fauci AS. Latent reservoirs of HIV: Obstacles to the eradication of virus. *Proc Natl Acad Sci U S A*, 1999;96:10958–10961.
9. Garcia F, Montserrat P, Vidal C, et al. Dynamics of viral load rebound and immunological changes after stopping effective antiretroviral therapy. *AIDS*, 1999;13:F79–F86.
10. Menno DJ, de Boer RJ, de Wolf F, et al. Overshoot of HIV-1 viremia after early discontinuation of antiretroviral treatment. *AIDS*, 1997;11:F79–F84.
11. Harrigan PR, Whaley M, Montaner JS. Rate of HIV-1 RNA rebound upon stopping antiretroviral therapy. *AIDS*, 1999;13:F59–F62.
12. Ruiz L, Martinez-Picado J, Romeu J, et al. Structured treatment interruption in chronically HIV-1 infected patients after long-term viral suppression. *AIDS*, 2000;14:397–403.
13. Davey RT Jr., Bhat N, Yoder C, et al. HIV-1 and T-cell dynamics after interruption of highly active antiretrovial therapy (HAART) in patients with a history of sustained viral suppression. *Proc Natl Acad Sci U S A*, 1999;96:15109–15114.
14. Deeks SG, Hecht FM, Swanson M, et al. HIV RNA and CD4 cell count response to protease inhibitor therapy in an urban AIDS clinic: response to both initial and salvage therapy. *AIDS*, 1999;13: F35–F43.
15. Paterson DL, Swindells S, Mohr J, et al. Adherence to protease inhibitor therapy and outcomes in patients with HIV infection. *Ann Intern Med*, 2000;133:21–30.
16. Kalams SA, Goulder PJ, Shea AK, et al. Levels of human immunodeficiency virus type 1-specific cytotoxic T-lymphocyte effector and memory responses decline after suppression of viremia with highly active antiretroviral therapy. *J Virol*, 1999; 73:6721–6728.
17. Ogg GS, Jin X, Bonhoeffer S, et al. Quantitation of HIV-1-specific cytotoxic T lymphocytes and plasma load of viral RNA. *Science*, 1998;279: 2103–2106.
18. Dalod M, Dupuis M, Deschemin JC, et al. Broad, intense anti-human immunodeficiency virus (HIV) ex vivo CD8(+) responses in HIV type 1-infected patients: comparison with anti-Epstein-Barr virus responses and changes during antiretroviral therapy. *J Virol*, 1999:73:7108–7116.
19. Ogg GS, Jin X, Bonhoeffer S, et al. Decay Kinetics of Human Immunodeficiency Virus-Specific Effector Cytotoxic T Lymphocytes after Combination Antiretroviral Therapy. *J Virol*, 1999;73:797–800.
20. Pitcher CJ, Quittner C, Peterson DM, et al. HIV-1-specific CD4 T cells are detectable in most individuals with active HIV-1 infection, but decline with prolonged viral suppression. *Nat Med*, 1999;5: 518–525.
21. Carr A, Samaras K, Burton S, et al. A syndrome of peripheral lipodystrophy, hyperlipidemia and insulin resistance in patients receiving HIV protease inhibitors. *AIDS*, 1998;12:F51–F58.
22. Mellors JW, Rinaldo CR, Gupta P, et al. Prognosis of HIV-1 infection predicted by the quantity of virus in plasma. *Science*, 1996;272:1167–1170.
23. Ho DD, Neumann AU, Perelson AS, et al. Rapid turnover of plasma virions and CD4 lymphocytes in HIV-1 infection. *Nature*, 1995;373:1236.
24. Wei X, Ghosh SK, Taylor ME, et al. Viral dynamics in human immunodeficiency virus type 1 infection. *Nature*, 1995;373:117–122.
25. Perelson AS, Neumann AU, Markowitz M, et al. HIV-1 dynamics in vivo: virion clearance rate, infected cell lifespan and viral generation time. *Science*, 1996;271:1582–1586.
26. Staszewski S, Miller V, Sabin C, et al. Determinants of sustainable CD4 lymphocyte count increases in response to antiretroviral therapy. *AIDS*, 1999; 13:951–956.
27. Chun TW, Engel D, Berrey MM, et al. Early establishment of a pool of latently infected, resting CD4(+) T-cells during primary HIV-1 infection. *Proc Natl Acad Sci USA*, 1998;95:8869–8873.
28. Kempf DJ, Rode RA, Xu Y, et al. The duration of viral suppression during PI therapy for HIV-1 infection is predicted by plasma HIV-1 RNA at the nadir. *AIDS*, 1998;12:F9–F14.
29. Lalezari J, Drucker R, Demasi R, et al. A Controlled Phase II Trial Assessing Three Doses of T-20 in Combination with Abacavir, Amprenavir, Low Dose Ritonavir and Efavirenz in Non-Nucleoside Naïve Protease Inhibitor Experienced HIV-1 Infected Adults. In: Program and Abstracts of the 8th Conference on Retrovirus and Opportunistic Infections; Feb 4–8, 2001; Chicago, Illinois, USA. Abstract LB5.
30. Tavel JA, Miller KD, Masur H. Guide to major clinical trials of antiretroviral therapy in human immunodeficiency virus-infected patients: Protease inhibitors, non-nucleoside reverse transcriptase inhibitors, and nucleotide reverse transcriptase inhibitors. *Clin Infect Dis*, 1999;28:643–676.
31. Truchis P, Force G, Welker Y, et al. An open-label study to evaluate efficacy and safety of a quadruple combination therapy without protease inhibitor (Combivir + abacavir + efavirenz) in antiretroviral therapy naïve adults (CNAF3008). In: Program and Abstracts of the XIII International AIDS Conference; July 9–14, 2001; Durban, South Africa. Abstract 3208.
32. Medina DJ, Tsai CH, Hsiung GD, et al. Comparison of mitochondrial morphology, mitochondrial DNA content, and cell viability in cultured cells treated with three anti-human immunodeficiency virus dideoxynucleosides. *Antimicrob Agents Chemother*, 1994;38:18248.

33. Brinkman K, ter Hofstede HJ, Burger DM, et al. Adverse effects of reverse transcriptase inhibitors: mitochondrial toxicity as common pathway. *AIDS*, 1998;12:1735–1744.
34. Copeland WC, Chen MS, Wang TS. Human DNA polymerases alpha and beta are able to incorporate anti-HIV deoxynucleotides into DNA. *J Biol Chem*, 1992;267:21459–21464.
35. Fortgang IS, Belitsos PC, Chaisson RE, et al. Hepatomegaly and steatosis in HIV-infected patients receiving nucleoside analog antiretroviral therapy. *Am J Gastroenterol*, 1995;90:14336.
36. Sundar K, Suarez M, Banogon PE, et al. Zidovudine-induced fatal lactic acidosis and hepatic failure in patients with acquired immunodeficiency syndrome: Report of two patients and review of the literature. *Crit Care Med*, 1997;25: 1425–1430.
37. Staszewski S, Keiser P, Gathe J, et al. Ziagen/combivir is equivalent to indinavir/combivir in antiretroviral therapy (ART) naive adults at 24 weeks (CNA3005). In: Program and abstracts of the 6th Conference on Retroviruses and Opportunistic Infections; January 31–February 4, 1999; Chicago, Illinois. Abstract 19.
38. Abacavir package insert. Research Triangle Park, NC: Glaxo Wellcome, 1998.
39. Walensky RP, Goldberg JH, Daily JP. Anaphylaxis after re-challenge with abacavir. *AIDS*, 1999;13: 999–1000.
40. Flexner C. HIV-protease inhibitors. *N Engl J Med*, 1998;338:128–192.
41. Collier A, Squires KE. Saquinavir. In: Dolin M, Masur H, Saag M, eds. *AIDS therapy*. New York: Churchill Livingstone, 1999:129–143.
42. Danner S. Ritonavir. In: Dolin M, Masur H, Saag M, eds. *AIDS therapy*. New York: Churchill Livingstone, 1999:144–159.
43. Gulick R. Indinavir. In: Dolin M, Masur H, Saag M, eds. *AIDS therapy*. New York: Churchill Livingstone, 1999:159–176.
44. Haubrich R, Havlir D. Nelfinavir. In: Dolin M, Masur H, Saag M, eds. *AIDS therapy*. New York: Churchill Livingstone, 1999:177–188.
45. Murphy R, Kilby M. Amprenavir. In: Dolin M, Masur H, Saag M, eds. *AIDS therapy*. New York: Churchill Livingstone, 1999:188–198.
46. Stein DS, Fish DG, Bilello JA, et al. A 24-week open label phase I/II evaluation of the HIV PI MK639. *AIDS*, 1996;10:485–492.
47. Markowitz M, Conant M, Hurley A, et al. A preliminary evaluation of Nelfinavir, an inhibitor of HIV-1 protease, to treat HIV infection. *J Infect Dis*, 1998;177:1523–1540.
48. Gulick R, Mellors J, Havlir D, et al. Simultaneous vs. sequential initiation of therapy with indinavir, AZT, and 3TC for HIV-1 infection: 10 week follow-up. *JAMA*, 1998;280:35–41.
49. Demeter L, Hughes M, Fischl M, et al. Predictors of virologic and clinical response to IDV + AZT + 3TC. In: Program and Abstracts of the 5th Conference on Retrovirus and Opportunistic Infections; February 1–5, 1998; Chicago, Illinois. Abstract 409.
50. Murphy RL, Brun S, Hicks C, et al. ABT-378/ ritonavir plus stavudine and lamivudine for the treatment of antiretroviral-naive adults with HIV-1 infection: 48-week results. *AIDS*, 2001;15: F1–F9.
51. Clumeck N, Colebunders B, Vandercam B, et al. Randomized comparative outcome trial of Indinavir and Ritonavir in protease naïve HIV patients with CD4 below 100 c/u. In: Program and Abstracts of the 5th Conference on Retrovirus and Opportunistic Infections; February 1–5, 1998; Chicago, Illinois, USA. Abstract 386.
52. Tantillo C, Ding J, Jacob-Milina A. Location of anti-AIDS drugs, binding sites and resistance mutations. *J Mol Biol*, 1994;243:369–387.
53. Eshleman SH, Mracna M, Guay G, et al. Selection of Nevirapine Resistance (NVPR) Mutations in Ugandan Women and Infants Receiving NVP Prophylaxis To Prevent HIV-1 Vertical Transmission (HIVNET-012). In: Program and Abstracts of the 8th Conference on Retrovirus and Opportunistic Infections; February 4–8, 2001; Chicago, Illinois. Abstract 516.
54. Fiske WD, Benedek JH, Joshi AS, et al. Summary of pharmacokinetic drug interaction studies with efavirenz. *Clin Infect Dis*, 1998;27:1008.
55. Barner A, Myers M. Neviripine and rashes. *Lancet*, 1998;35:1133.
56. Carr A, Vella S, deJong MA, et al. A controlled trial of nevirapine plus AZT versus AZT alone in p24 antigenaemic HIV-infected patients: The Dutch–Italian-Australian nevirapine study group. *AIDS*, 1996;10:635–641.
57. Van Der Horst C, Sanne I, Wakeford C, et al. Two Randomized, Controlled, Equivalence Trials of Emtricitibine (FTC) to Lamivudine (3TC). In: Program and Abstracts of the 8th Conference on Retrovirus and Opportunistic Infections; Feb 4–8, 2001; Chicago, Illinois. Abstract 18.
58. Staszewski S, Morales-Ramirez J, Tashima KT, et al. Efavirenz plus Zidovudine and Lamivudine, Efavirenz plus Indinavir, and Indinavir plus Zidovudine and Lamivudine in the Treatment of HIV-1 Infection in Adults. *N Engl J Med*, 1999;341:1865–1873.
59. Charache S, Terrin ML, Moore, RD, et al. Effect of Hydroxyurea on the Frequency of Painful Crises in Sickle Cell Anemia. *New Engl J Med*, 1995;332: 1317–1322.
60. Lori F, Malykh A, Cara A, et al. Hydroxyurea as an Inhibitor of Human Immunodeficiency Virus-type 1 Replication. *Science*, 1994;266:801–804.

61. Wen YG, Cara A, Gallo RC, et al. Low levels of deoxynucleotides in peripheral blood lymphocytes: A strategy to inhibit human immunodeficiency virus type 1 replication. *Proc Natl Acad Sci USA*, 1993;90:8925–8928.
62. Vila J, Biron F, Nugier F, et al. 1-Year follow-up of the use of hydroxycarbamide and didanosine in HIV infection. *Lancet*, 1996;348:203–204.
63. Vila J, Nugier F, Bargues G, et al. Absence of viral rebound after treatment of HIV-infected patients with didanosine and hydroxycarbamide. *Lancet*, 1997;350:636–636.
64. Zala C, Rouleau D, Montaner JS. Role of Hydroxyurea in the treatment of disease due to human immunodeficiency virus infection. *Clin Inf Dis*, 2000;30(suppl 2):S143–S150.
65. Rutschmann OT, Opravil M, Iten A, et al. A placebo-controlled trial of didanosine plus stavudine, with and without hydroxyurea for the HIV infection. *AIDS*, 1998;12:F71–F77.
66. Lori, F, Foli A, Lisziewicz J, et al. Long-term Suppression of HIV-1 by Hydroxyurea and Didanosine. *JAMA*, 1997;227:1437–1438.
67. Hogg RS, Yip B, Wood E, et al. Diminished Effectiveness of Antiretroviral Therapy among Patients Initiating Therapy with CD4+Cell Counts Below 200/mm^3. In: 8th Conference on Retrovirus and Opportunistic Infections; Feb 4–8, 2001; Chicago, Illinois. Abstract 342.
68. Kaplan J, Hanson D, Karon J, et al. Late Initiation of Antiretroviral Therapy (at CD4+Lymphocyte Count <200 Cells/mL) Is Associated with Increased Risk of Death. In: 8th Conference on Retrovirus and Opportunistic Infections; Feb 4–8, 2001; Chicago, Illinois. Abstract 520.
69. Opravil M, Ledergerber B, Furrer H, et al. Clinical Benefit of Early Initiation of HAART in Patients with Asymptomatic HIV Infection and CD4Counts >350/mm^3. In: 8th Conference on Retrovirus and Opportunistic Infections; Feb 4–8, 2001; Chicago, Illinois. Abstract LB6.
70. Sterling TR, Chaisson RE, Bartlett JG, et al. CD4+ Lymphocyte Level Is Better than HIV-1 Plasma Viral Load in Determining When To Initiate HAART. In: 8th Conference on Retrovirus and Opportunistic Infections; Feb 4–8, 2001; Chicago, Illinois. Abstract 519.
71. Safe and Effective use of antiretroviral treatments in adults with particular references to resource limited settings. In: Muneri P, Praag EV, Vella S, eds. *World Health Organization Initiative on HIV/AIDS and Sexually Transmitted Infections*. Geneva: World Health Organization, 2000.
72. Chaisson RE, Keruly JC, Moore RD. Association of initial CD4 cell count and viral load with response to highly active antiretroviral therapy. *JAMA*, 2000; 284:3128–3129.
73. Casado JL, Perez Elias MI, Antela A, et al. Predictors of long-term response to protease inhibitor therapy in a cohort of HIV-infected patients. *AIDS*, 1998;12:F131–F151.
74. Deeks SG, Hecht FM, Swanson M, et al. HIV RNA and CD4 cell count response to protease inhibitor therapy in an urban AIDS clinic: Response to both initial and salvage therapy. *AIDS*, 1999;13:F35–F43.
75. Lucas GM, Chaisson RE, Moore RD. Highly active antiretroviral therapy in a large urban clinic: Risk factors for virologic failure and adverse drug reactions. *Ann Intern Med*, 1999;131:81–87.
76. Ledergerber B, Egger M, Opravil M, et al. Clinical progression and virological failure on highly active antiretroviral therapy in HIV-1 patients: A prospective cohort study. Swiss HIV Cohort Study. *Lancet*, 1999;353:863–868.
77. Deeks SG, Wrin T, Liegler T, et al. Virologic and immunologic consequences of discontinuing combination antiretroviral-drug therapy in HIV-infected patients with detectable viremia. *New Engl J Med*, 2001;334:472–480.
78. Hammer SM, Squires KE, Hughes MD, et al. A controlled trial of two nucleoside analogs plus indinavir in persons with human immunodeficiency virus infection and CD4 cell counts of 200 per mm or less. *New Engl J Med*, 1997;337:725–733.
79. Kaufmann D, Pantaleo G, Sudre P, et al. CD4-cell count in HIV-1-infected individuals remaining viraemic with highly active antiretroviral therapy (HAART). Swiss HIV cohort study. *Lancet*, 1998; 351:723–724.
80. Egger M. Opportunistic infections in the era of HAART. In: Program and Abstracts of the XII International Conference on AIDS; June 29–July 3, 1998; Geneva, Switzerland. Abstract 78.
81. Cohen C, Hunt S, Sension M, et al. Phenotypic Resistance Testing Significantly Improves Response to Therapy: A Randomized Trial (VIRA3001). In: 7th Conference on Retrovirus and Opportunistic Infections; January 30–February 2, 2000; San Francisco, California, USA. Abstract 237.
82. Baxter JD, Mayers DL, Wentworth DN, et al. CPCRA 046 Study Team. A pilot study of the short-term effects of antiretroviral management based on plasma genotypic antiretroviral resistance testing (GART) in patients failing antiretroviral therapy. In: 6th Conference on Retroviruses and Opportunistic Infections; January 31–February 4, 1999; Chicago, Illinois, USA. Abstract LB8.
83. Little SJ, Routy JP, Daar ES, et al. Antiretroviral drug susceptibility and response to initial therapy among recently HIV-infected subjects in North America. In: Program and abstracts of the 8th Conference on Retroviruses and Opportunistic Infections; February 4–8, 2001; Chicago, Illinois, USA. Abstract 756.

84. Havlir DV, Hellmann NS, Petropoulos CJ, et al. Drug susceptibility in HIV infection after viral rebound in patients receiving indinavir-containing regimens. *JAMA*, 2000;283:229–234.
85. Furrer H, Egger M, Opravil M, et al. Discontinuation of primary prophylaxis against Pneumocystis carinii pneumonia in HIV-1-infected adults treated with combination antiretroviral therapy. Swiss HIV Cohort Study. *N Engl J Med*, 1999;340:1301–1306.
86. Altfeld M, Rosenberg ES, Shankarappa R, et al. Cellular Immune Responses and Viral Diversity in Individuals Treated during Acute and Early HIV-1 Infection. *J Exp Med*, 2001;193:169–180.
87. Carmona A, Knobel H, Guelar A, et al. Factors influencing survival in HIV-infected patients treated with HAART. In: Program and Abstracts of the XIII International AIDS Conference; July 9–14, 2000; Durban, South Africa. Abstract TuOrB417.
88. Walsh JC, Hertogs K, Gazzard B. Viral drug resistance, adherence and pharmacokinetic indices in HIV-1 infected patients on successful and failing protease inhibitor based HAART. In: Program and Abstracts of the 40th Interscience Conference of Antimicrobial Agents and Chemotherapy; September 17–20, 2000; Toronto, Canada. Abstract 699.
89. Valdez H, Lederman NM, Woolley I, et al. Human immunodeficiency virus 1 protease inhibitors in clinical practice. *Arch Intern Med*, 1999;159: 1771–1776.
90. Lucas G, Chaisson RE, Moore RD. Highly active antiretroviral therapy in a large urban clinic: risk factors for virologic failure and adverse drug reactions. *Ann Intern Med*, 1999;131:81–87.
91. Wit F, van Leeuwen R, Weverling GJ, et al. Outcome and predictors of failure of highly active antiretroviral therapy: one year follow up of a cohort of human immunodeficiency virus type 1-infected persons. *J Infect Dis*, 1999;179:790–798.
92. Espinal MA, Laszlo A, Simonsen L, et al. Global trends in resistance to antituberculosis drugs. *New Engl J Med*, 2001:344:1294–1303.
93. Fischl M, Castro J, Monroig R, et al. Impact of Directly Observed Therapy on Long-Term Outcomes in HIV Clinical Trials. In: Program and Abstracts of the 8th Conference on Retrovirus and Opportunistic Infections; Feb 4–8, 2001; Chicago, Illinois. Abstract 528.
94. United States Department of Health and Human Services and Henry J. Kaiser Family Foundation. Guidelines for the use of antiretroviral agents in HIV-infected adults and adolescents; Released February 5, 2001. HIV/AIDS Treatment Information Service web site. Available at: *http://www.hivatis.org*. Accessed October 10, 2001.

20

HIV-1 Drug Resistance

Mark A. Wainberg and Bluma G. Brenner

McGill University AIDS Centre, Lady Davis Institute–Jewish General Hospital, Montréal, Québec, Canada H3T 1E2.

The use of antiretroviral drugs (ARVs) has been minimal in Africa. However, use has been increasing recently as a result of more countries undertaking mother-to-infant chemoprophylaxis programs and of the decreases in the costs of these drugs. The use of ARVs for postexposure prophylaxis, disease treatment, and, perhaps, in vaginal microbicides is likely to increase in Africa. Most of our current knowledge of ARV use and drug resistance is based on information gathered in the United States and Europe. It is important that fundamental questions about HIV-1 resistance to ARVs also be addressed in the context of their use among candidate populations in Africa, where factors such as viral and host genetics, stage of disease diagnosis, treatment options, health care services, and compliance might introduce unforeseen differences.

The reverse transcriptase (RT) and protease (PR) enzymes of HIV-1 are important targets in antiviral chemotherapeutic strategies. A number of important molecules have been developed that antagonize the function of RT by causing chain termination of elongating strands of viral DNA. In this manner, nucleoside analogs function as competitive inhibitors of naturally occurring nucleosides for incorporation into RT-catalyzed viral DNA strands. A different family of drugs, nonnucleoside RT inhibitors (NNRTIs), act as noncompetitive inhibitors of RT by directly interacting with its active site. Finally, a family of protease inhibitors (PIs) has also been developed that blocks the activity of the viral PR enzyme by competitive inhibition. Unfortunately, resistance to each of these drugs has occurred in every instance of their use owing to a series of mutations in each of the RT and PR genes that result in altered proteins that discriminate against the binding of the antiviral compounds. These mutations are located in different regions of the viral enzymes and, in some cases, cause cross-resistance among various members of the respective families of nucleoside RT inhibitor (NRTI), NNRTI, or PI compounds. The inevitability of drug resistance to ARVs in Africa and other developing country settings makes it essential to monitor this problem carefully and to establish surveillance programs that will provide insight into the extent of drug resistance. This is an important component of public health responsiveness to the HIV epidemic.

BIOLOGIC BASIS FOR DRUG RESISTANCE

The challenges in the clinical management of HIV disease include the need to prevent or overcome HIV-1's ability to develop resistance to drugs that antagonize the function of its RT and PR enzymes. The RT of the virus has a replication error rate or mutation rate of approximately 10^{-4}, which is several orders of magnitude higher than those of cellular polymerases. This rate makes it likely that mutations will occur during each replication cycle of the 9.2 kb retroviral genome. Because mutagenesis is an ongoing process in both the viral RT and PR genes, the virus is readily able to develop resistance to single antiviral agents that are designed to interfere with its replication. However, not all mutations will produce this result. Some, such as silent mutations in which no substitution in amino acid sequence occurs, may go unnoticed, while other mutations may themselves be lethal to the virus.

Drug resistance and HIV mutagenesis can be effectively recognized under the conditions of selective pressure that are imposed by ARV treatment of an infected individual. Thus, it can be inferred that all single point mutations that aid viral survival are within the viral quasispecies in the body before treatment with ARVs is even commenced. Of course, natural selection can also be exerted by the body's immune system, resulting in mutant HIV variants whose immunologic epitopes are not recognized by neutralizing and other antibodies and/or by cytotoxic T-lymphocytes. Selective pressure creates an environment in which mutated forms of HIV can predominate the quasispecies. One implication of this is that HIV variants that contain single point mutations associated with drug resistance are only a tiny minority of the virus population in untreated patients and are unable to replicate as quickly as wild-type viruses.

REVERSE TRANSCRIPTASE INHIBITORS

The RT enzyme is responsible for the transcription of double-stranded proviral DNA from viral genomic RNA. Two families of drugs have been developed to block RT: nucleoside analogs (known as ddNTPs) that act as competitive inhibitors of RT to arrest DNA chain elongation, and the NNRTIs that act as noncompetitive antagonists of RT's activity by binding to its catalytic site.

NRTIs are administered to patients as precursor compounds that become active when phosphorylated to their triphosphate form by cellular enzymes. These NRTIs lack a 3′ hydroxyl group necessary for elongation of viral DNA. These analogs can compete effectively with naturally occurring dNTP substrates to bind to RT and to incorporate into viral DNA (1,2).

The activity of NNRTIs is less understood but has been found to involve their binding to a hydrophobic pocket located close to the catalytic site of RT (3,4). NNRTI inhibition reduces the rate of polymerization without affecting nucleotide binding or nucleotide-induced conformational change (5). NNRTIs are particularly active at template positions where the RT enzyme naturally pauses. NNRTIs do not seem to influence the competition between ddNTPs and dNTPs for insertion into the growing proviral DNA chain (6).

Both types of anti-RT drugs have been shown to diminish plasma viral burden of HIV-1–infected subjects. However, monotherapy with any drug has led to viral resistance to that drug. By contrast, patients who receive combinations of three or more drugs are less likely to develop resistance because these "drug cocktails" can suppress viral replication with much greater efficiency. Although resistance conferring mutagenesis is less likely to occur with cocktail treatment, it is not impossible. The emergence of breakthrough viruses, in fact, has been demonstrated in patients receiving highly active antiretroviral therapy (HAART) (7,8). The persistence of reservoirs of latently infected cells represents another major impediment to currently applied anti-HIV chemotherapy (9). Replication of HIV might recur once therapy is stopped or interrupted (10). In addition, the eradication of a latent reservoir of 10^5 virus-infected cells could take as long as 60 years (9).

Nucleoside Reverse Transcriptase Inhibitors

Resistance to lamivudine (3TC) develops quickly, whereas resistance to other nucleoside analogs usually appears after about 6 months of therapy. Phenotypic resistance is detected by comparing the IC_{50} (that is, the drug concentration at which viral replication is decreased 50%) of pretreatment viral isolates with those obtained after therapy. Thus, higher IC_{50} values obtained after several months of treatment reflect a loss in viral susceptibility to ARVs. Selective polymerase chain reaction (PCR) analysis of the RT genome confirms that the number of mutations associated with drug resistance increases concomitantly with increases in IC_{50} values (10).

Mutations associated with drug resistance have been reported in response to the use of any single RT inhibitor from any drug class (Table 1) (11). However, not all drugs elicit the same mutagenic response; a drug's sensitivity and resistance patterns must be considered on an individual basis. For example, patients on 3TC monotherapy may develop high-level (1000-fold) resistance within weeks, whereas they may develop only a 50- to 100-fold decrease in sensitivity to zidovudine (ZDV) after 6 months or more.

In contrast, HIV may appear to remain reasonably sensitive, even after prolonged monotherapy, to four other commonly used nucleoside analogs: didanosine (ddI), zalcitabine (ddC), stavudine (d4T), and abacavir (ABC). In the case of ZDV, increases in IC_{50} below three-fold are regarded as nonsignificant, 10- to 50-fold increases are interpreted as partial resistance, and increases above 50-fold are considered to denote high-level resistance. In addition, viral resistance to nucleoside analogs often develops independent of dosage.

Tissue-culture data have shown that HIV-1 resistance against any NRTI, NNRTI,

TABLE 1. Major Mutations that Encode HIV Resistance to Nucleoside Analogs

Amino acid			Drugs against which resistance has been demonstrated using[a]	
Position	Wild-type[b]	Mutant[b]	Viral replication assay	Cell-free RT assay
41	Met (M)	Leu (L)	AZT	
62	Ala (A)	Val (V)	AZT, ddI, ddC, d4T, ddG	AZTTP
65	Lys (K)	Arg (R)	ddC, 3TC, ddI, PMEA	ddCTP, 3TCTP, ddATP, ddITP PMEApp, AZTTP
67	Asp (D)	Asn (N)	AZT	
69	Thr (T)	Asp (D)	ddC	
70	Lys (K)	Arg (R)	AZT	
74	Leu (L)	Val (V)	ddI, ddC	ddATP, ddCTP, AZTTP
75	Val (V)	Thr (T)	d4T	
75	Val (V)	Ile (I)	AZT, ddI, ddC, d4T, ddG	AZTTP
77	Phe (F)	Leu (L)	AZT, ddI, ddC, d4T, ddG	AZTTP
89	Glu (E)	Gly (G)	Not applicable	ddGTP
116	Phe (F)	Tyr (Y)	AZT, ddI, ddC, d4T, ddG	AZTTP
151	Gln (Q)	Met (M)	AZT, ddI, ddC, d4T, ddG	AZTTP
184	Met (M)	Val/Ile (V/I)	ddI, ddC, 3TC	3TCTP
215	Thr (T)	Tyr/Phe (Y/F)	AZT	
219	Lys (K)	Gln (Q)		AZT

[a]AZT indicates azidothymidine (zidovudine); AZTTP, AZT 5′-triphosphate; ddATP, 2′,3′-dideoxyadenosine triphosphate; ddC, 2′,3′-dideoxycytidine (zalcitabine); ddCTP, ddC triphosphate; ddG, 2′,3′ dideoxyguanosine; ddGTP, ddG triphosphate; ddI, 2′,3′ dideoxyinosine (didanosine); ddITP, ddI triphosphate; d4T, 2′,3′-didehydro-3′-deoxythymidine (stavudine); PMEA, 9(2-phosphonylmethoxyethyl)adenine; PMEApp, PMEA diphosphate; 3TC, 2′,3′-dideoxy-3′-thiacytidine (lamivudine); 3TCTP, 3TC triphosphate.
[b]Three-letter and single-letter abbreviations given.

or PI can be easily demonstrated by gradually increasing the concentration of the selected drug in the tissue-culture medium (12,13). Cell lines are especially useful in this regard, since HIV replication occurs very efficiently in such hosts. Tissue-culture selection provides an effective preclinical measure of HIV mutagenesis, especially because the same resistance conferring mutations that arise in cell culture also appear clinically.

Drug-resistant variants of the virus may also be selected for (rather than induced) by pharmacologic pressure. Owing to the high turnover and mutation rate of HIV-1, the retroviral quasispecies will include defective particles and singly mutated drug-resistant variants prior to ARV therapy. Because time is required to accumulate multiple mutations within a single viral genome, multiply mutated variants appear later. In addition, these variants are not commonly found in the retroviral pool of untreated patients. Patients with advanced infection have a higher viral load and possibly a broader range of quasispecies than newly infected individuals. Such patients are often immunosuppressed and may also have diminished ability to immunologically control viral replication, which possibly leads to more rapid development of drug resistance (7,8).

Site-directed mutagenesis has shown that a variety of RT mutations encode HIV resistance to both NRTIs and NNRTIs. Crystallographic and biochemical data have demonstrated that mutations conferring resistance to NNRTIs are found in the peptide residues that make contact with these compounds within their binding pocket (3,4).

Resistance-encoding mutations to NRTIs are found in different regions of the RT enzyme, probably because of the complex, multistep process by which nucleosides become incorporated. Such mutations can decrease RT susceptibility to nucleoside analogs. A summary of prominent mutations is found in Table 1 and elsewhere (11).

Resistance to some NRTIs can also be encoded by the following five RT mutations: A62V (alanine → valine), V75I (valine → isoleucine), F77L (phenylalanine → leucine), F116Y (phenylalanine → tyrosine), and Q151M (glutamine → methionine). These mutations were observed in viral isolates from patients taking ZDV plus either ddI or ddC for more than one year. These isolates were not found to have other substitutions associated with resistance against each of ZDV, ddI, or ddC in monotherapy (7).

It has also been shown that a family of insertion and deletion mutations between codons 67 and 70 can confer resistance to a variety of NRTIs including ZDV, 3TC, ddI, ddC, and d4T. Usually, the insertion and deletion mutations occurring within this range of codons confer multidrug resistance in a ZDV-resistant background.

Nonnucleoside Reverse Transcriptase Inhibitors

Diminished sensitivity to NNRTIs appears quickly both in culture selection protocols and in patients (6,14–16). NNRTIs share a common binding site, and mutations that encode NNRTI resistance are located within the binding pocket that makes drug contact (3,4,6–17). This explains data showing extensive cross-resistance among all currently approved NNRTIs, although synergy among NNRTIs has occasionally been reported (17,18).

A substitution at codon 181 (Y181C; tyrosine → cysteine) is a common mutation that encodes cross-resistance among many NNRTIs (14,19,20). Replacement of Y181 by a serine or a histidine also confers HIV resistance to NNRTIs (21). This residue is located on the floor of the NNRTI binding pocket.

A mutation at codon 236 (P236L; proline → leucine), which confers resistance to a class of NNRTIs [such as bis-heteroarylpiperazine (BHAP) compounds like delavirdine], can diminish resistance to thiobenzimidazolone (TIBO), nevirapine, and pyridinones that are encoded by Y181C, if both mutations are present in the same virus (22).

A substitution at codon 188 (Y188H; tyrosine → histidine) confers resistance to TIBO and pyridinone, while replacement of tyrosine by cysteine (Y188C) encodes resistance to TIBO, pyridinone, and nevirapine (19,21,22). Thus, nevirapine apparently interacts with RT through different mechanisms.

A mutation at codon 103 (K103N; lysine → asparagine) is another common substitution that encodes resistance to almost all classes of NNRTIs (14,19,20). The amino acid K103 is located on the β5-β6 connecting loop, distant from the polymerase active site of the enzyme (23,24). The RT crystal structure positions the side chain of K103 as pointing out at the entrance of the NNRTI binding pocket, thus enabling drug contact to occur. The K103N substitution alters interactions between NNRTIs and RT. This mutation shows synergy with Y181C for resistance to NNRTIs (25). A mutation at codon 138 (E138K; glutamic acid → lysine) confers resistance only to some NNRTIs (20,26) owing to changes that affect the p51 rather than the p66 subunit.

Resistance to NNRTIs is also observed in cell-free enzyme assays (19,21,27,28). Both Y181I (tyrosine → isoleucine) and Y188L (tyrosine → leucine) mediated decreased sensitivity to NNRTIs without affecting either substrate recognition or catalytic efficiency. This corroborates the theory that resistance to NNRTIs is attributable to the diminished ability of these drugs to be bound by RT. A mutation at L100I caused a 15-fold decrease in sensitivity to pyridinone derivatives and a two-fold increase in IC_{95} in tissue-culture studies. However, L101E (leucine → glutamic acid) had only a minimal effect on RT in cell-free assays in regard to sensitivity to pyridinones but showed a 10-fold increase in IC_{95} in tissue culture (19). Therefore, a variety of factors contribute directly or indirectly to interactions between NNRTIs and RT.

PROTEASE INHIBITORS

Drug-resistant viruses have been observed for all PIs developed to date (29). In addition, some strains of HIV have displayed cross-resistance to a variety of PIs after either clinical use or in-vitro drug exposure (29). In general, the patterns of mutations observed with PIs are more complex than those observed with RT antagonists. First, a greater number of mutations within the PR gene are involved. This also involves greater variability in temporal patterns of appearance of different mutations and in the manner in which different combinations of mutations give rise to phenotypic resistance. These data suggest that PR can adapt more easily than RT to pressures exerted by antiviral drugs. At least 40 mutations in PR have been identified as responsible for resistance to PIs (29).

Certain mutations within the PR genes are more important than others and can confer resistance, virtually on their own, to certain PIs (29). One mutation, D30N (aspartic acid → asparagine), is probably specific to nelfinavir, a potent anti-PR drug. However, a variety of other mutations may confer cross-resistance among multiple drugs within the PI family. In addition, a wide assortment of secondary mutations has been observed. When combined with primary mutations, these secondary mutations can cause increased levels of resistance. On the other hand, the singular presence of certain secondary mutations may not lead to drug resistance, and, in this context, certain amino acid changes should be considered to represent naturally occurring polymorphisms. It should also be noted that resistance to PIs can result from mutations within the substrates of the PR enzyme, the *gag* and *gag-pol* precursor proteins of HIV. Various studies have shown that mutations at cleavage sites within these substrates can be responsible for drug resistance, both in tissue culture as well as in clinical analyses (29). However, the full clinical significance of cleavage site mutations to PR resistance is not yet understood.

At present, HIV therapeutics is faced with the question of how to treat patients who have failed multiple PI-containing regimens because of PI cross-resistance (30). It is hoped that certain newer PIs, including ABT-378, may not be as susceptible to this sort of failure (31,32). Indeed, there is now abundant data to suggest that viral strains that are resistant to all previously developed PIs may remain susceptible to ABT-378 as well as to other, newer drugs of this class. An additional breakthrough has come through the understanding that combinations of ritonavir (RTV) with either indinavir (IDV) or saquinavir (SQV) can result in significantly elevated drug levels of the latter compounds (33,34). In this context, viral strains that may initially display resistance to IDV, SQV, or both because of cross-resistance at low plasma concentrations may revert to full sensitivity when plasma concentrations are elevated through combination with RTV. These effects are attributable to the fact that the latter compound is an effective antagonist of cytochrome P450 metabolic pathways, activity that can serve to delay the clearance of coadministered IDV or SQV from the blood (34).

TECHNIQUES FOR DETERMINING HIV'S RESISTANCE TO ANTIRETROVIRALS

The emergence of resistance to ARVs can be demonstrated by assays of viral genotype or phenotype. Genotypic assays for drug resistance determine the nucleotide sequence of genes encoding the RT and PR enzymes so as to identify specific amino acid changes that confer resistance to particular ARVs or cross-resistance to NRTIs, NNRTIs, or PIs (11,19,29). Genotyping involves amplification of RT and PR genes from reverse-transcribed plasma viral RNA or PCR-amplified proviral DNA. Direct sequencing is then performed using any of a number of automated systems. Alternately, hybridization-based assays can simultaneously probe for a limited number of wild-type codons or for point mutations conferring resistance to NRTIs (ZDV, 3TC, ddI) or PIs (35).

Phenotypic assays monitor the cumulative effects of resistance mutations on susceptibility of viral quasispecies to a given concentration of varying ARV drug (12,13). The conventional phenotypic assay monitors the replicative properties of viral isolates in the presence of increasing concentrations of drug. Phenotypic drug susceptibility is defined as the concentration of drug that inhibits viral production, that is, either RT activity or p24 antigen, by 50% (IC_{50}) or 90% (IC_{90}). Phenotypic resistance can also be expressed in the context of drug toxicity monitored by cell viability, known as the $TCID_{50}$ values, which gives a therapeutic index that is the ratio of $IC_{50}/TCID_{50}$. Direct phenotyping, while highly reflective of emerging drug resistance, requires the initial preparation of high-titer viral stocks that require 4 to 8 weeks of coculture of virus with peripheral blood mononuclear cells activated with phytohemagglutinin (PHA).

However, phenotypic recombinant assays provide a more rapid (2 week) approach to assess drug susceptibility. PR and RT sequences are amplified from plasma viral RNA by PCR and are inserted into viral vectors that contain indicator genes such as luciferase. Vectors are transfected into host cell lines to monitor luciferase activity in the presence and absence of ARVs.

Genotypic and phenotypic resistance assays provide complementary information (36). Genotypic assays rapidly detect all mutations in RT and PR that occur prior to the onset of phenotypic resistance. Phenotypic assays assess the combined effects of accumulated mutations on drug response. However, phenotypic assays are less accessible, time-consuming, and expensive. To offset these problems, "virtual phenotyping" of sequences generated by automated genotyping has been introduced. This technique can predict phenotypic susceptibility by using databases that correlate viral sequence to expected phenotype.

Drug-resistance testing enhances clinical decision making power. Indeed, several randomized trials have shown genotypic testing to be of significant benefit in improving virologic suppression (37–38). Resistance testing can provide information useful in selecting an initial ARV regimen, changing a regimen in treatment failure, verifying patient adherence to regimens, ensuring adequate drug potency, and identifying salvage treatment strategies.

TRANSMISSION OF DRUG-RESISTANT VARIANTS OF HIV-1

The widespread use of ARV agents has led to an increase in the transmission of drug-resistant viruses to previously uninfected individuals. Four primary HIV-1 infection cohorts in Geneva, New York, Montreal, and San Diego, California, have shown transmission of at least one resistant variant in 20% to 25% of newly infected individuals (39–42). As reflected in the Montreal cohort (n = 105), transmission of viral strains resistant to at least one drug was present in 5.7% of new cases. Single-class cross-resistance to NRTIs, NNRTIs, or PIs occurred in 8.5% of new cases, while dual- or triple-class multidrug resistance (MDR) was noted in 8.5% of new cases. Early reports suggest that newly infected individuals may not respond to drugs for which they harbor resistance (41–43). Recent studies in our laboratory show the MDR variants transmitted in primary infection represent the predominant quasispecies that can persist for at least 1 year in the presence or absence of ARV treatment (unpublished results). In the absence of archival wild-type viruses, MDR primary infections may have long-term treatment consequences. Similarly, vertical transmission of ZDV resistance after monotherapy showed the emergence of ZDV-resistant variants in 7% to 29% of pregnant mothers and in 5% to 21% of newly infected infants (44).

HIV-1 SUBTYPES AND DRUG RESISTANCE

Whereas combination chemotherapy has stabilized rates of clade B infections present in North America and Europe, worldwide epidemics with HIV-1 group M (non-B, A through J) and O clades are expanding. The epicenters of HIV-1 infection are currently in Africa (69% of new infections comprise clades C, A, D, G, and O) and Southeast Asia (19% of new infections comprise clade E and C). Particularly troublesome are escalating rates of clade C infections (48% of new HIV-1 infections). However, most of our knowledge of drug resistance is limited to the clade B model. Although there are overall similarities in the genomic arrangement of all HIV-1 subtypes, RT regions of African isolates show 9.3% to 20.1% divergence from clade B with 3.8% to 5.8% intraclade divergence (45,46).

Early studies show that clade diversity leads to altered drug susceptibility of nonclade B isolates. HIV-1 group O and simian immunodeficiency virus have been shown to be intrinsically resistant to all NNRTIs owing to the presence of amino acids 181C and 181I in wild-type RTs (47). Similarly, clades F and C may display impaired susceptibility to NNRTIs (48). In addition to genotypic diversity in the RT and PR regions, viral subtypes may differ in promotor regions that affect transcriptional regulation of replication, which is important in drug response. For example, subtype C long terminal repeat regions (LTRs) have three to four NF-κB sites, subtype B LTRs have two NF-κB sites, and subtype E LTRs have just one such site (49). Recently, it has been reported that non-B subtypes were statistically associated with more rapid progression to resistance after HAART treatment (50).

SURVEILLANCE OF RESISTANCE TESTING

Because HIV drug resistance is a growing and worldwide problem, it is essential to establish facilities and laboratories to monitor this issue, particularly in developing countries. This will require that laboratories are built wherever appropriate and that trained personnel are hired to carry out programs related to resistance testing. Of course, it also follows that the standard of care of triple-drug therapy should be applied as broadly as possible in both developed and developing countries. This is key toward minimizing the extent to which drug resistance will be likely to occur.

In addition to establishing regional laboratory infrastructure, it is necessary to educate physicians, patients, drug dispensers, health ministry employees, and others about the problem of HIV drug resistance (51). This need will become more clear should resistance begin to be found following use of antiretroviral therapy to prevent mother-to-infant transmission of HIV-1.

The issue of simplifying drug regimens in developing countries is also important. It is vital that adherence be maximized to prevent the development of resistance, and it is likewise essential for both patients and clinicians to understand that full adherence is required to maintain high drug levels as a means to minimize viral replication and the occurrence of resistance (51). It follows as well, that cost–benefit research is needed to counter the assumption that use of a two-drug regimen is less expensive than use of a three-drug regimen. This assumption is not necessarily true since the development of resistance is a consequence of long-term use of substandard antiretroviral therapy. It also follows that research into the clinical benefits for individuals as well as populations as a whole is essential. This can be carried out, at least in part, through mathematical modeling. Clearly, if resistance becomes a major problem among individuals on substandard therapeutic regimens, the consequences for populations may become devastating. Accordingly, budgets for treatment should include resistance testing for patients from the outset of their treatment regimens. Long-term follow-up should be included wherever short-term interventions are planned in these efforts and should include international organizations and pharmaceutical companies as well as local and national governments.

It will be essential to perform resistance testing on-site and to determine the extent to which resistance may have occurred in untreated individuals in different countries and, wherever possible, in individuals undergoing primary infection. The implementation of resistance testing will require appropriate quality assurance programs as well as essential data management at the local level. This implies that regional infrastructure must support both HIV awareness and education at the local level. These initiatives should take into account the need to monitor polymorphisms as well as the treatment-related incidence of resistance conferring mutations. It should be emphasized that these infrastructures will benefit future intervention and prevention programs, such as those associated with use of anti-HIV vaccines. However, at the same time, adequate budgets will be required to provide for such things as sample storage and freezer space.

Physicians will need to be taught the consequences of drug resistance as well as how to interpret polymorphisms and the primary mutations associated with drug resistance. Patients will need to understand the importance of optimal treatment and adherence. Research into culture-related adherence issues is urgently needed. Regional and national public health policy decision makers need to be provided with the data necessary to implement these recommendations.

CONCLUSION

These issues also impact the question of postexposure prophylaxis in the occupational setting; resistance considerations in this context should not be ignored. One special subject, widely practiced at this time, is the use of drugs to prevent mother-to-infant transmission of HIV-1. Clearly, there is a need to balance the benefits of prevention of such transmission against the potential for development of resistant strains by use of single antiretroviral agents such as nevirapine. In addition, the simplicity of any given regimen needs to be balanced against the likelihood that resistance may occur. The importance of HIV drug resistance also needs to be considered in relation to its potential pathogenetic impact on other infectious diseases such as tuberculosis.

Thus, there are now compelling reasons for the introduction of widespread resistance testing wherever ARVs are being used. The introduction of resistance testing must be accompanied by local capacity building and must reflect regional considerations such as the nature of viral subtypes prevalent in any given geographic locale.

REFERENCES

1. Furman PA, Fyfe JA, St Clair MH, et al. Phosphorylation of 3′-azido-3' deoxythymidine and selective interactions of the 5′-triphosphate with human immunodeficiency virus reverse transcriptase. *Proc Natl Acad Sci USA*, 1986;83:8333–8337.
2. Hart GJ, Orr DC, Penn CR, et al. Effects of (-) 2′-deoxy-3′-thiacytidine (3TC) 5′-triphosphate on human immunodeficiency virus reverse transcriptase and mammalian DNA polymerases alpha, beta and gamma. *Antimicrob Agents Chemother*, 1992;37:918–920.
3. Ding J, Das K, Moereels H, et al. Structure of HIV-1 RT/TIBO R 86183 complex reveals similarity in the binding of diverse non-nucleoside inhibitors. *Nature Struct Biology*, 1995;2:407–415.
4. Wu JC, Warren TC, Adams J, et al. A novel dipyridodiazepinone inhibitor of HIV-1 reverse transcriptase acts through a nonsubstrate binding site. *Biochemistry*, 1991;30:2022–2026.
5. Spence RA, Kati WM, Anderson KS, et al. Mechanism of inhibition of HIV-1 reverse transcriptase by non-nucleoside inhibitors. *Science*, 1995; 267:988–992.
6. Gu Z, Quan Y, Li Z, et al. Effects of non-nucleoside inhibitors of human immunodeficiency virus type 1 in cell-free recombinant reverse transcriptase assays. *J Biol Chem*, 1995;270:31046–31051.
7. Gunthard HF, Wong JK, Ignacio CC, et al. Human immunodeficiency virus replication and genotypic resistance in blood and lymph nodes after a year of potent antiretroviral therapy. *J Virol*, 1998;72:2422–2428.
8. Palmer S, Shafer RW, Merigan TC. Highly drug-resistant HIV-1 clinical isolates are cross-resistant to many antiretroviral compounds in current clinical development. *AIDS*, 1999;13:661–7.
9. Finzi, D, Blankson J, Siliciano JD, et al. Latent infection of CD4+ T cells provides a mechanism for lifelong persistence of HIV-1, even in patients on effective combination therapy. *Nature Medicine*, 1997;5:512–517.
10. Wong, JK, Hezareh M, Gunthard HF, et al. Recovery of replication-competent HIV despite prolonged suppression of plasma viremia. *Science*, 1997;278(5431):1291–1295.
11. Schinazi R, Larder B, Mellors J. Mutations in retroviral genes associated in drug resistance. *Intl Antiviral News*, 1997;5:129–142.
12. DAIDS Virology Manual for HIV Laboratories: National Institute for Allergy and Infectious Disease, January 1997.
13. Japour AJ, Mayers DL, Johnson VA, et al. A standardized peripheral mononuclear assay for determination of drug susceptibilities of clinical human immunodeficiency virus type 1 isolates. *Antimicrob Agents Chemother*, 1993;37:1095–1101.
14. Richman D, Shih CK, Lowy I, et al. Human immunodeficiency virus type 1 mutants resistant to non-nucleoside inhibitors of reverse transcriptase arise in cell culture. *Proc Natl Acad Sci USA*, 1991; 88:11241–11245.
15. Vandamme AM, Debyser Z, Pauwels R, et al. Characterization of HIV-1 strains isolated from patients treated with TIBO R82913. *AIDS Res Hum Retroviruses*, 1994;10:39–46.
16. Chong KT, Pagano PJ, Hinshaw RR. Bisheteroarylpiperazine reverse transcriptase inhibitor in combination with 3′-azido-3′-deoxythymidine or 2',3′-dideoxycytidine synergistically inhibits human immunodeficiency virus type 1 replication in vitro. *Antimicrob Agents Chemother*, 1994;38:288–293.
17. Esnouf R, Ren J, Ross C, et al. Mechanism of inhibition of HIV-1 reverse transcriptase by non-nucleoside inhibitors. *Nature Struct Biol*, 1995;2:303–308.
18. Fletcher RS, Arion D, Borkow G, et al. Synergistic inhibition of HIV-1 reverse transcriptase DNA polymerase activity and virus replication in vitro by combinations of carboxanilide non-nucleoside compounds. *Biochemistry*, 1995;34:10106–10112.
19. Byrnes VW, Sardana VV, Schleif WA, et al. Comprehensive mutant enzyme and viral variant assessment of human immunodeficiency virus type 1 reverse transcriptase resistance to non-nucleoside inhibitors. *Antimicrob Agents Chemother*, 1993; 37:1576–1579.
20. Balzarini J, Karlsson A, Perez-Perez MJ, et al. Treatment of human immunodeficiency virus type 1

(HIV-1)-infected cells with combinations of HIV-1–specific inhibitors results in different resistance pattern than does treatment with single-drug therapy. *J Virol,* 1993;67:5353–5359.
21. Sardana VV, Emini EA, Gotlib L, et al. Functional analysis of HIV-1 reverse transcriptase amino acids involved in resistance to multiple non-nucleoside inhibitors. *J Biol Chem,* 1992;267:17526–17530.
22. Dueweke TJ, Pushkarskaya T, Poppe SM, et al. A mutation in reverse transcriptase of bis(hetroaryl1) piperazine-resistant human immunodeficiency virus type 1 that confers increased sensitivity to other non-nucleoside inhibitors. *Proc Natl Acad Sci USA,* 1993;90:4713–4717.
23. Jacobo-Molina A, Ding J, Nanni RG, et al. Crystal structure of human immunodeficiency virus type 1 reverse transcriptase complexed with double-stranded DNA at 3.0 Å resolution shows bent DNA. *Proc Natl Acad Sci USA,* 1993;90:6320–6324.
24. Kolstaedt LA, Wang J, Friedman JM, et al. Crystal structure at 3.5 Å resolution of HIV-1 reverse transcriptase complexed with an inhibitor. *Science,* 1992;256:1783–1790.
25. Nunberg JH, Schleif WA, Boots EJ, et al. Viral resistance to human immunodeficiency virus type 1–specific pyridinone reverse transcriptase inhibitors. *J Virol,* 1991;65:4887–4892.
26. Jonckheere H, Taymans JM, Balzarini J, et al. Resistance of HIV-1 reverse transcriptase against [2′,5′-bis-O-(tert-butyldimethylsilyl-3′-spiro5″-(4″amino-1″,2″-oxathiole-2″,2″-dioxide)] (TSAO) derivatives is determined by the mutation Glu138 (Lys on the p51 subunit. *J Biol Chem,* 1994;269: 25255–25258.
27. Loya S, Bakhanashvili M, Tal R, et al. Enzymatic properties of two mutants of reverse transcriptase of human immunodeficiency virus type 1 (tyrosine 181(isoleucine and tyrosine 188(leucine), resistant to nonnucleoside inhibitors. *AIDS Res Hum Retroviruses,* 1994;10:939–946.
28. Boyer PL, Currens MJ, McMahon JB, et al. Analysis of non-nucleoside drug-resistance variants of human immunodeficiency virus type 1 reverse transcriptase. *J Virol,* 1993;67:2412–2420.
29. Condra J. Virologic and clinical implications of resistance to HIV-1 protease inhibitors. *Drug Resistance Updates,* 1998;1:292–299.
30. Deeks SG. Failure of HIV-1 protease inhibitors to fully suppress viral replication. Implications for salvage therapy. *Adv Exptl Med Biol,* 1999;458: 175–182.
31. Murphy RI. New antiretroviral drugs part I: PIs. *AIDS Clin Care,* 1999;11:35–37.
32. Sham HL, Kempf DJ, Molla A, et al. ABT-378, a highly potent inhibitor of human immunodeficiency virus protease. *Antimicrob Agents Chemother,* 1998;42:3218–3224.
33. Parades R, Puig T, Amo A, et al. High-dose saquinavir plus ritonavir: long-term efficacy in HIV-positive protease inhibitor-experienced patients and predictors of virologic response. *J AIDS,* 1999;22:132–138.
34. Reiser M, Salzberger B, Steipel A, et al. Virological efficacy and plasma drug concentrations of nelfinavir plus saquinavir as salvage therapy in HIV-infected patients refractory to standard triple therapy. *Eur J Med Res,* 1999;4:54–58.
35. Stuyver L, Wyseur A, Rombout A, et al. Line probe assay for rapid detection of drug-selected mutations in the human immunodeficiency virus type 1 reverse transcriptase gene. *Antimicrob Agents Chemother,* 1997;4:284–291.
36. Merigan T. Viral resistance testing: practical issues and future opportunities. *AIDS Treat News,* 1999;316:1–6.
37. Durant J, Clevenbergh P, Halfon P, et al. Drug resistance genotyping in HIV-1 therapy; the VIRADAPT randomized controlled trial. *Lancet,* 1999;353: 2195–2199.
38. Van Vaerenbergh K, Van Laethem K, Van Wijngaerden E, et al. Baseline HIV type 1 genotypic resistance to a newly added nucleoside analog is predictive of virologic failure of the new therapy. *AIDS Res Hum Retroviruses,* 2000;16:529–537.
39. Salomon H, Wainberg MA, Brenner BG, et al. Prevalence of HIV-1 viruses resistant to antiretroviral drugs in 81 individuals newly infected by sexual contact or intravenous drug use. *AIDS,* 2000;14: F17–F23.
40. Yerly S, Kaiser L, Race E, et al. Transmission of antiretroviral-drug-resistant HIV-1 variants. *Lancet,* 1999;354:729–733.
41. Boden D, Hurley A, Zhang L, et al. HIV-1 drug resistance in newly infected individuals. *JAMA,* 1999;282:1135–1141.
42. Little SJ, Daar ES, D'Aquila RT, et al. Reduced drug susceptibility among patients with primary HIV infection. *JAMA,* 1999;282:1142–1149.
43. Hecht GM, Grant RM, Petropoulos CJ, et al. Sexual transmission of an HIV-1 variant resistant to multiple reverse-transcriptase and protease inhibitors. *N Engl J Med,* 1998;339:307–311.
44. Brenner BG, Wainberg MA. The role of antiretrovirals and drug resistance in vertical transmission. *Annals NY Acad Sci,* 2000;918:9–15.
45. Quinones ME, Arts EJ. Recombination in HIV: Update and implications. *AIDS Rev,* 1999;1:89–100.
46. Jansens W, Buve A, Nkengasong JN. The puzzle of HIV-1 subtypes in Africa. *AIDS,* 1997;11:705–712.
47. Descamps D, Collin G, Letourneur F, et al. Susceptibility of human immunodeficiency virus type 1 group O isolates to antiretroviral agents: in vitro phenotypic and genotypic analysis. *J Virol,* 1997;71:8893–8898.

48. Apetrei C, Descamps D, Collin, et al. Human immunodeficiency virus subtype F reverse transcriptase sequence and drug susceptibility. *J Virol,* 1998;72:3534–3538.
49. Montano MA, Novitsky VA, Blackard JT, et al. Divergent transcriptional regulation among expanding human immunodeficiency virus type 1 substypes. *J Virol*, 1997;71:8657–8665.
50. Caride E, Hertogs, Larder B, et al. Genotyping and phenotyping analysis of B and non-B HIV-1 subtypes from Brazilian patients under HAART. *Antiviral Ther,* 2000;5:128.
51. Wainberg MA, Friedland G. Public health implications of antiretroviral therapy and HIV drug resistance. *JAMA,* 1999;279:1977–1983.

21

Opportunistic Infections

*Robert Colebunders, †Patrick K. Kayembe, and ‡Ann Marie Nelson

**Department of Clinical Sciences, Institute of Tropical Medicine and University of Antwerp, Antwerp, Belgium.*
†Kinshasa School of Medicine and School of Public Health, University of Kinshasa, Democratic Republic of Congo.
‡Department of Infectious and Parasitic Disease Pathology, Armed Forces Institute of Pathology, Washington, DC, USA.

Many opportunistic infections that are listed in the AIDS case definition of the U.S. Centers for Disease Control and Prevention (CDC) cannot be diagnosed in Africa because of limited diagnostic facilities and trained personnel. However, even when a specific etiology for a particular disease state cannot be confirmed, a clinical diagnosis is often possible, allowing patients to be treated empirically.

This chapter deals with the opportunistic infections and diseases associated with HIV infection, the differential diagnoses, and strategies for treatment in African field conditions. Infections are grouped by category rather than by organ involvement. Tuber-culosis (TB), the most frequently occurring opportunistic infection, is discussed in Chapter 22 (*this volume*). Table 1 shows the frequency of opportunistic infections among hospitalized patients in Côte d'Ivoire (1), Kenya (2), and Senegal (3), and among the subjects of two autopsy studies in Côte d'Ivoire (4) and the Democratic

TABLE 1. Spectrum of Disease in Hospitalized HIV-Infected Adults in African Countries[a]

Type of Data	Morbidity				Mortality	
Country (Reference)	Côte d'Ivoire (1)	Kenya (2)	Senegal (3)		Côte d'Ivoire (4)	Democratic Republic of Congo (5)
Population	Infectious disease ward admissions	Medical ward admissions	HIV-1–infected	HIV-2–infected	Medical ward admissions	Hospital deaths with suspected AIDS
Number of HIV^+ Patients	199	95	599	137	247	63
Bacteremia	20%	26%	—	—	16%	—
HIV wasting	16%	—	—	—	—	13%
Meningitis	14%	—	3%–1%	0%	5%	—
Tuberculosis	13%	18%	30%	26%	38%	41%[d]
Isosporiasis	10%	—	3%	7%	—	—
Cerebral toxoplasmosis	7%	—	1%	0%	15%	11%[e]
Bacterial enteritis	7%	—	8%	18%	—	—
Nonspecific diarrhea	7%	15%	—	—	10%[c]	—
Esophageal candidiasis	3%	—	—	—	—	31%[f]
Pneumonia	1%[b]	16%	3%	1%	30%	34%
Cryptococcosis	3%	1%	—	—	3%	19%
Cytomegalovirus	—	—	—	—	18%	13%
Kaposi's sarcoma	1%	2%	1%	1%	9%	16%
PCP	—	—	—	—	3%	<2%

[a]PCP indicates *Pneumocystis carinii* pneumonia; —, data not available; Note: patients could have more than one diagnosis.
[b]Patients with respiratory symptoms were underrepresented in this study.
[c]Nonspecific enteritis.
[d]Mycobacterial disease, extrapulmonary; no data for pulmonary tuberculosis given.
[e]One cerebral toxoplasmosis, others disseminated; only two brains were available for examination.
[f]Esophageal or tracheal candidiasis.

Republic of Congo (5). Tuberculosis, pneumonia, and cerebral toxoplasmosis are the most prevalent opportunistic diseases or conditions among patients dying in African hospitals. The disease progression of HIV-2 is slower that that of HIV-1 (6), but may also lead to the development of AIDS and opportunistic infections (7). Based on data from a limited number of studies, it appears that opportunistic infections in HIV-2 infection are similar to those in HIV-1 infection (4,8).

For each infection, clinical and epidemiologic characteristics will be described, followed by differential diagnosis and therapeutic considerations. Readers are referred to infectious disease textbooks for detailed descriptions of infectious agents and specialized laboratory diagnostic methods.

PARASITIC INFECTIONS

Toxoplasmosis

Even though *Toxoplasma gondii* is ubiquitous, the prevalence of cerebral toxoplamosis among people with AIDS is relatively low in Africa—5% to 15% (9). However, this condition is probably underdiagnosed because adequate laboratory and radiology support are often lacking. Toxoplasmosis in most AIDS patients is generally believed to result from the reactivation of a latent infection. The central nervous system is the site most frequently involved. Other sites of infection reported in patients with AIDS include the eyes (retinochoroiditis), heart, and lungs.

The clinical manifestations of central nervous system toxoplasmosis, although variable, include headache, fever, and focal neurologic abnormalities such as hemiparesis, hemianopsia, cerebellar or sensitive disturbances, confusion, and lethargy. Focal or generalized seizures occur. A lumbar puncture excludes other etiologies such as cryptococcal meningitis, but cerebrospinal fluid (CSF) findings or serologic tests for toxoplasmosis are generally of little value in the diagnosis of cerebral toxoplasmosis. A lumbar puncture is contraindicated if clinical symptoms or a funduscopy suggest intracranial hypertension. Cerebral toxoplasmosis is more often observed in patients with IgG toxoplasmosis serum antibodies. In developed countries, the diagnosis of cerebral toxoplasmosis is made on the basis of computerized tomography (CT) scan findings (Figure 1). On CT scan, single or multiple hypodense ring-enhanced lesions (after contrast injection) are generally seen. A differential diagnosis should also include a cerebral lymphoma or an abscess caused by mycobacteria or cryptococci. In Africa, the diagnosis should be considered when the patient exhibits fever, headache, or a focal neurologic defect and is negative for cryptococcosis. Toxoplasmosis should also be considered in patients with myocarditis. Toxoplasmic chorioretinitis was observed in 3% of patients in a prospective survey in Togo (10).

Antitoxoplasmosis treatment should be started in HIV-infected patients who have focal neurologic deficits. Primary treatment consists of pyrimethamine (75 mg the first day and 50 mg/day the following days), sulfadiazine (4 to 6 g/day in four divided doses) and leucovorin (10 mg/day). Clinical improvement should be observed in patients with cerebral toxoplasmosis after one week of treatment. If such improvement occurs, treatment should be continued for at least 3 to 5 weeks, followed by secondary prophylaxis with pyrimethamine (25 mg/day) and sulfadiazine (2 to 4 g/day) and leucovorin (10 mg/day). Possible side effects include fever, rash, anemia, leukopenia, and thrombocytopenia. An alternative treatment is pyrim-ethamine and clindamycin.

Cryptosporidiosis

Cryptosporidiosis is reported in 4% to 28% of AIDS patients in Africa who have chronic diarrhea (11–13) (Table 2). Cryptosporidia, transmitted by fecal–oral contamination, causes diarrhea that is generally

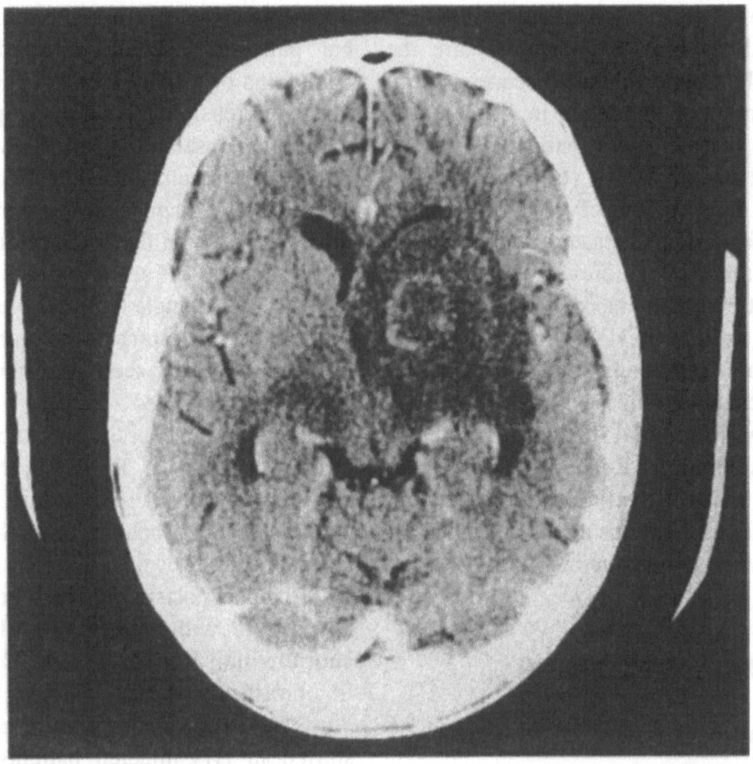

FIGURE 1. Cerebral abscess caused by a toxoplasmosis infection. Computerized tomography scan after contrast injection, with ring enhancement of the contrast. The abscess is surrounded by cerebral edema, causing compression of the lateral ventricle.

liquid and profuse and may be associated with abdominal pain, flatulence, bloating, nausea, and anorexia. The infection may resolve spontaneously, but in patients with end stage HIV disease the diarrhea is usually persistent. Cryptosporidia can be identified in stools after special staining with Ziehl-Neelsen carbol-fuchsin (Kinyoun technique). Cryptosporidiosis of the biliary tract is frequent and causes cholangitis and cholecystitis. Cryptosporidia have also been found in the respiratory tract.

There is no approved effective treatment for cryptosporidiosis, but cryptosporidia may disappear during immune reconstitution with highly active antiretroviral treatment (HAART). An experimental drug, nitazoxanide, was shown to be effective in certain African patients (14). Patients should be treated symptomatically to avoid dehydration and abdominal discomfort. To prevent spread of cryptosporidia infection, good hygiene with enteric precautions such as hand washing and proper disposal of contaminated material is essential.

Cyclospora

Cyclospora cayetanensis is a newly recognized cause of diarrhea in immune incompetent persons and AIDS patients (15). Its prevalence among HIV-infected individuals in Africa remains unknown.

Isosporiasis

Isospora belli is reported in 7% to 13% of African AIDS patients with chronic

TABLE 2. Parasitic Intestinal Pathogens among HIV-Infected Adults with Diarrhea in Africa[a]

Country (Reference)	Democratic Republic of Congo (12)	Burundi (16)	Zambia (17)	Ethiopia (11)	Zimbabwe (13)
Population	HIV-infected	AIDS[b]	HIV-infected	HIV-infected	AIDS
Duration of Diarrhea	>1 month	NS	>1 month	Chronic	>1 month
Number of HIV^+ Patients	106	100	124	147	82
Cryptosporidia	22%	15%	6%	26%	9%
Isospora belli	7%	20%	8%	1%	2%
Microsporidia	2%[c]	—	—	—	18%[e]
Giardia lamblia	0	1%	2%	4%	2%
Entamoeba histolytica					
cysts	3%	16%[d]	2%	8%[d]	—
trophozoites	2%		1%		—
Strongyloides stercoralis	5%	10%	3%	3%	—

[a]NS indicates not specified; —, data not available.
[b]Investigation included upper gastrointestinal endoscopy; in other studies, the only investigation was stool examination.
[c]Later electron microscopic studies by the investigators (Nelson, et al.) revealed three cases of microsporidiosis.
[d]Not specified whether cysts or trophozoites.
[e]18% by microscopy, 51% by PCR.

diarrhea (16,17). Clinically this diarrhea is similar to that associated with cryptosporidia. Isosporiasis is treatable with trimethoprim (320 mg), and sulfamethoxazole (1600 mg) twice daily for 2 to 3 weeks. Relapses are common so secondary prophylaxis with trimethoprim (160 mg) and sulfamethoxazole (800 mg) should be given twice daily.

Microsporidiosis

Microsporidia are frequently observed in the stools of HIV-infected patients with chronic diarrhea (18–21). The microsporidan associated with infection of the small intestine is *Enterocytozoon bieneusi*. A study in Mali documented a 32% prevalence of *E. bieneusi* in HIV-positive patients and a 27% rate in HIV-negative patients who presented with diarrhea and weight loss (21). *Encephalitozoon intestinalis* also causes severe diarrhea and may disseminate to lungs and sinuses (22). *Encephalitozoon cuniculi* may cause disseminated infections, including keratoconjunctivitis, hepatitis, and peritonitis.

Microsporidia can be identified using tissue Gram stains, immunofluorescent stains on stool samples, or by electron microscopy. Albendazole may be useful for the treatment of *E. intestinalis*, but its effect on *E. bieneusi* infection is variable (23).

Malaria

Initial cross-sectional studies found no association between malaria and HIV infection, except that in the early phases of the HIV epidemic, many children with severe malaria-induced anemia acquired HIV infection by transfusion of unscreened blood (24). Later studies showed that HIV-positive individuals with malaria had higher malaria parasitemia than HIV-negative individuals with malaria (25). Parasitemia may be particularly high in individuals with HIV infection and severe immune deficiency, suggesting that *Plasmodium falciparum* acts as an opportunistic agent in persons with HIV (26). Recent investigations have shown that infant mortality is higher among babies born to mothers who are coinfected with placental malaria and HIV-1 infection (27).

Trypanosomiasis

Limited data are available on the interaction of trypanosomiasis and HIV infection. The increase in prevalence of trypanosomiasis in areas of the Democratic Republic of Congo is due to lack of treatment and vector control, and probably not to HIV infection. To date, no unusual clinical presentations of African trypanosomiasis have been reported (28). A case control study conducted in Côte d'Ivoire found no statistical difference between the prevalence of HIV infection among trypanosomiasis patients and controls (29).

Leishmaniasis

Both cutaneous and visceral forms of leishmaniasis occur in desert and savannah areas of northern and sub–Saharan Africa. Many cases of HIV-associated visceral leishmaniasis have been reported from those parts of the world where the disease is endemic (30–33). Fever, hepatosplenomegaly, and hematologic abnormalities (due to bone marrow involvement) are the most common findings, but clinical features are often atypical. For example, not all patients with leishmaniasis have splenomegaly, and interstitial pneumonia is frequent in some areas. Pulmonary leishmaniasis must be differentiated from *Pneumocystis carinii* pneumonia (PCP). Diagnosis is made by bone marrow aspirate or biopsy of the affected organ. Serology is frequently negative in patients with immune suppression. Failure to respond to initial treatment with stibogluconate, 20 mg/kg/day, occurs in as many as 20% of HIV-infected patients. Because relapses are common and often fatal, patients should receive secondary prophylaxis.

Helminthiasis

Helminthic infections are extremely frequent among African populations in general. It has been suggested that chronic immune activation due to helminthic infections could increase susceptibility for HIV infection, increase HIV plasma viral load, and favor HIV disease progression (34). This remains, however, a hypothesis. In general, helminths are not considered to cause opportunistic infections except strongyloidiasis. Severe infection with *Strongyloides stercoralis* has been reported in African patients with AIDS (35, 36), but such infection is exceptional. One study showed HIV-infected onchocerciasis patients to have impaired antibody response to *Onchocerca volvulus* (37).

Scabies

Sarcoptes scabiei often causes severe, generalized eruptions in HIV-infected patients. Typically pruritic, red papules are found in the intertriginous areas, the wrists, and may also spread to the face and scalp. Severe forms of *S. scabiei* infection in persons with HIV infection are called Norwegian scabies (38). A prurigo-nodularis–type postscabietic dermatitis occurs even in patients who have been successfully treated with 1% gamma benzene hexachloride applications.

Intestinal Protozoa

There are few data on the possible interaction between HIV infection and amebiasis or giardiasis. These diseases do not appear to be more prevalent among individuals who are HIV-positive than those who are HIV-negative. The clinical symptoms of these diseases in HIV-positive people appear to be similar to those described in HIV-negative people.

FUNGAL INFECTIONS

Pneumocystis carinii Pneumonia

Pneumocystis carinii pneumonia is less frequent in people with AIDS in Africa than in those living in Europe and the United States (39, 40). In adult autopsy studies, reported PCP prevalence rates were 12% in

Côte d'Ivoire (4), 5% in Uganda (41), and 2% in the Democratic Republic of Congo (5). Studies utilizing bronchoalveolar lavage and/or induced sputum reported prevalence rates of 0% in Zambia (42) and Uganda (43), and 11% in Congo (44). Both transbronchial biopsies and bronchoalveolar lavage were done among sputum-smear Ziehl-negative patients with pulmonary symptoms, revealing PCP prevalence rates of 7% among study participants in Rwanda (45) and 22% among those in Zimbabwe (46). In a study from South Africa of 67 HIV-infected patients whose sputum smears were negative for TB and who had a fiberoptic bronchoscopic evaluation, PCP was diagnosed in 27% of those of African origin and in 59% of those of European origin (47). The reasons for these different PCP prevalence rates are unclear.

Pneumocystis carinii pneumonia can be diagnosed by bronchoalveolar lavage, sputum induction, or transbronchial biopsy, although transbronchial biopsy is generally not needed to diagnose PCP. Sputum induction is slightly less sensitive than bronchoalveolar lavage (39). In Africa, these diagnostic procedures are not available in most health care settings, a situation which may contribute to infrequent reports of PCP in Africa. *Pneumocystis carinii* is certainly prevalent in Africa; it had been diagnosed in infants with kwashiorkor prior to the AIDS epidemic (48). A recent serologic study in Gambia documented a high prevalence of PCP antibodies among children (49). Other studies have shown a high prevalence of PCP in infants and young children (31% in Côte d'Ivoire and 44% in South Africa) (50,51). One of the most accepted explanations for the lower prevalence of PCP in adult AIDS patients in Africa is that African patients generally die of infections caused by more virulent pathogens, such as TB or pneumonia, when their $CD4^+$ lymphocyte count is still relatively high. Some AIDS patients in Africa may also develop very low $CD4^+$ lymphocyte counts, but in general do not live for long with such severe immune suppression. It is unlikely that there are differences in genetic susceptibility to PCP, as PCP has been well documented in African patients living in Europe (52). The mode of acquisition of PCP is poorly understood. Initially it was thought that a person with HIV developed PCP because of reactivation of a latent infection. Some reports, however, have suggested that person-to-person transmission may also occur (53). It has also been suggested that certain African strains of PCP have a lower pathogenicity than strains found in the United States and Europe (54).

Clinically, PCP is characterized by a nonproductive cough and dyspnea. The patient often presents with low-grade fever and may occasionally complain of chest pain. Cyanosis can occur in severe cases; the onset is usually insidious. The chest x-ray may be normal initially, but bilateral interstitial infiltrates often develop in untreated patients (Figure 2). Infiltrates may also be unilateral, lobar, or nodular. Pleural effusions are extremely rare, and hilar adenopathy is not seen in patients who are infected with PCP only. Spontaneous pneumothorax occasionally occurs. If the chest x-ray is normal, pulmonary function tests showing decreased diffusing capacity of carbon monoxide, blood gas abnormalities, and increased lactate dehydrogenase serum levels (>350 IU) may suggest a PCP diagnosis.

Diagnosis of PCP must be differentiated from pulmonary *Mycobacterium tuberculosis*, atypical mycobacteriosis, mycosis (pulmonary cryptococcosis), cytomegalovirus (CMV) infec-tion, bacterial pneumonia caused by *Strepto-coccus pneumoniae* or *Hemophilus influenza*, and pulmonary Kaposi sarcoma. The diagnosis of pulmonary mycobacteriosis can be made by examining sputum for acid-fast bacilli. The differential diagnosis of TB with atypical mycobacteria infection requires the capability to perform mycobacterial cultures. Sometimes empirical therapy helps in making the diagnosis.

The recommended therapy for PCP is high-dose cotrimoxazole (20 mg trimethoprim + 100 mg sulfamethoxazole/kg/day) for

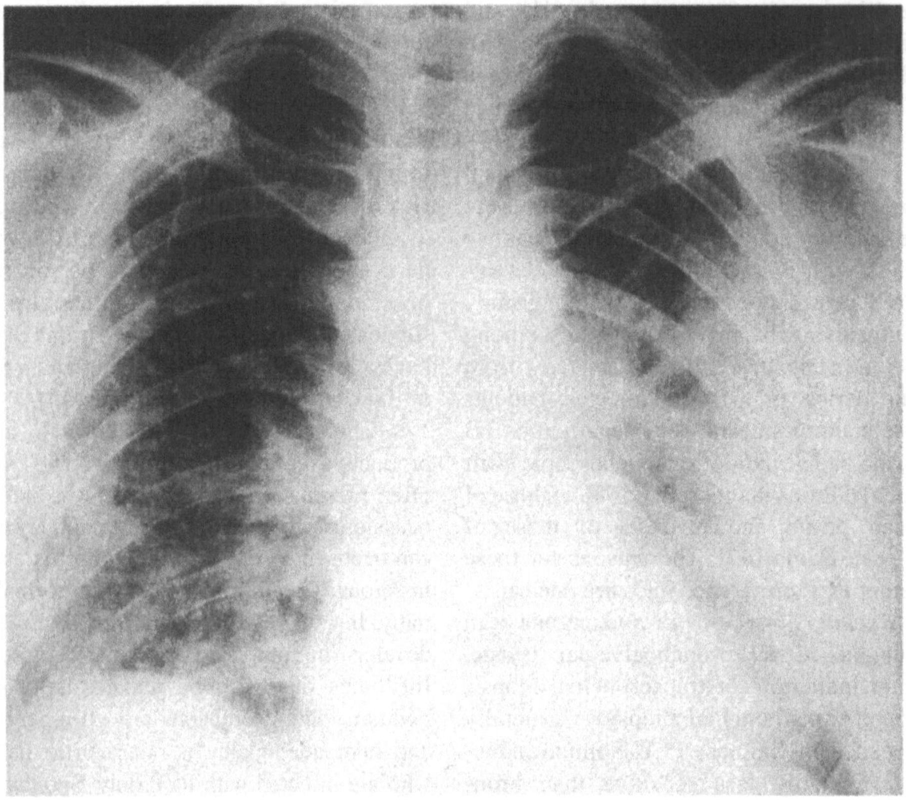

FIGURE 2. *Pneumocystis carinii* pneumonia bilateral pulmonary infiltrates.

3 weeks. Many patients will develop side effects during cotrimoxazole treatment, such as fever, rash, neutropenia, and hepatitis. If severe side effects occur, patients can be treated intravenously (i.v.) with pentamidine (4 mg/kg/day), or with pentamidine inhalations (for the less severe cases), or with a combination of trimethoprim (20 mg/kg/day) and dapsone (100 mg/day).

Secondary prophylaxis for PCP should follow initial therapy. Cotrimoxazole is also the first choice for secondary prophylaxis of PCP. Other prophylactic agents are dapsone (100 mg twice weekly) or pentamidine inhalations (300 mg every 4 weeks).

Candidiasis

Almost everyone with HIV infection will develop candidiasis during their course of disease. People with AIDS have developed a number of forms of oral candidiasis, including pseudomembranous (thrush), atrophic and hypertrophic, and angular cheilitis (55). Onychomycosis and chronic vulvovaginitis are other common manifestations of *Candida* infection in immunosuppressed patients.

Oral candidiasis can be easily diagnosed by examining the patient's mouth for the characteristic white spots (Figure 3). If adequate treatment is not available, oral candidiasis often progresses to *Candida* esophagitis. In some patients, *Candida* esophagitis may occur without oral candidiasis. Disseminated systemic candidiasis is rare in AIDS patients. Meningitis caused by *Candida albicans* has been reported (56).

Many antifungal drugs are available for the treatment of candidiasis. The least expensive are topical drugs such as nystatin,

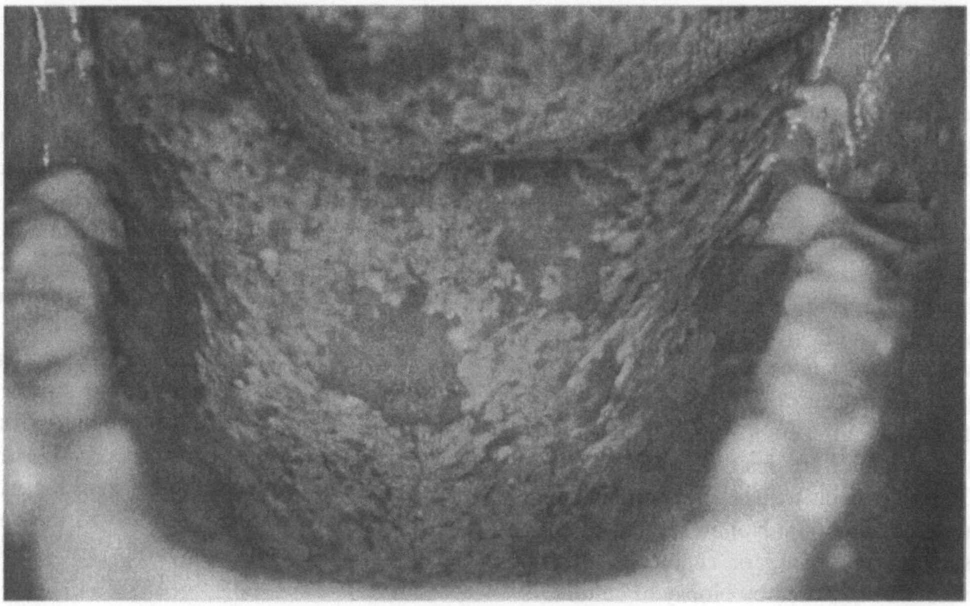

FIGURE 3. Oral candidiasis.

miconazole, clotrimazole, and gentian violet. A study in the Democratic Republic of Congo showed that gentian violet was as effective as ketoconazole in treating oral candidiasis (57), but its violet color may stigmatize patients. Systemic antifungals need to be given when topical treatment fails. *Candida* esophagitis is best treated with 400 mg of ketoconazole daily for about 14 days. If the patient does not improve, amphotericin B, fluconazole, or itraconazole should be used. Oral candidiasis often recurs after completion of therapy, especially in patients with severe immunodeficiency.

Cryptococcosis

Cryptococcosis is an opportunistic infection that can easily be diagnosed in Africa because it requires no sophisticated diagnostic methods or equipment. The prevalence of cryptococcal meningitis is high among AIDS patients in central and southern Africa (58,59) but seems to be lower among those in West Africa (60,61). Cryptococcal meningitis was the initial AIDS-defining illness in 84% of 44 patients with cryptococcal meningitis in Durban, South Africa (62). Meningitis is the most common clinical presentation of cryptococcal infection. The lungs, lymph nodes, liver, and spleen are also commonly involved; any organ may be involved in disseminated infection (63). People with cryptococcal meningitis may be totally asymptomatic, but usually complain of headache and fever (64). Neck stiffness is often absent. Patients with very severe forms may experience altered consciousness. Neurologic signs, particularly cranial nerve palsies and papilla edema, are observed relatively frequently (62). Cryptococcal meningitis is a complication of advanced HIV disease with pronounced immunodeficiency. Prognosis is poor.

Cutaneous lesions occur in 10% to 15% of patients with cryptococcal infection. The presentation varies from small waxy nodules (similar to molluscum contagiosum) to herpetiform papulovesicles to pustules, abscesses, vegetative plaques, and large ulcers (65).

The diagnosis of cryptococcal meningitis is simple: by direct examination of the CSF using Indian ink coloration. The CSF is clear and in general, there is no increase in the white blood cell count. Serology for cryptococcal antigen (by the latex agglutination test) in the CSF and serum, as well as fungal cultures, can also be used to diagnose cryptococcal meningitis. In more than 90% of India ink coloration-positive cases, cryptococcal antigen is found in serum and CSF (66). In some cases the cryptococcal antigen test may be positive before cryptococci can be isolated from the CSF. Cerebrospinal fluid, blood, and urine cultures are positive in 100%, 75%, and 30% of patients with cryptococcal meningitis, respectively (66). Nonmeningeal infections, such as pulmonary or cutaneous infections, must be diagnosed by biopsy or culture.

Cryptococcal meningitis can be treated with amphotericin B (0.4–1 mg/kg/day) or high doses of fluconazole (400 to 600 mg/day) for at least 6 weeks. Afterward, suppressive therapy with 100 to 200 mg/day of fluconazole is recommended. Such treatment is very expensive, however, and not often available in Africa (67).

Histoplasmosis

Disseminated *Histoplasma capsulatum* infection accounts for less than 2% of the opportunistic diseases reported in the United States (68) and Africa (69–72). Clinically, patients present with fever, polyadenopathy, hepatosplenomegaly, skin lesions, or an interstitial pneumonia similar to PCP. Diagnosis is made by microscopic examination for histoplasma in lymph nodes, blood, bone marrow, or lungs. Itraconazole is the apparent treatment of choice for patients with histoplasmosis.

Histoplasma capsulatum var *duboisii*, the cause of African histoplasmosis, has been reported from patients in Congo and the Democratic Republic of Congo (71,72). Lesions are seen in the skin, bone, lymph nodes, and, in the severely immunosuppressed, may be disseminated.

Other Fungal Infections

Cutaneous fungal infections, such as tineas, are common complications of HIV infection. They tend to be multifocal, recurrent, or chronic. The feet, inguinal areas, and scalp are the sites that are most frequently involved. Diagnosis is made by examining skin scrapings with potassium hydroxide solution. Lesions are often resistant to topical application of antifungal preparations. If warranted, systemic griseofulvin or ketoconazole can be used. In a study from Dar es Salaam, Tanzania, 81% of patients with a fungal keratitis were HIV-positive while only 33% of those with nonfungal keratitis were HIV-positive. *Fusarium solani* was the most common organism, accounting for 75% of cases of fungal keratitis (73).

BACTERIAL INFECTIONS

The depletion of the immune system renders HIV-positive people vulnerable to a wide variety of pathogens. Most likely B-lymphocyte dysfunction and neutropenia are responsible for the occurrence of severe bacterial infections and septicemia. Blood culture studies conducted in Africa among hospitalized HIV-infected adults with fever revealed clinically significant bacteria in 15% to 30% of patients (1,74). Gram-negative bacilli, particularly nontyphoid salmonella and *Streptococcus pneumoniae*, were the organisms most frequently isolated. Bloodstream infection studies in hospitals in Malawi and Tanzania that looked for bacteria and mycobacteria found 28% to 39% prevalence rates of *Mycobacterium tuberculosis* (74–76).

Atypical Mycobacterial Infections

Atypical mycobacterial infections are difficult to diagnose without blood or tissue culture. Infections with *Mycobacterium avium-intracellulare* complex (MAC) occur in very advanced stages of HIV infection and are frequently observed among AIDS patients in developed countries. The true prevalence of MAC infection in developing countries is unknown, although in studies in which cultures were performed, MAC infections were rare (77). Clinical manifestations associated with MAC infection are persistent fever, weight loss, anorexia, anemia, and sometimes diarrhea. Treatment of MAC consists of clarithromycin, ethambutol, and rifabutin.

Buruli ulcer, a destructive lesion of the skin and soft tissue caused by *Mycobacterium ulcerans*, is common in central and West Africa, but has not been reported as a complication of HIV infection.

Leprosy and HIV Infection

It has been suggested that infection with HIV may increase the incidence or severity of leprosy among individuals with subclinical infection with *Mycobacterium leprae*, either through shortening the incubation period or by increasing disease penetrance (78). As yet, no clear association between HIV infection and leprosy has been demonstrated (79,80). Studies indicate that the prevalence of HIV infection in persons with leprosy is similar to that in the general population (80,81). Pathology studies however, suggest that lesions tend to be multibacillary in patients with advanced immunosuppression (82).

Salmonella Septicemia

Salmonella septicemia in patients with HIV infection is generally caused by a non-typhoid *Salmonella* infection. Such infections are characterized by sudden onset of high fever and chills. Gastrointestinal symptoms are often lacking. The types of *Salmonella* generally involved are *S. typhimurium* and *S. enteritidis* (1,2). Studies conducted in Kenya and Malawi found *S. typhimurium* to be the dominant pathogen (74), whereas in Côte d'Ivoire, it was *S. enteritidis* (1). Typhoid fever caused by *S. typhi* does not seem to occur more frequently in HIV-seropositive patients than in HIV-seronegative patients. *Salmonella* septicemia in HIV-seropositive patients has a tendency to relapse. Treatment consists of ampicillin (4 g/day orally or i.v.) or chloramphenicol (2–3 g/day orally or i.v.). In the case of recurrent *Salmonella* septicemia episodes, maintenance antibiotic treatment should be considered.

Bacterial Pneumonia

Bacterial pneumonia is a frequent complication in patients with HIV infection in Africa and often occurs prior to the onset of full-blown AIDS. If untreated, severe bacterial pneumonias may lead to early mortality. *Streptococcus pneumoniae* was the pathogen most frequently isolated in Ethiopia (83), Zimbabwe (84), Rwanda (85), and Kenya (2). Fever, cough, and occasionally pleuritic pain are the presenting features. Pneumonia caused by *Rhodococcus equi* has also been reported (86). Streptococcal pneumonia should be treated with penicillin G (6 million units/day i.v.). *Haemophilus* pneumonia can be treated with ampicillin for susceptible strains, or amoxicillin and clavulanic acid, or cotrimoxazole. In Kenya, empiric oral ampicillin was found to be very effective in HIV-infected patients with bronchitis but not in those with pneumonia (87).

Nocardiosis has been found at autopsy in Uganda, the Democratic Republic of Congo, and Côte d'Ivoire (3). It is clinically and radiologically similar to TB. Pleural and chest wall involvement occurs in 10% of cases. Dissemination to the central nervous system and soft tissue is also common. Sputum for acid-fast bacilli are negative, Gram stain may show long filamentous organisms with variable staining.

Sexually Transmitted Infections

Syphilis, gonorrhea, chlamydia, chancroid (*Haemophilus ducreyi*), and other sexually transmitted bacterial infections are discussed in detail in Chapter 14 (*this volume*).

If available, rapid plasma reagin (RPR) and Treponema pallidum hemagglutination assay (TPHA) tests should be performed in all persons with HIV infection; however, both false positive and false negative reactions have been reported (88).

The recommended treatment of syphilis is benzathine benzylpenicillin, 2.4 million IU intramuscularly (1.2 million IU in each buttock), once a week for 3 weeks. If penicillin is not available, or for nonpregnant patients who are allergic to penicillin, the recommended treatment is tetracycline (500 mg four times daily for 21 days).

Other Bacterial Infections

Bacterial meningitis is common in both adults and children. *Streptococcus pneumoniae*, *Neisseria meningitidis*, *Haemophilus influenzae*, and *Mycobacterium tuberculosis* are the most common bacteria isolated (89). *Treponema pallidum* may also cause meningitis (90). Other bacterial infections include those caused by *Pseudomonas* and *Staphylococcus* species: pyomyositis, sinusitis, otitis, erysipelas, furunculosis, pustular dermatitis, impetigo, and hydradenitis suppurativa.

Bacillary angiomatosis is a newly recognized infectious disease observed in people with HIV infection. The putative agent of this disease is a Gram-negative organism, *Bartonella henselae*. Bacillary angiomatosis may involve the skin and lymph nodes. It may cause peliosis hepatis and other visceral lesions (91). The cutaneous lesions resemble Kaposi sarcoma or pyogenic granulomas. To date, only one case of suspected bacillary angiomatosis has been reported from Africa (in an HIV-seropositive child from Zimbabwe) (92). Another case with disseminated cutaneous lesions was seen in the Democratic Republic of Congo (personal observation, Nelson). A biopsy is needed for differential diagnosis. Erythromycin therapy is recommended for a minimum of 4 weeks.

VIRAL INFECTIONS

Several viral infections are frequently observed in people with HIV, including CMV, herpes simplex virus (HSV), herpes zoster, and human papillomavirus (HPV) infections. Although of interest in Africa because of its association with Burkitt lymphoma, the prevalence of Epstein-Barr virus infection among people with HIV is unknown.

Cytomegalovirus Infection

Cytomegalovirus infection is a major cause of morbidity and mortality in AIDS patients. Generalized CMV infection usually occurs in the advanced stages of illness. The sites most commonly involved are the retina, gastrointestinal and biliary tracts, lungs, and adrenal glands, although any organ can be involved. Cytomegalovirus retinitis, colitis, and cholangitis are the most frequent clinical manifestations. In contrast with patients in the United States and Europe (pre–HAART), CMV infection seems to occur less frequently among AIDS patients in Africa (93). Prevalence of CMV infection was 13%, and 11%, in autopsy series in the Democratic Republic of Congo, and Côte d'Ivoire, respectively (4,5). In one prospective study in Togo, CMV retinitis was diagnosed in 27% of AIDS patients (26). Cytomegalovirus pneumonia and hepatitis were high in infant autopsies in South Africa (21).

The diagnosis of CMV infection is made by identifying viral inclusion bodies in tissue specimens. Culturing the virus from an organ alone is not sufficient. The diagnosis of CMV retinitis can be made clinically by funduscopy, which shows a typical pattern of perivascular exudates and hemorrhages. Untreated, CMV retinitis may lead to blindness. Most adult patients with AIDS have antibodies against CMV. Cytomegalovirus serology is therefore not a useful diagnostic tool. Treatment of CMV infection consists of foscarnet, ganciclovir, or cidofovir.

Herpes Simplex Virus Infection

Recurrent or chronic ulcerations caused by HSV infection are observed in 5% to 10% of AIDS patients in Africa. Ulcerations are generally localized in the anogenital region, but may also occur on the tongue or gingival, and can be very painful. The diagnosis of an HSV genital or oral ulceration should be considered when a painful ulceration does not respond to antibiotic treatment. However, HSV ulcerations should be distinguished from other ulcerative lesions such as those caused by chancroid and syphilis. Severe HSV esophagitis and encephalitis are much less common than genital or oral ulcerations.

In most cases a presumptive diagnosis of HSV infection can be made by clinical history and examination. A simple diagnostic method is the Tzanck test, which shows the multinucleated giant cells that are typical of HSV. Biopsy, Pap smear, and culture can also be used, but are not always available.

The recommended therapy for HSV infection is 200 mg of acyclovir administered orally five times a day for 5 to 10 days or until lesions heal. Parenteral acyclovir may be needed for severe extensive lesions or for herpes esophagitis or encephalitis. Acyclovir-resistant strains have been reported. Patients with such strains can be treated with foscarnet.

Herpes Zoster Infections

Herpes zoster infection generally appears in the early stages of HIV infection (94, 95) and develops in 5% to 10% of people with HIV. In regions where HIV infection is highly prevalent, it has a high predictive value for HIV infection (96). Herpes zoster generally involves one to three dermatomes, but extensive multidermatomal zoster or disseminated zoster can occur. Most infections resolve spontaneously over 1 to 3 weeks, leaving scars in most people. Herpes zoster infection of the trigeminal dermatome (ophthalmic zona) may lead to corneal ulcerations. Many patients develop postherpetic neuralgias. If financial resources are limited, only symptomatic treatment may be possible. High-dose acyclovir, if available, should be started as soon as possible using 800 mg daily for 5 to 10 days or until the lesions have healed. Herpes zoster is recurrent in 10% to 20% of cases.

Human Papillomavirus

Human papillomavirus infection has been associated with cervical and other squamous neoplasias and invasive carcinomas. These associations and complications are discussed in Chapter 23 (*this volume*). Condyloma acuminatum and other warts are common in people with HIV. The lesions are most frequent on the face, hands, feet, and anogenital areas. They can be flat and filiform or large and vegetating, and are often resistant to treatment. Treatment consists of the local application of podophyllin/podophyllotoxin, 20% solution one or two times per week until cleared. Trichloroacetic acid can also be applied. If available, cryotherapy can be used. Surgical excision may be required. Recurrence rates are very high.

Hepatitis B

Coinfection of hepatitis B virus (HBV) and HIV is very common in Africa (97). In persons with HIV infection, HBV infection is frequently chronic (98). Several reports have described the reappearance of hepatitis surface antigen in HIV-infected patients previously thought to be immune to HBV (99). The impact of HIV on the severity of chronic HBV infection is not clear (98). In certain studies it has been suggested that HIV–HBV coinfected patients develop milder clinical liver disease than those with only HBV (100), but in other studies, a significantly shorter survival time has been observed among among coinfected patients (101).

Hepatitis C

Hepatitis C is mainly transmitted through the parenteral mode. In developed countries it is mainly observed among intravenous drug users, but in Africa, hepatitis C is also transmitted through the use of contaminated needles in the health care setting and via unscreened blood transfusions (102, 103). The natural history of hepatitis C virus (HCV) infection is accelerated in immunocompromised patients, and a high prevalence of liver failure has been seen in HIV-coinfected individuals (104). The risk of developing chronic liver disease caused by HCV increases with HIV disease progression (104). In patients treated with HAART, hepatitis C infection may also have a negative impact on their recovery from immune deficiency (105).

Molluscum Contagiosum

Molluscum contagiosum presents as waxy, flesh-colored, and umbilicated papules. In immunosuppressed people, the lesions may be disseminated, or coalesce to form large ulcerated plaques. Biopsy or smears of the lesion to demonstrate molluscum bodies are required to differentiate molluscum contagiosum from disseminated cryptococcus or histoplasmosis. Lesions may be treated by pricking with a needle and touching with phenol solution. Cryotherapy or excision can also be used. Recurrence is common.

Hairy Leukoplakia

Hairy leukoplakia has been associated with Epstein-Barr virus. It usually presents as a corrugated white plaque on the lateral margin of the tongue. It has been reported in both HIV-1– and HIV-2–infected patients from Africa, but its prevalence is not well described. In one large study in South Africa, the prevalence was 20% (106).

Progressive Multifocal Leukoencephalopathy

Progressive multifocal leukoencephalopathy is caused by a papovavirus (JC) infection of the central nervous system that results in a progressive demyelinization. Its prevalence in Africa is not known. Diagnosis requires a CT scan and brain biopsy. Cidofovir could have a beneficial effect in some patients (107).

CONCLUSION

Because HAART may not become available in the near future for many people with HIV infection in Africa, opportunistic infections will continue to occur. Therefore, prevention and early treatment of opportunistic infections are probably the best available methods to decrease morbidity and early mortality of HIV infection in Africa.

REFERENCES

1. Grant AD, Djomand G, Smets P, et al. Profound immunosuppression across the spectrum of opportunistic disease among hospitalized HIV-infected adults in Abidjan, Côte d'Ivoire. *AIDS*, 1997;11: 1357–1364.
2. Gilks CF, Otieno LS, Brindle RJ, et al. The presentation and outcome of HIV-related disease in Nairobi. *Q J Med*, 1992;82:25–32.
3. Ndour M, Sow PS, Coll-Seck AM, et al. AIDS caused by HIV-1 and HIV-2 infection: are there clinical differences? Results of AIDS surveillance 1986–1997 at Fann Hospital in Dakar, Senegal. *Trop Med Int Health*, 2000;5:687–691.
4. Lucas SB, Odida M, Wabinga H. The pathology of severe morbidity and mortality caused by HIV infection in Africa. *AIDS*, 1991;5(suppl 1):S143–S148.
5. Nelson AM, Perriens JH, Kapita B, et al. A clinical and pathological comparison of the WHO and CDC case definitions for AIDS in Kinshasa, Zaïre: is passive surveillance valid? *AIDS*, 1993;7: 1241–1245.

6. Marlink R, Kanki P, Thior I, et al. Reduced rate of disease development after HIV-2 infection as compared to HIV-1. *Science*, 1994;265: 1587–1590.
7. De Cock KM, Odehouri K, Colebunders RL, et al. A comparison of HIV-2 and HIV-1 infection in hospitalized patients in Abidjan, Côte d'Ivoire. *AIDS*, 1990;4:443–448.
8. Sow PS, Faye MA, Diouf G, et al. Opportunistic infections in HIV-2 infected patients in Dakar (Senegal). In: Program and abstracts of the Xth International Conference on AIDS; August 7–12, 1994; Yokohama, Japan. Abstract PA0128.
9. Perriens JH, Mussa M, Luabeya MK, et al. Neurological complications of HIV-1-seropositive internal medicine in patients in Kinshasa, Zaïre. *J Acquir Immune Defic Syndr*, 1992;5:333–340.
10. Balo KP, Amoussou YP, Bechetoille A, et al. Cytomegalovirus retinitis and ocular complications in AIDS patients in Togo. *J Fr Opthalmol*, 1999;22:1042–1046.
11. Fisseha B, Petros B, WoldeMichael T. Cryptosporidium and other parasites in Ethiopian AIDS patients with chronic diarrhoea. *East Afr Med J*, 1998;75:100–101.
12. Colebunders R, Francis H, Mann JM, et al. Persistent diarrhoea, strongly associated with HIV infection in Kinshasa, Zaïre. *Am J Gastroenterol*, 1987;82:859–864.
13. Gumbo T, Sarbah S, Gangaidzo IT, et al. Intestinal parasites in patients with diarrhea and human immunodeficiency virus infection in Zimbabwe. *AIDS*, 1999;13:819–821.
14. Doumbo O, Rossignol JF, Pichard E, et al. Nitazoxanide in the treatment of cryptosporidial diarrhea and other intestinal parasitic infections associated with acquired immunodeficiency syndrome in tropical Africa. *Am J Trop Med Hyg*, 1997;56:637–639.
15. Wurtz R. Cyclospora: a newly identified intestinal pathogen of humans. *Clin Infect Dis*, 1994;18: 620–623.
16. Floch JJ, Laroche R, Kadende P, et al. Parasites, etiologic agents of diarrhoeas in AIDS-patients in Burundi. Interest of the aspirated duodenal liquid examination [in French]. *Bull Soc Pathol Exot*, 1989;82:316–320.
17. Khumalo-Ngwenya B, Luo NP, Chintu C, et al. Gut parasites in HIV-seropositive Zambian adults with diarrhoea. *East Afr Med J*, 1994;71:379–383.
18. Kelly P, Davies SE, Mandanda B, et al. Enteropathy in Zambians with HIV-related diarrhoea: regression modelling of potential determinants of mucosal damage. *Gut*, 1997;41:811–816.
19. Drobniewski F, Kelly P, Carew A, et al. Human microsporidiosis in African AIDS patients with chronic diarrhea. *J Infect Dis*, 1995;171: 515–516.
20. Van Gool T, Luderhoff E, Nathoo KJ, et al. High prevalence of Enterocytozoon bieneusi infections among HIV-positive individuals with persistent diarrhoea in Harare, Zimbabwe. *Trans R Soc Trop Med Hyg*, 1995;89:478–480.
21. Maiga I, Doumbo O, Dembele M, et al. Human intestinal microsporidiosis in Bamako (Mali): the presence of Enterocytozoon bieneusi in HIV seropositive patients. *Sante*, 1997;4:257–262.
22. Kelly P, McPhail G, Ngwenya B, et al. Septata intestinalis: a new microsporidian in Africa [letter]. *Lancet*, 1994;344:271–272.
23. Goodgame R. Understanding intestinal spore-forming protozoa: cryptosporidia, microsporidia, isospora and cyclospora. *Ann Intern Med*, 1996;124:429.
24. Greenberg AE, Nguyen-Dinh P, Mann JM, et al. The association between malaria, blood transfusions, and HIV seropositivity in a pediatric population in Kinshasa, Zaïre. *JAMA*, 1988;259: 545–549.
25. Verhoeff FH, Brabin BJ, Hart CA, et al. Increased prevalence of malaria in HIV-infected pregnant women and its implications for malaria control. *Trop Med Int Health*, 1999;4:5–12.
26. Whitworth J, Morgan D, Quigley M, et al. Effect of HIV-1 and increasing immunosuppression on malaria parasitaemia and clinical episodes in adults in rural Uganda: a cohort study. *Lancet*, 2000;356: 1051–1056.
27. Bloland PB, Wirima JJ, Steketee RW, et al. Maternal HIV infection and infant mortality in Malawi: evidence for increased mortality due to placental malaria infection. *AIDS*, 1995;9:721–726.
28. Louis JP, Jannin J, Hengy C, et al. Absence d'interrelations entre les retroviroses à VIH et la trypanosomiasis humaine Africain (THA). *Bull Soc Path Exot Filiales*, 1991;84:25–29.
29. Meda HA, Doua F, Laveissiere C, et al. Human immunodeficiency virus infection and human African trypanosomiasis: a case control study in Côte d'Ivoire. *Trans R Soc Trop Med Hyg*, 1995;89:639–643.
30. Ndiaye PB, Develoux M, Dieng MT, et al. Diffuse cutaneous leishmaniasis and acquired immunodeficiency syndrome in a Senegalese patient. *Bull Soc Pathol Exot*, 1996;89:282–286.
31. Berhe N, Hailu A, Wolday D, et al. Ethiopian visceral leishmaniasis patients co-infected with human immunodeficiency virus. *Trans R Soc Trop Med Hyg*, 1995;89:205–207.
32. Pharoah PD, Ponnighaus JM, Chavula D, Lucas SB. Two cases of cutaneous leishmaniasis in Malawi. *Trans R Soc Trop Med Hyg*, 1993;87:668–670.
33. Marlier S, Menard G, Gisserot O, et al. Leishmaniasis and human immunodeficiency virus: an emerging co-infection? *Med Trop*, 1999;59:193–200.
34. Bentwich Z, Maartens G, Torten D, et al. Concurrent infections and HIV pathogenesis. *AIDS*, 2000;14:2071–2081.

35. Fleming AF. Opportunistic infections in AIDS in developed and developing countries. *Trans R Soc Trop Med Hyg*, 1990;84(suppl 1):1–6.
36. Genta RM. Global prevalence of strongyloidiasis: critical review with epidemiologic insights into the prevention of disseminated disease. *Rev Infect Dis*, 1989;11:755–767.
37. Tawill SA, Gallin M, Erttmann KD, et al. Impaired antibody responses and loss of reactivity to Onchocerca volvulus antigens by HIV-seropositive onchocerciasis patients. *Trans R Soc Trop Med Hyg*, 1996;90:85–89.
38. Rau RC, Baird IM. Crusted scabies in a patient with acquired immunodeficiency syndrome. *J Am Acad Dermatol*, 1986;15:1058–1059.
39. Lucas SB. Missing infections in AIDS. *Trans R Soc Trop Med Hyg*, 1990;84(suppl 1):34–38.
40. Lucas SB, Hounnou A, Peacock C, et al. The mortality and pathology of HIV infection in a west African city. *AIDS*, 1993;7:1569–1579.
41. Rana SF, Hawken MP, Mwachari C, Bhatt SM, et al. Autopsy study of HIV-1 positive and HIV-1 negative adult medical patients in Nairobi, Kenya. *J Acquir Immune Defic Syndr Hum Retrovirol*, 2000;24:23–29.
42. Elvin KM, Lumbwe CM, Luo NP, et al. Pneumocystis carinii is not a major cause of pneumonia in HIV infected patients in Lusaka, Zambia. *Trans R Soc Trop Med Hyg*, 1989;83:553–555.
43. Lucas S, Goodgame R, Kocjan G, Serwadda D. Absence of Pneumocystis in Ugandan AIDS patients. *AIDS*, 1989;3:47–48.
44. Carme B, Mboussa J, Andzin M. Pneumocystis carinii is rare in AIDS in Central Africa. *Trans R Soc Trop Med Hyg*, 1991;85:80.
45. Batungwanayo J, Taelman H, Lucas S, et al. Pulmonary disease associated with the human immunodeficiency virus in Kigali, Rwanda. A fiberoptic bronchoscopic study of 111 cases of undetermined etiology. *Am J Respir Crit Care Med*, 1994;149:1591–1596.
46. McLeod DT, Neill P, Gwanzura L, et al. Pneumocystis carinii pneumonia in patients with AIDS in Central Africa. *Respir Med*, 1990;84:225–228.
47. Mahomed AG, Murray J, Klempman S, et al. Pneumocystis carinii pneumonia in HIV infected patients from South Africa. *East Afr Med J*, 1999;76:80–84.
48. Bwibo NO, Owor R. *Pneumocystis carinii* pneumonia in Ugandan African children. *W Afr Med J*, 1970;19:184–185.
49. Wakefield AE, Stewart TJ, Moxon ER, et al. Infection with Pneumocystis carinii is prevalent in healthy Gambian children. *Trans R Soc Trop Med Hyg*, 1990;84:800–802.
50. Lucas SB, Peacock CS, Hounnou A, et al. Disease in children infected with HIV in Abidjan, Côte d'Ivoire. *BMJ*, 1996;312:335–338.
51. Jeena PM, Coovadia HM, Chrystal V. Pneumocystis carinii and cytomegalovirus infections in severely ill HIV-infected African infants. *Ann Trop Paediatr*, 1996;16:361–368.
52. Del Amo J, Petruckevitch A, Phillips A, et al. Spectrum of disease in Africans with AIDS in London. *AIDS*, 1996;10:1563–1569.
53. Jacobs JL, Libby DM, Winters RA, et al. A cluster of Pneumocystis carinii pneumonia in adults without predisposing illnesses. *N Engl J Med*, 1991;324:246–250.
54. Vermund SH, Lucas S, Bartlett, et al. Molecular and clinical evidence of PCP strains of low pathogenicity from Africa compared to US/ Europe/ Australia. In: Program and abstracts of the 12th World AIDS Conference; June 28–July 3, 1998; Geneva, Switzerland. Abstract 22177.
55. Mayanja B, Morgan D, Ross A. The burden of mucocutaneous conditions and the association with HIV-1 infection in a rural community in Uganda. *Trop Med Int Health*, 1999;4:349–354.
56. Munoz J, Teira R, Zubero Z, et al. Meningitis caused by Candida albicans in a patient with AIDS: treatment with fluconazole. *Enferm Infect Microbiol Clin*, 1990;8:590–591.
57. Nyst MJ, Perriens JH, Kimputu L, et al. Gentian violet, ketoconazole and nystatin in oropharyngeal and esophageal candidiasis in Zaïrian AIDS patients. *Ann Soc Belg Med Trop*, 1992;72:45–52.
58. Bogaerts J, Rouvroy D, Taelman H, et al. AIDS-associated cryptococcal meningitis in Rwanda (1983–1992): epidemiologic and diagnostic features. *J Infect*, 1999:39:32–37.
59. Heyderman RS, Gangaidzo IT, Hakim JG, et al. Cryptococcal meningitis in human immmunodeficiency virus-infected patients in Harare, Zimbabwe. *Clin Infect Dis*, 1998;26:284–289.
60. Frimpong EH, Lartey RA. Study of the aetiologic agents of meningitis in Kumasi, Ghana, with special reference to Cryptococcal neoformans. *East Afr Med J*, 1998;75:516–519.
61. Grant AD, Djomand G, De Cock KM. Natural history and spectrum of disease in adults with HIV/AIDS in Africa. *AIDS*, 1997;11:S43–S54.
62. Moosa MY, Coovadia YM. Cryptococcal meningitis in Durban, South Africa: a comparison of clinical features, laboratory findings, and outcome for human immunodeficiency virus (HIV)-positive and HIV-negative patients. *Clin Infect Dis*, 1997;24: 131–134.
63. Mitchel TG, Perfect JR. Cryptococcosis in the era of AIDS—100 years after the discovery of *Cryptococcus neoformans*. *Clin Microbiol Rev*, 1995;8:515–548.
64. Castro Guardiola A, Ocana Rivera I, Gasser Laguna I, et al. Sixteen cases of infection by Cryptococco-sis neoformans in patients with AIDS. *Enferm Infect Microbiol Clin*, 1991;9:90–94.

65. Zalla MJ, Su WP, Fransway AF. Dermatologic manifestations of human immunodeficiency virus infection. *Mayo Clin Proc*, 1992;67:1089–1108.
66. Desmet P, Kayembe KD, De Vroey C. The value of cryptococcal serum antigen screening among HIV-positive/AIDS patients in Kinshasa, Zaïre. *AIDS*, 1989;3:77–78.
67. Denning DW. Cost implications of alternative treatments for AIDS patients with cryptococcal meningitis. *J Infect*, 1992;24:212–213.
68. Graybill JR. Histoplasmosis and AIDS. *J Infect Dis*, 1988;158:623–626.
69. Pillay T, Pillay DG, Bramdev A. Disseminated histoplasmosis in a human immunodeficiency virus-infected African child. *Pediatr Infect Dis J*, 1997;16:417–418.
70. Pakasa M, Nsiangana Z. Histoplasmosis due to Histoplasma Duboisii (five new cases): possible association with schistosoma mansoni. *J Mycol Med*, 1991;1:306–309.
71. Chandenier J, Goma D, Moyen G, et al. African histoplasmosis due to Histoplasma capsulatum var duboisii: relationship with AIDS in recent Congolese cases. *Sante*, 1995;5:227–234.
72. Geffray L, Veyssier P, Cevallos R, et al. African histoplasmosis: clinical and therapeutic aspects, relation to AIDS. Apropos of 4 cases, including a case with HIV-1-HTLV-1 co-infection. *Ann Med Interne*, 1994;145:424–428.
73. Mselle J. Fungal keratitis as an indicator of HIV infection in Africa. *Trop Doct*, 999;29: 133–135.
74. Graham SM, Walsh AL, Molyneux EM, et al. Clinical presentation of non-typhoidal Salmonella bacteremia in Malawian children. *Trans R Soc Trop Med Hyg*, 2000;94:31–314.
75. Archibald LK, McDonald C, Nwanyanwu O, et al. A hospital-based prevalence survey of bloodstream infections (BSI) in febrile patients in Malawi: Implications for diagnosis and therapy. *J Infect Dis*, 2000;181:1414–1420.
76. Archibald LK, den Dulk MO, Pallangyo KJ, et al. Fatal Mycobacterium tuberculosis bloodstream infections in febrile hospitalized patients in Dar es Salaam, Tanzania. *Clin Infect Dis*, 1998;26:290–296.
77. Okello DO, Sewankambo N, Goodgame R, et al. Absence of bacteremia with *Mycobacterium avium-intracellulare* in Ugandan patients with AIDS. *J Infect Dis*, 1990;162:208–210.
78. Ponnighaus JM, Mwanjasi LJ, Fine PE, et al. Is HIV infection a risk factor for leprosy? *Int J Lepr Other Mycobact Dis*, 1991;59:221–228.
79. Munyao TM, Bwayo JJ, Owili DM, et al. Human immunodeficiency virus-1 in leprosy patients attending Kenyatta National Hospital, Nairobi. *East Afr Med J*, 1994;71:490–492.
80. Leonard G, Sangare A, Verdier M, et al. Prevalence of HIV infection among patients with leprosy in African countries and Yemen. *J Acquir Immune Defic Syndr*, 1990;3:1109–1113.
81. Kawuma HF, Bwire R, Adatu-Engwau F. Leprosy and infection with the human immunodeficiency virus in Uganda; a case-control study. *Int J Lepr Other Mycobact Dis*, 1994;62:521–526.
82. Moran CA, Nelson AM, Tuur SM, et al. Leprosy in five human immunodeficiency virus-infected patients. *Mod Pathol*, 1995;8:662–664.
83. Aderaye G. Community acquired pneumonia in adults in Addis Ababa: etiologic agents and the impact of HIV infection. *Tuber Lung Dis*, 1994;75:308–312.
84. Afolabi OA, Pozniak A, Mutetwa S, et al. The impact of HIV in community acquired pneumonia in Africa. In: Program and abstracts of the XI International Conference on AIDS/IV STD World Congress; June 6–11, 1993; Berlin, Germany. Abstract WS-B19-3.
85. Taelman H, Batungwanayo J, Bogaerts J, et al. Lobar pneumonia and HIV-1 infection in Central Africa. In: Program and abstracts of the IX International Conference on AIDS and STDs in Africa; December 1995; Kampala, Uganda. Abstract TuB169.
86. Colebunders R, De Roo A, Verstraeten T, et al. Rhodococcus equi infection in 3 AIDS patients. *Acta Clin Belg*, 1996;51:101–105.
87. Meier A, Meier AS, Mwachari C, et al. Respiratory tract infection in HIV-1 infected adults in Nairobi, Kenya: evaluation of risk factors and the WHO treatment algorithm. In: Program and abstracts of the XIII International AIDS Conference; July 9–14, 2000; Durban, South Africa. Abstract TuPeB3129.
88. Rompalo AM, Cannon RO, Quinn TC, et al. Association of biologic false-positive reactions for syphilis with human immunodeficiency virus infection. *J Infect Dis*, 1992;165:1124–1126.
89. Wanyoike MN, Waiyaki PG, McLiegeyo SO, et al. Bacteriology and sensitivity patterns of pyogenic meningitis at Kenyatta National Hospital, Nairobi, Kenya. *East Afr Med J*, 1995;72:658–660.
90. Silber E, Sonnenberg P, Koornhof HJ, et al. Dual infective pathology in patients with cryptococcal meningitis. *Neurology*, 1998;51:1213–1215.
91. Perkocha LA, Geaghan SM, Yen TS, et al. Clincal and pathological features of bacillary peliosis hepatitis in association with human immunodeficiency virus infection. *N Engl J Med*, 1990;323: 1581–1586.
92. Chitsike I, Muronda C. Bacillary angiomatosis in an HIV positive child. First case report in Zimbabwe. *Cent Afr J Med*, 1997;43:238–239.
93. Jaffar S, Ariyoshi K, Frith P, et al. Retinal manifestations of HIV-1 and HIV-2 infections among hospital patients in The Gambia, West Africa. *Trop Med Int Health*, 1999;4:487–492.
94. Van de Perre P, Bakkers E, Batungwanayo J, et al. Herpes zoster in African patients: an early

manifestation of HIV infection. *Scand J Infect Dis*, 1988;20:277–282.

95. Tyndall MW, Nasio J, Agoki E, et al. Herpes zoster as the initial presentation of human immunodeficiency virus type 1 infection in Kenya. *Clin Infect Dis*, 1995;21:1035–1037.
96. Colebunders R, Mann JM, Francis H, et al. Herpes zoster in African patients: a clinical predictor of human immunodeficiency virus infection. *J Infect Dis*, 1988;157:314–318.
97. Ahmed SD, Cueval SE, Brabin BJ, et al. Seroprevalence of hepatitis B and C and HIV in Malawian pregnant women. *J Infect*, 1998;37: 248–251.
98. Lazizi Y, Grangeot-Keros L, Delfraissy J. Reappearance of hepatitis B virus in immune patients infected with the human immunodeficiency virus type 1. *J Infect Dis*, 1988;158: 666–667.
99. Scharschmidt B, Held M, Hollander H. Hepatitis B in patients with HIV infection: relationship to AIDS and patient survival. *Ann Intern Med*, 1992;117:837.
100. Housset C, Pol S, Carnot F, et al. Interactions between human immunodeficiency virus-1, hepatitis delta virus and hepatitis B virus infections in 260 chronic carriers of hepatitis B virus. *Hepatology*, 1992;15:578–583.
101. Pawlotsky JM, Belec L, Gresenguet G, et al. High prevalence of hepatitis B, C, and E markers in young sexually active adults from the Central African Republic. *J Med Virol*, 1995;46:269–272.
102. Matee MI, Lyamuya EF, Mbena EC, et al. Prevalence of transfusion-associated viral infections and syphilis among blood donors in Muhimbili Medical Centre, Dar es Salaam, Tanzania. *East Afr Med J*, 1999;76:167–171.
103. Eyster ME, Diamondstone LS, Lien JM, et al. Natural history of hepatitis C virus infection in multitransfused hemophiliacs: effect of coinfection with human immunodeficiency virus. The Multicenter Hemophilia Cohort Study. *J Acquir Immune Defic Syndr Hum Retrovirol*, 1993;6:602–610.
104. Wright T, Hollander H, Pu X. Hepatitis C in HIV-infected patients with and without AIDS: prevalence and relationship to patient survival. *Hepatology*, 1994;20:1152–1155.
105. Greub G, Ledergerber B, Battegay M, et al. Clinical progression, survival, and immune recovery during antiretroviral therapy in patients with HIV-1 and hepatitis C virus coinfection: the Swiss HIV Cohort Study. *The Lancet*, 2000;356:1800–1805.
106. Arendorf TM, Bredekamp B, Cloete CA, et al. Oral manifestations of HIV infection in 600 South African patients. *J Oral Pathol Med*, 1998;27: 176–179.
107. Berenguer J, Mallolas J. Intravenous cidofovir for compassionate use in AIDS patients with cytomegalovirus retinitis. Spanish Cidofovir Study Group. *Clin Infect Dis*, 2000;30:182–184.

22

Tuberculosis

*Renée Ridzon and †Harriet Mayanja-Kizza

*Division of Tuberculosis Elimination, Centers for Disease Control and Prevention, Atlanta, Georgia, USA.
†Faculty of Medicine, Makerere University, Kampala, Uganda.

The burden of tuberculosis (TB) disease in Africa is closely linked to the AIDS pandemic. TB is one of the leading causes of HIV-related morbidity and mortality throughout Africa. In sub–Saharan Africa, TB is the leading cause of death among people with HIV infection, and worldwide, TB accounts for about one-third of AIDS deaths (1). In 1993, prompted by escalating rates of TB in Africa and other parts of the world, the World Health Organization (WHO) designated the disease a global public health emergency. HIV infection is the greatest known risk factor for reactivation of latent infection with *Mycobacterium tuberculosis*, as well as for progression of new infection or reinfection to active TB disease. Further, HIV infection alters the natural history and clinical manifestations of TB, as well as paradigms for its management and control (2). Because TB is transmissible to both persons with and without HIV infection, rising TB rates in Africa affect the public health of the population as well the health of individuals (3).

MICROBIOLOGY

Bacteria of the genus *Mycobacterium* are slow-growing, rod-shaped, obligate aerobic organisms. These organisms are characterized by a lipid-rich cell wall that, when stained, is resistant to decolorization with acid-alcohol treatment—thus the designation acid-fast bacilli (AFB) (4). *Mycobacterium tuberculosis* complex comprises four species: *M. tuberculosis, M. bovis, M. microti*, and *M. africanum*. These organisms are collectively referred to as the tubercle bacilli. The majority of TB cases in humans are caused by *M. tuberculosis*, followed by *M. bovis*; however, in Africa, *M. africanum* is reported to be the cause of 10% to 20% of TB cases. Although *M. tuberculosis* complex can cause disease in some animals (*M. tuberculosis* in primates and *M. bovis* in cattle), TB, for the most part, is transmitted only from humans to other humans.

The tubercle bacillus is distinguished from other mycobacteria by means of phenotypic examination, biochemical testing, or genetic probes. The speciation of specific organisms within the *M. tuberculosis* complex is more difficult and requires testing methodologies, such as chromatography, that are only available in specialized laboratories (5). For practical purposes, however, speciation is not of primary importance, since the majority of TB cases are caused by the species *M. tuberculosis*, and there is little difference in treatment or outcome based on species.

TRANSMISSION

Although *M. bovis* is usually transmitted through ingestion of contaminated, unpasteurized dairy products, TB is normally transmitted person-to-person by the airborne spread of *M. tuberculosis* or *M. africanum* organisms that are present in infected respiratory secretions (6). Infection can occur when a person inhales droplet nuclei containing tubercle bacilli. These droplets are produced when someone with infectious pulmonary TB coughs or otherwise forcefully expels air. When inhaled, these droplets may escape the host's upper airway defenses and reach the alveoli, where primary infection may result (6).

The infectiousness of a person with TB is dependent on the number of tubercle bacilli he or she expels into the air, which in turn is dependent on the presence of disease in the lungs, cavitation on chest radiograph, disease in the airways or larynx, the number of organisms on smear examination of sputum, and the forcefulness of cough. Crowded conditions, poor air movement and circulation, and lengthy exposure to an infectious individual, enhance transmission of *M. tuberculosis*. The period of infectiousness of a patient can be prolonged due to delayed diagnosis, poor adherence with medications, or inappropriate treatment of TB that is caused by drug-resistant organisms. For the most part, children are far less infectious than adults, although transmission attributed to young children has been described (7). Data have shown that TB patients with HIV infection are no more infectious than TB patients without HIV infection (8).

EPIDEMIOLOGY

It is estimated that one-third of the world's population, or approximately 2 billion persons, are infected with *M. tuberculosis* (9). Annually, eight million persons develop TB disease and two million die from it (9). Tuberculin skin test surveys that were performed in Africa before the HIV pandemic indicated that 30% to 70% of adults were infected with *M. tuberculosis* (10). In 1999, the WHO was notified of 644,972 new cases of TB in Africa; of these, approximately 50% were sputum smear-positive pulmonary cases (11). In the world, there are an estimated 34 million persons infected with HIV. Of these, approximately 15 to 16 million persons are coinfected with *M. tuberculosis* (12,13). Up to 70% of these dually infected persons live in sub–Saharan Africa (14).

The AIDS pandemic has had a profound effect on TB in Africa and is responsible for dramatic increases in the prevalence of TB. TB is the most common opportunistic infection seen in Africans with HIV infection, and is the leading cause of death in persons with HIV infection. There are two factors responsible for the HIV-related increase in TB cases: HIV-infected individuals are at increased risk of reactivation of latent *M. tuberculosis* infection; and HIV-infected individuals who are recently infected, or reinfected with *M. tuberculosis* develop active TB and progress to disease at an accelerated rate.

In a study of the spectrum of HIV-related disease in which autopsies were performed, TB was present in approximately 40% of persons with HIV infection, and attributed as the primary cause of death in 32% (15). Other studies have shown that patients with HIV infection and active TB were at twice the risk of death than were those with HIV infection alone (16). Even when their $CD4^+$ cell counts were similar, the rate of death for patients with both HIV infection and TB was higher than that for patients with HIV infection alone (17).

There is increasing incidence of TB in all sub–Saharan African countries. This dramatic rise in incidence has lead to changes in the epidemiology of TB as well as to the destabilization of already overburdened national TB control programs. Data obtained from 18 African nations in 1999 showed that HIV prevalence in adults aged 15 to 49 was

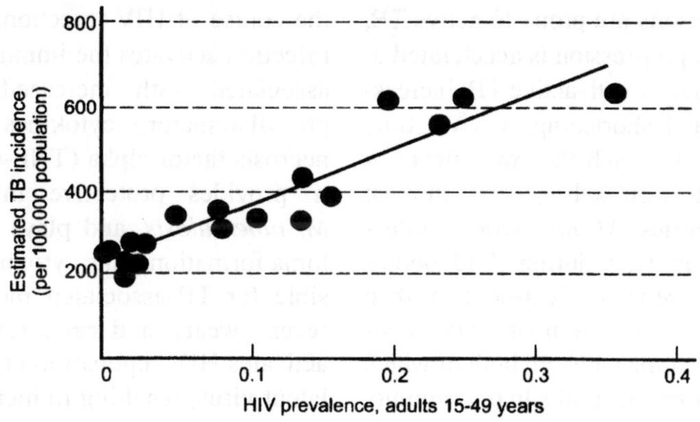

FIGURE 1. Relationship between estimated incidence of TB (all forms) and HIV prevalence in adults for 18 African countries in 1999 (11).

directly correlated to TB incidence (11) (Figure 1). According to the WHO, TB case notification rates for Africa nearly doubled from 1981 to 1998 (59.3 per 100,000 to 107.5 per 100,000) (18). Of the 23 countries in the world with the greatest number of TB cases, nine are in sub–Saharan Africa. Listed in order of number of cases, they are: Nigeria, Ethiopia, South Africa, The Democratic Republic of Congo, Kenya, Tanzania, Mozambique, Uganda, and Zimbabwe. In each of these countries, the estimated incidence of TB in 1999 was over 300 cases per 100,000 persons (11). Rates of HIV coinfection among African TB patients are significant. In countries where HIV is highly endemic, such as Uganda, Burundi, Malawi, and Zimbabwe, 57% to 74% of patients with active TB are found to also have HIV infection (19–21). In the countries of West Africa, where HIV is not as highly endemic, 3% to 43% of TB cases occur in persons with HIV infection (19–21).

In African nations with high HIV prevalence, the estimated number of TB cases occurring in 2005 will be nearly double that which occurred in 1999 (11). It is projected that the total number of TB cases worldwide and in Africa will continue to increase over the coming decades, as will the proportion of cases with HIV coinfection.

PATHOGENESIS

Primary infection with *M. tuberculosis* occurs when tubercle bacilli are inhaled and grow intracellularly in the host's alveolar macrophages. This occurrence is followed by the recruitment of new macrophages and lymphocytes, and the formation of a tuberculous granuloma. Primary TB disease, which occurs in about 5% of those infected as a result of the hematogenous or lymphatic spread of tubercle bacillus, may present as perihilar lymphadenopathy and pulmonary infiltrates. In some persons, particularly children, more serious forms of disease, such as miliary disease or meningitis, may occur at this stage. In over 90% of HIV-uninfected persons, however, primary TB infection is contained and enters a clinically latent stage that may persist for decades or the lifetime of the host. Persons with latent TB infection are neither sick nor infectious. Persons at increased risk of progressing from latent infection to reactivation disease include those with certain medical conditions such as diabetes mellitus, renal failure, some malignancies, immunosuppressive therapy, or HIV infection (22). Of these risks, HIV infection is by far the greatest, by several orders of magnitude (23).

HIV and *M. tuberculosis* infections interact, each affecting the other adversely.

HIV-infected persons are prone to active TB, and HIV disease progression is accelerated in HIV-infected persons with active TB, increasing morbidity and shortening survival time (24). The order in which the two infections occur has an effect on pathogenesis. In most developing countries, *M. tuberculosis* infection usually occurs first, during childhood or adolescence, before HIV infection. HIV then gradually causes a reduction of $CD4^+$ cells and interferon-gamma (IFN-γ), both of which are key mediators of protective immunity against the development of active TB. This reduction of immune protection results in an increased rate of reactivation of latent infection. The risk of reactivation in those with HIV and latent *M. tuberculosis* infection is estimated to be 5% to 10% annually, far exceeding the estimated lifetime risk of reactivation in those without HIV infection (2% to 7%) (25). When reactivation TB occurs early in HIV infection, while immunity is relatively well preserved, cavitary pulmonary disease may be present. However, when immunodeficiency is advanced, pulmonary findings may be atypical, and there is an increased rate of extrapulmonary disease (2).

Primary infection or reinfection with *M. tuberculosis* may occur in those already infected with HIV. When *M. tuberculosis* infection occurs in advanced HIV disease ($CD4^+ < 200$ cells/mm^3), progression to TB disease is rapid, findings on chest radiograph are atypical, and rates of extrapulmonary and disseminated disease are increased (26). Atypical findings associated with pulmonary disease include lower-lobe infiltrates, hilar lymphadenopathy, and miliary spread. Extrapulmonary disease may involve the pleura, meninges, peritoneum, kidneys, or lymph nodes. Histologically, rather than the formation of granulomas and tissue breakdown with cavities, the hallmark of extrapulmonary TB is the presence of foamy epithelioid cells which are in fact, macrophages laden with AFB (15).

While HIV may worsen the course of TB, the development of TB also profoundly affects the course of HIV infection. *M. tuberculosis* infection activates the immune system and is associated with increased expression of proinflammatory cytokines such as tumor necrosis factor-alpha (TNF-α) (27,28). TNF-α provides protective immunity against *M. tuberculosis*, and plays a role in granuloma formation. This cytokine is also responsible for TB-associated morbidity, such as fever, sweats, and cachexia. In addition, it activates HIV replication in cells that harbor latent virus, resulting in increased viral load, increased frequency of other opportunistic infections, accelerated decline of $CD4^+$ cells, and shortened survival time (24,29).

CLINICAL MANIFESTATIONS OF TUBERCULOSIS IN HIV INFECTION

Pulmonary Tuberculosis

Pulmonary disease is the most common presentation of TB in persons with HIV infection and is seen with or without extrapulmonary involvement (30). Persons with early HIV infection present with the typical picture of cavitating, upper lobe pulmonary TB. The symptoms, which are similar to those seen in persons with TB who do not have HIV infection, include cough, chest pain, hemoptysis, fever, night sweats, and weight loss. HIV-infected TB patients have smaller numbers of bacilli in sputum smears, and a smaller proportion have sputum smear-positive disease than TB patients who are not infected with HIV (31).

Extrapulmonary Tuberculosis

Extrapulmonary disease is more common in persons with HIV infection than in those without HIV infection. In Zambia, extrapulmonary TB, with or without pulmonary disease, was found in 60% of HIV-infected patients compared to 28% of those without

HIV infection (32). The occurrence of extrapulmonary TB and mycobacteremia increases with the level of immunosuppression (2). In many forms of extrapulmonary TB, symptoms are nonspecific, and extrapulmonary disease should be considered when a patient with HIV infection presents with fever of unknown origin. Because the majority of patients with extrapulmonary TB also have pulmonary TB, a chest radiograph demonstrating pulmonary disease may be helpful in the diagnosis of extrapulmonary TB.

The sites most commonly affected by extrapulmonary TB include the pleura, abdominal viscera, lymph nodes, meninges, pericardium, and bones and joints. Pleural TB is the most common of these and is manifested by exudative effusions. Persons with abdominal TB may present with complaints of pain, diarrhea, and vomiting. Pathologic findings include intra-abdominal lymphadenopathy, or parenchymal involvement of the liver, spleen or kidneys. On clinical examination, there may be mild to moderate ascites, associated with abdominal tenderness and enlargement of the liver or spleen. Persons with renal TB may present with pyelonephritis with sterile pyuria. In HIV-infected persons, tuberculous lymphadenitis may manifest as enlarged, tender lymph nodes and presentation may be acute, mimicking pyogenic infection. In advanced HIV disease, lymph node aspirate may show a multitude of AFB on Ziehl-Neelsen stain. Tuberculous meningitis should be suspected in any patient with chronic constitutional symptoms of days' to weeks' duration and features of meningitis. The prognosis of such patients is poor, especially if the diagnosis is suspected late, after multiple courses of antibiotics and antimalarials (in endemic regions) for unremitting fevers and headache. Some patients with central nervous system infection may present with brain tuberculomas and features of intracerebral space-occupying lesions. Such lesions are usually unilateral (33). Miliary TB is more common among patients with advanced immunosuppression, and tuberculous pericarditis may present as chest pain and cardiac failure (2,13).

Pediatric Tuberculosis

As in adults, the clinical manifestations of TB in HIV-infected children are dependent on the stage of immunosuppression. The signs of TB in children with early HIV infection are similar to those seen in children without HIV infection. During later stages of HIV infection, disseminated disease, tuberculous meningitis, and widespread tuberculous adenitis become more common (14). Studies in Africa have reported a high prevalence of HIV infection in children with TB. In one study conducted in Malawi, the prevalence of HIV was 57.8% in children with probable TB, and 71% in those with confirmed TB (34–36).

DIAGNOSIS

Mycobacterium tuberculosis Infection

The tuberculin skin test is a diagnostic tool used to detect *M. tuberculosis* infection. The Mantoux technique, using purified protein derivative, is the preferred method of administering tuberculin skin tests. This test is not useful for the diagnosis of active TB disease in many parts of Africa because people in high-prevalence populations will have high rates of latent infection and test positive, regardless of their disease status. Thus, tuberculin skin testing should be utilized only for the diagnosis of latent TB infection when treatment for this is being considered. Bacille Calmette-Guérin (BCG) vaccination is used widely in Africa, which may also complicate the interpretation of the tuberculin skin test because BCG may produce a false positive test. This situation should not contraindicate the use of tuberculin skin testing as a general rule. However, a negative tuberculin skin test does not rule out infection with *M. tuberculosis*, especially in HIV-infected persons who may not be able to mount a positive skin test due to immunosuppression.

Tuberculosis Disease

Pulmonary Tuberculosis

Examination of acid-fast smears of sputum using the Ziehl-Neelsen staining method is the primary method for the diagnosis of pulmonary TB in Africa. This method is inexpensive, and can be performed in remote areas with a microscope using sun-reflected lighting. A concentration of 10^4 organisms/ml must be present in a specimen in order to demonstrate organisms on the smear. Technicians must be properly trained to obtain high quality readings of smears. The International Union against TB and Lung Disease recommends that, on average, a technician should process and examine a maximum of 20 slides per day. Unfortunately, due to overload of diagnostic facilities and lack of staff, many technicians process an excess of slides or combine smear examination with other diagnostic procedures, and the quality of readings may suffer as a result.

In most African settings, a positive sputum smear is used as diagnostic evidence of pulmonary TB and prompts initiation of treatment. In addition to diagnosis, sputum smears are used to judge the degree of infectiousness and to evaluate the patient's response to treatment.

Sputum can be induced with nebulized hypertonic saline to increase the yield of sputum smears. Smear examination of lavage fluid obtained by bronchoscopy is a higher-yield diagnostic option, but it is costly and only available in selected settings. In settings where sputum induction or bronchoscopy is used, appropriate infection control measures should be in place to protect health-care workers and patients from the infectious aerosols generated by these procedures (37).

Fluorescent staining, if available, increases the sensitivity of smear examination. Sputum testing with polymerase chain reaction-based diagnostics is both highly sensitive and specific for the detection of *M. tuberculosis*. This type of testing, however, is costly and requires a well-equipped laboratory.

Mycobacterial cultures are not routinely performed throughout most of Africa because of prohibitive cost and the lack of proper laboratory facilities in many regions. If available, cultures may be warranted for certain purposes, such as to evaluate prolonged fever in patients who do not show localizing signs of disease, to survey for drug resistance in communities, to obtain drug-susceptibility results for selected individuals, or to diagnose patients with abnormal chest radiographs and negative sputum smears. When cultures are performed, solid media is usually used. Results are generally not available for 6 to 8 weeks, limiting the usefulness of this media. The more rapid culture systems that use liquid media are not available in most African settings.

Chest radiography is a useful adjunct for the diagnosis of pulmonary TB, especially in cases of smear-negative disease. Chest radiography is available in referral and district-level hospitals, but may not be available at rural health posts. In areas where chest radiography is not available, HIV-infected persons for whom there is a strong clinical suspicion of pulmonary TB may be started empirically on anti-TB treatment. In patients with endobronchial TB and disease in those with advanced immunosuppression, chest radiograph findings may be minimal or absent, even if they have highly smear-positive sputum specimens. In patients with HIV infection, therefore, a normal chest radiograph does not exclude infectious pulmonary TB.

Extrapulmonary Tuberculosis

Diagnosis of extrapulmonary TB may be definitive or presumptive. Ultrasonography, computerized tomography (CT) scans and magnetic resonance imaging (MRI) may aid diagnosis. The pleural fluid of patients with extrapulmonary TB is exudative; cell counts will show lymphocytic predominance; and smears may occasionally demonstrate AFB. The yield of pleural fluid culture is generally not as high as that of sputum. Pleural biopsy may show granulomatous changes. In cases of abdominal TB, ultrasonography may demonstrate ascites with enlargement of nodes. Other diagnostic considerations include lymphoma, and rarely, Kaposi's sarcoma. Smears and cultures of peritoneal fluid generally have a low yield. Biopsies of liver may demonstrate granulomas. Tuberculous adenitis may be diagnosed by lymph node aspiration; positive smears are common in patients with advanced HIV infection. When the smear of an aspirate is negative, a biopsy should be performed to distinguish TB from lymphoma. Confirmation of tuberculous meningitis is difficult because both smears and cultures of cerebrospinal fluid have low yields. Therefore, treatment is generally based on clinical findings. Pericarditis due to TB is also difficult to diagnose. However, precordial chest pain and congestive heart failure may be important findings leading to the diagnosis. On echocardiography, there may be pathognomonic fibrous strands between the thickened pericardium and the heart.

Since TB is the first HIV-related opportunistic infection to occur in many cases, patients may be unaware of their HIV infection at the time that TB is diagnosed. Because of this, all persons with newly diagnosed TB should receive HIV counseling and testing, and if positive, be referred to AIDS programs. Clinicians should be aware that the diagnosis of TB may be interpreted as a sign of HIV infection and lead to stigmatization of patients.

TREATMENT

The successful treatment of TB requires the extended use of several agents that are active against *M. tuberculosis*. Since drug-susceptibility results are not available in many African settings, physicians will often have to choose treatment regimens empirically. Treatment of TB is divided into two phases: an initial intensive phase followed by a continuation phase. Ideally, the entire treatment regimen should be delivered in a supervised manner in which ingestion of medications is directly observed. This approach optimizes patient adherence and cure, and minimizes the risk of developing drug resistance. To limit the development of resistance, treatment should be supervised at least during the intensive phase for all new smear-positive pulmonary cases, and throughout both phases for all retreatment cases or for those taking rifampin-containing regimens (14). In cases of treatment of active disease with self-administered therapy, it is recommended that approved fixed-dose combination formulations be used to decrease the risk of drug resistance.

The WHO recommends three possible treatment regimens for new patients with smear-positive pulmonary TB, extensive smear-negative pulmonary disease, or severe extrapulmonary disease (Table 1). Each regimen starts with 2 months of daily or thrice-weekly intensive-phase therapy, followed by 4 to 6 months of continuation-phase therapy. For new patients with tuberculous meningitis, miliary TB, or spinal TB with neurologic signs, an extended continuation-phase of daily therapy with isoniazid and rifampin for 7 months may be preferred.

In several studies, TB patients with HIV infection experienced higher rates of cure of TB and lower rates of TB recurrence and death with the use of short-course rifampin-containing regimens compared with non- rifampin-containing regimens (38–41). The optimal duration of TB therapy for those with HIV infection is controversial (39,42,43). In resource-poor settings, cost may prohibit the use of rifampin throughout both phases of treatment; ethambutol is substituted for rifampin in the continuation-phase need to keep consistent with use of

TABLE 1. WHO-Recommended Regimens for the Treatment of Tuberculosis (14)

Patient diagnosis	Treatment regimen options[a] Intensive-phase, dosed daily or 3 times per week	Continuation phase
New smear-positive pulmonary TB New smear-negative pulmonary TB with extensive parenchymal involvement New cases of severe forms of extrapulmonary TB	2 EHRZ (SHRZ)	6 HE, 4 HR, or 4 H_3R_3
Sputum smear-positive: Relapse Treatment failure Treatment after interruption	2 SHRZE + 1 HRZE	5 $H_3R_3E_3$ or 5 HRE
New smear-negative pulmonary TB (other than listed above) New less severe forms of extrapulmonary TB	2 HRZ	6 HE, 4 HR, or 4 H_3R_3

[a]The standard code for TB treatment regimens is as follows: S indicates streptomycin; H, isoniazid; R, rifampin; Z, pyrazinamide; and E, ethambutol. A regimen consists of 2 phases: intensive and continuation. The number before the regimen indicates the duration of that phase in months (e.g. 2 EHRZ indicates 2 months of ethambutol, isoniazid, rifampin, and pyrazinamide). A number in subscript after a letter indicates the number of doses of that drug per week (e.g. H_3 indicates three doses of isoniazid per week). If there is no number in subscript after a letter, treatment with that drug is daily. An alternative drug (or drugs) appears as a letter or letters in parentheses.

continuation-phase and intensive-phase of some regimens. In such cases, continuation-phase therapy should last for at least 6 months and total treatment, for at least 8 months. Although regimens that substitute ethambutol for rifampin in the continuation phase are less expensive, one study reported a relapse rate of 8% in TB patients with HIV infection who received treatment with ethambutol. This rate was higher than that of historical controls who were treated with rifampin throughout both phases of treatment (43).

In the past, thiacetazone-containing regimens were used in Africa because of their low cost. However, thiacetazone has been associated with severe, often fatal, cutaneous reactions in persons with HIV infection (38). Because of this, the WHO recommends that this drug not be used to treat persons with known or suspected HIV infection. If possible, all TB patients should be treated with nonthiacetazone-containing regimens, and should receive rifampin at least during the 2 months of intensive-phase therapy (14).

Treatment regimens often cannot be tailored to individual drug-susceptibility results because the availability of drug-susceptibility testing in Africa is limited at best. Thus, those who are at risk for acquired drug resistance should receive expanded therapy; expanded empiric regimens are recommended for patients with positive sputum smears that result from treatment failure, interruption, or relapse. An increased number of drugs are used for expanded therapy. The duration of intensive-phase therapy with an expanded regimen is 3 months, and the continuation-phase is 5 months (Table 1). If susceptibility testing demonstrates that a patient has developed multidrug resistance (resistance to at least isoniazid and rifampin), therapy must be individualized and continued for at least 18 months (44).

A modified regimen may be used for cases of smear-negative pulmonary disease that is not extensive, or for less severe forms of extrapulmonary disease (Table 1). Streptomycin should only be used in settings that have the capability to sterilize the needles and syringes used for its administration (14). Dosages and adverse effects of first-line anti-TB drugs are listed in Table 2. Because HIV infection is a risk factor for isoniazid-associated peripheral neuropathy, persons

TABLE 2. WHO-Recommended Dosages for Adults and Children, and Adverse Effects of Anti-TB Medications (14)

Drug	Oral dose (mg/kg),[a] (Maximum dose) Daily	Three times per week[b]	Adverse effects
Isoniazid	5, (300)	10[c]	Rash Peripheral neuropathy Hepatic enzyme elevation Hepatitis Central nervous system effects Elevation of phenytoin and carbamazepine levels
Rifampin	10, (600)	10, (600)	Rash Gastrointestinal distress Hepatic enzyme elevation Hepatitis Fever Thrombocytopenia Flu-like symptoms Orange-colored body fluids Decreased levels of many drugs, including: methadone, warfarin, glucocorticoids, oral hypoglycemics, anticonvulsants, dapsone, cyclosporin, digitalis, oral contraceptives, certain protease inhibitors and nonnucleoside reverse transcriptase inhibitors
Pyrazinamide	25	35	Flushing of skin Gastrointestinal distress Rash Hyperuricemia with arthralgias, gout (rare) Hepatitis
Ethambutol	15	30	Optic neuritis (decreased red–green discrimination, decreased visual acuity)
Streptomycin	15	15	Ototoxicity (hearing loss and vestibular dysfunction) Nephrotoxicity Sterile abscesses

[a]Some TB control programs recommend higher doses per kg of certain anti-TB medications for the treatment of children (23).
[b]Twice-weekly dosages are used in a number of TB control programs in developed countries, but are not currently recommended by the WHO or the International Union Against TB and Lung Disease.
[c]Some TB control programs recommend an isoniazid dose of 15 mg/kg (maximum dose 900 mg) for thrice-weekly dosing (23).

with HIV infection should receive 10 mg of pyridoxine daily while receiving isoniazid treatment (14).

Response to treatment should be assessed for all patients with smear-positive pulmonary disease by monitoring sputum smears. At a minimum, sputums should be checked at the end of the intensive-phase, during the continuation-phase, and at the end of treatment; at least two sputum samples should be obtained each time. Chest radiography is not recommended for routine monitoring because of its cost. For patients with sputum smear-negative or extrapulmonary disease, clinical monitoring should be performed (14). Clinical monitoring of all patients is also important to detect adverse effects of anti-TB drugs (14). A patient who remains sputum smear-positive 5 months or longer after starting anti-TB therapy is considered a treatment failure and needs to be restarted on an expanded treatment regimen (Table 1).

Up to 30% of persons in sub–Saharan Africa who are coinfected with HIV and TB may die within 12 months of starting anti-TB therapy (3,45). In many, if not most cases, the cause of death is advanced HIV infection or other opportunistic infections rather than progressive or refractory TB. The case fatality rate in all TB patients is closely linked to HIV prevalence. Even among TB patients without HIV infection, TB case fatality rates are greater in high HIV-prevalence settings than in low HIV-prevalence settings (45). This increased rate is probably a result of poorer health service performance in areas where HIV-related disease is overburdening health care systems. Research is needed to better define the cause of death in persons with HIV infection and TB and to determine interventions to prevent fatalities in these patients.

To treat coinfected individuals effectively, both their TB and HIV infections must be addressed. Ideally, this would mean that coinfected TB patients receive antiretroviral therapy and prophylaxis for HIV-related opportunistic infections, in addition to appropriate TB treatment—an ideal that requires cooperation between TB and AIDS programs. TB program sites can be used to deliver HIV prevention messages, HIV counseling and testing, and cotrimoxazole prophylaxis for opportunistic infections. AIDS programs and voluntary counseling and testing sites can provide valuable TB case finding information.

Of the standard first-line drugs used for treatment, only rifampin has the potential for significant interactions with other drugs. This potential will become increasingly important with the introduction of highly active antiretroviral therapy (HAART) in Africa. There are significant drug–drug interactions between rifampin and certain protease inhibitors and nonnucleoside reverse transcriptase inhibitors (46). Rifabutin has been recommended as a substitute for rifampin. Guidelines have been published that recommend specific regimens and dose adjustments when HAART is used concomitantly with anti-TB medications (46).

When HIV patients who are coinfected with TB begin HAART, their TB symptoms may worsen as a result of immune restoration. The clinical course may consist of worsening fever, pulmonary infiltrates, and lymphadenopathy; symptoms typically start within days to weeks after the initiation of HAART. Treatment of TB symptoms resulting from immune restoration is generally supportive, although in some cases corticosteroids have been used (47).

PREVENTION

Treatment for latent TB infection, also known as chemoprophylaxis or preventive therapy, can prevent the progression of *M. tuberculosis* infection to active disease. This treatment has been recommended for use in children in Africa who are household contacts of persons with infectious TB (13). Several controlled trials have demonstrated the efficacy of treatment for *M. tuberculosis* infection in preventing TB in persons with HIV infection and a reactive tuberculin skin test (48–52). As a result, the WHO has recommended the use of 6 months of isoniazid preventive therapy for HIV-infected individuals who have latent TB infection (53). However, most African countries lack the resources to perform the screening tuberculin skin tests and chest radiographs needed to implement this intervention. In settings where the prevalence of *M. tuberculosis* infection is over 30%, isoniazid has been recommendations for use in HIV-infected individuals, even if tuberculin skin testing is not performed. When resources are limited, priority for isoniazid preventive therapy should be given to populations at particularly high risk, such as HIV-infected health care workers, prisoners, and miners (53).

Truly effective prevention of TB will depend on the development of a safe vaccine that is more effective than BCG. Unfortunately, no such vaccine currently exists, but several candidates are under development.

OTHER ISSUES

Infection Control Issues

Particularly in highly endemic areas, nosocomial transmission of *M. tuberculosis* may occur, placing health care workers, laboratory workers, and patients at risk for infection or reinfection with *M. tuberculosis* (37,54). In one South African study, nosocomial transmission of multidrug-resistant TB to HIV-infected persons who were hospitalized for the treatment of drug-susceptible TB was documented (55). Efforts should be made to control TB transmission in health care settings. Although some infection control measures, such as the use of isolation rooms and respiratory protection, are not feasible in low-income settings, other controls can be effective. These controls include maximizing ventilation, separating those with TB from other patients, and performing cough-generating procedures such as sputum-specimen collection in either outdoor or well-ventilated spaces that are removed from other patients (37,56). To prevent nosocomial transmission of drug-resistant TB to patients, it may be useful to separate those with newly diagnosed TB from treatment failure and re-treatment patients.

Drug-Resistant Tuberculosis

Because drug-susceptibility results are not available on an individual basis, national surveys for drug resistance among *M. tuberculosis* isolates are important. In a recent worldwide survey, rates of drug resistance from 1996 through 1999 were examined in a number of countries, including eight African countries. For new TB cases, resistance to isoniazid and multidrug resistance ranged from 2.7%–7.9% and 0.5%–3.5%, respectively. For retreatment cases, rates for isoniazid resistance were 16.0%–61.5%, and for multidrug resistance, 3.3%–28.1% (57). In a study examining the drug susceptibility of *M. tuberculosis* isolates from notified TB cases in the United States from 1993 through 1996 among persons aged 25 to 44 years, the risk of drug-resistant TB was higher among persons with known HIV infection. There was a significantly higher rate of TB caused by isolates that were resistant to at least isoniazid, at least isoniazid and rifampin, or rifampin alone, in those with HIV infection (23).

Persons with TB caused by isolates that are resistant to isoniazid alone, rifampin alone, or at least isoniazid and rifampin have higher treatment failure rates than those with TB caused by organisms that are susceptible to all first-line anti-TB drugs (58). A program known as directly observed therapy, short course, plus (DOTS plus) has been proposed by the WHO to offer optimal treatment for cases of drug-resistant TB and to prevent increasing rates of drug resistance. This program consists of culture and drug-susceptibility testing for patients, with regimens tailored to drug-susceptibility results (59). The feasibility of such a program in Africa, however, remains to be established.

CONCLUSION

TB is a disease that threatens all persons, regardless of immune status. Increased rates of TB disease, combined with its airborne transmission, pose a public health threat to all persons and not only to those with HIV infection. Unfortunately, a large burden of the world's TB morbidity and mortality has been and will continue to be borne by those with HIV infection. The HIV pandemic has changed the natural history, clinical manifestations, and paradigms for controlling TB in individuals, institutions and the general population, and aggressive efforts for its control are desperately needed. In Africa, HIV infection and TB cases are integrally linked. Thus, prevention and control efforts aimed at each disease must take the other into consideration. This may be best accomplished by integrating TB and AIDS activities in African nations. The scope of TB control should be expanded to include broad case finding and wide-scale implementation of DOT to guarantee effective treatment of all TB patients. Among those with HIV infection, latent TB infections must be treated; measures to prevent HIV transmission must be implemented; and HAART must be provided. Only when these measures are in place, can there be both decreased morbidity and mortality in persons coinfected with HIV and *M. tuberculosis*, and effective control of TB in Africa.

REFERENCES

1. UNAIDS. Report on the global HIV/AIDS epidemic. Geneva: UNAIDS, June 2000.
2. Havlir DV, Barnes PF. Tuberculosis in patients with human immunodeficiency virus infection. *N Engl J Med*, 1999;340:367–373.
3. Harries AD, Hargreaves NJ, Kemp J, et al. Deaths from tuberculosis in sub-Saharan African countries with a high prevalence of HIV-1. *Lancet*, 2001;357:1519–1523.
4. Kubica GP, Wayne LG. *The Mycobacteria: A Source Book*. New York: Marcel Dekker, 1984: 38–41.
5. Hanna BA. Diagnosis of tuberculosis by microbiologic techniques. In: Rom W, Garay S, eds. *Tuberculosis*, 1st ed. Boston: Little, Brown and Company, 1996:149–159.
6. Riley RL. Airborne infection. *Am J Med*, 1974;57: 466–475.
7. Curtis A, Ridzon R, Ferry J, et al. Extensive transmission of *M. tuberculosis* from a child. *N Engl J Med*, 1999;341:1491–1495.
8. Cauthen GM, Dooley SW, Onorato IM, et al. Transmission of *Mycobacterium tuberculosis* from tuberculosis patients with HIV infection or AIDS. *Am J Epidemiol*, 1996;144:69–77.
9. Dye C, Scheele S, Dolin P, et al. Consensus Statement. Global burden of tuberculosis: estimated incidence, prevalence, and mortality by country. *JAMA*, 1999;282:677–686.
10. Styblo K. The global aspect of tuberculosis and HIV infection. *Bull Int Union Tuberc Lung Dis*, 1990;65:28–32.
11. World Health Organization. *Global Tuberculosis Control, WHO Report 2001*. WHO/TB/2001.287. Geneva: World Health Organization, 2001.
12. Report on the Global HIV/AIDS Epidemic. UNAIDS/00.13E. UNAIDS: Geneva, 2000.
13. Harries AD, Maher D. *TB/HIV: A Clinical Manual*. Geneva: World Health Organization, 1996;126–127.
14. Maher D, Chaulet P, Spinaci S, et al. *Treatment of tuberculosis: guidelines for national programmes*, 2nd ed. Geneva: World Health Organization, 1997.
15. Lucas SB, Hounnou A, Peacock C, et al. The mortality and pathology of HIV infection in a West African city. *AIDS*, 1993;7:1569–1579.
16. Whalen C, Horsburgh CR, Hom D, et al. Accelerated course of human immunodeficiency virus infection after tuberculosis. *Am J Respir Crit Care Med*, 1995;151:129–135.
17. Whalen C, Okwera A, Johnson J, et al. Predictors of survival in HIV-infected patients with pulmonary tuberculosis. Makerere University-Case Western Reserve University Research Collaboration. *Am J Respir Crit Care Med*, 1996;153:1977–1981.
18. World Health Organization. *Global Tuberculosis Control. WHO Report 2000*. WHO/CDS/TB/2000. 275. Geneva: World Health Organization, 2000.
19. Raviglione MC, Harries AD, Msiska R, et al. Tuberculosis and HIV: current status in Africa. *AIDS*, 1997;11(suppl B):S115.
20. Kenyon TA, Mwasekaga MJ, Huebner R, et al. Low levels of drug-resistance amidst rapidly increasing tuberculosis and human immunodeficiency virus co-epidemics in Botswana. *Int J Tuberc Lung Dis*, 1999;3:4–11.
21. Eriki PO, Okwera A, Aisu T, et al. The influence of human immunodeficiency virus infection on tuberculosis in Kampala, Uganda. *Am Rev Respir Dis*, 1991;143:185–187.
22. Centers for Disease Control and Prevention. Targeted tuberculin testing and treatment of latent tuberculosis infection. *MMWR*, 2000;49(No. RR-6):7–10.
23. Centers for Disease Control and Prevention. Prevention and treatment of tuberculosis among patients infected with human immunodeficiency virus: principles of therapy and revised recommendations. *MMWR*, 1998;47(RR-20):1–58.
24. Whalen CC, Nsubuga P, Okwera A, et al. Impact of pulmonary tuberculosis on survival of HIV-infected adults: a prospective epidemiologic study in Uganda. *AIDS*, 2000;14:1219–1228.
25. Selwyn PA, Hartel D, Lewis VA, et al. A prospective study of the risk of tuberculosis among intravenous drug users with human immunodeficiency virus infection. *N Engl J Med*, 1989;320: 545–550.
26. Perlman DC, El-Sadr WM, Nelson ET, et al. Variation of chest radiographic patterns in pulmonary tuberculosis by degree of human immunodeficiency virus-related suppression. *Clin Infect Dis*, 1997;25:242–246.

27. Wallis RS, Vjecha M, Amir-Tahmasseb M, et al. Influence of tuberculosis on human immunodeficiency virus (HIV-1); enhanced cytokine expression and elevated beta 2-microglobulin in HIV-1-associated tuberculosis. *J Infect Dis*, 1993; 167:43–48.
28. Vanham G, Edmonds K, Qing L, et al. Generalized immune activation in pulmonary tuberculosis: co-activation with HIV infection. *Clin Exp Immunol*, 1996;103:30–34.
29. Badri M, Ehrlich R, Wood R, et al. Association between tuberculosis and HIV disease progression in a high tuberculosis prevalence area. *Int J Tuberc Lung Dis*, 2001;5:225–232.
30. Theuer CP, Hopewell PC, Elias D, et al. Human immunodeficiency virus infection in tuberculosis patients. *J Infect Dis*, 1990;162:8–12.
31. Elliott AM, Namaambo K, Allen BW, et al. Negative sputum smear results in HIV-positive patients with pulmonary tuberculosis in Lusaka, Zambia. *Tuberc Lung Dis*, 1993;74:191–194.
32. Elliott AM, Halwiindi B, Hayes RJ, et al. The impact of human immunodeficiency virus on presentation and diagnosis of tuberculosis in a cohort study in Zambia. *J Trop Med Hyg*, 1993;96:1–11.
33. Thonell L, Pendle S, Sacks L. Clinical and radiologic features of South African patients with tuberculomas of the brain. *Clin Infect Dis*, 2000;31: 619–620.
34. Sassan-Morokro M, De Cock KM, Ackah A, et al. Tuberculosis and HIV infection in children in Abidjan, Cote d'Ivoire. *Trans R Soc Trop Med Hyg*, 1994;88:178–181.
35. Chintu C, Bhat G, Luo C, et al. Seroprevalence of human immunodeficiency virus type 1 infection in Zambian children with tuberculosis. *Pediatr Infect Dis J*, 1993;12:499–504.
36. Kiwanuka J, Graham SM, Coulter JB, et al. Diagnosis of pulmonary tuberculosis in children in an HIV-endemic area, Malawi. *Annals of Tropical Paediatrics*, 2001:21:5–14.
37. Granich R, Binkin NJ, Jarvis WR, et al. *Guidelines for the prevention of tuberculosis in health care facilities in resource-limited settings*. WHO/CDS/TB/99.269. Geneva: World Health Organization, 1999.
38. Okwera A, Whalen C, Byekwaso F, et al. Randomised trial of thiacetazone and rifampicin-containing regimens for pulmonary tuberculosis in HIV-infected Ugandans. *Lancet*, 1994;344:1323–1328.
39. Perriens JH, Colebunders RL, Karahunga C, et al. Increased mortality and tuberculosis treatment failure among human immunodeficiency virus (HIV) seropositive compared with HIV seronegative patients with pulmonary tuberculosis treated with "standard" chemotherapy in Kinshasa, Zaire. *Am Rev Respir Dis*, 1991;144:750–755.
40. Hawken M, Nunn P, Gathua S, et al. Increased recurrence of tuberculosis in HIV-1-infected patients in Kenya. *Lancet*, 1993;342:332–337.
41. Elliott AM, Halwiindi B, Hayes RJ, et al. The impact of human immunodeficiency virus on mortality of patients treated for tuberculosis in a cohort study in Zambia. *Trans R Soc Trop Med Hyg*, 1995;89:78–82.
42. Pulido F, Pena JM, Rubio R, et al. Relapse of tuberculosis after treatment in human immunodefiency virus-infected patients. *Arch Intern Med*, 1997;157:227–232.
43. Johnson JL, Okwere A, Nsubuga P, et al. Efficacy of unsupervised 8-month rifampicin-containing regimen for treatment of pulmonary tuberculosis in HIV-infected adults. *Int J Tuberc and Lung Dis*, 2000;4:1032–1040.
44. Iseman MD. Treatment of multidrug-resistant tuberculosis. *N Engl J Med*, 1993;329:784–791. [erratum appears in N Engl J Med 1993 Nov 4;329(19):1435].
45. Mukadi YD, Maher D, Harries A. Tuberculosis case fatality rates in high HIV prevalence populations in sub-Saharan Africa. *AIDS*, 2001;15:143–152.
46. Centers for Disease Control and Prevention. Updated guidelines for the use of rifabutin or rifampin for the treatment and prevention of tuberculosis among HIV-infected patients taking protease inhibitors or nonnucleoside reverse transcriptase inhibitors. *MMWR*, 2000;49:185–189.
47. Narita M, Ashkin D, Hollender ES, et al. Paradoxical worsening of tuberculosis following antiretroviral therapy in patients with AIDS. *Am J Respir Crit Care Med*, 1998;158:157–161.
48. Whalen CC, Johnson JL, Okwera A, et al. A trial of three regimens to prevent tuberculosis in Ugandan adults infected with human immunodeficiency virus. Uganda-Case Western Reserve University Research Collaboration. *N Engl J Med*, 1997; 337:801–808.
49. Hawken MP, Meme HK, Elliot LC, et al. Isoniazid preventive therapy for tuberculosis in HIV-infected adults: results of a randomized controlled trial. *AIDS*, 1997;11:875–882.
50. Mwinga AG, Hosp M, Godfrey-Faussett P, et al. Twice weekly tuberculosis preventive therapy in HIV infection in Zambia. *AIDS*, 1998;12: 2447–2457.
51. Gordin FM, Mats JP, Miller C, et al. A controlled trial of isoniazid in persons with anergy and human immunodeficiency virus infection who are at high risk for tuberculosis. *N Engl J Med*, 1997;5: 315–320.
52. Pape JW, Jean SS, Ho JL, et al. Effect of isoniazid prophylaxis on the incidence of active tuberculosis and progression of HIV infection. *Lancet*, 1993;243:268–272.

53. World Health Organization. Preventive therapy against tuberculosis in people living with HIV. *Weekly Epidemiological Record*, 1999;74:385–400.
54. Rivero A, Marquez M, Santos J, et al. High rate of tuberculosis reinfection during a nosocomial outbreak of multidrug-resistant tuberculosis caused by *Mycobacterium bovis* strain B. *Clin Infect Dis*, 2001;32:159–161.
55. Sacks LV, Pendle S, Orlovic D, et al. A comparison of outbreak- and nonoutbreak-related multidrug-resistant tuberculosis among human immunodeficiency virus-infected patients in a South African hospital. *Clin Infect Dis*, 1999; 29:96–101.
56. Harries AD, Maher D, Nunn P. Practical and affordable measures for the protection of health care workers from tuberculosis in low-income countries. *Bull WHO*, 1997;75:477–489.
57. Espinal MA, Lazlo A, Simonsen L, et al. Global trends in resistance to antituberculosis drugs. *N Engl J Med*, 2001;344:1294–1303.
58. Espinal MA, Kim SJ, Suarez PG, et al. Standard short-course chemotherapy for drug-resistant tuberculosis treatment outcomes in 6 countries. *JAMA*, 2000;283:2537–2545.
59. World Health Organization. Guidelines for establishing DOTS-plus pilot projects for the management of MDR-TB. 2000; WHO/CDS/TB/2000:279.

23

HIV Infection and Cancer

*Robert Newton, †Freddy Sitas, ‡Martin Dedicoat, and §John L. Ziegler

**Cancer Research UK Epidemiology Unit, Radcliffe Infirmary, Oxford, United Kingdom.*
†Cancer Epidemiology Research Group, National Cancer Registry, South African Institute for Medical Research, Johannesburg, South Africa.
‡Liverpool School of Tropical Medicine and the Africa Centre & Hlabisa Hospital, KwaZulu Natal, South Africa.
§Cancer Risk Program, UCSF Comprehensive Cancer Center, University of California San Francisco, San Francisco, California, USA.

The human immunodeficiency virus (HIV) is distinguished from other cancer-causing viruses in that there is little evidence that it plays a direct oncogenic role in the development of a specific cancer. Instead, via its effects on the immune system, it appears to facilitate the development of a number of cancers, all of which are either known, or thought, to be caused by other infectious agents. For the purposes of this chapter, therefore, "causality" is defined simply on the premise that elimination of HIV infection would lead to a reduced risk of developing such cancers. The abbreviation "HIV" is used throughout and refers specifically to infection with HIV-1; reports on the association of cancers with HIV-2 are infrequent.

Even though the first cases of HIV disease were reported as recently as 1981, prevalence rates have quickly escalated and the World Health Organization (WHO) and UNAIDS currently estimate that over 36 million people are infected, the majority of whom are in sub–Saharan Africa (updates are available at www.unaids.org). Despite a high prevalence of HIV, information from Africa on the association between HIV infection and cancer is sparse. Cancers that are known to be HIV-associated, such as Kaposi's sarcoma (KS) and Burkitt's lymphoma, were endemic in some parts of Africa even before the advent of acquired immunodeficiency syndrome (AIDS) (1–4). Cervical cancer and hepatocellular carcinoma, both of which are caused by infectious agents, are also relatively frequent in parts of Africa (5). HIV-associated immunosuppression may increase the risk of other cancers caused by infectious agents (6). It is possible, therefore, that the HIV epidemic will have a profound effect on the patterns of cancer across the continent.

CANCERS ASSOCIATED WITH HIV INFECTION

Although many cancers have been reported to be increased in people with HIV infection, for only a few is the evidence sufficiently strong and consistent to decisively conclude that there is an increased risk. It is well recognized that infection with HIV is causally associated with KS, non-Hodgkin's lymphoma, and, in light of recent data emerging from sub–Saharan Africa, with conjunctival squamous cell carcinoma. Recent evidence for two other cancers in western populations—Hodgkin's disease and in children, leiomyosarcoma—also suggests an increase in risk associated with HIV infection (7–9). HIV infection may increase incidence of other cancers but, if so, such cancers are probably rare, or the relative risks associated with HIV are not very high.

Kaposi's Sarcoma

Clinical Manifestations

The clinical characteristics of KS that were described in homosexual men at the outset of the HIV epidemic differed markedly from those of the usually indolent condition, which generally affects the skin of the lower limbs of elderly men, that had been described previously (10). Although identical histologically, HIV-associated KS often presents with multiple lesions that affect both the skin and internal organs. Untreated HIV-infected individuals with KS survive for about 14 to 18 months, while individuals without HIV may live with KS for 10 to 15 years (11,12). However, an aggressive form of KS has occasionally been seen in both HIV-seronegative and HIV-seropositive children in Africa (Figure 1) (13,14). In children, the disease sites that are predominantly affected are the mucous membranes and draining lymph nodes of the head and neck, and the inguinal and genital areas (13).

Geographic Distribution before HIV

Before the HIV epidemic, incidence of KS showed a greater geographic variation than that of most other cancers. It was as common in parts of sub–Saharan Africa, such as Uganda and eastern Zaire (now the Democratic Republic of Congo), as colon cancer is in Europe and the United States, representing up to 9% of all cancers in men (1–4). Narrow belts of relatively high incidence stretched westward across the former Zaire to the coast of Cameroon and southward down the rift valley into Malawi and parts of South Africa (Figure 2) (1,15). Kaposi's sarcoma was also endemic, although much rarer, in

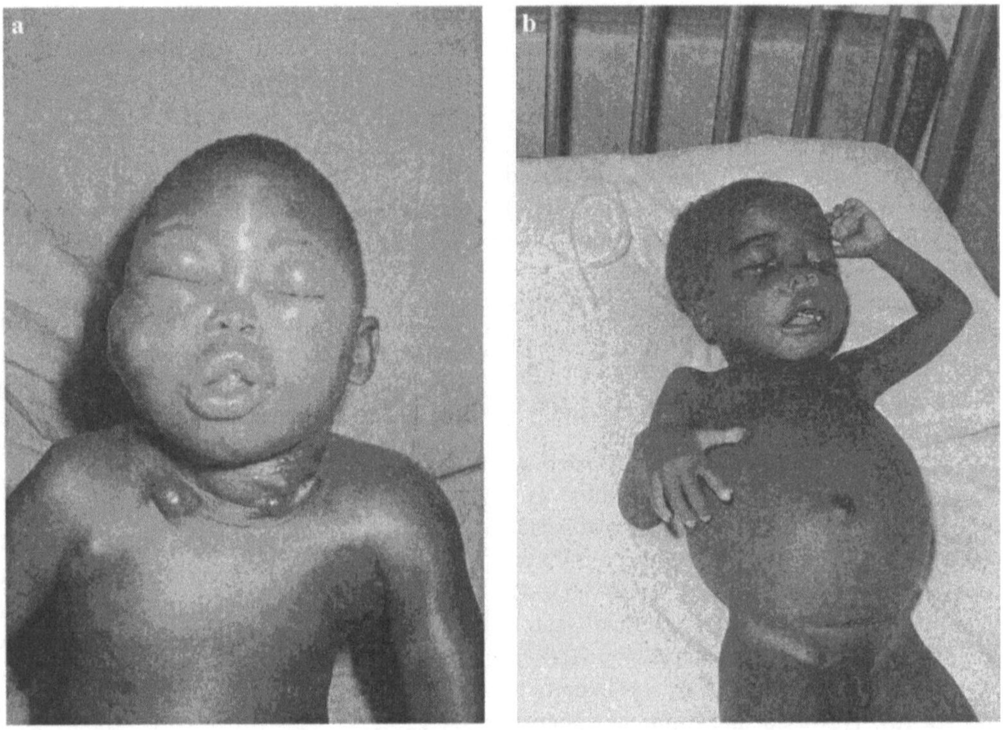

FIGURE 1. HIV-infected Ugandan children with Kaposi's sarcoma (photographs by John Ziegler).

countries around the Mediterranean—particularly Italy, Greece, and the Middle East—but was almost nonexistent elsewhere in the world, except in immigrants from the endemic countries (16–18). In all of these areas, KS was considerably more common in men than in women (1). The geographic variation in incidence correlates broadly with the distribution of human herpesvirus-8 (HHV-8), the principle cause of KS.

HIV and Kaposi's Sarcoma

The appearance of aggressive forms of KS in the United States in the early 1980s heralded the onset of the HIV epidemic in western countries. Although the incidence of KS has increased in populations at high risk for HIV infection in northern Europe and the United States, it had been so low before the onset of the HIV epidemic that it remains a relatively rare tumor in these areas (16,19). In contrast, an explosion in the incidence of KS has occurred in those parts of Africa where the prevalence of HIV is high and where KS was relatively common even before the AIDS epidemic. In the last 10 to 15 years, the incidence of KS has increased about 20-fold in Uganda and Zimbabwe, such that it is now the most common cancer in men and the second most common in women in these countries (20,21). Similarly, between 1988 and 1996, the incidence of KS increased at least 3-fold in South Africa, and continues to increase as the HIV epidemic worsens (22). Results from case-control studies conducted in Africa confirm that the epidemic increases in the incidence of KS are due to the spread of HIV infection (5,23–26).

Data from the South African National Cancer Registry show that between 1992 and

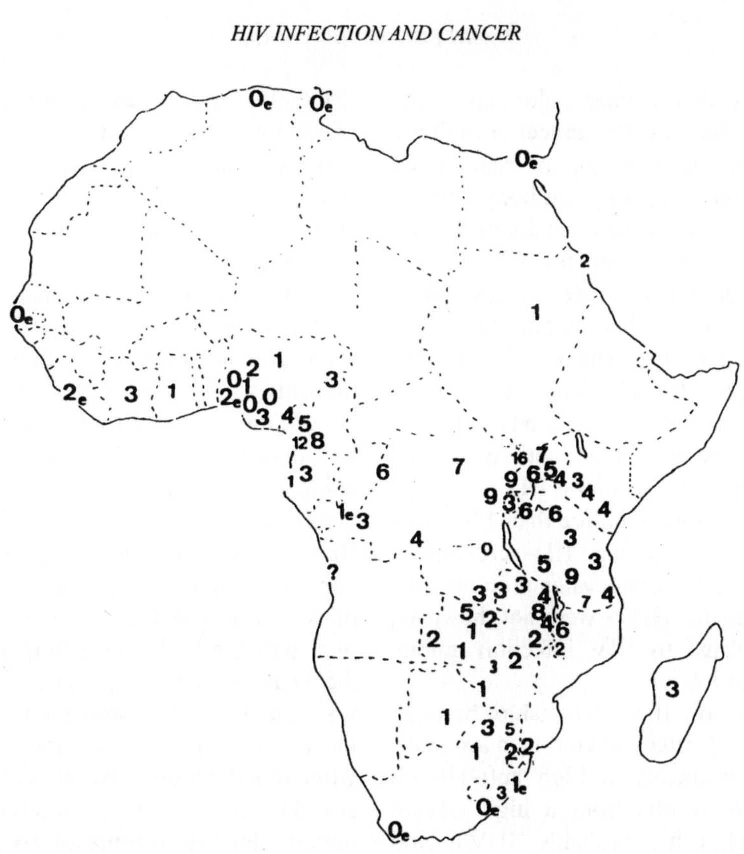

FIGURE 2. Estimated cumulative incidence rates per 1000 (age 0–64) for Kaposi's sarcoma in men, before the onset of the HIV epidemic. Subsript "e" refers to centers where estimates of cumulative incidence rest on specific assumptions, as outlined in the reference (1).

1996, the incidence of KS doubled in men, but increased about 7-fold in women, such that the male-to-female ratio of KS, which was 7 : 1 in 1988, is now 2 : 1 (22). Applying the age-specific incidence rate of KS, estimated by the Kampala Cancer Registry (20), to the black South African population, suggests that an additional 8000 cases of KS will occur annually in South Africa as a result of the HIV epidemic and that the overall population lifetime risk (0–74 years) of developing a cancer will increase from about 1 in 4 to 1 in 3.5 (22).

HHV-8 and Kaposi's Sarcoma

Human herpesvirus-8 (HHV-8), a newly discovered human herpesvirus (27), has been consistently associated with KS and is now considered to be the principal cause of the disease (28). Genomic sequences of HHV-8 are present in the tumor cells of KS lesions in virtually all patients (29), and its presence in peripheral blood, detected by polymerase chain reaction or serology, predicts the subsequent development of the tumor (30,31). Furthermore, HHV-8 is most prevalent in groups or populations that are at highest risk of developing KS, such as HIV-infected men who have sex with men in the United States, or populations in parts of Africa where the tumor has long been endemic (1,32,33).

A recent case-control study of black cancer patients from Johannesburg and Soweto, South Africa found that infection with HHV-8 was strongly associated with

KS, but not with any other major cancer site or type, including prostate cancer or multiple myeloma (34). In addition, the risk of KS increased with increasing antibody titer to HHV-8 (measured by the intensity of the fluorescent signal). However, for a given titer, this risk was much greater among HIV-seropositive patients than among those who were HIV-seronegative. The most intense fluorescent signal for HHV-8, which corresponded to a median antibody titer of 1:208,400, was associated with a 12-fold increase in risk of KS among HIV-seronegative patients, but with a more than 1600-fold increase in risk among HIV-seropositive patients. HHV-8 seroprevalence rates and antibody titers to HHV-8 were not, however, markedly related to HIV infection among those without KS.

No data on the relationship between HHV-8 antibody titer and viral load are available, but presumably, a high anti–HHV-8 antibody titer results from a high HHV-8 viral load. Thus, it is probably HHV-8 viral load, rather than antibody titer, that primarily determines the risk of KS. The excess risk of KS in HIV-seropositive individuals may mean that for a given anti–HHV-8 antibody titer, viral load in those coinfected with HIV is higher than in those who are not coinfected with HIV. Alternatively, high-titer HHV-8 infection could result from a high level of expression of an antigenically important gene product. Nevertheless, the relationship between high HHV-8 antibody titer and KS is similar to that between Epstein-Barr virus (EBV), a related gamma herpesvirus, and African Burkitt's lymphoma and nasopharyngeal cancer; individuals with high EBV antibody titers appear to be at highest risk of developing these cancers (35,36).

Epidemiology and Transmission of HHV-8

The modes of HHV-8 transmission have yet to be fully elucidated. In the West, sex between men, which is the main behavioral risk factor for KS, may be an important route of HHV-8 transmission (37,38,39). There is weak evidence of sexual transmission of HHV-8 among heterosexuals from a study conducted in South Africa, although the increase in risk with increasing number of sexual partners was not great (34). Furthermore, there was no difference in the seroprevalence of HHV-8 among study participants with or without HIV infection.

In three South African studies, the seroprevalence of HHV-8 was relatively high compared with that in the United States, and has been found to increase steadily with age (from birth, through childhood, and into adult life) and decrease with increasing level of education (34,40,41). Among black hospital patients in Johannesburg and Soweto, the standardized seroprevalence of HHV-8 was just over 30%, compared to 20% among black blood donors and about 5% among white blood donors; this rate did not vary by sex (34). In a rural, black South African population, HHV-8 seroprevalence rates were even higher (40). Similar findings have been reported from other parts of Africa where HHV-8 seroprevalence is also high and increases with age. These findings suggest that the virus is not a newly introduced sexually transmitted infection in Africa, as it may be in the United States (42). Furthermore, the lower seroprevalence of HHV-8 in whites compared to blacks in South Africa, and the decrease in seroprevalence with increasing education, implies that factors associated with poverty contribute to transmission of the virus (34).

The presence of anti HHV-8 antibodies in infants is evidence that HHV-8 is likely to be transmitted from mother to child (40). A study of South African mothers and their children found that about 30% of the children (under 10 years of age) of HHV-8–seropositive mothers were HHV-8 seropositive, whereas none of the children of HHV-8–seronegative mothers were HHV-8–seropositive (41). Furthermore, the proportion of children who were seropositive for HHV-8 increased in relation to their mothers' HHV-8 antibody titer. Although the data are inconclusive, HHV-8–seropositive mothers with high-titer infection may be about twice as likely to have HHV-8–seropositive children as mothers with low-titer infections (43).

The steady increase in the prevalence of HHV-8 infection throughout childhood, and the occurrence of KS in children in parts of sub–Saharan Africa before the AIDS epidemic, suggest that other nonsexual transmission of HHV-8 from person to person must occur (40,42). A recent study in Uganda showed that HHV-8 seropositivity in children was correlated with the presence of antibodies to hepatitis B core antigen (42). Hepatitis B is known to be transmitted from person to person and this correlation may suggest a similar route for HHV-8 (44).

Other Risk Factors for Kaposi's Sarcoma in Africa

The main determinant of KS risk throughout the world, both in people with and without HIV, is infection with HHV-8 (28). In the West, KS is so rare in HIV-uninfected people that it has never been adequately studied among them. Thus, much more is known about the characteristics of KS in people with HIV infection than is known about the disease in people without HIV. The main behavioral risk factor for HIV-associated KS in western populations is sex between men (45). Whether sex between men is also a risk factor for KS in HIV-negative individuals in western populations is unknown. Certainly, KS was far more common in men than in women before the HIV epidemic and thus it is possible that HHV-8 was transmitted sexually between men in the past, even though its prevalence in most countries was probably low.

The epidemiology of KS in Africa is different than that in the West. Although HHV-8 seropositivity is associated with poor education and low social class in South Africa, studies from Uganda show that the development of KS in both HIV-seronegative and HIV-seropositive individuals is associated with markers of high social class, such as better education and wealth (46,47). Furthermore, despite the fact that HHV-8 is very prevalent in Uganda, KS is a relatively uncommon manifestation of HIV disease, occurring in fewer than 7% of cases (20). The interpretation of these findings is difficult. Perhaps high social status protects an individual from early infection with HHV-8, and the age at which infection occurs (or even the route of infection) affects the subsequent risk of KS. This hypothesis is reminiscent of the effect of infection in adult life with EBV in relation to the risk of infectious mononucleosis.

Immunosuppression is another important risk factor for KS (5). In people who have received transplants, or who are infected with HIV, the cause of the immunosuppression is clear. In the absence of these factors, there is no evidence that those who develop KS are overtly immunosuppressed by other factors. It has been suggested that exposure to fine soil particles, which might pass through the skin of barefoot individuals and block the lymphatic system, may cause local immunosuppression, a suggestion that may explain the characteristic distribution of KS lesions on the lower limbs of HIV-uninfected individuals (48). One report from Uganda indicated that among HIV-seronegative individuals, those who went barefoot were at a higher risk of KS than those who regularly wore shoes, but this finding has not yet been confirmed by other studies (47).

Summary and Future Research

There is little doubt that HHV-8 is responsible for most, if not all, cases of KS. Many questions remain unanswered, however, about the etiology of this tumor. Why, for example, is KS more common in men than in women in Africa, when the prevalence of HHV-8 is the same in both sexes?

What are the cofactors that facilitate the development of the disease? The association between high anti–HHV-8 antibody titers and KS risk is clear, but it is not known whether these antibody titers are persistently high prior to the diagnosis of the tumor. Nor are the determinants of high antibody titers fully understood. Although anti–HHV-8 antibody titers presumably reflect HHV-8 viral load, there is little direct evidence for this and, for a given HHV-8 titer, the exact mechanism by which HIV has such a dramatic impact on the risk of KS is not clear.

Kaposi's sarcoma is one outcome of infection with HHV-8, in both HIV-seropositive and -seronegative adults and children. In children, it is possible that the tumor may be a manifestation of primary infection with HHV-8, but this is speculative. In adults, all the available evidence suggests that KS occurs after primary infection with HHV-8 (28). Almost no data are available on the clinical manifestations, if any, of primary infection with HHV-8 and therefore, the importance of such manifestations in terms of morbidity is not understood. In a recent case report, transient angiolymphoid hyperplasia was found to occur as part of an HHV-8 sero-conversion syndrome in an HIV-infected adult (49).

In South Africa, about one-third of children born to HHV-8 seropositive mothers are also HHV-8 seropositive, but the determinants of HHV-8 transmission from mother to child are unknown. Maternal anti–HHV-8 antibody titers may be important and probably reflect the level of viral load, although this needs clarification. The role of other factors that may affect transmission, such as coinfection with HIV, maternal age at delivery, mode and place of delivery, and length of breastfeeding, have yet to be investigated. It is not known if HHV-8 is present in breast milk, although it has been identified in saliva (50). If person-to-person transmission occurs via nonsexual route, other than from a mother to her child, nothing is known about the mechanism or outcome of this.

Finally, there have been increased reports of KS among HIV-seronegative men who have sex with men in New York, and among HIV-seronegative children in Africa (13,14,51). If the recent spread of HIV in the African population has also led to an increase in the spread of HHV-8 infection, the incidence of KS may increase even among people who are HIV-uninfected.

Non-Hodgkin's Lymphoma

In the West, people diagnosed with AIDS are about 60 times more likely than people without HIV to have some form of non-Hodgkin's lymphoma, and 1000 times more likely to have Burkitt's lymphoma or central nervous system lymphomas (52). The magnitude of this increased risk is similar to that in immunosuppressed transplant recipients, and increases with increasing level of immunosuppression (53,54). Non-Hodgkin's lymphoma is the AIDS-defining condition in about 3% of cases (less in pediatric cases), although as many as 10% of those with HIV infection may go on to develop the disease at some stage during their illness (52,55,56). The prevalence of non-Hodgkin's lymphoma in autopsy studies of HIV-infected individuals can be as high as 20% (57).

HIV-associated non-Hodgkin's lymphomas, although histologically heterogeneous, are characterized by an aggressive clinical course. High-grade disease is common and extranodal sites are often involved. Central nervous system lesions are virtually unknown to occur except in immunosuppressed individuals. In general, three broad types of HIV-associated non-Hodgkin's lymphoma can be distinguished by their clinical, histologic and epidemiologic features. The most common type is a B-cell immunoblastic tumor, the risk of which increases steadily with age (51). About one-fifth of lymphomas in AIDS patients in the West are of the second type—primary cerebral lymphomas—and a fifth are of the third type, Burkitt's

TABLE 1. Summary of Studies Comparing the Risk of Non-Hodgkin's Lymphoma in HIV-Seropositive and HIV-Seronegative Individuals in Africa

Study site (reference)	# HIV-seropositive/n (%)	Odds ratio (95% confidence limit)[a]
Rwanda (24)	7/19 (37%)	12.6 (2.2–54.4)
South Africa (23)	27/40 (68%)	4.8 (1.5–14.8)
South Africa (25)	23/105 (22%)	5.0 (2.7–9.5)
Uganda (26)	13/21 (62%)	6.2 (1.9–19.9)

[a]In the United States and Europe, the odds ratio is approximately 50–100 (6).

lymphomas. The risk of cerebral lymphomas in HIV-infected individuals does not change with age and that of Burkitt's lymphomas peaks between 10 and 19 years of age, mirroring the epidemiologic pattern of sporadic Burkitt's lymphoma in the United States (52). For all types of non-Hodgkin's lymphomas, the risk of disease is twice as high in men than in women.

Much less is known about HIV-associated non-Hodgkin's lymphomas occurring in Africa. To date, four case-control studies have compared the risk of non-Hodgkin's lymphoma in HIV-seropositive and -seronegative individuals in Africa, and in each study, the relative risk among the HIV-seropositive individuals was considerably less than would be expected in the West (Table 1) (23–26). The reasons for this geographic difference are not clear. Data from the West suggest that among those with HIV, the risk of non-Hodgkin's lymphoma increases with the patient's level of immunosuppression; many HIV-infected Africans may die of other causes before reaching high levels of immunosuppression. Also, the accurate diagnosis of a lymphoma requires relatively sophisticated technology that is unavailable in many African countries, a situation that suggests that some cases in Africa may go unreported. However, even careful autopsy studies of HIV-infected individuals have identified fewer cases of non-Hodgkin's lymphoma in Africa than have been identified in similar studies in the West. In contrast with the explosion in the incidence of KS in Africa, cancer registry data from African countries with high HIV prevalence show that there have been only very slight increases in the incidence of non-Hodgkin's lymphoma (20,21,55,58). Furthermore, HIV-infected people in the United States who were born in Africa or the Caribbean, are at a lower risk of developing non-Hodgkin's lymphoma than other HIV-infected people (52). This suggests that HIV-infected black Africans may indeed be at a lower risk of developing non-Hodgkin's lymphoma than HIV-infected people in the West. Although these differences in the risk of non-Hodgkin's lymphoma by race and HIV transmission group are not great, they may point to the importance of genetic factors, or more likely, socioeconomic factors in the etiology of the disease. Although speculative, it is possible that people of lower socioeconomic status are exposed to an infectious agent at a younger age, offering them some protection against the subsequent development of non-Hodgkin's lymphoma.

Still less is known about the histologic subtypes of lymphoma that occur in HIV-infected Africans. As in the West, the predominant type would appear to be immunoblastic tumors, and cerebral lymphomas have been identified at autopsy (58). There is some evidence that Burkitt's lymphoma, which is endemic in parts of sub-Saharan Africa, is associated with HIV infection there, although data are sparse (25,26).

Conjunctival Squamous Cell Carcinoma

Conjunctival squamous cell carcinoma is an extreme form of a spectrum of conditions collectively known as "ocular surface epithelial dysplasias," which range in severity from mild dysplasia, to carcinoma in situ, and ultimately, to invasive carcinoma (Figure 3). Although rare in Europe, Templeton noted that conjunctival squamous cell carcinoma was relatively common in parts of sub–Saharan Africa during the 1960s, and suggested that exposure to solar ultraviolet radiation might be a cause (59). Lee et al. reported that the risk of ocular surface epithelial dysplasias was related to lifetime exposure to solar ultraviolet light (60). The strongest risk factor in this study was a past history of skin cancer (OR, 15; 95% CI, 2–114), although other factors, such as having been outdoors for more than 50% of the time during the first 6 years of life, fair skin, pale irides, and propensity to burn on exposure to sunlight, were also important. In addition, Newton et al. found that the incidence of squamous cell carcinoma of the eye increased by 29% per unit increase in exposure to ambient solar ultraviolet radiation ($p < 0.0001$), equivalent to a 49% increase in incidence with each 10° decline in latitude (61). Ultraviolet-B radiation is known to damage DNA in human epithelial cells and thus it is a plausible cause of the disease (62).

Two case reports of conjunctival squamous cell carcinoma in HIV-seropositive males in the United States (63,64), coupled with a dramatic increase in the number of tumors seen by ophthalmologists in at least two African centers (65,66), led to the suggestion that the disease could be associated with HIV. Four studies from Africa and one from the United States have confirmed this suggestion (26,65–68). Although each study was small, their results were remarkably consistent (Table 2). A recent report from Uganda indicated that the incidence rate of conjunctival cancer increased three-fold during the 1990s, presumably as a result of the HIV epidemic (69).

In other immunosuppressed groups, such as transplant recipients, there has been no suggestion of an increased risk of conjunctival squamous cell carcinoma, although a thorough literature review has yielded one case report of this cancer, which occurred as a second primary in a patient with malignant lymphoma who was on chemotherapy (70). The absence of many reports of conjunctival squamous cell carcinoma is not surprising though, given its rarity in Western populations (61).

Several types of squamous carcinoma are associated with human papillomavirus (HPV) infection, most notably cancer of the uterine cervix, which is induced largely by HPV-16 and -18. Squamous carcinoma of the skin has also been associated with HPV-5 and -8 in immunosuppressed individuals (71). The evidence of an association between HPV and conjunctival squamous cell carcinoma is conflicting. In several studies of ocular surface epithelial dysplasias, the proportion of lesions in which HPV (predominantly type 16, but also types 6, 11, and 18) was detected was variable (72).

Little is known about other potential risk factors for conjunctival squamous cell carcinoma, but ocular trauma may also be important (59,73). Of particular relevance is the existence of "cancer eye" in cattle, which could be a useful animal model. This cancer is a conjunctival squamous cell carcinoma that has been associated with both ultraviolet radiation and bovine papillomavirus infection (71).

In summary, there is strong epidemiologic evidence that solar ultraviolet radiation is an important cause of conjunctival squamous cell carcinoma. HIV infection is another established risk factor, although it is not clear if HIV acts directly, or via immunosuppression, to activate potentially oncogenic viruses. The role of other factors, particularly conjunctival papillomavirus infection, has yet to be resolved.

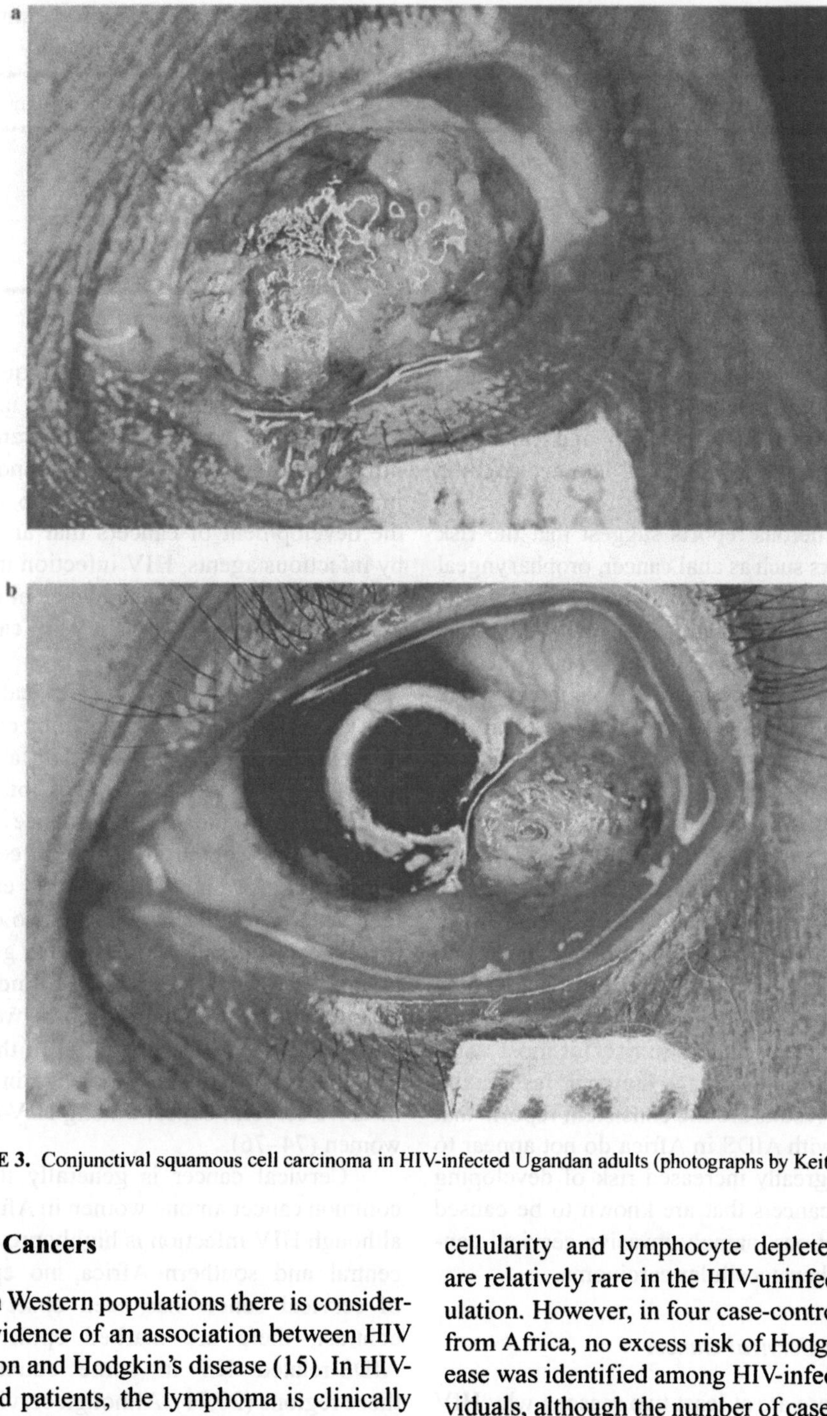

FIGURE 3. Conjunctival squamous cell carcinoma in HIV-infected Ugandan adults (photographs by Keith Waddell).

Other Cancers

In Western populations there is considerable evidence of an association between HIV infection and Hodgkin's disease (15). In HIV-infected patients, the lymphoma is clinically unusual, generally presenting at a late stage, often with extranodal dissemination. The predominant histologic subtypes are mixed cellularity and lymphocyte depleted, which are relatively rare in the HIV-uninfected population. However, in four case-control studies from Africa, no excess risk of Hodgkin's disease was identified among HIV-infected individuals, although the number of cases studied was small (23–26). Similarly, although there are reports of leiomyosarcoma occurring with increased frequency among HIV-infected

TABLE 2. Summary of Studies Comparing the Risk of Conjunctival Squamous Cell Carcinoma in HIV-Seropositive and HIV-Seronegative Individuals

Study site (reference)	# HIV-seropositive/n (%)	Odds ratio (95% confidence limit)
Rwanda (65)	9/11 (82%)	13.0 (2.2–76.9)
Uganda (66)	36/48 (75%)	13.0 (4.5–39.4)
Uganda (67)	27/38 (71%)	13.1 (4.7–37.6)
USA (68)	4 observed/0.3 expected	13.0 (4.0–34.0)
Uganda (26)	17/22 (77%)	10.9 (3.1–37.7)

children in the United States (15), only one study from Africa has considered the association between HIV infection and cancer in children, and no cases of leiomyosarcoma were identified (26).

Numerous reports suggest that the risk of cancers such as anal cancer, oropharyngeal cancers, and plasma cell tumors, might be increased in association with HIV infection. With the possible exception of anal cancer in the West, the evidence of HIV-associated risk for these tumors is scant, and there is no evidence of excess risk among HIV-infected individuals in Africa (15,23–26). Conversely, HIV infection has been linked to cancer of the vulva in South Africa (23,25), and to cancer of the penis in Uganda (26), although the number of cases is very small.

Results from descriptive, cohort and case-control studies, indicate that people with HIV infection and AIDS are not experiencing large increases in risk for most types of cancer (51). Perhaps the most fascinating of these results are the consistent reports that people with AIDS in Africa do not appear to be at a greatly increased risk of developing certain cancers that are known to be caused by infections, namely invasive cervical cancer and hepatocellular carcinoma.

Invasive Cervical Cancer

There are at least two reasons why HIV infection might be associated with an increased risk of invasive cervical cancer. First, cervical cancer is known to be caused by a sexually transmitted agent or agents, namely HPV (71). Women who acquire HIV by heterosexual contact are at an increased risk of contracting other sexually transmitted infections, including HPV. Second, since immunosuppression is believed to enhance the development of cancers that are caused by infectious agents, HIV infection might be expected to increase the incidence of invasive cervical cancer in women who carry the causal agent.

Even though invasive cervical cancer was classified as an AIDS-defining condition in 1993, there are very few data about the disease in the West. This lack of data is chiefly due to the low prevalence of HIV infection in women in western countries. Furthermore, women in western countries tend to have regular Pap smears, so cases of preclinical cervical neoplasia are generally treated early. However, the few studies that have looked at the relationship between cervical cancer and HIV infection in the West, have shown a moderate increase in risk of invasive cervical cancer among HIV-infected women (74–76).

Cervical cancer is generally the most common cancer among women in Africa, and although HIV infection is highly prevalent in central and southern Africa, no epidemic of cervical cancer has been observed. By contrast, there are marked epidemics of AIDS-related KS in some countries of those regions (20,21). Although cervical cancer incidence in Uganda has increased moderately since the 1960s, this increase has been uniform across all age groups and is not restricted to those most affected by HIV.

Table 3 summarizes the relative risks for invasive cervical cancer in HIV-seropositive patients compared to HIV-seronegative patients from five case-control studies conducted in different African countries (23–26, 77). The results do not indicate a large increase in risk of invasive cervical cancer in Africa. It has been suggested that HIV-infected women in Africa may die of other causes before developing invasive cervical cancer. However, cervical cancer is so common in Africa that many women must have premalignant cervical lesions or even in situ cancer, prior to becoming infected with HIV. If HIV-associated immunosuppression hastens the clinical course of cervical cancer in such women, it is surprising that no epidemic of the disease has been seen in Africa and that a more dramatic increase in the risk of invasive cervical cancer has not been found among HIV-infected individuals.

Hepatocellular Carcinoma

The incidence of hepatocellular carcinoma might be expected to be higher among HIV-infected individuals than among those who are HIV-uninfected. Hepatocellular carcinoma is primarily caused by infection with hepatitis B, which can be transmitted sexually (78). An increased risk of hepatocellular carcinoma has been identified in immunosuppressed transplant recipients. However, this risk may be the result of such patients having received hepatitis B-infected blood products, rather than a result of their immunosuppression; the excess risk among these patients was reported before the introduction of blood screening for hepatitis B and has not been found with more recent data (56,79).

There is little evidence that hepatocellular cancer incidence has increased in populations in the United States with a high prevalence of HIV infection, nor have increases in incidence been seen in African countries with a high prevalence of both HIV and hepatitis viruses (19–21). Data from three case-control studies of HIV and hepatocellular carcinoma in Africa show no higher risk of the tumor in HIV-seropositive patients than in HIV-seronegative patients (Table 4) (23,24,26). Potential difficulties in diagnosing hepatocellular carcinoma in Africa might contribute to the absence of an observed association, but even in western populations, the evidence for a strong association with HIV infection is scant (15).

MECHANISMS BY WHICH HIV FACILITATES THE DEVELOPMENT OF CANCER

There is no consistent evidence that HIV has direct oncogenic effects. The specific mechanism of carcinogenesis for HIV-associated malignancies may be different for each cancer type. Nonetheless, much of the increased cancer risk found in people with HIV is similar to that found in immunodeficient

TABLE 3. Summary of Studies Comparing the Risk of Invasive Cervical Cancer in HIV-Seropositive and HIV-Seronegative Individuals in Africa

Study site (reference)	# HIV-seropositive/n (%)	Odds ratio (95% confidence limit)
Rwanda (24)	0/23 (0%)	0.0 (0.0–5.4)
South Africa (23)	7/180 (4%)	0.6 (0.2–1.9)
Cote d'ivoire (77)	2/13 (15%)	1.3 (0.2–8.2)
South Africa (25)	167/1323 (13%)	1.6 (1.1–2.3)
Uganda (26)	21/65 (62%)	1.6 (0.7–3.6)

TABLE 4. Summary of Studies Comparing the Risk of Hepatocellular Carcinoma in HIV-Seropositive and HIV-Seronegative Individuals in Africa

Study site (reference)	# HIV-seropositive/n (%)	Odds ratio (95% confidence limit)
Rwanda (24)	1/35 (3%)	0.9 (0.1–6.1)
South Africa (23)	4/64 (6%)	0.9 (0.3–2.9)
Uganda (26)	4/19 (21%)	1.2 (0.3–4.2)

children and in transplant recipients, suggesting that it is the impairment of immune function that is the major factor leading to the appearance of these tumors (5). Furthermore, risk of KS and non-Hodgkin's lymphoma increases with increasing immunosuppression, suggesting that this is the principle mechanism favoring the development of these cancers (51). In general, any form of immunosuppression—congenital, therapeutic, or HIV-associated—appears to lead to the selective development of certain cancers that are caused by infectious agents. Some of the cancers that have been found in people with HIV but not in transplant recipients are probably explained by the fact that HIV has infected such a broad range of people from different parts of the world, while transplants are performed in more limited groups. For example, conjunctival squamous cell carcinoma is common in equatorial Africa, where HIV infection is also common, but tissue transplantation is rare. Also, leiomyosarcoma appears to occur exclusively as a rare complication of HIV infection in children, and few children have been given long-term immunosuppressive therapy.

Immunosuppression in the absence of HIV is associated with an increased risk of KS and, as with HIV-associated KS, the cancer risk varies depending on the country of origin of the patients. Studies from Europe, North America, and Australasia show that KS represents between 1% and 4% of all cancers in immunosuppressed transplant recipients, whereas in a study from Saudi Arabia, nearly 90% of tumors diagnosed in renal transplant recipients were KS (79–84). This broadly reflects the incidence of KS in each country prior to the HIV epidemic and presumably also reflects background differences in the prevalence of HHV-8 infection in each population. In addition, the clinical manifestations of KS in people with HIV-associated and other types of immunosuppression are similar, and there are reports of spontaneous regression of disease in transplant recipients if immunosuppressive therapy is withdrawn (85).

Whether HIV has a growth-promoting effect on KS lesions is debatable. HIV's Tat protein (a regulatory protein produced by the HIV *tat* gene) can promote the growth of *in vitro* cell cultures derived from the tumor (86). In addition, KS-like lesions have been found by some investigators, but not by others, to develop in mice transgenic for HIV-1 *tat* (87) and HIV-associated KS lesions do not contain high levels of HIV-infected cells (88). In West Africa, where HHV-8 is common but KS is infrequent, almost all cases of the tumor are associated with HIV-1 rather than HIV-2 infection, even when standardized for $CD4^+$ count (89). Therefore, HIV-1 *tat* may play a contributory role in the development of KS lesions *in vivo*, although, it seems that the increased risk of KS in HIV-infected individuals is largely mediated by immunosuppression, rather than by the virus itself. It is noteworthy that KS grows more aggressively and is more widespread in the skin and viscera in AIDS patients than in HIV-uninfected individuals. It was this aggressive manifestation that was a salient feature of the early phase of the African HIV epidemic (90).

Non-Hodgkin's lymphoma is the most commonly reported tumor in most studies of immunosuppressed transplant recipients and children with rare congenital defects of the immune system, such as X-linked gamma globulinemia or ataxia telangiectasia. The clinical course of non-Hodgkin's lymphomas in transplant recipients can be as aggressive as in HIV-infected individuals (although there are some differences in the histologic subtypes of lymphoma commonly found in each group); spontaneous remission has been reported with the cessation of immunosuppressive therapy (91).

Consistent failure to detect HIV sequences within the tumor clone indicates that the virus does not directly cause transformation of B-lymphocytes. All these factors suggest that the role of HIV in lymphomagenesis is indirect and related to its effects on immunoregulation. Interestingly, however, HIV-associated non-Hodgkin's lymphomas differ in some respects from those lymphomas occurring in immunosuppressed transplant recipients, perhaps because the nature of the immunosuppression is different.

B-cell immunoblastic lymphoma is the most common subtype of non-Hodgkin's lymphoma in both HIV-infected individuals and immunosuppressed transplant recipients. Post-transplant immunoblastic lymphomas are nearly always associated with EBV and probably represent the end result of an EBV-driven lymphoproliferation in the absence of effective T-cell immunity. However, EBV sequences are detectable in only about 50% of cases of HIV-associated immunoblastic lymphomas (although in 100% of primary cerebral lymphomas), suggesting that other factors may also be important (92). It has been suggested that several nonspecific host factors may play a role in lymphomagenesis in HIV-infected individuals, such as disrupted immunosurveillance, chronic antigenic stimulation, and cytokine dysregulation, all of which could be responsible for expanding the B-cell population from which a lymphoma subsequently develops. A small subset of these cancers, called "primary effusion lymphomas" have been associated with infection with HHV-8, although many of them contain EBV sequences as well (28).

Burkitt's lymphoma occurs at an increased frequency in HIV-seropositive individuals, but not in immunosuppressed transplant recipients. It is unclear whether this occurs as a result of HIV-specific immune dysfunction. HIV-associated Burkitt's lymphoma resembles the sporadic form of the disease found in the West. Sequences of EBV DNA can be found in about half of these cases and most have a characteristic c-myc/immunoglobulin gene translocation (92). The increased B-cell activation that accompanies HIV infection may increase the likelihood of such mutational events. However, c-myc/immunoglobulin gene translocations can be found in circulating B-cells in the peripheral blood of otherwise healthy HIV-seropositive individuals and their presence does not appear to correlate with the subsequent development of a lymphoma (93). This suggests that further oncogenic steps are involved in the development of Burkitt's lymphoma.

IMPACT OF HIV INFECTION ON CANCER INCIDENCE

It is estimated that, in 1990, there were about 52,000 cases of cancer that were a consequence of HIV infection, the majority of which occurred in sub–Saharan Africa (94). This conservative estimate is based on the known impact of HIV infection on only the two cancers with which it has been most clearly linked: KS and non-Hodgkin's lymphoma. The estimate does not take into account the possible effects of HIV on other cancers, such as conjunctival squamous cell carcinoma, Hodgkin's disease, or pediatric leiyomyosarcoma, but the number of cases of such cancers is very small.

The impact of the HIV epidemic on cancer incidence in populations with a high prevalence of HIV infection is clearly reflected in cancer registry statistics. However, if KS and non-Hodgkin's lymphoma are excluded from such statistics, there is little evidence that the incidence of all other cancers combined has increased. In Uganda and Zimbabwe the incidence of KS has increased between 10- and 20-fold since the HIV epidemic began (1,20,21). The incidence of non-Hodgkin's lymphoma in these countries, however, has changed little.

The impact of highly active antiretroviral therapy (HAART) on the incidence of HIV-associated cancers is significant. Since the widespread introduction of HAART in Western populations during the mid-1990s, the incidence of KS and non-Hodgkin's lymphoma has declined by about 50% and 30%, respectively (95). The critical importance of immunosuppression in the etiology of these tumors in HIV-infected individuals is clear and anything that reduces the level of immunosuppression is likely to reduce the risk of cancer. However, in developing countries, where such treatment has been prohibitively expensive and therefore not yet widely available, the incidence of HIV-associated cancers is likely to increase in relation to the spread of the HIV epidemic.

CONCLUSION

The control and prevention of HIV-associated cancers must involve adequate control of HIV infection itself, and control of the infections, such as HHV-8, that are known to cause HIV-associated cancers. Controlling the impact of HIV infection on cancer incidence requires limiting the onset of immunosuppression in HIV-infected individuals (with antiretroviral drugs) and minimizing HIV transmission.

Because infectious agents are a significant and theoretically preventable cause of cancer, the identification of additional cancers with an infectious etiology has important public health implications. Immunosuppression leads to the selective development of certain cancers that are known (or thought) to be caused by infections. Although tragic, the fact that millions of people are now infected with HIV has provided an unprecedented opportunity to investigate the role of the immune system in the etiology of cancer, and to identify new cancers with infectious causes.

There is good evidence that immunosuppression associated with HIV infection increases the risk of KS, non-Hodgkin's lymphoma, conjunctival squamous cell carcinoma, Hodgkin's disease, and leiomyosarcoma in children. Most of these cancers are thought to be caused by specific human herpesviruses. Few other cancers show any increase in risk associated with HIV infection, although relatively small increases for rare tumours cannot be excluded.

There is mounting evidence that causal factors in the etiology of HIV-associated cancers are similar to those for the same cancers occurring in the general population and likewise, the personal characteristics of those who develop a specific cancer are similar among HIV-infected and HIV-uninfected individuals with the same tumor.

The main determinant of KS risk is known to be infection with HHV-8 and this infection is identified in both HIV-seropositive and HIV-seronegative adults and children. Case-control studies from Uganda show that the personal characteristics of those who develop KS show striking similarities between those with and without HIV infection and that these individuals are distinguished by features of wealth and high social status.

Viral genomes and viral gene products of EBV have been found in tumor tissue of subjects with non-Hodgkin's lymphoma, but they tend to be found more often in immunosuppressed people than in the immunocompetent. The implications of this are unclear, but there is evidence that the viral load of both HHV-8 and EBV increases with increasing levels of immune impairment, which in turn would make the virus easier to detect with current technology (28,96). This has important implications for research on HIV-associated cancers. The same factors that are important in the etiology of cancer in those with HIV infection are probably also important in the etiology of cancer in those without HIV infection. Furthermore, an infectious cause is likely to be easier to identify in the immuno-suppressed than in the immuno-competent. Thus, the study of HIV-associated cancers will be of relevance to the population as a whole.

There may be other cancers whose incidence is increased in association with HIV infection but, if so, they are probably rare and the associated relative risks are not likely to be large. Further research is needed to clarify which other tumours are and are not, increased in people with HIV and, if so, the magnitude of the associated relative risk. In particular, there is a need for further record linkage studies in populations where HIV prevalence is low, and for further case-control studies in populations where HIV prevalence is high. In the meantime, because the numbers of specific cancers reported in any single study tends to be small, it would be valuable to combine the results from existing studies.

Understanding why immunosuppression increases the risk of certain, but not all, cancers that are known to be caused by infectious agents may lead to important insights into the carcinogenic process. Understanding why certain viruses can be found in association with tumors in HIV-seropositive subjects but not in similar tumors in HIV-seronegative subjects may clarify the role of these infections in the etiology of cancer in the general population. With the prospect of improved survival for HIV-infected people and the wider relevance of such research, it will become increasingly important to know more about the risk of cancer in these individuals.

REFERENCES

1. Cook-Mozaffari P, Newton R, Beral V, et al. The geographical distribution of Kaposi's sarcoma and of lymphomas in Africa before the AIDS epidemic. *Br J Cancer*, 1998;78:1521–1528.
2. Oettlé AG. Geographical and racial differences in the frequency of Kaposi's sarcoma as evidence of environmental or genetic causes. *Acta unio int contra cancrum*, 1962;18:330–363.
3. Templeton AC. Kaposi's sarcoma. In: Sommers SC, Rosen PP, eds. *Pathology Annual*. New York, Appleton: Century-Crofts, 1981;315–336.
4. Hutt MSR. Classical and endemic form of Kaposi's sarcoma. A review. *Antibiot Chemother*, 1984; 32: 12–17.
5. Parkin DM, Muir CS, Whelan SL, et al. Cancer Incidence in Five Continents. *IARC Scientific Publication*, 1992; volume 6: No. 20.
6. Beral V, Newton R. Overview of the epidemiology of immunodeficiency-associated cancers. *Monogr Natl Cancer Inst*, 1998:23;1–6.
7. Pollock BH, Jenson HB, McClain KL, et al. Risk factors for HIV-related malignancies in children. *J Aquir Immune Defic Syndr Hum Retrovirol*, 1997;14:A17.
8. Grulich A, Wan X, Law M, et al. Rates of non-AIDS defining cancers in people with AIDS. *J Aquir Immune Defic Syndr Hum Retrovirol*, 1997;14:A18.
9. Rabkin C. Epidemiology of malignancies other than Kaposi's sarcoma and non-Hodgkin's lymphoma in HIV infection. *J Aquir Immune Defic Syndr Hum Retrovirol*, 1997;14:A12.
10. Dorffel J. Histogenesis of multiple idiopathic hemorrhagic sarcoma of Kaposi. *Arch Dermatol Syph*, 1932;26:608–634.
11. Tappero JW, Conant MA, Wolfe SF, et al. Kaposi's sarcoma. Epidemiology, pathogenesis, histology, clinical spectrum, staging criteria and therapy. *J Am Acad Dermatol*, 1993;28:371–395.
12. Casabona J, Salas T, Salinas R. Trends and survival in AIDS-associated malignancies. *Eur J Cancer*, 1993;29A:877–881.
13. Ziegler JL, Katongole-Mbidde E. Kaposi's sarcoma in childhood: an analysis of 100 cases from Uganda and relationship to HIV infection. *Int J Cancer*, 1996;65:200–203.
14. Mbulaiteye SM, Ziegler JL, Katongole-Mbidde E, et al. Kaposi's sarcoma study group. Risk factors for childhood Kaposi's sarcoma in Uganda: a case-control study. Abstract 7. *J Aquir Immune Defic Syndr Hum Retrovirol*, 1997;14:A18.
15. Newton R, Beral V, Weiss R. Human Immunodeficiency Virus Infection and Cancer. In: Newton R, Beral V, Weiss R, eds. *Infections and Human Cancer*. Cancer Surveys Series, volume 33. Cold Spring Harbor: Cold Spring Harbor Laboratory Press, 1999.
16. Biggar RJ, Horm J, Fraumeni JF, et al. Incidence of Kaposi's sarcoma and mycosis fungoides in the United States including Puerto Rico, 1973–1981. *J Natl Cancer Inst*, 1984;73:89–94.

17. Grulich AE, Beral V, Swerdlow AJ. Kaposi's sarcoma in England and Wales before the AIDS epidemic. *Br J Cancer*, 1992;66:1135–1137.
18. Hjalgrim H, Melbye M, Pukkala E, et al. Epidemiology of Kaposi's sarcoma in the Nordic countries prior to the AIDS epidemic. *Br J Cancer*, 1996;74:1499–1502.
19. Rabkin CS, Biggar RJ, Horm JW. Increasing incidence of cancers associated with the human immunodeficiency virus epidemic. *Int J Cancer*, 1991;47:692–696.
20. Wabinga HR, Parkin DM, Wabwire-Mangen F, et al. Cancer in Kampala, Uganda, in 1989–91: Changes in incidence in the era of AIDS. *Int J Cancer*, 1993:54:26–36.
21. Bassett MT, Chokunonga E, Mauchaza B, et al. Cancer in the African population of Harare, Zimbabwe in 1990–92. *Int J Cancer*, 1995;63:29–36.
22. Sitas F, Madhoo J, Wessie J. *Incidence of histologically diagnosed cancer in South Africa, 1993–1995*. Johannesburg: National Cancer Registry of South Africa, South African Institute of Medical Research, 1998.
23. Sitas F, Bezwoda WR, Levin V, et al. Association between human immunodeficiency virus type 1 infection and cancer in the black population of Johannesburg and Soweto, South Africa. *Br J Cancer*, 1997;75:1704–1707.
24. Newton R, Grulich A, Beral V, et al. Cancer and HIV infection in Rwanda. *Lancet*, 1995;345: 1378–1379.
25. Sitas F, Pacell-Norman R, Carrara H, et al. The spectrum of HIV-1 related cancers in South Africa. *Int J Cancer*, 2000;88:489–492.
26. Newton R, Ziegler J, Beral V, et al. Uganda Kaposi's Sarcoma Study Group. A case-control study of human immunodeficiency virus infection and cancer in adults and children residing in Kampala, Uganda. *Int J Cancer*, 2001;92:622–627.
27. Chang Y, Cesarman E, Pessin MS, et al. Identification of Herpesvirus-like DNA sequences in AIDS-associated Kaposi's sarcoma. *Science*, 1994;266:1865–1869.
28. Boshoff C. Kaposi's sarcoma associated herpesvirus. In: Newton R, Beral V, Weiss R, eds. *Infections and Human cancer*. Cancer Surveys Series Volume 33. Cold Spring Harbor: Cold Spring Harbor Laboratory Press, 1999.
29. Boshoff C, Schulz TF, Kennedy MM, et al. Kaposi's sarcoma-associated herpesvirus infects endothelial and spindle cells. *Nat Med*, 1995;1:1274–1278.
30. Whitby D, Howard MR, Tenant-Flowers M, et al. Detection of Kaposi's sarcoma-associated herpesvirus in peripheral blood of HIV-infected individuals and progression to Kaposi's sarcoma. *Lancet*, 1995;346:799–802.
31. Gao SJ, Kingsley L, Hoover DR, et al. Seroconversion of antibodies to Kaposi's sarcoma-associated herpesvirus-related latent nuclear antigens prior to onset of Kaposi's sarcoma. *New Engl J Med*, 1996;335:233–241.
32. Gao SJ, Kingsley L, Li M, et al. Seroprevalence of Kaposi's sarcoma-associated herpesvirus antibodies among Americans, Italians and Ugandans with and without Kaposi's sarcoma. *Nat Med*, 1996;2:925–928.
33. Simpson GR, Schulz TF, Whitby D, et al. Prevalence of Kaposi's sarcoma associated herpesvirus infection measured by antibodies to recombinant capsid protein and latent immunofluorescence antigen. *Lancet*, 1996;348:1133–1138.
34. Sitas F, Carrara H, Beral V, et al. Antibodies against human herpesvirus 8 in black South African patients with cancer. *New Engl J Med*, 1999;340: 1863–1871.
35. de Thé G, Geser A, Day NE, et al. Epidemiological evidence for causal relationship between Epstein-Barr Virus and Burkitt's lymphoma from a Ugandan prospective study. *Nature*, 1978;274:751–761.
36. de Thé G, Lavoue MF, Muenz L. Differences in EBV antibody titres of patients with nasopharyngeal carcinoma originating from areas of high, intermediate and low incidence areas. In: de Thé G, Ito Y, eds. *Nasopharyngeal Carcinoma: Etiology and Control*. Lyon: International Agency for Research on Cancer, 1978. (IARC Scientific Publication no. 20).
37. Martin JN, Ganem DE, Osmond DH, et al. Sexual transmission and the natural history of Human Herpesvirus-8 infection. *New Engl J Med*, 1998;338:948–954.
38. Melbye M, Cook PM, Hjalgrim H, et al. Risk factors for HHV-8 seropositivity and progression to Kaposi's sarcoma in a cohort of homosexual men, 1981–96. *J Aquir Immune Defic Syndr Hum Retrovirol*, 1997;14:A16 S1.
39. Grulich A, Olsen S, Hendry O, et al. Route of transmission of Kaposi's sarcoma associated herpesvirus. *J Aquir Immune Defic Syndr Hum Retrovirol*, 1997;14:A16 S2.
40. Wilkinson D, Sheldon, J, Gilks C, et al. Prevalence of infection with Human Herpesvirus 8 (HHV-8)/Kaposi's sarcoma herpesvirus (KSHV) in rural South Africa. *S Afr Med J*, 1999;89:554–557.
41. Bourboulia D, Whitby D, Boshoff C, et al. Serologic evidence for mother to child transmission of Kaposi sarcoma associated herpesvirus infection. *JAMA*, 1998;280:31–32.
42. Mayama S, Cuervas LE, Sheldon J, et al. Prevalence and transmission of Kaposi's sarcoma associated herpesvirus (Human herpesvirus 8) in Ugandan children and adolescents. *Int J Cancer*, 1998;77:817–820.
43. Sitas F, Newton R, Boshoff C. Probability of mother-to-child transmission of HHV-8 increases with increasing maternal antibody titre for HHV-8. *New Engl J Med*, 1999;340:1923.

44. Abdool-Karim SS, Coovadia HC, Windsor IM, et al. The prevalence and transmission of Hepatitis B virus infection in urban, rural and institutional black children of Natal/KwaZulu, South Africa. *Int J Epidemiol*, 1988;17:168–173.
45. Beral V, Peterman TA, Berkelman RL, et al. Kaposi's sarcoma among persons with AIDS: a sexually transmitted infection? *Lancet*, 1990;335: 123–128.
46. Ziegler JL, Newton R, Katongole-Mbidde E, et al. Risk factors for HIV-associated Kaposi's sarcoma in Uganda: a case-control study of 1026 adults. *AIDS*, 1997;11:1619–1626.
47. Ziegler J and the Uganda Kaposi's Sarcoma Study Group. Wealth and soil exposure are risk factors for endemic Kaposi's sarcoma in Uganda. *J Aquir Immune Defic Syndr Hum Retrovirol*, 1998; 17:A12.
48. Ziegler JL. Endemic Kaposi's sarcoma in Africa and local volcanic soils. *Lancet*, 1993;342:1348–1351.
49. Oksenhendler E, Cazals-Hatem D, Schulz TF, et al. Transient angiolymphoid hyperplasia and Kaposi's sarcoma after primary infection with human herpes virus 8 in a patient with Human immunodeficiency virus infection. *New Engl J Med*, 1998;338: 1585–1590.
50. Vieira D, Hunag L, Koelle D, et al. Transmissible Kaposi's-associated herpesvirus (Human herpesvirus 8) in saliva of men with a history of Kaposi's sarcoma. *J Virol*, 1997;71:7083–7087.
51. IARC monograph on the evaluation of carcinogenic risks to humans. *Human immunodeficiency viruses and human T-cell lymphotropic viruses*. Volume 67. Lyon, France: IARC, 1996.
52. Beral V, Peterman TA, Berkelman R, et al. AIDS-associated non-Hodgkin lymphoma. *Lancet*, 1991;337:805–809.
53. Kinlen LJ, Sheil AG, Peto J, et al. Collaborative United Kingdom-Australasian study of cancer in patients treated with immunosuppressive drugs. *Br Med J*, 1979;2:1461–1466.
54. Pluda JM, Venzon DJ, Tosato G, et al. Parameters affecting the development of non-Hodgkin's lymphoma in patients with severe human immunodeficiency virus infection receiving anti-retroviral therapy. *J Clin Oncol*, 1993;11:1099–1107.
55. Serraino D, Salamina G, Franceschi S, et al. The epidemiology of non-Hodgkin's lymphoma in the World Health Organization European Region. *Br J Cancer*, 1992;66:912–916.
56. Lyter D, Besley D, Thackeray R, et al. Incidence of malignancies in the Multicenter AIDS Cohort Study (MACS). *Proceedings ASCO*, 1994;13:50. Abstract A2.
57. Wilkes MS, Felix JC, Fortwin AH, et al. Value of necropsy in acquired immunodeficiency syndrome. *Lancet*, 1988;2:85–88.
58. Lucas SB, Diomande M, Hounnou A, et al. HIV-associated lymphoma in Africa: an autopsy study on Côte D'Ivoire. *Int J Cancer*, 1994;59: 20–24.
59. Templeton AC. Tumours of the eye and adnexa. *Recent Results Cancer Res*, 1973;41:203–214.
60. Lee GA, Williams G, Hirst LW, et al. Risk Factors in the Development of Ocular Surface Epithelial Dysplasia. *Ophthalmol*, 1994;101:360–364.
61. Newton R, Ferlay J, Reeves G, et al. Incidence of squamous cell carcinoma of the eye increases with increasing levels of ambient solar ultraviolet radiation. *Lancet*, 1996;347:1450–1451.
62. IARC monograph on the evaluation of carcinogenic risks to Humans. Volume 55. *Solar and Ultraviolet Radiation*. Lyon: IARC, 1992.
63. Winward KE, Curtin VT. Conjunctival squamous cell carcinoma in a patient with human immunodeficiency virus infection. *Am J Ophthalmol*, 1989; 107:554–555.
64. Kim RY, Seiff SR, Howes EL Jr, et al. Necrotizing scleritis secondary to conjunctival squamous cell carcinoma in acquired immunodeficiency syndrome. *Am J Ophthalmol*, 1990;109:231–233.
65. Kestelyn P, Stevens AM, Ndayambaje A, et al. HIV and conjunctival malignancies. *Lancet*, 1990;336: 51–52.
66. Ateenyi-Agaba C. Conjunctival squamous cell carcinoma associated with HIV infection in Kampala, Uganda. *Lancet*, 1995;345:695–696.
67. Waddell KM, Lewallen S, Lucas SB, et al. Carcinoma of the conjunctiva and HIV infection in Uganda and Malawi. *Br J Ophthalmol*, 1996;80:503–508.
68. Goedert JJ, Coté TR. Conjunctival malignant disease with AIDS in USA. *Lancet*, 1995;ii:257–258.
69. Parkin DM, Wabinga H, Nambooze S, et al. AIDS-related cancers in Africa: maturation of the epidemic in Uganda. *AIDS*, 1999;13:2563–2570.
70. Kushner FH, Mushen RL. Conjunctival squamous cell carcinoma combined with malignant lymphoma. *Am J Ophthalmol*, 1975;80:503–506.
71. IARC monograph on the evaluation of carcinogenic risks to Humans. Volume 64. Human papillomaviruses. Lyon: IARC, 1995.
72. Newton R. A review of the aetiology of squamous cell carcinoma of the conjunctiva. *Br J Cancer*, 1996;74:1511–1513.
73. Margo CE, Groden LR. Squamous cell carcinoma of the cornea and conjunctiva following a thermal burn of the eye. *Cornea*, 1986;5:185–188.
74. Franceschi S, Dal Maso L, Arniani S, et al. Cancer and AIDS Registry Linkage Study. Risk of cancer other than Kaposi's sarcoma and non-Hodgkin's lymphoma in persons with AIDS in Italy. *Br J Cancer*, 1998;78:966–970.
75. Goedert JJ, Coté TR, Virgo P, et al. AIDS-Cancer Match Study Group. Spectrum of AIDS-associated malignant disorders. *Lancet*, 1998;351:1833–1839.

76. Selik RM, Rabkin CS. Cancer death rates associated with Human Immunodeficiency Virus infection in the United States. *J National Cancer Institute*, 1998;90:1300–1302.
77. La Ruche G, You B, Mensah-Ado I, et al. Human papillomavirus and human immunodeficiency virus infections: relation with cervical dysplasia-neoplasia in African women. *Int J Cancer*, 1998;74:480–486.
78. IARC monograph on the evaluation of carcinogenic risks to Humans. Volume 59. *Hepatitis viruses*. Lyon: IARC, 1994.
79. Birkland SA, Storm HH, Lamm LU, et al. Cancer risk after renal transplantation in the Nordic countries, 1964–1986. *Int J Cancer*, 1995;60:183–189.
80. Klepp O, Dahl O, Stenwig JT. Association of Kaposi's sarcoma and prior immunosuppressive therapy. *Cancer*, 1978;42:2626–2630.
81. Harwood AR, Osoba D, Hofstader SL, et al. Kaposi's sarcoma in recipients of renal transplants. *Am J Med*, 1979;67:759–765.
82. Penn I. Kaposi's sarcoma in organ transplant recipients. *Transplantation*, 1979;27:8–11.
83. Sheil AG, Flavel S, Disney AP, et al. Cancer incidence in renal transplant patients treated with azathioprine or cyclosporin. *Transplant Proc*, 1987;19: 2214–2216.
84. Qunibi W, Akhtar M, Sheth K, et al. Kaposi's sarcoma: the most common tumour after renal transplantation in Saudi Arabia. *Am J Med*, 1988;84: 25–232.
85. Frances C, Farge D, Boisnic S. Syndrome de Kaposi des transplantes. *J Mal Vasc*, 1991;16:163–165.
86. Ensoli B, Gendelman R, Markham P, et al. Synergy between basic fibroblast growth factor and HIV-1 Tat protein in induction of Kaposi's sarcoma. *Nature*, 1994;371:674–680.
87. Vogel J, Hinrichs SH, Reynolds RK, et al. The HIV *tat* gene induces dermal lesions resembling Kaposi's sarcoma in transgenic mice. *Nature*, 1988;335:606–611.
88. Roth WK, Brandstetter H, Sturzl M. Cellular and molecular features of HIV-associated Kaposi's sarcoma. *AIDS*, 1992;6:895–913.
89. Ariyoshi K, Schim van der Loeff M, Cook P, et al. Kaposi's sarcoma in the Gambia, West Africa is less frequent in Human Immunodeficiency Virus type 2 than in Human Immunodeficiency Virus type 1 infection despite a high prevalence of Human Herpes Virus 8. *J Hum Virol*, 1998;1:193–199.
90. Bayley AC, Cheinsong-Popov R, Dalgleish AG, et al. HTLV-III serology distinguishes atypical and endemic Kaposi's sarcoma in Africa. *Lancet*, 1985;I:359–361.
91. Starzl TE, Porter KA, Iwatsuki S, et al. Reversibility of lymphomas and lymphoproliferative lesions developing under cyclosporin-steroid therapy. *Lancet*, 1984;I:583–587.
92. Herndier BG, Kaplan LD, McGrath MS. Pathogenesis of AIDS lymphomas. *AIDS*, 1994;8: 1025–1049.
93. Muller JR, Janz S, Goedert JJ, et al. Persistence of immunoglobulin heavy chain/c-myc recombination-positive lymphocytes clones in the blood of human immunodeficiency virus-infected homosexual men. *Proc Natl Acad Sci USA*, 1995;92: 6577–6581.
94. Parkin DM, Pisani P, Munoz N, et al. The global health burden of infection associated cancers. In: Newton R, Beral V, Weiss R, eds. *Infections and Human Cancer*. Cancer Surveys Series, volume 33. Cold Spring Harbor: Cold Spring Harbor Laboratory Press, 1999.
95. International Collaboration on HIV and Cancer. The impact of highly active anti-retroviral therapy on the incidence of cancer in people infected with the Human Immunodeficiency Virus. *J National Cancer Institute*, 2000;92:1823–1830.
96. Rickinson A. The role of herpesviruses in immune deficiency-associated lymphomas. *J Acquir Immune Defic Syndr Hum Retrovirol*, 1997;14:A15.

24

Challenges and Opportunities for Nurses

Sheila D. Tlou

University of Botswana, Gaborone, Botswana.

In Africa, HIV and AIDS are systematically wiping out all the gains that have been made in people's quality of life by the adoption of primary health care practices and the betterment of health care delivery systems. This chapter provides an overview of the current challenges and issues facing nurses in Africa in their efforts at HIV and AIDS prevention and care, and their work to alleviate the impact HIV and AIDS are having on individuals, families, and communities.

In most African countries, health care systems are organized in levels of increasing complexity, starting from the most basic health post or mobile health stop to major referral hospitals. In all these facilities, nurses are the backbone to health care delivery. Health consultations, nutrition care, health education, maternal health, patient education, and immunization of infants and children against communicable diseases are nursing responsibilities and included within the discipline and practice of nursing. Nursing has, therefore, earned itself a special place in the national health care systems of the nations of Africa.

Nurses in Africa are involved in caring for increasing numbers of people living with HIV or AIDS. They are expected to counsel, test, and provide care and support to infected and affected people as well as implement public health education programs aimed at preventing the spread of the infection. HIV and AIDS, however, are relatively new diseases, and few practicing nurses have learned about treatment and care of HIV-infected patients during their preservice training. They, therefore, need education and support in order to function effectively in the health promotion, preventive, curative, and rehabilitative aspects of HIV and AIDS.

NURSES AND HIV AND AIDS PREVENTION

Primary prevention is the most important component in controlling the spread of HIV and AIDS, and nurses play a critical role in educating individuals, families, and communities toward that goal. So far, nurses in Africa have been able to develop models of care by adapting the International Council of Nurses (ICN) and World Health Organization (WHO) "Guidelines for Nursing Management of People Infected with the Human Immunodeficiency Virus (HIV)" (1). Each country's National Nurses Association has based its own guidelines and standards of care on this set of guidelines, but there is no documented evidence of successful HIV and AIDS care models that can be used across countries and cultures. Baylor College of Medicine in Houston, Texas, in the United States was among the first institutions to develop a nursing curriculum for HIV and

AIDS prevention and care that is currently being tested for its applicability in other cultures, especially those in African countries. This curriculum was developed because of a realization that although almost all nurses are expected to provide HIV and AIDS care and to counsel clients for voluntary HIV counseling and testing, very few have received any relevant training. The main premise is that education for nurses on HIV and AIDS is crucial for them not only as caregivers but also as people whose behavior and occupation could place them at risk for HIV infection (2).

The increasing number of AIDS-related deaths and the high job turnover rate associated with AIDS burnout among nurses are causes for concern in African countries, given the already inadequate number of medical and other health care personnel. Personal risk assessment, assertiveness, and empowerment to reduce personal risk are issues that need to be incorporated into all nursing curricula on HIV and AIDS. One curriculum being developed by the Botswana-Harvard Partnership in HIV/AIDS Research and Education seeks to empower nurses in their roles as caregivers, educators, and counselors. It includes modules targeting nursing personnel and ensuring that HIV and AIDS education for nurses is as comprehensive and as culturally relevant as possible.

NURSING CARE FOR PEOPLE LIVING WITH HIV OR AIDS

HIV and AIDS are life-threatening conditions that evoke fear among populations including the caregiving population. Negative attitudes and beliefs about HIV/AIDS have been shown to limit caregivers' abilities to provide holistic and effective care to those living with HIV or AIDS and to their families (Lebaka N, unpublished data, 1998). The dominant mode of transmission of HIV and its prognosis continue to contribute to a fear of contagion among health workers, especially among nurses who do the "hands on" care of people with AIDS. Fear of contagion is an emotional reaction to the threat of AIDS. Some studies have found that higher educational attainment can be associated with lower levels of fear (3).

In some instances, medical personnel who perceived themselves as being inadequately prepared for the management of HIV infection in children cited a lack of education and a lack of proper management guidelines as reasons behind their inadequate level of preparation. Many expressed a high level of fear of contracting HIV from a patient, a feeling that made many less inclined to do invasive diagnostic investigations and procedures (4). Nurses in Africa experience the same feelings of fear of contagion because of ignorance, but also because of a lack of clear guidelines on management protocols in most countries. In Zambia, a study was done among 69 nurses to determine if their decisions to leave bedside nursing were influenced by their fear of occupational exposure to HIV (5). They gave as their major reasons for leaving poor conditions of service, inconsistent or awkward hours, and lack of materials and equipment appropriate for the care of AIDS patients.

In order to meet the need for education and information, workshops and training programs conducted for nurses in Africa have focused on caring for individuals living with HIV or AIDS in health care facilities and in private homes, as well as on counseling and health education for HIV-infected individuals and their families.

In 2000, the WHO, UNAIDS, and ICN developed and distributed comprehensive guidelines entitled "Fact Sheets on HIV/AIDS for Nurses and Midwives." These guidelines are intended to help health care providers care for people living with HIV and AIDS (6).

PSYCHOSOCIAL CARE OF PERSONS LIVING WITH HIV OR AIDS

HIV and AIDS continue to generate fear, stigma, intolerance, and discrimination among people throughout the world mainly because of their association with topics such as sex, sexual orientation, and death and dying, topics that are taboo in many cultures, including cultures in Africa. Because of these circumstances, people are often reluctant to access care and support services such as voluntary counseling and testing programs, to adopt preventive strategies such as use of condoms, to seek treatment for sexually transmitted infections, or to disclose their HIV status. Health professionals are as vulnerable to these feelings as others and, thus, often do not avail themselves of the counseling services provided by their own colleagues.

Conferences on AIDS in Africa are characterized by lack of scientific presentations on sexual orientation and AIDS mainly because heterosexuality is considered the main mode of HIV transmission. There is a need, however, for nurses to educate people of all sexual orientations about safer sexual practices. In Africa, as elsewhere, the stigma associated with being gay brings lesbians and men who have sex with men, as well as their relatives, severe psychosocial stress and discrimination, even from health professionals. In one study, nurses were found to react more negatively to patients who were diagnosed with AIDS than to patients who had leukemia. The study participants felt that they should have a right to refuse to work with people living with AIDS, and some, in fact, indicated they would not work with homosexual men (7).

Despite such attitudes and behavior, nurses in Africa are often the only health professionals available to offer social and psychologic support to clients of all sexual orientations who experience fear, loneliness, and depression when confronting their own death. They also have to provide individual and family counseling for caregivers of terminally ill patients. Anecdotal evidence indicates that nurses in Africa need proper training in counseling in order to provide emotional and spiritual support to individuals, families, and communities affected by HIV and AIDS. There are some best practices in this area that can be looked to. In Uganda, to ensure quality of care for persons living with HIV or AIDS, nationwide efforts were made as early as 1989 to prepare nurses to provide appropriate psychosocial care, including counseling, for clients and their families, and a manual of nursing care and guidelines was developed and evaluated (8).

For most African countries, the importance of psychosocial issues in HIV and AIDS care was not emphasized until the implementation of community home-based care programs. These programs were developed out of the need to provide nursing care on a long-term basis to clients who were discharged from health institutions to relieve overcrowding. With the advent of this method of nursing practice, African nurses were able to see first-hand the interaction between HIV and AIDS and social conditions such as poverty, illiteracy, unemployment, gender inequality, the plight of orphans and street children, and the need for a holistic approach to care that addresses all these issues (9).

HIV AND AIDS: WHEN THE NURSE IS AT RISK

Health care workers are at risk for HIV infection because they can regularly come in contact with blood and body fluids. Estimates of their risk for needlestick exposure to HIV-infected blood, derived from prospective studies, are in the order of 1 in 300. As HIV prevalence in the general population increases, so does the percentage of patients who have HIV infection. Workplace conditions, such as poor lighting, lack of appropriate protective materials and disinfectants, and outdated techniques such as needle recapping, increase the risk of injury to health care workers. A study conducted in Zambia showed increasing mortality rates among female nurses over three consecutive periods (10). However, these rates were not compared to mortality rates in other occupational groups.

In many settings, however, health care workers are at greater risk of becoming infected with HIV through personal behavior than professional risk. Most nurses are women, and in most African countries, legal systems and cultural norms reinforce gender-based systems that discriminate against women. Men are given control over productive resources; most marriage laws subordinate wives to their husbands; there is tolerance for gender-based violence; and inheritance customs make men the principal beneficiaries of family property. This still occurs despite the fact that most African countries have ratified the United Nations Convention on the Elimination of All Forms of Discrimination Against Women (CEDAW). Female nurses suffer the same gender inequality as other women in society. If they are not in a position to negotiate or insist on safer sex, they are placed at risk for HIV infection.

Although little is known about the magnitude of risk for HIV infection among traditional birth attendants or health care workers, accessible and appropriate precautionary measures should be taken to address their concerns.

As early as 1988, some hospitals in Europe and the United States started to offer zidovudine (ZDV) to health care workers as treatment against occupational exposure to HIV, such as for needlestick injuries, as well as to women who were victims of rape or sexual violence (11). Very few countries in Africa have made similar provisions for their health care workers, and those that have only recently implemented such policies. Botswana, for example, started providing antiretroviral drugs for rape survivors and postneedlestick injury prophylaxis in 2000.

In 1994, the ICN issued a position statement calling upon all member associations to collaborate with their respective governments to ensure that relevant, up-to-date knowledge on HIV and AIDS and on safer sexual practices were made available to all health care providers (12). The statement stressed observance of universal precautions that include careful handling of "sharps" such as needles, hand washing with water and soap before and after all procedures, proper handling of soiled linen, safe disposal of waste contaminated with blood and body fluids, proper disinfection of instruments, and use of gloves and plastic aprons. The ICN also called upon nurses to rise to the challenge presented by HIV and AIDS and to accept their responsibilities in promoting prevention, as well as in caring for those infected and affected by HIV.

NURSING RESEARCH ON HIV AND AIDS

Most interventions and policies on HIV and AIDS in Africa are implemented on the basis of intuition rather than on evidence provided by scientific research. In fact, the situation concerning nursing research in Africa is characterized by a lack of forums for interaction between nurse researchers, policymakers, and clinical nurses. Very few clinical nurses undertake research and what research does occur is conducted in universities by lecturers and students as part of research training. This "ivory tower" type of research is usually limited in scope and appreciation and does not address policy needs (13). Even where major large-scale studies are undertaken, the dominant model is that nurse researchers from resource-rich countries identify problems, send researchers and intervention specialists to the resource-scarce countries where they "learn" and then transfer their learning to health care workers in these poorer countries. The researchers in resource-scarce countries "collaborate" with those in resource-rich countries and are invited to participate in further research. This model does very little to improve research capacity in resource-scarce countries and, therefore, does not lead to the development of culturally appropriate interventions and policies, especially in such areas as HIV and AIDS prevention and care.

FUTURE DIRECTIONS: NURSING PARTNERSHIPS FOR HIV AND AIDS PREVENTION AND CARE

As the HIV epidemic in Africa grows, so does the challenge to nurses in Africa. The theme for the 1998 International Nurses Day emphasized collaboration for the prevention and control of HIV and AIDS. The ICN encouraged nurses from all over the world to form partnerships with local, regional, and international governmental bodies, non-governmental organizations, and the private business sector to defend human rights, curtail the spread of HIV and AIDS, and reduce the devastation the epidemic is having on families and communities.

The positive responses to this call by nurses, especially from nurses in Africa, remain undocumented but very often such partnerships are lacking and urgently need to be established. A study of traditional healers and formal health workers, including nurses, found that all the healers and only half of the formal health workers were keen to collaborate on training and care for people living with AIDS (14). Yet such collaboration is important. Throughout Africa, many people with symptoms of sexually transmitted infections prefer to consult traditional doctors and healers because the traditional healers are perceived to be more holistic in their approach to health and healing than modern health care workers.

The following are specific groups of people or stakeholders that nurses in Africa need to collaborate with in order to overcome the epidemic.

Men have, until recently, been the almost invisible part of the solution to the HIV and AIDS epidemic, even though it has been widely documented that their socialization and behavior do much to determine how and to whom the virus is transmitted (15). However, labeling men, especially African men, as irresponsible, violent, predatory, and fast transmitters of the virus does not facilitate their involvement, and it ignores the fact that the majority of men in Africa are good, caring, responsible, loving, and very gender-sensitive individuals. It is only recently that many stakeholders realize that the qualities of these good men can be tapped and used as role models of appropriate behaviors for men who have the wrong perception of "masculine" behavior. Nurses need to collaborate and form partnerships with men who can be role models.

Civil society needs to be involved not just as actors but as decision makers, planners, and designers of programs on HIV and AIDS prevention and the reduction of its impact. Most government programs fail because they lack community-based experience and expertise. For example, poverty reduction cannot be accomplished through antipoverty programs alone. It needs to be addressed democratically and with changes in economic structures that give all people access to resources and opportunities that enhance their quality of life. Community health nurses in Africa see these problems in their daily work and need to document them for use in such civil efforts.

Older persons are important stakeholders because they are increasingly taking on unrecognized, unappreciated, and unremunerated social and economic responsibilities of caring for the sick and for children orphaned by HIV and AIDS, often at the expense of their own health and well-being (16). Nurses should, therefore, ensure that HIV and AIDS interventions, including information, education and support, also target this segment of the population.

People living with HIV and AIDS are a good resource for help and advice on HIV and AIDS education, counseling, and support efforts. Their involvement can ensure that they have equal access to food, sanitation, education, housing and health care, including the provision of antiretroviral drugs. Nurses need to actively work to eradicate stigma and discrimination toward persons living with HIV or AIDS.

Nursing networks already exist in Africa, with regional bodies such as the East, Central, and Southern African College of

Nursing (ECSACON) collaborating to advance nursing and improve patient care. Similar networks or associations of nurses working in HIV and AIDS care can be formed. Such groups can focus can focus on holding conferences, workshops, and continuing education programs that will advance African nurses' knowledge of HIV infection and care for those infected with the virus or living with AIDS.

Finally, African nurses need to undertake research that can quantify and, therefore, validate the magnitude of the HIV and AIDS epidemic that exists in some countries. For example, although most African states agree that young people have the right to develop their capacities; to access a range of services and opportunities; to live, learn, and earn in a safe and supportive environment; and to participate in decisions and actions that directly affect them, institutions such as schools, nongovernmental organizations, the media, the private sector, and governments are, in fact, doing very little to support these rights. Access to information relating to sexual health is still a controversial issue despite extensive research showing that school-based life skills education empowers youth and does not increase their sexual activity (17). African nurses can use such information to create youth-friendly environments in their communities and health facilities.

In conclusion, nurses are the front-line health workers in all African countries, yet preservice and in-service education on HIV and AIDS prevention and care for themselves and their patients is still lacking. Their empowerment with information on HIV and AIDS and the development of research skills would go a long way toward ensuring the development and documentation of efforts to reduce and alleviate the impact of HIV and AIDS on communities and nations in Africa.

REFERENCES

1. WHO and ICN. *Guidelines for Nursing Management of People Infected with the Human Immunodeficiency Virus (HIV)*. Geneva: WHO, 1993.
2. Baylor College of Medicine. *HIV Nursing Curriculum*. Houston: Baylor College of Medicine, 2001.
3. Meisenhelder, J. Contributing factors to fear of HIV contagion in registered nurses. *Image: Journal of Nursing Scholarship*, 1994;26:65–69.
4. Fransman D, McCullogh M, Lavies D, et al. Doctors' attitudes to the care of children with HIV in South Africa. *AIDS Care*, 2000;12:89–96.
5. Chime J. The impact of the occupational risk of HIV/AIDS on retention of bedside nurses in Zambia. In: ICN, ed. *On the Continuum of HIV/AIDS Care*. Geneva: ICN, 1994;57–66.
6. WHO, UNAIDS, ICN. *Fact Sheets on HIV/AIDS for nurses and midwives*. Geneva: WHO, 2000.
7. Huerta S, Oddi L. Refusal to care for patients with Human immunodeficiency virus/acquired immunodeficiency syndrome: issues and responses. *Journal of Professional Nursing*, 1992;8:221–230.
8. Byahuka E. Research in Quality of AIDS Care. In: ICN, ed. *On the Continuum of HIV/AIDS Care*. Geneva: ICN, 1994:75–78.
9. Ngcongco NV. Nurses fighting the HIV/AIDS epidemic in Africa. *International Nursing Review*, 1998;45:85–88.
10. Buve A, Foster SD, Mbwili C, et al. Mortality among female nurses in the face of the AIDS epidemic: a pilot study in Zambia. *AIDS*, 1994;8:396.
11. Henderson DK. Postexposure chemoprophylaxis for occupational exposure to the human immunodeficiency virus. *JAMA*, 1999;281:931–936.
12. ICN. *Reducing the impact of HIV/AIDS on nursing/midwifery personnel: guidelines for National Nurse's Association and others*. Geneva: ICN, 1996.
13. Tlou SD. Women, the girl child and HIV/AIDS. In: Program and Abstracts of the 45th Session of the United Nations Commission on the Status of Women; March 6–16, 2001; New York, United States.
14. Burnett A, Baggaley R, Ndovi-MacMillan M, et al. Caring for People Living with HIV in Zambia: Are Traditional Healers and Formal Health Workers Willing to Work Together? *AIDS Care*, 1999;11:481–491.
15. Panos. *AIDS and Men: Old Problem, New Angle*. London: Panos, 1998.
16. Tlou SD. Empowering Older Women in AIDS Prevention and Care. *Southern African Journal of Gerontology*, 1996;92:27–32.
17. Kirby D, Short L, Collins J, et al. School-based Programs to Reduce Sexual Risk Behaviours: A Review of Effectiveness. *Public Health Reports*, 1994;109:339–360.

25

Home-Based Care

*†Quarraisha Abdool Karim, ‡Samuel Kalibala, §Elly T. Katabira and †Zena A. Stein

*Department of Community Health, University of Natal, Durban, South Africa. †Division of Epidemiology, Mailman School of Public Health, Columbia University, New York, USA. ‡Population Council, Nairobi, Kenya. §World Health Organization, Harare, Zimbabwe.

The introduction of highly active antiretroviral therapy (HAART) has transformed HIV infection in individuals in the developed world into a manageable, if chronic, disease. In contrast, in those parts of the world where HAART is virtually unavailable, the number of symptomatic people in need of care continues to escalate unabated (1–3). Sub–Saharan Africa is, unfortunately, an outstanding example of the latter.

The people of sub–Saharan Africa continue to bear a disproportionate 70% of the global burden of HIV infection (4). Since the first reported cases of AIDS in central and eastern Africa in the early 1980s (5) no part of the continent has been left untouched by HIV. About 11.5 million people have died of HIV-related illnesses in sub–Saharan Africa, representing 83% of the world's total HIV/AIDS-related deaths (4). The number of individuals with HIV disease or AIDS is growing rapidly (6,7,8). Even if HIV infection rates decline steeply in the near future, the plight of those already infected, and that of their families and communities will not be averted. The full force of the growing burden of caregiving will be felt as the millions who are infected with the virus progress to HIV disease and AIDS.

In resource-scarce countries, existing health care delivery systems, with few exceptions, remain inadequate for the delivery of even basic care (9). When one patient on HAART in a developed country may spend several thousands of U.S. dollars per annum on medication alone, it is hard to realize that the average annual per capita health expenditure in most sub–Saharan countries is less than US$3 (10). While most sub–Saharan countries are transforming their health care delivery systems in the direction of greater access and equity, decades-old economic and social policies (11) have resulted in dysfunctional, overburdened, and underresourced health infrastructures. The advancing HIV epidemic in sub–Saharan Africa is further eroding this weak system by imposing new demands. Many health care facilities report a dramatic rise to 70% or 80% in bed occupancy for persons with HIV-related conditions (12,13). In addition, health care workers are, like the rest of the population they serve, succumbing to HIV disease and AIDS (14). The additional demand on inadequate health care infrastructure together with the declining number of providers presents a major challenge for health care delivery systems throughout Africa.

The epidemics of HIV and AIDS are also bringing new users to the overburdened health services system: the young and economically active sector of the population. Although these individuals have not traditionally placed demands on these services, their needs now must be considered. A number of countries are exploring ways to provide care for people with AIDS outside of the formal health care setting. A variety of innovative care initiatives have emerged (15–17). Home-based care is prominent among them.

The concept of caring for patients at home is not new. In the past, home-based care was used extensively (and, in many instances, successfully) for the care of the elderly and of individuals with chronic disease, mental illness, cancer, or infectious diseases such as tuberculosis (18–22). Care provided at home is best suited to those with long-term care needs, those who require the type of nursing a family member can be trained to provide, and those who regard their home as the most supportive, therapeutic setting for their care (23,24). Further motivation for home-based care can be found among family members who wish to keep a disabled and sick relative in the home and to play a central role in providing the required care. In Africa, there is a strong tradition of the extended family being involved in all matters affecting the family, including the care of its sick and disabled members (25,26).

Three additional factors have bolstered initiatives in Africa for home-based care for patients with HIV disease and AIDS. First, HIV is increasingly associated with poverty (27). Problems related to poverty at home and in the community, in addition to those related to HIV disease and AIDS, often compound one another. In such circumstances, even a home-based care service that is limited to providing food supplements and counseling may help reduce HIV-related morbidity. Second, the demand for clinic- and hospital-based care, both in out-patient and in-patient service, is vast, while the combined capacity of these services remains relatively meager. Establishing a solid system for home-based care, and thereby expanding the capacity for care within the community, could be a step toward building a more acceptable and sustainable care delivery system. Third, as HIV is being transmitted disproportionately among young and economically active adults, HIV disease and AIDS is depleting the ranks of the professional caregivers in society.

MODELS FOR HIV AND AIDS HOME-BASED CARE

In Africa, access to voluntary HIV counseling and testing facilities remains limited, and the majority of individuals who are infected with HIV remain unaware of their status (24). In many instances, individuals first visit a traditional or spiritual healer to understand their symptoms (28,29). Most learn their HIV status only after they visit a health care facility and find out their symptoms are the result of their being infected with HIV. Even in these settings, laboratory diagnostic facilities remain limited, and diagnosis is, in most instances, based on clinical presentation (30).

New initiatives for patient care have been proposed by hospitals, nongovernmental organizations (NGOs), or community-based organizations (31–33). These new initiatives generally provide care outside of the formal health care delivery system, and are most commonly referred to as home-based care initiatives. Diversity among these proposed services is considerable and reflects different aims, priorities, and limitations.

Hospital-initiated programs represent a type of home-based care that is usually delivered by individuals, teams of health care workers, or multidisciplinary teams which could include nurses, doctors, social workers, and spiritual leaders. Factors that could limit the size and composition of a team include the availability of resources (human and financial) and the degree to which staff are motivated to participate. The type of care delivered may include medical treatment of minor ailments, nursing, pastoral care, counseling, and social support. In the hospital-initiated model, the home-care team trains and instructs the family of the patient on how to care for simple ailments and when to seek outside help. In addition, education on preventing HIV infection is provided, and family members are given an opportunity to ask questions relating to HIV and AIDS. The hospital serves as the nucleus for the home-based service and patient referral to the home or hospital is part of the service.

Home-care programs delivered by NGOs or community-based groups are usually funded by international donor agencies and staffed by volunteers from the community and/or by service professionals. In these programs, home-based care usually involves providing assistance with chores, spiritual and psychologic support, food parcels, some nursing care, and palliative care. Drawbacks to such programs can include the lack of smooth referral processes for sick patients (especially true when programs are not linked with formal health care providers), and the potential nonsustainability of resources (a factor for programs dependent upon donor funds which may be arbitrarily reduced or withdrawn).

Whether hospital- or community-initiated, each program uses its own approach and sets its own goal. Some program teams provide a nurse and driver; some treat opportunistic infections; some provide drugs for prophylaxis and pain relief; some train volunteers; and some focus on improving the skills of the home caregiver.

One successful HIV home-based care program (which is used as a model for many new hospital-initiated programs), was begun by the Salvation Army at Chikankata Hospital in Mazabuka, Zambia (32). About ten years ago, bed occupancy rates at Chikankata Hospital grew as a result of increasing cases of HIV disease. In an effort to understand how to best handle the increase, staff interviewed patients about where they would prefer to receive their care. About 90% of those interviewed said they would prefer to live at home and to be visited monthly by a team of health workers from the hospital. The home-based care program that was subsequently established had as its goal the provision of care that would meet the physical, psychologic, spiritual, and social needs of each patient. Additional objectives included contact tracing of sexual partners, counseling and education of family members on HIV and AIDS, and fostering community acceptance of those living with HIV or AIDS.

Another successful home-based care program is that begun at Monze Hospital in Ndola, Zambia. Monze Hospital is a 252-bed Catholic Mission district-level hospital. It is a nucleus for 14 rural health centers. Since the early 1980s this hospital has worked to strengthen the delivery of primary health care services by training staff and outreach workers, an effort that, to date, has produced 96 community health workers and traditional birth attendants. When demand for care started to increase in Monze, the program added an objective that dealt with "the promotion of family and community involvement in the care of persons with AIDS" (32).

Individuals enter the Monze home-care program when they are discharged from the hospital. Each participant is escorted to the rural health facility closest to his or her home and introduced to the staff. Family members also meet at the facility, are counseled by the staff, and are provided with basic information on how to care for the patient at home. The system of referral, under which the family first contacts the community health worker and then the rural health center staff, when required, is also carefully explained.

To further alleviate the demand for hospital care brought on by the epidemic, the Monze community builds and furnishes "village-type" homes that are close to the rural health center. Under this initiative, the houses serve as wards and are used by patients who need supervised care or treatment.

A recent evaluation of home-based care initiatives in Zambia identified the Monze model as the one most appropriate for this country and recommended its adoption throughout Zambia (32). The Monze model reflects a true partnership between community and formal health services, one that includes indigenous solutions for providing care.

Among NGO-initiated programs, the program begun by The AIDS Support Organisation (TASO) is an outstanding example (33). TASO was established in Uganda in 1987, the outgrowth of a support group for people living with HIV or AIDS and their families. The group's initial goal of providing psychosocial support expanded rapidly to include voluntary testing and counseling. Prevention activities and medical and nursing care for opportunistic infections were made available at seven centers throughout Uganda, each center affiliated with a government-run district hospital. In 1996 alone, TASO served a cumulative client base of 22,000.

Another NGO-initiated home-based care program is FOCUS (Families, Orphans, and Children Under Stress). FOCUS was established by the Family AIDS Caring Trust (FACT) in Zimbabwe (34). This program establishes networks for, and trains and supervises women from local church groups, as they identify needy households and provide services that range from nursing and orphan care to the distribution of food parcels. This program emphasizes community ownership and the use of existing community resources to ensure sustainability. Rather than participating in the direct delivery of specific care services, FOCUS acts as a catalyst to facilitate and support community-based care provision efforts.

WHAT HAVE WE LEARNED FROM HOME-BASED CARE INITIATIVES?

While systematic evaluations of home-based care programs for individuals with HIV disease or AIDS in Africa remain rare, much can be gleaned from experiences documented over the past decade. Because traditions, needs, and resources differ between communities and countries, no one model will suit all circumstances. Comparisons, however, will still provide lessons to the planner.

A Continuum of Services

Home-based care has to be viewed as one component in a continuum of care and services necessary for optimal health care service delivery to individuals with HIV disease or AIDS. Among home-care services, those that provide a link or mechanism of referral to a formal health care provider are more successful and sustainable than those that do not. In instances where such links do not exist, care provision often results in instances of neglect, since referrals for appropriate care cannot be made (23,31–34).

An Alternative to Hospital Care?

While several home-based care programs were started to serve as alternatives to hospital- or facilities-based care, the limitations of this approach became rapidly apparent (31,33,35,36). An individual who is not visited by a home team or by a caregiver may delay seeking care at a health facility. However, a person who is visited regularly by a home team is more likely to be identified to be in need of facilities-based care services and be referred to a health facility. Thus, the home-based programs structured to ensure the person the right care at the right time actually can result in an increase in the use of hospitals or care facilities.

Coverage

Little data exists on the average number of clients covered by home-care programs. In most instances, the number of clients served is determined by resources available (human, facility, and financial) rather than by demand (15). In some instances, service may be restricted to individuals living within a fixed distance of a health facility (32,34). In other instances, the physical distance between clients is the rate limiting step to enrollment (31). In addition to such physical restrictions, certain characteristics of the client population may limit use of the services. Potential clients may lack knowledge of their HIV status, or of the existence of service; they may be uncertain of new service, or of its acceptability (23,32,33,35).

In situations where coverage could be estimated or modeled, it was low, between 2% and 23% of those in need of care (34). One fact that makes it difficult to estimate coverage is that the number of people needing care grows much faster than does the number of services that can provide that care. For example, a study conducted in Zimbabwe (34) reported that, in 1991, about 1,000 people living with AIDS had access to health services whereas by 1995, this number had increased to 3,000. However, the number of people in need of home care during the same time period increased from 3,000 to 50,000, indicating an actual decline in coverage from 33% to 6%.

Costs of Home Care

Several cost-analysis and cost-effectiveness studies of home-based care services have been undertaken (35–37). Usually, the cost of a home care visit is compared to the cost of a hospital in-patient visit. While these comparisons showed no clear winner, they did indicate some interesting breakdowns of how funds and time are spent. A costing study conducted in Zambia (35) demonstrated that an average home visit could cost between US$14 and US$26, compared to between US$7 and US$25 for a one-day stay at the hospital. Transportation costs accounted for 44% of the home-care costs. On average, however, individuals receiving home care required 2 fewer days hospitalization compared to individuals not receiving home care, an effective savings of between US$14 and US$50. While an average home-care visit took 68 minutes, only 15 minutes of that was spent on caregiving.

No data exist on the costs to the family or household for providing home care. Since the quality and type of care delivered through the home and family differs from that available at a health care facility (either as an out- or in-patient) and given the complementarity of all services on the patient's well-being, such head-to-head comparisons can create a misperception of the actual costs and quality of the respective services. Nevertheless, economic estimates that take into account the context are in order.

Stigma, Discrimination, and Disclosure

Home-care services reach families and communities that hospital services do not. These services provide prevention and counseling activities that hospital services cannot. In addition, these services can enhance prevention efforts at a community level and can help families and communities reduce the social stigma and discrimination so often associated with HIV and AIDS.

In most cases, unless supporting voluntary disclosure of HIV infection is a target of a service group's program, the scope of community educational activities carried out by a service group is limited to a relatively small client group. Although it is important to respect the right of a patient to choose whether to disclose his or her HIV status, maintaining confidentiality has posed numerous dilemmas for health care workers and to home-care teams working with individuals who have not disclosed their HIV status to the home caregiver or spouse.

A few home-care initiatives have adopted a novel approach known as "shared confidentiality" (33,34). Using this approach, the individual is requested during pre-test counseling to choose which two or three significant individuals he or she would like to tell about the decision to have an HIV test and share the results of that test. These individuals then also receive counseling both before the test is given and when the results become available. Although no formal evaluation of this approach has been undertaken, anecdotal data suggest that shared confidentiality has enhanced the way patients and their families deal and cope with HIV-related issues including home care.

The vignette below captures what home services can achieve in this regard and that simply cannot happen in a hospital or clinic.

> "I was so scared of catching the infection that I even denied her children social contact with her. The first thing I asked (the team) was how to live and care for her. The team helped me a great deal with information on HIV infection and AIDS, after that I felt very much at ease to talk and relate to her. Her father reacted very angrily upon hearing her diagnosis ... but because of the support from the teams we have both accepted her. The team has helped me to understand how to accept, support and care for my daughter" (31).

Gender

Sub–Saharan Africa is unusual in being the only region of the world where more women than men are infected with HIV (4). Here as elsewhere, knowledge of their HIV status often leads to loss of security, violence, ostracism and/or stigma (38,39). Yet despite bearing a disproportionate burden of the epidemic, most caregivers, both in formal settings and in homes and communities, are women (40). Thus, HIV can have a two-fold effect on women; it can make them both the caregiver and the one needing care.

CHALLENGES AND RECOMMENDATIONS

Home-based care should be developed as one component of a linked set of activities for HIV prevention and care for people living with HIV or AIDS. It should be targeted to those it can best serve; HIV-infected individuals who are symptomatic, even occasionally those who are critically ill, bedridden, or terminally ill, if the home environment can keep the individual comfortable. Asymptomatic individuals should not require home-based care but can be counseled and treated prophylactically as appropriate. Hospital beds should be used only under predetermined circumstances, for example, when special equipment or medications that may control suffering cannot be administered by home caregivers, even with training.

Thus, strategies for increasing the capacity of services and of communities must change from an approach in which only direct help and care is provided, to one that supports the whole care process within the household and community. For example, a pool of home care equipment for loan to client families would be useful in many settings. Establishing support systems for caregivers within the home and within the teams will enable them to sustain their work without "burning out." Additional types of community workers and traditional healers must be included in the program, and the skills and resources to train families to perform care activities must be developed.

Since so much of the success of home-based care depends on the existence of community support for its members living with HIV, it is crucial to know and understand community views concerning HIV and AIDS and home-based care. It is also important to understand people's desires, reactions, and consequences to dying at home. Incorporating the views of all caregivers—religious leaders, traditional healers, home caregivers, those needing care, and members of the home-based care team—are crucial to the design of a successful program.

Because the majority of the cost-analysis studies of home-based care programs have been undertaken from the perspective of the service provider, it would be useful and informative to examine the cost implications of different services from the perspective of HIV-infected persons and their households.

There should be an integration of HIV home-based care services with other community outreach services, such as those for tuberculosis. This could increase the number of people served and reduce the costs of delivering home-based care. While respecting the wishes of HIV-infected clients, home-based care teams should ensure that adequate counseling is given to their clients' sexual partners and caregivers. Finally, equal care for all patient groups—whether an HIV-infected person cared for at home or an AIDS sufferer cared for in a hospital—requires ongoing vigilance of health care needs and services.

Just as the HIV epidemic has highlighted issues such as poverty, discrimination, and marginalization as factors critical to the disproportionate spread of HIV infection in some communities and countries, the provision of care to those with HIV disease has highlighted the vast inequities that exist concerning access to basic, good quality health care around the globe.

Global efforts have increased substantially in the past six months to explore strategies for increasing access to good quality, basic health care, including access to antiretrovirals for the millions of young adults already infected with HIV. As has been the case with directly observed therapy for tuberculosis, the home and the community, with additional support and training for family and community members, will be important venues for the use of antiretrovirals and enhancing adherence.

REFERENCES

1. Van Praag E, Perriens JH. Caring for patients with HIV and AIDS in middle income countries: Preventing transmission from mother to child is far more cost-effective than treating symptomatic infection. *BMJ* 1996;313:440.
2. Muller O, Corrah T, Katabira E, et al. Antiretroviral therapy in sub-Saharan Africa. *Lancet* 1998;351:68.
3. Hearst N, Mandel JS. A research agenda for AIDS prevention in the developing world. *AIDS* 1997;11 (Suppl 1):S1–S4.
4. Joint United Nations Programme on HIV/AIDS and World Health Organisation. *AIDS Epidemic update:December 2000.* Geneva:UNAIDS/WHO; 2001.
5. Fontanet A, Piot P. State of our knowledge:the epidemiology of HIV/AIDS. *Health Transition Rev* 1994;4:11–23.
6. Timaeus IM. Impact of the HIV epidemic on mortality in sub-Saharan Africa:evidence from national surveys and censuses. *AIDS* 1998;12:S15–S27.
7. Dondero TJ, Curran JW. Excess deaths in Africa from HIV:confirmed and quantified. *Lancet* 1994;343:989–990.
8. Abdool Karim Q, Abdool Karim SS. South Africa:Host to a new and emerging HIV epidemic. *Sexually Transmitted Infections* 1999;75:139–147.
9. Gilks CF, Katabira E, De Cock KM. The challenge of providing care for HIV/AIDS in Africa. *AIDS* 1997;11(Suppl B):S99–S106.
10. Mann J, Tarantola D. *AIDS in the World II.* Cambridge:Oxford University Press;1996;536–544.
11. Sanders D, Sambo A. AIDS in Africa:the implications of economic recession and structural adjustment. *Health Pol Plann* 1991;6:157–165.
12. Foster S. The impact of HIV on the University Teaching Hospital, Lusaka, Zambia. *World Hosp Health Serv* 1995;31:18–21.
13. Anderson S. Community responses to AIDS. *Int Nurs Rev* 1994;41:57–60.
14. Buve A, Foster SD, Mbwili C, et al. Mortality among female nurses in the face of the AIDS epidemic:a pilot study in Zambia [letter]. *AIDS* 1994;8:396.
15. Russell M, Schneider H. *A Rapid Appraisal of Community-based Care and Support Programmes in South Africa.* Johannesburg: Centre for Health Policy, University of Witwatersrand; January 2000.
16. Panos Institute. *Home-based care, not home-based neglect.* AIDS Information Sheet No 10;July 1996.
17. Almedal C. HIV and AIDS. Home care project in Rwanda. *Sykepl Fag* 1993;81:34.
18. Fernandez Navarro JM, Pozuelo Munoz B, Orti Martinez P, et al. Evaluation of a home care program for children with cancer. *An Esp Paediat* 2000;52:41–46.
19. Crome P, Malham A, Baker D, et al. Domiciliary visits to the old and mentally ill:how valuable? *JR Soc Med* 2000;93:187–190.
20. Maher D, Hausler HP, Raviglione MC. Tuberculosis care in community care organisations in sub-Saharan Africa:practice and potential. *Int J of Tuberculosis and Lung Disease* 1997;1:276–283.
21. Johnson B, Montgomery P. Chronic mentally ill individuals re-entering the community after hospitalisation. Phase II:The urban experience. *J Psychiatr Ment Health Nurs* 1999;6:445–451.

22. Faison KJ, Faria SH, Frank D. Caregivers of chronically ill elderly:perceived burden. *J Community Health Nurs* 1999;16;243–253.
23. Jackson H, Kerkhoven R. Developing AIDS care in Zimbabwe:a case for residential community centre. *AIDS Care* 1995;7:663–673.
24. Kalibala S, Rubaramira R, Kaleeba N. Non-governmental organisations and community responses to HIV/AIDS and the role of HIV-positive persons in prevention and care. *AIDS* 1997;11(Suppl B): S151–S157.
25. Ankrah EM. The impact of HIV/AIDS on the family and other significant relationships:the African clan revisited. *AIDS Care* 1993;5:5–22.
26. Seeley J, Kajura E, Bachengana C, et al. The extended family and support for people with AIDS in a rural population in south west Uganda:a safety net with holes? *AIDS Care*. 1993;5:117–122.
27. Danziger R. The social impact of HIV/AIDS in developing countries. *Soc Sci Med* 1994;39:905–917.
28. Katabira E, Kamya MR, Mubiru FX, et al. HIV Infection:Diagnostic and treatment strategies for Healthcare Workers. Second Edition. Uganda:STD and AIDS Control Programme;2000.
29. Baleta A. South Africa to bring traditional healers into mainstream medicine. *Lancet* 1998;352:554.
30. Katabira E, Wabitsch KR. Management issues for patients with HIV infection in Africa. *AIDS* 1991;5 (Suppl 1):S149–S155.
31. Soldan K, Abdool Karim Q, Abdool Karim SS. Home-based care for AIDS-evaluation of the KwaZulu pilot programme. South Africa:South African Medical Research Council;1993.
32. Chela CM, Siankanga ZC. Home and community care:the Zambia experience. *AIDS* 1991;5:(Suppl 1):S157–S161.
33. Kaleeba N, Kalibala S, Kaseje M, et al. Participatory evaluation of counselling, medical and social services of The AIDS Support Organisation (TASO) in Uganda. *AIDS Care* 1997;9:13–26.
34. Osborne CM, van Praag E, Jackson H. Models of care for patients with HIV/AIDS. *AIDS* 1997;11 (Suppl B):S135–S141.
35. Chela CM, Msiska R, Sichone M, et al. Cost and Impact of Home based care for people living with HIV/AIDS in Zambia. Report prepared for the Ministry of Health, Zambia;1994.
36. Hansen K, Woelk G, Jackson H, et al. The cost of home-based care for HIV/AIDS patients in Zimbabwe. *AIDS Care* 1998;10:751–759.
37. Buwalda P, Kruijthoff DJ, de Bruyn M, et al. Evaluation of a home care/counselling AIDS Programme in Kgatleng district, Botswana. *AIDS Care* 1994;6:153–160.
38. Seidel G, Ntuli N. HIV, confidentiality, gender and support in rural South Africa. *Lancet* 1996;347:469.
39. Temmerman M, Ndinya-Achola J, Ambani J, et al. The right not to know HIV test results. *Lancet* 1995;345:969–970.
40. Taylor L, Seeley J, Kajura E. Informal care for illness in rural southwest Uganda:the central role that women play. *Health Transit Rev* 1996;6:49–56.

26

Nutrition and HIV Infection

*Annamaria K. Kiure, †Gernard I. Msamanga, and ‡Wafaie W. Fawzi

*Department of Nutrition, Harvard School of Public Health, Boston, Massachusetts, USA.
†Community Health Department, Muhimbili University College of Health Sciences, Dar es Salaam, Tanzania.
‡Departments of Nutrition and Epidemiology, Harvard School of Public Health, Boston, Massachusetts, USA.

Severe undernutrition impairs immune function and thus reduces resistance to infections (1). Similarly, the pathogenesis of human immunodeficiency virus (HIV) infection leading to acquired immunodeficiency syndrome (AIDS) may be accelerated in individuals with specific nutrient deficiencies, coexisting infections, and suppressed immune function. In this chapter we will review studies that have examined the potential effects of nutritional status on immune function, viral load, and disease progression among HIV-infected individuals. Potential mechanisms of nutrition in slowing progression to clinical AIDS will be discussed. In addition, the potential role of nutritional status in HIV vertical transmission and its relationship to maternal and child health will be presented.

PREVALENCE OF UNDERNUTRITION AMONG PERSONS WITH HIV INFECTION

Nutritional disorders are common among persons living with HIV infection in sub–Saharan Africa and other parts of the world. Early in the HIV epidemic, malnutrition in the form of "slim disease" was described among adult populations in Uganda (2). The prevalence of wasting was reported to be 40.3% in adult AIDS patients in Burundi (3) and 44% in HIV-seropositive subjects in an autopsy study in Côte d'Ivoire (4). In Côte d'Ivoire, the body mass index (BMI) of 67% of the study participants was low ($< 21.5\ kg/m^2$), while 13% were very thin ($BMI < 18.0\ kg/m^2$) (5). In this study more men than women were found to have a low BMI. Baseline serum albumin levels were found to be abnormally low in 23% of the HIV-infected men who participated in the prospective Multicenter AIDS Cohort Study (MACS) in the United States (6).

Micronutrient deficiencies are also common among persons living with HIV infection. Table 1 shows the prevalence of low levels of serum or plasma micronutrients in HIV-infected individuals at different locations, including deficiencies in vitamins A, B_6, B_{12}, E, C, riboflavin (B_2), and in folate, zinc, and selenium (6–19). The prevalence rates of low blood levels of riboflavin (26%) and copper (74%) were higher among asymptomatic HIV-1–seropositive men who have sex with men (MSM) than among HIV-1–seronegative controls in Miami (11). Other studies have reported low blood levels of vitamin C (20), vitamin E (20,21,22),

TABLE 1. The Prevalence of Selected Micronutrient Deficiencies among HIV-Infected Individuals

Nutrient	Criteria to determine deficiency	Site	Prevalence[a] (% Deficient)	Reference
Carotenoids	<1.50 μmol/L	USA, New Jersey	26	7
	<1.44 μmol/L	USA, New Jersey	31	8
	<0.88 μmol/L	Germany, Berlin	77	9
Vitamin A	<1.36 μmol/L	USA, Baltimore/Washington	10	6
	<1.05 μmol/L	USA, Baltimore	15	10
	<1.05 μmol/L	USA, Miami	18	11
	<1.05 μmol/L	USA, Baltimore	29	12
	<0.70 μmol/L	Kenya	24	13
	<0.70 μmol/L	Tanzania	34	14
	<1.05 μmol/L	Malawi	65	15
Vitamin B_6	<30.00 ng/ml	USA, New Jersey	17	8
	AC > 1.70[b]	USA, Miami	53	11
Vitamin B_{12}	<177.60 pmol/L	USA, Miami	23	11
	<185.00 pmol/L	USA, Los Angeles	36	16
	<132.00 pmol/L	Canada, Montreal	30.5	17
Vitamin E	<14.00 μmol/L	USA, New Jersey	4	7
	<0.60 mg/dl	USA, New Jersey	12	8
	<11.60 μmol/L	USA, Baltimore/Washington	22	6
	<6.00 μg/dl	USA, Miami	27	11
Vitamin C	<34.50 μmol/L	USA, Miami	10	11
	<23.00 μmol/L	USA, New Jersey	20	7
	<23.00 μmol/L	USA, New Jersey	27	8
Riboflavin	AC > 1.25[c]	USA, Miami	26	11
Folate	<11.25 nmol/L	USA, New Jersey	3	8
	<11.00 nmol/L	USA, New Jersey	15	7
Zinc	<10.70 μmol/L	USA, New Jersey	4	7
	<8.42 μmol/L	USA	29	18
	<11.50 μmol/L	USA, Miami	50	11
Selenium	<85.00 μg/l	USA, Miami	11	19

[a]Measurements on serum or plasma.
[b]Erythrocyte transaminase assay, activity coefficient (AC) > 1.70 for deficiency.
[c]Erythrocyte glutathione reductase assay, activity coefficient (AC) > 1.25 for deficiency.

β-carotene (20,22), and selenium (20,23) in HIV-positive individuals in Canada, the United States, and Italy. Semba et al. (24) and Antelman et al. (25) recently reported the prevalence of anemia among asymptomatic HIV-infected pregnant women in urban clinic centers in Malawi and Tanzania to be 73.1% and 83%, respectively.

Macronutrient and micronutrient deficiencies commonly coexist in HIV-infected individuals. High prevalence of wasting and specific micronutrient deficiencies such as vitamin A and carotene (26), vitamin B_{12} (16), folate (26,27), and zinc (28) have been reported in HIV-infected individuals. Results from cross-sectional studies are limited by failure to establish a temporal relationship between HIV infection and specific nutrient deficiencies. HIV infection could lead to nutritional deficiency through decreased dietary nutrient intake, malabsorption, and increased utilization and excretion of nutrients (5,29,30). On the other hand, nutrient deficiencies may contribute to faster HIV disease progression by impairing immune function.

FUNCTIONS OF MACRONUTRIENTS AND MICRONUTRIENTS

Macronutrients are related to wasting and energy balance in HIV-infected patients, while micronutrients play different roles in immune function. In this section we will discuss the functions of macronutrients, followed by a review of animal and human studies on selected micronutrients and immune function. Macronutrients include carbohydrates, proteins, fat, and fiber. Carbohydrates are a major dietary constituent, making up 50% to 70% of a person's total energy intake (31). However, energy intake may be low in some parts of sub–Saharan Africa because the composition of dietary carbohydrates available varies from one region to another due to food production and distribution differences and sociocultural factors such as certain food taboos. The main function of carbohydrates is to provide energy for several metabolic processes in the body. Dietary fat provides approximately 15% to 20% of a person's total energy intake in Africa, whereas in the United States and Europe, fat intake contributes between 30% and 45% of total energy intake (31). Dietary fat is a source of energy and provides the structural component of cell membranes (32). Energy stored in adipose tissue becomes available during periods of starvation, an important mechanism for patients with reduced food intake. Amino acids are building blocks for proteins that are required for the growth and transport of nutrients in the blood. Supplementation of several amino acids has been suggested as a method for reducing weight loss among HIV-infected individuals. A combination of three amino acids known as HMB/Gln/Arg—beta-hydroxy-beta-methylbutyrate (HMB); a metabolite of leucine, L-glutamine (Gln); and L-arginine (Arg)—given for 8 weeks to patients with HIV-associated wasting resulted in significant weight gain for patients in the treatment arm compared with those receiving placebo (33). Improvements in gut function leading to absorption of supplemented and other nutrients may have contributed to weight gain in patients in the treatment arm.

Micronutrients include fat-soluble vitamins A, D, E, and K, and water-soluble vitamins such as B_1 (thiamin), B_2 (riboflavin), B_3 (niacin), B_5 (pantothenic acid), B_6 (pyridoxine), biotin, B_{12} (cyanocobalamin), folic acid, and vitamin C. Major mineral micronutrients include iron, zinc, selenium, and iodine. Micronutrients with immunologic and epithelial maintenance functions will be reviewed based on existing in-vitro animal and human studies.

Beta-carotene is a provitamin A carotenoid that may enhance T-cell and B-cell immune function possibly through conversion to vitamin A or by acting as an antioxidant (34,35). Daily supplementation of β-carotene among elderly volunteers has led to an increase in number of T-lymphocytes and cells with interleukin-2 (IL-2) receptors (34). Increased number of natural killer cells in HIV-infected children has also been observed following vitamin A supplementation in South Africa (36). In a meta-analysis, vitamin A supplementation among children whose HIV status was not determined resulted in significant reductions in total mortality and in the severity of measles and diarrhea (37).

Vitamin E is required for immune function and to protect the body's cells from oxidative damage. In mice infected with murine AIDS, vitamin E supplementation was associated with significant improvements in IL-2 production and natural killer cell cytotoxicity as well as reduced production of the proinflammatory cytokines such as tumor necrosis factor-alpha (TNF-α) and interleukin-6 (IL-6) (38). Vitamin E deficiency has been shown to impair T-cell–mediated function including delayed-type hypersensitivity (DTH) response, lymphocyte proliferation, and IL-2 production in animal and human studies (39). Supplementation with vitamin E in healthy elderly people significantly improved lymphocyte proliferation, IL-2 production, DTH, and response to T-cell–dependent vaccines, and reduced the incidence of self-reported infections (40,41).

Vitamin C acts as an antioxidant and plays a role in immune function and formation of connective tissues. Proliferation of T-lymphocytes and B-lymphocytes increased following vitamin C supplementation in some human studies (42), and increased levels of vitamin C were associated with a lower rate of infection (43).

Several B-complex vitamins have been observed to have roles in immune function. Vitamin B_6 deficiency in healthy elderly individuals significantly reduced the total number of lymphocytes, lymphocyte proliferation, and IL-2 production in response to T-cell mitogens; these defects were corrected following B_6 repletion (44). Among HIV-infected individuals, vitamin B_6 deficiency was associated with reduced natural killer cell cytotoxicity and impaired mitogen-induced lymphocyte proliferation (45). Riboflavin deficiency has been shown to impair the ability to generate humoral antibodies in response to test antigens, but research on its effects on cell-mediated immunity is limited (46). Data from clinical studies show that patients with low serum vitamin B_{12} had impaired neutrophil function, while in-vitro and animal studies indicate that vitamin B_{12} supplements are associated with enhanced antibody function and mitogenic responses (46).

Selenium is required for proper activity of the enzyme glutathione peroxidase (GSH-Px) (47), which is involved in cellular antioxidant systems. Selenium deficiency is associated with immune dysfunction leading to impaired phagocytic cell function, decreased $CD4^+$ T-lymphocytes and the occurrence of opportunistic infections. In-vitro (48) and animal studies (49) showed increased GSH-Px activity in HIV-infected T-lymphocytes and murine AIDS models respectively, following selenium supplementation. In another in-vitro study, selenium supplementation for 3 days prior to exposure to TNF-α suppressed TNF-α–induced HIV-1 replication in acutely infected human monocytes, but not in T-lymphocytes or in chronically infected T-lymphocytic or monocytic cell lines (50). Selenium supplementation as parenteral nutrition improved immune response in patients with chronic gut failure whose HIV status was not determined (51).

Zinc plays an important role in the growth, development, and function of natural killer cells, macrophages, neutrophils, and T- and B-lymphocytes (52). Zinc was found to inhibit HIV-1 RNA transcription in an in-vitro study (53) and to possibly slow HIV-1 replication in humans (54). Zinc supplementation resulted in significant reductions in the severity of diarrhea, malaria, and acute respiratory infections among children whose HIV status has not been determined (55).

CAUSES OF NUTRITIONAL PROBLEMS IN HIV-INFECTED INDIVIDUALS

Nutritional deficiencies may contribute to increased immune suppression leading to increased progression of HIV disease. Advanced HIV disease, in turn, worsens nutritional status (56). The etiologic factors for undernutrition in HIV-infected patients include inadequate dietary intake (30,57), nutrient malabsorption (58), and disturbances related to weight loss and increased energy expenditure (57,59).

Inadequate dietary intake is common among HIV-infected patients and may be the result of anorexia or of dysphagia and painful swallowing caused by gastrointestinal *Candida* infection (30,5). Low energy intake ($<67\%$ of the recommended daily allowance [RDA]) was found among 24.7% of HIV-1–infected patients studied in South Africa (60). The prevalence of inadequate protein intake in this study was 12.3%. Low intake of vitamins A, B_6, C, and D, as well as of calcium, iron, and zinc were also reported (60). Low intake of micronutrients was associated with a predominantly maize-based diet; maize is a poor source of such nutrients. Among HIV-infected children with growth failure, the mean daily energy intake was lower than that among HIV-infected children without growth failure (61). Among HIV-infected men in the MACS study in the United States, the prevalence of low (below the RDA) total nutrient intake (from both food and supplements) was 29% for vitamin A and 27% for vitamin E (6). In contrast, Baum et al. found the mean total intake of vitamins A, B_6, B_{12}, E, and zinc to be significantly higher in HIV-positive MSM compared to HIV-negative MSM in the United States (62).

The relationship between weight loss, infection, energy intake, and energy expenditure has been described for HIV-infected individuals. The presence of infection may increase utilization of energy and nutrients thus leading to decreased nutrient stores, a condition that may be followed by weight loss. Wasting among HIV-infected patients has been described to occur in the presence of specific symptoms, such as diarrhea (63). In HIV-infected patients with opportunistic infections, resting energy expenditures are elevated to levels that are frequently accompanied by weight loss during disease progression (57,59,64). Some studies have suggested that it is reduced energy intake, rather than increased energy expenditure that is primarily responsible for the HIV-wasting syndrome in adults (30,57) and growth failure in HIV-infected children (61,65). Metabolic changes and increased utilization of nutrients in HIV-infected patients have been associated with increased levels of blood lipids and increased catabolism of carbohydrates and proteins (57,66,67).

Nutrient malabsorption may occur because of impaired gut mucosal function caused by repeated episodes of infectious diarrhea. Loss of intestinal absorptive surface [measured by permeability to lactulose and mannitol and absorption of D-xylose (68)], fat malabsorption (69), and abnormal Schilling tests indicating vitamin B_{12} malabsorption (70,71) was commonly found in HIV-infected patients with or without diarrhea. Furthermore, increased loss of nutrients in urine among HIV-infected patients may lead to nutrient deficiencies. HIV-infected patients are at a higher risk of developing renal disease leading to low molecular mass proteinuria with loss of retinol, retinol-binding protein, and albumin in the urine (72,73).

THE POTENTIAL ROLE OF MACRONUTRIENTS IN HIV DISEASE PROGRESSION

Disease progression may be accelerated in HIV-infected individuals who are undernourished as a result of macronutrient-related disorders. Evidence from epidemiologic studies that describe the relationship between macronutrient-related undernutrition and immunologic markers, viral load, and clinical outcomes among HIV-infected individuals will be discussed in this section.

Macronutrients and Immunologic and Virologic Markers in HIV-Infected Individuals

$CD4^+$ cell counts, $CD8^+$ cell counts, and $CD4^+/CD8^+$ ratios are immunologic markers commonly used to predict survival and prognosis of HIV-infected patients. Undernutrition owing to macronutrient deficiencies has been associated with low $CD4^+$ cell counts in HIV-infected patients. HIV-infected individuals with low mean weight and low arm and muscle circumference (5), and HIV-infected children with growth impairment (65) were shown to have low $CD4^+$ cell counts.

Studies have examined the relationship between viral load, energy intake, free fat mass, and growth velocity among children. In a cross-sectional study, high viral load, high IL-6, and decreased total serum proteins were more likely to be found in HIV-infected children with growth impairment than in HIV-infected children with normal growth (65). However, the temporal relationship between nutritional status and immunologic and virologic markers cannot be established in cross-sectional studies.

Data from longitudinal studies that have examined the association between immunologic markers and macronutrient status are scarce. In a longitudinal study from Miami that followed HIV-infected individuals for 3.5 years, 73% of women with $CD4^{+}$ count $<200/mm^3$ were more likely to have lower levels of plasma prealbumin than men (24%) with similar $CD4^{+}$ counts (74). Few longitudinal studies have examined the relationship between macronutrient-related disorders and viral load among HIV-infected children. In follow-up studies, low mean daily energy intake, free fat mass and low 12-month growth velocity (61), and low linear growth from 3 months of age (75), were associated with increased plasma concentration of HIV RNA in HIV-infected children with growth failure (75) compared to those with no growth failure. In the latter study, infants who had a high viral load in the first 6 months of life were significantly more likely to have severe growth failure.

Macronutrients and Clinical Outcomes

Observational studies using anthropometric indicators have shown that mortality is increased among HIV-infected individuals in states of macronutrient-related undernutrition. Wasting, particularly loss of lean body mass, was demonstrated to be associated with early mortality (76,77) and susceptibility to opportunistic infections among participants of the Community Programs for Clinical Research in AIDS in the United States (77). In a case-control study nested within a follow-up study, HIV-infected injection drug users (IDUs) with wasting (more than 10% loss of weight from baseline to last visit before death; mean follow-up, 2.4 years) had approximately eight-fold higher risk of mortality compared with controls, after adjusting for $CD4^{+}$ cell counts (78). Predisposing factors for wasting in this study were reported as oral thrush, diarrhea, and hospitalization, which may indicate reduced nutrient intake, and malabsorption.

Few longitudinal studies have examined the association between biochemical indicators of macronutrient status and mortality among HIV-infected individuals. The adjusted hazard ratio for mortality was significantly threefold higher for HIV-infected women in the lowest serum albumin category (<35 g/L) compared with those in the highest category (≥ 42 g/L) in the United States (79). In this study, baseline serum albumin level was reported to be an independent predictor of mortality during 3 years of follow-up. Low lean body mass index (LBMI), and high plasma levels of C-reactive proteins were also significant predictors of mortality among HIV-infected individuals followed for 42 months before the use of protease inhibitors (80). After controlling for $CD4^{+}$ counts; levels of C-reactive protein, albumin, and prealbumin; and other clinical factors, the hazard for death was threefold higher among individuals with low LBMI (<14.5) compared to those with higher LBMI (≥ 14.5). In another 5-year follow-up study of HIV-1 vertically infected children, HIV RNA and serum albumin levels, and baseline $CD4^{+}$ cell counts were predictors of survival (81). Lower levels of serum albumin and hemoglobin were commonly observed in HIV-infected children who died compared with survivors.

Inconsistent results were observed in two intervention studies that examined the effect of macronutrient supplementation on weight gain among HIV-infected individuals with weight loss. In a randomized placebo-controlled study, supplementation with HMB/Gln/Arg for 8 weeks resulted in weight gain of about 3.0 kg for patients in the treatment arm and 0.37 kg for those in the placebo arm (33). However, in another randomized trial, supplementation of two different caloric diets and a noncaloric diet (multivitamins and minerals only) for 4 months did not result in a significant percentage change in weight among HIV-infected individuals (82).

THE POTENTIAL ROLE OF MICRONUTRIENTS IN HIV DISEASE PROGRESSION

Micronutrient deficiency may be associated with increased HIV disease progression owing to the impairment of the immune system and increase in viral replication (measured by immunologic markers and viral load). The reduced level of $CD4^+$ cells in HIV-infected individuals may be a result of exhaustion of the immune system caused by the destructive effects of HIV, other chronic infections, and overstimulation of inflammatory processes. Low levels of antioxidant micronutrients in the blood and increased levels of oxidation products may increase HIV replication in HIV-infected individuals, allowing new virions to infect more $CD4^+$ cells. Supplementation of β-carotene or vitamin A is associated with enhanced cellular immunity measured by $CD4^+$ and $CD8^+$ cell counts in both human (34,83,84) and animal studies (85). In addition, vitamin-A enhanced humoral immunity has been demonstrated by antibody response to disease antigens such as those containing tetanus (86) and measles (87).

Increased oxidative stress in states of micronutrient deficiency may be related to increased viral load. Excess reactive oxygen species can induce cellular injury, lysis, and activation of nuclear factor-κB (NF-κB), a factor involved in the transcription of HIV-1 and its replication (88). It has been suggested that supplementation of antioxidant micronutrients (such as vitamins A, C, E, and selenium) may reduce oxidative stress and hence reduce viral replication in HIV-infected patients. However, the mechanism by which selenium may suppress TNF-α–induced HIV-1 replication *in vitro* is not fully understood. Suppression may be mediated through increased activity of cellular antioxidants such as selenoproteins and GSH-Px (50).

Micronutrients and Immunologic Markers in HIV-Infected Individuals

Cross-sectional studies have examined biochemical markers of nutrient status and immunologic markers of HIV disease progression such as $CD4^+$ cell counts. In Thailand, HIV-1–infected pregnant women in the first trimester with $CD4^+$ counts <200 cells/mm^3 had mean serum vitamin A and β-carotene levels 37% lower than those in HIV-uninfected individuals (89). Plasma zinc and magnesium levels were shown to be significant predictors of $CD4^+$ cell count among HIV-1–infected individuals in a cross-sectional study in the United States (90).

In a longitudinal study in Miami, HIV-1–infected women with $CD4^+$ counts <200/mm^3 were more likely to have lower levels of plasma selenium and vitamin A and E than men with similar $CD4^+$ cell counts (74). Development of vitamin A or B_{12} deficiency was significantly associated with a decline in $CD4^+$ cell count in a longitudinal study of HIV-infected MSM (91). In this study, normalization of vitamin A, vitamin B_{12}, and zinc was significantly associated with higher $CD4^+$ cell count, a finding that was unaffected by the use of zidovudine. Findings from these studies were adjusted for factors such as baseline clinical signs and symptoms that describe HIV disease stage and $CD4^+$ cell counts. However, confounding resulting from unmeasured and unknown factors such as the duration of HIV infection and time to development of nutritional deficiencies cannot be ruled out. In addition, biochemical indicators of nutrient status such as vitamin A, zinc, and selenium are not reliable since blood levels of these nutrients are reduced in response to infection even in the absence of deficiency. Dietary intake of micronutrients has also been assessed prospectively in relation to immunologic markers of HIV infection. In a study conducted in San Francisco, higher dietary intake of zinc, thiamine, niacin, and riboflavin were positively related to $CD4^+$ cell counts (92).

Randomized trials are better suited to the examination of epidemiologic associations because randomization minimizes confounding exposure variables. In a small randomized crossover study, daily supplementation with 180 mg of β-carotene for 4 weeks was associated with a small increase in total white blood cell count, an increase in $CD4^+$ cell count, and a beneficial change in $CD4^+/CD8^+$ ratio compared with study participants receiving a placebo. These parameters decreased when participants in the β-carotene arm were switched to the placebo arm (93). However, this effect was not observed in another study by the same investigators in which 5,000 international units (IU) of vitamin A and 180 mg of β-carotene were used (94). A single high dose of vitamin A (200,000 IU) given to IDUs in the United States had no significant effect on $CD4^+$ lymphocyte count measured at 2 and 4 weeks after treatment (95). A large, double-blind, placebo-controlled, randomized trial of vitamins (with a 2×2 factorial design of placebo, vitamin A alone, multivitamins excluding vitamin A, or multivitamins including vitamin A) among HIV-infected pregnant women in Tanzania showed a significant increase in $CD4^+$, $CD8^+$, and CD3 cell counts in the group supplemented with multivitamins, but no beneficial effect in a group supplemented with vitamin A (14). Findings from a clinical trial among children with AIDS in South Africa showed that 60 mg of retinol equivalents of vitamin A given on two consecutive days could increase circulating $CD4^+$ and natural killer cell counts 1 month after supplementation (36). In a small, randomized trial with partial cross-over design, a combination of N-acetylcysteine (NAC) and sodium selenite resulted in a nonsignificant increase in $CD4^+$ counts at 6 weeks following supplementation (96).

Micronutrients and Viral Load

Micronutrient deficiency may be associated with an increase in HIV viral load. In a longitudinal study from Rwanda, lowered levels of serum retinol were associated with increased viral load among HIV-1–infected women in the late stages of disease progression (97). A few randomized trials have examined the effects of antioxidant micronutrient supplements on viral load but have not found a significant association. Supplementation of retinol and β-carotene to HIV-infected pregnant women in South Africa (98), and of vitamin A to HIV-infected IDUs (95) and HIV-infected nonpregnant and nonbreastfeeding women (99) in Baltimore, United States, did not result in significant change in viral load. Daily supplementation with selenium or β-carotene for 1 year led to significant increases in GSH-Px activity at 3 and 6 months among adult HIV-infected men and women in France whose routes of infection were blood transfusion, injection drug use, or sexual (both MSM and heterosexuals) (100). Levels of GSH-Px activity were much higher in the selenium group than in the β-carotene group and were significantly different from those of the placebo group, although viral load was not measured in this study. In a small, randomized trial with partial crossover design, daily supplementation with NAC and sodium selenite did not result in reduced viral load at the end of 24 weeks (96). However, in another small, randomized, placebo-controlled, double-blind study in Canada, a significant reduction in viral load was achieved after 3 months of supplementation with large daily doses of vitamins C and E (101). Vitamins C and E may reduce oxidative stress in HIV-infected individuals, leading to reductions in viral load. Beneficial effects of vitamins C and E may be mediated by a mechanism in which vitamin C regenerates vitamin E during an antioxidant defense process (102).

Micronutrients and Clinical Outcomes

Micronutrient deficiencies are associated with faster HIV disease progression (103). Therefore, it may be argued that improving nutritional status and dietary intake of nutrients may help reduce progression to AIDS and morbidity and mortality among HIV-infected persons. Observational studies have examined the relationship between nutritional factors and HIV disease progression by assessing nutrient status using biochemical markers and dietary intake. In a case-control study nested in the MACS study, patients who progressed to AIDS had significantly lower levels of serum zinc compared with nonprogressors and HIV-uninfected participants (104). Inconsistent results were seen in two studies of the association between serum retinol levels and progression to AIDS; a significant association was reported from the study conducted in Rwanda (97) but not in the study conducted in the Unites States (6). Low baseline serum retinol levels, however, were observed in the study from Rwanda, while in the U.S. study, these levels were within the normal range. In the U.S. study, HIV-infected individuals in the highest quartile of serum vitamin E levels had a significant, 35% lower risk of progression to AIDS than those whose levels were in the lowest quartile (6). In the same study population, low serum vitamin B_{12} levels were associated with a twofold increase in risk for progression (105).

Observational studies have also examined the relationship between biochemical indicators of nutrient status and mortality. In a nested case-control study, HIV-infected individuals with vitamin A deficiency had an approximately fourfold higher risk of death than controls after adjusting for $CD4^+$ cell counts (78). In a longitudinal study among HIV-infected IDUs in Baltimore, low serum retinol levels were also associated with a fourfold increase in risk for mortality after adjusting for $CD4^+$ cell counts and other clinical markers (10). Higher likelihood of survival was noted among HIV-infected women with higher serum retinol levels in Rwanda (97). Selenium deficiency in HIV-1–infected individuals has been observed to increase risk of mortality among adults (106,107) and among HIV-1 vertically infected children (108). These biochemical studies are limited since serum levels of nutrients such as vitamin A, selenium, and zinc may be reduced in response to infection even in the absence of tissue depletion (104,109). Therefore, blood levels of these nutrients may act as a proxy for disease stage, although the possibility of a causal relationship to disease progression cannot be excluded.

Because individuals fighting infections may demonstrate low blood levels of certain nutrients despite adequate body stores, studying the effects of nutrients from dietary sources rather than from blood levels may be more informative. In the MACS study, there was a U-shaped relationship between dietary vitamin A intake and progression to AIDS, with poor outcomes in the lowest and highest quartiles of intake (110). In the MACS study (110) and in a study in and San Francisco (92), high levels of vitamin C, thiamin, or niacin intake were associated with a reduced risk of disease progression to AIDS. In addition, increased intake of iron, vitamin E, and riboflavin significantly reduced the hazard for AIDS (92). In the MACS study, the highest quartiles of dietary intake of vitamins B_1, B_2, B_6, and niacin were associated with increased survival time of up to 1.3 years (111). Although zinc intake is considered to be beneficial to immune function, results from epidemiologic studies of the risk for progression to AIDS have been inconsistent. Increased risk for developing AIDS was associated with higher zinc intake from dietary sources alone and from total intake (both food and supplements) among HIV-infected

MSM in the MACS study (110). Higher levels of total zinc intake were also associated with poor survival (111). However, in a study conducted in MSM in San Francisco, there was no association between higher dietary zinc intake and progression to AIDS (92).

Results from studies of the effects of dietary nutrient intake on HIV disease progression and mortality may be limited by confounding factors such as opportunistic infections, time since seroconversion, drug treatment, and existing nutritional deficiencies. Furthermore, dietary and biochemical studies are limited by the fact that reverse causality may partly explain the positive association between nutrient deficiencies and HIV disease progression: HIV infection may cause reduced nutrient intake, reduced nutrient absorption, and subsequently, low plasma nutrient levels.

Results from clinical trials among children have shown that supplementation of vitamin A is beneficial in populations deficient in the vitamin. In a trial conducted in South Africa, vitamin A supplementation in maternally infected children was shown to reduce HIV disease progression and diarrhea by about 50% (112). In a large trial in Tanzania, we reported an overall 50% reduction in mortality among both HIV-infected and -uninfected children, with the benefits greater among the HIV-positive children (113). In the same study, among children who were admitted with pneumonia, vitamin A supplementation significantly reduced diarrheal morbidity in those with HIV and in those with wasting disease (114). These results indicate the potential role of micronutrients in improving the health of children who are undernourished and have infections and of children born to HIV-infected women, particularly those who become vertically infected.

To date, there is no evidence of the effect of micronutrient supplementation on clinical outcomes among HIV-infected adults. In a randomized, placebo-controlled trial in Zambia, low serum levels of vitamin A and E (before supplementation with vitamins A, C, E, and selenium and zinc) were strong predictors of early mortality among patients with AIDS diarrhea-wasting syndrome (115). However, these supplements did not reduce duration of diarrhea or time to death during the first month of follow-up. Malabsorption during persistent diarrhea may have contributed to these results. Results from a vitamin A trial in South Africa among pregnant women showed no significant beneficial effects on HIV disease progression as measured by reports of either HIV- or pregnancy-related symptoms during the prenatal or postnatal period (116). In a small trial in San Diego, daily supplements of selenium to HIV-infected adults with AIDS led to improvement of HIV-related symptoms from pulmonary, gastrointestinal, skin, and neurologic disorders in 74% of patients (117).

NUTRITION, HIV TRANSMISSION, AND CHILD HEALTH

The potential role of micronutrients in reducing vertical transmission of HIV has been recently reviewed (118,119). Enhanced humoral and cellular immune function, slowed maternal disease progression, and enhanced integrity of placental, lower genital tract, and mammary duct epithelial linings following micronutrient supplementation have been described as possible mechanisms to reduce risk of vertical transmission.

The relationship between humoral and cellular mucosal immunity in the lower genital tract and vertical transmission of HIV has been described. Secretions in the lower genital tract have been shown to contain anti–HIV cytokines, antibodies, and other immunologic factors (120). Nutritional deficiencies may result in weak mucosal immunity, risk of increased viral load, risk of other genital infections, and impaired integrity of placental and genital epithelial linings. These conditions may facilitate in-utero and intrapartum transmission of HIV. The finding that vitamin A deficiency in rats was associated with reduced placental integrity (121) and impaired integrity of the genital epithelia (122,123) may explain its potential role in increased vertical transmission of HIV. Vitamin A deficiency may be associated with a higher risk of desquamation of the cervix, and possible injury and bleeding of the vaginal mucosa, exposing the fetus to HIV-infected blood and tissues during delivery. This potential mechanism of increasing risk of intrapartum HIV transmission is further supported by reports from a study in Kenya in which low plasma vitamin A was associated with a higher risk of HIV shedding in secretions of the lower genital tract (13,124).

Impaired mucosal barrier and immunity in mammary ducts may increase risk of HIV transmission to infants by the desquamation and shedding of HIV-infected epithelial cells or free-floating HIV virus into breast milk. Local infection and inflammation of breast tissue increases permeability of blood vessels, which in turn increases shedding of virus into breast milk. Infant infection may be facilitated by impaired gut mucosal barrier in the presence of mucosal breaches during diarrhea diseases, gut candidiasis, and in states of vitamin A deficiency that may impair mucosal immune response.

In a study conducted in Kenya, low plasma vitamin A levels were associated with a higher risk of viral shedding in breast milk among HIV-infected women during pregnancy (125). These results suggest that maternal vitamin A status before and after delivery is an important factor for breast milk transmission of HIV. However, because of the observational nature of this study, limitations reviewed earlier should be considered, as should the limitation presented by using serum vitamin A as a marker of vitamin A status. The effect of micronutrient intake on transmission of HIV-1 through breastfeeding is yet to be determined fully.

The relationship between micronutrient deficiencies and viral load in breast milk and subclinical mastitis (defined by high sodium/potassium ratio in breast milk) has been examined. Low serum levels of vitamin A and subclinical mastitis in women in Malawi (126) and South Africa (127) have been associated with high viral load in breast milk and an increased risk of HIV transmission through breast milk.

Longitudinal studies have examined the relationship between nutritional status and vertical transmission of HIV. In Malawi, higher serum retinol among HIV-infected pregnant women was associated with a reduced risk of vertical transmission (15). In Rwanda, low levels of serum vitamin A among HIV-infected women were associated with increased risk of infant death or perinatal HIV-transmission (128). Inconsistent results for serum vitamin A levels and vertical transmission were seen in studies conducted in the United States (129–131).

Intervention trials have examined the association between nutrient intake from supplements and the risk of vertical transmission of HIV. Prenatal vitamin A supplementation to HIV-infected pregnant women in Malawi had no effect on HIV transmission at 6 weeks or by 12 months compared to placebo (132). In a large trial in Tanzania, supplementation with both vitamin A and multivitamins in pregnant women did not significantly affect the risk of vertical transmission in utero or during the intrapartum and early breastfeeding periods (up to 6 weeks) (133). The effect of vitamin supplements on breast milk transmission of HIV and on clinical progression of HIV disease, however, has yet to be ascertained in this study, since women continued to take the supplements while breastfeeding. In South Africa, among HIV-infected women receiving supplements of preformed vitamin A and β-carotene or receiving placebo during the prenatal period, the risks of HIV infection in infants by 3 months of age were similar (134).

Improved birth outcomes among HIV-infected pregnant women have been described in Tanzania, where multivitamin supplementation significantly reduced fetal loss by 39%, low birth weight by 44%, severe preterm birth (<34 weeks of gestation) by 39%, and small size for gestation age at birth by 43%, compared to birth outcomes among women who received no multivitamins (14).

CONCLUSION

There is adequate evidence that vitamin A supplementation reduces morbidity from diarrheal diseases and all-cause mortality among HIV-infected children born to HIV-seropositive women. There is no conclusive data on the effect of other micronutrients on the health of children born to HIV-infected women, although cross-sectional studies suggest that there is a deficiency of nutrients such as vitamin E and β-carotene among these children. There is some evidence that micronutrient supplementation among adults may increase $CD4^+$ cell counts and reduce viral loads. However, data from randomized studies on the effect of micronutrients on clinical outcomes are limited.

Results from a large randomized trial in Tanzania suggest that supplementation of vitamin A and other vitamins during prenatal and postpartum periods are unlikely to have a beneficial effect on vertical intrauterine and intrapartum transmission. Results from randomized trials in Malawi and South Africa showed no effect of vitamin A on HIV transmission. The possibility that doses higher than those used in these trials may have beneficial effect on vertical transmission cannot be excluded. However, the doses used in the Tanzanian and South African studies were already several-fold greater than the RDA. In addition, the majority of women in the trials in Malawi, South Africa, and Tanzania started receiving supplements at their first prenatal visit, which took place, on average, at about 20 weeks of gestation. This may explain the lack of a beneficial effect on transmission since the supplements may have not been provided early enough to positively affect formation of the fetal immune system. Such a scenario has been shown in mice; zinc deficiency during early gestation resulted in immunodeficiency that persisted for three generations in spite of adequate zinc diets in the second and third generations (135). The effects of vitamin A and multivitamins on HIV transmission through breastfeeding has yet to be determined. The roles of other micronutrients such as selenium and zinc in vertical HIV transmission have not been examined.

The effects of multivitamins on adverse pregnancy outcomes were observed in the trial from Tanzania, where reductions in fetal loss, low birth weight, and prematurity were found among the infants of HIV-1–infected pregnant women. These beneficial effects may be largely mediated through improvements in immune function and hematologic status that are particular to HIV-infected women. Given these protective effects, micronutrient supplementation to HIV-infected pregnant women is recommended.

In areas where antiretroviral drugs are unavailable or unaffordable, supplementation with micronutrients may act as a low-cost adjunct intervention together with prevention and treatment of opportunistic infections. Low-cost and short-course antiretroviral drugs have been found to be effective in reducing vertical transmission of HIV in Uganda (136) and other parts of the world (137). These findings may necessitate the provision of these drugs to HIV-infected pregnant women in sub–Saharan Africa where resources are poor. However, the implementation of HIV voluntary counseling and testing services and the costs of sustaining the supply of antiretroviral drugs are major concerns in this region. Given the efficacy of these interventions, attention should be shifted toward examining the means of reducing transmission through breastfeeding. It is important to consider the role of nutritional supplements in maintaining child health and survival in settings where early weaning or formula feeding are considered.

REFERENCES

1. Scrimshaw NS, SanGiovanni JP. Synergism of nutrition, infection, and immunity: an overview. *Am J Clin Nutr*, 1997;7:464S–477S.
2. Serwadda D, Mugerwa RD, Sewankambo NK, et al. Slim disease: a new disease in Uganda and its association with HTLV-III infection. *Lancet*, 1985;2: 849–852.
3. Niyongabo T, Henzel D, Ndayishimyie JM, et al. Nutritional status of adult inpatients in Bujumbura, Burundi (impact of HIV infection). *Eur J Clin Nutr*, 1999;53:579–582.
4. Lucas SB, De Cock KM, Hounnou A, et al. Contribution of tuberculosis to slim disease in Africa. *Br Med J*, 1994;308:1531–1533.
5. Castetbon K, Kadio A, Bondurand A, et al. Nutritional status and dietary intakes in human immunodeficiency virus (HIV)-infected outpatients in Abidjan, Côte D'Ivoire, 1995. *Eur J Clin Nutr*, 1997;51:81–86.
6. Tang AM, Graham NMH, Semba RD, et al. Association between serum vitamin A and E levels and HIV-1 disease progression. *AIDS*, 1997;11: 613–620.
7. Skurnick JH, Bogden JD, Baker H, et al. Micronutrient profiles in HIV-1–infected heterosexual adults. *J Acquir Immune Defic Syndr Hum Retrovirol*, 1996;12:75–83.
8. Bogden JD, Baker H, Frank O, et al. Micronutrient status and human immunodeficiency virus infection. *Ann N Y Acad Sci*, 1990;587:189–195.
9. Ullrich R, Schneider T, Heise W, et al. Serum carotene deficiency in HIV-infected patients. Berlin Diarrhoea/Wasting Syndrome Study Group. *AIDS*, 1994;8:661–665.
10. Semba, RD, Graham NMH, Caiaffa WT, et al. Increased mortality associated with vitamin A deficiency during human immunodeficiency virus type 1 infection. *Arch Intern Med*, 1993;153:2149–2154.
11. Beach RS, Mantero-Atienza E, Shor-Posner G, et al. Specific micronutrient abnormalities in asymptomatic HIV-1 infection. *AIDS*, 1992;6: 701–708.
12. Semba RD, Farzadegan H, Vlahov D. Vitamin A levels and human immunodeficiency virus load in injection drug users. *Clin Diagn Lab Immunol*, 1997;4:93–95.
13. John GC, Nduati RW, Mbori-Ngacha D, et al. Genital shedding of human immunodeficiency virus type 1 DNA during pregnancy: association with immunosuppression, abnormal cervical or vaginal discharge, and severe vitamin A deficiency. *J Infect Dis*, 1997;175:57–62.
14. Fawzi WW, Msamanga GI, Spiegelman D, et al. Randomized trial of effects of vitamin supplements on pregnancy outcomes and T cell counts in HIV-1–infected women in Tanzania. *Lancet*, 1998;351:1477–1482.
15. Semba RD, Miotti PG, Chiphangwi JD, et al. Maternal vitamin A deficiency and mother-to-child transmission of HIV-1. *Lancet*, 1994;343:1593–1597.
16. Burkes RL, Cohen H, Krailo M, et al. Low serum cobalamin levels occur frequently in the acquired immune deficiency syndrome and related disorders. *Eur J Haematol*, 1987;38:141–147.
17. Paltiel O, Falutz J, Veilleux M, et al. Clinical correlates of subnormal vitamin B_{12} levels in patients infected with the human immunodeficiency virus. *Am J Hematol*, 1995;49:318–322.
18. Koch J, Neal EA, Schlott MJ, et al. Zinc levels and infections in hospitalized patients with HIV/AIDS. *Nutrition*, 1996;12:515–518.
19. Mantero-Atienza E, Sotomayor MG, Shor-Posner G, et al. Selenium status and immune function in asymptomatic HIV-1 seropositive men. *Nutr Res*, 1991;11:1237–1250.
20. Allard JP, Aghdassi E, Chau J, et al. Oxidative stress and plasma antioxidant micronutrients in humans with HIV infection. *Am J Clin Nutr*, 1998;67:143–147.
21. Pacht ER, Diaz P, Clanton T, et al. Serum vitamin E decreases in HIV-seropositive subjects over time. *J Lab Clin Med*, 1997;130:293–296.
22. Mastroiacovo P, Ajassa C, Berardelli G, et al. Antioxidant vitamins and immunodeficiency. *Int J Vitam Nutr Res*, 1996;66:141–145.
23. Look MP, Rockstroh JK, Rao GS, et al. Serum selenium, plasma glutathione (GSH) and erythrocyte glutathione peroxidase (GSH-Px)-levels in asymptomatic versus symptomatic human immunodeficiency virus-1 (HIV-1) infection. *Eur J Clin Nutr*, 1997;51:266–272.
24. Semba RD, Kumwenda N, Hoover DR, et al. Assessment of iron status using plasma transferrin receptor in pregnant women with and without human immunodeficiency virus infection in Malawi. *Eur J Clin Nutr*, 2000;54:872–877.
25. Antelman G, Msamanga GI, Spiegelman D, et al. Nutritional factors and infectious disease contribute to anemia among pregnant women with Human Immunodeficiency Virus in Tanzania. *J Nutr*, 2000;130:1950–1957.
26. Coodley GO, Coodley MK, Nelson HD, et al. Micronutrient concentrations in the HIV wasting syndrome. *AIDS*, 1993;7:1595–1600.
27. Smith J, Howells DW, Kendall B, et al. Folate deficiency and demyelination in AIDS. *Lancet*, 1987;2:215.
28. Falutz J, Tsoukas C, Gold P. Zinc as a cofactor in human immunodeficiency virus-induced immunosuppression. *JAMA*, 1998;259:2850–2851.
29. Keusch GT, Farthing MJG. Nutritional aspects of AIDS. *Annu Rev Nutr*, 1990;10:475–501.

30. Macallan DC, Noble C, Baldwin C, et al. Energy expenditure and wasting syndrome in human immunodeficiency virus infection. *New Engl J Med*, 1995;333:83–88.
31. Ziegler EE, Filer LJ. *Present Knowledge in Nutrition* 7th ed. Washington, DC: International Life Sciences Institute (ILSI); 1996.
32. Murray RK, Granner DK, Mayes PA, et al. *Harper's Biochemistry* 25th ed. Connecticut: Appleton & Lange; 2000.
33. Clark RH, Feleke G, Din M, et al. Nutritional treatment for acquired immunodeficiency virus-associated wasting using beta-hydroxy beta-methylbutyrate, glutamine, and arginine: a randomized, double-blind, placebo-controlled study. *JPEN*, 2000;24:133–139.
34. Watson RR, Prabhala RH, Plezia PM, et al. Effect of β-carotene on lymphocyte subpopulations in elderly humans: evidence for a dose-response relationship. *Am J Clin Nutr*, 1991;53:90–94.
35. Ross AC, Stephenson CB. Vitamin A and retinoids in antiviral responses. *FASEB J*, 1996;10:979–985.
36. Hussey G, Hughes J, Potgieter S, et al. Vitamin A status and supplementation and its effects on immunity in children with AIDS. In: Program and Abstracts of the XVII International Vitamin A Consultative Group Meeting; 1996; Guatemala City, Guatemala. Washington, DC: International Life Sciences Institute: pages 6, 81.
37. Fawzi WW, Chalmers TC, Herrera MG, et al. Vitamin A supplementation and child mortality: a meta-analysis. *JAMA*, 1993;269:898–903.
38. Wang Y, Huang DS, Lian B, et al. Nutritional status and immune response in mice with murine AIDS are normalized by vitamin E supplementation. *J Nutr*, 1994;124:2024–2032.
39. Meydani SN, Wu D, Santos MS, et al. Antioxidants and immune response in the aged: overview of present evidence. *Am J Clin Nutr*, 1995;62:1462S–1476S.
40. Meydani SN, Barklund PM, Liu S, et al. Vitamin E supplementation enhances cell-mediated immunity in healthy elderly subjects. *Am J Clin Nutr*, 1990;52:557–563.
41. Meydani SN, Meydani M, Blumberg JB, et al. Vitamin E supplementation enhances in vivo immune response in healthy elderly: A dose-response study. *JAMA*, 1997;277:1380–1386.
42. Bendich A. Antioxidant vitamins and immune responses. In: Chandra RK, Alan R, eds. *Nutrition and Immunology*. New York: Liss, Inc., 1988:125–147.
43. Hemila H. Vitamin C and infectious diseases. In: Pacler L, Fuchs J, eds. *Vitamin C in Health and Disease*. New York: Marcel Dekker, Inc., 1997.
44. Meydani SN, Ribaya-Mercado JD, Russell RM, et al. Vitamin B-6 deficiency impairs interleukin-2 production and lymphocyte proliferation in elderly adults. *Am J Clin Nutr*, 1991;53:1275–1280.
45. Baum MK, Mantero-Atienza E, Shor-Posner G, et al. Association of vitamin B-6 status with parameters of immune function in early HIV-1 infection. *J Acquir Immune Defic Syndr*, 1991;4:1122–1132.
46. Bendich A, Cohen M. B vitamins: effects on specific and non-specific immune responses. In: Chandra RK, Alan R, eds. *Nutrition and Immunology*. New York: Liss, Inc.; 1988:101–123.
47. Rotruck JT, Pope AL, Ganther HE, et al. Selenium: biochemical role as a component of glutathione peroxidase. *Science*, 1973;179:588–590.
48. Sappey C, Legrand-Poels S, Best-Belpomme M, et al. Stimulation of glutathione peroxidase activity decreases HIV type 1 activation after oxidative stress. *AIDS Res Hum Retroviruses*, 1994;10:1451–1461.
49. Chen C, Zhou J, Xu H, et al. Effect of selenium supplementation on mice infected with LP-BM5 MuLV, a murine AIDS model. *Biol Trace Elem Res*, 1997;59:187–193.
50. Hori K, Hatfield D, Maldarelli F, et al. Selenium supplementation suppresses tumor necrosis factor alpha-induced human immunodeficiency virus type 1 replication in vitro. *AIDS Res Hum Retroviruses*, 1997;13:1325–1332.
51. Peretz A, Neve J, Duchateau J, et al. Effects of selenium supplementation on immune parameters in gut failure patients on home parenteral nutrition. *Nutrition*, 1991;7:215–221.
52. Shankar AH, Prasad AS. Zinc and immune function: the biological basis of altered resistance to infection. *Am J Clin Nutr*, 1998;68:447S–463S.
53. Haraguchi Y, Sakurai H, Hussain S, et al. Inhibition of HIV-1 infection by zinc group metal compounds. *Antiviral Res*, 1999;43:132–133.
54. Baum MK, Shor-Posner G, Campa A. Zinc status in human immunodeficiency virus infection. *J Nutr*, 2000;130:1421S–1423S.
55. Black RE. Therapeutic and preventive effects of zinc on serious childhood infectious diseases in developing countries. *Am J Clin Nutr*, 1998;68:476S–479S.
56. Semba RD, Tang AM. Micronutrients and the pathogenesis of human immunodeficiency virus infection. *Br J Nutr*, 1999;81:181–189.
57. Grunfeld C, Pang M, Schimizu L, et al. Resting energy expenditure, caloric intake, and short-term weight change in human immunodeficiency virus infection and the acquired immunodeficiency syndrome. *Am J Clin Nutr*, 1992;55:455–460.
58. Gillin JS, Shike M, Alock N, et al. Malabsorption and mucosal abnormalities of the small intestine in the Acquired Immunodeficiency Syndrome. *Ann Intern Med*, 1985;102:619–622.
59. Melchior JC, Salmon D, Rigaud D, et al. Resting energy expenditure is increased in stable, malnourished HIV-infected patients. *Am J Clin Nutr*, 1991;53:437–441.

60. Dannhauser A, van Staden AM, van der Ryst E, et al. Nutritional status of HIV-1 seropositive patients in Free State Province of South Africa: Anthropometric and dietary profile. *Eur J Clin Nutr*, 1999;53:165–173.
61. Arpadi SM, Cuff PA, Kotler DP, et al. Growth velocity, fat-free mass and energy intake are inversely related to viral load in HIV-infected children. *J Nutr*, 2000;130:2498–2502.
62. Baum M, Cassetti L, Bonvehi P, et al. Inadequate dietary intake and altered nutrition status in early HIV-1 infection. *Nutrition*, 1994;10:16–20.
63. Macallan DC, Noble C, Baldwin C, et al. Prospective analysis of patterns of weight change in stage IV human immunodeficiency virus infection. *Am J Clin Nutr*, 1993;58:417–424.
64. Melchior JC, Raguin G, Boulier A, et al. Resting energy expenditure in human immunodeficiency virus-infected patients: Comparison between patients with and without secondary infections. *Am J Clin Nutr*, 1993;57:614–619.
65. Johann-Liang R, O'Neill L, Cervia J, et al. Energy balance, viral burden, insulin-like growth factor-1, interleukin-6 and growth impairment in children infected with human immunodeficiency virus. *AIDS*, 2000;14:683–690.
66. Grunfeld C, Kotler DP, Hamadeh R, et al. Hypertriglyceridemia in the acquired immunodeficiency syndrome. *Am J Med*, 1998;86:27–31.
67. Coodley GO, Loveless MO, Merrill TM. The HIV wasting syndrome: A review. *J Acquir Immune Defic Syndr*, 1992;7:681–694.
68. Pernet P, Vittecoq D, Kodjo A, et al. Intestinal absorption and permeability in human immunodeficiency virus-infected patients. *Scand J Gastroenterol*, 1999;34:29–34.
69. Koch J, Garcia-Shelton YL, Neal EA, et al. Steatorrhea: a common manifestation in patients with HIV/AIDS. *Nutrition*, 1996;12:507–510.
70. Harriman GR, Smith PD, Horne MK, et al. Vitamin B12 malabsorption in patients with acquired immunodeficiency syndrome. *Arch Intern Med*, 1989;149:2039–2041.
71. Ehrenpreis ED, Carlson SJ, Boorstein HL, et al. Malabsorption and deficiency of vitamin B12 in HIV-infected patients with chronic diarrhea. *Dig Dis Sci*, 1994;39:2159–2162.
72. Kabanda A, Vandercam B, Bernad A, et al. Low molecular weight proteinuria in human immunodeficiency virus-infected patients. *Am J Kidney Dis*, 1996;27:803–808.
73. Jolly PE, Moon TD, Mitra AK, et al. Vitamin A depletion in hospital and clinic patients with acquired immunodeficiency syndrome—a preliminary report. *Nutr Res*, 1997;17:1427–1441.
74. Baum MK, Shor-Posner G, Zhang G, et al. HIV-1 infection in women is associated with severe nutritional deficiencies. *J Acquir Immune Defic Syndr Hum Retrovirol*, 1997;16:272–278.
75. Pollack H, Glasberg H, Lee E, et al. Impaired early growth of infants perinatally infected with human immunodeficiency virus: Correlation with viral load. *J Pediatr*, 1997;130:915–922.
76. Kotler DP, Tierney AR, Wang J, et al. Magnitude of body-cell-mass depletion and the timing of death from wasting in AIDS. *Am J Clin Nutr*, 1989;50: 444–447.
77. Wheeler DA, Gilbert CL, Launer CA, et al. Weight loss as a predictor of survival and disease progression in HIV infection. Terry Beirn Community Programs for Clinical Research on AIDS. *J Acquir Immune Defic Syndr Hum Retrovirol*, 1998;18: 80–85.
78. Semba RD, Caiaffa WT, Graham NMH, et al. Vitamin A deficiency and wasting as predictors of mortality in human immunodeficiency virus-infected injection drug users. *J Infect Dis*, 1995;171:1196–1202.
79. Feldman JG, Burns DN, Gange SJ, et al. Serum albumin as a predictor of survival in HIV-infected women in the Women's Interagency HIV study. *AIDS*, 2000;14:863–870.
80. Melchior JC, Niyongabo T, Henzel D, et al. Malnutrition and wasting, immunodeficiency, and chronic inflammation as independent predictors of survival in HIV-infected patients. *Nutrition*, 1999;15:865–869.
81. Shearer WT, Easley KA, Goldfarb J, et al. Evaluation of immune survival factors in pediatric HIV-1 infection. *Ann N Y Acad Sci*, 2000;918: 298–312.
82. Gibert CL, Wheeler DA, Collins G, et al. Randomized, controlled trial of caloric supplements in HIV infection. Terry Beirn Community Programs for Clinical Research on AIDS. *J Acquir Immune Defic Syndr*, 1999;22:253–259.
83. Prabhala RH, Garewal HS, Hicks MJ, et al. The effects of 13-cis-retinoic acid and beta-carotene on cellular immunity on humans. *Cancer*, 1997;67: 1556–1560.
84. Semba RD, Muhilal, Ward BJ, Griffin DE, et al. Abnormal T-cell proportions in vitamin A-deficient children. *Lancet*, 1993;341:5–8.
85. Bendich A, Shapiro SS. Effects of beta-carotene and canthaxanthin on the immune responses of the rat. *J Nutr*, 1996;116:2254–2262.
86. Semba RD, Muhilal, Scott AL, et al. Depressed immune response to tetanus in children with vitamin A deficiency. *J Nutr*, 1992;122:101–107.
87. Coutsoudis A, Kiepiela P, Coovadia H, et al. Vitamin A supplementation enhances specific IgG antibody levels and total lymphocyte numbers while improving morbidity in measles. *Pediatr Infect Dis J*, 1992;11:203–209.

88. Pace GW, Leaf CD. The role of oxidative stress in HIV disease. *Free Radic Biol Med*, 1995;19: 523–528.
89. Phuapradit W, Chaturachinda K, Taneepanichskul S, et al. Serum vitamin A and beta-carotene levels in pregnant women infected with human immunodeficiency virus-1. *Obstet Gynecol*, 1996;87:564–567.
90. Bogden JD, Kemp FW, Han S, et al. Status of selected nutrients and progression of human immunodeficiency virus type 1 infection. *Am J Clin Nutr*, 2000;72:809–815.
91. Baum MK, Shor-Posner G, Lu Y, et al. Micronutrients and HIV-1 disease progression. *AIDS*, 1995;9:1051–1056.
92. Abrams B, Duncan D, Hertz-Picciotto I. A prospective study of dietary intake and acquired immune deficiency syndrome in HIV-seropositive homosexual men. *J Acquir Immune Defic Syndr*, 1993;6:949–958.
93. Coodley GO, Nelson HD, Loveless MO, et al. Beta-carotene in HIV infection. *J Acquir Immune Defic Syndr*, 1993;6:272–276.
94. Coodley GO, Coodley MK, Lusk R, et al. Beta-carotene in HIV infection: an extended evaluation. *AIDS*, 1996;10:967–973.
95. Semba RD, Lyles CM, Margolick JB, et al. Vitamin A supplementation and human immunodeficiency virus load in injection drug users. *J Infect Dis*, 1998;177:611–616.
96. Look MP, Rockstroh JK, Rao GS, et al. Sodium selenite and N-acetylcysteine in antiretroviral-naive HIV-1–infected patients: a randomized, controlled pilot study. *Eur J Clin Invest*, 1998;28: 389–397.
97. Camp WL, Allen S, Alvarez JO, et al. Serum retinol and HIV-1 RNA viral load in rapid and slow progressors. *J Acquir Immune Defic Syndr Hum Retrovirol*, 1998;18:401–406.
98. Coutsoudis A, Moodley D, Pillay K, et al. Effects of vitamin A supplementation on viral load in HIV-1–infected pregnant women. *J Acquir Immune Defic Syndr Hum Retrovirol*, 1997;15:86–87.
99. Humphrey JH, Quinn T, Fine D, et al. Short-term effects of large-dose vitamin A supplementation on viral load and immune response in HIV-infected women. *J Acquir Immune Defic Syndr Hum Retrovirol*, 1999;20:44–51.
100. Delmas-Beauvieux MC, Peuchant E, Couchrouron A, et al. The enzymatic antioxidant system in blood and glutathione status in human immunodeficiency virus (HIV)-infected patients: effects of supplementation with selenium or β-carotene. *Am J Clin Nutr*, 1996;64:101–107.
101. Allard JP, Aghdassi E, Chau J, et al. Effects of vitamin E and C supplementation on oxidative stress and viral load in HIV-infected subjects. *AIDS*, 1998;12:1653–1659.
102. Niki E, Noguchi N, Tsuchihashi H, et al. Interaction among vitamin C, vitamin E, and beta-carotene. *Am J Clin Nutr*, 1995;62:1322S–1326S.
103. Semba RD. Vitamin A and HIV infection. *Proc Nutr Soc*, 1997;56:459–569.
104. Graham NM, Sorenson D, Odaka N, et al. Relationship of serum copper and zinc levels to HIV seropositivity and progression to AIDS. *J Acquir Immune Defic Syndr*, 1991;4:976–980.
105. Tang AM, Graham NMH, Chandra RK, et al. Low serum vitamin B-12 concentrations are associated with faster human immunodeficiency virus type 1 (HIV-1) disease progression. *J Nutr*, 1997;127: 345–351.
106. Allavena C, Dousset B, May T, et al. Relationship of trace element, immunological markers, and HIV-1 infection progression. *Biol Trace Elem Res*, 1995;47:133–138.
107. Baum MK, Shor-Posner G, Lai S, et al. High risk of HIV-related mortality is associated with selenium deficiency. *J Acquir Immune Defic Syndr Hum Retrovirol*, 1997;15:370–374.
108. Campa A, Shor-Posner G, Indacochea F, et al. Mortality risk in selenium-deficient HIV-positive children. *J Acquir Immune Defic Syndr Hum Retrovirol*, 1999;20:508–513.
109. Filteau SM, Morris SS, Abbott RA, et al. Influence of morbidity on serum retinol of children in a community-based study in northern Ghana. *Am J Clin Nutr*, 1993;58:192–197.
110. Tang AM, Graham NMH, Kirby AJ, et al. Dietary micronutrient intake and risk of progression to Acquired Immunodeficiency Syndrome (AIDS) in Human Immunodeficiency Virus type 1 (HIV-1)-infected homosexual men. *Am J Epidemiol*, 1993;138:937–951.
111. Tang AM, Graham NMH, Saah AJ. Effects of micronutient intake on survival in human immunodeficiency virus type 1 infection. *Am J Epidemiol*, 1996;143:1244–1256.
112. Coutsoudis A, Bobat RA, Coovadia HM, et al. The effects of vitamin A supplementation on the morbidity of children born to HIV-infected women. *Am J Pub Health*, 1995;85:1076–1081.
113. Fawzi WW, Mbise RL, Hertzmark E, et al. A randomized trial of vitamin A supplements in relation to mortality among human immunodeficiency virus-infected and uninfected children in Tanzania. *Pediatr Infect Dis J*, 1999;18:127–133.
114. Fawzi WW, Mbise R, Spiegelman D, et al. Vitamin A supplements and diarrheal and respiratory tract infections among children in Dar es Salaam, Tanzania. *J Pediatr*, 2000;137:660–667.
115. Kelly P, Musonda R, Kafwembe E, et al. Micronutrient supplementation in the AIDS diarrhoea wasting syndrome in Zambia: A randomized controlled trial. *AIDS*, 1999;13:495–500.

116. Kennedy CM, Coutsoudis A, Kuhn L, et al. Randomized controlled trial assessing the effect of vitamin A supplementation on maternal morbidity during pregnancy and postpartum among HIV-infected women. *J Acquir Immune Defic Syndr*, 2000;24:37–44.
117. Olmsted L, Schrauzer GN, Flores-Arce M, et al. Selenium supplementation of symptomatic human immunodeficiency virus infected patients. *Biol Trace Elem Res*, 1989;20:59–65.
118. Fawzi WW, Hunter DJ. Vitamins in HIV disease progression and vertical transmission. *Epidemiology*, 1998;9:457–466.
119. Fawzi, W. Nutritional factors and vertical transmission of HIV-1. Epidemiology and potential mechanisms. *Ann N Y Acad Sci*, 2000;918:99–114
120. Anderson, DJ, Politch JA, Tucker LD, et al. Quantitation of mediators of inflammation and immunity in genital tract secretion and their relevance to HIV type 1 transmission. *AIDS Res Hum Retroviruses*, 1998;14:43S–49S.
121. Noback CR, Takahashi YI. Micromorphology of the placenta of rats reared on marginal vitamin-A-deficient diet. *Acta Anat (Basel)*, 1978;102:195–202.
122. Wolbach SB, Howe PR. Tissue changes following deprivation of fat-soluble A vitamin. *J Exp Med*, 1925;42:753–777.
123. Kuhn RH. Effect of locally applied vitamin A and estrogen on the rat vagina. *Am J Anat*, 1954;95: 309–328.
124. Mostad SB, Overbaugh J, De Vange DM, et al. Hormonal contraception, vitamin A deficiency, and other risk factors for shedding of HIV-1 infected cells from the cervix and vagina. *Lancet*, 1997;350:922–927.
125. Nduati RW, John GC, Richardson BA, et al. Human immunodeficiency virus type 1-infected cells in breast milk: association with immunosuppression and vitamin A deficiency. *J Infect Dis*, 1995;172:1461–1468.
126. Semba RD, Kumwenda N, Hoover DR, et al. Human immunodeficiency virus load in breast milk, mastitis, and mother-to-child transmission of human immunodeficiency virus type 1. *J Infect Dis*, 1999;180:93–98.
127. Willumsen JF, Filteau SM, Coutsoudis A, et al. Subclinical mastitis as a risk factor for mother-infant HIV transmission. *Adv Exp Med Biol*, 2000;478:211–223.
128. Graham N, Bulterys M, Chao A, et al. Effect of maternal vitamin A deficiency on infant mortality and perinatal HIV transmission. Paper presented at the National Conference on Human Retroviruses and Related Infection; December 12–16, 1993; Baltimore, Maryland, USA.
129. Greenberg BL, Semba RD, Vink PE, et al. Vitamin A deficiency and maternal-infant transmissions of HIV in two metropolitan areas in the United States. *AIDS*, 1997;11:325–332.
130. Burns DN, FitzGerald G, Semba R, et al. Vitamin A deficiency and other nutritional indices during pregnancy in human immunodeficiency virus infection: prevalence, clinical correlates, and outcome. Women and Infants Transmission Study Group. *Clin Infect Dis*, 1999;29:328–334.
131. Burger H, Kovacs A, Weister B, et al. Maternal serum vitamin A levels are not associated with mother-to-child transmission of HIV-1 in the United States. *J Acquir Immune Defic Syndr Hum Retrovirol*, 1997;14:321–326.
132. Semba R. Nutritional interventions: vitamin A and breastfeeding. Paper presented at the III International symposium on Global Strategies to Prevent Perinatal HIV Transmission; November 9–10, 1998; Valencia, Spain.
133. Fawzi WW, Msamanga G, Hunter D, et al. Randomized trial of vitamin supplements in relation to vertical transmission of HIV-1 in Tanzania. *J Acquir Immune Defic Syndr*, 2000;23:246–254.
134. Coutsoudis A, Pillay K, Spooner E, et al. Randomized trial testing the effect of vitamin A supplementation on pregnancy outcomes and early mother-to-child HIV-1 transmission in Durban, South Africa. South African Vitamin A Study Group. *AIDS*, 1999;13:1517–1524.
135. Beach RS, Gershwin ME, Hurley LS. Gestational zinc deprivation in mice: persistence of immunodeficiency for three generations. *Science*, 1982;218: 469–471.
136. Guay LA, Musoke P, Fleming T, et al. Intrapartum and neonatal single-dose nevirapine compared with zidovudine for prevention of mother-to-child transmission of HIV-1 in Kampala, Uganda: HIVNET 012 randomised trial. *Lancet*, 1999;354:795–802.
137. Mofenson LM. Short course zidovudine for prevention of perinatal infection. *Lancet*, 1999;353: 766–767.

27

Access to HIV and AIDS Care

*Kirthana Ramanathan, †Daniel Tarantola, and *Richard G. Marlink

*Harvard AIDS Institute, Boston, Massachusetts, USA.
†Director General's Office, World Health Organization, Geneva, Switzerland.

In sub–Saharan African countries access to health care continues to be affected by financial and health infrastructure constraints. Since 1978, when 134 countries declared their commitment to achieving "health care for all by the year 2000" (1), the best approach to improving the capacity and distribution of health infrastructure, and hence access to care, has been a subject of continued debate. Over the last 2 decades, the onset and escalation of the HIV epidemic in sub–Saharan Africa has highlighted a critical need to address deficiencies in health systems. In particular, with the prospect of more affordable generic or patented combination anti-retroviral therapies in sub–Saharan African countries, there is renewed interest in improving the health infrastructure required for HIV and AIDS prevention and care.

Integrated community-based health care systems are of particular importance for HIV and AIDS care and prevention because of the complex medical, social, and psychologic needs of persons and communities affected by the epidemic. Especially without treatment, persons living with HIV face the prospect of progressive physical decline through wasting, multiple infections, malignancies, and pain (2). They may face stigmatization and risk ostracism from their families and communities. Their illness may lead to unemployment, deepening poverty (3), and the prospect of leaving orphaned children. With advancing disease, their increasing needs for medical care, public assistance, and spiritual guidance require a comprehensive range of interventions.

In most sub–Saharan African countries, however, the current capacity of health infrastructure is limited. There is inadequate availability of outpatient and inpatient facilities (4), a lack of trained health workers (5), and incomplete drug distribution systems (6), especially in rural areas. In addition, the AIDS epidemic has taken a significant toll on health personnel; HIV-related illness, overwork and burnout, and the need to stay home from work to care for family members with HIV and AIDS have resulted in a loss of trained staff (7).

Due to the limitations of the formal health infrastructure in many countries, a number of alternative models of care have evolved over the course of the epidemic. These models have aimed to improve access to care by bridging the gap between the services available and the health care needs of persons living with HIV or AIDS. Nongovernmental organizations (NGOs), religious groups, families, and communities have played a prominent role in the organization and operation of such alternative models.

In this chapter, we discuss the barriers affecting access to HIV and AIDS care in sub–Saharan Africa. We describe the capacity and distribution of existing health care systems, and their effect on current levels of access to HIV and AIDS care. The extent to which infrastructure must be improved to provide comprehensive HIV and AIDS care, including antiretroviral therapy, is discussed. International and national attempts to improve access to HIV and AIDS care are reviewed.

FACTORS AFFECTING ACCESS TO HIV AND AIDS CARE

Access to comprehensive health care for people in sub–Saharan African countries with HIV, AIDS, or other health problems, is determined by a complexity of geopolitical, social, and economic factors.

Individual utilization of existing health services for HIV or AIDS may be affected by social barriers such as stigma, discrimination, and the inequitable status of women in some societies (8). Members of marginalized populations that are especially vulnerable to HIV infection, such as sex workers or migrant workers, may also be affected by societal and institutional barriers to health care (9). Factors such as high rates of illiteracy may affect treatment-seeking behaviors (5,10). Lastly, deepening poverty, often a result of HIV-related illness, can affect the ability to pay for health care (11,12).

The capacity and distribution of public health infrastructure affects the system's ability to provide the wide range of health services required for HIV and AIDS care at the population level. While in most sub–Saharan African countries the private sector, including traditional practice, plays an important role in health care provision, the role of the state has been prominent in the delivery of modern pharmacopea to the vast majority who cannot afford private medical care (13). In the early 1990s, of all medical facilities in Cameroon only 34% were private; in Senegal this figure was 30%, in Botswana, 20%, and in Ethiopia and Burkina Faso, only a few facilities were private (14). Private medical care mostly serves people in urban areas in African countries, and due to high costs, is available mostly to the elite or to workers employed by private companies (13). Hence, for the vast majority, access to care is determined by the level of public investment in health services. This investment is in turn affected by political and economic realities, such as burgeoning debt (13), other governmental priorities, and declines in social spending associated with structural adjustment programs (15–17). In addition, geopolitical factors such as conflict, civil unrest, and intermittent natural disasters, may result in disruptions to existing health services. Provision of health services to populations living in rural areas may be further obstructed by the costs associated with transport over long distances and harsh terrain (18).

In most sub–Saharan African countries per capita public health expenditure is on average USD$20[a] annually. Government health expenditure in Burundi, Ethiopia, and the Democratic Republic of Congo was less than 10 international dollars per person annually in 1997 (19). These figures are in enormous contrast to the average per capita public expenditure of 1,500 international dollars in the United States, Japan, and western European countries. The disparity in public health spending between these high-income countries and sub–Saharan African countries with high HIV prevalence is shown in Figure 1.

Inadequate health expenditure, compounded by meager investment in education and unattractive salaries for health personnel, has contributed to low levels of staffing by medically qualified personnel in health facilities. While high-income countries report on average 200 doctors and 500 to 1,000 nurses per 100,000 people in the population, sub–Saharan African countries average only 16 doctors and 75 nurses per 100,000 people (Figure 2). Poor public expenditure on health has also resulted in lower proportions of the population with physical access to care. For

[a]Unless otherwise specified, all dollar amounts are in U.S. dollars.

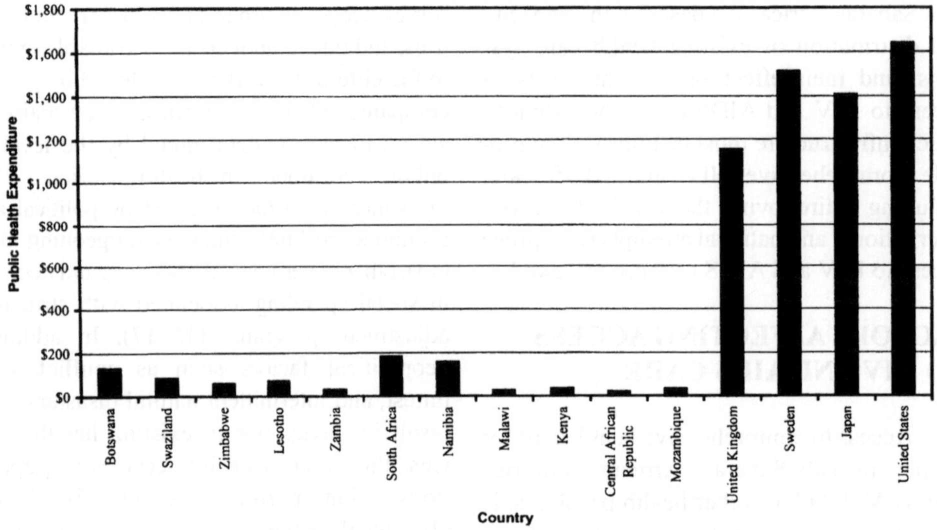

FIGURE 1. Per capita public expenditure on health in international dollars (1997) for sub–Saharan African and high-income countries (19).

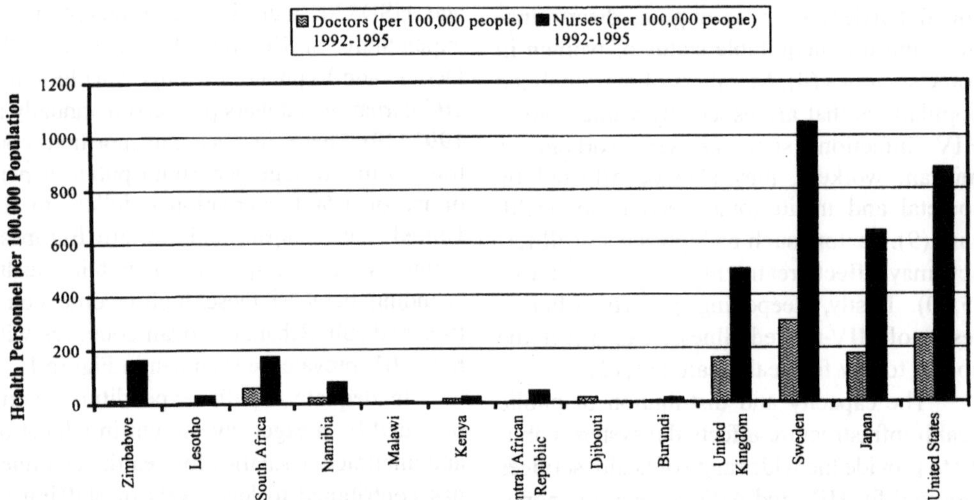

FIGURE 2. Availability of health personnel in sub–Saharan African and high-income countries (1992–1995) (5). Data also available at: http://www3.who.int/whosis/health_personnel/health_personnel.cfm?path=whosis,health_personnel&language=english. Accessed: February 7, 2002.

example, from 1990 to 1995, the percentage of the population with access to health services in sub–Saharan Africa ranged from 40% to 50%, with lower levels in rural areas (20), as shown in Figure 3.

Public health systems that were developed in sub–Saharan African countries during colonization were mostly curative in orientation, urban-based, and dependent on imported drugs. These biases have largely continued post-independence, with large proportions of limited health budgets (40% to 60%) spent on a few urban hospitals in capital cities (13). For example, in Zimbabwe in

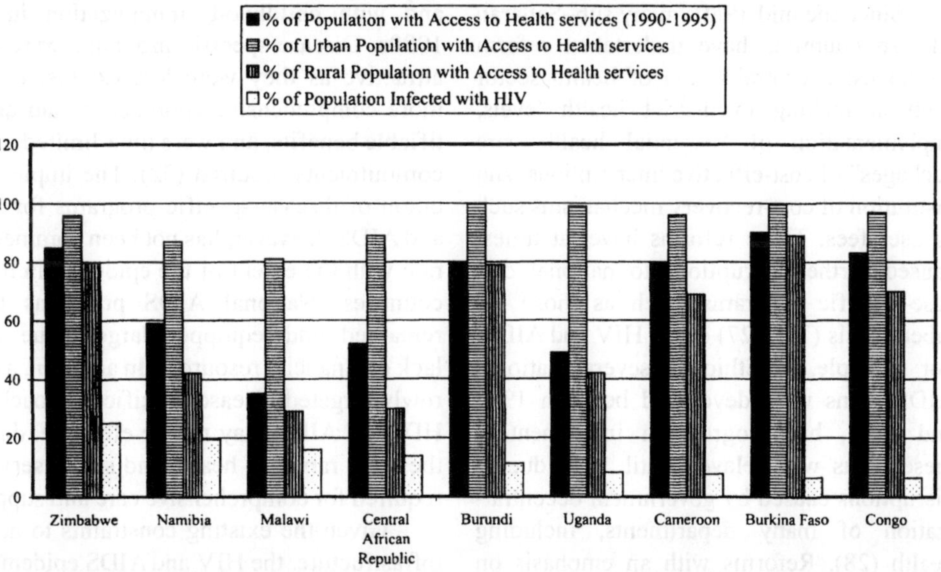

FIGURE 3. Percent of population with access to health services in urban and rural areas in selected sub–Saharan African countries (1990–1995) (20, 24).

1980, 44% of public funds for health services went to urban hospitals that served 15% of the population, whereas 24% of funds were allocated to the rural areas occupied by 77% of the population (21).

Over the last 2 decades, however, increased priority has been given to the development of community-based integrated systems of care. For example, in Senegal, health huts and health posts have been constructed in semi-urban and rural areas, and training has been provided for large numbers of community health workers (22). Similarly, in Somalia in the early 1980s, the Ministry of Health began primary health programs to reach the 90% of the rural and nomadic population that lacked access to national health services (23). Despite these attempts, rural and urban disparities in infrastructure persist (Figure 3). These disparities are a significant weakness in African public health systems, given that up to 70% of the population in African countries may live in rural areas. Addressing the disparities in the availability of health services is especially important to curbing the AIDS epidemic, as rates of HIV infection in the semi-urban and rural areas of some countries, such as Senegal (24) and Botswana (25), are increasing. The lack of health services such as prevention counseling or sexually transmitted disease (STD) management in these areas may be a contributing factor to increasing rates of HIV infection.

Access to and appropriate utilization of secondary and tertiary levels of care, especially in urban or semi-urban areas, is affected by ineffective referral systems. For example, an assessment of the referral system north of Harare, Zimbabwe, through retrospective review of 500 patients who had malaria or acute lower respiratory infection (ALRI), showed that all levels of hospital care had similar mixes of patients; 54% of malaria patients and 58% of ALRI patients with mild illness presented directly to the highest levels of care. Proximity to care was the greatest determinant of utilization of a particular level of care (21). Similarly, in a study of 148 HIV-infected patients attending a teaching and referral hospital clinic in Cape Town, South Africa, 69% of visits to the referral hospital were considered suitable for primary care by the practicing clinicians (26).

Since the mid 1980s many sub–Saharan African countries have undertaken reform initiatives: decentralization of health sector decision making to district health levels, implementation of "essential health care packages" of cost-effective interventions, and institution of cost-recovery mechanisms such as user fees. These reforms have, at times, caused further disruptions to national disease-specific programs, such as those for tuberculosis (TB) (27) or for HIV and AIDS. For example, in Ethiopia, several national AIDS plans were developed between 1987 and 1991, but progress in implementing these plans was delayed until 1998 due to disruptions caused by government decentralization of many departments, including health (28). Reforms with an emphasis on user financing may have resulted in a growing exclusion of the poor from available services. The institution of user fees has been shown to reduce health service utilization rates in a sustained fashion especially among the poor and children; user fees were associated with a 32% decrease in use of government health facilities in Swaziland, a 50% decrease in use of primary health care units in Mozambique, and a 64% drop in outpatient attendance in Zambia, especially in the poorest neighborhoods (29). Such exclusion of the most vulnerable in society is of particular significance for HIV and AIDS care, since these individuals are often at greater risk for HIV infection (9).

Donor-driven, vertically structured, and disease-specific programs implemented in sub–Saharan African countries over the last few decades have contributed little to the development of effective and integrated health systems (30). These programs have been organized as distinct entities, with strong centralized control, particularly due to the weaknesses and poor coverage of existing national health infrastructure in many countries (31). Disease control programs were attractive to donors because of the initial successes achieved, for example, with malaria control or smallpox in the 1960s and 1970s, and with childhood immunization in the 1980s. Disease-specific programs were also attractive as they were less expensive than more comprehensive approaches, had quantifiable benefits, and were time-limited in the commitments required (32). The implementation of disease-specific programs for HIV and AIDS, however, has not been commensurate with the extent of the epidemic in many countries. National AIDS programs have remained underequipped largely due to a lack of financial resources. In addition, a narrowly targeted disease-specific approach for HIV and AIDS may not be effective, due to the wide range of health and social services required for comprehensive care and support.

Given the existing constraints to health infrastructure, the HIV and AIDS epidemic is placing a tremendous burden on the health sector. With the rise in HIV-related illnesses such as TB, pneumonia, and diarrheal disease, there is an increase in demand for health services and medications (33). At present, most care is sought in secondary and tertiary institutions (34), with 40% to 70% of hospital beds occupied by patients with HIV and AIDS in some sub–Saharan countries (7). Poorly functioning and understaffed primary health systems, lack of essential medicines in peripheral facilities, ineffective referral systems, fear of recognition at local facilities (34), or initial presentation with advanced HIV-related illness, contribute to care being pursued at these higher levels where care is costly and difficult to sustain. In South Africa, for example, estimates suggest that up to 75% of the South African health budget could be utilized for HIV-related illness by 2005 if treatment continues to be provided mainly at referral hospitals (26).

On the supply side, existing health systems are being further weakened by the loss of health personnel, due to the direct impact of HIV- and AIDS-related illness and death among health workers (7). Rising rates of TB among health care workers have been observed and attributed to coinfection with HIV. For example, in one study of health workers in a South African district hospital, a 5-fold rise in annualized incidence rates of TB was found in the years 1993–1996 compared with 1991–1992 (35). In addition, many health personnel face burnout as they struggle to meet demands beyond their capacity (33,36). The cost to the health sector is heightened by absenteeism, reduced productivity, additional staffing needs, and an increased necessity to train new personnel (7). There are also many that cannot report to work as they are the care providers for family members with HIV or AIDS (37,38).

In summary, the limited capacity and distribution of public health systems, poor availability and affordability of the private sector services, inadequately funded programs for HIV and AIDS, and the direct or indirect impact of HIV on the health work force, significantly limit the provision of comprehensive HIV and AIDS care (39). These limitations are compounded by a number of socioeconomic barriers that prevent individuals with HIV infection from utilizing health services and accessing the treatments that could augment the duration and quality of their lives. Against the background of insufficient prevention efforts and increasing rates of HIV infection, these barriers to care translate into the severely reduced life expectancy and increased mortality currently being seen in sub–Saharan Africa.

EXISTING SYSTEMS OF CARE

A number of systems of care have evolved over the course of the epidemic to address the gap between the needs of communities affected by HIV and AIDS and the available formal health care services. These systems of care have largely been driven by the mobilization of persons living with HIV or AIDS, family members, community groups, religious groups, and a multitude of indigenous and international NGOs.

Many of these organizations became engaged in the response to HIV and AIDS through prevention programs, focusing their efforts on information, education, and behavior change, as part of the global emphasis on halting progression of the epidemic. With continued HIV transmission and increasing burden of illness however, there was growing realization that exclusively preventive activities were insufficient. The result was the proliferation of systems of care mainly based in patients' homes, which provided basic medical care, welfare support, and supportive counseling.

Nongovernmental organizations have been especially important in understanding and advocating for community needs. For example, in Uganda, The AIDS Support Organisation (TASO) has been intensively involved in prevention and care activities since 1987 (40). The Society for Women and AIDS in Kenya (SWAK) is an organization with a membership of 6,000 women from all eight provinces in Kenya, that has led the mobilization of women at a grass-roots level, through information about HIV and AIDS prevention and care, networking, and advocacy activities (41). Though NGOs have played an active role in responding to the epidemic, they too suffer from human, financial, and technical resource constraints. Networks of NGOs have therefore evolved. For example, the Network for AIDS Research in East and Southern Africa (NARESA) was formed by a group of AIDS researchers in 1989 to promote research in the region, share information, and develop appropriate control strategies (42). The African Council of AIDS Services Organization (AFRICASO) linked NGOs active in both prevention and care. The International HIV/AIDS Alliance aims to enhance the capacity and self-reliance of country-based partner NGOs. The Red Cross and Red Crescent movement has benefited from support and guidance from its Federation. Multiple faith-based groups have extended prevention and care services to the communities in which they were rooted and beyond. Many of these networks continue to focus their work on HIV prevention activities, but there has been a gradual shift toward focusing their advocacy and devoting more attention and resources to care issues.

Estimates suggest that traditional health care systems are used by between 60% and 80% of individuals in developing countries (43). Cultural practices, proximity, and the deterring effects of some health sector reforms (such as user financing) are contributing factors to the choice of these systems of care. For example, in Uganda, estimates suggest that one biomedical doctor exists per 20,000 people, whereas one traditional health practitioner (THP) exists for every 200 to 400 people (43).

The high level of use of traditional health care has prompted attempts to improve collaboration between the traditional and biomedical sectors. In Uganda, South Africa, Zambia, and Mozambique, collaboration is being promoted especially for HIV prevention (44). In South Africa, 1,510 THPs reached 850,000 clients with AIDS/STD prevention messages, and in Mozambique, 81% of THPs who were educated about HIV transmission promoted condom use to their STD patients (43).

Comprehensive HIV and AIDS care is yet to fully benefit from the assistance of traditional healers, although Uganda can be cited as a country in which increasing efforts are being made in this direction. In Uganda in 1992, Traditional and Modern Health Practitioners Together Against AIDS (THETA) was established to research traditional medicines against HIV-related illness, and to promote collaboration between traditional and biomedical sectors. The traditional practitioners involved were subsequently trained in HIV prevention, counseling, and clinical diagnostic skills. An evaluation of the program in 1998 showed that 60% to 80% of trained healers provided condoms, counseling, and AIDS community education, and 97% referred patients to the biomedical sector (45).

Faith-based organizations have made important contributions to care services. For example, the Catholic Diocese in Ndola, Zambia runs a home-based care program for chronic illnesses including HIV, AIDS, and TB. Social support and nursing care is provided by church volunteers and community health workers, with close links to local health facilities (34). In Zambia, the Salvation Army has been a forerunner in the provision of HIV/AIDS care (46). In Tanzania, a comparison of health facilities suggested that church-based facilities had higher drug and commodity availability, better delivery services, and better working conditions than government hospitals and health centers (47).

The corporate sector has to date demonstrated a delayed recognition of the threat posed by HIV/AIDS to their productivity, operations, and profits (48, 49). Companies that have acknowledged the epidemic have implemented HIV prevention programs such as AIDS education for employees and their families, condom distribution and STD treatment, and have extended benefits to employees affected by AIDS (50). However, corporate contributions to the provision of HIV and AIDS care are inadequate in general, and many companies use avoidance strategies to reduce costs associated with HIV care. These strategies include reducing the benefits available to infected workers, or avoiding the hire of new employees who are infected or thought to be in high-risk groups (51).

HIV and AIDS care projects, at present, tend to be isolated and small-scale. Greater integration of community-based programs and national health systems would help ensure appropriate treatment and referral protocols, avoid duplication of efforts, and improve the availability of drugs and commodities. There is some evidence of increasing collaboration between these isolated or distinct systems of care. The National AIDS Control Program (NACP) in Zimbabwe collaborated with the country's essential drugs action program to develop cost-effective STD treatment protocols. In Zambia, counseling courses and training materials were developed through cooperation between the

Ministry of Health, Zambia's NACP, and church-based organizations (52,53). Further collaboration among NGOs and community groups, the traditional sector, religious institutions, the corporate sector, and national AIDS programs, is a necessary step toward expanding access to more comprehensive HIV and AIDS care.

COMPREHENSIVE MODELS OF CARE

Comprehensive care must satisfy the diverse and changing needs of persons living with HIV or AIDS. As HIV infection progresses, medical needs change, and the level of infrastructure required to provide medical care (for example for severe opportunistic infections) may increase. In addition, there may be increasing financial burdens, spiritual needs, and other requirements for supportive counseling, as well as the need to care for caregivers (34). These services are also required for the optimal delivery of antiretroviral therapy to ensure adherence, to prevent the development of drug resistance, and to provide patient care in the event of antiretroviral treatment failure.

In order to meet these diverse patient needs, a comprehensive system of care may include the ten components described in Table 1. These 10 areas of care were evaluated and deemed critical for an effective HIV and AIDS care system through consultations with local AIDS care experts, HIV researchers, AIDS care practitioners, government and nongovernment public health experts, and persons living with HIV or AIDS in five diverse regions worldwide for the Enhancing Care Initiative[a].

The development of such an ideal and comprehensive system of HIV and AIDS care will depend on the adequacy of existing health infrastructure in a specific region. National priorities and resources will also determine the best way to scale up HIV and AIDS care.

TABLE 1. Ten Components of a Health System for the Provision of HIV and AIDS Care[a]

- Voluntary HIV counseling and testing programs (VCT)
- Basic medical services, including services for HIV/STD prevention
- Laboratory and diagnostic services
- HIV and AIDS clinical case management, including opportunistic infection prophylaxis and treatment programs
- New therapies including combination antiretroviral therapy
- Community-based care initiatives, including traditional and complementary therapies
- Social services
- Care education, training, and information dissemination programs
- Supportive and palliative care
- Care for the caregiver

[a]Adapted from the Enhancing Care Initiative, Harvard AIDS Institute, Boston, Massachusetts, USA. Visit http://www.eci.harvard.edu for more information.

One suggested approach to developing a comprehensive care system in resource-constrained settings, is to divide care and prevention interventions into three levels, according to the health infrastructure required for their provision (Figure 4). This model suggests that even with basic or minimal health infrastructure, such as simple outpatient facilities, populations could access voluntary HIV counseling and testing (VCT), psychosocial support, and palliative care. They also could access prevention information and education, and STD management services. With an intermediate level of health infrastructure, such as primary hospitals and basic diagnostic services, treatment and prophylaxis for opportunistic infections, home-based care, and antiretroviral drugs for the prevention of mother-to-child transmission and postexposure prophylaxis for health workers could be provided. An advanced level of infrastructure would allow safe and effective use of highly active antiretroviral therapy (HAART), advanced care for certain HIV-related diseases, and specialists' advice for referrals and training.

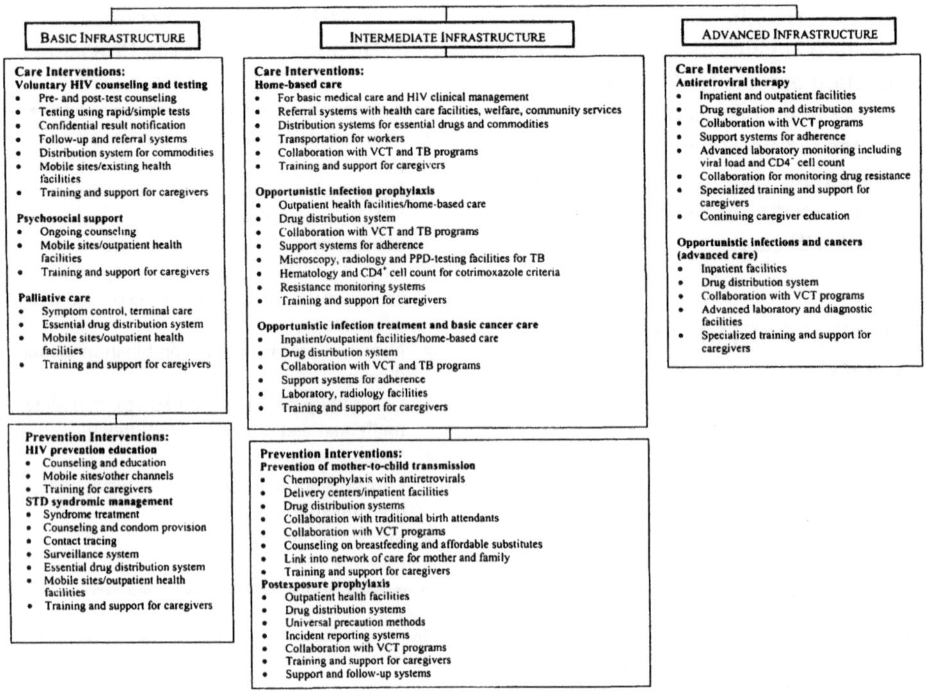

FIGURE 4. An example of a comprehensive approach to HIV and AIDS care.

LACK OF ACCESS TO SELECTED COMPONENTS OF COMPREHENSIVE HIV AND AIDS CARE

Unfortunately, despite the increased response of formal health systems to HIV and AIDS and the mobilization of many organizations at the community level, access to even basic levels of HIV and AIDS care remains poor. An indication of the current levels of access to specific HIV and AIDS care services is difficult to assess at a country level. Most national health surveys, such as the Demographic and Health Survey (54), provide some indication of the state of HIV prevention—levels of knowledge regarding HIV prevention, or access to HIV prevention methods.

By describing access to general health services and reviewing the coverage and quality of selected HIV and AIDS programs, an understanding of the current state of access to HIV and AIDS care in sub–Saharan African countries can be gained. In addition, an overview of the technical and structural resources required for the provision of comprehensive HIV and AIDS care (Figure 4), is presented to highlight the extent to which infrastructure must be improved in order to enhance access to care.

Voluntary HIV Counseling and Testing

Voluntary HIV counseling and testing is vital to the identification of individuals living with HIV to facilitate their entry into a care system. Voluntary counseling and testing is also important for HIV prevention efforts because it influences risk behaviors.

Access to VCT services in sub–Saharan African communities is affected by difficulties in achieving adequate coverage and quality of testing services, especially in rural areas (7). The use of mobile test clinics may improve availability of testing services for rural populations, but, may delay HIV test results due to the need to transport specimens to laboratories for HIV serology. This may create difficulties in continuity of care, obstructing or delaying result notification, follow-up counseling, and linkage with care and prevention services (55).

The use of rapid HIV testing systems has been shown to improve both coverage and quality of follow-up. For example, in a rural South African hospital, rapid on-site testing was found to dramatically reduce the waiting period for test results, and hence increased rates of follow-up counseling (56). When used in confirmatory sequences, rapid HIV tests have achieved comparable sensitivities and specificities to traditional HIV ELISA assays (57). Rapid HIV tests are feasible for use in rural areas because they require no formal laboratory facilities, may not require refrigeration, and can be performed by staff with little formal laboratory training, suggesting applicability in rural African settings.

Stigma and discrimination associated with HIV testing and the disclosure of HIV-positive status constrain the use of existing HIV testing services. Women in particular, have been found to face violence and the loss of food, shelter, and relationships upon disclosure of their HIV status (58). In addition, lack of access to treatment interventions represents an important barrier preventing many from seeking HIV testing. Those who are faced with no prospect of enhanced care, such as opportunistic infection prophylaxis or antiretroviral therapy, lack incentives to undergo HIV testing (59).

Uganda is an example of a country that has achieved some success in providing access to quality VCT services. In the mid 1980s, in response to demands for HIV testing after national awareness campaigns, many organizations collaborated with the Ugandan national AIDS program to open VCT services in Kampala and surrounding districts. In 1992 operations began in peri-urban and rural areas. Mobile counselors and phlebotomists traveled to the sites weekly or twice a month, to transport samples to laboratory facilities in Kampala. They returned to sites 2 to 4 weeks later to give test results. There were problems, however, including high costs of transporting samples, complex routing of blood samples, and the consequent delays in follow-up and notification. Many clients were not available on the day of follow-up or could not be traced (55).

These types of difficulties demonstrated the need for a decentralized approach that would allow VCT to be performed locally and patients to be notified promptly. As a result, VCT services were expanded through integration with existing hospitals and health centers at the district level, training for district personnel, and the initiation of a pilot program for the use of rapid HIV test kits. Trials in 1995 and 1996 showed that the same-day services made possible by the use of rapid HIV test kits were desired by clients, preferred by staff, and feasible to implement, even at rural sites. By 1998, 35 VCT sites were operating at hospitals and health centers and more than 5,000 people had received VCT (55,60). Widespread access to voluntary HIV testing through the use of rapid tests, with pre- and post-test counseling, therefore, appears to be a feasible strategy with great potential for improving access to this component of HIV care.

Palliative Care and Essential Drugs

Palliative care, including symptom control, psychosocial support, and terminal care is important in all stages of HIV-related illness, but especially with advancing disease (61).

At present a large proportion of the population in sub–Saharan African countries lack access to basic palliative care services. The most significant barriers include a lack of access to essential drugs for pain and palliation, as well as a scarcity of trained human resources for patient care (5). The World Health Organization has estimated that less than 50% of the sub–Saharan African population have access to essential drugs, including basic palliative drugs (6). The shortage of drugs is due not only to a lack of financial resources, but also to inefficient drug supply and distribution systems in the public sector, unregulated procurement and dispensation in the private sector, and waste due to overuse by some providers. The shortage results in poor availability of low-cost drugs in public health facilities and high prices for drugs in the private sector, affecting access to essential drugs especially for the poor (62).

In 1984 the World Health Organization launched its Essential Drugs Program to regulate drugs in the private sector and provide safe, effective, and low-cost drugs through the public sector (63). Many sub–Saharan countries subsequently developed national drug policies and adopted lists of essential drugs that would meet principle country needs. Ongoing management problems and insufficient financial and manpower resources continue to limit drug availability, however, especially at the peripheral levels of the health system (62).

In an attempt to improve health services and drug availability, especially in rural areas, programs that promote cost recovery through community financing, such as the Bamako Initiative, have been implemented in several sub–Saharan African countries. The Bamako initiative was sponsored by African Ministers of Health, the WHO, and UNICEF at a meeting in 1987 and was implemented in several countries, including Burundi, Gambia, Kenya, Senegal, and Uganda over the last decade (64). Most schemes were structured to allow health services in rural communities to be financed through the sale of essential drugs, with financial resources managed by community committees. In some countries, however, the costs recovered were often not enough to cover the costs of running the health facilities. Management capacity was inadequate, and there was an incentive to increase drug sales inappropriately. Furthermore, drugs for the rural poor, although at lower cost than those sold in the private sector, remained out of financial reach for many (64,65). Drug supply and distribution, therefore, remains an important area for improving access to even basic levels of HIV and AIDS care in many countries.

Home-Based Care

The delivery of organized basic medical and psychologic support for patients in their homes may have several advantages for patients and their families. These advantages may include reduced hospital and transport costs and reduced isolation from family and friends. For health services, advantages may include reduction in the frequency and duration of hospital admissions, improved referral mechanisms, and better access to information about socioeconomic conditions at the patient's home (66,67). In addition, home-based care programs offer an opportunity to provide AIDS education for family members and to help reduce stigma among families and communities (68,69).

While organized home care has many benefits, at present, in sub–Saharan African countries, coverage is often very low due to inadequate financial resources and inadequate support for caregivers. As caseloads escalate, outreach workers may find it difficult to meet client needs due to increased traveling times and costs, which may result in reduced frequency and duration of visits and poor coverage of services (70). For the family, caring for the patient at home may mean a heavy workload. For example, in a study in Zimbabwe, it was found that caregivers spent 2.5 to 3.5 hours a day on routine patient care (70). Women often carry much of the burden of care, in addition to other family responsibilities (37,38). Due to adverse socioeconomic factors patients may also be nursed in overcrowded and impoverished conditions (71). Furthermore, families and communities may be reluctant to provide care due to stigma and negative attitudes (72,73).

Infrastructure requirements for optimal home-based care include referral systems linking the home with clinic and hospital facilities and social services, and transportation for home-based caregivers based in clinics or hospitals (Figure 4). To be sustainable and effective, models of home care must be in accordance with the capacity of the family and community to provide home-based care, and developed with support from formal medical services (74).

Examples of selected home-based care programs illustrate some of the constraints to achieving quality and coverage of services. At the Church of Scotland Hospital in KwaZulu-Natal, South Africa, a home-based care program relies on community health volunteers who reside close to patients' homes, to provide basic medical care and access to social support services. Volunteers receive referral support from the hospital. However, financial constraints make it difficult to access drugs for simple infections and palliative care. There are also difficulties in retention and sustainability due to the lack of incentives for volunteers. There are two similar programs in the same province of South Africa, but widespread services are not available at present (75).

In Zimbabwe, multiple home-based care schemes have evolved, with many using clinic and hospital staff, in collaboration with NGOs. Well-developed hospital–home outreach programs include those based in mission hospitals in rural areas, with NGOs and local authorities involved predominantly in urban areas. The escalation of the AIDS epidemic has resulted in increasing referrals to the services, and it has been difficult to achieve an appropriate level of coverage (67).

In Uganda, NGOs and community-based organizations have been intensively involved in home-based care operations. For example, TASO has eight centers in various parts of Uganda and provides comprehensive home care services using trained home care teams (76). There are also mobile programs operated by several mission hospitals such as Kitovu Mission Hospital in Masaka, Nsambya Hospital in Kampala, and the Jinja Diocese. At present though, the patients requiring care outnumber the services available, especially in rural areas (40).

In most other sub–Saharan African countries, the levels of home-based care or outreach systems described in these examples, are not available or functional at present.

Opportunistic Illness Treatment and Prophylaxis

Opportunistic infections, particularly TB (2), are the leading causes of AIDS-related mortality and morbidity in sub–Saharan African countries, a situation that makes access to treatment and prophylaxis for opportunistic infections an important concern.

Most opportunistic infections are treatable with prompt recognition and appropriate management in community and peripheral health facilities. Treatment may occasionally require admission to secondary or tertiary facilities. Constraints to the safe and effective treatment of opportunistic infections include poor availability of essential drugs and commodities, lack of skills among care providers at peripheral health facilities, and inadequate laboratory access for diagnosis and monitoring, in addition to the limited availability of health facilities to serve the populations in need.

Safe and effective treatment of opportunistic infections requires rational selection and use of the drugs that are affordable, sustainable financing systems, and reliable supply and delivery systems. Early treatment and prevention of opportunistic infections is enhanced by VCT programs, home-based care for ongoing therapy, adherence support systems, and training and support for caregivers. These requirements and enhancing factors are summarized in Figure 4. Some opportunistic illnesses such as cytomegalovirus infection, lymphomas, and advanced Kaposi's sarcoma require advanced health infrastructure and specialized care that may be available only in tertiary referral facilities.

While HAART remains the most effective strategy for reducing morbidity and mortality related to opportunistic infections, antibiotic prophylaxis has emerged as an important preventive measure. In sub–Saharan African countries, cotrimoxazole prophylaxis can prevent multiple infections. In two randomized controlled trials in Côte d'Ivoire, cotrimoxazole prophylaxis, compared with placebo, resulted in fewer hospitalizations and fewer cases of enteritis, pneumonia, isosporiasis, nontyphoidal salmonella and septicemia, and in one study there was a decrease in mortality (77,78).

At present, cotrimoxazole is widely used for bacterial infections in developing countries. It is listed as an essential drug, and it is inexpensive. Based on a review of evidence by a WHO/UNAIDS consultation in March 2000, it was recommended that cotrimoxazole prophylaxis be offered to HIV-positive adults (including pregnant women after the third trimester), children who are symptomatic and those who are asymptomatic with a low $CD4^+$ T-cell count, and to infants born to HIV-infected mothers. Although concerns were raised about resistance to this antibiotic, the relationship between widespread cotrimoxazole prophylaxis and the development of drug resistance is not known at present (79). According to the WHO/UNAIDS recommendations, the system required for widespread administration of cotrimoxazole prophylaxis includes VCT services, $CD4^+$ T-cell count facilities, and a system for monitoring antimicrobial resistance. These requirements, therefore, limit access to cotrimoxazole prophylaxis in most countries at present.

In most sub–Saharan African countries, treatment for TB is available through national TB control programs. Poor collaboration between HIV testing programs and TB programs, however, may limit access to TB treatment and prophylaxis for those infected with HIV. Poor collaboration may also prevent those with TB from obtaining appropriate HIV testing, counseling, and care (80).

The Côte d'Ivoire National TB program is an example of successful integration of TB and HIV programs. This program implemented a free VCT program for patients with newly diagnosed TB in two TB centers in Abidjan, and later in six district sites. Patients with TB were provided with HIV counseling and offered free testing during initial presentation. During the scheduled two-month TB follow-up visit, patients were given HIV test results and post-test HIV counseling. Of the 19,500 patients who were offered HIV testing, 91.8% consented and 43.2% were HIV-seropositive. Those who were HIV-seropositive were offered ongoing psychosocial support, and TB center staff received training and drug supplies from the Ministry of Health to provide HIV-related illness symptom relief and treatment of opportunistic infections other than TB (81).

Currently, there are a number of uncertainties regarding the value of universal TB prophylaxis for HIV-positive individuals in settings with high incidence of TB. In an analysis of four trials from Haiti, Kenya, Uganda, and the United States, preventive therapy was found to reduce risk of TB by 43%, with a 68% reduction in risk in purified protein derivative (PPD)-positive individuals, but only an 18% reduction in PPD-negative individuals (82). The data is conclusive regarding benefit in PPD-positive individuals. However, in PPD-negative individuals the appropriate role of TB prophylaxis in TB endemic countries is not well established. On the one hand, prophylaxis for all HIV-positive people may be appropriate because PPD tests lack specificity due to confounding by previous vaccination or anergy in advanced HIV. Alternatively, PPD tests help to identify those who may benefit the most from TB prophylaxis. WHO guidelines recommend prophylaxis for PPD-positive individuals without active TB. Where PPD testing is not feasible, prophylaxis can be considered for all HIV-infected individuals living in populations with TB prevalence rates of at least 30%, health workers, household contacts of

TB patients, and other selected high-risk groups (83).

In all cases, active TB must be clinically excluded. Therefore, the main constraint to widespread TB prophylaxis is the need for VCT, followed by sputum microscopy and chest radiographs. Botswana, however, is an example of a country with this required infrastructure that is proceeding with a national program of isoniazid prophylaxis in collaboration with the national TB program. The program will not determine eligibility by PPD-testing, due to the lack of specificity of the test, and due to the high incidence of TB in the population (84).

Important areas for further research include whether to initiate TB prophylaxis in early or late HIV disease, the appropriate duration of prophylaxis, and the long-term effects on drug resistance (80). Given these uncertainties, infrastructure requirements, and costs involved, prophylactic therapy for TB in HIV-infected patients is not widely available in most sub–Saharan countries at present.

Antiretroviral Therapy

The present global situation in terms of access to antiretrovirals is one of immense inequity, in which most of the population affected by HIV or AIDS remain without access to HAART. Among the factors preventing widespread access to antiretroviral therapy are inadequate health infrastructure and the high cost of antiretroviral drugs, despite the recent reductions in prices of both generic and patented products. Mobilizing resources to build infrastructure for antiretroviral therapy delivery, as well as defining better ways to operationalize treatment in resource-scarce settings, are necessary to improve access to antiretroviral therapy. While the costs of drugs and health infrastructure for antiretroviral delivery may be high, the benefits of this therapy—costs saved due to illnesses averted, economic benefits due to productivity gains, and improvements to quality and length of life—must be factored into the economic equation, and require further evaluation.

Amongst the key infrastructure requirements for the provision of HAART, laboratory facilities for measuring viral load and $CD4^+$ T-cell counts, and facilities for monitoring drug resistance are significant contraints in many sub–Saharan African countries. Systems to regulate drug procurement, distribution, and dispensation are also essential aspects of antiretroviral provision. The potential for drug resistance to develop as a result of suboptimal treatment or nonadherence justifies the need for appropriate viral load monitoring, support systems for patients on treatment, and drug resistance monitoring. Due to the rapidly evolving field of antiretroviral treatment, the complexity of drug regimens, and the threat of adverse drug interactions and reactions, thorough training of clinicians and staff must be provided, along with a system for updating guidelines for clinical and laboratory practice. Requirements for the institution of antiretroviral therapy are summarized in Figure 4.

Given these infrastructure requirements, antiretrovirals, while present in many of the poorest countries, are accessible only to a minority. Individuals who can afford these drugs may access them from private pharmacies or unregulated sources, facing risks that include ineffective therapy and the development of drug resistance. Government-initiated pilot programs for antiretroviral therapy are currently being planned or conducted in several sub–Saharan countries, including Botswana, Côte d'Ivoire, Gabon, Nigeria, Rwanda, Senegal, and Uganda. These countries have achieved drug price reductions through negotiations with pharmaceutical companies (85,86).

The antiretroviral pilot program conducted in Senegal represents an example of successful preparation for antiretroviral therapy. In response to the epidemic, in 1998, the government of Senegal initiated and supported a small pilot program of antiretroviral therapy, to assess the feasibility of treatment in the country. Due to the high costs of therapy, only 70 patients could be included. Negotiations with pharmaceutical companies and a grant from the French National AIDS Research Association, made it possible for patients to receive free viral load and $CD4^+$ T-cell quantification; antiretroviral drugs were purchased at reduced prices. A circuit for the supply and distribution of drugs was successfully organized. Interim analysis in May 1999 demonstrated good clinical, virologic, and immunologic efficacy of antiretroviral therapy, and 93.9% of patients were compliant with at least 80% of doses (87). The pilot program demonstrated the feasibility and effectiveness of antiretroviral therapy in Senegal. Due to strong political commitment, and negotiations for reduced prices, initiatives are currently underway to expand access to the program.

In Côte d'Ivoire, an antiretroviral program was commenced in August 1998, when UNAIDS and the Côte d'Ivoire Ministry of Health launched the HIV Drug Access Initiative. Through negotiations with pharmaceutical companies, antiretrovirals were obtained at reduced prices, and six treatment centers were operationalized in Abidjan to provide antiretroviral therapy. Patients would pay according to a scale reflecting their income, with subsidies for those eligible supported by a $1 million Ivorian government fund. By March 2000, 1,874 antiretroviral-naïve patients had been screened for eligibility. However, 40% did not return for the results of their screening; their reasons for not returning are currently under evaluation. Of the 1,080 patients who returned, only 39% (422 patients) received antiretroviral therapy, mainly due to a pending decision regarding subsidies, or ineligibility due to abnormal serum chemistry or to virologic and immunologic parameters. Either HAART or a dual NRTI regimen (in cases of financial constraint) was prescribed. After a 20-month follow-up, 71% of those who received therapy initially were still active on therapy, 19% were lost to follow-up, and 7% had died. There was good virologic and immunologic efficacy in the HAART group (50% had undetectable viral loads at 120 days), but lower efficacy in the dual therapy group (20% had undetectable viral load at 120 days), with few severe adverse events (88).

In Uganda, antiretrovirals became available in 1992 through a clinical trial undertaken at the Joint Clinical Research Center (JCRC) in Kampala to determine the lowest effective dose of zidovudine (89). In 1996, HAART regimens became available in the private sector, but due to high costs only a few patients who could afford to pay had access to therapy (personal communication, Cissy Kityo-Mutuluuza, May 2001).

In August 1998, the UNAIDS drug access program was operationalized in Uganda, and several treatment centers were equipped to deliver antiretrovirals. Through this program approximately 905 patients accessed antiretroviral treatment (out of an estimated 1.5 million persons with HIV infection). Most patients recruited had an advanced stage of disease. Both dual NRTI regimens and HAART were used, with those on HAART demonstrating greater and more sustained responses to therapy. The greatest barrier to treatment was affordability of drugs, with currency devaluations resulting in increased costs to patients, and treatment interruptions at times. The other costs associated with monitoring and treatment were supported by outside agencies in this program. If these costs were to be transferred to the patient over the longer term however, the financial burden would likely impact access to therapy (90).

Recent drug price reductions, due to competition from generic manufacturers have further lowered drug costs, and may assist more patients in accessing treatment in Uganda. To date, in the country, approximately 3,000 individuals have accessed antiretrovirals through the JCRC since 1996 or through the UNAIDS access initiative treatment centers and private practitioners. In a recent meeting about HIV and AIDS care issues in Africa held in Kampala, Uganda, April 18–20, 2001, His Excellency the President of Uganda pledged that the government would provide funding to subsidize antiretrovirals (personal communication, Cissy Kityo-Mutuluuza, May 2001). This commitment may further expand access to HAART therapy in Uganda.

In Botswana, it is estimated that 2,000 HIV-infected individuals have access to HAART through the private sector. Most antiretroviral regimens are available to these individuals at reduced prices (compared to high-income countries). The therapy is financed through out-of-pocket payments, Medical AID schemes, or private insurance schemes, at a cost of 1,100 pula per month (or approximately $200). This amount however, is not affordable for many, and the choice of drug regimen is often limited to those drugs that can be bought within the total amount covered by the schemes (personal communication, Drs. Diana Dickenson, Kgosidialwa Mompati, April 2001).

In recent months, the government of Botswana has embarced on the national provision of HAART through the public health sector. The government has achieved reductions in antiretroviral drug prices through negotiations with multinational pharmaceutical companies, and commenced programs for strengthening the human and technical infrastructure required for antiretroviral therapy delivery. Activities include the creation of a national antiretroviral implementation team and assessments of the infrastructure requirements for the delivery of antiretrovirals in several locations throughout the country.

In summary, current pilot programs have achieved promising results in improving virologic, immunologic, and clinical markers of HIV disease. The programs demonstrate success in operationalizing antiretroviral treatment in sub–Saharan African countries. They highlight the need for further evaluation and research to enable the delivery of this therapy at lower costs and at lower levels of infrastructure. Inadequate availability of resources to finance widespread antiretroviral treatment is a critical barrier that limits the expansion of these pilot projects to a national scale, as discussed in the next section.

ATTEMPTS TO IMPROVE ACCESS TO HIV AND AIDS CARE

International attempts to improve access to HIV care have suffered from inadequate global financial commitments. For much of the last 2 decades, while African countries have struggled under the dual burdens of debt and AIDS, international relief efforts have been highly disappointing. According to donor country reports of official development assistance, total international aid (excluding loans) to sub–Saharan African countries for HIV and AIDS programs averaged $61 million annually, from 1990 to 1998 (91). This level of international aid is highly incommensurate with the estimated $9 billion now estimated to be required annually for global HIV and AIDS care and prevention efforts (92).

In the declaration of commitment to HIV and AIDS adopted by the United Nations General Assembly at the Special Session on HIV and AIDS in June 2001, industrialized countries were urged to provide 0.7% of their gross national product in overall official development assistance to developing countries (93). As depicted in Figure 5, countries such as Denmark, Norway, and Sweden met or exceeded this target amount in 1999, but many other nations, including the United States, spend well below this target (94). Other initiatives specifically focused on HIV and AIDS, such as the LIFE initiative of the U.S. government, have provided approximately $200 million annually to countries in sub–Saharan Africa and India for HIV, TB, and malaria (95).

Insufficient resources helped lead to the launch of a global fund by Secretary-General

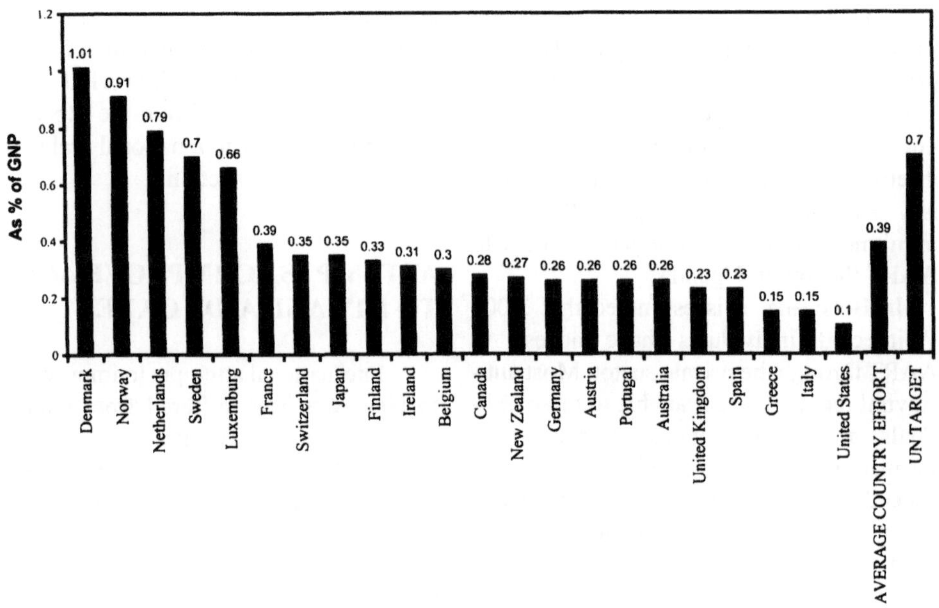

FIGURE 5. Net official development assistance as a percentage of GNP in 1999 (94).

Kofi Annan to address the HIV and AIDS epidemic, as well as the burdens of TB and malaria in developing countries. To date contributions to the fund by public and private pledges amount to $1.7 billion (96). The operational structure of the fund is yet to be fully established and the ways in which this initiative will help meet global resource needs for these diseases presently remains to be seen.

International organizations have limited resources for HIV and AIDS activities. The total operations of UNAIDS were within a budget of $140 million for 1998–1999, and the request for 2000–2001 from cosponsoring UN agencies represents no increase over this level. In addition, only 41% of this total will be spent on activities related to Africa (97). Lending for HIV and AIDS programs globally by the World Bank from 1986 to 1998 amounted to $595.4 million. Average annual lending was $117 million from 1992 to 1995, and despite the escalation of the HIV epidemic, World Bank lending from 1995 to 1998, declined to an average of $30 million annually (97).

In addition, these relatively scant international resources donated toward initiatives for HIV and AIDS have largely focused on prevention interventions. During the initial decade of the AIDS epidemic, prior to the advent of antiretroviral treatments, difficult choices were made to commit scarce international and national resources to HIV prevention programs, while those already infected faced a rapidly fatal course of disease (7). Even after the advent of highly effective combination antiretroviral therapies in the mid-1990s, very little has changed. Support for specific HIV and AIDS care interventions has remained at extremely low levels. For example, USAID global priorities for AIDS programs remain HIV prevention education, condom promotion, and STD management (95). These priorities, while critical to controlling and reducing HIV transmission, do not focus on HIV or AIDS care.

In recent years, the private sector has provided increased resources to address the epidemic, and resources have also been allocated to HIV and AIDS care. For example, recent grants to sub-Saharan African programs from the Bill and Melinda Gates foundation total over $150 million (98) for initiatives that include strengthening various prevention programs, improving AIDS orphan care, palliative care, and comprehensive HIV/AIDS care and prevention. Other foundations are responding to a lesser degree.

National attempts to improve access to HIV and AIDS care have also suffered from financial constraints, and resources that have been allocated for HIV and AIDS have predominantly funded prevention activities. In a survey of National AIDS program managers from 1990 to 1991, it was found that an average of 70.2% of resources were allocated to prevention, 43.4% to blood safety, and 11.4% to HIV and AIDS care, in Côte d'Ivoire, Cameroon, Tanzania, Ethiopia, and Nigeria (99). This trend appears to have continued in some more recent national AIDS program budgets. For example, in Tanzania, from 1998 to 2002, a total of $88,250 (including VCT) was budgeted for HIV and AIDS care activities. However, $4,232,875 has been budgeted for HIV prevention programs (100). In Uganda, from 2000 to 2006, a total of $11,934,538 has been budgeted for care, and $16,741,536 has been budgeted for prevention activities (101). It should be noted that conclusions drawn from direct comparisons between prevention and care expenditures through national AIDS programs may be limited because spending on HIV and AIDS care is largely through general health expenditures, rather than through national HIV and AIDS programs. Nevertheless, the data suggest that spending on HIV and AIDS care through both general health expenditure (Figure 1) and national AIDS programs has been inadequate to meet population needs.

International agencies, donors and governments are now beginning to realize the importance of HIV and AIDS care, not only to relieve human suffering but also to complement prevention efforts. With the prospect of more affordable antiretroviral drugs, and pilot programs in sub–Saharan African countries demonstrating the feasibility of administering HAART, there has been increasing attention to improving the health infrastructure required for providing optimal HIV and AIDS care. However, given the state of health systems and insufficient resources, a significant and rapid escalation of current international and national efforts is required.

CONCLUSION

In sub–Saharan African countries at present, access to even elementary components of a comprehensive care system is inadequate for most of the population infected with HIV. This situation is due to a complexity of contemporary and historic, economic, social and geographic barriers, which continue to limit the provision and utilization of health services. Current levels of access to health care in sub–Saharan Africa are inadequate to stem the social, demographic and economic crisis due to HIV and AIDS. Review of the international response and financial resource commitments to date confirm that a significant and rapid escalation of these efforts is required. The HIV and AIDS epidemic has highlighted the need to invest in the capacity and distribution of national health infrastructure, and on reducing the societal and economic barriers that continue to prevent access to health care in Africa.

Since 1996, when scientific evidence of the efficacy of triple combination antiretroviral therapy became available, there has been a gradual shift in the paradigm applied to the response to HIV/AIDS. From interventions largely focused on prevention, national responses are now expanding, to include actions and resources geared to providing care and support to people living with HIV/AIDS. This shift is occurring amidst a continuing controversy around the wisdom of allocating a substantial amount of resources to HIV when other health and social priorities receive little attention. Yet the severity of the impact of AIDS, now clearly visible and measurable in most African countries, commands unusual, probably unprecedented measures. The debate and resolution of the United Nations General Assembly Special Session on AIDS, held in New York in 2001 emphasized the need to respond to the challenge of AIDS with a comprehensive set of actions encompassing prevention and care. Such a response is clearly not going to be easy, given the magnitude of the issues at stake and the uncertainty about the capacity to raise the national and international resources to match the needs. Yet some form of care, including antiretroviral therapy, exists to some extent in every country in Africa, often supported fully or in part by out-of-pocket expenditure and implemented through ad-hoc procurement of medicines. Every country, therefore, has the opportunity to learn from ongoing experiences and draw the lessons needed to expand access to care to its maximum capacity, striving toward equitable, quality, and sustained care. Starting small, making treatment available rapidly through the existing services, however limited in their outreach, may be possible for most countries in Africa. Furthering mechanisms to make drugs and diagnostics more available while building a health system capacity that can support expansion and reach out to all sections of society is the true challenge of coming years.

REFERENCES

1. Apel H. [The WHO/UNICEF Conference on Primary Health Care, Alma-Ata, September 6–22, 1978]. *Zeitschrift fur die Gesamte Hygiene und Ihre Grenzgebiete*, 1979;25:498–504.
2. Grant AD, Djomand G, De Cock KM. Natural history and spectrum of disease in adults with HIV/AIDS in Africa. *AIDS*, 1997;11:S43–S54.
3. World Bank. *Intensifying Action Against HIV/AIDS in Africa, Responding to a Development Crisis.* Washington, DC: World Bank Group; 1999.
4. Bos E, Hon V, Maeda A. *Health, Nutrition, and Population Indicators*. Washington, DC: The World Bank; 1998.
5. UNDP. UNDP Human Development Report 2000. Available at http://www.undp.org/hdro/highlights/past.htm. Accessed: October 31, 2001.
6. WHO. *Removing Obstacles to Health Development: Report on Infectious Diseases*. Geneva: World Health Organization; 1999.
7. UNAIDS. *Report on the Global HIV and AIDS Epidemic*. UNAIDS/00.13E. Geneva: UNAIDS; 2000.
8. The Voluntary HIV-1 Counseling and Testing Efficacy Study Group. Efficacy of voluntary HIV-1 counselling and testing in individuals and couples in Kenya, Tanzania, and Trinidad: a randomised trial. *Lancet*, 2000;356:103–112.
9. Mann J. Assessing Vulnerability to HIV Infection and AIDS. In: Mann J, Tarantola D, Netter T, eds. *AIDS in the World: A Global Report*. Cambridge: Harvard University Press, 1992:577–602.
10. Addai I. Determinants of use of maternal-child health services in rural Ghana. *J Biosoc Sci*, 2000; 32:1–15.
11. Menon R, Wawer M, Konde-Lule J. The Economic Impact of Adult Mortality on Households in Rakai District, Uganda. In: Ainsworth M, Fransen L, Over M, eds. *Confronting AIDS: Evidence from the Developing World*. Washington, DC: The World Bank, 1998:325–339.
12. Bechu N. The Impact of AIDS on the Economy and Families of Cote d'Ivoire: Changes in Consumption Among AIDS-affected Households. In: Ainsworth M, Fransen L, Over M, eds. *Confronting AIDS: Evidence from the Developing World*. Washington, DC: The World Bank, 1998:341–348.
13. Alubo SO. Debt crisis, health and health services in Africa. *Soc Sci Med*, 1990;31:639–648.
14. Ogbu O, Gallagher M. Public expenditures and health care in Africa. *Soc Sci Med*, 1992;34: 615–624.
15. Pinstrup-Anderson P, Jaramillo M, Stewart F. The Impact on Current Expenditure. In: Jolly R, ed. *Adjustment with a Human Face*. Oxford: Clarendon Press, 1987.
16. Davies R, Saunders D. Stabilization policies and the effect on child health in Zimbabwe. *Review of African Political Economics*, 1987;38:3–23.
17. Anyinam C. The Social Costs of the IMF's Adjustment Programs: The Case Study of Health Development in Ghana. *Int J Health Serv*, 1989;19:531–547.
18. Over M. The effect of scale on cost projections for a primary health care program in a developing country. *Soc Sci Med*, 1986;22:351–360.
19. WHO. The World Health Report. Available at http://www.who.int/whr/2000/en/report.htm. Accessed: April 13, 2001.
20. UNICEF. *The State of the World's Children*. Oxford: Oxford University Press; 1997.

21. Sanders D, Kravitz J, Lewin S, et al. Zimbabwe's hospital referral system: does it work? *Health Policy Plan*, 1998;13:359–370.
22. Diallo I, Molouba R, Sarr LC. Primary health care: from aspiration to achievement. *World Health Forum*, 1993;14:349–355.
23. Bentley C. Primary health care in northwestern Somalia: a case study. *Soc Sci Med*, 1989;28: 1019–1030.
24. UNAIDS. UNAIDS Regional Fact Sheets June 2000, Africa: Senegal. Available at http://www.unaids.org/hivaidsinfo/statistics/june00/fact_sheet/africa.html. Accessed: October 31, 2001.
25. Botswana Ministry of Health. *Sentinel Surveillance Report*. Gaborone: Botswana Ministry of Health; 1999.
26. Metrikin AS, Zwarenstein M, Steinberg MH, et al. Is HIV/AIDS a primary-care disease? Appropriate levels of outpatient care for patients with HIV/AIDS. *AIDS*, 1995;9:619–623.
27. Chaulet P. After health sector reform, whither lung health? *Int J Tuberc Lung Dis*, 1998;2:349–359.
28. Stover J, Johnston A. *The Art of Policy Formulation: Experiences from Africa in Developing National HIV/AIDS Policies*. Washington, DC: The POLICY Project (USAID); 1999.
29. Reddy D, Vandermoortele J. *User Financing of Basic Social Services: A Review of Theoretical Arguments and Empirical Evidence*. New York: UNICEF Office of Evaluation, Policy, and Planning; 1996.
30. Smith DL, Bryant JH. Building the infrastructure for primary health care: an overview of vertical and integrated approaches. *Soc Sci Med*, 1988;26: 909–917.
31. Gish O. The political economy of primary care and "health by the people": an historical exploration. *Soc Sci Med*, 1979;13C:203–211.
32. Mills A. Vertical vs. horizontal health programmes in Africa: idealism, pragmatism, resources and efficiency. *Soc Sci Med*, 1983;17:1971–1981.
33. Floyd K, Reid RA, Wilkinson D, et al. Admission trends in a rural South African hospital during the early years of the HIV epidemic. *JAMA*, 1999;282: 1087–1091.
34. Osborne CM, van Praag E, Jackson H. Models of care for patients with HIV/AIDS. *AIDS*, 1997;11: S135–S141.
35. Wilkinson D, Gilks CF. Increasing frequency of tuberculosis among staff in a South African district hospital: impact of the HIV epidemic on the supply side of health care. *Trans Royal Soc Trop Med Hyg*, 1998;92:500–502.
36. Arthur G, Bhatt SM, Muhindi D, et al. The changing impact of HIV/AIDS on Kenyatta National Hospital, Nairobi from 1988/89 through 1992 to 1997. *AIDS*, 2000;14:1625–1631.
37. Mushonga R. Family Caregivers of HIV/AIDS Patients in Rural Zimbabwe. In: Abstracts of the XII International Conference on AIDS; June 28–July 3, 1998; Geneva. Abstract 24391.
38. Weinreich S, Mphanza J, Taraking M. Community Based Home Care and Women's Empowerment. In: Program of the XII International Conference on AIDS; June 28–July 3, 1998; Geneva. Abstract 264/34102.
39. WHO Initiative on HIV/AIDS and Sexually Transmitted Infections. Safe and Effective Use of Antiretroviral Treatments in Adults with Particular Reference to Resource Limited Settings. WHO/HSI/2000.04.0 Available at http://www.who. int/HIV_AIDS/WHO_HSI_2000.04_1.04/index.htm. Accessed: October 31, 2001.
40. UNAIDS. Knowledge is Power: Voluntary HIV Counseling and Testing in Uganda. A Case Study. UNAIDS/99.8E. Available at http://www.unaids.org/publications/documents/health/counselling/knowledgecse.pdf. Accessed: November 2, 2001.
41. WeCareToo Website: Society for Women and AIDS in Kenya page. Available at http://www.wecaretoo. com/Organizations/KEN/swak. html. Accessed: January 30, 2002.
42. USAID. USAID African Partners. Available at http://www.usaid.gov/regions/afr/. Accessed: October 31, 2001.
43. Green EC. The participation of African traditional healers in AIDS/STD prevention programmes. *Tropical Doctor*, 1997;27:56–59.
44. UNAIDS. Collaboration with Traditional Healers in HIV/AIDS Prevention and Care in Sub-Saharan Africa: A Literature Review. UNAIDS/00.29.E. Available at http://www.unaids.org/publications/documents/care/general/JC299-TradHeal-E.pdf. Accessed: November 2, 2001.
45. *THETA Participation Evaluation Report, Innovation or Re-awakening? Roles of Traditional Healers in the Management and Prevention of HIV/AIDS in Uganda*. October 1998.
46. Campbell I. Chikankata hospital AIDS care and prevention, 'products' of home and hospital care, October 1990–September 1991. In: Program of the Presentation to the Congressional Forum on HIV/AIDS; June, 1992; Washington, DC.
47. Gilson L, Magomi M, Mkangaa E. The structural quality of Tanzanian primary health facilities. *Bull WHO*, 1995;73:105–114.
48. Whiteside A. AIDS and the Private Sector. *AIDS Analysis Africa*, 2000;10:1–6.
49. Aventin L, Huard P. HIV/AIDS and Manufacturing in Abidjan. *AIDS Analysis Africa*, 1997;7:2–4.
50. Roberts N, Rau B. *Private Sector AIDS Policy African Workplace profiles: Case studies of Business Managing HIV/AIDS*. Durham: Family Health International/AIDSCAP; 1997.

51. Simon J, Rosen S, Whiteside A. The Response of African Businesses to HIV/AIDS. In: Program of the XIII International AIDS Conference; 9–24 July, 2000; Durban, South Africa.
52. Matomora MK, Lamboray JL, Laing R. Integration of AIDS program activities into national health systems. *AIDS*, 1991;5:S193–S196.
53. Martin AL, Van Praag E, Misiska R. An African model of home based care. In: Mann J, Tarantola D, eds. *AIDS in the World II*. New York: Oxford University Press, 1996:410.
54. Demographic and Health Survey. Available at www.measuredhs.com. Accessed: May 1, 2001.
55. Kassler WJ, Alwano-Edyegu MG, Marum E, et al. Rapid HIV testing with same-day results: a field trial in Uganda. *Int J STD AIDS*, 1998;9:134–138.
56. Wilkinson D, Wilkinson N, Lombard C, et al. On-site HIV testing in resource-poor settings: is one rapid test enough? [see comments]. *AIDS*, 1997; 11:377–381.
57. Anonymous. The importance of simple/rapid assays in HIV testing. *Weekly Epidemiological Record*, 1998;73:321–326.
58. Temmerman M, Ndinya-Achola J, Ambani J, et al. The right not to know HIV-test results. *Lancet*, 1995;345:969–970.
59. Campbell CH, Marum ME, Alwano-Edyegu M, et al. The role of HIV counseling and testing in the developing world. *AIDS Educ Prev*, 1997;9:92–104.
60. Downing RG, Otten RA, Marum E, et al. Optimizing the delivery of HIV counseling and testing services: the Uganda experience using rapid HIV antibody test algorithms. *J Acquir Immune Defic Syndr*, 1998;18:384–388.
61. Lo B, Snyder L. Care at the end of life: guiding practice where there are no easy answers. *Ann Internal Med*, 1999;130:772–774.
62. Foster S. Supply and use of essential drugs in sub–Saharan Africa: some issues and possible solutions. *Soc Sci Med*, 1991;32:1201–1218.
63. UNAIDS. Access to Drugs: UNAIDS Technical Update. WC 503.2. Available at http://www.unaids.org/publications/documents/health/access/accestue.pdf. Accessed: October 31, 2001.
64. McPake B, Hanson K, Mills A. Community financing of health care in Africa: an evaluation of the Bamako initiative. *Soc Sci Med*, 1993;36:1383–1395.
65. Jallow MT. Essential drugs in the Gambia. *World Health Forum*, 1993;14:136–139.
66. Fakande I, Malomo O. Home care of AIDS patients from the Medical and nursing viewpoint – A project in Ife-Ijesa Zone, Osun State, Nigeria. In: Program of the XII International Conference on AIDS; June 28–July 3, 1998; Geneva.
67. Jackson H, Kerkhoven R. Developing AIDS care in Zimbabwe: a case for residential community centres? *AIDS Care*, 1995;7:663–673.
68. Corrigan C, Jannetta P, Mashangra R. AIDS Education Programme Targeting Adult Family Members During Home Based Care. In: Program of the XI International Conference on AIDS; July 7–22, 1996; Vancouver.
69. Reijer P. The Effect of Community Based Home Care Programmes for People Living with HIV/AIDS and Peer Educators Programmes on Knowledge, Attitude, and Practice on HIV/AIDS in the Community. In: Program of the XII International Conference on AIDS; June 28–July 3, 1998; Geneva.
70. Hansen K, Woelk G, Jackson H, et al. The cost of home-based care for HIV/AIDS patients in Zimbabwe. *AIDS Care*, 1998;10:751–759.
71. Seeley J, Kajura E, Bachengana C, et al. The extended family and support for people with AIDS in a rural population in south west Uganda: a safety net with holes? *AIDS Care*, 1993;5:117–122.
72. Olenja JM. Assessing community attitude towards home-based care for people with AIDS (PWAs) in Kenya. *J Community Health*, 1999;24:187–199.
73. Nfila B. Home Based Care: A Viable Option for the Care of AIDS and Other Terminally Ill Patients in Botswana. In: Program of the XI International Conference on AIDS; July 7–22, 1996; Vancouver.
74. McDonnell S, Brennan M, Burnham G, et al. Assessing and planning home-based care for persons with AIDS. *Health Policy Plan*, 1994;9: 429–437.
75. Gathiram V, Mtinjana A. Establishing a continuum of HIV Care and enhancing home-based care in rural and urban resource-poor settings in Kwa-Zulu Natal (KZN). In: Program of the XIII International AIDS Conference; 9–24 July, 2000; Durban, South Africa.
76. Mawejje D, Gitta P, Kiwanuka R, et al. Community's ability in the provision of home-based care: the TASO experience. In: Program of the XI Conference on AIDS; July 7–22, 1996; Vancouver.
77. Anglaret X, Chene G, Attia A, et al. Early chemoprophylaxis with trimethoprim-sulphamethoxazole for HIV-1–infected adults in Abidjan, Cote d'Ivoire: a randomised trial. Cotrimo-CI Study Group. *Lancet*, 1999;353:1463–1468.
78. Wiktor SZ, Sassan-Morokro M, Grant AD, et al. Efficacy of trimethoprim-sulphamethoxazole prophylaxis to decrease morbidity and mortality in HIV-1–infected patients with tuberculosis in Abidjan, Cote d'Ivoire: a randomised controlled trial. *Lancet*, 1999;353:1469–1475.
79. *Use of Cotrimoxazole Prophylaxis in Adults and Children living with HIV/AIDS in Africa, Recommendations and Operational Issues*. Harare, Zimbabwe: UNAIDS/WHO Consultation, March 2000.
80. De Cock KM, Binkin NJ, Zuber PL, et al. Research issues involving HIV-associated tuberculosis in

resource-poor countries. *JAMA*, 1996;276: 1502–1507.
81. Abouya L, Coulibaly IM, Wiktor SZ, et al. The Cote d'Ivoire national HIV counseling and testing program for tuberculosis patients: implementation and analysis of epidemiologic data. *AIDS*, 1998;12:505–512.
82. Wilkinson D, Squire SB, Garner P. Effect of preventive treatment for tuberculosis in adults infected with HIV: systematic review of randomised placebo controlled trials. *BMJ*, 1998;317:625–629.
83. Anonymous. Preventive therapy against tuberculosis in people living with HIV. *Weekly Epidemiological Record*, 1999;74:385–398.
84. WHO. Global Tuberculosis Control: WHO Report 1999. WHO/TBI99.259. Available at http://www.who.int/gtb/publications/globrep99/index.html. Accessed: October 31, 2001.
85. Cipla in the News web site. Available at http://www.cipla.com/whatsnew/ciplanews.htm. Accessed: May 1, 2001.
86. Zuniga J. Out of Africa: Uganda and UNAIDS advance a bold experiment. *J Int Assoc Physicians AIDS Care*, 1999;5:48–60.
87. Sow P, Diakhate N, Toure Kane N. Clinical, Immunological, and Virological Effectiveness of Antiretroviral Therapy in a Resource-Poor Setting: the Senegalese Experience. In: Program of the 8th Conference on Retroviruses and Opportunistic Infections; 2001; Chicago.
88. Djomand G, Roels T, Chorba T. HIV/AIDS DRUG ACCESS INITIATIVE Preliminary report Covering the period August 1998–March 2000. Available at http://www.unaids.org/publications/ documents/care/unaids_dai/cote_ivoire_drug_access_initiative.doc. Accessed: January 30, 2002.
89. Ochola D, Weidle P, Malamba S, et al. Preliminary Report Uganda Ministry of Health—UNAIDS HIV/AIDS Drug Access Initiative August 1998–March 2000. Available at http://www.unaids.org/publications/documents/care/unaids_da/uguanda_drug_access_initiative.doc. Accessed: January 30, 2002.
90. Uganda Ministry of Health. *UNAIDS HIV/AIDS Drug Access initiative: Preliminary Report, August 1998–March 2000.* Kampala: Uganda Ministry of Health; 2000.
91. Attaran A, Sachs J. Defining and refining international donor support for combating the AIDS pandemic. *Lancet*, 2001;357:57–61.
92. Schwartlander B, Stover J, Walker N, et al. AIDS. Resource needs for HIV/AIDS. *Science*, 2001;292: 2434–2436.
93. United Nations. Declaration of commitment on HIV/AIDS. Available at http://www.un.org/ga/aids/ coverage/FinalDeclarationHIVAIDS.html. Accessed: November 1, 2001.
94. Organization for Economic Cooperation and Development. Net ODA in 1999—as a Percentage of GNP. Available at http://www1.oecd.org/ dac/images/ODA99per.jpg. Accessed: October 31, 2001.
95. USAID. HIV/AIDS Undoing Decades of Development. *Front Lines*, 2000;40:1–5.
96. The Global Fund to Fight AIDS, Tuberculosis, and Malaria. Contributions Web Site. Available at http://www.globalfundatm.org/contribute.html. Accessed: January 31, 2002.
97. UNAIDS. UNAIDS Proposed Unified Budget and workplan for 2000–2001. UNAIDS/UWB/2000–01. Available at http://www.unaids.org/about/governance/governance.html. Accessed: March 12, 2001.
98. Bill and Melinda Gates Foundation Web Site. Available at http://www.gatesfoundation.org. Accessed: May 6, 2001.
99. Cameron C, Shepard J. The Cost of AIDS Care and Prevention. In: Mann J, Tarantola D, Netter T, eds. *AIDS in the World 1992: A Global Report.* Cambridge: Harvard University Press, 1992: 477–509.
100. National AIDS Control Programme of the United Republic of Tanzania. *Strategic Framework for the Third Medium Term Plan, 1998–2002.* Dar Es Salaam: Tanzania Ministry of Health; 1998.
101. Uganda AIDS Commission. *The National Strategic Framework for HIV/AIDS Activities in Uganda: 2000/1 to 2005/6.* Kampala: Government of Uganda, UNAIDS; 2000.

28

Diagnosis of Pediatric HIV Infection

*Chewe Luo and †Brian Coulter

*UNICEF Botswana, Gaborone, Botswana.
†Liverpool School of Tropical Medicine, Liverpool, United Kingdom.

Human immunodeficiency virus (HIV) infection is a major problem in many pediatric care facilities in sub–Saharan Africa, with up to 45% of HIV-infected children rapidly developing AIDS and dying within their first 2 years of life (1). The clinical presentation of pediatric HIV disease in African children often lacks specificity and usually mimics clinical entities that are commonly observed in children who are not HIV-infected. Pediatric AIDS diagnosis is extremely difficult for many health care providers in Africa, especially in situations where front-line workers may lack specific clinical algorithms, and laboratory and diagnostic facilities are limited. The majority of pediatric AIDS deaths in Africa, therefore, occur without confirmation that they are indeed HIV-related.

Because 95% of pediatric HIV infections result from mother-to-child transmission (MTCT) and because progression of HIV disease in children can be much more rapid than in adults, the process of diagnosing pediatric HIV infection should begin with identifying maternal HIV infection before or during pregnancy. In addition to the implications for maternal care, the identification of HIV-infected pregnant women provides an opportunity to reduce the risk of HIV infection to babies through the provision of preventive antiretroviral therapy (ART) during pregnancy and/or at delivery. Confirmation of maternal HIV status also allows clinicians to identify at-risk babies who will require laboratory testing for HIV infection. Early diagnosis of children who are HIV-infected helps facilitate close clinical monitoring and, where possible, early preventive therapy for opportunistic infections such as *Pneumocystis carinii* pneumonia (PCP), and provision of ART from early infancy.

In Africa, HIV voluntary counseling and testing (VCT) is not universally available to pregnant women. Where HIV testing is available, it is generally performed for routine confirmation of a clinical HIV diagnosis and for blood screening. In children born to HIV-infected mothers, maternally acquired HIV antibodies (IgG) persist for up to 15 to 18 months after birth. A positive antibody test in a child under 18 months of age, therefore, only confirms exposure to maternal infection. The DNA polymerase chain reaction (PCR) test, now recommended for early diagnosis of pediatric HIV, is not only expensive, but it requires both sophisticated equipment and experienced technologists. The outcomes of not being able to confirm maternal and/or infant HIV status, a common situation in African health care settings, are described in Table 1.

TABLE 1. Constraints in Diagnosing HIV Infection in Mothers and Children in Developing Countries and the Outcomes of Unknown HIV Status[a]

Constraints	Typical outcomes
Maternal HIV Status is Unknown • Mother is not willing to be tested[b] • Antenatal HIV test is not available	No ARVs to prevent MTCT No planned maternal HIV management and care No preventive therapy for PCP or TB (isoniazid and cotrimoxazole) No counseling on infant feeding options No counseling on family planning Late diagnosis of pediatric HIV if infant is infected by MTCT Missed diagnosis in early infant deaths that result from HIV infection No close monitoring of children for possible opportunistic infections
Maternal Status is Known; Infant Status is Unknown • PCR is not available	Overdiagnosis of HIV infection in infants who may be uninfected No PCP prophylaxis to HIV-infected infants, except in situations where all HIV-exposed children receive PCP prophylaxis HIV-infected infants may die of missed opportunistic infections before serologic confirmation of their HIV status is possible (at 15–18 months) Late presentation with HIV-related disease in infants who are infected by MTCT Usually no follow-up
Mother with HIV Breastfeeds HIV-Uninfected Infant	Infant is exposed to HIV for the duration of breastfeeding PCR tests required for infant during lactation period PCP prophylaxis is required for breastfed infant, regardless of HIV status, due to persistent exposure

[a]PCR indicates polymerase chain reaction; ARVs, antiretroviral agents; MTCT, mother-to-child transmission; PCP, *Pneumocystis carinii* pneumonia; TB, tuberculosis.
[b]Unwillingness to be tested is often due to fear of stigma and/or family break-up.

CLINICAL OUTCOME AND PRESENTATION

Children with HIV appear to follow a more severe and rapid course of disease than HIV-infected adults, although a small proportion of children may be slow progressors and remain asymptomatic for prolonged periods. In a study in Rwanda, the estimated risk of death among HIV-infected children at 1 year of age was 260 per 1,000 live births (95% CI, 160 to 410) (1). In contrast, mortality of the uninfected children born to HIV-positive mothers in this study was only 20 per 1,000 (95% CI, 10 to 70), a rate that was not significantly different from that of children born to HIV-negative mothers (50 per 1,000; 95% CI, 30 to 90). Infant mortality rates among HIV-infected children in Uganda and South Africa—330 and 350 per 1,000 live births, respectively—were much higher than those among HIV-negative children—107 and 59 per 1,000, respectively (2,3).

Because the clinical presentation of pediatric HIV infection in Africa is usually nonspecific, and existing classification systems are not particularly useful without supportive diagnostic facilities, diagnosis is a challenge for most health care providers. Systems for classifying pediatric HIV infection and AIDS are described in the following sections.

CDC Classification System for Children Under 13 Years of Age and Its Applicability in Africa

The Centers for Disease Control and Prevention (CDC) classification system for pediatric HIV infection, which was revised in 1994 (4), is the most widely used in industrialized countries. However, in its current format it is not appropriate for most facilities in Africa. In this system, children are grouped according to clinical categories (N, A, B, and C) and immune categories (1, 2, and 3) (Table 2) (4). This system also uses age-specific $CD4^+$ cell count or percentage as a marker of immune status (Table 3). $CD4^+$ quantification requires complicated and expensive equipment that is not widely available in Africa.

Although the HIV-related clinical events that are observed in African children may not differ significantly from those seen in children in industrialized countries, diagnoses in African health facilities are likely to be missed, especially those defined in CDC clinical category C (Table 2). These missed diagnoses are often a result of a widespread lack of laboratory and other diagnostic facilities such as those used for microbiology, virology, echocardiography, and radiology. Furthermore, diseases that are considered indicators of HIV infection, such as pneumonia, diarrhea, anemia, wasting, and meningitis, are also frequently observed in young African children who are not HIV-infected. The prevalence of these diseases among both HIV-infected and -uninfected children in Africa reduces their usefulness as HIV indicators. The etiologic agents and the frequency and severity of these diseases are what distinguish them in children with HIV infection compared to their HIV-uninfected counterparts.

Respiratory tract infections occur more frequently in HIV-infected children than in HIV-uninfected children (5,6,7). Malaria does not appear to be more common in HIV-infected than HIV-uninfected children (8). Pediatric autopsy data from Africa has also shown that respiratory diseases are dominant causes of death among HIV-infected children; such diseases have been found to be significantly more common in HIV-positive children than in HIV-negative children (9–12).

Malnutrition or wasting that is not a result of undernutrition may be an indicator of HIV infection. It is not unusual for children in Africa to suffer from both HIV infection and malnutrition. These children are often identified in malnutrition units for failure to respond to routine management.

Pneumocystis carinii is a frequent and severe cause of pneumonia affecting HIV-infected young infants in industrialized countries. Earlier reports indicated that PCP was less common among HIV-infected children in African countries than in those from more developed countries (13,14). More recently, however, both autopsy and clinical studies have shown that PCP is common in sub–Saharan Africa (9,10,15,16). A clinical diagnosis of PCP should be strongly considered in an infant less than 6 months of age who has severe pneumonia characterized by marked hypoxia and does not respond to standard antibiotics (ampicillin or chloramphenicol). Laboratory confirmation of PCP is difficult. Immunofluorescent techniques on nasopharyngeal aspirates may be useful, but tend to underestimate disease frequency (16,17).

HIV-infected African children commonly present with chronic respiratory symptoms, which are usually difficult to classify or diagnose. Many of these children may have HIV-related lymphoid interstitial pneumonia (LIP) but the diagnosis is usually confused with pulmonary tuberculosis (TB)

TABLE 2. Centers for Disease Control Pediatric HIV Classification System (4)

	Clinical categories[a]			
Immune categories	N No signs/symptoms	A Mild signs/symptoms	B Moderate signs/symptoms	C Severe signs/symptoms
1. No evidence of suppression	N1	A1	B1	C1
2. Evidence of moderate suppression	N2	A2	B2	C2
3. Severe suppression	N3	A3	B3	C3
	N: Children who have no signs or symptoms considered to be the result of HIV infection or who have only one of the conditions listed in category A.	A: Children with two or more of the following conditions but none of the conditions listed in categories B or C: Lymphadenopathy (≥0.5 cm at more than two sites; bilateral = one site); Hepatomegaly; Splenomegaly; Dermatitis; Parotitis; Recurrent or persistent upper respiratory infection, sinusitis, or otitis media.	B: Children who have symptomatic conditions other than those listed for category A or category C that are attributed to HIV infection. Examples include but are not limited to the following: Anemia (<8 g/dL), neutropenia (<1,000/mm^3), or thrombocytopenia (<100,000/mm^3) persisting for 30 days or longer; Bacterial meningitis, pneumonia, or sepsis (single episode); Candidiasis, oropharyngeal, persisting for longer than 2 months; Cardiomyopathy; CMV infection with onset before 1 month of age; Diarrhea, recurrent or chronic; Hepatitis; HSV stomatitis, recurrent	C: Children who have any condition listed in the 1987 surveillance case definition for AIDS (38), with the exception of LIP (which is a category B condition), including: Multiple or recurrent severe bacterial infections; Esophageal or pulmonary candidiasis; Disseminated coccidiomycosis; Extrapulmonary cryptococcosis; Cryptosporidiosis or isosporiasis; CMV disease at more than 1 month of age; Encephalopathy; HSV infection causing a mucocutaneous ulcer that persists for longer than 1 month or bronchitis, pneumonitis, or esophagitis for any duration in a

Continued

TABLE 2. *Continued*

	Clinical categories[a]			
Immune categories	N No signs/symptoms	A Mild signs/symptoms	B Moderate signs/symptoms	C Severe signs/symptoms
1. No evidence of suppression	N1	A1	B1	C1
2. Evidence of moderate suppression	N2	A2	B2	C2
3. Severe suppression	N3	A3	B3	C3
			(more than two episodes within 1 year); HSV bronchitis, pneumonitis, or esophagitis with onset before 1 month of age; Herpes zoster (shingles) involving at least two distinct episodes or more than one dermatome; Leiomyosarcoma; LIP or PLH complex; Nephropathy; Nocardiosis; Fever lasting longer than 1 month; Toxoplasmosis with onset before 1 month of age; Varicella, disseminated (complicated chickenpox)	child older than 1 month of age; Disseminated histoplasmosis; Kaposi's sarcoma; Primary lymphoma of the brain; Burkitt's or immunoblastic lymphoma; Disseminated or extrapulmonary TB; Disseminated other or unspecified *Mycobacteria* spp.; Disseminated *M. avium*; PCP; PML; Recurrent salmonella (nontyphoid) septicemia; Toxoplasmosis of the brain at more than 1 month of age; Wasting syndrome

[a]CMV indicates cytomegalovirus; HSV, herpes simplex virus; LIP, lymphoid interstitial pneumonia; PLH, pulmonary lymphoid hyperplasia; TB, tuberculosis; PCP, *Pneumocystis carinii* pneumonia; PML, progressive multifocal leukoencephalopathy.

TABLE 3. Centers for Disease Control Immunologic Categories Based on Age-Specific $CD4^+$ T-Lymphocyte Counts and Percent of Total Lymphocytes (4)

	Age of the child					
	<12 months		1–5 years		6–12 years	
Immune category	$CD4^+/mm^3$	% $CD4^+$	$CD4^+/mm^3$	% $CD4^+$	$CD4^+/mm^3$	% $CD4^+$
1. No immunosuppression	≥1500	≥25	≥1,000	≥25	≥500	≥25
2. Moderate immunosuppression	750–1,499	15–24	500–999	15–24	200–499	15–24
3. Severe immunosuppression	<750	<15	<500	<15	<200	<15

TABLE 4. 1985 WHO Case Definition for Pediatric AIDS (18)

Major signs:
Weight loss or failure to thrive
Chronic diarrhea lasting longer than 1 month
Prolonged fever lasting longer than 1 month

Minor signs:
Generalized lymphadenopathy
Oropharyngeal candidiasis
Repeated common infections
Generalized dermatitis
Confirmed maternal HIV infection

Pediatric AIDS is suspected in a child presenting with at least two major signs and two minor signs in the absence of known causes of immunosuppression.

because of the radiologic features of interstitial infiltrates with hilar prominence. Other causes of chronic chest disease include Kaposi's sarcoma and bronchiectasis, and less commonly, cardiac disorders.

World Health Organization Case Definition for Pediatric AIDS

For AIDS surveillance purposes, in 1985 the World Health Organization (WHO) defined clinical diagnosis criteria for settings with limited laboratory facilities (18) (Table 4). These criteria include conditions that are categorized as "major" or "minor" signs of AIDS. Because many health facilities were unable to conduct HIV tests, confirmation of maternal HIV infection with antibody testing was considered a minor sign. This definition has major limitations in its applicability to clinical settings.

The 1985 WHO definition was evaluated in various African countries, using HIV antibody testing as a gold standard for comparison (19–21). The accuracy of antibody testing is limited by its low specificity in children less than 15 months of age. The definition was found to have low sensitivity and positive predictive value. However, with country-specific modifications, the definition may be made more useful. In Zambia, country-specific criteria were developed, taking account of commonly observed clinical entities in children who are not HIV-infected. Diarrhea and malnutrition, classified as "major" in the WHO definition, but more frequently observed in HIV-uninfected Zambian children, were reclassified as "minor" (21). The sensitivity, specificity, and positive predictive value of the definition using the Zambian criteria were 79.3%, 91.4%, and 86.8%, respectively, compared to 69%, 64%, and 38% using the unmodified WHO/Bangui definition.

Ghent Classification

In 1992, a working group on MTCT convened in Ghent, Belgium and developed guidelines to standardize criteria for estimating transmission rates in various studies and surveillance systems (Table 5) (22).

TABLE 5. HIV-Related Signs and Symptoms, Ghent 1992 (22)

Persistent diarrhea lasting longer than 15 days
Oral candidiasis beyond the neonatal period
Generalized lymphadenopathy (enlarged nodes in at least 2 independent anatomical sites)
Failure to thrive (no weight gain for a period of 3 months or crossing two percentile lines on the growth chart)
Chronic parotitis lasting longer than 1 month
Herpes zoster (shingles)
Recurrent pneumonia (2 or more episodes)

HIV-related signs and symptoms of pediatric AIDS were agreed upon for use with confirmation of an HIV antibody test at 15 months of age. Without laboratory confirmation, the individual clinical entities defined by the Ghent group, although common in HIV-infected children, lack specificity and are not useful for decision-making in clinical settings particularly because: PCP without prompt treatment is usually fatal on the first episode; and the etiology of lymph node enlargement in an HIV-infected child includes HIV-related nonspecific hyperplasia, TB, Kaposi's sarcoma, and lymphoma.

LABORATORY DIAGNOSIS OF PEDIATRIC HIV

There is a range of methods for diagnosing HIV infection in pregnant women and infants. An algorithm for HIV testing of pregnant women and their infants in industrialized countries is outlined in Figure 1.

Industrialized Countries

Increased uptake of HIV screening and the administration of antiretroviral agents (ARVs) during the antenatal period have dramatically reduced HIV infection in at-risk infants in the United States and Europe. However, there are still a proportion of HIV-infected women who present at delivery without prior screening. For this group, it has been proposed that rapid HIV serologic testing be undertaken at delivery to facilitate advice regarding avoidance of breastfeeding and the administration of ARVs to mother and infant during delivery and the postnatal period. Also, an HIV-exposed infant can be screened soon after delivery and during the early neonatal period to confirm HIV infection.

Approximately two-thirds of MTCT cases occur at or around the time of birth. However, tests for HIV infection at birth are only positive in 30% to 50% of babies whose HIV infection is subsequently confirmed. By 4 to 6 weeks of age, virtually all HIV-infected infants may be diagnosed. At this stage PCP prophylaxis may be commenced, and multiple ARVs introduced, if indicated. Intrauterine exposure is assumed to be the cause of infection if PCR or HIV viral culture is positive within 48 hours of birth. Intrapartum exposure is assumed to be the cause of infection if diagnostic tests are negative in first 48 hours but positive after 1 week (23,24). PCR results are not affected by antenatal ARVs. All HIV-infected mothers are advised not to breastfeed, so postnatal transmission is rarely an issue. Final confirmation of infant HIV status is undertaken by HIV enzyme-linked immunosorbent assay (ELISA) after 18 months when it is presumed that all passively acquired antibodies will have disappeared. A false-negative HIV ELISA could occur in an infant with advanced disease and low immunoglobulins; however, such a case would be an exception to the rule.

African Countries

Very few countries to date have fully implemented national programs to prevent MTCT of HIV. One of the elements of the Botswana program is VCT for all pregnant women. In some other countries, pilot projects have been implemented to assess the feasibility of integrating the prevention of MTCT into routine antenatal care services. Acceptability of VCT is still a major problem;

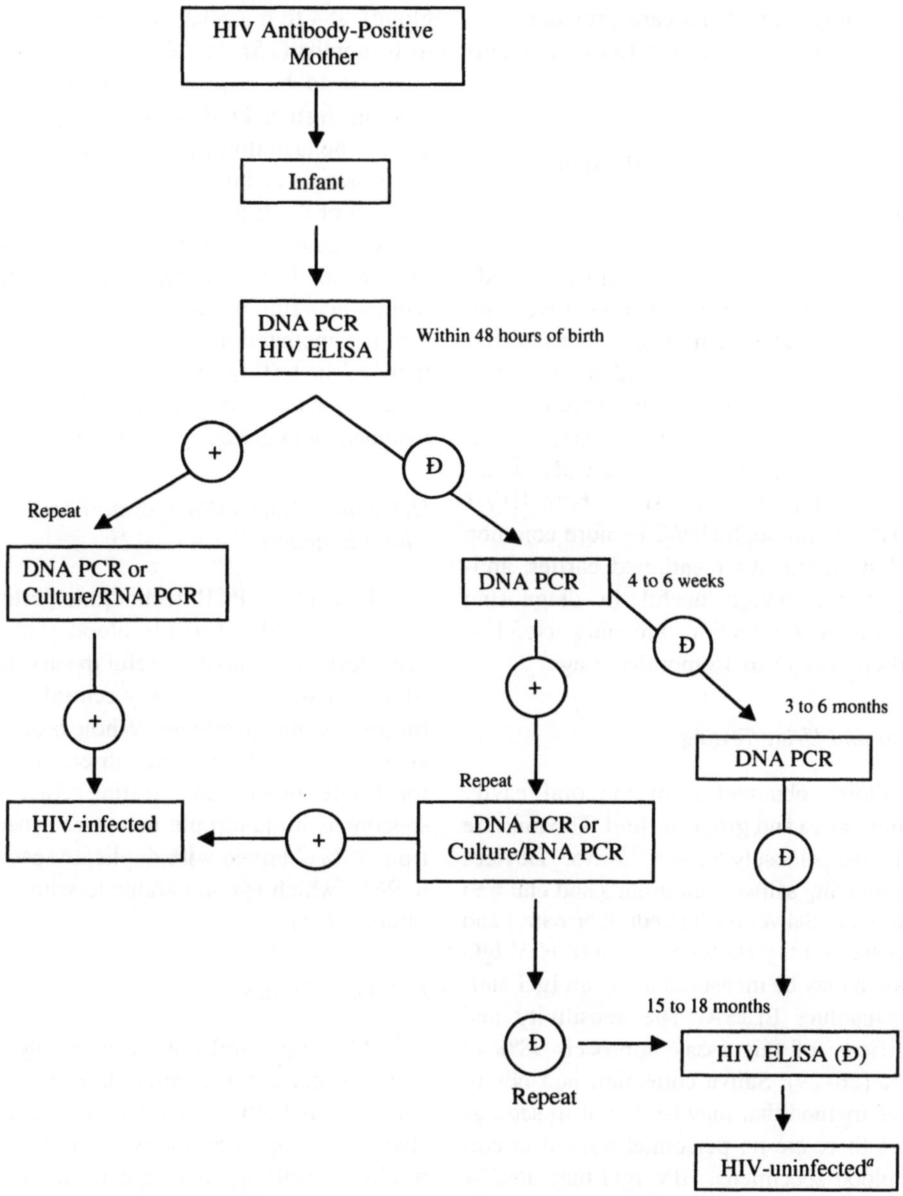

FIGURE 1. Diagnosis of perinatal HIV-infected infants less than 18 months of age. [a]Infant remains at risk for HIV as long as mother breastfeeds. Adapted from (25).

the majority of pregnant women in many African countries present in labor with unknown HIV status.

For the newborns of women whose HIV status is known, the PCR test for confirming infant infection is usually unavailable because of cost and the expertise required to perform the test. In Zambia, PCR testing and viral culture is limited to research specimens in one teaching hospital where the work is undertaken by a trained virologist. The situation is probably similar in many other African countries. Diagnosis of pediatric HIV infection in Africa is therefore dependent on the clinical judgment of the care provider, supported by an antibody test at 15 to 18 months of age.

Diagnostic Tests for HIV Infection

Antibody Serology

A highly sensitive HIV ELISA antibody test is used for screening and, if positive, confirmation is undertaken using either a different type of HIV ELISA of higher specificity or Western Blot or immunofluorescent assays (25). Cheaper, rapid serologic tests, such as those using a dipstick method, are also available. It is important to test for both HIV-1 and HIV-2, although HIV-2 is more common in West Africa. As mentioned earlier, antibody tests, though useful in diagnosing maternal HIV infection, are only useful in children over 15 to 18 months of age.

Saliva and Urine Testing

Fluids obtained from the oral cavity include saliva and gingival fluid. The mixture of the two is loosely termed "saliva." Devices for collecting saliva from infants and children include the Salivette (Sarstedt, Germany) and Orapette (Trinity Biotech, Ireland). HIV IgG in saliva may be measured using an IgG antibody capture ELISA. The sensitivity and specificity of this assay approach 98% to 100% (26–29). Saliva collection is a noninvasive method that may be useful in settings where there are no personnel trained to collect blood specimens. HIV IgG may also be detected in urine; urine tests yield comparable results to those performed with serum and saliva, depending on the laboratory technique used (26,27,30).

Polymerase Chain Reaction

Qualitative HIV DNA PCR is the standard method of confirming pediatric HIV infection. In industrialized countries it is commonly performed at birth (peripheral blood), at 4 to 6 weeks, and if necessary, at 3 to 6 months (25). In Africa, where children continue to be exposed because of breastfeeding, further PCR tests are required both during the lactation period and 6 weeks after the cessation of breastfeeding. In addition to the cost of the test and the laboratory expertise it requires, the lack of subtype-specific primers for HIV-1 subtypes A, D, C, and O (common in sub–Saharan Africa and Southeast Asia), is another drawback, reducing the sensitivity of the test. Quantitative HIV RNA PCR is used for measuring viral load, response to treatment, and disease progression.

HIV Filter Paper DNA Polymerase Chain Reaction

HIV DNA PCR techniques performed directly from dried whole blood spots have been developed and are useful in surveillance studies or settings with only central facilities for processing specimens. Whole blood spots are obtained on filter paper, dried, and stored for future processing. Testing filter paper specimens in quadruple increases sensitivity from 88% obtained with duplicate specimens to 96%, which is comparable to whole blood samples (31).

HIV Viral Culture

Although viral culture is highly sensitive and specific, it is rarely used for routine testing. It is both labor intensive and expensive, and results are not available for 2 to 4 weeks. Sensitivity and specificity of HIV viral culture is similar to that of PCR.

p24 Antigen

High levels of HIV IgG may form complexes with p24 antigen, reducing the sensitivity of p24 antigen assays. This can be overcome by incubation with acid, a process that dissociates immune complexes, termed immune complex disssociation (ICD) (24,25,32,33). Sensitivity is low in the first few weeks of life and there may be false-positive results (24). After 2 months, sensitivity may reach 88% and specificity, 100%. The test is relatively inexpensive compared to PCR and viral culture and it is suitable for use in developing countries. However, the sensitivity of less than 90% limits its use as a definitive test.

HIV IgA

HIV-1–specific IgA has been investigated as a marker for early diagnosis of HIV infection (33–37). Techniques for IgA detection include IgA ELISA, immunoblotting, and capture enzyme immunoassays. In most HIV-infected infants, HIV IgA is not detected in serum until after 3 months of age. However, HIV IgA may be detected in infants less than 1 month of age if their HIV infection is the result of intrauterine exposure. At 6 months of age, 85% to 100% of HIV-infected infants may have detectable HIV IgA; by 12 to 18 months, this percentage is 90% to 95%. However, after 6 to 9 months, HIV IgA levels may decrease in some infants, especially in those progressing to AIDS. Thus, HIV IgA does not necessarily reach 100% sensitivity even in older children or adults.

In the first month of life, specificity of IgA detection techniques may be low. It is presumed that this is due to the infant's exposure to maternal IgA. After 1 month, specificity is around 96% to 100%. High levels of IgG (due to polyclonal stimulation) may interfere with HIV IgA analysis by inhibiting binding of serum IgA to test antigen. Pretreatment with protein G to remove IgG increases sensitivity. The sensitivity of HIV IgA assays in most studies does not generally exceed 95%; this level may be lower for assays performed with samples from immunosuppressed children with hypogammaglobulinaemia. Furthermore, analysis of IgA detection is difficult due to the need for dissociation of IgA from IgG. For these reasons, HIV IgA alone cannot be recommended as a routine marker for diagnosing HIV infection in developing countries.

HIV IgM

HIV IgM has lower sensitivity than HIV IgA. In intrauterine infection, HIV IgM may peak and fall early and thus not be detected postnatally, or IgM may not be produced in detectable amounts at all in some HIV-infected infants (25,32).

CONCLUSION

The high prevalence of HIV in African adults fuels the pediatric epidemic. While programs aimed at preventing mother-to-child HIV transmission are going to scale, clinicians urgently need improved clinical and diagnostic tools to provide the much needed care for those children who are already HIV-infected.

REFERENCES

1. Spira R, Lepage P, Msellati P, et al. Natural history of HIV type 1 infection in children: a five-year prospective study in Rwanda. *Pediatrics*, 1999;104:e56.
2. Lepage P, Spira R, Kalibala S, et al. Care of human immunodeficiency virus infected children in developing countries—Report of a workshop for clinical research. *Pediatr Infect Dis J*, 1998;17:581–586.
3. World Health Organisation. *The World Health Report 1999—Making a difference*. Geneva, 1999.
4. Centers for Disease Control and Prevention Classification System for human immunodeficiency virus (HIV) infection in children under 13 years of age. *MMWR*, 1994;43:1–17.
5. Vetter K, Djomand G, Zadi F, et al. Clinical spectrum of human immunodeficiency virus in children in a West African city. *Pediatr Infect Dis J*, 1996; 15:438–442.
6. Westwood ATR, Eley BS, Gilbert RG, et al. Bacterial infection in children with HIV: a prospective study from Cape Town, South Africa. *Ann Trop Paediatr*, 2000;20:193–208.
7. Bobat R, Moodley D, Coutsoudis A, et al. The early natural history of vertically transmitted HIV-1 infection in African children in Durban, South Africa. *Ann Trop Paediatr*, 1998;18:187–196.
8. Kalyesuba I, Mudido-Musoke P, Marum L, et al. Effect of malaria infection on human type-1 infected Ugandan children. *Pediatr Infect Dis J*, 1997:16:876–888.

9. Lucas SB, Peacock CS, Hounnou A, et al. Disease in children infected with HIV in Abidjan, Cote d'Ivoire. *Br Med J*, 1996;312:335–338.
10. Ikeogu M, Wolf B, Mathe S. Pulmonary manifestations of HIV seropositivity and malnutrition in Zimbabwe. *Arch Dis Child*, 1997;76:124–128.
11. Jeena P, Coovadia H, Chrystal V. *Pneumocystis carinii* and cytomegalovirus infections in severely ill HIV infected African infants. *Ann Trop Paediatr*, 1996;16:361–368.
12. Ansari NA, Kombe AH, Kenyon TA, et al. Mortality and pulmonary pathology of children with HIV infection in Francistown, Botswana. *Int J Tuberc Lung Dis*, 1999;3 (Suppl 1):S201.
13. Fleming A. Opportunistic infections in AIDS in developed and developing countries. *Trans R Soc Trop Med Hyg*, 1990;84:1–6.
14. Abouya Y, Beaumel A, Lucas S, et al. *Pneumocystis carinii* pneumonia. An uncommon cause of death in African children infected with HIV. *JAMA*, 1991;265:1693–1697.
15. Smyth A, Tong CY, Carty H, et al. Impact of HIV on mortality from acute lower respiratory infection in rural Zambia. *Arch Dis Child*, 1997;77:227–230.
16. Graham SM, Mtitimila EL, Kamanga HS, et al. The clinical presentation and outcome of *Pneumocystis carinii* pneumonia in Malawian children. *Lancet*, 2000;355:369–373.
17. Kamiya Y, Mtitimila E, Graham SM, et al. *Pneumocystis carinii* pneumonia in Malawian children. *Ann Trop Paediatr*, 1997;17:121–126.
18. World Health Organisation. Acquired immunodeficiency syndrome (AIDS). WHO/CDC case definition for AIDS. *Wkly Epidemiol Rec*, 1985;61:69–76.
19. Colebunders RI, Greenburg A, Nguyen-Dinh, et al. Evaluation of clinical case definition of AIDS in African children. *AIDS*, 1987;1:151–153.
20. Lepage P, Van de Perre P, Dabis F, et al. Evaluation and simplification of the World Health Organisation clinical case definition for paediatric AIDS. *AIDS*, 1989;3:221–225.
21. Chintu C, Malek A, Nyumbu M, et al. Case definition of paediatric AIDS: the Zambian experience. *Int J STD AIDS*, 1993;4:83–85.
22. Dabis F, Msellati P, Dunn D, et al. Estimating the rate of mother to child transmission of HIV: report of a workshop on methodological issues, Ghent (Belgium), February 17 to 20, 1992. *AIDS*, 1993;7:1139–1148.
23. Bryson YJ, Luzuriaga K, Wara D. Proposed definition of in utero versus intra-partum transmission of HIV-1. *New Engl J Med*, 1992;327:1246–1247.
24. Nesheim S, Lee F, Kalish ML, et al. Diagnosis of perinatal human immunodeficiency virus infection by polymerase chain reaction and p24 antigen detection after immune complex dissociation in an urban community hospital. *J Infect Dis*, 1997;175: 1333–1336.
25. Nielsen K, Bryson YJ. Diagnosis of HIV infection in children. In: *HIV/AIDS in Infants, Children and Adolescents, Pediatric Clinics of North America*. Philadelphia: W.B. Saunders, 2000;47:39–63.
26. Gershy-Damet GM, Koffi K, Abouya L, et al. Salivary and urinary diagnosis of human immunodeficiency viruses 1 and 2 infection in Cote d'Ivoire, using two assays. *Trans R Soc Trop Med Hyg*, 1992;86:670–671.
27. Holme-Hansen C, Constantine NT, Haukenes G. Detection of antibodies to HIV in homologous sets of plasma, urine and oral mucosal transudate samples using rapid assays in Tanzania. *Clin Diagn Virol*, 1993;1:207–214.
28. Tamashiro H, Constantine NT. Serological diagnosis of HIV infection using oral fluid samples. *Bull WHO*, 1994;72:135–143.
29. Tess B, Granato C, Parry JV, et al. Salivary testing for human immunodeficiency virus type 1 infection in children born to infected mothers in Sao Paulo, Brazil. *Pediatr Infect Dis J*, 1996;15:787–790.
30. Sterne JA, Turner AC, Connell JA, et al. Human immunodeficiency virus: GACPAT and GACELISA as diagnostic tests for antibodies in urine. *Trans R Soc Trop Med Hyg*, 1993;87:181–183.
31. Panteleeff DD, John G, Nduati R, et al. Rapid method for screening dried blood samples on filter paper for human immunodeficiency virus type 1 DNA. *J Clin Microbiol*, 1999;37:350–353.
32. Valente P, Sever JL. Early diagnosis and immunological changes in HIV-1 infected pregnant women and their children. *Isr J Med Sci*, 1994;30: 421–430.
33. Bredberg-Raden U, Urassa E, Grankvist O, et al. Early diagnosis of HIV-1 infection in infants in Dar-es-Salaam, Tanzania. *Clin Diagn Virol*, 1995;4:163–173.
34. Quinn TC, Kline RL, Halsey N, et al. Early diagnosis of perinatal HIV infection by detection of viral-specific IgA antibodies. *JAMA*, 1991;266:3439–3442.
35. Parekh BS, Shaffer N, Coughlin R, et al. Human immunodeficiency virus 1-specific IgA capture enzyme immunoassay for early diagnosis of human immunodeficiency virus 1 infection in infants. *Pediatr Infect Dis J*, 1993;12:908–913.
36. Livingston RA, Hutton N, Halsey NA et al. Human immunodeficiency virus-specific IgA in infants born to human immunodeficiency virus-seropositive women. *Arch Pediatr Adolesc Med*, 1995;149: 503–507.
37. Moodley D, Coovadia HM, Bobat RA, et al. HIV-1 specific immunoglobulin A antibodies as an effective marker of perinatal infection in developing countries. *J Trop Pediatr*, 1997;43:80–83.
38. Centers for Disease Control. Revision of the CDC surveillance case definition for acquired immunodeficiency syndrome. *MMWR*, 1987;36(Suppl 1s):1S.

29

Treatment of HIV in Children Using Antiretroviral Drugs

*Gabriel M. Anabwani and †Mark W. Kline

*Princess Marina Hospital, Gaborone, Botswana.
†Baylor College of Medicine, Houston, Texas, USA.

The turning point in the control of pediatric HIV can be attributed to the Pediatric AIDS Clinical Trials Group (PACTG) protocol 076, the landmark study showing the potent effect of zidovudine (ZDV) in preventing mother-to-infant transmission of HIV (1). Since then, rates of perinatal HIV transmission have been dramatically reduced in many parts of the world. Furthermore, better understanding of the biology of HIV and the development of newer and more potent anti-retroviral drugs have enabled physicians to convert HIV infection from a progressively fatal disease to a more chronic, treatable viral infection. In resource-rich countries, these treatment developments have improved the prognosis of pediatric HIV and the quality of life of many HIV-infected children. However, in African countries, where 80% of the world's HIV-infected children live, access to such treatments is limited at best (2).

There is little data on the survival of HIV-infected children who do not receive antiretroviral treatment. Literature from industrialized countries suggests that survival is bimodal: 10% to 20% of those infected progress rapidly and die before reaching the age of 5, while 80% to 90%, like their adult counterparts, survive for a mean of 9 to 10 years following infection (3). Little is known about disease progression in HIV-infected African children, as longitudinal studies have not been conducted. However, because HIV-uninfected African children experience higher infant and child mortality rates than their counterparts in resource-rich countries, it is commonly believed that the proportion of HIV-infected children in Africa who survive 9 to 10 years is significantly less.

The HIV epidemic in Africa paints a very bleak picture. The main obstacles to care are poor health infrastructures that are severely limited by their capacity to serve the people in need. Other obstacles include long distances between health facilities, poor roads and transport systems, weak economies, socio-cultural factors, and, in some cases, inadequate political leadership. However, important changes are taking place. There has been outstanding political leadership at the national level in some countries (notably Uganda, Senegal, and Botswana). The recently launched Bristol-Myers Squibb Company's initiative, Secure the Future, and the Merck Foundation and the Bill and Melinda Gates' donations have provided much needed financial support to certain African countries. Moreover, calls from the United Nations Secretary-General have led to the release of a joint statement of intent in which five pharmaceutical companies (Boehringer Ingelheim GmbH, Bristol-Myers Squibb Company, Glaxo-Wellcome PLC, Merck & Company, and Roche Holding AG) have created programs that aim to reduce prices of antiretrovirals and to increase access to treatment in developing countries. Many international institutions and organizations are active in Africa, working in partnership with governments, local societies, and institutions to find better and more effective ways to ameliorate the ongoing devastation caused by the epidemic. Thus, treatment of HIV in African children using antiretroviral drugs may not be as far-fetched an idea as it would have been just a few years ago.

Guidelines for antiretroviral treatment continue to evolve with new clinical trial data and better understanding of the pathogenesis of HIV. However, because most clinical trials have been done in industrialized countries where there are few HIV-infected children, data on treatment for children continue to lag behind that for adults. This chapter discusses the principles of drug treatment of HIV in children and suggests ways in which they might be applied in African settings. Due to the paucity of clinical trial data from Africa, these suggestions are adapted from current international recommendations, especially those of the United-States-based Working Group on Antiretroviral Therapy and Medical Management of HIV-Infected Children. Their recommendations and others are available online from the HIV/AIDS Treatment Information Service: http://www.hivatis.org (4).

ANTIRETROVIRAL AGENTS CURRENTLY AVAILABLE FOR TREATMENT OF PEDIATRIC HIV INFECTION

In the United States, any drug that is approved by the Food and Drug Administration (FDA) for use in adults can also be prescribed for children. However, most pediatricians are careful to use only those drugs for which appropriate pediatric doses have been established, and safety in children has been demonstrated. In addition, pediatric formulations of some antiretroviral agents are unavailable, largely eliminating their use in children who are unable to swallow tablets or capsules.

Three main classes of antiretroviral agents are currently in use. Within each class, there are various individual agents that are used in various combinations. Currently, monotherapy of any kind is not recommended in HIV treatment.

Nucleoside Reverse Transcriptase Inhibitors

The nucleoside reverse transcriptase inhibitors (NRTIs) undergo intracellular activation to an active 5′-triphosphate form. Viral RNA is used as a template for synthesis of proviral DNA. The active triphosphate derivatives of the NRTIs compete with endogenous deoxynucleotide triphosphates for incorporation into proviral DNA, a process regulated by viral reverse transcriptase. Once incorporated, there is premature termination of elongation of the proviral DNA chain. Generally in combination with one another, NRTIs provide the backbone for most of the combination treatment regimens in use today.

Six NRTIs are being prescribed for children: zidovudine (ZDV), didanosine (ddI), stavudine (d4T), lamivudine (3TC), zalcitabine (ddC), and abacavir (ABC). The formulations, dosing, and common side effects or adverse events of NRTIs are shown in Table 1.

Zidovudine is usually given three or four times daily, but twice-daily dosing is also used. The drug can suppress bone marrow, causing neutropenia or anemia. Reducing the dose or temporarily stopping treatment with ZDV usually manages this side effect.

TABLE 1. Formulations, Side Effects/Adverse Events, and Dosing of NRTIs for Children

Drug	Formulation(s)	Side effects/Adverse events	Dosing
ZDV	Capsule, strawberry-flavored syrup	Bone marrow suppression with neutropenia or anemia[a]	90–180 mg/m^2 body surface area three or four times daily (maximum 200 mg four times daily)
ddI[b]	Chewable orange-flavored tablet, pediatric powder for oral solution	Pancreatitis[c], peripheral neuropathy[d]	90–120 mg/m^2 body surface area twice daily (maximum 200–250 mg twice daily)
d4T	Capsule, oral liquid solution	Peripheral neuropathy[d] (rare in children)	1 mg/kg of body weight twice daily (maximum 40 mg twice daily)
3TC	Tablet, strawberry-banana-flavored liquid	Pancreatitis[c], peripheral neuropathy[d]	4 mg/kg of body weight twice daily (maximum 150 mg twice daily)
ddC[e]	Tablet	Peripheral neuropathy[d], oral ulcers	0.005–0.01 mg/kg of body weight three times daily (maximum 0.75 mg three times daily)
ABC	Tablet, strawberry-banana-flavored liquid	Hypersensitivity reactions	8 mg/kg of body weight twice daily (maximum 300 mg twice daily)

[a]ZDV-associated bone marrow suppression is usually treated by temporarily stopping treatment with the drug, reducing the dose, or giving another medicine to help boost bone marrow activity.
[b]ddI should be administered on an empty stomach and taken with water or apple juice only. Administration of ddI with other liquids or foods reduces absorption by the stomach. The other approved NRTIs may be taken with or without food.
[c]Pancreatitis (inflammation of the pancreas) is a potentially severe, even life-threatening, side effect of therapy with either ddI or 3TC. Symptoms of pancreatitis include abdominal pain and vomiting.
[d]Symptoms of peripheral neuropathy include numbness, pain, or tingling, usually of the arms, legs, hands, or feet. Peripheral neuropathy usually improves or goes away when use of the drug is stopped.
[e]Not approved for use in children younger than 13 years.

Generally, ddI is given twice daily, but some clinicians recommend once-daily dosing for children. Rare side effects of ddI therapy include pancreatitis and peripheral neuropathy. If one of these side effects occurs, it may be necessary to permanently discontinue ddI treatment.

Stavudine is given twice daily. The drug is remarkably well-tolerated and safe for use in HIV-infected children. Although peripheral neuropathy occurs occasionally among HIV-infected adults treated with d4T, this side effect has been observed only rarely among HIV-infected children.

Lamivudine is given twice daily. In combination with ZDV or d4T, 3TC is an important component of several first-line therapies for HIV-infected children. It is generally well tolerated and safe, but some patients have experienced pancreatitis and peripheral neuropathy.

Zalcitabine has not been studied extensively in children. Reported side effects include peripheral neuropathy and oral ulcers.

Abacavir is given twice daily. Approximately 5% of individuals treated with ABC experience signs and symptoms of hypersensitivity or allergic-type reactions, which can include fever, nausea, vomiting, diarrhea, rash, and respiratory distress (4). If such a reaction occurs, treatment with ABC must be permanently discontinued. Administering ABC to an individual who has experienced this reaction can be dangerous or life-threatening.

Nonnucleoside Reverse Transcriptase Inhibitors

Nonnucleoside reverse transcriptase inhibitors (NNRTIs), similar to NRTIs, target the reverse transcriptase enzyme. They directly bind and inhibit the activity of the enzyme, as opposed to NRTIs, which mimic the nuclei acid building blocks of DNA utilized by the enzyme. Because of this synergistic mode of action, NNRTIs have been used in combination with NRTIs and protease inhibitors, and have been found to be generally well tolerated and safe. However, NNRTIs commonly cause skin rashes, including, occasionally, Stevens–Johnson syndrome. This side effect usually develops during the first several weeks following the initiation of NNRTI therapy. In most cases, the rash disappears within a few days, but serious—even life-threatening—rashes can also occur. Viral resistance to one NNRTI generally confers cross-resistance to other members of the class. Formulations and dosing guidelines for the NNRTIs are listed in Table 2.

Protease Inhibitors

The HIV protease inhibitors are active at a late step in viral replication, preventing maturation of infectious virions. Their target is the viral protease enzyme, which is ordinarily responsible for cleavage of large viral polyproteins into smaller, functional units.

TABLE 2. Formulations and Dosing of NNRTIs for Children[a]

Drug	Formulation(s)	Dosing
Nevirapine[b]	Tablet, Suspension	7 mg/kg (age 2 months to 8 years) or 4 mg/kg (age 8 years or older) twice daily (maximum 200 mg twice daily)
Efavirenz	Capsule	200–600 mg according to body weight once daily (maximum 600 mg once daily)
Delavirdine	Tablet	Pediatric dosing guidelines are unavailable

[a]Recommended doses are based on available information from pediatric studies. Dosing may change as additional information becomes available. All of the NNRTIs can cause serious or even life-threatening rashes.

[b]Nevirapine is often given at reduced dose (4 mg/kg/day) for the first 14 days of treatment to help reduce the risk of rash.

Protease inhibitors, like all antiretrovirals, must be taken in the correct doses and on precise schedules. Missed doses can lead to viral resistance and drug failure, possibly limiting future treatment options. In general, viral resistance to one protease inhibitor, like viral resistance to an NNRTI, confers cross-resistance to other members of the class.

All of the protease inhibitors interact pharmacologically with many other agents that are metabolized by the hepatic cytochrome P450 enzyme system. Physicians should exercise extreme caution and carefully review the prescribing information concerning drug interactions before prescribing a protease inhibitor with any other drug.

The formulations, dosing, and common side effects of the protease inhibitors are shown in Table 3. Four protease inhibitors, ritonavir, nelfinavir, amprenavir, and a combination of lopinavir and ritonavir (Kaletra), are available in pediatric formulations. Two others, indinavir and saquinavir, are available only in adult capsules.

Ritonavir is given twice daily and must be taken with food. The liquid form of ritonavir has a very bitter taste, which may be masked by eating peanut butter or drinking chocolate milk before and after taking the drug. In pediatric studies, nausea, vomiting, and hepatitis have caused some children to stop taking the drug (5,6). To help prevent nausea and vomiting, ritonavir may be given in gradually increased doses over a period of 5 days, until the full dosage is reached.

Nelfinavir, available in tablet and powder preparations, is generally given three times daily. Nelfinavir tablets can be crushed or pulverized for children who are unable to swallow pills. The crushed tablets and powder dissolve poorly in liquids, so they should be given suspended in a liquid (such as water, formula, or milk) or mixed with a soft food (such as pudding). Nelfinavir should not be given with citrus juices or in applesauce.

Amprenavir is given twice or three times daily. It is not recommended for children less than 4 years of age (4). Amprenavir can be taken with or without food, but should not be taken with a high-fat meal because of adverse effects on bioavailability.

Kaletra, recently approved by the FDA, is given twice daily with food. Kaletra is a coformulation of the protease inhibitors lopinavir and ritonavir; the latter is present in only a small amount to reduce metabolism and increase plasma levels of lopinavir. Kaletra is available in capsule-form or as an

TABLE 3. Comparing Protease Inhibitors for Children[a]

Drug	Formulation(s)	Side effects	Dosing
Ritonavir	Capsule oral liquid	Nausea, vomiting	400 mg/m^2 body surface area twice daily (maximum 600 mg twice daily)
Nelfinavir	Tablet, powder	Diarrhea	30 mg/kg of body weight three times daily (maximum 750 mg three times daily)
Amprenavir	Capsule, oral liquid	Diarrhea	22.5 mg/kg of body weight twice daily or 17 mg/kg three times daily (maximum daily dose, 2,800 mg)
Lopinavir/ Ritonavir	Capsule, oral liquid	Diarrhea	12/3 mg/kg (7 to <15 kg) or 10/2.5 mg/kg (15 to 40 kg) twice daily (maximum 400/100 mg twice daily)
Indinavir	Capsule	Nausea, vomiting, hematuria, kidney	500 mg/m^2 body surface area every 8 hours (maximum 800 mg every 8 hours)
Saquinavir	Capsule	Diarrhea	50 mg/kg three times daily (maximum 1200 mg three times daily)

[a]Note: Recommended doses are based on available information from pediatric studies. Dosing may change as additional information becomes available. Recommended doses are different when protease inhibitors are used in combination with one another. Always check with a knowledgeable health professional before giving any new medicine to a child who is taking a protease inhibitor.

oral solution. Adverse events observed in children treated with Kaletra are similar to those observed with ritonavir therapy.

Indinavir is usually given every 8 hours on an empty stomach. The drug is available only in capsules; attempts to develop a formulation for young children have been unsuccessful. Most young children will not tolerate the very bitter taste of the contents of indinavir capsules. Some young children may take indinavir capsule contents in applesauce, which can help mask the taste. In pediatric studies of indinavir, some children experienced nausea and vomiting or hematuria (7,8). Crystallization of indinavir in the renal tubules can cause nephrolithiasis. The risk of hematuria and kidney stones can be reduced by encouraging and helping children to drink fluids copiously throughout the day.

Saquinavir is generally used only in combination with another protease inhibitor, such as ritonavir or nelfinavir, to boost its concentration in the blood. The soft gel capsule formulation has better bioavailability than the hard gel capsule. Saquinavir must be given with food. Saquinavir has been safe and well tolerated in initial pediatric studies (9).

Hydroxyurea

Hydroxyurea (HU) is an anticancer drug in widespread use since the 1960s. It was first proposed for the treatment of HIV infection because of its ability to inhibit a cellular protein, ribonucleoside reductase, which represents the rate-limiting step in synthesis of deoxynucleotide triphosphates. These compounds are intracellular competitors of the NRTIs. By reducing their concentrations, HU promotes incorporation of nucleoside analogs into viral DNA by reverse transcriptase, thereby blocking DNA synthesis. This effect appears to be particularly powerful when HU is combined with ddI, probably because of the competition of ddI with deoxyadenosine triphosphate, which HU depletes more completely than other deoxynucleotides. However, HU also enhances the *in vitro* anti-HIV activity of thymidine or cytidine nucleoside analogs by increasing their intracellular phosphorylation (activation), providing a possible rationale for combination therapy with HU and drugs like d4T or 3TC.

Hydroxyurea has several potential advantages over existing ARVs. First, because it targets a cellular rather than viral protein, mutational resistance to the drug is unlikely to occur. Second, there is evidence that HU can compensate for ddI resistance, possibly restoring the drug's activity. This could be a particularly important consideration in the child with extensive ARV experience and few or no remaining therapeutic options. Finally, HU is remarkably inexpensive, which could make the drug particularly valuable in the developing world, where highly active antiretroviral therapy (HAART) is currently prohibitively expensive.

Controlled studies have demonstrated superior reduction in plasma HIV RNA concentrations for HIV-infected adults treated with HU in combination with ddI or d4T/ddI, as compared to those treated with ddI or d4T/ddI alone. Neutropenia or thrombocytopenia, pancreatitis, and peripheral neuropathy have been observed in some adults treated with HU in combination with NRTIs.

Recent advisories have cautioned against the use of HU in combination with d4T plus ddI because of hepatotoxicity and fatal cases of pancreatitis in adults (10). There is very little published experience on the use of HU in HIV-infected children, but one early study found the drug to be well tolerated and safe (11). Additional safety and efficacy data are needed before firm recommendations can be made for the use of HU in HIV-infected adults or children.

CURRENT INDICATIONS FOR TREATMENT OF PEDIATRIC HIV INFECTION

Antiretroviral therapy is rarely initiated in newborns, except in the clinical research

TABLE 4. Indications for Initiation of Antiretroviral Therapy in Children with HIV Infection (4)

- Clinical symptoms associated with HIV infection—CDC clinical categories A, B, or C (see chapter 28, Table 2, *this volume*).
- Evidence of moderate or severe immune suppression, indicated by $CD4^+$ T-lymphocyte absolute number or percentage—immune category 2 or 3 (see chapter 28, Table 3, *this volume*).
- Age less than 12 months, regardless of clinical, immunologic, or virologic status.
- For asymptomatic children aged 1 year or older with normal immune status, two options can be considered:
  (1) Preferred Approach: Initiate therapy, regardless of age or symptom status.
  (2) Alternative Approach: Defer treatment in situations in which the risk for clinical disease progression is low (such as in patients with low viral load and high $CD4^+$ cells) and other factors (for example concern for the durability of response, safety, or adherence) favor postponing treatment. In such cases, the health care provider should regularly monitor virologic, immunologic, and clinical status and should consider initiating therapy if the patient exhibits the following:
    - High or increasing HIV RNA copy number;
    - Rapidly declining $CD4^+$ T-lymphocyte number or percentage to values approaching those indicative of moderate immune suppression—immune category 2 (see chapter 28, Table 3, *this volume*);
    - Clinical symptoms.

setting or as prophylaxis against vertical transmission. Symptoms and signs of HIV infection are rarely present at birth or in the first few weeks of life. Nevertheless, use of direct HIV diagnostic tests, such as DNA PCR, can permit confirmation of HIV infection in the first months of life. Although there have been no controlled studies, strong theoretical arguments favor initiation of treatment as early as possible in newborns to suppress early viral replication.

Current indications for initiating antiretroviral therapy in HIV-infected children in the United States are shown in Table 4. The clinical symptoms and $CD4^+$ T-lymphocyte count value thresholds that are used in determining a patient's need for treatment are outlined in Chapter 28, Tables 2 and 3, *this volume*. The concentration of plasma HIV RNA that is indicative of increased risk for disease progression is not well defined in young children. However, any child with more than 100,000 HIV RNA copies/mL is at high risk for mortality, and antiretroviral therapy should be considered, regardless of age, or clinical or immune status. Physicians may consider initiating treatment in asymptomatic children older than 30 months whose plasma HIV RNA levels are greater than 10,000 or 20,000 copies/mL, levels at which treatment is recommended for adults. In addition, any child whose test results repeatedly demonstrate a substantial increase in plasma HIV RNA level (more than a 0.7 $\log_{10}$, or five-fold, increase in children aged less than 2 years, and more than a 0.5 $\log_{10}$, or three-fold, increase in those aged over 2 years) should be considered for therapy regardless of clinical or immune status, or absolute plasma HIV RNA level.

Table 5 shows the antiretroviral regimens recommended by the Working Group on Antiretroviral Therapy and Medical Management of HIV-Infected Children (4). Triple combination therapy is recommended for most HIV-infected infants and children because of its potential to produce long-term suppression of viral replication, preserve immune function, and delay disease progression. The preferred regimens generally consist of two NRTIs and one protease inhibitor. However, dual NRTI regimens may be suitable alternatives to triple combination therapy in many resource-scarce environments. Well-controlled pediatric studies of these two-drug regimens (ZDV plus 3TC, ZDV plus ddI, or d4T plus ddI) document their safety and efficacy (12–14). Monotherapy of any

TABLE 5. Recommended Antiretroviral Regimens for Initial Therapy for HIV Infection in Children (4)

Strongly recommended:
Based on evidence of clinical benefit and/or sustained suppression of HIV replication in clinical trials in HIV-infected adults and/or children.

- One highly active protease inhibitor plus two NRTIs.
  - The preferred protease inhibitors for infants and children who cannot swallow pills or capsules are nelfinavir or ritonavir. The alternative for those who can swallow pills or capsules is indinavir.
  - Recommended dual NRTI combinations: most data on use in children are available for the combinations of ZDV and ddI, and for ZDV and 3TC. Data that are more limited are available for the combinations of d4T and ddI, d4T and 3TC, and ZDV and ddC.
- Alternative for children who can swallow capsules: Efavirenz plus 2 NRTIs, or efavirenz plus nelfinavir plus 1 NRTI.

Recommended as an alternative:
Based on clinical trial evidence of suppression of HIV replication, but (*i*) durability may be less in adults and/or children than with strongly recommended regimens; or (*ii*) the durability of suppression is not yet defined; or (*iii*) evidence of efficacy may not outweigh potential adverse consequences (including toxicity, drug interactions, and cost).

- Nevirapine plus 2 NRTIs.
- Abacavir plus ZDV plus 3TC.

Offer only in special circumstances:
Clinical trial evidence of limited benefit for patients or data are inconclusive.

- Two NRTIs.
- Amprenavir plus 2 NRTIs or abacavir.

kind, with the exception of ZDV to prevent vertical HIV transmission, is not recommended.

MONITORING PEDIATRIC ANTIRETROVIRAL THERAPY

The activity of an antiretroviral drug regimen may be monitored by routine clinical and neurodevelopmental evaluations, laboratory testing for drug toxicity, and virologic and immunologic testing. In general, long-term (6 months or longer) observations of weight-growth velocity are more meaningful than short-term fluctuations in weight. Marked changes in plasma HIV RNA levels or $CD4^+$ T-lymphocyte count should be confirmed by repeat testing.

CHANGING ANTIRETROVIRAL THERAPY IN CHILDREN

Several circumstances may indicate the need to change a patient's antiretroviral regimen: (*i*) intolerance or toxicity of the current regimen, (*ii*) failure of the current regimen, or (*iii*) evidence that another regimen offers superior results (Table 6). In the instance of treatment failure, a careful evaluation to rule out nonadherence and, when possible, drug resistance, is warranted.

ANTIRETROVIRAL THERAPY: SPECIAL CONSIDERATIONS FOR AFRICAN COUNTRIES

HIV clinicians making treatment decisions in resource-poor settings must consider several additional factors, such as the cost, availability, and sustainability of antiretroviral regimens. These decisions often require finding a balance between what is currently ideal and what may be adequate.

Protease-sparing regimens deserve favorable consideration because the high cost of protease inhibitors places them out of reach for patients with limited financial

TABLE 6. Considerations for Changing Antiretroviral Therapy in HIV-Infected Children (4)

Virologic considerations[a]

- Less than a minimally acceptable virologic response after 8 to 12 weeks of therapy. For children receiving ARV therapy of two NRTIs and a protease inhibitor, such a response is defined as a less than ten-fold (1.0 $\log_{10}$) decrease from baseline HIV RNA levels. For children who are receiving less potent antiretroviral therapy, such as dual NRTI combinations, an insufficient response is defined as a less than five-fold (0.7 $\log_{10}$) decrease in HIV RNA levels from baseline.
- HIV RNA is not suppressed to undetectable levels after 4 to 6 months of ARV therapy.[b]
- Repeated detection of HIV RNA in children who initially responded to ARV therapy with undetectable levels.[c]
- A reproducible increase in HIV RNA copy number among children who have had a substantial HIV RNA response but still have low levels of detectable HIV RNA. Such an increase would warrant change in therapy if, after initiation of the therapeutic regimen, a greater than three-fold (0.5 $\log_{10}$) increase in copy number is observed among children aged 2 years or older, or a greater than five-fold (0.7 $\log_{10}$) increase is observed among children aged less than 2 years.

Immunologic considerations[b]

- Change in immunologic classification (see Chapter 28, Table 3, *this volume*).[d]
- For children with $CD4^+$ T-lymphocyte percentages of less than 15% (those in immune category 3), a persistent decline of five percentiles or more in $CD4^+$ cell percentage (for example, from 15% to 10%).
- A rapid and substantial decrease in absolute $CD4^+$ T-lymphocyte count (for example, a greater than 30% decline in less than 6 months).

Clinical considerations

- Progressive neurodevelopmental deterioration.
- Growth failure defined as persistent decline in weight-growth velocity despite adequate nutritional support and without other explanation.
- Disease progression defined as advancement from one pediatric clinical category to another (for example, from clinical category A to clinical category B).[e]

[a]At least two measurements, taken 1 week apart, should be performed before considering change in therapy.
[b]The initial HIV RNA level of the child at the start of therapy and the level achieved with therapy should be considered when contemplating potential drug changes. For example, an immediate change in therapy may not be warranted if there is a sustained 1.5- to 2.0-$\log_{10}$ decrease in HIV RNA copy number, even if RNA remains detectable at low levels.
[c]More frequent evaluation of HIV RNA levels should be considered if the HIV RNA increase is limited. For example, when using an HIV RNA assay with a lower limit of detection of 1,000 copies/mL, there is a $\leq$0.7 $\log_{10}$ increase from undetectable to approximately 5,000 copies/mL in an infant aged less than 2 years.
[d]Minimal changes in $CD4^+$ T-lymphocyte percentile that may result in change in immunologic category (for example, from 26% to 24%, or 16% to 14%) may not be as worrisome as a rapid substantial change in $CD4^+$ percentile within the same immunologic category (such as a drop from 35% to 25%).
[e]In patients with stable immunologic and virologic parameters, progression from one clinical category to another may not represent an indication to change therapy. Thus, in patients whose disease progression is not associated with neurologic deterioration or growth failure, virologic and immunologic considerations are important in deciding whether to change therapy.

means. The role of HU as a cost-saving agent in children needs further research and definition.

Initiating Antiretroviral Therapy in African Settings

Antiretroviral therapies are largely unavailable in many African settings due to a lack of resources. Before widespread antiretroviral therapy is initiated in such settings, however, public health officials must evaluate the preparedness of health systems to meet the needs of HIV-infected individuals. In general, antiretroviral therapy should not be started without ensuring that facilities for counseling, diagnosis, and laboratory monitoring are in place; that the supply of antiretroviral drugs in the country is adequate; and that a critical number of health professionals have been trained in the management of HIV/AIDS.

Clinicians must be prepared to assess the readiness of patients and their families to begin antiretroviral therapy. The following are some key questions to be considered:

(*i*) Do the patient and his or her family members fully comprehend what is involved? The need for prolonged and probably life-long, costly treatment must be understood from the outset. The importance of adherence to regimens likely to cause unpleasant side effects must be explained. Similarly, the patient must understand the effect that HIV treatment regimens may have on lifestyle, including the need for regular consultations to monitor therapy.

(*ii*) Having understood what is involved, are the patient and family members fully committed to the treatment?

(*iii*) What financial resources are available to the patient and family? Personal finances, insurance, and medical aid opportunities should be considered, as appropriate.

(*iv*) Are any other members of the family infected with HIV or ill, and how does this impact the family's financial resources?

(*v*) How stable is the family?

(*vi*) What social support is available (for example, extended family, friends, school system)?

(*vii*) How accessible is the local health system physically, socioculturally, and financially?

If, after considering these questions, a clinician concludes that a patient or family are not ready for antiretroviral therapy, initiation of treatment should be delayed or postponed.

Issues of Adherence

Adherence is crucial to the success of antiretroviral therapy (15,16,17). Poor adherence results in subtherapeutic drug levels, which lead to the emergence of viral drug resistance that may render entire classes of drugs ineffective. In children, however, adherence poses special challenges (17). First, infants and young children are dependent on others for drug administration. Second, palatable liquid formulations that are appropriate for young children are often unavailable. Third, developmental and psychologic factors associated with adolescence pose additional problems.

A comprehensive assessment of adherence issues should be undertaken with all children for whom antiretroviral therapy is planned, including an evaluation of the caregiver's capacity and willingness to administer a complex regimen, the child's willingness to take the drugs, the availability of potential social support systems, and the availability of a safe place to store the drugs in the home. Disclosure of the child's HIV status should also be discussed. When caregivers keep a child's HIV status secret due to fear of stigma, adherence may be compromised by their reluctance to administer medications in the presence of other members of the family, friends or visitors; reluctance to fill prescriptions in their own neighborhoods; or reluctance to ask others to administer the medications in their absence, such as when the child is in school. Openness about the child's illness can therefore enhance adherence.

Psychologic, social, developmental, and emotional factors that are often associated with adolescence can pose a major hindrance to adherence. These factors include lack of familiarity with local health care systems, misinformation, low self-esteem, rebelliousness, unstructured or chaotic lifestyles, peer pressure, and inadequate social support from the immediate or extended family. Such issues should be explored in a sensitive, compassionate, and culturally appropriate manner before therapy is initiated. Members of a multidisciplinary team may be required to address specific adherence issues. If a complete evaluation is not possible during the first consultation, it should be done in subsequent consultations.

To ensure compliance with prescribed medications, such evaluations should be part of an intensive education program for infected children and their caregivers. Caregivers should be guided in developing individualized plans for drug administration, and encouraged to use appropriate cues and reminders to avoid missed doses. Close follow-up, including pill counts and the monitoring of virologic response are essential in ensuring that adherence is maintained.

Considerations for Stopping Antiretroviral Therapy

Poor adherence or the emergence of life-threatening toxicity warrant discontinuation of antiretroviral therapy. There is little point in continuing treatment in a situation of poor adherence as this increases the risk of drug resistance without any clinical benefits to the patient. Therefore, treatment should be discontinued until the factors leading to poor adherence have been thoroughly evaluated and addressed. When adherence cannot be assured, only follow-up is advised.

Irrespective of a regimen's clinical or virologic efficacy, emergence of life-threatening toxicity contraindicates continuation of treatment. Toxicities should be managed on an individual basis according to specific prescription information.

CONCLUSION

Much needed refinements to the drug management of the HIV-infected child in Africa will depend on the extent to which studies can yield data that are relevant and specific to African pediatric populations and settings. Strategies that simplify drug management regimens to once-daily dosages of fewer pills could improve adherence and minimize the emergence of resistance. Looking to the future, several developments (scientific, economic, and political) are likely to significantly impact the drug management of HIV.

REFERENCES

1. Connor EM, Sperling RS, Gelber R, et al. Reduction of maternal-infant transmission of human immunodeficiency virus type 1 with zidovudine treatment. *N Engl J Med*, 1994;331:1173–1180.
2. AIDS Epidemic Update: December 2000. UNAIDS Web site. Available at: *http://www.UNAIDS.org*. Accessed April 12, 2001.
3. Rogers MF, Lindegren ML, Simonds RJ, et al. Pediatric HIV Infection in the United States. In: Pizzo PA, Wilfert CM, eds. *Pediatric AIDS: The Challenge of HIV Infections in Infants, Children, and Adolescents*. Baltimore: Williams and Wilkins, 1998:3–11.
4. Working Group on Antiretroviral Therapy and Medical Management of HIV-Infected Children. Guidelines for the Use of Antiretroviral Agents in Pediatric Infection. HIV/AIDS Treatment Information Service Web site. Available at: *http://www.hivatis.org*. Accessed April 15, 1999.
5. Mueller BU, Nelson RP Jr, Sleasman J, et al. A phase I/II study of the protease inhibitor ritonavir in children with human immunodeficiency virus infection. *Pediatrics*, 1998;101(3 Pt 1):335–343.
6. Nachman SA, Stanley K, Yogev R, et al. Nucleoside analogs plus ritonavir in stable antiretroviral therapy-experienced HIV-infected children: a randomized controlled trial. Pediatric AIDS Clinical Trials Group 338 Study Team. *JAMA*, 2000;283:492–498.
7. Kline MW, Fletcher CV, Harris AT, et al. A pilot study of combination therapy with indinavir, stavudine (d4T), and didanosine (ddI) in children infected with the human immunodeficiency virus. *J Pediatr*, 1998;132(3 Pt 1):543–546.
8. Mueller BU, Sleasman J, Nelson RP Jr., et al. A phase I/II study of the protease inhibitor ritonavir in children with HIV infection. *Pediatrics*, 1998; 102(1 Pt 1):101–109.
9. Kline MW, Brundage RC, Fletcher CV, et al. Combination therapy with saquinavir soft gelatin capsules in children with human immunodeficiency virus infection. *Pediatr Infect Dis J*, 2001;20: 666–671.
10. DdI, d4T, Hydroxyurea: new pancreatitis warning. *AIDS Treat News*. November 19, 1999;331:1–3.
11. Kline MW, Calles NR, Simon C, et al. Pilot study of hydroxyurea in human immunodeficiency virus-infected children receiving didanosine and/or stavudine. *Pediatr Infect Dis J*, 2000;19:1083–1086.
12. Englund JA, Baker CJ, Raskino C, et al. Zidovudine, didanosine, or both as the initial treatment for symptomatic HIV-infected children. AIDS Clinical Trials Group (ACTG) Study 152 Team. *New Engl J Med*, 1997;336:1704–1712.
13. McKinney RE Jr., Johnson GM, Stanley K, et al. A randomized study of combined zidovudine-lamivudine versus didanosine monotherapy in children with symptomatic therapy-naïve HIV-1 infection. The Pediatric AIDS Clinical Trials Group Protocol 300 Study Team. *J Pediatr*, 1998;133:500–508.
14. Kline MW, Van Dyke RB, Lindsey JC. Combination therapy with stavudine (d4T) plus didanosine (ddI)

in children with human immunodeficiency virus infection. The Pediatric AIDS Clinical Trials Group 327 Team. *Pediatrics*, 1999;103:e62.
15. Centers for Disease Control. Guidelines for the use of antiretroviral agents in HIV-infected adults and adolescents. *MMWR*, 1998;47(RR-5):42–82.
16. Yoved R, Gould E. Acquired Immunodeficiency Syndrome (Human Immunodeficiency Virus). In: Behrman RE, Kliegman RM, and Jenson HB, eds. *Nelson Textbook of Pediatrics*, 16th ed. Philadelphia: WB Saunders, 2000:1029.
17. Working Group on Antiretroviral Therapy and Medical Management of HIV-Infected Children. Guidelines for the Use of Antiretroviral Agents in Pediatric HIV Infection. HIV/AIDS Treatment Information Service Web Site. Available at: *http://www.hivatis.org*. Accessed January 10, 2001.

30

Pediatric Opportunistic Infections

*Shahin Lockman and †Kenneth McIntosh

**Department of Immunology and Infectious Diseases, Harvard School of Public Health, Boston Massachusetts, USA.*
†Division of Infectious Diseases, Children's Hospital/Harvard Medical School, Boston Massachusetts, USA.

SPECTRUM OF PEDIATRIC OPPORTUNISTIC INFECTIONS IN AFRICA

Data describing the etiology of pediatric opportunistic infections (OIs) in Africa are limited, and often derive from studies of hospitalized children rather than cohorts of prospectively followed HIV-infected infants. Although the term "opportunistic infection" is used, "opportunistic disease" might be more appropriate, as some of the disorders that disproportionately affect both HIV-infected children and adults have noninfectious etiologies (such as some malignancies). There is also an element of uncertainty in many of the published series, since the determination of pediatric HIV status is often based at least in part on serology, which is known to be inaccurate during the first 15 to 18 months of life.

The studies that have been conducted generally find that HIV-infected children in Africa suffer most frequently from pneumonia, diarrhea, bacteremia, failure to thrive, and lymphadenopathy. A study of consecutively hospitalized children in Côte d'Ivoire found that respiratory infections (26%) and malnutrition (26%) were the most common diagnoses among 338 HIV-1 antibody-positive children, and these diagnoses were significantly more common among the HIV-positive children than among the HIV-negative children admitted to the same hospital (1). In another study from Durban, South Africa, 48 children with vertically transmitted HIV infection were followed for a mean of 26 months, and diarrhea (78%), pneumonia (76%), and lymphadenopathy (70%) were the most frequent findings (2). Twenty-five of these children died during follow-up at a mean age of 10 months (but up to 48 months) of age; the most common diagnoses at the time of death were diarrhea, pneumonia, failure to thrive, and severe thrush, with 71% of the deaths associated with diarrhea or respiratory infection (3).

Mortality is consistently higher among hospitalized children who are HIV-positive than among those who are HIV-negative. The mortality rate among 354 hospitalized, HIV-positive, Zambian children between 6 months and 5 years of age was 19%, a rate significantly higher than that among the study's 912 hospitalized HIV-negative children (9%) ($p < 0.0001$) (4). A study conducted in Côte d'Ivoire also found a higher mortality rate among hospitalized children who were HIV-positive (21%) than among those who were HIV-negative (9%) (relative risk, 2.4; 95% CI, 1.9–3.1), with the highest death rate in children less than 15 months of age (1).

The following subsections will describe the most commonly identified OIs in HIV-infected children in Africa, and are divided into general body systems and their associated OIs.

Pulmonary Diseases and Tuberculosis

Pediatric autopsy studies have provided valuable information about the etiology of severe disease in HIV-infected children. One pediatric autopsy study from Côte d'Ivoire found that respiratory tract infections were more common in 78 HIV-positive children (94%) than in 77 HIV-negative children (68%), and median ages at death were 18 and 21 months, respectively ($p<0.05$) (5). *Pneumocystis carinii* was detected in 31% of HIV-positive children aged less than 15 months, but in none of the HIV-negative children (5). A second study from Zimbabwe, where HIV status is determined almost entirely by serology, reported the results of autopsies performed on 184 children less than 5 years of age who died at home: 122 children (64%) were HIV–antibody-positive, and among them, *P. carinii* pneumonia (PCP) was present in 19 (16%), probable cytomegalovirus (CMV) pneumonia in nine (7%), lymphoid interstitial pneumonitis (LIP) in 11 (9%), tuberculosis (TB) in six (5%), and a potential bacterial pathogen (detected by lung aspirate) in 106 (87%) (6); among the 62 HIV–antibody-negative children, TB was identified in two (3%), and a bacterial pathogen in 46 (74%) (6). Malnutrition was found in 58% of all the children, and was associated with bacterial lung infection in both HIV-positive and HIV-negative children (6). A third autopsy study, conducted in Botswana among 46 children with a median age of 10 months, found evidence of respiratory tract infection in more HIV-positive than HIV-negative children (97% versus 64%, $p = 0.007$) (7). Thirty-two of the children (70%) were HIV-positive; PCP was responsible for 31% of overall deaths in the HIV-positive children, and for 48% of deaths in those less than 12 months of age. Tuberculosis was found in 13% of HIV-positive children; the median age at death of HIV-positive children with TB was 36 months, compared with 4 months for children with PCP ($p=0.02$) (7). Interstitial pneumonitis was seen in 63% of HIV-positive children, and was ascribed to CMV, respiratory syncytial virus (RSV), LIP, and adenovirus in 25%, 13%, 6%, and 3%, respectively (7). These autopsy studies found PCP to be virtually confined to infants under 1 year of age. *Pneumocystis carinii* pneumonia was also more common in young children than in adults in Africa, an observation that has implications for both treatment of pulmonary disease and prophylaxis against PCP in infants in Africa.

Other studies have evaluated children prospectively. A South African study followed 194 children with respiratory symptoms lasting for more than 1 month, 138 (71%) of whom were HIV-infected (8). Twenty-eight of the HIV-infected children underwent invasive investigation because their symptoms persisted for more than 3 months despite treatment. Of these, 16 (57%) had LIP, four (14%) had other forms of interstitial pneumonia, and eight (29%) had TB. Among 14 HIV-negative children with symptoms lasting for more than 3 months, four (29%) had interstitial pneumonitis, four (29%) had TB, and three (21%) had bronchiectasis (8). A different report from South Africa describes the results of lymph node aspirate and biopsy in 45 children with lung disease lasting for at least 1 month as well as generalized lymphadenopathy (9). Twenty-seven (60%) of these children were HIV-positive. Tuberculosis was the final diagnosis in 11 (41%) of the 27 HIV-positive children and in 12 (67%) of the 18 HIV-negative children undergoing lymph node biopsies (9).

As discussed earlier, mortality among HIV-positive children is greater than that among HIV-negative children, including among those with pulmonary disease. Of 132 children admitted to a rural Zambian hospital with acute lower respiratory tract infection (ALRI), 14 (11%) were HIV-positive and 21 (16%) died; the relative risk for death in the HIV-positive compared to the HIV-negative children was 2.6 ($p = 0.08$) (10).

These studies describe the general spectrum of various respiratory diseases among HIV-infected children in Africa. Other investigators have studied specific pathogens, and in some instances evaluated the clinical presentation of these pathogens in HIV-positive compared with HIV-negative children. The following is a brief summary of these data.

Tuberculosis, the most important OI among HIV-infected adults in Africa, is difficult to diagnose in infants, and the strength of association between pediatric HIV and TB remains somewhat unclear, as do differences in the clinical presentation of TB in pediatric patients with and without HIV infection. Surveillance in the United States has shown that rates of pediatric TB are rising concomitantly with rates of HIV in some locales (11). Furthermore, cross-sectional studies in children with TB have found high (11% to 64%) HIV infection rates relative to the rates in children without TB (12,13). Studies of birth cohorts of infants infected with HIV perinatally have not, however, shown higher rates of TB in comparison to HIV-negative children, and the TB cases that were found in such studies were usually in children older than 15 months of age (2,14). These differences may arise from the difficulty of diagnosing TB in children as well as from study design. Clinical presentation was not found to differ significantly between HIV-infected and -uninfected children with TB in a study conducted among 237 Zambian children between 1 month and 14 years of age. Eighty-eight of them were HIV-positive, and pulmonary TB was the predominant clinical presentation in both HIV-positive and HIV-negative children (90% and 85%, respectively) (13). Another study of children with TB, conducted in Abidjan, Côte d'Ivoire, did not detect differences in chest x-ray (CXR) findings, general site of TB disease, or site of extrapulmonary TB among children with and without HIV (15). Differences in the clinical presentations of HIV-positive versus HIV-negative children with TB were seen, however, among 161 hospitalized children with TB in South Africa: lung cavities and miliary TB on CXR and chronic weight loss were more common in HIV-positive children, and the mortality rate among HIV-positive children (13%) was higher than that among HIV-negative children (2%) during the study period ($p = 0.03$) (16).

As noted, PCP is relatively common in children in Africa. A prospective study in Malawi of children aged 2 months to 5 years admitted to an urban hospital with radiologically proven severe pneumonia identified

P. carinii by immunofluorescent stain of nasopharyngeal aspirate (NPA) in 16 (11%) of 150 children; all 16 children with PCP were HIV-positive (17). Upon admission, children with PCP had lower oxygen saturation ($p = 0.003$), fewer focal findings on lung exam ($p = 0.003$), more interstitial infiltrates ($p = 0.0006$) and hyperinflation ($p = 0.006$) on CXR, and less consolidation on CXR ($p = 0.004$) than children with bacterial pneumonia. All children with PCP were between 2 and 5 months of age, and, despite treatment with high-dose oral cotrimoxazole, a larger proportion (63%) of them died before discharge compared with children with bacterial pneumonia (29%) ($p = 0.04$). In analysis, the authors found that the effects of HIV status and PCP on mortality were independent (17).

Viruses and their clinical presentation have rarely been evaluated in HIV-infected children with pneumonia in Africa. One group in South Africa tested nasopharyngeal aspirates of 990 children aged 2 months to 5 years, who were admitted to the hospital with severe lower respiratory tract infection, for RSV, influenza A and B, parainfluenza 1–3, and adenovirus antigens (18). Forty-seven percent of the children were HIV-positive. The relative risk of the development of severe lower respiratory tract infection associated with viruses was more than six times higher for HIV-infected than for HIV-uninfected children less than 2 years of age, but viruses were a proportionally less common cause of severe pneumonia in the HIV-positive children. Respiratory syncytial virus was the most common viral pathogen isolated in HIV-negative children, while parainfluenza virus and RSV were isolated with approximately equal frequency in HIV-positive children. The in-hospital mortality rate was greater for HIV-infected (14%) than HIV-negative children (2%) ($p < 0.0001$) overall, and was also greater for HIV-infected (8%) than HIV-uninfected (0%) children with viral-associated pneumonia ($p = 0.001$) (18).

Detailed information on the etiology of bacterial pneumonia in children in Africa with HIV is not available, although bacterial pneumonia in these individuals is not rare. In general, when children with pneumonia have had blood cultures performed in Africa, *Streptococcus pneumoniae*, *Haemophilus influenzae* species, *Staphylococcus aureus*, and *Escherichia coli* have been most frequently identified, including in a study of severe pneumonia among children ages 2 to 60 months admitted to a hospital in South Africa (19). It is also important to mention that in this same study, 60% of the *S. aureus* and 86% of the *E. coli* isolates were resistant to methicillin and cotrimoxazole, respectively. In an autopsy study from Zimbabwe, *Klebsiella* was the most frequently isolated organism from postmortem lung aspirates in both HIV-infected and -uninfected infants (6).

Fungal pneumonias (including cryptococcal and histoplasma) and CMV pneumonia have not yet been specifically and systematically sought in HIV-infected children in Africa. Fungal pneumonias are likely to be quite rare.

Gastrointestinal Diseases and Nutritional Disorders

HIV-infected children in Africa have significantly higher rates of acute and persistent (at least 14 days) diarrhea than HIV-negative children, as described in a study among 238 Zairian infants, 22% of whom were HIV-positive (20). Persistent diarrhea in both HIV-infected and -uninfected infants was also associated with symptomatic maternal HIV infection in the same study. More persistent and severe diarrhea, often accompanied by evidence of malnutrition, has also been associated with HIV-seropositivity in infants elsewhere in sub–Saharan Africa (21–24). HIV-infected infants with diarrhea are more likely to die from diarrheal illness than HIV-negative infants (20, 24).

The prevalence of specific stool pathogens is generally similar in both HIV-positive and HIV-negative children, even though the clinical outcome is usually worse among those infected with HIV (20,23). This statement applies to various species of enteropathogenic *E. coli* as well as other bacterial diarrheas (22,25).

The presence of intestinal parasites in children from Africa with and without HIV infection has been evaluated. In a Tanzanian study among children aged 15 months to 5 years, intestinal parasites were detected in approximately 50% of HIV-positive and HIV-negative children with chronic diarrhea as well as in controls without diarrhea (26). The most common diarrhea-associated pathogens found in these children were *Entamoeba histolytica*, *Cryptosporidium parvum*, and *Giardia lamblia*; rates of detection of these pathogens did not differ between HIV-positive and HIV-negative children (26). Rates of cryptosporidiosis, microsporidiosis, and cyclosporiasis among 74 children with acute or chronic diarrhea in Tanzania were also similar in the HIV-positive and -negative children (27). However, somewhat higher rates of *Cryptosporidium* were found in HIV-positive (14%) than HIV-negative (6%) children hospitalized with diarrhea in Zambia ($p = 0.01$), and in HIV-positive children with chronic diarrhea (21%) compared with HIV-positive children with acute diarrhea (5%) (28). Among 18 HIV-positive children hospitalized with diarrhea in Zimbabwe, none had *Enterocytozoon bieneusi* detected in their stools (although *E. bieneusi* was detected in 10% of the 202 adult patients with HIV and diarrhea) (29).

Few studies have looked for viruses associated with pediatric diarrhea in Africa. In Zambia, among 537 children hospitalized for diarrhea, 132 (25%) were found to have both HIV and rotavirus infection. Rotavirus infection was neither more common nor more severe in the HIV-positive than in the HIV-negative children (30). In a more recent study from South Africa however, rotavirus was the most common pathogen isolated from the stools of 176 children admitted to the hospital with diarrhea, and trended toward being more common among HIV-positive (36%) than HIV-negative (15%) children ($p = 0.06$) (25).

Reports on the presence of *Mycobacterium tuberculosis*, *Isospora belli*, and viruses other than rotavirus in HIV-infected children with diarrhea in Africa were not found. *Mycobacterium tuberculosis* has been isolated in 13% of stools of HIV-infected adults with diarrhea in Kenya (31), however, and *I. belli* is associated with chronic, severe diarrhea in South America. It would be useful to look for these pathogens in HIV-infected infants with diarrhea in Africa.

Oral thrush is common among HIV-infected infants. Children with HIV were found to be more likely to have oral thrush in Zimbabwe (odds ratio, 2.7; 95% CI, 1.2–6.4) (32) and Nigeria (33) than HIV-negative children. *Candida*, herpes simplex, and CMV esophagitis presumably exist in immunosuppressed children in Africa, as elsewhere in the world, but studies on these entities have not been published. HIV-infected children are also at risk of recurrent herpes simplex gingivostomatitis.

Malnutrition among children with HIV is common. Twenty-five percent of African children with malnutrition are HIV-infected, and the pattern of malnutrition in HIV-positive and HIV-negative children cannot be distinguished (34). Studies of the etiology of pediatric malabsorption in HIV-infected children suggest that lactose and carbohydrate malabsorption may occur even in the absence of enteric infection (35) and are perhaps due to a direct impact of HIV on the gastrointestinal tract.

Bacteremia and Other Systemic Infections

Bacteremia is fairly common among hospitalized, HIV-infected children in Africa. Among 309 children admitted to a hospital in Zimbabwe at a median age of 5 months, 168 (54%) of whom were diagnosed with HIV infection, those with HIV had an increased risk of bacteremia (40% vs. 20%; odds ratio

2.7; 95% CI, 1.6–4.6), and children with bacteremia had a higher rate of mortality (odds ratio, 2.0; 95% CI, 1.1–5.4) (36). The most common organisms identified were *S. aureus* (22 children), *S. pneumoniae* (20 children), nontyphoidal *Salmonella* (10 children), *E. coli* (four children), and *Klebsiella* species (four children) (36). In 212 infants less than 5 years of age who died at home in Zimbabwe, 122 (58%) of whom were HIV-positive, bacteremia was present in 92 (43%) blood cultures taken within 3 hours of death, and was associated with the presence of malnutrition, but was not associated with HIV infection when the analysis was corrected for malnutrition (37). *Klebsiella* species and *E. coli* were the most frequently isolated organisms (37). A prospective hospital-based study conducted in South Africa identified 49 patients less than 13 years of age with *S. pneumoniae* bacteremia, 25 (51%) of whom were HIV-positive (38). The incidence of *S. pneumoniae* bacteremia was 37 times higher in HIV-positive than in HIV-negative children (38).

These studies did not culture for fungus and mycobacteria. *Mycobacterium tuberculosis* may be the most common cause of bacteremia in febrile hospitalized adult patients (39), and it would be useful to evaluate HIV-infected children in Africa for mycobacteremia.

Measles is not frequently described in large series of HIV-infected children. When it occurs, however, it appears to be somewhat more severe than in HIV-uninfected children. In one autopsy series from Côte d'Ivoire, it was seen in 19% of older HIV-infected children, compared to 4% of HIV-uninfected children ($p < 0.06$) (5).

It should be noted that thus far, there is no evidence that malaria is more common or more severe among children with HIV.

Neurologic Diseases

Central nervous system (CNS) involvement in children with HIV can present in an acute or subacute fashion, and may be due to CNS infection with OIs or common CNS pathogens, malignancy, HIV encephalopathy, or stroke. Much of the CNS disease associated with HIV infection in children, however, cannot be directly ascribed to specific causes, and occurs gradually (either as a progressive encephalopathy with motor, cognitive, and behavioral deficits, or in a more static fashion with delay in development of motor, cognitive, and language skills) (40–42). There is good evidence that HIV itself infects the CNS and can cause neuropathologic changes.

The prevalence and etiology of neurologic diseases in HIV-infected infants in Africa have not been well elucidated. Sixty-one HIV-infected infants followed from birth to 24 months in Uganda were found to have lower mental and motor development scores than 234 HIV-uninfected infants of HIV-positive mothers and 115 infants of HIV-negative mothers (43). In a pediatric autopsy study in Côte d'Ivoire, the neuropathology of 76 HIV-infected and 77 HIV-negative children was compared: among the HIV-positive children, HIV encephalitis was found in four (5%), CMV in two (3%), toxoplasmosis in three (4%), lymphocytic meningitis in 24 (32%), and measles encephalitis in one (1%) (44). None of the HIV-negative children were found to have toxoplasma or CMV encephalitis, and none of the children in either group had CNS lymphoma (44).

In this and another study conducted in the same city, meningitis was equally common in both HIV-positive and HIV-negative children (1,35). A retrospective study of the etiology and cerebrospinal fluid findings of South African children with bacterial meningitis reported that HIV-infected children had significantly more *S. pneumoniae* and less *H. influenzae* and *Neisseria meningitidis* isolated than HIV-negative children; *S. pneumoniae* replaced *H. influenzae* type b as the dominant cause of meningitis in South Africa (45).

The clinical and radiologic features of tuberculous meningitis in 30 HIV-negative and 10 HIV-positive children were compared in South Africa (46). Those infected with HIV were younger, had a shorter duration of symptoms, and a greater degree of ventricular and gyral enhancement and cerebral atrophy on computed tomography (CT) of the brain; they also suffered a worse outcome than the HIV-negative children (three of the 10 died while none of the 30 HIV-negative children died ($p = 0.01$) (46).

Neither descriptions of other causes of meningitis in HIV-infected children in Africa, such as cryptococcal or toxoplasma meningitis, nor reports of primary CNS lymphoma in HIV-positive children in Africa have been published.

Dermatologic Diseases

The following is a summary of the more important dermatologic OIs that have been described in children in Africa.

Kaposi's sarcoma (KS), a vascular malignancy associated with human herpesvirus-8 (HHV-8) infection, is more common in HIV-positive persons, although it can also be found in HIV-negative individuals. A retrospective study conducted in Zambia found that 85 (9%) of the 915 histopathologically confirmed cases identified between 1980 and 1992 were in children 14 years of age or younger; the number of annual cases increased toward the end of the study period (47). The youngest child with KS was 7 months old, the mean age was 5.6 years, the male:female ratio was 1.8:1, and 78% initially presented with lymph node KS (47). Children with blood transfusion-related HIV had cutaneous or lymphocutaneous disease. Another report from Uganda of 100 cases of KS in children under 15 years of age found that their median age was 4 years, the male:female ratio was also 1.8:1, and 78% of the cases were HIV-positive (48). Kaposi's sarcoma tumors in these children had lymphadenopathic and mucocutaneous distributions, with an orofacial pattern in 79% and an inguinal-genital pattern in 13%; these patterns suggest mucosal routes of HHV-8 entry, possibly during breastfeeding. DNA sequences of HHV-8 were found in all of the eight cases tested (48).

It is difficult to distinguish bacillary angiomatosis (BA) from KS on physical exam; BA, caused by the bacterium *Bartonella henselae*, can cause vascular skin lesions and lesions in other organs that appear similar to those of KS. Thus far, one report of pediatric BA in Africa has been published from Zimbabwe (49).

Recurrent herpes zoster is frequent among adult patients with HIV in many parts of the world, including Africa, and reports of herpes zoster in children in Africa do exist. For example, among 200 consecutive patients with herpes zoster in Tanzania, age ranged from 10 months to 80 years, and all seven of the children less than 7 years of age were found to be HIV-positive (50). Molluscum contagiosum has been rarely reported in HIV-infected children in Africa; these lesions tend to be more widespread and larger in HIV-positive than in HIV-negative children.

Cancer

The most common tumors associated with pediatric HIV infection in Africa are non-Hodgkin's lymphoma (NHL) and KS (discussed earlier) (51,52). Investigators in Zambia looked retrospectively at the histopathologic records of children with cancer in 1990–1992 compared with 1980–1982 (pre-HIV epidemic). They found a very significant increase in the numbers of KS cases ($p < 0.0001$), an increase in retinoblastoma ($p = 0.02$), and increasing trends in NHL, nasopharyngeal carcinoma, and rhabdomyosarcoma (53). Among 78 HIV-positive children who died while hospitalized in Côte d'Ivoire and underwent autopsies (with a median age of 17 months), however, none had NHL (54).

DIAGNOSIS OF PEDIATRIC OPPORTUNISTIC INFECTIONS IN AFRICA

General

This section outlines some general approaches to the diagnosis of the etiology of the most common presenting syndromes in children suspected of having HIV in Africa. It is recognized that many laboratory and radiology techniques that optimize the ability to diagnose some of these conditions are not readily available in many African settings.

Pulmonary Diseases

Patient history and physical examination will help determine whether or not a child has very severe disease, severe ALRI, non-severe ALRI, or is not very ill, by World Health Organization (WHO) criteria. In severe or very severe cases, CXR should also be obtained where available. The diagnosis of the etiology of ALRI in infants and children is notoriously difficult, and the causative role of potential pathogens that are isolated is uncertain. Sputum samples of good quality are rarely available from children. Nevertheless, particularly with the aid of more recent laboratory techniques, a reasonable diagnostic evaluation can be performed for pediatric ALRI.

Bacterial ALRI usually presents with focal consolidation on CXR. Lung puncture and aspiration is the most sensitive and specific method for identifying bacterial pathogens associated with pediatric ALRI, but is labor-intensive and may carry excessive risk to the infant, making blood culture a more appropriate although less sensitive diagnostic approach. Large studies of children with ALRI have revealed rates of blood culture positivity of 9% to 18% (55–59), with higher rates in HIV-infected children (19). The close association between nasopharyngeal pneumococcal colonization and incidence of invasive pneumococcal disease has been established (although its presence does not always mean causation) (60). It is helpful, where possible, to obtain one aerobic blood culture from a child with suspected ALRI prior to starting antibiotics.

Mycobacterium tuberculosis, a pathogen of great importance in sub-Saharan Africa among both HIV-infected and -uninfected children, poses a significant diagnostic challenge in infants. The diagnosis of pediatric TB often relies on history of close exposure to a person with active TB, clinical history, Mantoux tuberculin skin test (TST), and CXR. Children with active TB often present with prolonged cough or fever (for at least 3 weeks), pneumonia not responding to antibiotic treatment, malnutrition, and large axillary or neck lymph nodes. It is worth checking a TST in a child with suspected TB, but it must be borne in mind that the TST is not a sensitive indicator of TB infection in an HIV-infected child. Although TSTs can be difficult to interpret in children who have received Bacille Calmette-Guérin (BCG) vaccination at birth (as occurs in most of Africa), a large TST survey among children 3 to 60 months of age in Botswana suggested that the TST remains helpful in diagnosing children who have been infected with *M. tuberculosis*, despite prior BCG vaccination (61). Chest x-rays of children with TB most often reveal adenopathy, but can also show consolidation, cavitation, or a miliary pattern, among others. Among 27 HIV-infected and 18 HIV-uninfected children studied in South Africa with persistent lung disease and generalized lymphadenopathy, dense patchy opacity with mediastinal adenopathy was the most frequently found CXR abnormality in children with TB, and was more common among children found to have TB in both groups than among those without TB (9). Early morning gastric lavage and aspirate remains the most useful tool in the diagnosis of pediatric TB in HIV-positive and -negative infants in Africa, with an estimated sensitivity of 32% to 50% (62–64), a rate higher than that of bronchoalveolar lavage (63,64). A recent study from South Africa reports that sputum induction was successfully performed on 142 out of 149 infants whose HIV-positive status was known or suspected, or who required intensive care unit support, and who were admitted with acute pneumonia (mean age 9 months, 70% HIV-infected) (65). Sputum induction was safe and had a slightly higher yield on *M. tuberculosis* culture than did gastric lavage (absolute difference 4%, $p = 0.08$). The rates of positive microscopy and bacteriology have been found to be similar in HIV-positive and HIV-negative children hospitalized with TB in South Africa (16).

Pneumocystis carinii pneumonia is common in infants who are not receiving PCP prophylaxis, but is extremely difficult to diagnose in children. Children often present with nonproductive cough, tachypnea, and tachycardia; auscultation of the chest may not reveal abnormal breath sounds. Among 151 HIV-infected children (median age 9 months) hospitalized with pneumonia in South Africa, 10% were found to have PCP on examination of induced sputum or bronchoalveolar lavage specimens; children with PCP were younger (3 vs. 10 months, $p < 0.001$) and had more severe pneumonia as reflected by a higher respiratory rate (63 vs. 50, $p < 0.001$), higher heart rate (160 vs. 140, $p = 0.03$), and greater incidence of cyanosis (53% vs. 25%, $p = 0.03$) compared with children without PCP (66). High serum lactate dehydrogenase was associated with PCP, but no CXR findings were diagnostic of PCP in these children (66). A separate article confirmed that children with PCP tend to be more ill at admission than children with pneumonia in whom *P. carinii* is not detected: among 150 children with radiographically proven severe pneumonia admitted to a hospital in Malawi, 16 had PCP, and those with PCP had a lower mean age, body temperature, and oxygen saturation than children with bacterial pneumonia, were less likely to have a focal abnormality on chest auscultation, and had much higher oxygen requirements (17). *Pneumocystis carinii* pneumonia often appears on CXR as a diffuse rapidly progressive alveolar-interstitial pattern with air bronchograms and interstitial infiltrates, but can also present with patchy (or no) abnormalities, air cyst, pneumothorax, pneumomediastinum, or pleural effusion. Final diagnosis of PCP versus another pathogen cannot be made by CXR. Definitive microbiologic diagnosis in children has traditionally relied upon invasive procedures such as lung aspirate or bronchopulmonary lavage, which cannot be routinely performed in most settings. Gomori methenamine-silver stain and toluidine blue stain have sensitivities of approximately 83% and monoclonal immunofluorescence assay (IFA) has a sensitivity of around 97% for PCP on induced sputa in adults, but induced sputa are difficult to obtain from infants. Immunofluorescence assay and polymerase chain reaction (PCR) of NPA have recently been investigated as alternatives to more invasive techniques. Immunofluorescence assay of NPA performed on 60 children aged 1 to 23 months who were hospitalized in Malawi with ALRI found PCP in five of them (67), but did not identify any of the 15 children with PCP among 151 HIV-positive children with ALRI in South Africa (66). The concordance of PCR and IFA for *P. carinii* is high for induced sputum (68) as well as for oral or nasopharyngeal wash specimens (69, 70). One study comparing induced sputum with NPA IFA results in 110 HIV-infected children less than 2 years of age admitted to the hospital with severe pneumonia in South Africa found PCP in 51% of the children: 50% of the children with PCP were diagnosed by induced sputum alone, 27% by NPA alone, and 23% using both techniques, leading the authors to conclude that induced sputum was more effective than NPA in diagnosing PCP in children ($p < 0.0001$), even in this group with a mean age of 5 months (71). Clinical judgment remains the most important diagnostic tool in most areas of the world. Experienced physicians can correctly predict PCP approximately 80% of the time in adults based on history, physical examination, and CXR (72), but this has not been confirmed to be true for diagnosis in children.

Children with LIP often present with nonproductive cough and slowly progressive hypoxia, with ventilatory failure sometimes occurring during what would otherwise have been a minor intercurrent respiratory illness. Diffuse symmetric interstitial and reticulonodular patterns are usually seen on CXR, occasionally with hilar or mediastinal adenopathy which can easily be mistaken for PCP or TB. It is difficult to diagnose LIP definitively without open lung biopsy.

The detection of specific viruses (for example CMV, RSV, parainfluenza viruses, etc.) is performed primarily for research purposes using antigen capture or PCR of bronchial wash specimens or NPA.

Gastrointestinal Diseases

Laboratory diagnosis of the etiology of persistent diarrhea consists of sending a stool sample (or rectal swab if no whole stool is available) to the laboratory for bacterial culture, and examination for ova and parasites for same-day processing. If sepsis is suspected, a blood culture should be sent as well. Plating on MacConkey agar will allow isolation of *Shigella*, *Salmonella*, and *E. coli*. Children with bloody diarrhea should have stool cultured for *Shigella* and examined for *E. histolytica*. Pathogenic *E. coli* will grow on MacConkey agar, but need specialized testing to be differentiated from nonpathogenic species, which will also readily grow on MacConkey plates. *Campylobacter* species can only be grown under special conditions. HIV-infected children with nonbloody chronic diarrhea can also have fresh stool examined for *Cryptosporidium* and *Isospora*. Modified acid-fast bacillus (AFB) stain will allow the detection of *Cryptosporidium* and wet mount or AFB stain will facilitate the detection of *Isospora*, which may need to be sought on multiple different specimens as *Isospora* parasites are shed in low numbers intermittently. Approximately two-thirds of HIV-infected children with persistent diarrhea will not have a pathogen associated with diarrhea found, despite this work up.

Oral thrush can usually be diagnosed clinically by the observation of white or beige pseudomembranous plaques and erythema on the oral mucosa. The plaques can be removed with difficulty to uncover a granular base that bleeds easily. The possibility of esophagitis should be entertained for an HIV-infected infant who appears unwilling to swallow. *Candida* esophagitis can occur in a child with or without evidence of oral thrush, although the presence of oral thrush should raise the question of possible *Candida* esophagitis if symptoms of dysphagia are present (73). Barium swallow may show a "moth-eaten" appearance when *Candida* esophagitis exists.

Neurologic Diseases

Children with acute onset of neurologic abnormalities such as depressed level of consciousness, meningismus, focal neurologic abnormalities, or seizures, should be evaluated immediately. If a child presents with a focal abnormality on neurologic exam or new-onset seizures, and access to CT exists, a CT scan should be obtained to look for focal brain lesions (which might suggest OIs such as toxoplasmosis, TB, or lymphoma) or stroke; however, antibacterial treatment should not be delayed while waiting for a CT scan if bacterial meningitis is possible. In most settings, diagnosis and treatment must proceed without radiologic imaging. In such circumstances, the WHO recommends performing lumbar puncture. Cerebrospinal fluid (CSF) should be sent for cell count and differential, protein, glucose, gram stain, bacterial culture, AFB stain, and, if enough fluid remains, for India ink stain to evaluate for *Cryptococcus*.

A recent study found that HIV-infected children with meningitis in South Africa had a lower median CSF neutrophil count (249 cells/ml vs. 400 cells/ml, $p = 0.02$) and lymphocyte count (29 cells/ml vs. 70 cells/ml, $p = 0.02$) than HIV-negative children, although their CSF bacterial gram stain (97% vs. 80%, $p = 0.002$) and culture (97% vs. 85%, $p = 0.02$) were more likely to be positive, suggesting a poor host response among the HIV-positive children (45). Analysis of the CSF will nevertheless provide the best guidance for therapy.

Children with tuberculous meningitis usually do not present with as rapid a course as those with bacterial meningitis, and can exhibit cranial nerve disturbances. In tuberculous meningitis, CSF protein is usually moderately elevated above normal, CSF glucose can be low (although this is not universally true), and lymphocytes usually predominate, particularly later in the course of disease. Acid-fast bacillus stain of CSF sediment detects less than one-third (74) and as few as 2% of cases of tuberculous meningitis (75), depending on the "gold standard" used for comparison. Sensitivity and specificity of *M. tuberculosis* PCR, using clinical suspicion of TB as the gold standard, are higher than AFB smear and TB culture, and have ranged between 37% to 90% and 88% to 100%, respectively (75–79). However, PCR for *M. tuberculosis* is not widely available nor yet approved for this use.

Dermatologic Diseases

The differential diagnosis of pediatric skin diseases will include both primarily HIV-associated disorders such as recurrent or extensive herpes zoster or herpes simplex stomatitis, KS, BA, and widespread molluscum contagiosum, as well as diseases that occur in children in the absence of HIV infection, including impetigo, folliculitis, dermatophytosis, seborrheic dermatitis, scabies, candidal rash, and drug eruption. Skin conditions that are not necessarily associated with HIV tend to be more severe and protracted in children with HIV.

Description of the presentation and appearance of these conditions is beyond the scope of this chapter. It may be difficult to distinguish KS and BA on clinical examination and results of histopathologic examination of a small (2 mm) skin punch biopsy will help to confirm the diagnosis, which can help guide treatment: *Bartonella* bacilli can be seen in BA on Warthin-Starry stain of a biopsy, and each entity has characteristic histopathology. Molluscum contagiosum usually presents with multiple skin-colored papules 2 mm to 4 mm in diameter, which commonly have central umbilication; diagnosis is usually clinical, although biopsy can confirm this diagnosis.

MANAGEMENT OF PEDIATRIC OPPORTUNISTIC INFECTIONS IN AFRICA

General

As is true for diagnostic approaches to ill children, the management of pediatric OIs in Africa will depend on the resources available. Furthermore, the definitive diagnosis of HIV infection in children in Africa can often not be made with certainty, as it requires PCR for children under 15 months of age. Empiric treatment will obviously vary depending on the local prevalence of certain pathogens (for example *N. meningitidis* among children with suspected acute bacterial meningitis). Choice of antibiotic should vary depending on local antibiotic resistance patterns, if these are known and if alternative antimicrobials are available.

Presented here are algorithms recommended by the WHO in resource-limited settings for management of syndromes and illnesses in HIV-infected children (80), as well as—in brief—the management of these illnesses where more resources are available.

Pulmonary Diseases

The WHO has recommended a 5-day course of either oral cotrimoxazole [trimethoprim (TMP) 4 mg/kg, sulfamethoxazole (SMX) 20 mg/kg every 12 hours] or amoxicillin for pneumonia in HIV-uninfected infants, and a 10-day course of cotrimoxazole in HIV-infected infants, with re-evaluation of the infant after 48 hours (80). The WHO recommends that children with severe pneumonia be admitted, undergo CXR, erythrocyte sedimentation rate, blood culture and TST. Children should be started on high-dose cotrimoxazole if PCP is suspected [TMP 5 mg/kg, SMX 25 mg/kg, IV (intravenously) every 6 hours for 21 days]; lower dose cotrimoxazole (TMP 4 mg/kg, SMX 20 mg/kg every 12 hours for 10 days) or IV chloramphenicol if they are 2 months of age or older and bacterial pneumonia is suspected; or IV penicillin and gentamicin if they are younger than 2 months of age (given the higher likelihood of group B *Streptococcus* infection in neonates). Given the clear evidence that PCP occurs almost exclusively in infants between 2 and 10 months of age, high-dose cotrimoxazole should probably be reserved for pneumonia in this age range.

In areas where third generation cephalosporins are available, ceftriaxone (50–75 mg/kg/day) or cefotaxime could be used instead of chloramphenicol or cotrimoxazole for suspected bacterial pneumonia, avoiding problems with toxicity and antimicrobial resistance of some pathogens. Antimicrobial treatment should be tailored to antibacterial sensitivities, when these are known.

If a child with suspected bacterial pneumonia does not improve on these regimens, addition of an anti-staphylococcal agent (such as cloxacillin) may be warranted, and other etiologies such as PCP, TB, LIP, and fungal or viral infections must be considered. In these cases, empiric treatment for PCP may be warranted if induced sputum for *P. carinii* cannot be obtained. This should be continued for a full 21-day course even if no improvement is seen within several days, as clinical improvement with PCP can be delayed, even with appropriate therapy. Children who have severe adverse reactions to cotrimoxazole can be treated with pentamidine (4 mg/kg/day IV for 2 to 3 weeks).

Anti–TB treatment should be considered in children with suspected HIV infection who do not respond to antibacterial and PCP treatment, or in whom clinical suspicion of TB is high. Tuberculin skin test and three early morning gastric lavages should be performed, if possible, to help make the diagnosis. Thiacetazone should be avoided due to increased rates of cutaneous hypersensitivity reactions among HIV-infected children (81). It is preferable to make the diagnosis of LIP on lung biopsy prior to initiation of steroid therapy, but this cannot always be done. Every effort should be made to rule out and treat TB and other pulmonary OIs before initiating empiric prednisone therapy (1–2 mg/kg/day for 2 to 3 weeks) for LIP.

Gastrointestinal Diseases and Nutritional Disorders

Causes of diarrhea and fever such as measles, otitis media, pneumonia, and malaria should be considered. If a specific stool pathogen is found, it should be treated accordingly. HIV-infected children with persistent diarrhea (generally defined as five or more stools per day lasting for at least 14 consecutive days in infants) or bloody diarrhea, should have the etiology of their diarrhea evaluated and, if dehydrated or severely malnourished, should be admitted to the hospital for treatment and evaluation if possible. Children who are being treated as outpatients should be sent home after their caretakers have been given and taught how to administer oral rehydration salts, and seen again after 2 days if they were initially dehydrated, are less than 1 year old, are not improving clinically at home, or are having persistently bloody stools.

Pending results of laboratory tests, or if laboratory testing is not available, the WHO recommends that children with bloody diarrhea be treated with cotrimoxazole (TMP 5 mg/kg, SMX 25 mg/kg orally twice daily for 5 days) to treat possible shigellosis, although high rates of cotrimox-azole-resistant *Shigella* have been documented in Africa (82). If local antibiotic sensitivities are known for *Shigella* species, these should be used to guide antibiotic choice. Nalidixic acid may be useful to treat very ill children with bloody diarrhea in areas with high rates of cotrimoxazole-resistant *Shigella*, as the benefits of quinolone use in this situation likely outweigh the risks.

Children who are not severely ill (i.e., do not have bloody stool, are afebrile, and are neither dehydrated nor malnourished) can be observed for a week while adequate nutrition is maintained. In non-exclusively breastfed infants the WHO recommends that the infant's diet should be modified by the following measures: (a) reduce cooked cereal by half and increase glucose or sucrose to compensate for this reduction, (b) remove animal milk from the diet and provide protein in the form of chicken meat or egg white, (c) add 2.5 cc oil per serving of food, and (d) maintain a total daily intake of 150 cal/kg in six divided feeds.

The WHO recommends the following treatment for ill HIV-infected children with symptomatic HIV and persistent diarrhea in whom certain stool pathogens are isolated. Non-typhoid or extraintestinal *Salmonella* is treated with ampicillin (25 mg/kg every 6 hours for 5 days). Enterotoxigenic and enteropathogenic *E. coli* (but not other strains of *E. coli*) and *Isospora* can be treated with cotrimoxazole (TMP 5 mg/kg, SMX 25 mg/kg every 12 hours for 5 days). *Campylobacter jejuni* can be treated with erythromycin (50 mg/kg/day in four divided doses per day for 5 days). *E. histolytica* is treated with metronidazole (30 mg/kg/day for 5 to 10 days), while *G. lamblia* is treated with half this dose of metronidazole (15 mg/kg/day) for 5 days. *Cryptosporidium* is difficult to treat; various regimens have been tried with little success. Acute diarrhea (less than 14 days) can occur in symptomatic HIV-infected children and can be managed using national or WHO (83) guidelines.

Children who are found to have oral thrush and who are feeding well can be treated with local application of gentian violet (1% aqueous solution) twice daily for 1 week, or with nystatin (100,000 units oral suspension four to six times daily for 1 week). Clotrimazole, miconazole gel, and amphotericin B suspension are other topical treatment options for oral thrush. Empiric treatment for *Candida* esophagitis of a child with oral thrush and difficulty feeding, consists of either ketoconazole (3–6 mg/kg daily orally for 1 week) or fluconazole (3 mg/kg daily orally for 1 week). Ketoconazole should be avoided in the presence of active liver disease. Esophagitis may resolve slowly even if clinical improvement is seen quickly, and prolonged therapy is often needed.

Neurologic Diseases

For children with subacute progressive or static HIV encephalopathy, antiretroviral therapy is the intervention most likely to improve CNS function, particularly if agents with good CNS permeability such as zidovudine are used (84,85). HIV-infected children with acute neurologic abnormalities should be rapidly evaluated at a hospital if possible. If this is not possible, empirical treatment of bacterial meningitis is recommended by the WHO—benzyl penicillin (40,000 international units (IU)/kg every 4 hours) and chloramphenicol (25 mg/kg every 6 hours) in children older than 1 month; and ampicillin and gentamicin in children less than 1 month old. If the child can be seen at a hospital, and fever and meningeal signs are present, lumbar puncture is recommended. The same empirical antibacterial therapy is started intravenously while awaiting laboratory results; treatment is then modified as necessary based on results of CSF analysis. As is true for pneumonia, where cefotaxime or ceftriaxone are available, these provide an easily administered and effective regimen for bacterial meningitis with fewer side effects than chloramphenicol and ampicillin. Children in whom CSF culture yields *H. influenzae* can be treated with ampicillin and chloramphenicol for 14–21 days. The WHO recommends treating *S. pneumoniae* meningitis with benzylpenicillin (50,000 IU/kg every 4 hours IV) for 14–21 days unless *S. pneumoniae* antimicrobial sensitivity patterns suggest otherwise.

If cryptococcus is identified in the CSF, treatment with amphotericin B (0.5–1 mg/kg daily every 6 hours for 6 weeks), followed by suppressive therapy with fluconazole (100 mg daily) indefinitely is recommended wherever possible. Cryptococcal meningitis is very uncommon in children, however.

In children in whom a bacterial, fungal, or mycobacterial pathogen is not identified in the CSF and who do not respond to antibacterials, a CT or magnetic resonance imaging scan becomes even more important to evaluate for focal lesions associated with toxoplasmosis, lymphoma, TB, or another process. If such focal lesions are seen, particularly hypodense ring-enhancing lesions in older children or encephalomalacia and calcification in neonates, empiric treatment for toxoplasmosis may be warranted (pyrimethamine 2 mg/kg for 2 days, then 1 mg/kg daily orally for 6 weeks plus sulfadiazine, 40 mg/kg orally every 12 hours for 6 weeks, and folinic acid 5 mg every 3 days orally while the child is receiving pyrimethamine). If the child responds clinically within 1 to 2 weeks, CNS toxoplasmosis was likely the cause of the acute neurologic deterioration, and daily suppressive therapy with lower-dose pyrimethamine and sulfadiazine plus folinic acid should be continued.

Dermatologic Diseases

The WHO guidelines recommend that children with herpes zoster lesions be treated symptomatically with calamine lotion. Acyclovir can be given for severe infection or to children with advanced HIV disease; oral absorption is poor, and acyclovir should be administered intravenously to children with severe herpes zoster. Children with severe herpes simplex lesions can also be treated with acyclovir (15–30 mg/kg daily orally or IV) for at least 1 week or until the lesions start to clear.

Children with severe molluscum contagiosum or condyloma acuminatum (warts) can be referred for cryotherapy, where this is available. Alternatively, topical podophyllin can be used for condyloma.

HIV-infected children with furunculosis, impetigo, or folliculitis can be treated with cloxacillin or erythromycin until lesions heal. Topical 2% mupirocin can also be tried.

Children with significant *Candida* skin lesions can be treated topically with gentian violet 1% aqueous solution or nystatin ointment twice daily for one week. Those with severe skin involvement who are not responding to topical treatment can receive oral ketoconazole or fluconazole. Dermatophytosis can be treated topically with miconazole cream, 2% twice daily until healed.

PROPHYLAXIS AGAINST PEDIATRIC OPPORTUNISTIC INFECTIONS IN AFRICA

Prophylaxis against *Pneumocystis carinii* pneumonia

Pneumocystis carinii pneumonia occurs in infants most often between 3 and 6 months of age. The HIV status of the vast majority of infants born to HIV-infected mothers in Africa will not be known at this age. Because of the morbidity and mortality associated with PCP in infants, cotrimoxazole prophylaxis against PCP is recommended by the WHO/UNAIDS for all HIV-exposed infants in Africa starting at 4 to 6 weeks of age, regardless of the infant's $CD4^+$ cell count, which is not predictive of the risk of PCP in infants less than 1 year of age (86). Infants who are first identified as being HIV-exposed anytime after 6 weeks of age should have prophylaxis initiated at the time of identification, unless the child has no symptoms of HIV infection and is found to be HIV-seronegative on two or more occasions over 6 months of age. PCP prophylaxis should be continued until at least 15 months of age in all infants known to be HIV-infected and in infants whose infection status has not yet been clearly determined. After 15 months of age, PCP prophylaxis should be continued in HIV-infected children who have had PCP in the past, have symptomatic HIV disease or have had an AIDS-defining illness, or have a $CD4^+$ cell count of less than 500 cells/mm^3 (if 1 to 5 years old), or a $CD4^+$ cell percentage of less than 15% (if less than 13 years old).

The regimen recommended by the WHO/UNAIDS Secretariat is cotrimoxazole syrup (or the equivalent dose of crushed tablet) once per day every day, at a dose of 150 mg/m^2/day of TMP and 750 mg/m^2/day of SMX (86). Alternative regimens include the same daily dose of TMP and SMX, but divided into two doses per day and given on three days per week rather than daily (either on consecutive days, or Mondays, Wednesdays, and Fridays) (87).

Children with severe cutaneous reactions or toxicity should have the cotrimoxazole stopped and may alternatively receive dapsone, 2 mg/kg/day (up to 100 mg/day) or aerosolized pentamidine (300 mg via inhaler once monthly) if the child is 5 or more years old.

Prophylaxis against Tuberculosis

In November 1999 the WHO issued a statement recommending that preventive therapy for TB should be part of a package of care for people living with HIV in settings where it is possible to exclude active TB, and where detection and appropriate treatment of active TB cases are already occurring (88). The WHO recommended targeting TB preventive therapy for HIV-infected persons with Mantoux TSTs $\geq$ 5 mm, groups at high risk for TB, and HIV-infected persons living in populations with an adult prevalence of tuberculous infection estimated to be greater than 30%.

This statement did not specifically address preventive therapy for TB in children. Many would agree, however, that infants with close exposure to AFB sputum smear-positive family members (especially breastfeeding infants of AFB smear-positive mothers) should be given 3 to 6 months of isoniazid (5 mg/kg/day) as prophylaxis against TB if there is no evidence that the infant is suffering from active TB, regardless of TST result.

CONCLUSION

This chapter reviews what is known about the more common OIs in HIV-infected children in Africa and discusses their diagnosis and management, which can be particularly challenging when health-related resources are limited. It is hoped that while our understanding of the optimal approaches to diagnosing and treating pediatric OIs in Africa will continue to increase, the number of new pediatric infections will decrease.

REFERENCES

1. Vetter KM, Djomand G, Zadi F, et al. Clinical spectrum of human immunodeficiency virus disease in children in a west African city. Project RETRO-CI. *Pediatr Infect Dis J*, 1996;15:438–442.
2. Bobat R, Moodley D, Coutsoudis A, et al. The early natural history of vertically transmitted HIV-1 infection in African children from Durban, South Africa. *Ann Trop Paediatr*, 1998;18:187–196.
3. Bobat R, Coovadia H, Moodley D, et al. Mortality in a cohort of children born to HIV-1 infected women from Durban, South Africa. *S Afr Med J*, 1999;89:646–648.
4. Chintu C, Luo C, Bhat G, et al. Impact of the human immunodeficiency virus type-1 on common

pediatric illnesses in Zambia. *J Trop Pediatr*, 1995;41:348–353.
5. Lucas SB, Peacock CS, Hounnou A, et al. Disease in children infected with HIV in Abidjan, Cote d'Ivoire. *BMJ*, 1996;312:335–338.
6. Ikeogu MO, Wolf B, Mathe S. Pulmonary manifestations in HIV seropositivity and malnutrition in Zimbabwe. *Arch Dis Child*, 1997;76:124–128.
7. Ansari NA, Kombe AH, Kenyon TA, et al. Mortality and pulmonary pathology of children with HIV infection in Francistown, Botswana. *30th IUATLD World Conference on Lung Health*; 14–18 September, 1999; Madrid, Spain. Abstract 484-PD.
8. Jeena PM, Coovadia HM, Thula SA, et al. Persistent and chronic lung disease in HIV-1 infected and uninfected African children. *AIDS*, 1998;12:1185–1193.
9. Jeena PM, Coovadia HM, Hadley LG, et al. Lymph node biopsies in HIV-infected and non-infected children with persistent lung disease. *Int J Tuberc Lung Dis*, 2000;4:139–146.
10. Smyth A, Tong CY, Carty H, et al. Impact of HIV on mortality from acute lower respiratory tract infection in rural Zambia. *Arch Dis Child*, 1997;77:227–230.
11. Gutman LT, Moye J, Zimmer B, et al. Tuberculosis in human immunodeficiency virus exposed or infected United States children. *Paediatr Infect Dis J*, 1994;13:963–968.
12. Sassan-Morokro M, De Cock KM, Ackah A, et al. Tuberculosis and HIV infection in children in Abidjan, Cote d'Ivoire. *Trans Roy Soc Trop Med Hyg*, 1994;88:178–181.
13. Chintu C, Bhat G, Luo C, et al. Seroprevalence of human immunodeficiency virus type 1 infection in Zambian children with tuberculosis. *Pediatr Infect Dis J*, 1993;12:499–504.
14. Ryder RW, Manzila T, Baende E, et al. Evidence from Zaire that breastfeeding by HIV-1 seropositive mothers is not a major route for perinatal HIV-1 transmission but does decrease morbidity. *AIDS*, 1991;5:709–714.
15. Mukadi YD, Wiktor SZ, Coulibaly IM, et al. Impact of HIV infection on the development, clinical presentation, and outcome of tuberculosis among children in Abidjan, Cote d'Ivoire. *AIDS*, 1997;11:1151–1158.
16. Madhi SA, Huebner RE, Doedens L, et al. HIV-1 co-infection in children hospitalised with tuberculosis in South Africa. *Int J Tuberc Lung Dis*, 2000;4:448–454.
17. Graham SM, Mtitimila EI, Kamanga HS, et al. Clinical presentation and outcome of *Pneumocystis carinii* pneumonia in Malawian children [published erratum appears in Lancet 2000 Mar 4;355(9206):850] [see comments]. *Lancet*, 2000;355:369–373.
18. Madhi SA, Schoub B, Simmank K, et al. Increased burden of respiratory viral associated severe lower respiratory tract infections in children infected with human immunodeficiency virus type-1. *J Pediatr*, 2000;137:78–84.
19. Madhi SA, Petersen K, Madhi A, et al. Increased disease burden and antibiotic resistance of bacteria causing severe community-acquired lower respiratory tract infections in human immunodeficiency virus type 1-infected children [In Process Citation]. *Clin Infect Dis*, 2000;31:170–176.
20. Thea DM, St. Louis ME, Atido U, et al. A prospective study of diarrhea and HIV-1 infection among 429 Zairian infants. *N Engl J Med*, 1993;329:1696–1702.
21. Esamai F, Buku GM. HIV seropositivity in children admitted with diarrhoea at Eldoret District Hospital, Kenya. *East Afr Med J*, 1994;71:631–634.
22. Pavia AT, Long EG, Ryder RW, et al. Diarrhea among African children born to human immunodeficiency virus 1-infected mothers: clinical, microbiologic and epidemiologic features. *Pediatr Infect Dis J*, 1992;11:996–1003.
23. Johnson S, Hendson W, Crewe-Brown H, et al. Effect of human immunodeficiency virus infection on episodes of diarrhea among children in South Africa. *Pediatr Infect Dis J*, 2000;19:972–979.
24. Keusch GT, Thea DM, Kamenga M, et al. Persistent diarrhea associated with AIDS. *Acta Paediatr Suppl*, 1992;381:45–48.
25. Johnson S, Crewe-Brown H, Dini L, et al. Differences in enteropathogens between HIV positive and negative children in Soweto, South Africa. In: Program and abstracts of the XIII International AIDS Conference; July 9–14, 2000; Durban, South Africa. Abstract MoPpB1090.
26. Cegielski JP, Msengi AE, Dukes CS, et al. Intestinal parasites and HIV infection in Tanzanian children with chronic diarrhea. *AIDS*, 1993;7:213–221.
27. Cegielski JP, Ortega YR, McKee S, et al. Cryptosporidium, enterocytozoon, and cyclospora infections in pediatric and adult patients with diarrhea in Tanzania. *Clin Infect Dis*, 1999;28:314–321.
28. Chintu C, Luo C, Baboo S, et al. Intestinal parasites in HIV-seropositive Zambian children with diarrhoea. *J Trop Pediatr*, 1995;41:149–152.
29. van Gool T, Luderhoff E, Nathoo KJ, et al. High prevalence of *Enterocytozoon bieneusi* infections among HIV-positive individuals with persistent diarrhoea in Harare, Zimbabwe. *Trans R Soc Trop Med Hyg*, 1995;89:478–480.
30. Oshitani H, Kasolo FC, Mpabalwani M, et al. Association of rotavirus and human immunodeficiency virus infection in children hospitalized with acute diarrhea, Lusaka, Zambia. *J Infect Dis*, 1994;169:897–900.
31. Mwachari C, Batchelor BI, Paul J, et al. Chronic diarrhoea among HIV-infected adult patients in Nairobi, Kenya. *J Infect*, 1998;37:48–53.

32. Ticklay IM, Nathoo KJ, Siziya S, et al. HIV infection in malnourished children in Harare, Zimbabwe. *East Afr Med J*, 1997;74:217–220.
33. Akpede GO, Ambe JP, Rabasa AI, et al. Presentation and outcome of HIV-1 infection in hospitalised infants and other children in north-eastern Nigeria. *East Afr Med J*, 1997;74:21–27.
34. Ball CS. Global issues in pediatric nutrition: AIDS. *Nutrition*, 1998;14:767–770.
35. Miller TL, Orav EJ, Martin SR, et al. Malnutrition and carbohydrate malabsorption in children with vertically transmitted human immunodeficiency virus 1 infection. *Gastroenterology*, 1991;100: 1296–1302.
36. Nathoo KJ, Chigonde S, Nhembe M, et al. Community-acquired bacteremia in human immunodeficiency virus-infected children in Harare, Zimbabwe [see comments]. *Pediatr Infect Dis J*, 1996;15:1092–1097.
37. Wolf BH, Ikeogu MO, Vos ET. Effect of nutritional and HIV status on bacteraemia in Zimbabwean children who died at home. *Eur J Pediatr*, 1995;154:299–303.
38. Jones N, Huebner R, Khoosal M, et al. The impact of HIV on *Streptococcus pneumoniae* bacteraemia in a South African population. *AIDS*, 1998;12: 2177–2184.
39. Archibald LK, den Dulk MO, Pallangyo KJ, et al. Fatal *Mycobacterium tuberculosis* bloodstream infections in febrile hospitalized adults in Dar es Salaam, Tanzania. *Clin Infect Dis*, 1998;26:290–296.
40. Epstein LG, Sharer LR, Oleske JM, et al. Neurologic manifestations of human immunodeficiency virus infection in children. *Pediatrics*, 1986;78:678–687.
41. Cooper ER, Hanson C, Diaz C, et al. Encephalopathy and progression of human immunodeficiency virus disease in a cohort of children with perinatally acquired human immunodeficiency virus infection. Women and Infants Transmission Study Group. *J Pediatr*, 1998;132:808–812.
42. Coplan J, Contello KA, Cunningham CK, et al. Early language development in children exposed to or infected with human immunodeficiency virus. *Pediatrics*, 1998;102:e8.
43. Drotar D, Olness K, Wiznitzer M, et al. Neurodevelopmental outcomes of Ugandan infants with HIV infection: an application of growth curve analysis. *Health Psychol*, 1999;18:114–121.
44. Bell JE, Lowrie S, Koffi K, et al. The neuropathology of HIV-infected African children in Abidjan, Cote d'Ivoire. *J Neuropathol Exp Neurol*, 1997;56: 686–692.
45. Madhi S, Madhi A, Peterson K, et al. Changing epidemiology of purulent meningitis in children due to HIV-1 infection. In: Program and Abstracts of the XIII International AIDS Conference; July 9–14, 2000; Durban, South Africa. Abstract WePpB1309.
46. Topley JM, Bamber S, Coovadia HM, et al. Tuberculous meningitis and co-infection with HIV. *Ann Trop Paediatr*, 1998;18:261–266.
47. Athale UH, Patil PS, Chintu C, et al. Influence of HIV epidemic on the incidence of Kaposi's sarcoma in Zambian children. *J Acquir Immune Defic Syndr Hum Retrovirol*, 1995;8:96–100.
48. Ziegler JL, Katongole-Mbidde E. Kaposi's sarcoma in childhood: an analysis of 100 cases from Uganda and relationship to HIV infection. *Int J Cancer*, 1996;65:200–203.
49. Chitsike I, Muronda C. Bacillary angiomatosis in an HIV positive child. First case report in Zimbabwe. *Cent Afr J Med*, 1997;43:238–239.
50. Naburi AE, Leppard B. Herpes zoster and HIV infection in Tanzania. *Int J STD AIDS*, 2000;11: 254–256.
51. Parkin DM, Wabinga H, Nambooze S, et al. AIDS-related cancers in Africa: maturation of the epidemic in Uganda [see comments]. *AIDS*, 1999;13:2563–2570.
52. Chitsike I, Siziya S. Seroprevalence of human immunodeficiency virus type 1 infection in childhood malignancy in Zimbabwe. *Cent Afr J Med*, 1998;44:242–245.
53. Chintu C, Athale UH, Patil PS. Childhood cancers in Zambia before and after the HIV epidemic. *Arch Dis Child*, 1995;73:100–104; discussion 104–105.
54. Lucas SB, Diomande M, Hounnou A, et al. HIV-associated lymphoma in Africa: an autopsy study in Cote d'Ivoire. *Int J Cancer*, 1994;59:20–24.
55. Barker J, Gratten M, Riley I, et al. Pneumonia in children in the Eastern Highlands of Papua New Guinea: a bacteriologic study of patients selected by standard clinical criteria. *J Infect Dis*, 1989;159:348–352.
56. Ghafoor A, Nomani NK, Ishaq Z, et al. Diagnoses of acute lower respiratory tract infections in children in Rawalpindi and Islamabad, Pakistan. *Rev Infect Dis*, 1990;12(Suppl 8):S907–914.
57. Tupasi TE, Lucero MG, Magdangal DM, et al. Etiology of acute lower respiratory tract infection in children from Alabang, Metro Manila. *Rev Infect Dis*, 1990;12(Suppl 8):S929–939.
58. Bahl R, Mishra S, Sharma D, et al. A bacteriological study in hospitalized children with pneumonia. *Ann Trop Paediatr*, 1995;15:173–177.
59. Falade AG, Mulholland EK, Adegbola RA, et al. Bacterial isolates from blood and lung aspirate cultures in Gambian children with lobar pneumonia. *Ann Trop Paediatr*, 1997;17:315–319.
60. Gray BM, Dillon HC Jr. Natural history of pneumococcal infections. *Pediatr Infect Dis J*, 1989;8: S23–S25.
61. Lockman S, Tappero JW, Kenyon TA, et al. Tuberculin reactivity in a pediatric population with

high BCG vaccination coverage. *Int J Tuberc Lung Dis*, 1999;3:23–30.
62. Lobato MN, Loeffler AM, Furst K, et al. Detection of *Mycobacterium tuberculosis* in gastric aspirates collected from children: hospitalization is not necessary. *Pediatrics*, 1998;102:E40.
63. Somu N, Swaminathan S, Paramasivan CN, et al. Value of bronchoalveolar lavage and gastric lavage in the diagnosis of pulmonary tuberculosis in children. *Tuberc Lung Dis*, 1995;76:295–299.
64. Abadco DL, Steiner P. Gastric lavage is better than bronchoalveolar lavage for isolation of *Mycobacterium tuberculosis* in childhood pulmonary tuberculosis. *Pediatr Infect Dis J*, 1992;11:735–738.
65. Zar HJ, Tannenbaum E, Apolles P, et al. Sputum induction for the diagnosis of pulmonary tuberculosis infection in infants and young children in an urban setting in South Africa. *Arch Dis Child*, 2000;82:305–308.
66. Zar HJ, Dechaboon A, Hanslo D, et al. *Pneumocystis carinii* pneumonia in South African children infected with human immunodeficiency virus [In Process Citation]. *Pediatr Infect Dis J*, 2000;19:603–607.
67. Kamiya Y, Mtitimila E, Graham SM, et al. *Pneumocystis carinii* pneumonia in Malawian children. *Ann Trop Paediatr*, 1997;17:121–126.
68. Mathis A, Weber R, Kuster H, et al. Simplified sample processing combined with a sensitive one-tube nested PCR assay for detection of *Pneumocystis carinii* in respiratory specimens. *J Clin Microbiol*, 1997;35:1691–1695.
69. Oz HS, Hughes WT. Search for *Pneumocystis carinii* DNA in upper and lower respiratory tract of humans. *Diagn Microbiol Infect Dis*, 2000;37:161–164.
70. Helweg-Larsen J, Jensen JS, Benfield T, et al. Diagnostic use of PCR for detection of *Pneumocystis carinii* in oral wash samples. *J Clin Microbiol*, 1998;36:2068–2072.
71. Ruffini DD, Madhi SA, Dahan E, et al. Induced sputum in the diagnosis of *Pneumocystis carinii* pneumonia (PCP) in HIV positive children using direct fluorescent antibody (DFA) techniques. In: Program and Abstracts of the XIII International AIDS Conference; July 9–14, 2000; Durban, South Africa. Abstract MoOrB117.
72. Sattler F, Nichols L, Hirano L, et al. Nonspecific interstitial pneumonitis mimicking *Pneumocystis carinii* pneumonia. *Am J Respir Crit Care Med*, 1997;156:912–917.
73. Wilcox CM, Straub RF, Clark WS. Prospective evaluation of oropharyngeal findings in human immunodeficiency virus-infected patients with esophageal ulceration [see comments]. *Am J Gastroenterol*, 1995;90:1938–1941.
74. Kennedy DH, Fallon RJ. Tuberculous meningitis. *JAMA*, 1979;241:264–268.
75. Nguyen LN, Kox LF, Pham LD, et al. The potential contribution of the polymerase chain reaction to the diagnosis of tuberculous meningitis. *Arch Neurol*, 1996;53:771–776.
76. Shankar P, Manjunath N, Mohan KK, et al. Rapid diagnosis of tuberculous meningitis by polymerase chain reaction. *Lancet*, 1991;337:5–7.
77. Ahuja GK, Mohan KK, Prasad K, et al. Diagnostic criteria for tuberculous meningitis and their validation. *Tuberc Lung Dis*, 1994;75:149–152.
78. Liu PY, Shi ZY, Lau YJ, et al. Rapid diagnosis of tuberculous meningitis by a simplified nested amplification protocol [see comments]. *Neurology*, 1994;44:1161–1164.
79. Bonington A, Strang JI, Klapper PE, et al. Use of Roche AMPLICOR *Mycobacterium tuberculosis* PCR in early diagnosis of tuberculous meningitis. *J Clin Microbiol*, 1998;36:1251–1254.
80. WHO. *Guidelines for the clinical management of HIV infection in children.* Geneva, Switzerland: World Health Organization Global Programme on AIDS, November 1993.
81. Chintu C, Luo C, Bhat G, et al. Cutaneous hypersensitivity reactions due to thiacetazone in the treatment of tuberculosis in Zambian children infected with HIV-I. *Arch Dis Child*, 1993;68: 665–668.
82. Shapiro R, Kumar L, Phillips-Howard P, et al. Antimicrobial-resistant bacterial diarrhea in rural western Kenya. *J Infect Dis*, 2001;183:1701–1704.
83. WHO. *Treatment and prevention of acute diarrhoea, Practical Guidelines, 2nd ed.* Geneva, Switzerland: World Health Organization, 1989.
84. DeCarli C, Fugate L, Falloon J, et al. Brain growth and cognitive improvement in children with human immunodeficiency virus-induced encephalopathy after 6 months of continuous infusion zidovudine therapy. *J Acquir Immune Defic Syndr*, 1991;4: 585–592.
85. Brouwers P, Moss H, Wolters P, et al. Effect of continuous-infusion zidovudine therapy on neuropsychologic functioning in children with symptomatic human immunodeficiency virus infection. *J Pediatr*, 1990;117:980–985.
86. UNAIDS. *Provisional WHO/UNAIDS Secretariat recommendations on the use of cotrimoxazole prophylaxis in adults and children living with HIV/AIDS in Africa.* Geneva, Switzerland: UNAIDS and WHO, 2000.
87. American Academy of Pediatrics Committee on Pediatric AIDS. Evaluation and medical treatment of the HIV-exposed infant. *Pediatrics*, 1997;99: 909–917.
88. WHO. Preventive therapy against tuberculosis in people living with HIV – Policy statement. *Weekly Epidemiological Record*, 1999;74:385.

31

Male Condoms and Circumcision

*Roger L. Shapiro and †Saidi H. Kapiga

**Department of Immunology and Infectious Diseases, Harvard School of Public Health, Boston, Massachusetts, USA.*
†Department of Population and International Health, Harvard School of Public Health, Boston, Massachusetts, USA.

The use of male condoms and the practice of male circumcision are among numerous strategies that have been examined as measures for preventing HIV infection. Condom use has been the mainstay of HIV prevention efforts since HIV was recognized as a sexually transmittable virus. Male circumcision, historically thought of as a ritual rather than a medical procedure, has only in recent years been considered as a potential preventive measure against HIV infection. However, with increasing evidence of its effectiveness and acceptability, male circumcision may soon become another valuable component of HIV prevention in Africa.

MALE CONDOMS

Condom Efficacy

The theoretical efficacy of latex condoms for preventing HIV transmission is 100%. Tests have confirmed that latex condoms do not leak HIV in the laboratory setting. In contrast, natural membrane condoms should not be used to prevent HIV infection because they may allow HIV transmission through small pores (1,2). Latex condoms may also prevent HIV infections by decreasing the incidence of other sexually transmitted diseases (STDs) that may facilitate HIV transmission (3,4).

Proper and consistent condom use has a proven record of effectiveness in the prevention of sexual transmission of HIV (5,6). In both Europe and Africa, studies have demonstrated up to a 90% reduction in HIV transmission among serodiscordant couples who reported consistent condom use (7,8). In a meta-analysis of 12 studies among serodiscordant couples, consistent condom use was 87% protective against HIV transmission compared with lack of condom use (9). Overreporting of condom use may account for some of the transmission reported in these studies. In a study conducted by the European Study Group on Heterosexual Transmission of AIDS, no HIV transmission occurred during 15,000 acts of intercourse among 124 serodiscordant couples who reported 100% use of latex condoms (7).

Male latex condoms have remained central to HIV prevention campaigns due to their proven bioefficacy in protecting sexual partners from HIV. Unfortunately, the efficacy of condoms based on reported use is much lower than their potential effectiveness, mainly due to inconsistent and improper use. In the previously mentioned European study of discordant couples, only 48% of all couples reported condom use at every act of intercourse, and those who reported inconsistent condom use had a seroconversion rate of 4.8 per 100 person-years (7). In Rwanda, a study of 51 serodiscordant couples found that only 18% reported condom use for every sexual act over a two-year period. The highest rates of seroconversion in this study were among those who never used condoms, and no seroconversion occurred among those reporting consistent condom use (10).

Condom Use in Africa

The low use efficacy of condoms is due primarily to non-use rather than incorrect use. As in many parts of the world, condom use in Africa tends to be low in many populations. Among high-risk adults in Nairobi, Kenya, only 3% reported using a condom with their last sexual partner (11), and in a multisite household survey performed in Benin, Cameroon, Kenya, and Zaire, only 21% to 25% of men reported that they always or often used condoms with nonspousal partners (12). In rural Lesotho, only 17% of the adult men surveyed had ever used a condom (13). In Rakai, Uganda, less than 14% of serodiscordant couples reported condom use during the previous year (14). In general, persons more likely to report condom use are younger males who are more educated, live in urban areas, and have more casual sexual partners than those who do not report condom use (11,15,16).

There are significant barriers to male condom use in many parts of the world, including throughout much of Africa. Such barriers include lack of female control over condom use, cost of condoms, limited availability of condoms, lack of knowledge about the effectiveness of condoms, fear or embarrassment associated with using condoms, lack of knowledge about HIV, perceived lack of HIV risk, decreased condom use in sexual acts following alcohol consumption, and culturally specific stigmas associated with condom use (11,16,17). A study in central Kenya demonstrated that over two-thirds of young women had never used a condom during sex. More than half of these women believed that HIV could pass through a condom or that a condom could get stuck inside their bodies (17). Misperceptions about condoms may discourage their use. Such misperceptions have been fostered, for example, by newspaper editorials that have claimed that condoms can actually spread HIV (17).

Strategies for Condom Promotion

Educational campaigns and social marketing techniques become very effective when access to free or low-cost condoms is increased. Such programs have been highly successful in Thailand, where condoms are now distributed and used in more than 90% of sexual acts in brothels as a result of the intensive government campaign requiring condom promotion in all commercial sexual transactions (18,19). In Cameroon, Kenya, and the Democratic Republic of Congo, high rates of condom use have been achieved among commercial sex workers (CSWs) who were intensively educated about condom use and provided with condoms (15,20,21). In Senegal, where condom promotion programs have been in place since the 1980s, two-thirds of male study participants reported condom use with nonregular partners, and peer education programs have demonstrated significant improvements in condom use (22,23). Peer educators from a community mobilization program in Carltonville, South Africa, distributed nearly 1.5 million free condoms in 1998 (24). In Uganda, where condom use had been infrequent in many areas (25), condom promotion, including the use of intensive media campaigns, has become an important component of a successful HIV prevention campaign (26). According to UNAIDS, condom use among teenage girls in Uganda tripled between 1994 and 1997, and the number of men reporting that they had ever used a condom during their lifetime doubled during this time period (17). Successful programs that integrate traditional educators such as a "senga," or paternal aunt, have also led to increased condom use among teenage girls in Uganda (27).

These examples demonstrate that the social marketing of condoms that combines expanded accessibility with consumer-specific promotion can increase condom sales and condom use in Africa. In the past 15 years, condom sales in sub–Saharan Africa have increased from less than 1 million to more than 200 million per year (28). However, broadly supported, appropriately targeted social marketing programs have the potential to further increase condom availability and use.

MALE CIRCUMCISION

Male Circumcision in Africa

Male circumcision was traditionally practiced in most Bantu-speaking regions of sub–Saharan Africa and remains a cultural practice throughout much of the region today (29). Circumcision is often used to mark the transition from boyhood to manhood either before or after puberty (29,30). Historically, circumcision was performed by traditional community leaders with no medical training, and frequently occurred under extreme conditions to test bravery. Over time, circumcision has become less common in some regions of Africa where it had been traditionally practiced; in some areas, medical practitioners and religious missionaries in the early twentieth century lobbied for the abandonment of circumcision (29,30). Non-circumcising areas now include almost all of Uganda, Rwanda, Burundi, Zambia, Malawi, Zimbabwe, and Botswana, and parts of western Kenya, western Tanzania, the Democratic Republic of Congo, Namibia, Mozambique, and South Africa (29,31). Thus, there are areas in Africa where circumcision may be culturally acceptable but no longer practiced.

Male Circumcision and HIV Risk

Lack of male circumcision was first implicated as a risk factor for HIV infection in the late 1980s. At least 38 cross-sectional studies have been performed that have evaluated the effect of circumcision on HIV prevalence (32–34); 27 studies from eight different countries demonstrated a significant association between lack of circumcision and HIV infection; five showed a trend toward an association; five showed no association; and one study reported increased risk among those circumcised. In a recent meta-analysis of 27 cohort, case-control, and cross-sectional studies conducted prior to April 1999, circumcision was found to be significantly protective against HIV infection by two-fold, and among men at high risk, there was over 70% protection (35).

Circumcision was associated with lower HIV infection rates in a recent multisite study performed in Kisumu, Kenya; Ndola, Zambia; Cotonou, Benin; and Yaounde, Cameroon between June 1997 and March 1998 (12). Approximately 1,000 participants per site were enrolled, and sexual behaviors did not differ significantly between sites. In multivariate analysis, being circumcised was associated with a lower risk of HIV infection. In Cotonou and Yaounde (lower HIV prevalence areas) nearly all men reported being circumcised, while in Ndola (high prevalence area) only 10% of men were circumcised. In Kisumu (high prevalence area), where the overall percentage of circumcised men was less than 30%, HIV prevalence was below 8% in men who were circumcised before becoming sexually active as compared with 25% in uncircumcised men.

At least eight prospective studies have evaluated a possible link between circumcision status and HIV infection (Table 1) (14,34,36–42); six of them associated lack of circumcision with increased HIV infection, and two found a trend toward increased infection. Seven of the studies determined HIV incidence in men directly, and one

TABLE 1. Prospective Studies Investigating the Association between Lack of Male Circumcision and Risk for HIV Infection (34)

Author (Reference)	Country	Year(s) of study	Population	Sample size	% Circumcised	Association[a]
Cameron et al. (36)	Kenya	1986–7	Male STD patients	293	73.0	RR = 8.2 95% CI, 3.0–23.0
Tyndall et al. (37)	Kenya	1990–1	Male genital ulcer disease patients	413	76.5	RR = 4.5 95% CI, 2.6–7.7
Telzak et al. (38)	USA	1990	Male STD patients (heterosexual, non-drug-using)	758	40.6	RR = 3.5 95% CI, 0.8–15.8
Mehendale et al. (39)	India	1993–5	Male STD patients	721	6.9	RR = 3.0 $p = 0.11$
Kassler et al. (40)	USA	1994–5	Male STD patients	Cases: 65 Controls: 131	Cases: 35.3 Controls: 61.8	RR = 2.9 95% CI, 1.3–6.3
Kapiga et al. (41)	Tanzania	1992–5	Women attending family planning clinics	1370	97.9[b]	RR = 3.4[c] 95% CI, 1.0–11.3
Lavreys et al. (42)	Kenya	1993–7	Male trucking company employees	746	87.3	HRR = 4.0 95% CI, 1.9–8.3
Quinn et al. (14)	Uganda	1994–8	Serodiscordant couples	187 partners of HIV^+ women	27.0	$p < 0.001$

[a]Reported associations are from multivariate analyses where conducted. RR indicates relative risk; CI, confidence interval, HRR, hazard rate ratio.
[b]% of male partners circumcised.
[c]RR for women with uncircumcised partners.

examined the HIV risk among female sexual partners of circumcised and uncircumcised men. The relative risks for infection among those who were uncircumcised range from 2.9 (95% CI, 1.3–6.3) to 8.2 (95% CI, 3.0–23.0). A study among HIV-serodiscordant couples in the Rakai district of Uganda demonstrated marked protection against seroconversion for men who were circumcised (14): 16.7 seroconversions per 100 person-years occurred among 137 uncircumcised men, whereas no seroconversions occurred among 50 circumcised men ($p < 0.001$).

One of the earliest prospective studies showing protection from HIV through circumcision was conducted by Cameron et al. in Nairobi between 1987 and 1988 (36). This study followed 293 men who were frequenting CSWs and were considered to be at high risk for HIV infection. Researchers documented an HIV seroconversion rate of 8.2% during the study period. By multivariate analysis, independent risk factors for seroconversion were lack of circumcision (risk ratio 8.2; 95% CI, 3.0 to 23.0), genital ulcers (risk ratio 4.7; 95% CI, 1.3 to 17.0), and regular CSW contact (risk ratio 3.2; 95% CI, 1.2 to 8.1); 53% of uncircumcised men with genital ulcers seroconverted, 29% of uncircumcised men without genital ulcers seroconverted, and only 3% of circumcised men without genital ulcers seroconverted.

Researchers in the Rakai district of Uganda have suggested that the protective effects of circumcision may depend on the age at which circumcision occurs, with maximum protection achieved through prepubertal circumcision (43,44). Other studies have found the opposite association between age at circumcision and protection (45), and one study demonstrated higher risk behavior among non-Muslim circumcised men than among uncircumcised men, suggesting that behavioral risk factors and the reasons for being circumcised (which may have included STD complications among the older group) may differ in men who are circumcised later in life (46). Biologically there is no apparent explanation for a gradation in protection because of age at circumcision, although increased risk for HIV acquisition is likely if sexual activity occurs in the weeks immediately following circumcision.

Mechanism of Protection

There are several plausible mechanisms to explain the observed association between lack of circumcision and HIV infection. The foreskin has a high density of Langerhans cells, which are potential entry sites for HIV. In-vitro evidence suggests that the use of Langerhans cells as a mechanism of entry may be particularly important for HIV-1C, the subtype dominant in much of Africa (47). The inner mucous surface of the foreskin is not keratinised and is rich in Langerhans cells, making it particularly susceptible to the virus (48). During intercourse the foreskin is pulled back down the shaft of the penis and the inner surface of the foreskin is exposed to vaginal secretions. The foreskin is also susceptible to epithelial disruption during intercourse, thus increasing transmission risk.

An intact foreskin may also increase the risk of ulcerative STDs such as chancroid, syphilis, and possibly herpes simplex virus type-2 (HSV-2) (34,42,49). These diseases are known cofactors for enhanced HIV transmission (36,50,51). The mechanism for this increased risk may stem from both epithelial cell disruption and increased shedding of HIV in the genital tract among those affected by STDs (14,52).

Male Circumcision and HIV Prevention

Although behavior change (abstinence, monogamy), condom use, and programs to prevent mother-to-child transmission have been the main focus of HIV prevention efforts in Africa, male circumcision could become an aspect of prevention efforts. Potential advantages of circumcision as an intervention include the fact that circumcision is currently available, affordable, permanent, requires no thought at the time of sexual activity, and may be culturally acceptable in much of Africa. In fact, some researchers have suggested circumcision as a potential explanation for the continued rates of fairly low HIV seroprevalence in some countries, particularly those in West Africa, while other countries with similar patterns of sexual behavior have very high prevalence (31,32). Although conclusive evidence is not available, studies such as the UNAIDS-sponsored multisite trial (12) suggest that the lack of circumcision may be an important cofactor fuelling the HIV epidemic in the worst affected areas of sub–Saharan Africa, and that circumcision may therefore be useful in preventive efforts.

The role of circumcision as an HIV intervention strategy remains a charged topic from a scientific, cultural, and behavioral perspective. Most experts agree that a randomized clinical trial may be required to resolve remaining questions about the efficacy of circumcision in preventing HIV, particularly to address issues of potential confounding by religion or behavioral factors that have been raised in previous studies. Such a study might also address the question of whether the age at which circumcision is performed affects protection, and this information, combined with regional and cultural considerations, may help determine the optimal age for a circumcision intervention. Any potential circumcision interventions—clinical trials or community-wide interventions—must be integrated into other aspects of HIV prevention. It should be understood that male circumcision is not a substitute for other preventive methods such as abstinence and condom use.

For any circumcision program, just as in any hospital where circumcision is offered, the risks and benefits of circumcision must be clearly elucidated for all participants. In addition to the probable benefit of HIV risk reduction, circumcision offers the following health benefits: ten-fold decreased risk of bladder infections during the first year of life (53); prevention of phimosis (constriction of the penis) by the foreskin, which affects about 0.3% to 0.9% of males worldwide (54); reduced chance of cancer of the penis later in life (between one in 600 and one in 900 uncircumcised men worldwide may develop penile cancer in their lifetime compared with virtually no circumcised men) (55); reduced cervical cancer among female sexual partners of circumcised men (56); improved hygiene; and reduced chance of contracting some STDs, particularly ulcerative diseases such as syphilis and chancroid (34,42,49).

Potential health risks and other concerns about circumcision must also be considered. Circumcision, as with any minor surgical procedure, has a small risk of bleeding and infection following the procedure. In safe hospital settings, about 0.1% to 1% have excessive bleeding and about the same number report minor infections following the procedure (56). Circumcision may be painful. Doctors can provide a local anesthetic or anesthetic cream to decrease pain, which is worse for older boys and men, but also occurs among newborns (56). Circumcision may not be acceptable to all ethnic groups, and traditional beliefs and customs about circumcision need to be considered. Circumcision may not be widely accepted by many communities and individuals.

CONCLUSION

This chapter has examined condoms and male circumcision as HIV preventive strategies in Africa. Condoms are a highly effective method of preventing HIV when used properly, and play a central role in HIV prevention programs in Africa. Although condom use remains low in many areas of Africa, condom accessibility and use can be improved dramatically through creative and culturally appropriate social marketing and education programs. Male circumcision may play a role in future HIV prevention programs; the weight of current evidence supports its effectiveness. However, a randomized clinical trial, as currently planned in western Kenya, may be needed to further elucidate issues of confounding and the impact of circumcision on reducing HIV transmission in the general population. Ultimately, the success of both condom promotion efforts and male circumcision programs will depend on their resonance at the local level.

REFERENCES

1. Judson F, Ehret J, Bodin G, et al. *In vitro* evaluations of condoms with and without nonoxynol-9 as physical and chemical barriers against *Chlamydia trachomatis*, herpes simplex virus type 2, and human immunodeficiency virus. *Sex Trans Dis*, 1989;16:51–56.
2. Rietmeijer C, Krebs J, Feorino P, et al. Condoms as physical and chemical barriers against human immunodeficiency virus. *JAMA*, 1988;259:1851–1853.
3. From the Centers for Disease Control and Prevention. Update: barrier protection against HIV infection and other sexually transmitted diseases. *JAMA*, 1993;270:933–934.
4. UNAIDS Technical Update. The male condom. Geneva, Switzerland: UNAIDS, 2000.
5. Ngugi EN, Plummer FA, Simonsen JN, et al. Prevention of transmission of human immunodeficiency virus in Africa: effectiveness of condom promotion and health education among prostitutes. *Lancet*, 1988;2:887–890.
6. Mann J, Quinn TC, Piot P, et al. Condom use and HIV infection among prostitutes in Zaire. *New Engl J Med*, 1987;316:345.
7. DeVincenzi I. A longitudinal study of human immunodeficiency virus transmission by heterosexual partners. *New Engl J Med*, 1994;331:341–346.
8. Bagurukira E, Kiwanuka A, Bakaki P, et al. Condom use between HIV serology discordant couples in Kampala. In: Abstracts of the XIII International Conference on AIDS; July 9–14, 2000; Durban, South Africa. Abstract ThOrD779.
9. Davis KR, Weller SC. The effectiveness of condoms in reducing heterosexual transmission of HIV. *Fam Plann Perspect*, 1999;31:272–279.
10. Allen S, Tice J, Van de Perre P, et al. Effect of serotesting with counseling on condom use and seroconversion among HIV discordant couples in Africa. *Br Med J*, 1992;304:1605–1609.
11. Ndinya-Achola, Ghee AE, Kihara AN, et al. High HIV prevalence, low condom use and gender differences in sexual behaviour among patients with STD-related complaints at a Nairobi primary health care clinic. *Intl J STD AIDS*, 1997;8:506–514.
12. UNAIDS. Differences in HIV spread in four sub–Saharan African cities: summary of the multi-site study. September 14, 1999. UNAIDS website. Available at: http://www.unaids.org/whatsnew/ press/ eng/pressarc99/lusaka14sep99.html. Accessed: November 24, 2001.
13. Colvin M, Sharp B. Sexually transmitted infections and HIV in a rural community in the Lesotho highlands. *Sex Transm Infect*, 2000;76:39–42.
14. Quinn TC, Wawer MJ, Sewankambo N, et al. Viral load and heterosexual transmission of human immunodeficiency virus type 1. *New Engl J Med*, 2000;342:921–929.
15. Laga M, Alary M, Nzila N, et al. Condom promotion, sexually transmitted diseases treatment, and declining incidence of HIV-1 infection in female Zairian sex workers. *Lancet*, 1994;344:246–248.
16. Allen S, Serufilira A, Bogaerts J, et al. Confidential HIV testing and condom promotion in Africa: impact on HIV and gonorrhea rates. *JAMA*, 1992; 268:3338–3343.
17. UNAIDS. Report on the Global HIV/AIDS epidemic, June 2000. Geneva, Switzerland: UNAIDS, 2000.
18. Celentano DD, Nelson KE, Lyles CM, et al. Decreasing incidence of HIV and sexually transmitted diseases in young Thai men: evidence for success of the HIV/AIDS control and prevention program. *AIDS*, 1998;12:F29–F36.
19. Rojanapithayakorn W, Hanenberg R. The 100% condom program in Thailand. *AIDS*, 1996;10:1–7.
20. Lawson L, Katzenstein D, Vermund S. Emerging biomedical interventions. In: Gibney L, DiClemente J, Vermund SH, eds. *Preventing HIV in Developing Countries: Biomedical and Behavioral Approaches*. New York: Kluwer Academic/Plenum, 1999:43–69.
21. Moses S, Plummer FA, Ngugi EN, et al. Controlling HIV in Africa: effectiveness and cost of an intervention in a high-frequency STD transmitter core group. *AIDS*, 1991;5:407–411.
22. Meda N, Ndoye I, M'Boup S, et al. Low and stable HIV infection rates in Senegal: natural course of the epidemic or evidence for success of prevention? *AIDS*, 1999;13:1397–1405.
23. Leonard L, Ndiaye I, Kapadia A, et al. HIV prevention among male clients of female sex workers in Kaolack, Senegal: results of a peer education program. *AIDS Educ Prev*, 2000;12:21–37.
24. Moema S, Neilsen G, Mzaidume Y, et al. Into the pocket, onto the penis: condom distribution in Carletonville, South Africa. In: Abstracts of the XIII International Conference on AIDS; July 9–14, 2000; Durban, South Africa. Abstract MoOrC249.
25. Stoneburner R. Analysis of HIV trend and behavioral data in Uganda, Kenya, and Zambia: prevalence declines in Uganda relate more to reduction

in sex partners than condom use. In: Abstracts of the XIII International Conference on AIDS; July 9–14, 2000; Durban, South Africa. Abstract ThOrC721.
26. Nakityo R, Mugyenyi D. The role of the media in HIV prevention in Uganda. In: Abstracts of the XIII International Conference on AIDS; July 9–14, 2000; Durban, South Africa. Abstract TuPeE3872.
27. Whitworth J, Muyinda H, Pool R. Harnessing traditional sex education institutions: the senga model in Uganda. In: Abstracts of the XIII International Conference on AIDS; July 9–14, 2000; Durban, South Africa. Abstract WePeD4704.
28. Goodridge GA, Lamptey PR. HIV prevention for the general population. In: Gibney L, DiClemente J, Vermund SH, eds. *Preventing HIV in Developing Countries: Biomedical and Behavioral Approaches*. New York: Kluwer Academic/Plenum, 1999: 331–362.
29. Marck J. Aspects of male circumcision in subequatorial African culture history. *Health Transit Rev*, 1997;7(Suppl):337–360.
30. Schapera I. *Tribal Innovators*. London: The Athlone Press; 1970.
31. Moses S, Bradley JE, Nagelkerke NJ, et al. Geographical patterns of male circumcision practices in Africa: association with HIV seroprevalence. *Int J Epidemiol*, 1990;19:693–697.
32. Halperin DT, Bailey RC. Male circumcision and HIV infection: 10 years and counting. *Lancet*, 1999;35:1813–1815.
33. Moses S, Plummer FA, Bradley JE, et al. The association between lack of male circumcision and risk for HIV infection: a review of the epidemiological data. *Sex Transm Dis*, 1994;21:201–210.
34. Moses S, Bailey RC, Ronald AR. Male circumcision: assessment of health benefits and risks. *Sex Transm Inf*, 1998;74:368–373.
35. Weiss HA, Quigley MA, Hayes RJ. Male circumcision and risk of HIV infection in sub-Saharan Africa: a systematic review and meta-analysis. *AIDS*, 2000;14:2361–2370.
36. Cameron BE, Simonsen JN, D'Costa LJ, et al. Female to male transmission of human immunodeficiency virus type 1: risk factors for seroconversion in men. *Lancet*, 1989;2:403–407.
37. Tyndall MW, Ronald AR, Agoki E, et al. Increased risk of infection with human immunodeficiency virus type 1 among uncircumcised men presenting with genital ulcer disease in Kenya. *Clin Infect Dis*, 1996;23:449–453.
38. Telzak ET, Chiasson MA, Bevier PJ, et al. HIV-1 seroconversion in patients with and without genital ulcer disease: a prospective study. *Ann Intern Med*, 1993;119:1181–1186.
39. Mehendale SM, Shepherd ME, Divekar AD, et al. Evidence for high prevalence and rapid transmission of HIV among individuals attending STD clinics in Pune, India. *Indian J Med Res*, 1996;104: 327–335.
40. Kassler WJ, Aral SO. Beyond risk groups: behavioral correlates of HIV seroconversion in sexually transmitted disease clinic patients. In: Abstract monograph, XI International Meeting of the International Society for STD Research; 27–30 Aug 1995; New Orleans, USA. Abstract 107.
41. Kapiga SH, Lyamuya EF, Lwihula GK, et al. The incidence of HIV infection among women using family planning methods in Dar Es Salaam, Tanzania. *AIDS*, 1998;12:75–84.
42. Lavreys L, Rakwar JP, Thompson ML, et al. Effect of circumcision on incidence of human immunodeficiency virus type 1 and other sexually transmitted diseases: a prospective cohort study of trucking company employees in Kenya. *J Infect Dis*, 1999; 180:330–336.
43. Kelly R, Kiwanuka N, Wawer MJ, et al. Age of male circumcision and risk of prevalent HIV infection in rural Uganda. *AIDS*, 1999;13:399–405.
44. Gray RH, Kiwanuka N, Quinn TC, et al. Male circumcision and HIV acquisition and transmission: cohort studies in Rakai, Uganda. *AIDS*, 2000;14: 2371–2381.
45. Quigley M, Munguti K, Grosskurth H, et al. Sexual behaviour patterns and other risk factors for HIV infection in rural Tanzania: a case-control study. *AIDS*, 1997;11:237–248.
46. Bailey RC, Neema S, Othieno R. Sexual behaviors and other HIV risk factors in circumcised and uncircumcised men in Uganda. *J Acquir Immune Defic Syndr*, 1999;22:294–301.
47. Soto-Ramirez LE, Renjifo B, McLane MF, et al. HIV-1 Langerhans' Cell Tropism Associated with Heterosexual Transmission of HIV. *Science*, 1996;271:1291–1293.
48. Szabo R, Short RV. How does male circumcision protect against HIV infection? *BMJ*, 2000;320: 1592–1594.
49. Cook LS, Koutsky LA, Holmes KK. Circumcision and sexually transmitted diseases. *Am J Public Health*, 1994;84:197–201.
50. Flemming DT, Wasserheit JN. From epidemiological synergy to public health policy and practice: the contribution of other sexually transmitted diseases to sexual transmission of HIV infection. *Sex Transm Infect*, 1999;75:3–17.
51. Orroth KK, Gavyole A, Todd J, et al. Syndromic treatment of sexually transmitted diseases reduces the proportion of incident HIV infections attributable to these diseases in rural Tanzania. *AIDS*, 2000;14:1429–1437.
52. Schoen EJ, Wiswell TE, Moses S. New Policy on Circumcision-Cause for Concern. *Pediatrics*, 2000; 105:620–623.

53. Wiswell TE, Hachey WE. Urinary tract infections and the circumcision state: an update. *Clin Pediat*, 1993;32:130–134.
54. American Academy of Pediatrics. Report of the task force on circumcision. *Pediatrics*, 1989;84: 388–391.
55. Kochen M, McCurdy S. Circumcision and risk of cancer of the penis. A life-table analysis. *Am J Dis Child*, 1980;134:484–486.
56. Wiswell TE. Circumcision circumspection. *N Engl J Med*, 1997;336:1244–1245.

32

Female Condoms and Microbicides

*Eka Esu-Williams and †Kelly Blanchard

*Population Council, Horizons Program,[a] Johannesburg, South Africa.
†Robert H. Ebert Program on Critical Issues in Reproductive Health, Population Council, Johannesburg, South Africa.

Prevention of HIV infection is a key component in the global response to the AIDS epidemic. This is particularly true in Africa where infection rates are still rising, and access to treatment and care for infected individuals is likely to remain limited to the wealthy for some time to come. In Africa in particular, and increasingly around the world, women are becoming infected with HIV at higher rates than men. This is due, in large part, to the fact that current strategies to prevent HIV and other sexually transmitted diseases (STDs) do not work or are not appropriate for many women. There are four major strategies for the prevention of HIV and other STDs: abstaining, using condoms, reducing number of sexual partners, and treating any STDs early. Globally, gender dynamics contribute to situations in which women are often not able to demand protective measures or refuse sex. Poverty is also a key risk factor, forcing many women to engage in sex for survival and reducing their ability to negotiate condom use with steady partners. Finally, for the fourth prevention strategy to be effective, all women must have access to health care services and know when they have an STD. Up to 75% of STDs in women are asymptomatic, and many women do not have access to treatment. New HIV/STD prevention strategies and technologies are urgently needed to help women protect themselves.

[a]Horizons is an HIV/AIDS operations research program supported by the United States Agency for International Development.

Female condoms and microbicides are safer sex products designed to be woman-initiated and woman-controlled. The Female Condom, the product currently approved for use in more than 60 developing countries, is a strong, loose-fitting, polyurethane sheath that functions similarly to the male condom except that it is inserted inside the vagina. A flexible inner ring is used to insert the female condom, and the soft outer ring remains outside the vagina during intercourse. The female condom protects the vagina, cervix, and external genitalia from infections.

Microbicides are vaginal or rectal products that could be formulated as creams, gels, or films, much like currently available spermicides. Although no microbicide has been proven effective, the idea is that the gel would be inserted into the vagina or rectum prior to sexual activity. While female condoms are designed to prevent both STDs and pregnancy, contraceptive and noncontraceptive versions of microbicides are under investigation.

Female-controlled products are an important addition to the current safer sex technology—male condoms. Such products offer women a chance to initiate discussion of safer sex; furthermore, a woman can offer to use the product instead of asking her partner to use a male condom. Both female condoms and microbicides provide women and couples with additional options for preventing infection with HIV and other STDs. Research on contraceptive use and STD prevention efforts show that more safer sex options lead to more protected acts of intercourse (1–3). Even a product that is less effective at preventing infection than a male condom on a per use basis, as is likely in the case of a microbicide, could significantly impact HIV/STD transmission, if found to be acceptable and widely used. Data on female condoms and potential microbicides suggest that these products will be appealing to at least some women and men. For example, in Zimbabwe, a study conducted among sex workers, urban female family planning clinic attendees, and rural women in long-term relationships showed that a large majority of the women liked the female condom and preferred it over the male condom (4). In a recent study in Zimbabwe that compared female condom users (n = 493), male condom users (n = 633), and nonusers of either method (n = 624), 15% of men and women reported that they always used the female condom (5). Among those who had used both the female and the male condom, 80% said they intended to continue to use either one, and 68% of women said they would use the female condom again. Women who participated in multicountry safety studies of two potential microbicides reported that they liked the product (6–8). Men in a three-country study who were asked about the idea of a microbicide reported that they thought women would use such a product (9).

PRODUCT AVAILABILITY AND CURRENT RESEARCH NEEDS

Female Condoms

The female condom is manufactured by the Female Health Company and is commercially available under several brand names (Reality, Femidom, Femy). It is also available though social marketing programs (*care*™ in Southern Africa) and public sector programs in developing countries (The Female Condom). The female condom is as effective as other barrier methods and has no side effects (10). Furthermore, a wide range of studies in many countries and in diverse populations show that use of the female condom is acceptable to a significant number of women (11). Yet in most countries, the female condom is not widely available for a variety of reasons. It is relatively more expensive than the male condom (public sector cost is USD$0.57, while one male condom costs approximately $0.05), and in many countries the product has either not been introduced or its availability has been limited to pilot acceptability studies, despite evidence for a growing demand. Only Brazil, Ghana, South Africa, and Zimbabwe have embarked on large-scale programs to promote widespread availability of the female condom. Increasing access to this technology in other countries should be prioritized.

Reuse of female condoms is another important issue that has implications for product cost and accessibility. The female condom is currently registered for single use, but reuse has been widely reported (12). Reliable data on reuse are scarce, but studies from South Africa, Bolivia, Zambia, Cameroon, Zimbabwe, Papua New Guinea, Bangladesh, and Côte d'Ivoire provide evidence of different levels and patterns of reuse (13). In South Africa, for example, as many as 80% of women studied reported that they would be prepared to reuse the female condom once or twice, and more than 60% reported that they would use it more than twice (14). Reuse in Zambia has been motivated by lack of supplies, cost, and coercion by male partners (15). The World Health Organization (WHO) and UNAIDS organized a consultation of scientists, programmers, condom production and quality assurance experts, and women's activists in June 2000 to examine the safety and feasibility of reuse. Results from the following two key trials conducted in South Africa and in the United States were reviewed. Rees et al. reported that after 10 washes with liquid detergent or bar soap and water followed by pat-drying there was no meaningful difference between washed and unwashed female condoms (14). A second part of this study examined multiple use, washing, drying, and relubrication. Approximately 50 female condoms were tested for leaks after each use and rewash. The presence of holes or leaks was similar between the rewashed and unused condoms until after the eighth wash. The study conducted in the United States found similar results: there was no significant difference with respect to the number of holes between female condoms that had been washed multiple times and those that had not been washed (16). The evidence presented from these studies was inadequate to determine whether microbial pathogens were inactivated or eliminated after washing with soap and water. Although disinfection with bleach could achieve this, the effect of such a procedure on the structural integrity of the female condom is unknown. There are no data on the effect of washed or disinfected female condoms on normal vaginal flora. A draft protocol for washing, disinfecting, drying, and relubricating female condoms was developed and is currently being tested. Further guidance on reuse is expected from the WHO and UNAIDS (17).

Microbicides

Unfortunately, no microbicide product has been proven to prevent the transmission of HIV and other STDs; however, research in this area has increased dramatically over the last decade. There are currently over 60 compounds being investigated as potential microbicides, and approximately 20 are in or are nearing small- to medium-scale clinical trials (18). Researchers are investigating compounds that might work in a variety of ways, including by destroying microorganisms, blocking pathogens from attaching to and thus infecting cells, boosting the natural defenses of the vagina, or inhibiting HIV replication and potentially preventing systemic infection (19). We will briefly describe each class of compounds.

Broad-Spectrum Microbicides

This class of compounds, which includes nonoxynol-9 (N9) and other surfactants, has been the most widely studied. These products generally work by disrupting the cell membrane of viruses and other pathogens. Unfortunately, these products are indiscriminate and may also disrupt the cells of the vaginal epithelium, potentially causing irritation that could actually increase HIV/STD transmission. Three large efficacy studies of N9 products have been conducted (Table 1). Studies of a sponge with N9 (20) and an N9 film (21) found that these products did not prevent HIV infection. In a recent study of an N9 gel (22), women who used N9 had a higher rate of HIV infection than women who used the placebo gel. Unfortunately it may be impossible to decipher whether N9 increased HIV acquisition, or if the placebo gel was actually a more effective microbicide. Discussions as to whether it is useful or indeed ethical to continue research on N9 are ongoing. One surfactant-containing compound, called SAVVY™, addresses this issue by using a compound that has been shown to work in vitro at low concentrations that do not affect normal healthy cells. This product is slated for small-scale human testing in the near future.

Blocking Agents

Products in this category are currently moving into larger-scale safety testing and will hopefully be ready for efficacy testing in the next year or two. These products generally contain large, highly-charged molecules that are believed to coat both the surface of the vaginal epithelium as well as viruses or other pathogens present in the vagina. The like electrical charges then prevent viruses or other pathogens from attaching to epithelial cells, and thus prevent infection. Some products in this category include Carraguard™ (PC-515), dextrin sulfate, and PRO2000™. These products have been shown to be effective at blocking a variety of pathogens both in vitro and in animal models (23–26). In addition, current data indicate that these products are likely to cause significantly less irritation than N9-containing products (27). Small-scale safety studies (Phase 1) have shown no significant adverse effects and indicate that women find the products acceptable (7,8). Carraguard™ is currently undergoing expanded safety trials (Phase II) and similar trials are planned for dextrin sulfate, and PRO2000™ in the near future.

Acid Buffers and Natural Products

The pH of a healthy vagina is naturally acidic and HIV and other pathogens cannot survive in an acidic environment. Two potential products, Buffergel and lactobacillus suppositories, act by maintaining or increasing the acidity of the vagina. These products also have the potential to treat bacterial vaginosis, a condition that has been found to be associated with risk for HIV infection (28, 29) and other complications, such as premature labor. Buffergel is a product that counters the neutralizing effect of semen, thus maintaining the natural acidity of the vagina. Small-scale safety studies have shown this product to be safe and acceptable to women (6); larger-scale safety studies are currently planned. Lactobacillus suppositories are designed to recolonize the vagina with this naturally occurring bacteria that produces hydrogen peroxide, thereby maintaining the acidic environment. Preliminary studies have been successful, and planned research will assess the effectiveness of this product for HIV prevention and treatment of bacterial vaginosis.

Inhibitors of Viral Replication

A number of proven treatments for HIV infection, including PMPA (tenofovir) and nevirapine, could potentially be formulated as topical vaginal or rectal microbicides. It is thought that they could prevent the replication of HIV once it has entered cells in the reproductive tract, or reduce the infectiousness of HIV, thus preventing systemic infection. To date, research of these products has been limited to *in vitro* tests (30). Potential barriers to widespread availability of such products include cost and potential systemic side effects. Although these products are further behind in the pipeline than others described previously, this is a promising area for future investigation.

ETHICAL CONSIDERATIONS FOR RESEARCH ON HIV/STD PREVENTION TECHNOLOGIES

Evaluating the efficacy of any HIV prevention technology is challenging. Many of

TABLE 1. Summary of Effectiveness Studies of Potential N9 Microbicides

Author (reference)	Product	n	Population/Location	Outcome
Kreiss et al. (20)	Sponge plus N9	138	Sex workers/Nairobi, Kenya	Sponge plus N9 led to increased rates of genital ulceration and vulvitis and did not protect against HIV infection.
Roddy et al. (21)	70 mg N9 film	1,292	Sex workers/Cameroon	N9 film did not protect against infection with HIV, chlamydia, or gonorrhea.
van Damme et al. (22)	52.5 mg N9 gel (Advantage-S)	990	Sex workers/Abidjan, Côte d'Ivoire; Durban and Johannesburg, South Africa; Cotonou, Benin; and Hat Yai and Bangkok, Thailand	Final data are not yet released. Rates of new HIV infections were higher in the N9 group than in the placebo group. N9 gel had no effect on chlamydia and gonorrhea.

these studies must be conducted among women at risk of HIV infection, who are often vulnerable. Counseling before and after HIV testing must be done, and women participating in trials need support to cope with positive HIV test results. Informed consent is particularly challenging due to the complexity of the studies and, in the case of microbicides, the difficulty of explaining the concept of the investigational agent and the fact that it may be only partially effective, if effective at all (31). Microbicide research has stimulated additional discussion and work on the definition and evaluation of informed consent. This work highlights the challenges of conducting complex clinical trials among vulnerable populations (32).

Finally, because it is ethically essential that women participating in microbicide trials be counseled to use condoms to protect themselves from HIV and other STDs (33–35), the analysis of microbicide efficacy in a trial setting is complex. The challenge for analysis though, can easily be managed with effective randomization, subgroup analysis (particularly of women who choose not to or cannot use condoms—which may be a significant proportion of participants in some settings), and other appropriate statistical techniques.

Local consultation with researchers, women's health advocates, potential trial participants, as well as equal collaboration with host country and local partners is necessary to develop effective and culturally appropriate strategies to address these issues. A number of such consultations on microbicide research have taken place and provide a model for broader research of HIV prevention technologies (36,37).

An additional concern expressed about the future of microbicides is that they may lead to reduced condom use. This is a question that needs more attention and research. Although more options are likely to lead to more protected sexual acts, messages that effectively explain where microbicides fit into the HIV/STD prevention scheme are crucial. A microbicide is likely to be less effective on a per-use basis than a condom, and messages about microbicides should emphasize that using a condom is still the best way to protect oneself from infection.

POLICY AND PROGRAM PRIORITIES

The efficacy of the female condom for disease prevention, its acceptability, and its role in initiating negotiation of safer sex has been documented. However, cost continues to be a major determinant of the extent of its distribution and use. Current efforts by UNAIDS and the Female Health Company are directed at increasing global sales volume to bring the price down. Such approaches will also be important to ensure access to other products such as microbicides in the future. Enhanced national and global advocacy is required to ensure that decision makers understand the public health benefits of the female condom and the need to invest in its introduction and availability so that the female condom may eventually be as readily available as male condoms. These efforts must include public sector service providers, as well as nongovernmental and community-based organizations that are well positioned to reach communities directly.

Although there is no microbicide product currently ready for endorsement as an HIV/STD prevention measure, work must begin now to ensure that an effective product will be available in the future. First, health policy makers worldwide need to familiarize themselves with microbicide research and its importance. Second, funding for research must be increased. Recent efforts in this area have been extremely successful, and funding is now two to three times the level of 3 years ago. To increase the chances of finding an effective and acceptable product, the number of products under investigation must be greatly increased. Third, purchase funds, which have been discussed for HIV vaccines, have also been discussed for microbicides and need further consideration and commitment. Fourth, women themselves need to be informed about the potential utility of a microbicide in preventing HIV and other STDs. This is most important in areas where microbicides will be tested. Although informing women prior to product availability could unreasonably raise expectations for a product that is still years away, advocacy and pressure from women's groups could be one of the most effective ways to mobilize support for future product development and distribution. Finally, research on effective distribution mechanisms and the diminution of potential barriers to access should begin now. The identification and development of strategies to deal with these issues beforehand will help to ensure that a product is in the hands of women as soon as possible. Such strategies include up-to-date training for health care providers on new technologies so they will be able to provide information to their clients and help them choose products that meet their needs. Further research on the appropriate training for providers and non-providers to increase awareness and use of safer sex technologies is critical.

CONCLUSION

One of the recurring themes in the fight against HIV and other STDs is the recognition that although many of the tools needed to control the spread of disease do exist, they are not widely used or available. The female condom is one such tool, and an effective microbicide will also add to the number of options at a woman's disposal. Ensuring that these tools are available to women and couples should be policy and program planning priorities. For women who are vulnerable and are unable to negotiate the use of male condoms or to refuse sex, the female condom and microbicides are vital options. To meet the needs of these women, we must ensure the allocation of adequate resources for microbicide development and trials, the procurement of female condoms, and the provision of the necessary support for women and men who choose to use these options.

REFERENCES

1. Akbar J, Phillips J, Koenig M. Trends in contraceptive method mix, continuation rates and failure rates in Matlab, Bangladesh: 1978–87. In: *Measuring the dynamics of contraceptive use.* New York: United Nations, 1990.
2. Pariani S, Heer D, Van Arsdol M. Continued contraceptive use in five family planning clinics in Surabaya, Indonesia. *Studies in Family Planning,* 1987;22:384–390.
3. Latka M, Gollub E, French P, et al. Male-condom and female-condom use among women after counseling in a risk-reduction hierarchy for STD prevention. *Sex Transm Dis,* 2000;27:431–437.
4. Ray S, Bassett M, Maposhere C, et al. Acceptability of the female condom in Zimbabwe: Positive but male-centered responses. *Reproductive Health Matters,* 1995;5:68–79.
5. Kerrigan D, Mobley S, Rutenberg N, et al. The Female Condom: Dynamics of Use in Urban Zimbabwe. New York: Population Council/Horizons Report, 2000.
6. Bentley ME, Morrow KM, Fullem A, et al. Acceptability of a novel vaginal microbicide during a safety trial among low-risk women. *Fam Plann Perspect,* 2000;32:184–188.
7. Elias CJ, Coggins C, Alvarez F, et al. Colposcopic evaluation of a vaginal gel formulation of iota-carrageenan. *Contraception,* 1997;57:387–389.
8. Coggins C, Blanchard K, Alvarez F, et al. Preliminary safety and acceptability of a carrageenan gel for possible use as a vaginal microbicide. *Sex Trans Inf,* 2000;76:480–483.
9. Coggins C, Blanchard K, Friedland B. Men's attitudes toward a potential vaginal microbicide in Zimbabwe, Mexico and the USA. *Reproductive Health Matters,* 2000;8:132–141.
10. World Health Organization. *The Female Condom: A review.* Geneva, Switzerland: WHO, 1997.
11. Cecil H, Perry M, Seal D, et al. The female condom: What we have learned thus far? *AIDS and Behavior,* 1998;2:241–256.
12. Rees H, Beksinska M, Mqoqi N, et al. Multiphased study to investigate the safety of re-use of the female condom. Johannesburg, South Africa: Reproductive Health Research Unit, Department of Obstetrics and Gynaecology, Baragwanath Hospital, February, 1999.

13. Neilsen G. Background Paper: Programmatic Issues. WHO/UNAIDS Consultation on the Safety and Feasibility of the Re-use of the Female Condom. Geneva: WHO/UNAIDS, June, 2000.
14. Rees H, Beksinska M, Dickson-Tetteh KE, et al. The re-use of the female condom in a multi-phased study. Technical Report to WHO Consultation. Unpublished paper. Geneva, Switzerland: World Health Organization, 2000.
15. Smith JB, Nkhama G, Sebastian P, et al. Qualitative research on condom research among women in two developing countries. North Carolina: Family Health International, 1999.
16. Joannis C, Latka M, Glover LH, et al. Structural Integrity of the Female Condom after a Single Use, Washing, Disinfection. Family Health. International, Draft, 2000.
17. Information Update: Consultation on Re-use of the Female Condom. Geneva, Switzerland: WHO and UNAIDS, 2000.
18. Alliance for Microbicide Development. Microbicides in development—complete listing. Alliance for Microbicide Development Web site. Available at: http://www.microbicide.org/products%20in%20dev.htm. Accessed January 24, 2002.
19. van Damme L, Rosenberg ZF. Microbicides and barrier methods in HIV prevention. *AIDS*, 1999;13(suppl A):S85–S92.
20. Kreiss J, Ngugi E, Holmes KK, et al. Efficacy of nonoxynol-9 contraceptive sponge use in preventing heterosexual acquisition of HIV in Nairobi prostitutes. *JAMA*, 1992;268:477–482.
21. Roddy RE, Zekeng L, Ryan KA, et al. A controlled trial of nonoxynol 9 film to reduce male-to-female transmission of sexually transmitted diseases. *N Engl J Med*, 1998;339:504–510.
22. van Damme L. Advances in topical microbicides. Plenary presentation at the XIII International AIDS Conference; July 9–14, 2000; Durban, South Africa. Abstract PL04.
23. Zaretsky FR, Pearce-Pratt R, Phillips DM. Sulfated polyanions block Chlamydia trachomatis infection of cervix derived human epithelia. *Infect Immunol*, 1995;63:3520–3526.
24. Pearce-Pratt R, Phillips DM. Sulphated polysaccharides inhibit lymphocyte-to-epithelial transmission of HIV. *Biol Reprod*, 1996;54:173–182.
25. Zacharopoulos V, Phillips DM. Vaginal formulations of carrageenan protect mice from herpes simplex virus infection. *Clin Diag Lab Immunol*, 1997; 4:465–468.
26. Bourne N, Bernstein DI, Ireland J, et al. The topical microbicide PRO2000 protects against genital herpes in a mouse model. *J Infect Dis*, 1999;180: 203–205.
27. Phillips DM, Zacharopoulos V. Nonoxynol-9 enhances rectal infection by herpes simplex virus in mice. *Contraception*, 1998;57:341–348.
28. Sewankambo N, Gray RH, Wawer MJ, et al. HIV-1 infection associated with abnormal vaginal flora morphology and bacterial vaginosis. *Lancet*, 1997;350:546–550.
29. Taha TE, Hoover DR, Dallabetta GA, et al. Bacterial vaginosis and disturbances of vaginal flora: associated with increased acquisition of HIV. *AIDS*, 1998;12:1699–1706.
30. Wainberg M. Future microbicides research should focus on specific anti-HIV approaches. Presentation at the XIII International AIDS Conference; July 9–14, 2000; Durban, South Africa.
31. Ramjee, G, Morar NS, Alary M, et al. Challenges in the conduct of vaginal microbicide effectiveness trials in the developing world. *AIDS*, 2000;14: 2553–2557.
32. Friedland B. Informed consent in microbicides testing. Presentation at Microbicides 2000; March 13–16, 2000; Washington, DC.
33. Potts M. Thinking about vaginal microbicide testing. *Am J Public Health*, 2000;90:188–190.
34. van de Wijgert J, Elias C, Ellertson C, et al. Condom promotion in microbicide trials. *Am J Public Health*, 2000;90:1153–1154.
35. de Zoysa I, Elias CJ, Bentley ME. Microbicide research and "the investigator's dilemma." *Am J Public Health*, 2000;90:1155.
36. Heise L, McGrory E, Wood S. Practical and ethical dilemmas in the clinical testing of microbicides: A report on a symposium. International Women's Health Coalition, New York, 1998.
37. Fonn S, McGrory E. Informing research on HIV prevention: A consultation. New York: Population Council, 1999.

33

Behavioral Change: Goals and Means

*Poloko Kebaabetswe and †Kathleen F. Norr

*Botswana–Harvard Partnership for HIV Research and Education, Gaborone, Botswana.
†College of Nursing, University of Illinois at Chicago, Chicago, Illinois, USA.

Understanding the behaviors that put individuals at risk of HIV infection, and identifying ways to change these behaviors, are important strategies to help halt the spread of HIV in Africa and other developing countries. It may be feasible for African countries to provide effective behavioral change interventions within the constraints of their economic and human resources. A major concern, however, is that a limited number of such interventions exist at a scale capable of containing the epidemic. In this chapter, we will review the goals and means of behavioral change for HIV prevention and the barriers to change, with special emphasis on Africa. We will also examine existing successful and well-evaluated interventions that hold promise for adaptation and application in Africa.

GOALS OF BEHAVIORAL CHANGE PROGRAMS

The ultimate goal of behavioral change intervention in HIV prevention is to reduce behaviors that increase the risk of HIV transmission and, thus, reduce the incidence of HIV. In Africa, where the primary route of transmission is heterosexual, there is widespread agreement that the most important goal of behavioral change programs should be to reduce unprotected sexual contact. However, there is debate regarding the selection of specific behaviors and populations to target.

Behaviors to Change

The "ABCs" (Abstinence, Being faithful, and Condom use) are widely recognized as key behaviors that reduce the risk of HIV transmission. Abstinence includes delay of first sexual experience for adolescents. Being faithful, which can apply to a monogamous or polygamous union, includes reducing the number of one's sexual partners, an especially important effort in situations where serial monogamy is common. For maximum effectiveness, male or female condoms must be used correctly and consistently. Experts generally agree that these three behaviors are effective ways to slow the spread of HIV. However, condom promotion continues to be debated in many African countries. Many religious leaders, as well as some politicians and citizens, believe that abstinence and faithfulness are the only morally acceptable solutions. Some also argue that promoting condom use encourages individuals to engage in high-risk sexual behavior or that using condoms does not effectively protect against HIV. In contrast, others believe that promotion of condom use is an important component of behavioral change programs.

Promoting condom use is more widely accepted in programs that target high-risk populations, such as commercial sex workers (CSWs), than in programs for the general population. Despite extensive research indicating that school-based sex education does not increase adolescent sexual activities (1, 2), condom promotion for young people is especially controversial, as shown by a recent editorial in a Botswana newspaper in which parents were described to be opposed to making condoms available to students at pre-tertiary schools (3).

Populations to Target for Behavioral Change

There are two different models guiding the selection of appropriate populations to target for behavioral change: the epidemiologic model and the holistic model. The epidemiologic model targets those populations with the highest risk of transmitting HIV, such as CSWs and their clients, migrant workers, and persons who already have another sexually transmitted disease (STD). An extension of the epidemiologic model expands high-risk groups to include vulnerable populations, such as adolescents and women. Young people are an especially important group in nearly all African countries, because HIV infection usually occurs during adolescence and young adulthood, especially among women (4,5).

The holistic or general population model targets the entire community or society. The World Health Organization's (WHO) primary health care model is the most widely recognized public health framework that includes this holistic approach (6). Although not all holistic approaches explicitly use a primary health care framework, primary health care emphasizes behavioral change interventions for the entire community with maximum community and multisectoral collaboration.

Proponents of the epidemiologic model argue that it is the most efficacious and cost-effective way to control any epidemic; mathematical modeling supports their argument (7,8). Ainsworth and Teokul argue that developing countries with limited economic and service-delivery capacities must be wary of broad programs that spread their resources too thin to achieve behavioral change (9). However, others argue that holistic, community-wide prevention programs provide more equitable access to prevention services and are thus more likely to gain political and popular support. The holistic approach also avoids reinforcing denial and stigmatization of individuals living with HIV or AIDS because it includes all members of a community (10–12). Sumartojo et al. (13) call for an integrated approach that combines both targeted and broad-based interventions appropriate for particular settings and stages of the HIV epidemic. However, there are few existing guidelines for the optimal program combination.

THE MEANS TO BEHAVIORAL CHANGE

Individual and Small Group Models

The first approaches to changing sexual behaviors were adapted from psychosocial models aimed at influencing a variety of behaviors. The health beliefs model identifies four key beliefs or perceptions related to behavioral change: threat, efficacy and benefits, barriers or negative effects, and cues to action, such as a mass media campaign (14, 15). The theory of reasoned action (16,17) identifies an individual's intention to behave a certain way as the best indicator of change. Intention is affected by an individual's attitude (perceived outcomes and evaluation of those outcomes) and social norms (expectations of other specific individuals and groups and the importance of meeting those expectations). Bandura's social learning model

(18,19) sees behavior change as a function of an individual's expectations of the outcome, and self-efficacy (confidence in his or her ability to change a risk behavior or adopt a new behavior). Self-efficacy can be increased through role-modeling, rehearsal, and support of specific new behaviors. Many HIV behavior change interventions merge elements of these three theories in their approaches to individual change.

The integrated social learning model, developed by the U.S. National Commission on AIDS (20), identifies eight key components needed for behavioral change: positive benefits/costs ratio, strong intent, necessary skills, high self-efficacy, expected positive emotional response, compatibility of the behavior with self-image, greater perceived social pressure to perform a behavior than not to perform it, and fewer environmental constraints to performing a behavior than not performing it.

There is strong empirical evidence that interventions based on the integrated social learning model can help change a variety of high-risk behaviors in many populations, including in men who have sex with men (21), adolescents (22,23), injection drug users (IDUs) and their sexual partners, (24–26), CSWs, and heterosexual women (27–30). Several reviews have noted that interventions that are guided by the integrated social learning model, interventions that are intensive and multidimensional, and interventions that are tailored specifically to the HIV prevention context of the target population, are more successful than those lacking such features (28,30,31).

Two models identify a specific process for changing individual behavior. The AIDS risk reduction model identifies three steps toward behavioral change: labeling one's behavior as high-risk, making a commitment to reduce high-risk behaviors, and taking action to perform the desired change. The transtheoretical model identifies five steps toward behavioral change: precontemplation, contemplation, preparation, action, and maintenance (32). Because individuals may relapse at any stage, ongoing reinforcement is critical. Previous attempts to change behavior are associated with later success, so a program with a high relapse rate may still be moving individuals toward eventual success. Matching the intervention message to the individual's readiness for change at a particular point increases chances of success, as documented in the United States by the Centers for Disease Control and Prevention's (CDC) multi-city study of community-based programs (33).

Community and Societal Models of Change

Community and societal models of change are distinguished by their emphasis on modifying structural barriers in the community, society, and culture. The goal of these modifications is to achieve more sustainable behavioral change through programs that are accessible and affordable to all members of the community (34). The diffuse influence of these models, the difficulty in identifying appropriate control groups, and the problems in measuring impact on structural factors or processes, make evaluation of interventions based on these models challenging (34,35). However, several approaches to introduce behavioral change beyond the individual level have been successful.

The diffusion of innovations theory (36, 37), originally developed for diffusion of agricultural innovations in rural community development, is based on the idea that most innovations spread gradually from innovators, who are usually influential and persuasive, to the rest of the community. This approach has been shown effective for HIV prevention programs. Peer group leaders (innovators) increased awareness of the need for safer sex and condom use among members of gay communities in a multisite study in the United States (21,38). In Africa, the diffusion of innovations approach, usually combined with a social learning model, has been used for transportation workers, bar girls, and CSWs (39–42).

Mass media campaigns incorporate a structural approach by using communication channels to influence societal awareness, knowledge, and norms. Communication channels include radio, television, newspapers, pamphlets, posters, dramas, and mass rallies (43). Merson highlights the success of mass media campaigns in containing the HIV epidemics in Switzerland, Australia, and New Zealand (25). In Switzerland, time-series data showed increased knowledge of HIV, condom sales, reported condom use, and HIV testing in the general population following an intensive mass media campaign (35,44,45).

Community empowerment (also called community organization, -mobilization, or -action research) is a strategy used in public health, behavioral sciences, and social movements to mobilize people to recognize structural barriers and to empower them to change these barriers (46–52). This approach is distinguished by its broad agenda for behavioral change—which addresses specific behaviors as well as underlying factors—and the active involvement of community members in designing, executing, and evaluating the empowerment project. Community involvement in evaluation directly contributes to capacity-building and increased awareness in the target community.

The CDC multisite community HIV prevention projects, which are directed at high-risk populations in the United States, are examples of successful community empowerment projects for HIV prevention. These projects use a stages of change theory (53) and a school-based intervention involving parents, teachers, and community members (54). In developing countries, several community empowerment interventions have been directed at CSWs in Nigeria, Kenya, Zimbabwe, and Ghana (39,42,55) and at community mobilization of women in Zaire (56) and Thailand (57). The Thai study has an especially clear description and evaluation of the community mobilization process (57).

Social marketing applies the principles of commercial marketing to promote behavioral change in individuals (58,59). This approach involves structural change because it usually changes social norms and reduces practical barriers, such as the availability and cost of condoms. A key component of social marketing is segmenting the market, which is similar to targeting and tailoring interventions for specific populations. Perhaps the most widespread and successful example of this approach is the social marketing of condoms, both in Africa and in other developing countries (60). A community coalition in the United States has also used social marketing to increase condom use among sexually active adolescents without negative community response (61).

Policy or infrastructure changes affect individual behavior indirectly by changing the structural factors that support high-risk behavior or prevent behavior change. The two best documented examples of these approaches include provision of clean injection equipment for IDUs and the establishment of a policy for 100% condom use in Thailand's brothels (25,62,63).

BARRIERS TO BEHAVIORAL CHANGE IN AFRICA

Despite much discussion about structural barriers to behavioral change, few strategies for eliminating these barriers have been produced (34,64–66). We will use the CDC intervention-oriented framework to systematically identify four types of structural barriers to behavioral change in Africa: economic, political, sociocultural, and organizational (34).

Economic Barriers

Poverty contributes to HIV transmission throughout Africa and serves as a barrier to sexual behavioral change (67). Economic pressures force many women and young girls into sex work. Some impoverished parents enlist their adolescent daughters into sex work to earn money for the family. In many African countries, sex work is episodic and casual, and therefore, difficult for public health officials to monitor. Women who periodically receive money for sex do not necessarily identify themselves as CSWs, nor do their casual partners necessarily categorize them as such. Despite the potential for behavioral change among people who engage in commercial sex work, the poverty level in Africa often necessitates this source of income. For example, CSWs in Zaire who had successfully changed their behavior to include increased condom use were unable to develop adequate alternative sources of income so that they could stop sex work altogether (56).

Initiatives for behavioral change are also hindered by the economic pressures that force many people to travel looking for work. Throughout sub–Saharan Africa, there is a long-standing tradition of male migration to cities, mines, and other industry sites in search of work. Migrant workers typically stay in dormitories and endure harsh working conditions while earning money to support their families (68,69). Male migrant workers, separated from their wives, may turn to relationships with CSWs or "second wives." Wives left at home may also have extramarital relationships, sometimes to earn money. When male migrant workers return home, they may shun the use of condoms, which would suggest unfaithfulness, and thus increase the risk of spreading HIV and other infections to their partners.

Prolonged separation of couples occurs at all social levels, for reasons such as education abroad or frequent, work-related transfers. Recently, for example, government workers in Botswana were required to accept frequent transfers, regardless of family disruption. Migration and family separation have also occurred in some areas of Africa because of famine and political conflict. Migration is a major contributing factor to the spread of HIV infection across the socioeconomic spectrum and to rural areas in many African countries.

Political Factors

Political factors play a significant role in facilitating or hindering behavioral change in individuals and communities. Perhaps the single most important factor related to national success in those developing countries where HIV incidence has declined, has been strong commitment to HIV prevention from the highest political levels (9).

In some African countries, weak or unstable governments, armed conflict, or health crises, such as famine or Ebola outbreaks, temporarily force HIV prevention to the bottom of the political agenda. In a resource-poor environment, funds devoted to HIV prevention inevitably mean fewer resources allocated for other, more popular programs. Additionally, widespread misinformation, denial, and the stigma of AIDS contribute to ambivalence about developing an HIV prevention policy. In such an environment, a politician who strongly supports HIV prevention risks causing controversy and losing political support.

In many countries, specific policies and laws, such as those barring the distribution of clean needles to injection drug users, are also barriers to behavioral change. Broad policy changes that are more difficult to accomplish include alleviating poverty, increasing access to education, raising hope for the future, and motivating health-seeking behavior. However, there are now signs of increasing awareness and political motivation at high levels in many African countries, such as the recent completion of a 5-year national strategic AIDS control plan in Malawi (4), the hosting of the *XIII International AIDS Conference* in South Africa, and the Mashi project in Botswana (a study of mother-to-child HIV prevention and the impact of combining feeding strategies with antiretroviral therapies on the rates of mother-to-child transmission of HIV).

Social and Cultural Barriers

HIV and AIDS have long been associated with stigma and denial worldwide (70). In Africa, these negative attitudes continue to be highly resistant to change except in very few countries, such as Uganda. Inaccurate information, including widespread rumors about the transmission of HIV, contributes to unfounded fears of casual, nonsexual contact with people living with HIV or AIDS, and further reinforces stigma. Failure to recognize personal risk, fear of open discussion of high-risk behaviors or prevention methods, reluctance to learn or disclose HIV status, and familial concealment of HIV status and AIDS-related deaths are examples of behaviors that are perpetuated by stigma and denial.

In most African countries, open discussion of sexuality is socially discouraged, especially between adults and youth, except during traditional rites of passage conducted by nonparental adults. In some areas, especially in towns, traditional initiation rites have nearly disappeared or have been supplanted by church-based ceremonies. Where the initiation ceremonies do continue, they rarely address HIV prevention. Some parents fear that these ceremonies may actually promote early sexual activity among youths (71). It is often difficult for parents to educate their children about the risk of HIV transmission because discussion of sex is taboo. Moreover, when parents reject sex education in schools, HIV prevention education is either minimal or unavailable to vulnerable young populations. Likewise, cultural taboos discourage partners from discussing sex and high-risk behaviors openly with one another.

Gender inequality is a barrier to HIV prevention and behavioral change at individual and societal levels worldwide. Africa is no exception. Traditional gender roles for African women deny them familial, economic, and political power, leaving them with limited access to resources. Therefore, they may be unable to negotiate safer sexual practices even when they know that their male partners are involved in high-risk sexual relationships (67). The acceptance of polygamy in many parts of Africa also confounds HIV prevention efforts (72).

Organizational Barriers

In many African countries, the ability to establish and maintain nationwide programs for behavioral change is limited, in part, due to the many economic, political, and sociocultural factors previously mentioned. Collaborative networks of both governmental and nongovernmental organizations must be strengthened and expanded, and larger groups of personnel need opportunities for training and professional growth (9). At present, competition over scarce resources, including educated personnel, remains a barrier to collaboration at every level (73). Additionally, although many behavioral change interventions have been evaluated, their comparative efficacy and the cost-effectiveness of their components are not well understood. Strategies for the expansion and cost-effective adaptation of existing interventions to new settings also require further study (12,34,35,67).

OVERCOMING STRUCTURAL BARRIERS

Structural barriers to behavioral change for HIV prevention in Africa are substantial, and some argue that reviewing these barriers may lead to despair rather than to action (74). Structural problems cannot be solved overnight, but there is evidence that many such barriers can be modified in progressive stages. Participants at the recent Southern Africa Development Community (SADC) conferences have recommended the development of regional policies on HIV in the workplace and are addressing other legal issues. Working with traditional leaders is effective in changing or reducing harm from their practices, as shown by efforts to help traditional healers in Botswana recognize AIDS and refer cases appropriately (75), and in working with Muslim leaders in Uganda to ensure safe funeral practices (76). Kotellos et al. discuss Family Health International's strategies for assessing and strengthening capacity-building at the individual, organizational, and institutional level (73). DiFranceisco et al. found that technical assistance in capacity-building is effective and welcomed by service organizations (77).

MODELS OF HOPE

Several recent, well-evaluated, individual projects and national programs have changed behaviors for HIV prevention in Africa and can serve as models for other African nations (Table 1). Two of these programs, based on the integrated social learning model, have influenced levels of knowledge, attitudes, and behaviors among students of a Tanzanian elementary school (78,79) and among students of a Namibian secondary school (80,81). Modified behaviors include delay of the onset of sexual activity among those not yet sexually active, and increased condom use among those who are sexually active. In Senegal and Tanzania, two programs based on the diffusion of innovations model trained peer leaders to discuss condom use and STD treatment with truck drivers and CSWs serving truck drivers (40, 41). Although it was difficult to reach this mobile group, both interventions successfully changed sexual behaviors, including increasing condom use.

Similarly, two successful programs have modified structural barriers. A mobile clinic which offered HIV testing, STD treatment, individual and group educational sessions, and condom instruction and distribution, was able to decrease STD incidence and increase condom use with CSWs among HIV-negative truckers in Kenya (82). A community mobilization program for CSWs in Côte d'Ivoire held community health meetings and trained CSWs to serve as peer educators (83). The program promoted HIV prevention through behavioral change in one-on-one and small group sessions, distributed condoms, and referred women to the clinic. The program reached more than half the CSWs in the target neighborhood and increased their condom negotiation skills and their use of condoms. The prevalence of HIV among CSWs, who were visiting the clinic for first-time testing, declined from 89% to 63% over 5 years.

At the national level, two developing countries, Thailand and Uganda, have succeeded in substantially reducing new HIV infections. Both national programs have received political support from the highest levels. Multiple models of behavioral change (social marketing of condoms, integrated social learning through peer groups and peer leaders, mass media campaigns, and structural changes) were implemented simultaneously. In Thailand, behavioral change efforts focused primarily on increasing use of condoms and clean injection equipment among people in high-risk groups, such as CSWs and their clients, IDUs, and army conscripts. A noteworthy innovation was the policy requiring all brothel owners to ensure 100% condom use, which eliminated customer refusal to use condoms and fear of competition from other brothels in which condoms were not required (62).

A more holistic approach in Uganda also shows clear signs of beginning to contain the epidemic. A cornerstone of Uganda's program has been its multisectoral approach that includes visible commitment from the president and widespread societal involvement. Uganda focused primarily on young people and emphasized abstinence for young people and faithfulness in established relationships, popularized in the "zero grazing" campaign, as well as condom promotion. As a result, the proportion of sexually active young men and women has declined, and the average age at initiation of sexual activity

TABLE 1. Models of Hope: Interventions that Changed Behaviors in Africa[a]

Conceptual model (reference)	Design	Country: Sample	Intervention	Outcomes	Comment
Integrated Social Learning (78)	Quasi-experimental: schools randomly assigned, pre-tests and post-tests 12 months later	Tanzania: urban and rural 6th graders, n = 814, 23% lost to follow-up	—Teachers gave class program in 2–3 months (20 hours) —Components: information, group discussion, student-created songs, dramas, etc. performed to younger students, community	—Significantly ↑ AIDS knowledge, positive attitudes, and discussion —However, # becoming sexually active was lower (6.6% vs. 16.5%), but not significant, perhaps due to the small # of cases	—Losses due mainly to school dropout; such students are probably also at higher risk —Condoms not included (not accepted in primary schools), but concept needs to be explored
Integrated Social Learning (80, 81)	Randomized longitudinal trial: pre-tests and post-tests at 6, 12 months after intervention	Namibia: 515 pupils at 10 secondary schools, 46% males	—14 sessions after school with teacher and PL (new graduate or teacher) —Focus on abstinence, condom use, skill-building, other risks	—Significantly ↑ knowledge, positive attitudes, self-efficacy —*Among virgins at intake:* females had less sexual activity or drinking; males had more condom use if sexually active	—Western social learning model effective in Africa —Both genders affected by intervention, but in different ways
Diffusion of Innovations Social Learning (40)	Longitudinal: pre-test and 2-year follow-up, no control	Senegal: 260 urban transport workers, 54% married	—PL selected by workers, trained, then weekly boosters —Good penetration: 2/3 of transport workers talked to PL	—*Among transport workers:* ↑ condom use and ↓ barriers to condom use, ↓ sex with CSWs —*Among CSWs:* ↑ condom use, but still unsafe sex	—PL can reach and change behavior of highly mobile group —Lack of control group, hard to verify sexual behaviors
Diffusion of Innovations Social Learning (41)	Longitudinal: pre-test and 2 surveys at 18 and 24 months, intensive (to 18 months), then maintenance, no control	Tanzania: truckers, women at truck stops, surveys have ≥ 198 men; 121 women	—Clients chose PLs —PLs trained, had regular visits & booster training —PLs talked, distributed and promoted condoms, and promoted STD treatment	- ↑ knowledge, perceived personal risk, reported STDs, and condom use; slight decline during maintenance period	—Documents impact both during intensive program and less intensive period of maintenance

Continued

TABLE 1. *Continued*

Conceptual model (reference)	Design	Country: Sample	Intervention	Outcomes	Comment
Structural Change (access to health care) (82)	Interrupted time series: pre-test and follow-up for 18 months, no control	Kenya: 556 male HIV-uninfected truck drivers, 25% not retained	—Initial VCT and on-site clinic visit weekly with VCT, STD treatment, group and individual discussion, condoms demonstrated and distributed	—Significantly ↓ extramarital sex, CSW contact, and STD incidence —However, no change in condom use for extramarital sex or with wives	—Only symptomatic STDs identified and treated —More travel related to higher risk, less follow-up
Community Mobilization Social Learning (PLs) (83)	Longitudinal cross-section surveys, since 1991	Cote d'Ivoire: Female CSWs; n=329, 1991 n=602, 1993 n=850, 1995	—Community health meetings —PLs teach groups and individuals, make clinic referrals, give condoms —Linked to clinic and condom social marketing program —Gradually expanded to clients, community	—CSW HIV prevalence ↓ from 89% initially to 63% among new clients at clinic —*Surveys found:* about half of the CSWs reached by the program; those reached had better negotiation skills, more condom use than those not in contact at all 3 surveys.	—Good example of sustainable program, integration of several approaches —CSWs change rapidly, difficult to maintain continuity and evaluate with survey —Program relies more and more on peer educators

[a]PL indicates Peer Leader; CSW, Commercial Sex Worker; STD, Sexually Transmitted Disease; VCT, Voluntary Counseling and Testing.

among young women is nearly two years later than it had been among earlier cohorts (84–86).

Thailand's national program illustrates a successful example of using an epidemiologic model, while Uganda's success is based on a holistic approach. Thailand's approach achieved relatively rapid behavioral change but has done little to address underlying social issues, such as the widespread commercial sex industry and the continued risk of HIV transmission among many CSWs (87, 88). Uganda's approach has begun to address some of the structural issues that underlie HIV transmission, such as social acceptance of adolescent sexual activity. Several researchers note that Thailand's approach has depended on a strong government; a highly centralized administration and health care system; a relatively homogeneous, tolerant, and pragmatic set of cultural values; and a national income substantially higher than that of most developing countries (67). Because few African countries have such an infrastructure, Uganda's approach may be more adaptable in other African nations than Thailand's approach.

CONCLUSION

This review has identified numerous barriers to behavioral change for HIV prevention in Africa. There are far too few intensive HIV prevention efforts being implemented, particularly in rural areas. However, there is strong evidence that the broad goals of behavioral change to reduce HIV transmission are widely accepted throughout Africa. The evidence from Uganda suggests that solutions feasible in Africa may include more emphasis on abstinence and faithfulness and less emphasis on condom use than has been characteristic in industrialized countries or in Thailand.

There is also substantial evidence that the means for changing behaviors to prevent HIV transmission are well developed. Important lessons can be learned from individual programs and countrywide models of success. Although theories on behavioral change may not apply to all cultures or populations, strong conceptual models can guide the transfer of effective programs from one setting to another. The effectiveness of interventions is enhanced by the use of multiple strategies, intensive contact, and continued reinforcement. When community members, parents, and teachers are involved, behavioral change programs can succeed in primary schools, before children are sexually active and when most are still in school. Strong evaluation designs are important because they provide the evidence of successes or failures that allows planners to select more effective interventions to promote behavioral change in the future.

With the lessons learned from Uganda and a growing international commitment to assist African nations in addressing the HIV epidemic, the path forward is now clear. As Winston Churchill declared during World War II, "It is not the end, it is not the beginning of the end, but it is the end of the beginning."

ACKNOWLEDGEMENTS

Poloko Kebaabetswe: I am grateful to Professor Max Essex, Chair of the Harvard AIDS Institute, and Professor Sheila Tlou of the University of Botswana for giving me an opportunity to share my thoughts on behavior change, and perhaps a window of hope in HIV Prevention, with my fellow Africans. My thanks to the Botswana-Harvard Partnership for HIV Research and Education team, especially Dr. Ibou Thior and Ria Madison for their constant encouragement, and to my family: Sethata, Tommie, Tullie, and Abigail, who through their patience and support reduced my stress while I increased theirs.

Dr. Norr would like to thank her many colleagues in AIDS prevention research in Africa, especially Dr. James Norr at the University of Illinois at Chicago, Dr. Sheila Tlou at the University of Botswana, and Dr. Chrissie Kaponda and her colleagues at

Kamuzu College of Nursing, all of whom have influenced her thinking about behavioral change in Africa.

We would like to acknowledge the bibliographic assistance of Kaoru Watanabe, MSN, doctoral candidate in nursing at the University of Illinois at Chicago.

REFERENCES

1. Kirby D, Korpi M, Adivi C, et al. An impact evaluation of project SNAPP: An AIDS and pregnancy prevention middle school program. *AIDS Educ Prev*, 1997;9(1 Supp):44–61.
2. Kirby D, Short L, Collins J, et al. School-based programs to reduce sexual risk behaviors: A review of effectiveness. *Public Health Rep*, 1994;109:339–360.
3. Kelebonye G. Condoms sow promiscuity. *The Voice Newspaper*. November 10, 2000-November 16, 2000;12–13.
4. National AIDS Control Programme. *Malawi's National Response to HIV/AIDS for 2000–2004: Combatting HIV/AIDS With Renewed Hope and Vigour in the New Millennium*. Malawi: Strategic Planning Unit, 1999.
5. AIDS/STD Unit Ministry of Health; *Sentinel Surveillance Report 1999.* Gaborone, Botswana: Ministry of Health, 1999.
6. World Health Organization. *Primary Health Care: Report of the International Conference on Primary Health Care, Alma-Ata.* Geneva, Switzerland: WHO, 1978.
7. Anderson RM. The role of mathematical models in the study of HIV transmission and the epidemiology of AIDS. *J Acquir Immune Defic Syndr*, 1988;1:241–256.
8. Bernstein RS, Sokal DC, Seiz ST, et al. Simulating the control of a heterosexual HIV epidemic in a severely affected East African city. *Interfaces*, 1998;28:101–126.
9. Ainsworth M, Teokul W. Breaking the silence: setting realistic priorities for AIDS control in less-developed countries. *Lancet*, 2000;356:55–60.
10. MacNeil JM, Anderson S. Beyond the dichotomy: linking HIV prevention with care. *AIDS*, 1998; 12(Suppl 2):S19–S26.
11. Kalichman S, Belcher L, Norris F, et al. Motivational enhancing and skills building HIV risk reduction counseling intervention for women. Paper presented at: XII International Conference on AIDS; June 28–July 3, 1998; Geneva, Switzerland.
12. Sumartojo E, Carey JW, Doll LS, et al. Targeted and general population interventions for HIV prevention: towards a comprehensive approach [editorial]. *AIDS*, 1997;11:1201–1209.
13. Conceptual basis and procedures for the intervention in a multisite HIV prevention trial. NIMH Multisite HIV Prevention Trial. *AIDS*, 1997; 11(Suppl 2):S29–S35.
14. Becker MH. AIDS and behavior changes. *Public Health Rev*, 1988;16(1–2):1–11.
15. Janz N, Becker MH. The health beliefs model and illness behavior. *Health Educ Monogr*, 1984;2: 387–408.
16. Ajzen I, Fishbein M. *Understanding Attitudes and Predicting Social Behavior*. Englewood, NJ: Prentice Hall; 1980.
17. Fishbein M, Ajzen I. *Belief, Attitude, Intention, and Behavior: An Introduction to Theory and Research.* Reading, MA: Addision-Wesley, 1975.
18. Bandura A. Human agency in social cognitive theory. *Am Psychol*, 1989;44:1175.
19. Bandura A. Social cognitive theory of mass communication. In: Bryan J, Zillman D, eds. *Media Effects: Advances in Theory and Research*. Hillsdale, NJ: Erlbaum, 1994.
20. National Commission on AIDS. *Behavioral and Social Sciences and the HIV/AIDS Epidemic.* Washington, DC: National Commission on AIDS, 1993.
21. Kelly JA, Murphy DA, Sikkema KJ, et al. Randomised, controlled, community-level HIV-prevention intervention for sexual-risk behaviour among homosexual men in US cities. Community HIV Prevention Research Collaborative. *Lancet*, 1997;350:1500–1505.
22. Jemmott JB, Jemmott LS, Fong GT. Abstinence and safer sex HIV risk-reduction interventions for African American adolescents: a randomized controlled trial. *JAMA*, 1998;279:1529–1536.
23. Rotheram-Borus MJ, Mahler KA, Rosario M. AIDS prevention with adolescents. *AIDS Educ Prev*, 1995;7:320–336.
24. Des Jarlais DC, Casriel C, Friedman SR, et al. AIDS and the transition to illicit drug injection: Results of a randomized trial prevention program. *Br J Addict*, 1992;87:493–498.
25. Merson MH. International perspective on AIDS prevention research. In: Program and abstracts of the NIH Consensus Development Conference on Interventions to Prevent HIV Risk Behavior; February 11–13, 1997; Bethesda, MD, USA. National Institutes of Health Online edition; 1997: 76–80.
26. McCusker J, Stoddard AM, Zapka JG, et al. Behavioral outcomes of AIDS educational interventions for drug users in short-term treatment. *Am J Public Health*, 1993;83:1463–1466.
27. Dancy BL, Marcantonio R, Norr K. The long-term effectiveness of an HIV prevention intervention for low-income African American women. *AIDS Educ Prev*, 2000;12:113–125.
28. Erhardt AA. Behavioral interventions with women. Paper presented at: NIH Consensus Development

Conference on Interventions to Prevent HIV Risk Behaviors; February 11–13, 1997; Bethesda, MD.
29. Sikkema KJ, Kelly JA, Winett RA, et al. Outcomes of a randomized community-level HIV prevention intervention for women living in 18 low-income housing developments. *Am J Public Health*, 2000;90:57–63.
30. Des Jarlais DC, Choopanya K, Vanichseni S, et al. AIDS risk reduction and reduced HIV seroconversion among injection drug users in Bangkok [see comments]. *Am J Public Health*, 1994;84:452–455.
31. Kalichman SC, Johnson BT, Carey MP. Prevention of sexually transmitted HIV infection: A meta-analytic review of the behavioral outcome literature. *Ann Behav Med*, 1996;18:6–15.
32. Prochaska JO. In search of how people change: Applications to addictive behaviors. *Am Psychol*, 1992;47:1102–1114.
33. Ellen JM, Kohn RP, Bolan GA, et al. Socioeconomic differences in sexually transmitted disease rates among black and white adolescents, San Francisco, 1990 to 1992. *Am J Public Health*, 1995;85:1546–1548.
34. Sumartojo E. Structural factors in HIV prevention: Concepts, examples, and implications for research. *AIDS*, 2000;14(Suppl 1):S3–S10.
35. O'Reilly KR, Piot P. International perspectives on individual and community approaches to the prevention of sexually transmitted disease and human immunodeficiency virus infection. *J Infect Dis*, 1996;174:S214–S222.
36. Rogers EM. *Diffusion of Innovations*. 1st ed. New York: Free Press; 1962.
37. Rogers EM. *Diffusion of Innovations*. 4th ed. New York: Free Press; 1995.
38. Kelly JA, St Lawrence JS, Stevenson LY, et al. Community AIDS/HIV Risk Reduction: The effect of endorsements by popular people in the three cities. *Am J Public Health*, 1992;82:1483–1489.
39. Asamoah-Adu A, Weir S, Pappoe M, et al. Evaluation of a targeted AIDS prevention intervention to increase condom use among prostitutes in Ghana. *AIDS*, 1994;8:239–246.
40. Leonard L, Ndiaye I, Kapadia A, et al. HIV prevention among male clients of female sex workers in Kaolack, Senegal: Results of a peer education program. *AIDS Educ Prev*, 2000;12:21–37.
41. Laukamm-Josten U, Mwizarubi BK, Outwater A, et al. Preventing HIV infection through peer education and condom promotion among truck drivers and their sexual partners in Tanzania, 1990–1993. *AIDS Care*, 2000;12:27–40.
42. Williams E, Lamson N, Efem S, et al. Implementation of an AIDS prevention program among prostitutes in the Cross River State of Nigeria [letter]. *AIDS*, 1992;6:229–230.
43. Family Health International. Behavior change through mass communication. Family Health International; n.d.
44. Hausser D, Zimmerman E, Dubois-Arber F, et al. *Evaluation of the AIDS Prevention Strategy in Switzerland: Third Assessment Report (1989–1990)*. Lausanne, Swizerland: Institut Universitaire de Medecine Sociale et Preventive, 1991.
45. Jeannin A, Dubois-Arber F, Paccaud F. HIV testing in Switzerland. *AIDS*, 1994;8:1599–1603.
46. Beeker C, Guenther-Grey C, Raj A. Community empowerment paradigm drift and the primary prevention of HIV/AIDS. *Soc Sci Med*, 1998;46: 831–842.
47. Drevdahl D. Coming to voice: the power of emancipatory community interventions. *Adv Nurs Sci*, 1995;18:13–24.
48. Fals-Borda O, Rahman MS, Eds. *Action and Knowledge: Breaking the Monopoly With Participatory Action Research*. New York: Intermediate Technology/Apex, 1991.
49. Freire P. *Pedagogy of the Oppressed*. New York: Seabury Press, 1970.
50. Henderson DJ. Consciousness raising in participatory research: method and methodology for emancipatory nursing inquiry. *Adv Nurs Sci*, 1995;17:58–69.
51. Stevens PE, Hall JM. Participatory action research for sustaining individual and community change: A model of HIV prevention education. *AIDS Educ Prev*, 1998;10:387–402.
52. Wallerstein N, Bernstein E. Introduction to community empowerment, participatory education, and health. *Health Educ Q*, 1994;21:141–148.
53. The CDC AIDS Community Demonstration Project Research Group. Community-level HIV intervention in 5 cities: Final outcome data from the CDC AIDS community demonstration projects. *Am J Public Health*, 1999;89:336–345.
54. Paikoff RL, Baptiste D. Training community women as co-facilitators of HIV-prevention family group. In: Program and Abstracts of the National Conference on Women and HIV; May 4–7, 1997; Pasadena, California, USA. Abstract no. 125.3.
55. Ngugi EN, Plummer FA, Mwongera M, et al. Decreased risky sexual behaviour following an integrated health service and community-based STD/AIDS intervention in Nairobi. *International Conference on AIDS*, 1993;9(1):87–96.
56. Schoepf BG. AIDS action-research with women in Kinshasa, Zaire. *Soc Sci Med*, 1993;37:1401–1403.
57. Elkins D, Maticka-Tyndale E, Kuyyakanond T, et al. Toward reducing the spread of HIV in northeastern Thai villages: evaluation of a village-based intervention. *AIDS Educ Prev*, 1997;9:49–69.
58. Lamptey PR, Price JE. Social marketing sexually transmitted disease and HIV prevention: a consumer-centered approach to achieving behavior change. *AIDS*, 1998;12(Supp 2):S1–S9.
59. Kotler P, Roberto EL. *Social Marketing: Strategies for Changing Public Behavior*. New York: Free Press; 1989.

60. World Health Organization; *Global Strategy for the Prevention and Control of AIDS*. WHA45.35. Geneva, Switzerland: WHO, 1992.
61. Kennedy MG, Mizuno Y, Seals BF, et al. Increasing condom use among adolescents with coalition-based social marketing. *AIDS*, 2000;14:1809–1818.
62. Rojanapithayakorn W, Hanenberg R. The 100% condom program in Thailand. *AIDS*, 1996;10:1–7.
63. Vlahov D. Role of needle exchange programs in AIDS prevention. In: Program and abstracts of the NIH Consensus Development Conference: Interventions to Prevent HIV Risk Behaviors; February 11–13, 1997; Bethesda, MD. National Institutes of Health; 1997:87–92.
64. Mann JM, Tarantola DJ. HIV 1998: The global picture. *Sci Am*, 1998;279:82–83.
65. Sweat MD, Denison JA. Reducing HIV incidence in developing countries with structural and environmental interventions. *AIDS*, 1995;9(Supp A): S251–S257.
66. Tawil O, Verster A, O'Reilly KR. Enabling approaches for HIV/AIDS prevention: can we modify the environment and minimize the risk? [editorial]. *AIDS*, 1995;9:1299–1306.
67. Parker RG, Easton D, Klein CH. Structural barriers and facilitators in HIV prevention: A review of international research. *AIDS*, 2000;14(Supp. 1):S22–S32.
68. UNAIDS, WHO. *AIDS Epidemic Update: December 1998*. Geneva, Switzerland: UNAIDS, 1998.
69. Campbell C, Williams B. Beyond the biomedical and behavioural: towards an integrated approach to HIV prevention in the southern African mining industry. *Soc Sci Med*, 1999;48:1625–1639.
70. Goldin CS. Stigmatization and AIDS: critical issues in public health. *Soc Sci Med*, 1994;39: 1359–1366.
71. Kamlongera CF. *Initiation Rites Among Yao Muslims in the Southern Region of Malawi: Jando and Nsondo From Machinga, Mangochi and Zomba, A Report*. Malawi; 1997.
72. Fidzani NH, Ntseane DM, Seloilwe ES. *HIV/AIDS in the North East District: Situation and Response Analysis*. Unpublished paper. Gaborone, Botswana, 2000.
73. Kotellos KA, Amon JJ, Benazerga WM. Field experiences: measuring capacity building efforts in HIV/AIDS prevention programmes. *AIDS*, 1998; 12(Supp 2):S109–S117.
74. Dowsett, G. The indeterminant macro-social: new traps for old players in HIV/AIDS social research. *Culture, Health and Sexuality*, 1999;1:95–102.
75. Ingstad B. The cultural construction of AIDS and its consequences for prevention in Botswana. *Med Anthropol Q*, 1990;4:28–37.
76. Kagimu M, Marum E, Wabwire-Mangen F, et al. Evaluation of the effectiveness of AIDS interventions in the Muslim community in Uganda. *AIDS Educ Prev*, 1998;10:215–228.
77. DiFranceisco W, Kelly JA, Otto-Salaj L, et al. Factors influencing attitudes within AIDS service organizations toward the use of research-based HIV prevention interventions. *AIDS Educ Prev*, 1999; 11:72–86.
78. Klepp KI, Ndeki SS, Seha AM, et al. AIDS education for primary school children in Tanzania: An evaluation study. *AIDS*, 1994;8:1157–1162.
79. Mnyika KS, Kvale G, Klepp KI. Perceived function of and barriers to condom use in Arusha and Kilimanjaro regions of Tanzania. *AIDS Care*, 1995; 7:295–305.
80. Fitzgerald AM, Stanton BF, Terreri N, et al. Use of Western-based HIV risk-reduction interventions targeting adolescents in an African setting. *J Adolesc Health*, 1999;25:52–61.
81. Stanton BF, Li X, Kahihuata J, et al. Increased protected sex and abstinence among Namibian youth following a HIV risk-reduction intervention: a randomized, longitudinal study. *AIDS*, 1998;12: 2473–2480.
82. Jackson DJ, Rakwar JP, Richardson BA, et al. Decreased incidence of sexually transmitted diseases among trucking company workers in Kenya: results of a behavioural risk-reduction programme. *AIDS*, 1997;11:903–909.
83. Tawil O, O'Reilly K, Coulibaly IM, et al. HIV prevention among vulnerable populations: outreach in the developing world. *AIDS*, 1999;13(Supp A):S239–S247.
84. Asiimwe-Okiror G, Opio AA, Musinguzi J, et al. Change in sexual behaviour and decline in HIV infection among young pregnant women in urban Uganda. *AIDS*, 1997;11:1757–1763.
85. Celentano DD, Nelson KE, Lyles CM, et al. Decreasing incidence of HIV and sexually transmitted diseases in young Thai men: evidence for success of the HIV/AIDS control and prevention program. *AIDS*, 1998;12:F29–F36.
86. Mulder D, Nunn A, Kamali A, et al. Decreasing HIV-1 seroprevalence in young adults in a rural Ugandan cohort. *BMJ*, 1995;311:833–836.
87. Kilmarx PH, Palanuvej T, Limpakarnjanarat K, et al. Seroprevalence of HIV among female sex workers in Bangkok: evidence of ongoing infection risk after the "100% condom program" was implemented. *J Acquir Immune Defic Syndr*, 1999;21: 313–316.
88. van Griensven GJ, Limanonda B, Ngaokeow S, et al. Evaluation of a targeted HIV prevention programme among female commercial sex workers in the south of Thailand. *Sex Trans Infect*, 1998;74: 54–58.

34

Voluntary Counseling and Testing

*Elizabeth Marum, †Carl H. Campbell, ‡Katawa Msowoya, §Augustine Barnaba, and †Beth Dillon

**Centers for Disease Control and Prevention, Nairobi, Kenya.*
†Centers for Disease Control and Prevention, Atlanta, Georgia, USA.
‡Malawi AIDS Counseling and Resource Organization, Blantyre, Malawi.
§Queen Elizabeth Central Hospital, Blantyre, Malawi.

GOALS AND DEFINITIONS OF VOLUNTARY COUNSELING AND TESTING

One of the most challenging features of the AIDS epidemic in Africa is that the majority of Africans infected with HIV do not know their HIV status, mainly as a result of the lack of HIV testing and counseling facilities. UNAIDS reports that the proportion of people who are unaware that they are HIV-infected is highest in the countries worst affected by the epidemic (1) and it is often estimated that in sub–Saharan African countries, less than 10% of persons infected with HIV are aware of their infection. As a result, most persons living with HIV in these countries are less likely to adopt behaviors which would prevent further transmission of HIV and they are unable to access care and services in the early stages of HIV disease. Voluntary counseling and HIV testing (VCT) programs are designed to provide easy access to HIV testing for persons who wish to know their serostatus, through an approach that emphasizes informed consent, pre- and post-test counseling, and referral to follow-up services.

The goal of VCT services is to enable individuals and couples to learn their test results voluntarily in a setting in which confidentiality is strictly maintained. In contrast to HIV testing that is ordered by a doctor or health worker for diagnostic purposes, VCT services are often characterized as "client-centered" because it is the client who requests the test voluntarily, often for non-medical reasons, and the counseling session is tailored to the client's unique risk issues, rather than a medical discussion of symptoms and treatment. Voluntary counseling and testing services strive to empower clients to use their test results to make informed decisions about important life events such as partner selection, marriage, pregnancy, and family finances, and to help clients reduce risk of HIV transmission.

ROLE OF VOLUNTARY COUNSELING AND TESTING IN AFRICA

Particularly in African countries with high HIV prevalence, it is of extreme importance that people learn their HIV status so that both prevention education and care services may be effectively utilized. AIDS education efforts have reached an increasing percentage of people in African populations. Surveys now find that 90% or more of the population in many countries is aware of AIDS and knowledgeable of risk factors, and as a result, there are increasing numbers of persons who want to learn whether they have been infected with HIV (2,3). For example, in Kenya, of those not yet tested, 63% of women and 66% of men surveyed indicated a desire for HIV testing (3). At the same time, in many African countries, health facilities are seriously congested, and laboratories and health workers are overwhelmed by patients with acute conditions. Scarce and unreliable supplies of HIV test kits and reagents have often forced medical institutions to "ration" HIV testing for blood donations and other critical needs. These hospitals and health facilities are often unable to devote personnel and laboratory materials for counseling and HIV tests for apparently healthy patients who request HIV testing for personal reasons, rather than by referral from a health worker for diagnostic reasons. To meet this demand for nonmedical HIV testing, VCT services have been developed and introduced in many African countries.

Until recently, early care for those who learned they were HIV-infected was limited to psychosocial services and supportive medical care, and the only programs for the prevention of mother-to-child HIV transmission (PMCT) and the prevention of tuberculosis (TB) and other opportunistic infections (OIs) were associated with research projects. Recent findings showing the effectiveness of these interventions in Africa (4–7) and the commitment of international donors to fund such projects have resulted in the introduction of these services on a wider scale in many countries; VCT is now seen as an entry point for these preventive services. Recent international efforts to lower the prices of antiretroviral drugs in developing countries have greatly increased motivation for persons to learn their serostatus before developing serious symptoms. As preventive and therapeutic services become more widely available, the demand for VCT will continue to increase in Africa, and the need to implement large-scale VCT services will become increasingly urgent. Although VCT may be requested more often in the future by persons wishing to access care, VCT will continue to offer a unique and powerful opportunity for prevention and support for all clients, both HIV-positive and -negative.

VOLUNTARY COUNSELING AND TESTING SERVICE MODELS

There are two basic models for VCT in Africa: stand-alone and integrated. "Stand-alone" or "free-standing" VCT centers are modeled after the "alternative test sites" developed in the United States in the mid- to late 1980s. Integrated VCT services are provided within an existing hospital or health facility, but as a separate service from the HIV testing that is done for medical diagnostic reasons. Within these models, there are two different ways to provide VCT test results, either with a waiting period, or as "same-day" services. Each of these models and approaches, and their relative merits, will be described.

Stand-alone VCT Centers

Stand-alone VCT centers in Africa were pioneered in Kampala, Uganda, where the AIDS Information Centre (AIC) was established in 1990. Located first in the basement of an office building in the central business district, AIC quickly established a reputation for providing confidential, reliable results, and demand for services at AIC grew rapidly. Over 60,000 clients were served in 1993 in centers in the four major cities of Uganda, and in over 20 mobile sites in rural areas (8). In 1997, AIC began assisting selected hospitals and health centers outside major urban areas, and by the end of 2000, there were 37 additional sites providing VCT services in Uganda. In Malawi, VCT services have been primarily provided by stand-alone centers in the two largest cities, and a stand-alone site has recently been developed in Harare, Zimbabwe.

In general, stand-alone VCT sites have had more success in attracting large numbers of clients, compared with integrated sites where VCT is offered along with other health services. For example, the Uganda VCT program has now served 512,126 clients in 12 years, a record unmatched in any other African country (AIC Project Reports). The VCT program in Zimbabwe opened nine integrated sites in 1999 and early 2000 and one stand-alone site in mid-2000. Within 2 months of opening, the stand-alone site was serving more than 150 clients daily, more clients than all nine integrated sites combined (Patrick Osewe, USAID Zimbabwe, personal communication, January 2001).

The ability to attract large numbers of clients who are not yet ill but may be HIV-infected or at risk for HIV infection is a great advantage of stand-alone sites, and confidentiality in these sites is more easily maintained than in integrated sites. Since all clients at stand-alone sites are requesting HIV testing, it is less likely that they will be stigmatized as members of a "high risk" group while they are waiting for the service. HIV prevention counseling is usually more strongly emphasized in stand-alone sites compared with sites in health facilities where issues of diagnosis and treatment may dominate the counseling session. Staff at stand-alone VCT sites devote their working hours to delivering VCT services, rather than to the myriad other tasks requiring the attention of staff in facilities that also provide medical care to patients with urgent problems. Stand-alone sites, however, are almost always heavily dependent on external donor funds, and the long-term sustainability of these programs is uncertain.

Integrated VCT Centers

Integrating VCT services within existing health facilities is believed to improve the likelihood that these services will be sustained over the long term. This approach is also thought to improve HIV-infected clients' access to other medical services, such as STD diagnosis and treatment, TB screening, PMCT, and general medical care. Integrated VCT services, because they use existing health facilities and personnel and are thus less costly to implement, can greatly increase access to VCT. Another potential advantage of integrated VCT services is that over time they may allow HIV testing to become an increasingly routine medical procedure, rather than a service distinct from other public health services.

Unfortunately, in many African countries, deteriorating public health infrastructure has led to poorly maintained facilities and chronic shortages of personnel, drugs, test kits (not only for HIV but for other diseases as well), and other supplies. Most importantly, in some African countries, health facilities are grossly inadequate to meet the urgent medical needs of the surrounding population, and the health workers in these sites may be able to devote only a few minutes to each sick patient. Thus, the ability of these institutions to attract VCT clients with no urgent medical problems, and to provide adequate risk reduction and counseling sessions is a major concern. For example, a project in Kenya piloting the introduction of VCT services in three existing government health facilities over 19 months has resulted in an average of less than four persons daily per site actually accepting VCT (9). In Tanzania, 59 VCT centers were set up in public hospitals throughout the country in 1998, but by 2000, few sites were operating, due to user fees that were perceived by clients to be too high, fear of lack of confidentiality, and lack of continued donor support (Janis Timberlake, USAID Tanzania, personal communication, January 2001). Most VCT providers working in Africa believe that it is important to offer both stand-alone and integrated VCT services, so that clients can choose the testing alternative most comfortable and affordable to them.

Waiting Period VCT Services

In both stand-alone and integrated VCT centers, the most common approach for serving clients is to conduct a pre-test counseling session, and if the client consents, a blood sample is drawn, and the client is then told to return for the results at a later date, usually after 1 or 2 weeks. A waiting period is usually needed because of laboratory procedures that may require samples to be "batched" until there is an adequate number to run a full plate of ELISAs (enzyme-linked immunosorbent assays—the most commonly used serologic HIV tests), and additional time may be needed to conduct confirmatory testing on the samples that initially test positive for HIV. Even when the VCT site is located in a health facility with a laboratory, a waiting period is often required to return results to the VCT providers. Many VCT counselors traditionally believed that a waiting period for reflection was beneficial to clients, allowing those who decide they are not ready to deal with their test results to elect not to return. However, many VCT clients have reported that the need to return for results after a waiting period is a deterrent to requesting VCT, especially for those who live some distance from the VCT site. As a result, most VCT sites find that between 20% and 30% of clients fail to return.

Same-Day VCT Services

VCT programs in Uganda and Malawi have introduced "same-day" VCT services, using simple, rapid HIV tests that are performed on-site. This method increases the percentage of clients who learn their results to almost 100%, and reduces the stress and anxiety associated with a waiting period. This approach, which was well received by both clients and counselors, was first introduced in Uganda in 1997, and quality assurance testing has documented a high rate of accuracy of results (10,11). The Malawi AIDS Counseling and Resource Organization (MACRO) introduced same-day results in January 2000, and this modification of services has resulted in a four-fold increase in utilization of VCT services, and a six-fold increase in the number of clients who learned their serostatus (12). Most clients report less stress and anxiety when they can learn their results immediately.

Confidentiality and Anonymity

Strict confidentiality is a hallmark of VCT programs. Some VCT sites record client names but have procedures in place to ensure that HIV test results are not divulged to anyone other than the client. Other VCT sites, especially stand-alone sites, offer anonymous testing whereby no names are recorded, and test results are linked to code numbers only. Anecdotal evidence from Uganda, Malawi, Kenya, Zambia, and elsewhere suggests that clients are attracted to VCT sites that offer anonymous testing, because of considerable fear of stigma, employment discrimination, and other forms of legal and human rights abuse of persons living with HIV. Many VCT clients are concerned not only that their results might be disclosed to others, but also that others may learn that they have sought HIV testing. Thus, VCT sites in more anonymous urban settings are often preferred over sites closer to home. The VCT site must be vigilant not only with record keeping, but also with general operating procedures to ensure confidentiality.

As preventive therapies become more available for TB, other OIs, and mother-to-child transmission, the need for referral to these services and to services for the detection and treatment of other sexually transmitted diseases (STDs) will pose challenges for anonymous VCT sites. Another concern is that emphasis on anonymity perpetuates the fear and silence surrounding

AIDS. VCT service providers are currently debating these issues, and it is likely that in the future, there will be more emphasis on confidential VCT, rather than anonymous VCT; sites may need to practice anonymity for VCT services and confidentiality for care and support referrals.

THE COUNSELING COMPONENT OF VCT SERVICES

The counseling component of VCT services is a tailored, highly focused, and relatively brief intervention. Counselors should focus on assessing and understanding the client's HIV risk behavior, developing a plan to reduce this risk, and identifying support resources. The intervention is client-centered in that it addresses the client's individual issues and circumstances related to HIV risk and risk reduction. In addition, counselors explore and address cultural customs and rituals that may impact risk. Educational information should only be provided to the extent that the client may be misinformed or does not understand essential HIV transmission and prevention issues. The session is designed to be interactive, exploring the issues and circumstances that contribute to risk, with opportunities for skill-building and role play. In both the rapid and the standard testing approaches, the total counseling time is between 25 and 60 minutes, determined by client needs and serostatus.

One commonly used counseling protocol for providing same-day results features eight components: (*i*) introduction and orientation to the session, (*ii*) risk assessment, (*iii*) prevention counseling, (*iv*) test-decision counseling, (*v*) test result counseling, (*vi*) negotiation of a risk reduction plan, (*vii*) partner disclosure, and (*viii*) support, referrals, and medical follow-up. The first four components are provided to each client and occur before testing. The relative emphasis of each of the second four components differs based on the client's test result.

For the HIV-negative client, the focus of the post-test component is on prevention of HIV infection, with an emphasis on establishing a realistic and specific risk reduction plan. The HIV-negative client is urged to ask partners to be tested. HIV-negative clients are encouraged to become community ambassadors for HIV prevention and for VCT. For the HIV-positive client, the focus is on coping and support issues, partner disclosure and referral, and medical follow-up. Counselors emphasize "living positively with HIV," taking care of one's health and emotional well-being in order to enhance life and stay well longer.

Counselor Training, Quality Assurance, and Supervision

The most important qualities in a VCT counselor are empathy, compassion, and a commitment to help prevent HIV. Both counselors with very limited formal education and those with more professional training can be excellent providers of VCT services. Candidates for VCT training should have completed training in general AIDS counseling. They must have a solid grasp of the fundamentals of HIV transmission and prevention and a basic understanding of HIV disease progression and clinical care. For those who are already trained counselors, the VCT-specific training is typically 3 to 5 days and focuses exclusively on learning the counseling protocol and the accompanying skills to conduct the intervention sensitively and effectively. Ideally the training is followed by opportunities for VCT session observation and mentoring from a senior VCT counselor.

The training and mentoring provide the counselor with the basic foundation for sound counseling services. Consistent and systematic application of quality assurance measures and ongoing supervision are crucial for sustaining the delivery of high quality and effective VCT services. Adherence to the counseling protocol and the use of appropriate counseling skills are critical. For this reason, supervisors are encouraged to routinely observe sessions, using a standardized quality assurance guide, and to provide feedback to counselors. Supervisors should also conduct case study conferences and convene staff meetings for counselors to share experiences, discuss challenging cases, role play, and develop advanced skills.

THE TESTING COMPONENT OF VCT SERVICES

Establishing a Testing Algorithm

In the past, most VCT sites relied on their local hospital laboratory for testing, so the testing algorithm used was simply whatever was being used in that laboratory. Because supply and distribution of HIV test kits continue to be inadequate in many African countries, VCT sites often experience delays in getting results, and at times, HIV-positive results are given to clients without confirmatory testing. The development of very simple, rapid HIV tests in the mid-1990s encouraged some VCT sites to begin conducting their own, on-site testing (8,9–11,13). Not only does this newer technology allow the VCT site to provide same-day services, it also permits the VCT provider to exercise more control over the selection of test kits, testing procedures, and quality assurance methods. Whether testing is done on or off-site, it is imperative for VCT sites to ensure that all positive samples are confirmed with an additional, different test before the results are released to the VCT client. Although the usual emphasis is on preventing false positive results from being given to clients, it is also important to reduce false negative results, as VCT clients make important life decisions based on their test results.

Traditionally, HIV testing algorithms have taken a serial approach, with one test being conducted first, and a second test being conducted only to confirm positive results. Some sites are now using a "parallel" approach in which two different tests are conducted on every sample. For example, in Malawi in early 2000, MACRO introduced same-day VCT using whole blood, rapid tests (13). Two different tests are used for every client, partly to avoid the need to collect another sample from those testing positive, and partly to increase public confidence in HIV testing. The simplicity of these tests, both to conduct and to interpret the results, and the portability of test strips, has meant that, with guidance from the counselor, VCT clients can see their test results themselves. Many clients and counselors have reported that these new procedures have greatly increased their confidence in the validity of the test results. In response to clients' and counselors' preference for this algorithm, MACRO decided to continue simultaneous parallel testing (two different tests performed on all samples) rather than change to the more typical serial procedures used in most laboratories whereby only HIV-positive samples are subjected to a second test. Other countries in Africa, including Kenya and Botswana, are now planning to use the parallel algorithm. These whole blood tests do not require electricity to run, and most need no refrigeration except in very hot climates, considerable advantages for VCT services in Africa where power supplies may be unavailable or unreliable.

The new, very accurate rapid tests using oral fluids will present a challenge to VCT services, as oral testing is likely to be more acceptable to clients, especially those who have fear of giving blood. Research will be needed to determine whether confirmation of positive oral fluid test results should be done with a different oral test or with a blood sample. Use of oral tests in VCT settings may create logistical problems; for example, collecting blood samples for confirmatory testing may compromise confidentiality for those testing positive. Careful operations research and evaluation will be needed before widespread use of oral tests can be advocated.

Assuring Quality of Testing

Many VCT sites, especially those receiving external funding and resources, assess the quality of HIV testing by subjecting random blood samples to additional testing, usually in a reference laboratory. In both Uganda and Malawi, for example, 5% of all samples are re-tested elsewhere for quality assurance. In most instances, re-testing is done with ELISA, although Western Blots are also used on selected samples, especially those with discordant results between the initial and confirmatory tests. In addition to random re-testing of samples, all VCT sites must conduct rigorous and regular review of record keeping systems to avoid recording errors. A disadvantage for anonymous VCT sites is that when incorrect results are discovered through quality assurance reviews, there is no way to notify the client of the correct results.

In Malawi, where finger-prick tests are used and thus no stored sera are available for quality control, filter paper samples are obtained from every client. In 2000, when finger prick testing was introduced, the 5% quality assurance testing documented 100% concordance with the results already given to the clients on the basis of the same-day rapid testing, indicating that the algorithm of two different, simultaneously performed rapid whole blood tests yields extremely accurate results.

When VCT is offered in existing local health facilities, there are unfortunately still many instances in which only one test is available at the facility, especially in rural areas, and therefore HIV-positive clients receive unconfirmed test results. Whether VCT is provided in a stand-alone center or as part of existing health services, all clients have the right to expect that HIV-positive results be confirmed with a second, different HIV test. All those involved in providing VCT in Africa must assiduously ensure that HIV-positive results are confirmed, and that systems are in place to monitor the quality of testing.

THE IMPACT OF VCT ON BEHAVIORAL CHANGE

VCT services are encouraged and supported in developing countries largely because knowledge of serostatus is believed to help clients reduce risk of HIV transmission. Studies of the impact of VCT have examined the association between VCT and behavioral change in Kenya, Tanzania, Zaire, Rwanda, and Uganda (8,14–18). In all of these studies, persons who received VCT services reported in subsequent follow-up sessions that they had reduced risky behaviors. In Kenya and Tanzania, the efficacy of VCT was studied using a randomized controlled trial that compared VCT to a health information session. This study found that among those in the VCT arm that enrolled as individuals rather than as couples, men reported a 35% reduction in unprotected sex with nonprimary partners, compared with a 13% reduction for those who received only health education; women reported a 39% reduction, compared with a 17% reduction after health education. This study also found that individual men and women who learned they were HIV-positive were more likely to reduce unprotected intercourse than were individuals who learned that they were not infected. Those who received VCT as couples were more likely to reduce unprotected sex with that partner than with sexual partners who did not participate in the study (18). Based on the results of these studies in multiple countries, it is now clear that learning serostatus helps individuals and couples reduce risk of HIV transmission, especially for those who learn they are infected and for those who learn their results together as a couple.

CARE AND SUPPORT AFTER VCT

Particularly in resource-poor settings, ensuring a reasonable level of care and support for VCT clients, especially for those who learn they are HIV-infected, poses a considerable challenge for VCT programs. The "Post-Test Club" model, first developed and described in Uganda (8,19), features long-term supportive services for all clients, regardless of serostatus. This model has now been replicated in a number of countries, including Malawi, Kenya, Zambia, and Zimbabwe. Services provided typically include ongoing counseling, peer support for maintaining behavior change, recreational facilities, and in some instances, basic medical care for HIV-positive club members. Club members are encouraged to participate in community outreach and volunteer service. HIV-positive clients who are symptomatic are commonly referred to other organizations for AIDS care. Club members have often become vocal advocates for an enhanced package of services for persons who learn they are infected through VCT programs. Many VCT programs are planning for additional services, such as prevention of TB and other OIs, and antiretroviral treatment.

LEGAL AND ETHICAL ISSUES

Organizations providing VCT services are often concerned about potential legal and ethical problems associated with HIV testing For example, the distinction may be unclear between purely voluntary HIV testing and other forms of HIV testing that are not voluntary, such as the testing of blood donors, pre-employment testing, and testing for purposes of immigration, insurance, and so forth. It is critical for VCT programs to emphasize and preserve the voluntary nature of their services, and to maintain strict confidentiality. To avoid the misuse of test results, some programs, such as in Uganda, do not give clients any form of written record of test results. In contrast, the VCT program in Malawi provides written results to clients, and to date, this has not resulted in violations of the rights of VCT clients. Counselors and managers of VCT programs must remain aware of the potential for misuse of test results, or for persons to be coerced into requesting VCT, and measures must be developed to avoid these problems. In addition, political commitment, country ownership, and community mobilization efforts can help create and support a legal and ethical framework to prevent potential abuses to individual human rights.

VCT SERVICES IN SPECIAL CIRCUMSTANCES

Prevention of Mother-to-Child Transmission (PMCT)

With the publication of research results in several countries in Africa and Asia (5,6, 20) showing that short-course antiretroviral therapies can contribute to PMCT, some countries in Africa are developing programs to implement these services. The entry points for prenatal care in most African countries are antenatal clinics (ANCs) in hospitals and health centers. Procedures are in place for routine collection of blood samples from pregnant women for syphilis and hemoglobin testing, and ANC services are working to introduce routine HIV testing. However, the provision of VCT will present an enormous challenge for these clinics, which are often overburdened with many patients and few staff. Most sites that offer PMCT services call for "voluntary" counseling and testing, and only pregnant women who consent to HIV testing can participate in the PMCT program. In some countries this has resulted in only a small fraction of eligible pregnant women actually being tested for HIV. This significantly reduces the potential benefits of PMCT programs, and these programs are now questioning the applicability of the typical "VCT model" for prenatal screening. In Zimbabwe, for example, two studies found that only 18% and 23% of eligible pregnant women accepted VCT (21,22). The debate regarding voluntary versus routine

HIV testing for pregnant women in African countries is the same as in developed countries, although very much complicated by the high HIV prevalence among pregnant women in Africa, combined with the lack of access to antiretroviral therapy after the birth of the infant.

Preventive Therapy for Tuberculosis and Opportunistic Infections (OIs)

Pilot programs, primarily sponsored by the World Health Organization (WHO), now exist in several African countries (Malawi, Uganda, Botswana) to introduce TB detection in VCT centers, and provide preventive TB therapy for HIV-positive clients who do not already have active TB. Research results from Côte d'Ivoire (4,7) have documented the ability of cotrimoxazole to prevent OIs. These findings have put pressure on VCT sites to offer this preventive therapy to their HIV-positive clients. Voluntary counseling and HIV testing sites are also being encouraged to provide family planning services and STD diagnosis and treatment. It is easier to introduce these services to integrated VCT sites than to stand-alone sites, which often have few, if any, medical staff, and laboratory facilities only for HIV testing, if at all. VCT providers that are accustomed to maintaining client anonymity may now need to change to confidential procedures to facilitate referral of their clients for these additional services.

VCT for Adolescents

The increasing documentation of a high incidence of HIV infection among young people, especially young women, has resulted in increasing interest in the provision of VCT services for adolescents. A recent study in Kenya found that 77% of untested youth indicated a desire for HIV testing in the future (23). In most African countries, few legal guidelines exist on the age of consent for medical testing, and there is considerable debate about the appropriateness of testing adolescents without parental consent, especially in cultures that emphasize family above individual rights. This is compounded by the fact that condom education, promotion, and distribution are routine services for all VCT clients, and yet condom promotion for adolescents remains just as controversial in African countries as it is in the United States. Lack of access to long-term therapies in Africa is also a challenge for VCT services for youth, as counselors find it extraordinarily difficult to convey positive test results to very young clients who have no hope of accessing antiretroviral drugs.

Premarital VCT

As knowledge of high HIV prevalence becomes more widespread in African populations, there is increasing pressure on families and the clergy to request premarital HIV testing. When young people are virtually required to be tested, the voluntary component of VCT erodes, and there is a high risk of negative outcomes for young people whose marriages are cancelled as a result of positive test results. Since HIV prevalence in Africa is usually much higher in young women than in young men, these negative outcomes are most likely to affect young women, who are often already disadvantaged in terms of access to legal and social protection. Providers and counselors of VCT must ensure that young people who request premarital testing consent voluntarily, and receive adequate counseling that addresses the consequences to their relationship should the results be discordant, and recommends follow-up services to cope with adverse outcomes.

Partner Notification and Couple Counseling

A major challenge for VCT services remains the issue of partner notification, and it is often very troubling for VCT counselors to maintain confidentiality when they know of HIV-positive clients who refuse to practice preventive behaviors. This is especially true for those working in cultures in which women have little control over their own sexual lives.

When couples come for VCT together, partner notification occurs naturally as part of the counseling session. Some VCT sites, especially in Uganda, Kenya, and Tanzania, have been successful in attracting a high percentage of their clients to come with their sexual partners. Voluntary counseling and HIV testing services targeted to couples require more promotion, and counselors will need additional training to deal effectively with the complex issues that arise, especially for discordant couples.

COSTS ASSOCIATED WITH VCT

Little is known about the true cost of providing integrated VCT, although a study in Kenya has estimated a cost of between USD$8 and $16 per person receiving VCT in a health facility (24). Costs associated with providing stand-alone VCT have been well studied in Uganda, Kenya, and Tanzania. In Uganda, the cost of providing VCT was relatively high when the VCT program was first introduced—more than $27 per client at low-volume sites. However, as demand increased, economies of scale were achieved, and the cost per client dropped to as low as $12 between 1994 and 1996, rising slightly in 1997 to $13.39 per client (8). Costs per client of $26.65 in Kenya and $28.93 in Tanzania have been reported from a recent study (25), although it should be noted that these costs were associated with relatively low-volume sites that had been in operation for less than 2 years. This study concluded that VCT is a cost-effective intervention, with a cost of $27.36 in Kenya and $45.03 in Tanzania per disability-adjusted life-year (DALY) saved (25). Since $50 per DALY saved is recommended as a guideline for public health interventions in developing countries, this research supports including VCT in national AIDS prevention programs.

In many sites, VCT is offered to clients at no charge, though some sites, including those in Uganda, Tanzania, and Kenya, have introduced "cost-sharing" or user fees. The rationale for charging these fees is to contribute to the sustainability of the programs, and to counteract any public perception that free services are not as high quality as those charging a fee. Some VCT programs offer "free days" to offer access to VCT to those who are unable to pay the normal fee. In both Uganda and Tanzania, these free days attract many more clients than usual, to the point of overwhelming service delivery, suggesting that the normal fees are a serious deterrent for many (Janis Timberlake, USAID Tanzania, personal communication, January 2001).

MONITORING AND EVALUATION OF VCT SERVICES

Considerable efforts have been undertaken to document, monitor, and evaluate VCT services, partly because many of them are supported by external donors and/or research projects (8,9,25,26). A standardized record-keeping form is recommended, along with both local and national monitoring of data. A major challenge for evaluating the impact of VCT has been the emphasis on anonymity, which makes it very difficult to collect follow-up data from VCT clients. Appropriate tools, including client satisfaction survey instruments and counseling quality assurance materials to monitor the content and delivery of VCT services should be incorporated into VCT program monitoring and evaluation protocols.

CONCLUSION

Despite the many challenges in implementing VCT services in Africa, it is clear that knowledge of serostatus is essential for individuals and couples to make informed decisions about medical care, and personal and family life. In African countries, especially those with very high HIV prevalence, ignorance of serostatus is a serious barrier to effective HIV prevention efforts. Lack of access to HIV testing also leads to missed opportunities for individuals to receive preventive therapies, supportive care, and counseling on appropriate risk reduction behaviors.

Voluntary counseling and HIV testing is an obvious and important entry point for HIV and AIDS care. In addition VCT as a prevention intervention has now been subjected to more rigorous analysis (both in terms of efficacy and cost-effectiveness) than many other HIV prevention interventions, such as community mobilization and peer education. The significant public health benefits and cost-effectiveness of VCT make it an important component of a comprehensive national response to the AIDS epidemic.

In the future, as antiretroviral therapies become more accessible in Africa, testing for HIV in clinical settings may become more routine. The prevention potential of VCT may hence be diluted in these settings as VCT providers will focus more on issues related to care. For this reason, stand-alone VCT services will continue to provide an alternative venue for many who are reluctant to be tested in health facilities, especially those who seek VCT for personal reasons. Particularly in light of the high HIV prevalence in many African countries, increasing the number of persons who know their serostatus by increasing access to VCT is of the highest priority. The implementation and maintenance of ample centers at both integrated and stand-alone sites is an essential part of this process.

REFERENCES

1. UNAIDS. *Report on the global HIV/AIDS epidemic, June 2000.* UNAIDS/00.13E, Geneva: United Nations Joint Programme on HIV/AIDS; 2000.
2. Bureau of Statistics [Tanzania] and Macro International Inc. *Tanzania Demographic and Health Survey 1996.* Calverton, Maryland: Bureau of Statistics and Macro International, 1997.
3. National Council for Population and Development (NCPD), Central Bureau of Statistics (CBS) (Office of the Vice President and Ministry of Planning and National Development [Kenya]), and Macro International Inc. (MI). *Kenya Demographic and Health Survey 1998.* Calverton, Maryland: NDPD, CBS, and MI, 1999.
4. Anglaret X, Chene G, Attia A, et al. Cotrimo-CI study group. Early chemoprophylaxis with trimethoprim-sulphamethoxazole for HIV-1-infected adults in Abidjan, Cote d'Ivoire: a randomized trial. *Lancet*, 1999;353:1463–1468.
5. Guay LA, Musoke P, Fleming T, et al. Intrapartum and neonatal single-dose nevirapine compared with zidovudine for prevention of mother-to-child transmission of HIV-1 in Kampala, Uganda: HIVNET 012 randomised trial. *Lancet*, 1999;354:795–802.
6. Wiktor S, Ekpini E, Karon J, et al. Short course oral zidovudine for prevention of mother-to-child transmission of HIV-1 in Abidjan, Cote d'Ivoire: a randomised trial. *Lancet*, 1999;353:781–785.
7. Wiktor S, Sassan-Morokro M, Grant A, et al. Efficacy of trimethoprim-sulphamethoxazole prophylaxis to decrease morbidity and mortality in HIV-1-infected patients with tuberculosis in Abidjan, Cote d'Ivoire: a randomized control trial. *Lancet*, 2000;353:1469–1475.
8. Alwano-Edyegu MG, Marum E. Knowledge is Power: Voluntary HIV counselling and testing in Uganda. *UNAIDS Best Practices Case Study.* Geneva: UNAIDS, June 1999.
9. Arthur G, Mutemi R, Odhiambo J, et al. Voluntary counseling and testing (VCT): improved access for the poor through integrating same day services into public primary health care clinics. In: Program and Abstracts of the XIII International Conference on AIDS; July 9–14, 2000; Durban, South Africa. Abstract MoPpC1028.
10. Downing R, Otten R, Marum E, et al. Optimizing the Delivery of HIV Counseling and Testing Services: The Uganda Experience Using Rapid HIV Antibody Test Algorithms. *J Acquir Immune Defic Syndr Hum Retrovirol*, 1998;18:384–388.
11. Kassler W, Alwano-Edyegu MG, Marum E, et al. Rapid HIV testing with same-day results: a field trial in Uganda. *Int J STD AIDS*, 1998;9:134–138.
12. Msowoya K, Marum E, Barnaba A, et al. Fourfold increase in utilization of voluntary HIV counseling and testing in Malawi with same day results and confirmed, rapid, fingerprick testing. In: Program and abstracts of the XIII International Conference

on AIDS; July 9–14, 2000; Durban, South Africa. Abstract LbPeA7012.

13. Marum E, Barnaba A, Feluzi H, et al. Whole blood, rapid HIV tests and same day counseling results in Malawi. In: Program and abstracts of the XIII International Conference on AIDS; July 9–14, 2000; Durban, South Africa. Abstract MoPeA2109.
14. Allen S, Tice J, Van de Perre P, et al. Effect of serotesting with counselling on condom use and seroconversion among HIV discordant couples in Africa. *Br Med J*, 1992;304:1605–1609.
15. Campbell C, Marum E, Alwano-Edwegu MG, et al. The role of HIV counseling and testing in the developing world. *AIDS Educ Prevention*, 1997; 9(Suppl.): B 92–104.
16. Heyward W, Barrer V, Malulu M, et al. Impact of HIV counseling and testing among child-bearing women in Kinshasa, Zaire. *AIDS*, 1993;7:1633–1637.
17. Kamenga M, Ryder R, Jingu M, et al. Evidence of marked sexual behavior change associated with low HIV-1 seroconversion in 149 married couples with discordant HIV-1 serostatus: Experience at an HIV counseling center in Zaire. *AIDS*, 1991;5:61–67.
18. Voluntary HIV-1 Counseling and Testing Efficacy Study Group. Efficacy of voluntary HIV-1 counseling and testing in individuals and couples in Kenya, Tanzania and Trinidad: a randomised trial. *Lancet*, 2000;356:103–112.
19. Marum E, Gumisiriza E, Moore M, et al. Impact of a Social Support Club following HIV Counseling and Testing, Uganda, 1993–1994. In: Program and abstracts of the X International Conference on AIDS; August 7–12, 1994; Yokohama, Japan. Abstract 240C.
20. Shaffer N, Chusachoowong R, Mock P, et al. Short-course zidovudine for perinatal HIV-1 transmission in Bangkok, Thailand: a randomised controlled trial. *Lancet*, 1999;353:773–780.
21. Martin-Herz S, Katzenstein D, Shetty A, et al. Predictors of acceptance of HIV testing and counseling by pregnant women in Zimbabwe. In: Program and abstracts of the XIII International Conference on AIDS; July 9–14, 2000; Durban, South Africa. Abstract ThPeC5313.
22. Moyo S, Mhazo M, Mateta P, et al. Acceptability of short-course AZT prevention regimen by HIV infected pregnant women: should VCT in the antenatal setting be modified? In: Program and abstracts of the XIII International Conference on AIDS; July 9–13, 2000; Durban, South Africa. Abstract TuPpB1158.
23. Population Council, HORIZONS Project. HIV voluntary counseling and testing among youth: Results from an exploratory study in Nairobi, Kenya and Kampala and Masaka, Uganda. October 2001.
24. Mutemi R, Forsythe S, Arthur G. Financial requirements of providing VCT throughout Kenya's health centers. In: Program and abstracts of the XIII International Conference on AIDS; July 9–14, 2000; Durban, South Africa. Abstract TuOrC310.
25. Sweat M, Gregorich S, Sangiwa G, et al. Cost-effectiveness of voluntary HIV-1 counselling and testing in reducing sexual transmission of HIV-1 in Kenya and Tanzania. *Lancet*, 2000;364:113–121.
26. Kalibala S, Geibel S, Kalule J, et al. Measuring integration of HIV into FP and STD services using checklists in four hospitals in Uganda. In: Program and abstracts of the XII International Conference on AIDS and STDs in Africa; December 9–13, 2001; Ouagadougou, Burkina Faso. Abstract 13DT1–3.

35

Prevention of Perinatal Transmission of HIV

*Sophie Le Coeur and †Marc Lallemant

*Institut National d'Études Démographiques, Paris, France.
†Institut de Recherche pour le Développement (IRD), Chiang Mai, Thailand.

UNAIDS estimates that among the 36.1 million persons who were living with HIV at the end of the year 2000, 1.4 million were children under 15 years of age (1). During the year 2000 alone, 600,000 new HIV infections and 500,000 deaths from AIDS occurred in children under the age of 15. Most of these pediatric infections were the result of mother-to-child transmission, and more than 90% occurred in sub–Saharan Africa. In countries where fertility is high and heterosexual transmission of HIV is predominant, many young women have become HIV-infected and the number of children at risk is expected to be high. Yet with the preventive methods available since 1994, most of these perinatal infections could have been avoided. This chapter briefly reviews what has been learned about the risks, timing, and mechanisms of perinatal transmission, and focuses on the results of the clinical trials that have radically changed the epidemiology of mother-to-child transmission where prevention programs have been implemented.

RATES, TIMING, AND RISKS OF MOTHER-TO-CHILD HIV TRANSMISSION

When, in the early 1980s, it became evident that infants could become infected with HIV through their mothers, the first questions to be asked were about the rate of transmission, its timing and mechanisms, and the risk factors associated with transmission (see Chapter 15, *this volume*).

Early studies showed that mother-to-child HIV transmission could occur during pregnancy, during labor and delivery, and during breastfeeding (2,3). In historic cohort studies of HIV-infected pregnant women in Africa, where most women subsequently breastfeed their infants, the rates of mother-to-child transmission varied from 25% to 43% (4,5). In contrast, in industrialized countries where most women formula-fed, the rates of mother-to-child transmission were much lower, ranging from 13% to 27% (6–8). Most of this differential was due to transmission through breastfeeding (2,9,10). In the absence of any intervention, about 35% of infants born to HIV-infected mothers become infected: 10% during the last weeks of pregnancy, 15% during labor and delivery, and 10% or more—depending on the age at weaning—during breastfeeding.

Factors associated with an increased risk of transmission were studied extensively in order to identify the most appropriate types of interventions to pursue for the prevention of vertical transmission. Numerous studies showed that the risk of transmission was increased when the mother was at an advanced stage of the disease, had impaired immunity, and/or had a micronutrient deficiency, such as vitamin A deficiency (11–16). In addition, high maternal viral load was associated with increased transmission in all studies where p24 antigenemia, HIV co-culture, or RNA/DNA PCR could be performed (17–21).

Published results of the influence of the level and specificity of maternal anti-HIV antibodies on perinatal transmission remain conflicting (22–26). The role of viral subtype or phenotype also remains unclear, although recent results from Tanzania suggest that subtype C is transmitted earlier than other subtypes (27).

The presence of HIV in the placenta does not usually correlate with infection in the infant (28). Given the very close contact between the maternal and the fetal circulation, the placenta acts as an extremely efficient barrier, but the mechanisms of protection are not known. In a model where the placenta is considered a mechanical barrier between mother and fetus, chorioamnionitis or STDs could disrupt the integrity of the placenta and facilitate HIV transmission by cell-free or cell-associated viruses (29). In contrast, if the placenta is considered to be the ultimate source of fetal infection, initial infection of the trophoblast, then of the endothelial cells, could allow the virus to enter the fetal blood stream (30, 31).

Little is known about fetal factors associated with mother-to-child HIV transmission. Fetal cell susceptibility to HIV may vary during gestation, and the fetal immune system may be more or less able to control HIV replication at different stages of development (32, 33).

Transmission during the intrapartum period may be a function of cervicovaginal viral load and local HIV-specific immune response (34). The infant's skin and mucosal surfaces are extensively exposed to maternal blood and secretions during delivery. Furthermore, the neonate's immature gastrointestinal tract may not be a significant enough obstacle to HIV in swallowed amniotic fluid, maternal secretions, or blood. Genetic factors may also play a role as suggested by a recent study in Kenya showing that the HLA supertype A2/6802 was associated with a decreased risk of perinatal transmission (35). Transmission is increased in women with a membrane rupture several hours before delivery, while cesarean section is associated with decreased transmission (36–38).

Lastly, in breastfed infants, the risk of transmission could be related to the duration of breastfeeding, the time of exposure, the infectiousness of the milk, and the presence of HIV-antibodies in the milk (39). A study conducted in Malawi showed that in breastfed infants found to be HIV-negative by PCR at 1 month of age (and whose only remaining risk factor was thus breastfeeding), the rate of infection was 5.2% at 6 months, 9% at 1 year, and 13.8% at 2 years (40).

STRATEGIES FOR INTERVENTION

While data on the timing and factors associated with transmission were accumulating, several prevention strategies were envisioned. Antiretrovirals could lower maternal viral load, prevent viral replication in the placenta, prevent viral replication in the fetus and/or the infant, or lower the viral load in the maternal genital tract (41–43). Passive immune therapy, and/or active immunization could enhance maternal and fetal/infant immune response (44). As a significant number of infants may be infected through mucosal exposure during the birth process, disinfection of the birth canal and elective caesarean section were also suggested as possible ways to reduce transmission (45–47). Correction of nutrient deficiencies, such as low maternal vitamin A level, could decrease the risk of transmission (15). Finally, in countries where breast-feeding was the rule, known HIV-infected mothers were advised not to breastfeed if safe infant formula feeding was feasible (10).

Antiretroviral Prophylaxis with Zidovudine: The First Success in the Prevention of Mother-to-Child Transmission of HIV

In the late 1980s, when the use of antiretrovirals was being considered for prevention of mother-to-child HIV transmission, zidovudine (ZDV) was the only drug that had been shown to have a clear antiretroviral effect and had been successfully used in clinical practice. Data on the timing of transmission were limited at the time. The Pediatric AIDS Clinical Trials Group Study 076 (PACTG 076) was the first trial to test the use of ZDV for prevention of mother-to-child transmission. To achieve maximum efficacy, all of the time periods when transmission of HIV from mothers to children might occur were covered (41, 48). Women participating in the study started taking oral ZDV between 14 and 34 weeks gestation and continued through the end of their pregnancy to prevent in-utero transmission. A ZDV intravenous infusion was administered to mothers during labor to prevent intrapartum transmission, and oral ZDV was given to the newborn for 6 weeks to ensure the presence of the drug in the infant in case any virus had passed into the infant's blood stream. All infants were formula-fed, eliminating the risk of infection through breast milk.

The trial was stopped at the first interim analysis because the transmission rate in the placebo group was significantly higher than that in the ZDV group. All women in the trial were then offered ZDV (41,48). The results of the trial, published in 1994, demonstrated a 67.5% (95% CI, 40.7%–82.1%) reduction of the transmission rate from 25.5% (95% CI, 18.4%–32.5%) in the placebo group to 8.3% (95% CI, 3.9%–12.8%) in the ZDV group ($p < 0.001$) (Table 1). All subsequent studies have confirmed the remarkable efficacy of ante-, intra-, and postpartum ZDV prophylaxis for the prevention of mother-to-child transmission (49–55). Zidovudine prophylaxis also appears to be very safe, the only short-term side effect being the occurrence of a mild anemia in infants treated with ZDV (41,56); the long-term safety of perinatal ZDV exposure is still unknown, however. Since the results of PACTG 076 became available in 1994, most industrialized countries have implemented prenatal HIV counseling and testing and ZDV prophylaxis, an intervention that has led to a dramatic decline in HIV incidence in children (57,58). In the United States, for example, the observed incidence of pediatric AIDS was reduced by more than 60% in the years following the establishment of prophylaxis programs (59).

In less developed countries, however, where more than 90% of perinatal HIV transmission occurs, it was immediately clear that programs to prevent mother-to-child HIV transmission would be difficult to integrate into existing health care systems. The provision of minimal maternal and child health care was already problematic within these systems and the prevention programs used in industrialized countries were complex and costly. The most critical issue therefore, was to find ways to apply the PACTG 076 trial results in settings where women had limited access to antenatal care, deliveries were performed under suboptimal conditions, women stayed in maternity hospitals for very short periods of time, and most infants were breastfed.

Short-Course Antiretroviral Therapy Trials

The goal of PACTG 076 was not to determine the timing or mechanism of perinatal transmission, but to test the treatment regimen that was believed to give the best chance of success in preventing transmission. However, by the time the results of this trial were known, more evidence on the timing of perinatal transmission had been obtained, indicating that most transmission occurred during the last weeks of pregnancy and

TABLE 1. Trials of Antiretrovirals to Prevent Mother-to-Child HIV Transmission[a]

Trial	Setting	Design and sample size	Feeding mode	Maternal regimen	Infant regimen	Transmission rate	Transmission rate reduction
ZIDOVUDINE							
PACTG 076	United States and France	Placebo-Controlled Placebo: $n=183$ ZDV: $n=180$	Artificial	AP: 100 mg × 5 per day orally from 14–34 weeks GA IP: IV infusion 2 mg/kg for 1 hour then 1 mg/hour until delivery	2 mg/kg × 4 per day orally for 6 weeks	Placebo: 25.5% ZDV: 8.3% $p < 0.001$	67.5%
U.S. CDC Bangkok Trial	Thailand	Placebo-Controlled Placebo: $n=194$ ZDV: $n=188$	Artificial	AP: 300 mg bid orally from 36 weeks GA IP: 300 mg orally every 3 hours	None	Placebo: 18.9% ZDV: 9.4% $p < 0.006$	50.1%
PHPT	Thailand	4 Arms Long-long: $n=401$ Short-short: $n=229$ Long-short: $n=340$ Short-long: $n=338$	Artificial	AP: 300 mg bid orally from 28 weeks GA (Long) *or* 35 weeks GA (Short) IP: 300 mg orally every 3 hours	2 mg/kg × 4 per day orally for 6 weeks (long) *or* for 3 days (short)	Long-long: 6.5% Short-short: 10.5% Long-short: 4.7% Short-long: 8.6%	
U.S. CDC Abidjan Trial	Côte d'Ivoire	Placebo-Controlled Placebo: $n=117$ ZDV: $n=123$	Breast	AP: 300 mg bid orally from 36 weeks GA IP: 300 mg orally every 3 hours	None	Placebo: 24.9% ZDV: 15.7% at 3 months of age	37%
DITRAME ANRS 049	Côte d'Ivoire and Burkina Faso	Placebo-Controlled Placebo: $n=186$ ZDV: n=182	Breast	AP: 300 mg bid orally from 36–38 weeks GA IP: 600 mg orally PP: 300 mg bid orally for 1 week	None	Placebo: 25.1% ZDV: 16.8% at 3 months of age	37%

ZIDOVUDINE + 3TC							
PETRA	South Africa, Uganda, and Tanzania	Placebo-Controlled Placebo: n=273 Arm A: n=359 (short AP + IP + PP treatment) Arm B: n=343 (IP + PP) Arm C: n=351 (IP)	Breast (70%) and Artificial (30%)	AP: ZDV 300 mg bid + 3TC 150 mg bid orally from 36 weeks GA IP: ZDV 300 mg every 3 hours + 3TC 150 mg bid orally PP: ZDV 300 mg bid + 3TC 150 mg bid orally for 1 week	ZDV 4 mg/kg bid orally + 3TC 2 mg/kg bid for 1 week	Placebo: 17.2% Arm A: 8.6% Arm B: 10.8% Arm C: 17.7% at 6 weeks of age	Arm A: 50% Arm B: 37%
NEVIRAPINE							
HIVNET 012	Uganda	2 Arms IP ZDV: n=308 Single-dose NVP: n=310	Breast	ZDV 600 mg at onset of labor followed by 300 mg every 3 hours orally *or* NVP 200 mg single dose orally at onset of labor	ZDV 4 mg/kg bid orally for 1 week *or* NVP 2 mg/kg single dose within 72 hours of birth	ZDV: 25.1% NVP: 13.1% at 14–16 weeks	47%
SAINT	South Africa	2 Arms Arm A: NVP Arm B: ZDV+3TC	Breast and Artificial	IP: NVP 200 mg *and* PP: NVP 200 mg 48–72 hours PP *or* IP: ZDV 300 mg every 3 hours + 3TC 150 mg bid orally *and* PP: ZDV 300 mg bid + 3TC 150 mg bid orally for 1 week	NVP 2 mg/kg 48–72 hours of birth *or* ZDV 4 mg/kg bid orally + 3TC 2 mg/kg bid for 1 week	Arm A: 12.7% Arm B: 9.5% at 10 weeks	
PACTG 316	USA, Brazil, France, and Bahamas	2 Arms Any antiretroviral treatment ± NVP Placebo: n=580 NVP: n=594	Artificial	NVP 200 mg single dose orally at onset of labor	NVP 2 mg/kg within 72 hours of birth	No NVP: 1.4% NVP: 1.5%	

[a]ZDV indicates zidovudine; AP, antepartum; GA, gestational age; IP, intrapartum; IV, intravenous; bid, twice daily; PP, postpartum; 3TC, lamivudine; NVP, nevirapine.

during delivery (60,61). In the years following the PACTG 076 results, several trials using short-course antiretroviral therapies were evaluated in several countries in Africa and Asia. Table 1 summarizes these trials.

Zidovudine Monotherapy

In 1997, a trial in Thailand by the U.S. Centers for Disease Control and Prevention (CDC) compared a ZDV regimen that started at 36 weeks of pregnancy (300 mg twice daily) and was followed by an oral loading dose during labor (300 mg every 3 hours), with a placebo (62). Women did not breastfeed. The rate of transmission was 18.9% (95% CI, 13.2%–24.2%) in the placebo group and 9.4% (95% CI, 5.2%–13.5%) in the ZDV group, $p = 0.006$, demonstrating a reduction of the transmission of HIV by 50.1% (95% CI, 15.4%–70.6%).

The CDC conducted another trial in Côte d'Ivoire, comparing the same regimens that had been studied in Thailand. However, in this study, more than 95% of women breastfed their infants (63). At 3 months of age, the transmission rates were 24.9% (95% CI, 16.8%–32.3%) in the placebo group and 15.7% (95% CI, 8.9%–21.9%) in the ZDV group. Transmission risk had been reduced by 37% (95% CI, −5.0%–63.0%). Although the efficacy was lower under these circumstances compared with the same regimen in nonbreastfeeding women in Thailand, this study confirmed the efficacy of ZDV in reducing mother-to-child transmission in breastfeeding women. While the relative efficacy of the treatment was reduced with the duration of breastfeeding, it was still at 23% after 2 years (64).

A short ZDV regimen was also tested in Burkina Faso and Côte d'Ivoire in the DITRAME ANRS 049 trial (65). Women were treated with ZDV from 36 to 38 weeks gestation (300 mg twice daily) until 7 days after delivery, with a 600 mg loading dose at the onset of labor. Most women breastfed their infants. At 3 months of age, the transmission rates were 25.1% (95% CI, 19.0%–31.3%) in the placebo group versus 16.8% (95% CI, 11.4%–22.1%) in the ZDV group. The efficacy of this regimen, estimated at 37% (95% CI, 1.0%–60%) at 3 months of age, was quite consistent with the efficacy found in the CDC trial in Côte d'Ivoire, indicating that the short postpartum maternal dosage may not provide additional efficacy when women are provided short antepartum and intrapartum prophylaxis. In this trial, the relative efficacy of ZDV was 30% after 15 months (66).

Finally, a large trial, the Perinatal HIV Prevention Trial (PHPT) was conducted by Harvard University and the Institut de Recherche pour le Developement (IRD) in collaboration with the Ministry of Public Health and Universities in Thailand to determine the most effective duration of maternal and infant treatment, and to answer a question that neither PACTG 076 nor the placebo-controlled trials mentioned earlier could answer: could an antiretroviral regimen such as PACTG 076, be simplified and shortened while still retaining full efficacy? One thousand, four hundred thirty-seven HIV-infected pregnant women were enrolled in this four-arm equivalence trial, comparing the safety and efficacy of maternal (300 mg twice daily) and infant (2 mg/kg every 6 hours) ZDV regimens administered for various periods of time as follows: starting at 28 weeks gestation in the mother and continuing for 6 weeks in the infant (Long-Long, the PACTG 076-like reference arm); starting at 35 weeks gestation in the mother and continuing for 3 days in the infant (Short-Short); Long-Short; and Short-Long. All mothers received 300 mg ZDV orally every 3 hours during labor. Infants were formula-fed. After its first interim analysis, the shortest ZDV regimen (Short-Short) had to be stopped because its transmission rate of 10.5% was clearly higher than the longer regimens (67). In the three other regimens the transmission rates were 6.5% (95% CI, 4.1%–8.9%) in the Long-Long regimen, 4.7% (95% CI, 2.4%–7.0%) in the Long-Short regimen, and

8.6% (95% CI, 5.6%–11.6%) in the Short-Long regimen (68). The benefit of giving mothers longer treatment was unequivocally established by the observation that in-utero transmission was much lower in the long maternal treatment arms, 1.6% (95% CI, 0.7%–2.6%) than in the short arms, 5.1% (95% CI, 3.2%–7.0%; $p < 0.001$). The study showed clearly that the extent of suppression of *in utero* transmission depends on the length of antiretroviral treatment during the latter part of pregnancy.

Whatever the type and the length of the antiretroviral regimen, in order to benefit from the prophylaxis, women needed to have access to antenatal care, be informed about AIDS, and be tested for HIV. When implementation of the PACTG 076 regimen began, it appeared that many women learned of their HIV status only at the very end of pregnancy, and sometimes at the maternity ward. It was not clear whether it was useful to start treatment in these women at that time and to then provide neonatal postexposure prophylaxis to their infants. One observational study in New York City (69) looked at the effect of ZDV prophylaxis in relation to the time of treatment initiation: the rate of transmission was 6.1% when the treatment began in the prenatal period, a rate consistent with the results of PACTG 076. Interestingly however, the rate was 10.0% when the treatment began during the intrapartum period and was continued in the child during the first 6 weeks of life. It was 9.3% when it began within the first 48 hours of life, 18.4% when it began on day 3 of life or later, and finally, in the absence of zidovudine prophylaxis, the rate was 26.6% (69). In the CDC-sponsored multicenter Perinatal AIDS Collaborative Transmission Study (PACTS) in the United States, the relative effectiveness of early neonatal ZDV treatment was 48% (70).

Zidovudine Plus 3TC

Because ZDV monotherapy often led to only a minimal decrease in viral load, the efficacy of short-course dual therapy regimens in reducing perinatal transmission was then tested. The UNAIDS-coordinated PETRA trial (71) used various durations of a combination of ZDV plus 3TC in predominantly breastfeeding populations in South Africa, Tanzania, and Uganda. The antenatal treatment was 300 mg oral ZDV plus 150 mg 3TC twice a day; intrapartum treatment was 300 mg oral ZDV every 3 hours plus 150 mg oral 3TC every 12 hours; postpartum treatment was 300 mg oral ZDV plus 150 mg 3TC twice a day for 1 week; and neonatal treatment was 4 mg/kg ZDV plus 2 mg/kg 3TC twice a day for 1 week. The reported early efficacy results at 6 weeks of age were as follows: where women were treated from 36 weeks gestation through labor and for 1 week postpartum, the rate of transmission was 8.6%; where women started treatment at onset of labor and continued for 1 week postpartum, the rate of transmission was 10.8%; and where women were treated during labor only, the transmission rate was 17.7%, a rate very similar to that in the placebo arm (17.2%). The intrapartum-only treatment was ineffective, but the intrapartum treatment together with postpartum and neonatal treatment significantly reduced transmission rates.

Intrapartum Nevirapine

In less developed countries, the proportion of women who come to deliver without having received any antenatal care can be extremely high, making the efficacy of intrapartum prophylaxis an especially critical issue. While several short ZDV or ZDV plus 3TC regimens were tested in Africa and Thailand, another trial assessed the efficacy of a single dose of nevirapine (NVP). Nevirapine is a very potent antiretroviral drug, characterized by a very fast oral absorption, rapid transplacental clearing, and a long half-life in the infant (72). In the early 1990s, the use of single-dose NVP was, therefore, extensively discussed as a means to decrease intrapartum HIV transmission.

The HIVNET 012 Clinical Trial in Uganda tested two different antiretroviral regimens during the intrapartum and neonatal period for the prevention of perinatal transmission (73). HIV-1–infected pregnant women were randomly assigned to receive 200 mg NVP orally at the onset of labor with 2 mg/kg to their infants 48 to 72 hours after birth, or 600 mg ZDV orally at the onset of labor followed by 300 mg ZDV every 3 hours until delivery and 4 mg/kg orally twice daily to infants for 7 days after birth. Virtually all infants were breastfed. HIV-1 transmission rates in the ZDV and NVP groups were respectively 10.4% and 8.2% at birth ($p = 0.354$), 21.3% and 11.9% by age 6–8 weeks ($p = 0.0027$), and 25.1% and 13.1% by age 14–16 weeks ($p = 0.0006$). These results showed that a single dose of NVP for mothers together with a single dose for infants can reduce intrapartum transmission by 48% (95% CI, 24%–65%) at 14–16 weeks of age. The results of this study brought hope for many developing countries: a simple and cheap way of reducing perinatal transmission of HIV was discovered. The single-dose NVP treatment, however, could have no impact on the in-utero transmission that might have already occurred, which was at about 8% to 10% in this study.

The results of HIVNET 012 were later confirmed by SAINT, a study conducted in South Africa, which compared a regimen of NVP (200 mg during labor and one dose to mother and infant 48–72 hours postdelivery), with one of the ZDV plus 3TC regimens tested in the PETRA study discussed earlier (multiple doses during labor and for 1 week to mother and infant postpartum) (74). Ten weeks after birth, the transmission rates were not significantly different in the two arms—12.7% in the NVP arm and 9.5% in the ZDV plus 3TC arm.

Antibody Therapy, Caesarean Section, and Other Combination Antiretroviral Therapies

HIV-Immunoglobulins

Although the role of anti-HIV antibodies in protecting the infant during natural infection was unclear, specific HIV Immunoglobulins prophylaxis was tested to reduce perinatal transmission. The PACTG 185 trial was designed to test the efficacy of HIV hyperimmune immunoglobulins (HIVIG) administered monthly during pregnancy and to the neonate at birth, in addition to standard ZDV prophylaxis (75, 76). The study failed to demonstrate any efficacy of HIVIG, with overall low transmission rates of 4.1% (95% CI, 1.5%–6.7%) in the HIVIG group and 6.0% (95% CI, 2.8%–9.1%) in the controls (75, 76).

Caesarean Section

It had been demonstrated that the risk of perinatal transmission was lower when the infant had been delivered less than 4 hours after the rupture of the membranes (36, 37) or when the infant had been delivered by caesarean section before the rupture of membranes or onset of labor (38). A randomized trial of modes of delivery demonstrated the efficacy of elective caesarean section for protecting infants (Table 2). In this trial, three of 170 infants (1.8%) born to women by caesarean section were infected, compared with 21 of 200 infants (10.5%) born to women by vaginal delivery ($p < 0.001$) (77). Elective caesarean section is now often proposed to HIV-infected pregnant women in industrialized countries. However, due to its cost (78), the risk of infection in potentially immunosuppressed women (79), and the risk of occupational exposure for the surgeons, caesarean section is not widely recommended in resource-poor countries.

Combination Antiretroviral Therapies

With the successes of combination antiretroviral therapy in adult patients, an increasing number of pregnant women, especially in industrialized countries, have been receiving multiple antiretroviral drugs as much for their own health as for the prevention of perinatal transmission. Because these regimens have a more pronounced effect in

TABLE 2. Trials of Interventions without Antiretrovirals[a]

Trial	Setting	Design and sample size	Feeding mode	Maternal regimen	Infant regimen	Transmission rate	Transmission rate reduction
Caesarean section							
European Collaboration	Europe	Randomized Trial Any ARV treatment ± C-section Elective C-section: $n=170$ Vaginal delivery: $n=200$	Artificial	Elective C-section at 38 weeks GA	None	C-section: 1.8% Vaginal: 10.5%	
Vaginal Disinfection							
	Malawi	Placebo-controlled Vaginal lavage: $n=505$ No lavage: $n=477$	Breast	Chlorhexidine (0.25% solution) IP Cotton swab cleansing procedure	Infant Bath	No lavage: 27.9% Lavage: 26.9% at 6–12 weeks	Efficacious when membranes were ruptured for > 4 hours
	Kenya	Placebo-Controlled Vaginal lavage: $n=309$ No lavage: $n=297$	Breast	Chlorhexidine (0.20%–0.40% solution) IP Douching procedure repeated every 3 hours	None	No lavage: 21.7% Lavage: 20.5% at 6–14 weeks	
Vitamin A							
Harvard Study	Tanzania	Placebo-Controlled Factorial Design, 4-arm Trial Vitamin A: $n=269$ MV excluding A: $n=269$ MV including A: $n=270$ Placebo: $n=267$	Breast	Vitamin A: AP (5,000 IU RP and 30 mg β-carotene/day) + IP (200,000 IU RP) MV excluding vitamin A: AP MV including vitamin A: AP + IP (200,000 IU RP)	None	MV: 10.1% No MV: 6.6% Vitamin A: 10.0% No vitamin A: 6.7% at birth	None, reduction of adverse pregnancy outcomes by MV including vitamin A
	Malawi	Placebo-controlled Placebo: $n=237$ Vitamin A: $n=233$	Breast	AP: Vitamin A (10,000 IU RP) 18 – 34 weeks GA PP: 200,000 IU RP (all mothers)	None	Placebo: 27.8% Vitamin A: 26.6% at 6 weeks	None, effect on reducing % of low birth weights
Durban Study	South Africa	Placebo-controlled Placebo: $n=360$ Vitamin A: $n=368$	Breast	AP: 5,000 IU RP and 300 mg β-carotene/day during third trimester IP: 200,000 IU RP	None	Placebo: 22.3% Vitamin A: 20.3% at 3 months	None, reduction among preterm infants
Artificial feeding							
	Kenya	Randomized trial of the mode of feeding Breastfeeding: $n=212$ Artificial feeding: $n=213$				Breast: 36.7% Artificial: 20.5% at 24 months	16.1% transmission through breastfeeding

[a]ARV indicates antiretroviral; GA, gestational age; IP, intrapartum; MV, multivitamin; RP, retinyl palmitate; AP, antepartum; IU, international unit; PP, postpartum.

reducing maternal viral load than ZDV monotherapy, it was likely that these regimens would be very effective in preventing perinatal transmission and indeed, the observed rates of transmission with these treatments have been extremely low (80).

In the French open-label study, ANRS 075, a ZDV plus 3TC regimen was offered to HIV-infected pregnant women and their infants: 250 mg ZDV to start, plus 150 mg 3TC twice daily orally added at 32 weeks gestation, ZDV infusion during labor, and 2 mg/kg ZDV every 6 hours plus 2 mg/kg 3TC every 12 hours orally for 6 weeks in the infant. The rate of transmission was 1.6% based on 445 mother–infant pairs (81). However, two cases of encephalopathy followed by death in two uninfected infants aged 13 months and 11 months were identified, raising concerns about the mitochondrial toxicity of this potent combination therapy (82). Shortly thereafter, the same French group discovered a few other cases of less severe mitochondrial dysfunction in infants who had been exposed to ZDV plus 3TC or ZDV alone. Because there was no control group, the relationship between the occurrence of mitochondrial anomalies and drug exposure remains unclear. Since then, there has been an extensive review of database records of children exposed to antiretroviral drugs during the neonatal period and no other cases have been found (83,84).

The large PACTG 316 study carried out in the United States, France, Brazil, and the Bahamas was designed to evaluate the additional efficacy of NVP on top of other antiretroviral treatment (85). Enrollment in that study was stopped because of the multiplicity of background treatments on top of which NVP was tested. One percent of the women had no background antiretroviral treatment; 23% were taking ZDV monotherapy; 28% were taking ZDV plus 3TC; and the others (49%) were taking other combinations with or without protease inhibitors. Thirty-four percent of women had elective caesarean section. The transmission rates were not significantly different between groups: 1.5% (95% CI, 0.7%–2.8%) in NVP group and 1.4% (95% CI, 0.6%–2.7%) in the placebo group, an impressively low transmission rate (85).

With ZDV monotherapy, intrapartum transmission remains relatively high (about 5%). Adding a single dose of a potent antiretroviral like NVP at onset of labor, when the risk of transmission is highest, may significantly reduce intrapartum and early postpartum transmission without adding significant cost or logistical complications. Based on this assumption, a large clinical trial of NVP added to ZDV is now being conducted in Thailand. In this study, women start ZDV prophylaxis as soon as possible after the 28th week of pregnancy and continue throughout delivery. In addition, they are randomized to one of three study arms: 200 mg NVP at onset of labor in mother plus 2 mg/kg NVP oral suspension 48 to 72 hours after birth in neonate (N-N); 200 mg NVP to mothers at onset of labor plus placebo in neonates (N-P); placebo in mothers and in neonates, the reference study arm (P-P).

Chemoprophylaxis for Breastfeeding Transmission

Recognizing that breastfeeding is beneficial to child health, and that in some situations it may not be possible to provide safe breastfeeding alternatives, several studies are looking at the benefit of providing antiretroviral prophylaxis to breastfed infants. This approach is currently being tested in a study by Harvard University in Botswana, comparing short-course antiviral regimens of one drug (ZDV) with two drugs (ZDV plus NVP). Women are randomized to receive either ZDV alone or ZDV plus NVP and to either breastfeed or formula-feed. Zidovudine is administered to all mothers starting at 34 weeks of pregnancy and NVP is given to one group of women during labor, as in the HIVNET 012 protocol. ZDV is administered to all babies for 7 days and NVP is given to one group of babies as in the

HIVNET 012 protocol. In addition, the study compares two postnatal interventions: ZDV prophylaxis to infants of breastfeeding mothers versus formula-feeding. Breastfeeding is stopped at 6 months after which the infants' caloric and nutritional needs can be met with other sources. The endpoints are postnatal HIV-1 transmission and infant morbidity and mortality.

As an alternative to chemoprophylaxis, a vaccine administered at birth to breastfed infants may be able to boost their immune systems enough to protect them during the most critical period of early breastfeeding. However, no prototype vaccine seems to be ready to be tested in this context. Detailed information on other methods for the prevention of breast milk transmission of HIV can be found in Chapter 36, *this volume*.

QUESTIONS STILL TO BE ANSWERED

The knowledge and the tools to prevent nearly all perinatal transmission now exist, but many questions remain to be answered, for example: how do ZDV and other antiretrovirals work; are these drugs safe in the short and long term; and are there efficacious universal preventive interventions that could be used when the HIV status of pregnant women is not known?

How Do ZDV and Other Antiretroviral Drugs Work?

In PACTG 076, transmission was observed at all maternal levels of viral load, including at undetectable levels. Decreased viral load, which was modest (0.24 log) in this study, explained only 11% of the observed treatment effect (41). In the CDC study conducted in Bangkok, however, the reduction of viral load (more than 0.50 log) could explain about 80% of the observed treatment effect (62). The absence of neonatal treatment in the CDC study or the different techniques used to measure viral load in the two studies could explain these discrepancies. The presence of ZDV in the fetus/infant prior to exposure to HIV may abort the first round of replication in the infant's cells and prevent infection from establishing itself.

Compared to ZDV, the effect of NVP on viral load is more obvious. In HIVNET 012, seven days after antiretroviral intake, maternal viral load was substantially reduced (1.03 log decrease) in the NVP group, whereas it was slightly increased (0.17 log increase) in the ZDV group ($p > 0.001$) (86). Although the risk of transmission was associated with baseline RNA level in this study, its decrease at seven days in the NVP group was also predictive of late transmission (intrapartum or postnatal). Because of the lack of activated lymphocytes to promote viral replication in fetuses, postexposure prophylaxis is most likely to benefit polymerase chain reaction (PCR)-negative infants at birth in whom the virus has passed during late gestation but remains unintegrated in the cells (87). As indicated in the Thai PHPT study of ZDV regimens, late initiation of antiretroviral prophylaxis may be partly compensated for by longer postexposure prophylaxis in the infant (68). Therefore, both decreased exposure of the fetus and infant through lower viral load in the mother (peripheral blood and vaginal secretions) and pre- and postexposure prophylaxis may explain the protective effects of ZDV and NVP (87–89).

Safety of In-Utero or Neonatal Antiretroviral Exposure

The risks associated with antiretroviral exposure have to be balanced with the benefits of being protected from HIV. The short-term risks associated with ZDV are limited to anemias, which are reversible at the end of treatment. In all placebo-controlled studies using ZDV, congenital anomalies, prematurity, and anthropometric parameters were similar in the placebo and ZDV groups. The biologic parameters were also similar, except for more frequent low hemoglobin levels and a few cases of severe but reversible anemias in the ZDV groups. In the DITRAME trial, however, there was an excess risk of neonatal death for infants in the ZDV group compared to those receiving placebo (4% versus 2%, $p = 0.04$), but this risk was no longer significant at 6 months of age (8.8% versus 13.6%) (65, 66).

The intermediate follow-up data are also reassuring: in children exposed to ZDV who were followed for up to 6 years in the PACTG 076 study, no significant differences in immunologic, developmental, or anthropometric parameters were observed (90). No tumors of any kind were observed among 727 children perinatally exposed to ZDV after a mean follow-up of 38 months (91).

A high rate of premature delivery was reported in a cohort of 30 pregnant women exposed to highly active antiretroviral therapy in Switzerland (92). However, these results were not confirmed in other studies (93,94).

Eight cases of mitochondrial dysfunction have been described in children perinatally exposed to nucleoside analog reverse transcriptase inhibitors (such as ZDV plus 3TC) in France (82). Five of these patients (two of whom died) presented with delayed neurologic symptoms and three had severe biologic or neurologic abnormalities. A retrospective review of perinatal exposure to antiretroviral drugs was initiated in the United States within the PACT study (94). Among 118 deaths, none were related to mitochondrial dysfunction, and among 1,954 living uninfected children, none of those perinatally exposed to antiretrovirals had signs or symptoms possibly related to mitochondrial dysfunction (94). In another review of 85 deaths among HIV-infected children in Newark, United States, mitochondrial dysfunction syndrome was not identified (95). Also, no cases suggestive of mitochondrial dysfunction were found among 14,000 uninfected children, including 33 who died (84). In the CDC trial in Bangkok and the PHPT study, among respectively 196 and 1,309 infants perinatally exposed to ZDV, no cases suggestive of mitochondrial toxicity were observed (68,96).

The major side effect of NVP is liver dysfunction and the development of rash, which occasionally develops into severe rash or Stevens-Johnson syndrome (97). In HIVNET 012, nine mothers developed maculopapular rash (4 in the ZDV group and 5 in the NVP group), but no case was serious (73). Eighteen babies had maculopapular rash (9 in the ZDV group and 9 in the NVP group); however, no cases were serious. The frequency and severity of biologic abnormalities was similar in the two groups. Similarly, in the SAINT study in South Africa, among 652 pregnant women and their infants who had each received a single dose of NVP, no episodes of liver toxicity or serious rash were reported (98). However, cases of severe liver failure, some of them fatal, were recently reported following postexposure prophylaxis with NVP-containing antiretroviral regimens in adults (99, 100). Although such cases have never been described after a single dose of NVP, this calls for close surveillance of hepatic parameters (101).

Nevertheless, when balancing the severe risk of death in cases of pediatric HIV infection with the high efficacy of antiretroviral prophylaxis, it is clear that antiretrovirals should be systematically offered to all HIV-infected pregnant women while safety is carefully assessed.

Are There Proposed Universal Preventive Interventions for Cases of Unknown HIV Status in Pregnant Women?

The rationale for testing shorter and simplified prophylactic regimens was that in most developing country situations, women have limited access to prenatal care and the long and complex PACTG 076 regimen appeared to be difficult to apply due to infrastructural and resource limitations. In some settings, women receive no antenatal care, are not offered HIV testing, and do not know about the risk of transmission of HIV to their infants. To decrease the risk of transmission in these settings, universal interventions likely to reduce perinatal transmission of HIV could be applied without HIV screening. Simple and inexpensive interventions such as vitamin A supplementation or vaginal disinfection have been tested for this purpose (Table 2).

Vaginal Disinfection

Because a significant number of infants are probably infected through mucosal exposure to HIV in the maternal secretions during the birth process, disinfection of the birth canal was envisioned as a strategy to reduce perinatal transmission of HIV. This intervention was expected to have an additional benefit in preventing other neonatal infections such as group B streptococcus infections (102).

In a study in Malawi, vaginal disinfection using chlorhexidine (0.25% solution) was shown to be ineffective in reducing mother-to-child transmission of HIV (103). The transmission rate at 6–12 weeks was 27.9% in the group of women with no disinfection compared to 26.9% in the group of women who had vaginal disinfection (Table 2). Vaginal disinfection was effective, however, in the subgroup of women who had a prolonged rupture of membranes. Overall neonatal morbidity and mortality from other causes was also significantly reduced in the intervention group. A lack of preventive effect of vaginal lavage by chlorhexidine (0.20%–0.40% solution) was also demonstrated in a study in Kenya (104). At 6–14 weeks, the overall transmission rates were not significantly different in the non-lavage (21.7%; 95% CI, 17.4%–27.4%) versus the lavage (20.5%; 95% CI, 16.0%–25.0%) groups. Finally, a phase II placebo-controlled study in Côte d'Ivoire and Burkina Faso using vaginal disinfection (one Benzalkonium vaginal suppository per day during the last month of pregnancy) and bathing of the neonate, confirmed the feasibility and acceptability of this kind of intervention but, because of its limited sample size, could not draw any conclusions about its efficacy in reducing perinatal transmission (105).

Vitamin A Supplementation

An association between the risk of perinatal transmission of HIV and vitamin A deficiency had been demonstrated in a study in Malawi (14). Vitamin A is relatively safe and inexpensive, and it is known for its beneficial effects as an anti-infectious agent: it reduces infant mortality by approximately 30% (106). For these reasons researchers envisioned using it to reduce perinatal transmission of HIV by providing it to all pregnant women regardless of their HIV status. Unfortunately, all trials have failed to demonstrate any efficacy of vitamin A in preventing perinatal transmission (Table 2).

For instance, in Malawi, a placebo-controlled trial could not demonstrate any efficacy of vitamin A supplementation (retinyl palmitate 10,000 international units [IU] per day) for the reduction of perinatal transmission, but showed a significant effect on decreasing the percentage of low birth weight infants (14.0% in the vitamin A group versus 21.1% in the control group) (107). In Durban, South Africa, 728 HIV infected women received either vitamin A (5,000 IU retinyl palmitate and 30 mg β-carotene during the third trimester of pregnancy and 200,000 IU retinyl palmitate at delivery) or placebo in a randomized trial (108). At 3 months of age, the transmission rates of HIV were not significantly different between the two groups: 20.3% (95% CI, 15.7%–24.9%) in the vitamin A group and 22.3% (95% CI, 17.5%–27.1%) in the placebo group. There was no difference in fetal or infant mortality rates between the two groups. Women receiving vitamin A supplements were, however, less likely to have a preterm delivery (11.4% in the vitamin A and 17.4% in the placebo group, $p = 0.03$) and among the 80 preterm deliveries, infants in the vitamin A group were less likely to be HIV-infected

(17.9%; 95% CI, 3.5%–32.2%) than those in the placebo group (33.8%; 95% CI, 19.8%–47.8%). Finally, in order to evaluate the efficacy of vitamin A and/or multivitamin (excluding vitamin A) supplement to reduce perinatal transmission of HIV, a large four-arm trial was performed in Tanzania. The study has demonstrated a clear benefit of multivitamins (including vitamin A) in decreasing adverse pregnancy outcomes (109), but not in reducing perinatal HIV transmission (110). At birth, the transmission rates were 10.1% in the multivitamin arm and 6.6% in the no-multivitamin arm ($p=0.08$), compared with 10.0% in the vitamin A arm and 6.7% in the no vitamin A arm ($p=0.11$). At 6 weeks of age, neither multivitamins nor vitamin A decreased the rate of transmission (111).

The failure of simple methods such as vitamin A supplementation or vaginal lavage to decrease mother-to-child transmission of HIV has been disappointing. By contrast, the impressive efficacy of a single dose of NVP, as demonstrated in the HIVNET 012 trial, has prompted a debate on the appropriateness of using NVP as a universal prophylactic treatment in circumstances where HIV testing is not available.

Ultra-Short Prophylactic Treatment: Intrapartum Counseling, Testing, and Antiretroviral Administration versus NVP Blanket Coverage

Because of its low cost and simplicity, the universal provision of NVP without previous counseling and testing was also envisioned for countries where HIV seroprevalence is very high (73). In a cost-effectiveness analysis, it was shown that in a hypothetical cohort of 20,000 pregnant women with 30% HIV-1 prevalence, the universal provision of the HIVNET 012 regimen would avert 603 cases of HIV-1 infection in babies and cost USD$83,333 (112). The associated cost-effectiveness ratio would be $138 per case averted or $5.25 per disability-adjusted life-year (DALY), an amount that is comparable to other public health interventions already in place, such as infant immunization. However, universal NVP coverage would deprive women of counseling and information about their HIV status and would make it impossible for them to make informed decisions about breastfeeding. Moreover, it would expose uninfected women and their infants to an unnecessary risk. Additional concerns about the emergence of possible resistance at individual and population levels (113) have hindered recommendations for widescale implementation of NVP for mother-to-child transmission prevention with or without prior HIV testing (110). Results from the PACTG 316 cohort confirm the occurrence of resistance mutations in about 10% of the women with detectable viral load (114,115). Follow-up data from HIVNET 012, however, indicate that one year after exposure to NVP, these resistance mutations are no longer detected (116). The clinical significance of these resistance mutations needs to be investigated.

For women who do not attend antenatal care, counseling and rapid HIV testing upon admission in the delivery room, followed by the administration of NVP to the women found to be HIV-positive, is now being tested by the CDC-funded Mother-Infant Rapid Intervention At Delivery (MIRIAD) Study. This approach seems feasible, although concerns about the appropriateness of pre- and post-test counseling in the delivery room have been raised (117,118).

CURRENT STRATEGIES TO REDUCE MOTHER-TO-CHILD TRANSMISSION

All efforts should be made to propose voluntary HIV counseling and testing to all pregnant women during the antenatal period and to recommend that they avoid breastfeeding when possible.

When women come to antenatal clinics early during pregnancy, HIV-positive women should be offered ZDV monotherapy or combination therapy depending on their clinical, immunologic, and virologic status, starting at least at 28 weeks gestation. Elective caesarean section should be offered as well and babies should be treated for 6 weeks.

When financial constraints exist, ZDV monotherapy should be started as soon after 28 weeks gestation as possible, followed by infant treatment for 3 days after birth. The PHPT study results suggest that, in a program that begins ZDV treatment for women at 28 weeks gestation, treatment of the infant beyond 3 days postpartum is unnecessary; however, when the mother starts ZDV later in pregnancy, 6 weeks of infant treatment may be beneficial. The 7-week increase in maternal treatment gained by starting at 28 weeks instead of 35 weeks prevents an important fraction of in-utero transmission and carries minimal additional cost. To bring the rate of infant infection closer to zero, an alternative approach to caesarean section would be to provide, in addition to ZDV monotherapy, a potent antiretroviral such as NVP during the perinatal period. This approach is now being tested by the Harvard group/IRD 054 in Thailand. Results should be available by the end of the year 2002.

When women attend prenatal care, but organizational issues within the health system may hinder their return for delivery, all HIV-positive women tested during pregnancy could be provided with a single dose of NVP to take at home at onset of labor and a single dose of NVP to give to their infants after birth. This regimen should be similar in efficacy to HIVNET 012, although in-utero transmission will not be prevented.

In settings where the majority of women do not attend prenatal care, voluntary HIV counseling and rapid testing of pregnant women in the delivery room should be offered, followed by the administration of a single dose of NVP as soon as HIV-positive status is confirmed. Infants of infected mothers should also be administered a single dose of NVP 48–72 hours after birth. In the HIVNET 012 study, women were advised to take the NVP at home at onset of labor. Therefore, it is expected that the efficacy of receiving the treatment at a later stage of labor in the delivery room will be less. An alternative option would be to follow the SAINT regimen and provide ZDV plus 3TC to the mother and the infant. The efficacy of this regimen is similar to NVP, but it is more expensive and the logistics are more complex.

Finally, when formula feeding is not an option, all efforts should be made to safely wean infants as early as possible. Exclusive breastfeeding has yet to demonstrate its benefit in a randomized clinical trial before it can be recommended. Weaning products could provide good alternatives to formula (119). They are cheaper and probably safer than formula. However, the feasibility of such an approach still needs to be demonstrated (see Chapter 36, *this volume*).

CONCLUSION

Using combinations of the existing tools, such as education, counseling, testing, antiretrovirals, caesarean section, and formula-feeding, the risk of mother-to-child transmission of HIV can be virtually eliminated. Yet many infants are still being infected. For many well-known reasons, preventive and curative interventions are rarely 100% successful and none ever cover 100% of the populations most in need. In the case of pediatric AIDS, this is often a result of the difficulty of incorporating the essential intervention components into existing mother–child health care systems. Without appropriate treatment, infected infants may die within a few years from a succession of infections and complications of HIV. Moreover, infected or not, infants born to HIV-infected mothers are likely to become orphans because of the death of their parents from AIDS in the absence of appropriate adult treatment. Therefore, providing comprehensive HIV care within the existing mother and child health services should be considered urgently. This is a challenge in industrialized countries, but also to a much greater extent in developing countries where health care systems are profoundly shaken by the AIDS epidemic, economic constraints and crises, and, in many cases, political unrest.

Efforts must now focus on implementing the results of the past 10 years of epidemiologic, basic scientific, and clinical research. This endeavor will require more political commitment, economic solidarity, and human rights advocacy than new scientific knowledge. No one is under the illusion that medical progress alone will solve the extraordinary societal problems raised by inequity, prejudice, and poverty. At the same time, research should proceed to identify and remove obstacles to the implementation of interventions known to be successful. It is the growing realization at the highest levels that the AIDS epidemic is a global threat, and that access to adequate care can no longer be withheld from those who need it most, that will allow the outstanding gains in AIDS research to become a reality worldwide.

REFERENCES

1. WHO/UNAIDS. *AIDS Epidemic Update, December 2000.* WHO/CDS/CSR/EDC/2000.9. Geneva: World Health Organization, 2000.
2. Lallemant M, Le Cœur S, M'Pelé P. Perinatal transmission of HIV in Africa. In: Essex M, Mboup S, Kanki P, Kalengayi M, eds. *AIDS in Africa*, 1st ed. New York: Raven Press, 1993:211–236.
3. Mofenson LM. Mother-child HIV-1 transmission: timing and determinants. *Obstet Gynecol Clin North Am*, 1997;24:759–784.
4. The Working Group on Mother-To-Child Transmission of HIV. Rates of mother-to-child transmission of HIV-1 in Africa, America, and Europe: results from 13 perinatal studies. *J Acquir Immune Defic Syndr Hum Retrovirol*, 1995;8: 506–510
5. Dabis F, Msellati P, Dunn D, et al. Estimating the rate of mother-to-child transmission of HIV. Report of a workshop on methodological issues, Ghent (Belgium). *AIDS*, 1993;7:1139–1148.
6. Blanche S, Rouzioux C, Guihard Moscato ML, et al., and the HIV Infection in Newborns French Collaborative Study Group. A prospective study of infants born to women seropositive for human immunodeficiency virus type 1. *N Engl J Med*, 1989;320:1643–1648.
7. European Collaborative Study. Children born to women with HIV-1 infection: natural history and risk of transmission. *Lancet*, 1991;337:253–260.
8. Andiman WA, Simpson BJ, Olson B, et al. Rate of transmission of human immunodeficiency virus type 1 infection from mother to child and short-term outcome of neonatal infection. Results of a prospective cohort study. *Am J Dis Child*, 1990; 144:758–766.
9. Dunn DT, Newell ML, Ades AE, et al. Risk of human immunodeficiency virus type 1 transmission through breastfeeding. *Lancet*, 1992;340:585–588.
10. UNAIDS. *HIV and Infant Feeding. A Review of HIV Transmission through Breastfeeding*. Geneva: WHO, June 1998.
11. Lepage P, Van De Perre P, Msellati P, et al. Mother-to-child transmission of human immunodeficiency virus type 1 (HIV-1) and its determinants: a cohort study in Kigali, Rwanda. *Am J Epidemiol*, 1993; 137:589–599.
12. Thomas PA, Weedon J, Krasinski K, et al. Maternal predictor of perinatal human immunodeficiency virus transmission. *Pediatr Infect Dis J*, 1994; 13:489–495.
13. Hague RA, Mok JY, Johnstone FD, et al. Maternal factors in HIV transmission. *Int J STD AIDS*, 1993; 4:142–146.
14. Semba RD, Miotti PG, Chiphangwi JD, et al. Maternal vitamin A deficiency and mother-to-child transmission of HIV-1. *Lancet*, 1994;343: 1593–1597.
15. Bridbord K, Willoughby A. Vitamin A and mother-to-child HIV-1 transmission. *Lancet*, 1994;343: 1585–1586.
16. Fawzi WW, Hunter DJ. Vitamins in HIV disease progression and vertical transmission. *Epidemiology*, 1998;9:457–466.
17. Borkowsky W, Krasinski K, Cao Y, et al. Correlation of perinatal transmission of human immunodeficiency virus type 1 with maternal viremia and lymphocyte phenotypes. *J Pediatr*, 1994;125:345–351.
18. Contopoulos-Ioannidis DG, Ioannidis JP. Maternal cell-free viremia in the natural history of perinatal HIV-1 transmission: a meta-analysis. *J Acquir Immune Defic Syndr Hum Retrovirol*, 1998;18: 126–135.
19. Mayaux MJ, Dussaix E, Isopet J, et al. Maternal virus load during pregnancy and mother-to-child

transmission of human immunodeficiency virus type 1: the French perinatal cohort studies. SEROGEST Cohort Group. *J Infect Dis*, 1997;175: 172–175.
20. Shaffer N, Roongpisuthipong A, Siriwasin W, et al. Maternal virus load and perinatal human immunodeficiency virus type 1 subtype E transmission, Thailand. Bangkok Collaborative Perinatal HIV Transmission Study Group. *J Infect Dis*, 1999;179: 590–599.
21. The European Collaborative Study. Vertical transmission of HIV-1: maternal immune status and obstetric factors. *AIDS*, 1996;10:1675–1681.
22. Devash Y, Calvelli TA, Wood DG, et al. Vertical transmission of human immunodeficiency virus is correlated with the absence of high-affinity/avidity maternal antibodies to the gp120 principal neutralizing domain. *Proc Natl Acad Sci USA*, 1990;87: 3445–3449.
23. Goedert JJ, Mendez H, Drummond JE, et al. Mother-to-infant transmission of human immunodeficiency virus type 1: association with prematurity or low anti-gp120. *Lancet*, 1989;2:1351–1354.
24. Rossi P, Moschese V, Broliden PA, et al. Presence of maternal antibodies to human immunodeficiency virus 1 envelope glycoprotein gp120 epitopes correlates with the uninfected status of children born to seropositive mothers. *Proc Natl Acad Sci USA*, 1989;86:8055–8058.
25. Lallemant M, Baillou A, Lallemant-Le Coeur S, et al. Maternal antibody response at delivery and perinatal transmission of human immunodeficiency virus type 1 in African women. *Lancet*, 1994;343:1001–1005.
26. Markham RB, Coberly J, Ruff AJ, et al. Maternal IgG1 and IgA antibody to V3 loop consensus sequence and maternal-infant HIV-1 transmission. *Lancet*, 1994;343:390–391.
27. Renjifo B, Fawzi W, Mwakagile D, et al. Differences in perinatal transmission among human immunodeficiency virus type 1 genotypes. *J Hum Virol*, 2001;4:16–25.
28. Anderson VM. The placental barrier to maternal HIV infection. *Obstet Gynecol Clin North Am*, 1997;24:797–819.
29. Burton GJ, O'Shea S, Rostron T, et al. Significance of placental damage in vertical transmission of human immunodeficiency virus. *J Med Virol*, 1996; 50:237–243.
30. Zachar V, Thomas RA, Jones T, et al. Vertical transmission of HIV: detection of proviral DNA in placental trophoblast. *AIDS*, 1994;8:129–140.
31. Lairmore MD, Cuthbert PS, Utley LL, et al. Cellular localization of CD4 in the human placenta. Implications for maternal-to-fetal transmission of HIV. *J Immunol*, 1993;151:1673–1681.
32. Brossard Y, Aubin J, Mandelbrot L, et al. Frequency of early in utero HIV infections: a blind DNA polymerase chain reaction study on 100 fetal thymuses. *AIDS*, 1995;9:359–366.
33. Mofenson LM. Epidemiology and determinants of vertical HIV transmission. *Sem Ped Inf Dis*, 1994;5:252–265.
34. Mandelbrot L, Burgard M, Teglas JP, et al. Frequent detection of HIV-1 in the gastric aspirates of neonates born to HIV-infected mothers. *AIDS*, 1999;13:2143–2149.
35. MacDonald KS, Embree JE, Nagelkerke NJ, et al. The HLA A2/6802 supertype is associated with reduced risk of perinatal human immunodeficiency virus type 1 transmission. *J Infect Dis*, 2001;183: 503–506.
36. The International Perinatal HIV Group. Duration of ruptured membranes and vertical transmission of HIV-1: a meta-analysis from 15 prospective cohort studies. *AIDS*, 2001;15:357–368.
37. Landesman SH, Kalish LA, Burns DN, et al. Obstetrical factors and the transmission of human immunodeficiency virus type 1 from mother to child. *N Engl J Med*, 1996;334:1617–1623.
38. The International Perinatal HIV Group. The mode of delivery and the risk of vertical transmission of human immunodeficiency virus type 1—a meta-analysis of 15 prospective cohort studies. *N Engl J Med*, 1999;340:977–987.
39. Embree JE, Njenga S, Datta P, et al. Risk factors for postnatal mother-child transmission of HIV-1. *AIDS*, 2000;14:2535–2541.
40. Miotti PG, Taha TE, Kumwenda NI, et al. HIV transmission through breastfeeding: a study in Malawi. *JAMA*, 1999;282:744–749.
41. Connor EM, Sperling RS, Gelber R, et al. for the Pediatric AIDS Clinical Trials Group Protocol 076 Study Group. Reduction of maternal-infant transmission of human immunodeficiency type I with zidovudine treatment. *N Engl J Med*, 1994;331: 1173–1180.
42. Newell ML, Peckham CS. Working towards a European strategy for intervention to reduce perinatal transmission of HIV. *Br J Obstet Gynaecol*, 1994;101:192–196.
43. Lallemant M, Le Coeur S, Tarantola D, et al. Preventing perinatal transmission. *Lancet*, 1994;343:1429–1430.
44. Ukwu HN, Graham BS, Lambert JS, et al. Perinatal transmission of HIV-1 and maternal immunization strategies for prevention. *Obstet Gynecol*, 1992;80: 458–468.
45. De Cock KM, Fowler MG, Mercier E, et al. Prevention of Mother-to-Child HIV transmission in resource-poor countries. Translating research into policy and practice. *JAMA*, 2000;283:1175–1182.
46. Dabis F, Leroy V, Castetbon K, et al. Preventing mother-to-child transmission of HIV-1 in Africa in the year 2000. *AIDS*, 2000;14:1017–1026.

47. Ioannidis JP, Abrams EJ, Ammann A, et al. Perinatal transmission of human immunodeficiency virus type 1 by pregnant women with RNA virus loads <1000 copies/mL. *J Infect Dis*, 2001; 183:539–545.
48. Sperling RS, Shapiro DE, Coombs RW, et al. Maternal viral load, zidovudine treatment, and the risk of transmission of human immunodeficiency virus type 1 from mother to infant. Pediatric AIDS Clinical Trials Group Protocol 076 Study Group. *N Engl J Med*, 1996;335:1621–1629.
49. Simpson BJ, Shapiro ED, Andiman WA. Reduction in the risk of vertical transmission of HIV-1 associated with treatment of pregnant women with orally administered zidovudine alone. *J Acquir Immune Defic Syndr*, 1997;14:145–152.
50. Matheson PB, Abrams EJ, Thomas PA, et al. Efficacy of antenatal zidovudine in reducing perinatal transmission of human immunodeficiency virus type 1. The New York City Perinatal HIV Transmission Collaborative Study Group. *J Infect Dis*, 1995;172:353–358.
51. Wade NA, Birkhead GS, Warren BL, et al. Abbreviated regimens of zidovudine prophylaxis and perinatal transmission of the human immunodeficiency virus. *N Engl J Med*, 1998;339:1409–1414.
52. Simonds RJ, Steketee R, Nesheim S, et al. Impact of zidovudine use on risk and risk factors for perinatal transmission of HIV. Perinatal AIDS Collaborative Transmission Studies. *AIDS*, 1998;12:301–308.
53. Therapeutic and other interventions to reduce the risk of mother-to-child transmission of HIV-1 in Europe. The European Collaborative Study. *Br J Obstet Gynaecol*, 1998;105:704–709.
54. Fowler MG, Mofenson L. Progress in prevention of perinatal HIV-1. *Acta Paediatr Suppl*, 1997;421: 97–103.
55. Mofenson LM. Reducing the risk of perinatal HIV-1 transmission with zidovudine: results and implications of AIDS Clinical Trials Group Protocol 076. *Acta Paediatr Suppl*, 1997;421:89–96.
56. Sperling RS, Shapiro DE, McSherry GD, et al. Safety of the maternal-infant zidovudine regimen utilized in the Pediatric AIDS Clinical Trial Group 076 Study. *AIDS*, 1998;12:1805–1813.
57. Connor EM, Mofenson LM. Zidovudine for the reduction of perinatal human immunodeficiency virus transmission: Pediatric AIDS Clinical Trials Group Protocol 076—results and treatment recommendations. *Pediatr Infect Dis J*, 1995;14:536–541.
58. Centers for Disease Control and Prevention. Recommendations of the U.S. Public Health Service Task Force on the use of zidovudine to reduce perinatal transmission of human immunodeficiency virus. *MMWR*, 1994;43:431–520.
59. Lindegren ML, Byers RH, Thomas P, et al. The perinatal HIV/AIDS epidemic in the United States: success in reducing perinatal transmission. *JAMA*, 1999;282:531–538.
60. Kuhn L, Stein ZA. Mother to infant HIV transmission: timing, risk factors and prevention. *Pediatr Perinatal Epidemiol*, 1995;9:1–29.
61. Rouzioux C, Costagliola D, Burgard M, et al. Estimated timing of mother-to-child human immunodeficiency virus type 1 (HIV-1) transmission by use of a Markov model. The HIV Infection in Newborns French Collaborative Study Group. *Am J Epidemiol*, 1995;142:1330–1337.
62. Shaffer N, Chuachoowong R, Mock PA, et al. Short-course zidovudine for perinatal HIV-1 transmission in Bangkok, Thailand: a randomised controlled trial. Bangkok Collaborative Perinatal HIV Transmission Study Group. *Lancet*, 1999;353:773–780.
63. Wiktor SZ, Ekpini E, Karon JM, et al. Short-course oral zidovudine for prevention of mother-to-child transmission of HIV-1 in Abidjan, Côte d'Ivoire: a randomised trial. *Lancet*, 1999;353:781–785.
64. Diaby L, Sibailly TS, Ekpini ER, et al. Effectiveness of a short-course oral zidovudine regimen in preventing mother-to-child transmission of HIV-1 in Abidjan, Côte d'Ivoire: long term follow-up in breast-feeding population. In: Program and Abstracts of the XI International Conference on AIDS and STDs in Africa; September 12–16, 1999; Lusaka, Zambia. Abstract 15PT38–15PT90.
65. Dabis F, Msellati P, Meda N, et al. 6-month efficacy, tolerance, and acceptability of a short regimen of oral zidovudine to reduce vertical transmission of HIV in breastfed children in Côte d'Ivoire and Burkina Faso: a double-blind placebo-controlled multicentre trial. DITRAME Study Group. Diminution de la Transmission Mere-Enfant. *Lancet*, 1999;353:786–792.
66. DITRAME ANRS 049 Study Group. 15-month efficacy of maternal oral zidovudine to decrease vertical transmission of HIV-1 in breastfed African children. *Lancet*, 1999;354:2050–2051.
67. Lallemant M, Jourdain G, Kim S, et al. and the Perinatal HIV Prevention Trial Group, Thailand. Perinatal HIV Prevention trial (PHPT), Thailand: DSMB recommends termination of short-short arm after first interim analysis. In: Program and Abstracts of the Second Conference on Global Strategies for the Prevention of HIV Transmission from Mothers to Infants; September 1–6, 1999; Montréal, Canada. Abstract 016.
68. Lallemant M, Jourdain G, Le Cœur S, et al. for the Perinatal HIV Prevention Trial (Thailand) Investigators. A trial of shortened zidovudine regimens to prevent mother-to-child transmission of Human Immunodeficiency Virus 1. *N Engl J Med*, 2000;343:982–991.
69. Wade NA, Birkhead GS, Warren BL, et al. Abbreviated regimens of zidovudine prophylaxis

and perinatal transmission of the human immunodeficiency virus. *N Engl J Med*, 1998;339:1409–1414.

70. Bulterys M, Orloff S, Abrams E, et al. Impact of zidovudine post-perinatal exposure prophylaxis on vertical HIV-1 transmission: a prospective cohort study in 4 US cities. In: Program and Abstracts of the 2nd Conference on Global strategies for the Prevention of HIV Transmission from Mothers to Infants; September 1–6, 1999; Montréal, Canada. Abstract 015.
71. Saba J for the PETRA Trial Study Team. Interim analysis of early efficacy of three short ZDV/3TC combination regimens to prevent mother to child transmission of HIV-1. In: Program and Asbtracts of the 6th Conference on Retroviruses and Opportunistic Infections; January 31–February 4, 1999. Chicago, Illinois, USA. Abstract S7.
72. Musoke P, Guay LA, Bagenda D, et al. A phase I/II study of the safety and pharmacokinetics of nevirapine in HIV-1–infected pregnant Ugandan women and their neonates (HIVNET 006). *AIDS*, 1999;13:479–486.
73. Guay LA, Musoke P, Fleming T, et al. Intrapartum and neonatal single-dose nevirapine compared with zidovudine for prevention of mother-to-child transmission of HIV-1 in Kampala, Uganda: HIVNET 012 randomised trial. *Lancet*, 1999;354:795–802.
74. Moodley D. The Saint Trial: Nevirapine (NVP) versus zidovudine (ZDV) + lamivudine (3TC) in prevention of peripartum HIV transmission. In: Program and Abstracts of the XIII International AIDS Conference; Durban, South Africa; July 9–14, 2000. Abstract LbOr2.
75. Stiehm ER, Lambert JS, Mofenson LM, et al. Efficacy of zidovudine and human immunodeficiency virus (HIV) hyperimmune immunoglobulin for reducing perinatal HIV transmission from HIV-infected women with advanced disease: results of Pediatric AIDS Clinical Trials Group Protocol 185. *J Infect Dis*, 1999;179:567–575.
76. Mofenson LM, Lambert JS, Stiehm ER, et al. Risk factors for perinatal transmission of human immunodeficiency virus type 1 in women treated with zidovudine. Pediatric AIDS Clinical Trials Group Study 185 Team. *N Engl J Med*, 1999;341:385–393.
77. The European Mode of Delivery Collaboration. Elective caesarean-section versus vaginal delivery in prevention of vertical HIV-1 transmission: a randomised clinical trial. *Lancet*, 1999;353: 1035–1039.
78. Chen KT, Sell RL, Tuomala RE. Cost-effectiveness of elective caesarean delivery in human immunodeficiency virus-infected women (1). *Obstet Gynecol*, 2001;97:161–168.
79. Read JS, Tuomala R, Kpamegan E, et al. Mode of delivery and postpartum morbidity among HIV-infected women: The Women and Infants Transmission Study. *J Acquir Immune Defic Syndr*, 2001;26:236–245.
80. Scott GB, Tuomola R. Combination antiretroviral therapy during pregnancy. *AIDS*, 1998;12:2495–497.
81. Mandelbrot L, Landreau-Mascaro A, Rekacewicz C, et al. Lamivudine-zidovudine combination for the prevention of maternal-infant transmission of HIV-1. *JAMA*, 2001;285:2129–2131.
82. Blanche S, Tardieu M, Rustin P, et al. Persistent mitochondrial dysfunction and perinatal exposure to antiretroviral nucleoside analogues. *Lancet*, 1999;354:1084–1089.
83. Bulterys M, Nesheim S, Abrams EJ, et al. Lack of evidence of mitochondrial dysfunction in the offspring of HIV-infected women. Retrospective review of perinatal exposure to antiretroviral drugs in the Perinatal AIDS Collaborative Transmission Study. *Ann N Y Acad Sci*, 2000;918:212–221.
84. Smith ME. US Nucleoside Safety Review Working Group. Ongoing nucleoside safety review of HIV-exposed children in US studies. In: Program and Abstracts of the 2nd Conference on Global Strategies for Prevention of HIV Transmission from Mothers to Infants; September 1–6, 1999; Montreal, Canada. Abstract 096.
85. Dorenbaum A, for the PACTG 316 Study Team. Report of results of PACTG 316: an international phase III trial of standard antiretroviral (ARV) prophylaxis plus nevirapine (NVP) for prevention of perinatal HIV transmission. In: Program and Abstracts of the 8th Conference on Retroviruses and Opportunistic Infections; Chicago, Illinois, USA; February 4–8, 2001. Abstract LB7.
86. Mmiro F, Fleming T, Desyve M, et al. Association of maternal HIV viral load and perinatal transmission in the HIVNET 012 trial. In: Program and Abstracts of the XIII International AIDS Conference; July 9–14, 2000; Durban, South Africa. Abstract TuPpB1231.
87. Kourtis AP, Bulterys M, Nesheim SR, et al. Understanding the timing of HIV transmission from mother to infant. *JAMA*, 2001,283:709–712.
88. Mofenson LM. Interaction between timing of perinatal human immunodeficiency virus infection and the design of preventive and therapeutic interventions. *Acta Paediatr Suppl*, 1997;421:1–9.
89. Aleixo LF, Goodenow MM, Sleasman JW. Zidovudine administered to women infected with human immunodeficiency virus type 1 and to their neonates reduces pediatric infection independent of an effect on levels of maternal virus. *J Pediatr*, 1997;130:906–914.
90. Culnane M, Fowler M, Lee SS, et al. Lack of long-term effects of in utero exposure to zidovudine among uninfected children born to HIV-infected women. Pediatric AIDS Clinical Trials Group Protocol 219/076 Teams. *JAMA*, 1999;281:151–157.

91. Hanson IC, Antonelli TA, Sperling RS, et al. Lack of tumors in infants with perinatal HIV-1 exposure and fetal/neonatal exposure to zidovudine. *J Acquir Immune Defic Syndr Hum Retrovirol*, 1999;20:463–467.
92. Lorenzi P, Spicher VM, Laubereau B, et al. Antiretroviral therapies in pregnancy: maternal, fetal and neonatal effects. *AIDS*, 1998;12: F241–F247.
93. Shapiro D, Tuomola R, Samelson R, et al. Antepartum antiretroviral therapy and pregnancy outcomes in 462 HIV-infected women in 1998–1999 (PACTG 367). In: Program and Abstracts of the 7th Conference on Retroviruses and Opportunistic Infections; January 31–February 2, 2000; San Francisco, California, USA. Abstract 664.
94. Bulterys M, Nesheim S, Abrams EJ, et al. Lack of evidence of mitochondrial dysfunction in the offspring of HIV-infected women. Retrospective review of perinatal exposure to antiretroviral drugs in the Perinatal AIDS Collaborative Transmission Study. *Ann N Y Acad Sci*, 2000;918:212–221.
95. Oleske J, Czarniecki L. Why and how children die of HIV infection: five-year mortality review from Newark, New Jersey. In: Program and Abstracts of the XIII International AIDS Conference; July 9–14, 2000; Durban, South Africa. Abstract MoPeC2488.
96. Chotpitayasunondh T, Chearskul S, Vanprapa N, et al. Safety of short-course antenatal zidovudine for children born to HIV-infected women, Bangkok, Thailand. In: Program and Abstracts of the XIII International AIDS Conference; July 9–14, 2000; Durban, South Africa. Abstract ThPeC5306.
97. Bardsley-Elliot A, Perry CM. Nevirapine: a review of its use in the prevention and treatment of paediatric HIV infection. *Paediatr Drugs*, 2000;2: 373–407.
98. Moodley D. Evaluation of safety and efficacy of two simple regimens for the prevention of mother to child transmission (MTCT) of HIV infection: nevirapine vs lamivudine and zidovudine used in a randomized clinical trial (the SAINT study). In: Program and Abstracts of the XIII International AIDS Conference; July 9–14, 2000; Durban, South Africa. Abstract TuOrB356.
99. Sha BE, Proid LA, Kessler HA, et al. Adverse effects associated with use of nevirapine in HIV postexposure prophylaxis for 2 health care workers. *JAMA*, 2000;284:2723.
100. Johnson S, Baraboutis JG. Adverse effects associated with use of nevirapine in HIV postexposure prophylaxis for 2 health care workers. *JAMA*, 2000;284:2722–2723.
101. Martinez E, Blanco JL, Arnaiz JA, et al. Hepatotoxicity in HIV-1 infected patients receiving nevirapine-containing antiretroviral therapy. *AIDS*, 2001;15:1261–1268.
102. Burman IG, Christensen P, Christensen K, et al. Prevention of excess neonatal morbidity associated with group B streptococci by vaginal chlorhexidine disinfection during labor. The Swedish Chlorhexidine Study Group. *Lancet*, 1992;340:65–69.
103. Biggar RJ, Miotti PG, Taha TE, et al. Perinatal intervention trial in Africa: effect of a birth canal cleansing intervention to prevent HIV transmission. *Lancet*, 1996;347:1647–1650.
104. Gaillard P, Mwanyumba F, Verhofstede C, et al. Vaginal lavage with chlorhexidine during labor to reduce mother-to-child HIV transmission: clinical trial in Mombasa, Kenya. *AIDS*, 2001;15:389–396.
105. Msellati P, Meda N, Leroy V, et al. Safety and acceptability of vaginal disinfection with benzalkonium chloride in HIV infected pregnant women in west Africa: ANRS 049b phase II randomized, double blinded placebo controlled trial. DITRAME Study Group. *Sex Transm Infect*, 1999;75:420–425.
106. Sommer A, West Jr KP. *Vitamin A deficiency: Health, Survival and Vision*. New York: Oxford University Press, 1996.
107. Semba R. Nutritional Interventions: Vitamin A and breast-feeding. In: Program of the 3rd International Symposium: Global Strategies to Prevent Perinatal HIV-1 Transmission; November 8–11, 1998; Valencia, Spain. ABSTRACT.
108. Coutsoudis A, Pillay K, Spooner E, et al. for the South African Vitamin A Study Group. Randomized trial testing the effect of vitamin A supplementation on pregnancy outcomes and early mother-to-child HIV-1 transmission in Durban, South Africa. *AIDS*, 1999;13:1517–1524.
109. Fawzi WW, Msamanga GI, Spiegelman D, et al. Randomised trial of effects of vitamin supplements on pregnancy outcomes and T cell counts in HIV-1–infected women in Tanzania. *Lancet*, 1998;351: 1477–1482.
110. WHO. Use of Nevirapine to Reduce Mother-to-Child Transmission of HIV (MTCT). WHO Review of Reported Resistance. Geneva: WHO, 24 March 2000.
111. Fawzi WW, Msamanga G, Hunter D, et al. Randomized trial of vitamin supplements in relation to vertical transmission of HIV-1 in Tanzania. *J Acquir Immune Defic Syndr*, 2000;23:246–254.
112. Marseille E, Kahn JG, Guay L, et al. Cost effectiveness of single-dose nevirapine regimen for mothers and babies to decrease vertical HIV-1 transmission in sub-Saharan Africa. *Lancet*, 1999;354:803–809.
113. Becker-Pergola G, Guay L, Mmiro P, et al. Selection of the K 103N nevirapine resistance mutation in Ugandan women receiving NVP prophylaxis to prevent HIV-1 vertical transmission

(HIVNET 006). In: Program and Abstracts of the 7th Conference on Retroviruses and Opportunistic Infections; San Francisco, California, USA; January 31–February 2, 2000. Abstract 658.

114. Chaix ML, Rekacewicz C, Bazin B, et al, and ANRS 083 Study Group French Perinatal Cohort. Genotypic resistance analysis in French women participating in PACTG316/ANRS 083. In: Program and Abstracts of the 8th Conference on Retroviruses and Opportunistic Infections; February 4–8, 2001; Chicago, Illinois, USA. Abstract 470.
115. Cunningham K, Britto P, Gelber R, et al. and the PACTG 316 Team. Genotypic resistance analysis in women participating in PACTG 316 with HIV-1 RNA >400 copies/ml. In: Program and Abstracts of the 8th Conference on Retroviruses and Opportunistic Infections; February 4–8, 2001; Chicago, Illinois, USA. Abstract 712.
116. Eshleman SH, Mracna M, Guay L, et al. Selection of nevirapine resistance (NVPR) mutations in ugandan women and infants receiving NVP prophylaxis to prevent HIV-1 vertical transmission (HIVNET-012). In: Program and Abstracts of the 8th Conference on Retroviruses and Opportunistic Infections; February 4–8, 2001; Chicago, Illinois, USA. Abstract 516.
117. Santos VV, Bastos FI, Nielsen K, et al. A prospective study of the feasibility of rapid HIV testing in pregnant women during the peripartum period in Rio de Janeiro, Brazil. In: Program and Abstracts of the 8th Conference on Retroviruses and Opportunistic Infections; February 4–8, 2001; Chicago, Illinois, USA. Abstract 695.
118. Smith L, Wade N, Warren B, et al. Expedited HIV testing of pregnant women at delivery in New York State (NYS). In: Program and Abstracts of the 8th Conference on Retroviruses and Opportunistic Infections; February 4–8, 2001; Chicago, Illinois, USA. Abstract 694.
119. Briend A, Lacsala R, Prudhon C, et al. Ready-to-use therapeutic food for treatment of marasmus. *Lancet*, 1999;353:1767–1768.

36

Prevention of Breast Milk Transmission of HIV

Balancing the Benefits and the Risks

Ruth Nduati and Dorothy Mbori-Ngacha

Department of Pediatrics, University of Nairobi, Nairobi, Kenya.

BREASTFEEDING

Benefits of Breastfeeding

The benefits of breastfeeding are well documented, particularly with regard to infectious disease prevention, nutritional gains, maternal–infant bonding, and contraception. Breast milk is the optimal source of nourishment for infants, meeting their nutritional requirements for the first 6 months of life, and continuing to be a major source of quality proteins for children well into the second year of life. Breast milk contains immunologic factors that provide vital protection against deadly childhood infections, particularly against diarrheal and respiratory infections. The complex mechanisms through which breast milk provides protection are not completely understood. However, it is clear that breastfeeding minimizes infection in infants by decreasing exposure to the enteropathogens that may contaminate food. In addition, breast milk contains immunoglobulins, cytokines, and immune active cells, such as macrophages, polymorphonuclear leukocytes, and lymphocytes, all of which act to provide both passive and active immunity against the pathogens that are a major cause of infant morbidity (1).

Breastfeeding and Infant Morbidity

Studies of morbidity associated with absence of breastfeeding, although observational in nature and sometimes limited by methodologic problems (2), have highlighted the benefits of breastfeeding. In a meta-analysis of results from 35 studies in 14 countries, breastfeeding was found to protect against diarrhea morbidity, especially during the first 6 months of life (3). Breastfeeding has also been found to be protective against pneumonia (4–6).

The role of breastfeeding in contraception results in additional benefits such as desirable birth intervals and improved child health. Breastfeeding also provides psychologic benefit by enhancing the maternal–infant bond.

Breastfeeding and Infant Mortality

Many studies have demonstrated that breastfeeding plays a major role in child survival. In a community-based study in Chile, the death rate of infants who were exclusively formula-fed during their first year of life was found to be three times higher than that of breastfed infants in the same age group (7). Subsequent studies conducted in Egypt and Rwanda documented similar results (5,8). A significant risk of death among infants who were not breastfed during infancy was also reported in a pooled analysis of breastfeeding and child mortality in resource-scarce countries (9). Infants less than 2 months old who were not breastfeeding faced the highest risk of death (OR, 5.8; 95% CI, 3.4 to 9.8) and infants in the next age group (2 to 3 months old) were still at a three-fold higher risk of death than their breastfeeding counterparts. Nicoll et al. (10) reported similar findings in their analysis of demographic health surveys (DHS) recently conducted in several African countries.

Risks Associated with Breastfeeding

Despite its benefits, breastfeeding is undoubtedly a route of HIV transmission. Therefore, the benefits of breastfeeding must be weighed against the risk of breast milk transmission of HIV and the consequential medical costs and emotional stress associated with caring for an HIV-infected child. The effects of breastfeeding on the health of HIV-infected mothers must also be considered.

Breastfeeding increases a woman's nutritional requirements. During a period of exclusive breastfeeding, the average woman produces 600 ml to 700 ml of milk per day, a process that requires a daily energy expenditure of approximately 630 kcal (11). Well-nourished women deposit adequate energy reserves during pregnancy to sustain lactation. Under-nourished pregnant women attain the energy required for lactation through breakdown of body fat and muscle, and further compromise their nutritional status if they continue to lactate without adequate nutritional intake (12). In sub–Saharan Africa many women do not gain adequate weight during pregnancy and are therefore nutritionally vulnerable during lactation (13).

Malnutrition is prevalent among women living with HIV. Researchers have documented vitamin A deficiency in approximately 50%, and anemia in 30% of pregnant HIV-infected women (14,15). Like other infections, HIV-1 infection increases basal metabolic rate, raising an infected individual's resting energy expenditure by about 150 kcal per day, a level approximately 10% above that of an uninfected individual. This expenditure is brought even higher when the individual is fighting opportunistic infections or has a high viral load (16). The combined metabolic burdens of HIV-1 infection and breastfeeding on malnourished populations could result in significant nutritional impairment and deterioration of maternal health. One study (an ad-hoc analysis of a randomized clinical trial of breastfeeding and formula-feeding) reported increased mortality among HIV-infected women who breastfed compared with those who formula-fed (17). A second cohort study reported to the contrary, but it was not sufficiently powered to answer this question (18,19).

BREAST MILK TRANSMISSION OF HIV

Breast milk transmission of HIV is estimated to account for one-third to one-half of the overall HIV transmission in breastfeeding babies (20). Formula-feeding, the most effective intervention against breast milk transmission of HIV is not entirely free of risk and may not be feasible in many situations despite high HIV prevalence. The selection of an intervention to prevent breast milk transmission of HIV must be based on a clear understanding of the magnitude, timing, and correlates of transmission. In addition, public health officials must consider regional and cultural variables in order to shape the successful implementation of such interventions.

Magnitude of Transmission

Evidence of breast milk transmission of HIV comes from many cohort studies and one randomized clinical trial. The most frequently quoted estimate of the risk of breast milk transmission of HIV, 14% (95% CI, 7% to 22%), is based on a meta-analysis of five studies carried out in populations that breastfed for only a short time and one in which babies were breastfed well into the second year of life (21). This estimate applies to the risk of transmission attributed to breast milk exposure, over and above that attributed to *in utero* or delivery-related exposure among women who acquire HIV infection prenatally. A subsequent meta-analysis included studies that had been part of the original meta-analysis along with recently published studies. Forty-seven percent of the infections in this analysis were attributable to breastfeeding (22). The risk of breast milk transmission of HIV was estimated to be 21% (95% CI, 10% to 33%) in cohorts breastfeeding for 3 months or longer, and 13% (95% CI 4% to 21%) in cohorts breastfeeding for less than 2 months. These results are comparable to rounded consensus estimates of the timing of mother-to-child transmission of HIV (20).

Similar estimates of breast milk transmission of HIV were documented in a randomized clinical trial of breastfeeding and formula-feeding among infants of HIV-infected women (23). Median duration of breastfeeding was 17 months in this study. At two years of age, 36.7% (95% CI, 29.4% to 44%) of the breastfed and 20.5% (95% CI, 14% to 27%) of the formula-fed infants were infected with HIV-1. Forty-four percent of the HIV-1 infections in the breastfeeding arm were attributable to breastfeeding. The estimated rate of breast milk transmission was 16.2% (95% CI, 6.5% to 25.9%). The findings of this study probably underestimate the true magnitude of breast milk transmission of HIV because 30% of those in the formula arm were not compliant compared to 4% in the breastfeeding arm (23).

The risk of breast milk transmission of HIV to the infants of antiretroviral-naïve African and Australian women who acquired HIV-1 postnatally was estimated to be 29% (95% CI, 16% to 42%) (21). In high HIV prevalence populations, up to 5% of women seroconvert in the year following a delivery and expose a significant number of babies to this high risk of HIV transmission (24). Outside of a study population, it is difficult to identify this group in time to prevent breast milk transmission of HIV. Antenatal voluntary counseling and testing (VCT) offers an opportunity to counsel women on ways to reduce their own risk of infection and protect their babies.

Breast Milk Transmission in Babies Exposed to Short-Course Antiretroviral Chemoprophylaxis

The additional risk of vertical HIV transmission posed by breastfeeding reduces the efficacy of antiretroviral drugs used to prevent mother-to-child transmission during late pregnancy and labor. Mother-to-child transmission of HIV was reduced by 50% in a study in which zidovudine was administered from 36 weeks of gestation through the intrapartum period in a nonbreastfeeding population in Thailand (25). Using a similar protocol in a breastfeeding population, the efficacy was 37% to 38% at 3 to 4 months, and declined to 28% at 24 months as babies continued to breastfeed (26–28). Figure 1 illustrates the reduced efficacy of antiretroviral drugs as babies continue to breastfeed; these data come from a combined analysis of two short-course zidovudine studies in Cote d'Ivoire (28).

In the PETRA study, babies breastfed for a median of 17 months (29). The benefits seen at 6 weeks of life following a short course of antenatal antiretroviral drugs were completely lost by 24 months of life (29, 30). A Ugandan study using single-dose nevirapine documented an efficacy of 47% at 14 to 16 weeks. Although this efficacy was maintained beyond this period, the absolute HIV infection rate in the intervention arm of this study was very high—approximately 20%. In this study babies were breastfed for an average of 6 months (31).

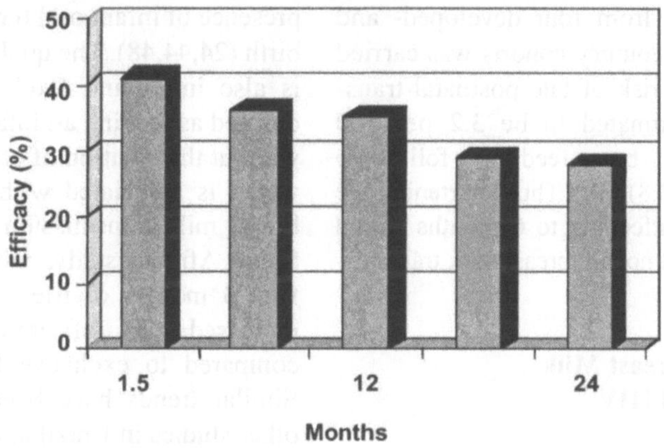

FIGURE 1. Efficacy over time of short-course zidovudine in a breastfeeding population. Data from (28).

Timing of Transmission

Breast milk transmission of HIV takes place during the time that babies are exposed to breast milk. Current HIV diagnostic tests are not able to distinguish the timing of infections that occur as a result of closely occurring points of mother–infant exposure: late pregnancy, delivery, or early breastfeeding. An infant diagnosed with HIV during the first 6 weeks of life could have acquired infection at any of these exposure points. Therefore, the easiest method of quantifying the risk of early postnatal transmission of HIV is by comparing the HIV-1 infection rates of exposed (breastfed) infants with those of unexposed (formula-fed) infants. Late postnatal transmission occurs in infants who are not infected at birth (determined by a reliable testing method such as DNA PCR) but subsequently become infected; this occurs predominantly through breastfeeding.

Early Postnatal Transmission

Most breast milk transmission takes place in the first few weeks of life. Evidence of early postnatal transmission comes from two clinical studies and mathematical modeling. In a randomized clinical trial comparing breastfeeding to formula-feeding in Nairobi, 63% of the risk difference had taken place by 6 weeks, 75% by 6 months, and 87% by 1 year (23). The findings of this study suggest that most transmission took place early during breastfeeding. In Malawi, 672 breastfed infants who were not infected at birth (confirmed by DNA PCR) were followed for up to 24.5 months. HIV incidence per month was 0.7% between months 1 and 5, 0.6% between months 6 and 11, 0.3% between months 12 and 17, and 0.2% between months 18 and 23. The decline in transmission was statistically significant (32). These findings are supported by two other studies, based on mathematical modeling, which found that breast milk transmission is nonlinear with transmission rates the highest during the first few weeks of life (33,34).

Late Postnatal Transmission

Reported risks of late postnatal transmission range from 4% to 12%, about one-third of the overall risk of breast milk transmission (35–39). Rates of late postnatal transmission vary according to the duration of breastfeeding and the point at which observations are made. For example, some studies of late postnatal transmission have observed babies from 6 months of age while others have begun at 2 to 3 months. In order to get a reliable estimate of the rate and timing of late postnatal transmission, a pooled analysis of data from four developed- and four developing-country cohorts was carried out. The overall risk of late postnatal transmission was estimated to be 3.2 per 100 child-years of breastfeeding follow-up (95% CI, 3.1 to 3.8) (40). Thus shortening the duration of breastfeeding to 6 months would prevent some, but not all, breast milk transmission of HIV.

Correlates of Breast Milk Transmission of HIV

Maternal Factors

The correlates of breast milk transmission can be categorized as maternal factors or infant factors. Maternal factors include maternal disease status and presence of breast disease. High maternal viral load, maternal immunosuppression, presence of HIV in breast milk and breast disease (including cracked or bleeding nipples, subclinical and clinical mastitis, and breast abscess) increase the risk of breast milk transmission of HIV (35,41–45). Subclinical mastitis, characterized by elevated levels of sodium in breast milk, is associated with breast milk stasis, systemic and local infection, as well as micronutrient deficiencies (46). Subclinical mastitis is also associated with elevated amounts of HIV in breast milk (43). Breast disease can be prevented through proper breastfeeding techniques that include appropriate latching-on of the baby to the breast and frequent emptying of the breasts. Vitamin A deficiency is also associated with elevated levels of HIV DNA in breast milk (15). However, vitamin A clinical trials have failed to demonstrate a reduced rate of mother-to-child transmission of HIV (15,43,45), and in one study, vitamin A was shown to be associated with an increased rate of breast milk transmission of HIV (RR 1.38; 95% CI, 1.09 to 1.76, $p = 0.009$) (47).

Infant Factors

Infant correlates of breast milk transmission of HIV include duration of breastfeeding, presence of infant oral thrush, and premature birth (24,44,48). The quality of breastfeeding is also important. Exclusive breastfeeding, defined as feeding an infant breast milk only without the addition of other milks, foods, or water, is associated with a reduced risk of breast milk transmission of HIV (45). In a South African study, mixed feeding in the first 3 months of life was associated with increased risk of infant HIV infection compared to exclusive breastfeeding (45). Similar trends have been observed in two other studies in Brazil and Kenya (48,49). In contrast, two earlier studies had compared mixed feeding to exclusive breastfeeding and found an insignificant reduction in breast milk transmission of HIV (50,51). Discrepancies in these findings probably result from lack of use of a uniform definition of breastfeeding across studies.

The mechanism by which exclusive breastfeeding may protect babies from HIV transmission is unknown, but there are several hypotheses:

i. The addition of foods other than breast milk to the diet of the young infant results in less frequent breastfeeding and incomplete emptying of the breast, leading to some degree of breast engorgement, a condition associated with subclinical mastitis.
ii. Antibodies and other anti-infective factors in breast milk may protect the baby from HIV infection, especially after the baby has been exposed to a large quota of virus during delivery. One observational cohort study documented a significantly lower rate of MTCT from breast milk containing HIV-specific IgM antibodies (42).
iii. The addition of other foods to the diet of the very young infant may result in gastrointestinal infection or allergic reaction causing increased vulnerability to HIV infection in the gastrointestinal tract. A recent study from the same group that reported on the increased risk of breast milk transmission of HIV for babies who are not exclusively breastfed has refuted this hypothesis. They were able to show

> that mixed feeding did not increase gut permeability or cause immune activation in young infants. In this study, increased gut permeability was demonstrated in babies who were subsequently shown to be HIV-1–infected (52).

All of the studies reporting a protective effect of exclusive breastfeeding are observational in nature, limiting researchers' abilities to determine the causal pathway. It is plausible that babies with an HIV seroconverting illness are fretful, prompting their mothers to add other foods to their diets.

PREVENTION OF BREAST MILK TRANSMISSION OF HIV

The most effective method of preventing breast milk transmission of HIV is complete avoidance of breastfeeding. Shortening the period of breastfeeding to 6 months prevents about one-third of the transmissions attributable to breastfeeding. However, as described earlier in this chapter, babies who are not breastfed are at increased risk of illness and death. Therefore, clear policy guidelines on infant feeding are essential to help health workers and mothers make informed decisions. Widespread, indiscriminate use of replacement feeding in resource-scarce settings would have a catastrophic effect on overall infant survival (53).

Policy on Infant Feeding

In 1996 the World Health Organization (WHO), the United Nations Children's Fund (UNICEF), and UNAIDS issued a joint policy statement on HIV and infant feeding (54). The statement's objective was to recommend key elements for the establishment of national policies and guidelines on HIV and infant feeding. The policy statement encourages the implementation of initiatives to prevent breast milk transmission of HIV that are accompanied by efforts to protect, promote, and support breastfeeding for HIV-uninfected women or women with unknown HIV status.

The policy statement endorses a human rights approach, affirming that men and women should have the right to determine the course of their reproductive health. The statement emphasizes the importance of counseling mothers on the benefits of breastfeeding, the risks of breast milk transmission of HIV, as well as the risks associated with replacement feeding. The statement identifies the following as key elements for establishing a policy on HIV and infant feeding: supporting breastfeeding, improving access to voluntary counseling and testing, ensuring informed choice, and preventing commercial pressure from manufacturers of infant foods.

The policy statement specifically states:

> "…it is mothers who are in the best position to decide whether to breast-feed particularly when they alone may know their HIV status and wish to exercise their right to keep that information confidential. It is therefore important that women be empowered to make fully informed decisions about infant feeding, and that they be suitably supported in carrying them out. This should include efforts to promote a hygienic environment, essentially clean water and sanitation, that will minimize health risks when a breast-milk substitute is used.
>
> When children born to women living with HIV can be assured uninterrupted access to nutritionally adequate breast-milk substitutes that are safely prepared and fed to them, they are at less risk of illness and death if they are not breast-fed. However, when these conditions are not fulfilled, in particular in an environment where infectious diseases and malnutrition are the primary causes of death during infancy, artificial feeding substantially increases children's risk of illness and death" (54).

A further technical consultation was convened by the WHO in October 2000 to review the policy statement because there were serious concerns about inappropriate use or spill-over of formula-feeding into the general population (19). The clarification states: (*i*) when replacement feeding is acceptable, feasible, affordable, sustainable and safe, avoidance of all breastfeeding by HIV-infected mothers is recommended; otherwise, exclusive breastfeeding is recommended during the first months of life; (*ii*) to minimize HIV transmission risk, breastfeeding should be discontinued as soon as feasible, taking into account local circumstances, the individual woman's situation and the risks of replacement feeding (including infections other than HIV and malnutrition); (*iii*) HIV-infected women should have access to information, follow-up clinical care and support, including family planning services and nutritional support (19).

Infant Feeding Options for HIV-Infected Women

Replacement feeding options include commercial formula, home-prepared formula, or modified full-cream powdered milk with the addition of nutritious, locally available, complementary or weaning foods after 6 months of age. Breastfeeding options include early cessation of exclusive breastfeeding, heat treatment of expressed breast milk, or wet nursing.

Breastfeeding Choices

The experience gained in initiating programs to prevent breast milk transmission of HIV has led to some modification of the guidelines recommended by UNAIDS. These refined interventions are "safer breastfeeding" and "modified breastfeeding" (55).

Safer Breastfeeding.

The majority of HIV-infected women in Africa breastfeed their infants well into the second year of life. Because voluntary counseling and testing is not readily available, many women are unaware of their HIV status. Safer breastfeeding is an optimal choice for uninfected women and should, to a certain extent, minimize breast milk transmission of HIV. Safer breastfeeding includes immediate exclusive breastfeeding; using good latch-on technique to avoid cracked nipples and engorgement; expressing and discarding breast milk from breasts with sores, abscesses, inflammation, or cracked nipples; seeking immediate medical attention for the latter conditions; and practicing safer sex (55). Mixed feeding is the norm in much of sub–Saharan Africa and it should not be assumed that women and health workers are familiar with safer breastfeeding. Therefore, counseling on safer breastfeeding should be one of the components of antenatal care provided to all women, regardless of their HIV status.

Modifications of Breastfeeding.

HIV-infected women may opt to breastfeed to maintain the confidentiality of their HIV status, to meet familial expectations, or to avoid the cost of replacement feeding. HIV-infected women who opt to breastfeed should be encouraged to practice safer breastfeeding and to shorten the duration of breastfeeding to 6 months. They should be informed of the estimated proportion of breast milk transmission that is prevented by these methods. Pasteurization of expressed breast milk or wet nursing are other possible modifications of breastfeeding. However, neither of these methods has been evaluated for feasibility at the household level.

Replacement Feeding Choices

Replacement feeding—defined as feeding an infant milk other than breast milk—can prevent breast milk transmission of HIV. Replacement feeding in combination with antiretroviral therapy is able to reduce the rate of mother-to-child transmission of HIV to less than 5% (56).

In the developed world, where formula-feeding is an established norm, it has been relatively safe and easy to implement replacement feeding. In the developing world, replacement feeding is a much more complex issue because of inadequate knowledge of the management of formula-feeding among mothers and health workers, and the stigma associated with not breastfeeding. Lack of knowledge may put babies at risk of infections and metabolic derangement because of poorly prepared formula. Stigma may translate into an unwillingness on the part of health workers to support a mother who chooses to formula-feed (57).

Health workers should assist women in carefully assessing their circumstances before recommending replacement feeding. The key requirements for successful replacement feeding are: access to clean water and adequate sanitation, access to adequate supplies of the replacement food, ability to prepare the foods properly, good personal hygiene, and ability to afford nutritious weaning foods. Women who are unable to meet these requirements are poor candidates for replacement feeding. A well-informed, counseled woman may be motivated to make the changes in her environment that will enable her to carry out replacement feeding safely. Identification of HIV-infected women early in the antenatal period offers health workers an opportunity to counsel on intervention options.

Modified Infant Formula. Infant formula that has been modified to mimic the biochemistry of breast milk is the optimal choice of replacement food. Infant formulas are made from modified cow's milk or Soya beans. In situations where there is access to clean water and adequate resources, formula-feeding is the optimal method of feeding the infant of an HIV-infected woman.

Home-modification of Animal Milk. Animal milk can be modified at home for infant feeding. This formulation requires the addition of micronutrient preparations that provide vitamin A, zinc and iron. In the first 3 months of life the milk should be diluted to reduce the protein and solute load to the infant and sugar should be added to increase the caloric content (Table 1) (58). Milk for a 3- to 6-month-old infant does not require dilution but still needs additional sugar to meet the caloric requirement.

The outcome of babies fed home-modified milk preparations has not been thoroughly evaluated. A study was carried out in Zambia to compare the cost and logistics of using formula versus home-modified animal milk (55). For the study population, which relied on purchasing both types of milk, the costs were similar. The investigators concluded that formula-feeding may be the preferred method in such populations because formula already contains the required nutrients and has a long shelf-life (55). However, if a mother is able to feed her infant with milk from her own cows, the home-modified milk preparation may be the more economic option.

TABLE 1. Home-Modification of Animal Milk

100 ml of full-cream animal milk (cow, camel, or goat)
50 ml of water
10 g of sugar
Micronutrient supplement

An infant needs 150 ml of milk per kg of body weight per day. An infant weighing 5 kg will thus require about 500 ml of cow's milk per day, plus dilution and sugar to make 750 ml of home-prepared formula.

Some mothers may find it difficult to conceptualize volume measurements. Simplified instructions are:
2 portions of milk
1 portion of water, plus sugar to taste
The milk should be boiled and then cooled before feeding the infant.

Unmodified animal milk has been proposed for women who want to carry out replacement feeding but cannot afford formula, do not have access to clean water, or are unable to learn how to carry out accurate milk dilutions.

Implementing Prevention of Breast Milk Transmission of HIV

Voluntary counseling and testing (VCT) for antenatal women is a starting point for the implementation of interventions to prevent mother-to-child transmission. Before 1998 in sub–Saharan Africa there was little incentive to provide antenatal HIV testing because there were no well-established interventions in place to provide treatment or to respond to the risks of perinatal transmission. Voluntary counseling and testing had been limited to

HIV research sites, blood donor service sites, or clinical care facilities. The discovery that short-course antiretrovirals could significantly reduce mother-to-child transmission of HIV was the first real incentive to set up VCT services in the antenatal setting. A number of African countries have initiated programs that integrate the prevention of mother-to-child transmission of HIV into existing antenatal services. Early results from evaluations of such programs indicate that there are many challenges to increasing access to services. Mothers' acceptance of VCT in these pilot programs is currently at approximately 50% with only 10% to 20% of the HIV-infected women receiving the complete package of services (59–63). Further research is necessary to provide insight into more effective ways to increase the use of VCT and other HIV prevention interventions.

CONCLUSION

Breastfeeding is responsible for one-third to one-half of the total number of cases of mother-to-child transmission of HIV in breastfeeding populations. Replacement feeding effectively prevents breast milk transmission of HIV. HIV-infected women should be informed to make choices about infant feeding based on both the efficacy of the methods and a clear understanding of the risks associated with replacement feeding. Safer breastfeeding is the optimal choice of infant feeding methods for many women in sub-Saharan Africa, but this should not rule out the option of replacement feeding for women who choose this method. Health workers must make use of the current guidelines available and stay well informed so that they can provide appropriate counseling to antenatal and lactating women.

REFERENCES

1. Lawrence R. *Breastfeeding: a guide for the medical profession*, 4th ed. St Louis: Mosby Year Book, Inc., 1994:149–180.
2. Sauls H. Potential effect of demographic and other variables in studies comparing morbidity of breast-fed and bottle-fed infants. *Pediatrics*, 1979;64: 523–527.
3. Feachem RG, Koblinsky MA. Interventions for the control of diarrheal diseases among young children: promotion of breast-feeding. *Bull WHO*, 1984;62:271–291.
4. Chandra RK: Prospective studies of the effect of breastfeeding on the incidence of infection and allergy. *Acta Paediatr Scand*, 1979;68:691–694.
5. Lepage P, Munyakazi C, Hennart P: Breastfeeding and hospital mortality in children in Rwanda. *Lancet*, 1981;2:409–411.
6. Cesar JA, Victora CG, Barros F, et al. Impact of breastfeeding on admission for pneumonia during postneonatal period in Brazil: nested case-control study. *BMJ*, 1999;318:1316–1320.
7. Plank SJ, Milanesi ML. Infant feeding and infant mortality in rural Chile. *Bull WHO*, 1973;48: 203–210
8. Janowitz B, Lewis JH, Parnell A, et al. Breast-feeding and child survival in Egypt. *J Biosoc Sci*, 1981;13:287–297.
9. WHO Collaborative Study Team on the Role of Breastfeeding on the Prevention of Infant Mortality. Effect of breastfeeding on infant and child mortality due to infectious diseases in less developed countries: a pooled analysis. *Lancet*, 2000;355:451–455.
10. Nicoll A, Newell ML, Peckham C, et al. Infant feeding and HIV-1 Infection (Review). *AIDS*, 2000;14(suppl 3):S57–S74.
11. Van Raaij JMA, Schonk CM, Vermaat-Miedema SH, et al. Energy cost of physical activity throughout pregnancy and the first year postpartum in Dutch women with sedentary lifestyles. *Am J Clin Nutr*, 1990;52:234–239.
12. Adair LS, Popkin BM. Prolonged breastfeeding contributes to depletion of maternal energy reserves in Filipino women. *J Nutr*, 1992;122:1643–1655.
13. Brewer MM, Bates MR, Vannay LP. Postpartum changes in maternal weight and body fat deposits in lactating vs. non-lactating women. *Am J Clin Nutr*, 1989;49:259–265.
14. Semba RD, Miotti PG, Chiphangwi JD, et al. Maternal vitamin A deficiency and mother-to-child transmission of HIV-1. *Lancet*, 1994;343: 1593–1597.
15. Nduati RW, John GC, Richardson BA, et al. Human immunodeficiency virus type 1-infected cells in breast milk: Association with immunosuppression and vitamin A deficiency. *J Infect Dis*, 1995;172: 1461–1468.
16. Melchior JC, Raguin G, Boulier A, et al. Resting energy expenditure in human immunodeficiency virus-infected patients: comparison between

patients with and without secondary infections. *Am J Clin Nutr*, 1993;57:614–619.

17. Nduati R, Richardson B, John G, et al. Effect of breastfeeding on mortality among HIV-1 infected women: a randomized trial. *Lancet*, 2001;357: 1651–1655.
18. Coutsoudis A, Coovadia H, Pillay K, et al. Are HIV-infected women who breastfeed at increased risk of mortality? *AIDS*, 2001;15:653–655.
19. World Health Organization. New data on the prevention of mother-to-child transmission of HIV and their policy implications: conclusions and recommendations. WHO Technical Consultation on behalf of the UNFPA/UNICEF/WHO/UNAIDS Inter-Agency Task Team on Mother-to-Child Transmission of HIV. Report WHO/RHR/01.28. Geneva: World Health Organization, 2001.
20. De Cock KM, Fowler MG, Mercier E, et al. Prevention of mother-to-child transmission in resource-poor countries. Translating research into policy and practice. *JAMA*, 2000;283:1175–1182.
21. Dunn DT, Newell ML, Ades AE, et al. Risk of human immunodeficiency type 1 transmission through breastfeeding. *Lancet*, 1992;340:585–588.
22. John CG, Richardson BA, Nduati RW, et al. Timing of breast milk HIV-1 transmission: a meta-analysis. *E Afr Med J*, 2001;78:75–79.
23. Nduati R, John G, Mbori-Ngacha DA, et al. Effect of breastfeeding and formula feeding on transmission of HIV-1: a randomized clinical trial. *JAMA*, 2000;283:1167–1174.
24. UNAIDS. HIV and infant feeding: a review of HIV transmission through breastfeeding. WHO/FRH/NUT/CHD/98.3, UNAIDS/98.5, UNICEF/PD/NUT/(J)98-3.
25. Shaffer N, Chuachoowong R, Mock PA, et al. Short-course zidovudine for perinatal HIV-1 transmission in Bangkok, Thailand: a randomised controlled trial. *Lancet* 1999;353:773–780.
26. Wiktor SZ, Ekpini E, Karon JM, et al. Short-course oral zidovudine fot prevention of mother-to-child transmission of HIV-1 in Abidjan, Cote d'Ivoire: a randomised trial. *Lancet*, 1999;353:781–785.
27. Dabis F, Msellati P, Meda N, et al. 6-month efficacy, tolerance, and acceptability of a short regimen of oral zidovudine to reduce vertical transmission of HIV in breastfed children in Côte d'Ivoire and Burkina Faso: a double-blind placebo-controlled multicentre trial. *Lancet*, 1999;353:786–792.
28. Wiktor SZ, Leroy V, Ekpini ER, et al. 24-month efficacy of short-course maternal zidovudine for the prevention of mother-to-child transmission in a breastfeeding population: a pooled analysis of two randomized clinical trials in West Africa. In: Program and abstracts of the XIII International AIDS Conference; July 9–14, 2000; Durban, South Africa. Abstract TuOrB354.
29. Gray G. The PETRA study: early and late efficacy of three short ZDV/3TC combination regimens to prevent mother-to-child transmission of HIV-1. In: Program and abstracts of the XIII International AIDS Conference; July 9–14, 2000; Durban, South Africa. Abstract LBOr5.
30. Lange JMA. PETRA trial study team. The PETRA study: early and late efficacy of three short ZDV/3TC combination regimens to prevent mother-to-child transmission of HIV-1. Paper presented at: Third Global Strategies for the Prevention of HIV Transmission from Mothers to Infants; September 9–13, 2001; Kampala, Uganda. Abstract 17.
31. Owor M, Deeyre M, Duefield C, et al. The one year safety and efficacy data of the HIVNET 012 randomized trial. In: Program and abstracts of the XIII International AIDS Conference; July 9–14, 2000; Durban, South Africa. Abstract LBOr1.
32. Miotti PG, Taha TET, Kumwenda MI, et al. HIV transmission through breastfeeding: a study in Malawi. *JAMA*, 1999;282:744–749.
33. Dunn DT, Tes BH, Rodrigues LC, et al. Mother-to-child transmission of HIV: implications of variation in maternal infectivity. *AIDS*, 1998;12: 2211–2216.
34. Richardson B, John G, Nduati R, et al. Breast milk infectivity of HIV-1 infected mothers. In: Program and abstracts of the XIII International AIDS Conference; July 9–14, 2000; Durban, South Africa. Abstract WeOrC492.
35. Ekpini ER, Wiktor SZ, Satten GA, et al. Late postnatal mother-to-child transmission in Abidjan, Cote d'Ivoire. *Lancet*, 1997;349:1054–1059.
36. Karlsson K, Massawe A, Urassa E, et al. Late postnatal transmission of human immunodeficiency virus type 1 infection from mother-to-infant in Dar-es-salaam, Tanzania. *Pediatr Infect Dis J*, 1997;16: 963–967.
37. Simonon A, Lepage P, Karita E, et al. An assessment of the timing of mother-to-child transmission of human immunodeficiency virus type 1 by means of polymerase chain reaction. *J Acquire Immune Defic Syndr*, 1994;7:952–957.
38. Bertolli J, St Louis ME, Simonds RJ, et al. Estimating the timing of mother-to-child transmission of human immunodeficiency virus in a breast-feeding population in Kinshasa, Zaire. *J Infect Dis*, 1996;174:722–726.
39. Datta P, Embree JE, Kreis JK, et al. Mother-to-child transmission of human immunodeficiency virus type 1: Report from the Nairobi study. *J of Infect Dis*, 1994;170:1134–1140.
40. Leroy V, Newell ML, Dabis F, et al. International multicentre pooled analysis of late postnatal mother-to-child transmission of HIV-1 infection. *Lancet*, 1998;352:597–600.

41. Wiktor S, Ekpini E, Nduati R. Prevention of mother-to-child transmission of HIV-1 in Africa. *AIDS*, 1997;11(suppl B):579–587.
42. Van de Perre P, Simonon A, Hitimana DG, et al. Infective and anti-infective factors of breast milk of HIV infected women. *Lancet*, 1993;341:914–918.
43. Semba RD, Kumwenda N, Hoover DR, et al. Human immunodeficiency virus load in breast milk, mastitis and mother-to-child transmission of human immunodeficiency virus type 1. *J Infect Dis*, 1999:180:93–98.
44. John G, Nduati RW, Mbori-Ngacha DA, et al. Correlates of mother-to-child human immunodeficiency virus type 1 (HIV-1) transmission; association with maternal plasma HIV-1 viral load, genital HIV-1 DNA shedding, and breast infections. *J Infect Dis*, 2001;183:206–212.
45. Coutsoudis A, Pillay K, Spooner E, et al. Influence of infant-feeding patterns on early mother-to-child transmission of HIV-1 in Durban, South Africa: a prospective cohort study. *Lancet*, 1999;354: 471–476.
46. Filteau SM, Lietz G, Mulokozi G, et al. Milk cytokines and subclinical breast inflammation in Tanzanian women: effects of dietary red palm oil or sunflower oil supplementation. *Immunology*, 1999; 97:595–600.
47. Fawzi WW, Masamanga G, Hunter D, et al. Randomized trial of vitamin supplements in relation to transmission of HIV-1 through breastfeeding and mortality in the first two years of life. Paper presented at: The Third Global Strategies for the Prevention of HIV Transmission from Mothers to Infants. September 9–13, 2001. Kampala, Uganda. Abstract 06.
48. Tess BH, Rodrigues LC, Newell ML, et al. Sao Paulo Collaborative Study for Vertical Transmission of HIV-1. Infant feeding and risk of mother-to-child transmission of HIV-1 in Sao Paulo State, Brazil. *J Acquire Immune Defic Syndr*, 1998; 19:189–194.
49. Taren D, Nahlen B, van Eijk A, et al. Early introduction of mixed feeding and postnatal HIV transmission. In: Program and abstracts of the XIII International AIDS Conference; July 9–14, 2000; Durban, South Africa. Abstract MoPeB2200.
50. Bobat R, Moodley D, Coutsoudis A, et al. Breastfeeding by HIV-1-infected women and outcome in their infants: a cohort study from Durban, South Africa. *AIDS*, 1997;11:1627–1633.
51. Ryder RW, Manzila T, Baende E, et al. Evidence from Zaire that breast-feeding by HIV-1-seropositive mothers is not a major route for perinatal HIV-1 transmission but does decrease morbidity. *AIDS*, 1991;5:709–714.
52. Rollins NC, Filteau SM, Coutsoudis A, et al. Feeding mode, intestinal permeability, and neopterin excretion: a longitudinal study in infants of HIV-1 infected South African women. *J Acquir Immune Defic Syndr*, 2001;28:132–139.
53. Kuhn L, Stein Z. Infant survival, HIV infection and feeding alternatives in less-developed countries. *Am J Public Health*, 1997;87:926–931.
54. UNAIDS. HIV and infant feeding: an interim statement. *Wkly Epidemiol Rec*, 1996;71:289–291.
55. Piwoz EG. HIV and infant feeding: Risks and realities in Africa. In: *Breastfeeding: Issues and Challenges in the New Millennium*. Washington DC: Academy for Educational Development, 2001.
56. Fowler MG, Simonds RJ, Roongpisuthipong A. Update on Perinatal HIV Transmission. *Pediatr Clin North Am*, 2000;47:21–38.
57. Seidel G, Sewpaul V, Dano B. Experiences of breastfeeding and vulnerability of HIV-positive women in Durban, South Africa. *Health Policy and Planning*, 2000;15:24–33.
58. UNAIDS. HIV and infant feeding: a guide for health-care managers and supervisors. WHO/FRH/NUT/CHD/98.2, UNAIDS/98.4. 1998. Available at: http://www.unaids.org/publications/ documents/mtct/infantguide.html. Accessed February 3, 2002.
59. Veloso V, Sudo EC, Vasconselos A, et al. Implementation of interventions to reduce HIV vertical transmission in Brazil. In: Program and abstracts of the XIII International AIDS Conference; July 9–14, 2000; Durban, South Africa. Abstract WeOrC548.
60. Sibailly TS, Ekpini ER, Kamelan-Tonoh A, et al. Impact of on-site rapid testing with same day post-test counseling on acceptance of short course zidovudine for prevention of mother-to-child transmission of HIV in Abidjan, Côte d'Ivoire. In: Program and abstracts of the XIII International AIDS Conference; July 9–14, 2000; Durban, South Africa. Abstract WeOrC549.
61. Mazhani L, Phiri L, Keapoletswe K, et al. Implementation of a population based pilot program to reduce mother-to-child HIV transmission, Botswana. In: Program and abstracts of the XIII International AIDS Conference; July 9–14, 2000; Durban, South Africa. Abstract WeOrC550.
62. Karita E, Uwamaliya H, Carmelinda S, et al. Acceptability and feasibility of the introduction of a short regimen of oral zidovudine (ZDV) to reduce mother-to-child transmission (MTCT) of HIV in Rwanda. In: Program and abstracts of the XIII International AIDS Conference; July 9–14, 2000; Durban, South Africa. Abstract WeOr551.
63. Mbori-Ngacha D, Nduati R, Kalibala S, et al. Utilization of services for the prevention of mother-to-child transmission (MTCT) of HIV-1 in 2 sites in Kenya. In: The Third Global Strategies for the Prevention of HIV Transmission from Mothers to Infants; September 9–13, 2001; Kampala, Uganda. Poster Abstract 330.

Postexposure Prophylaxis for Occupational Exposure and Sexual Assault

*Elisabeth Bouvet, †Anne Laporte, and ‡Arnaud Tarantola

*Hôpital Bichat-Claude Bernard, Paris, France.
†Institut de Veille Sanitaire, Saint-Maurice, France.
‡World Health Organization, Genera, Switzerland.

Antiretrovirals are increasingly used for prophylaxis of HIV infection following occupational exposure to HIV or sexual assault. This chapter will discuss the risks related to HIV infection following occupational exposure or sexual assault; the scientific rationale for the use of postexposure prophylaxis (PEP); the implementation of PEP systems, including exposure prevention methods; and the management of PEP in health personnel and victims of sexual assault.

RISK OF HIV TRANSMISSION FOLLOWING OCCUPATIONAL BLOOD EXPOSURE

Heath care workers (HCWs) throughout history have been faced with the risk of occupational infections following percutaneous, nonintact skin, or mucosal contact with blood that may be contaminated with viruses, bacteria, or parasites. The HIV epidemic has renewed awareness of this risk and has increased interest in the use of antiviral drugs for PEP. Although the risk associated with a single accidental blood exposure (ABE) to HIV-infected blood may be low, the overall risk associated with repeated exposures to HIV-infected blood throughout the professional career of a HCW may be significantly higher (1–3). Existing data from various countries around the world, including African countries (4,5), have not shown a higher HIV prevalence among HCWs than that found in the general population. The data from Africa, however, are from the mid- to late 1980s, and little is known about the cumulative occupational risk or specific HIV prevalence in African HCWs in the current context of a much more severe epidemic. Few data are available regarding the occupational risks and HIV prevalence among other exposed health workers of particular importance in African countries, such as birth attendants (6,7), traditional healers, or forensic personnel (8).

The average risk of HIV-1 transmission following a single percutaneous exposure to HIV-infected blood is estimated to be 0.29% (95% CI, 0.13%–0.70%) (9), while the risk associated with a single nonintact skin or mucosal exposure to infected blood has been estimated to be approximately 0.03% (10). The HIV-1 strains that are prevalent in southern Africa may be more easily transmitted than others, but this has not been formally documented. There are no data on the probability of HIV-2 transmission following ABE. The factors that determine the risk of HIV-1 transmission following a single parenteral exposure in industrialized countries have been more accurately ascertained in a case-control study, conducted by the U.S. Centers for Disease Control and Prevention (CDC), which will be discussed later in this chapter (11).

The overall risk of infection by ABE is determined not only by the characteristics of a single exposure, but also by the frequency of such exposures. Accidental blood exposure incidence rates are significantly higher in African countries than in Western countries, such as France, for example (14,15) (Table 1). The overall risk of occupational HIV infection varies according to the incidence and severity of ABEs, patients' HIV seroprevalence and viral load, the transmissibility of HIV, as well as post–ABE management (Table 2). The incidence of ABE is higher in understaffed and insufficiently equipped facilities, and among overworked and/or insufficiently informed or trained HCWs (16). These facility and staffing issues are of particular relevance in resource-poor countries. A study carried out by Gumudoka et al. (12), for instance, provided valuable insight into the challenges faced by HCWs in Tanzania.

Available data show that the overall risk of occupational HIV infection is much higher in African countries than in the West (1,3, 29). Lack of access to safety devices and protective wear in African health care settings contributes to a high overall risk of occupational exposure (12). Most HCWs in African facilities do not have access to blood-drawing safety devices or adequate sharps containers (12,30). The risk of exposure is higher for surgical personnel if they do not use blunt suture needles (31), or if they do not wear two pairs of gloves (32–34). These high-risk circumstances are created by lack of information, willingness, or in most cases, lack of a regular supply of appropriate equipment (1,2,35). While no specific study on double-glove wearing has been conducted in Africa, this prevention method has been shown elsewhere to reduce the risk of perioperative

TABLE 1. Incidence of Accidental Blood Exposure in Some African Countries and in France

Country	Reference	Incidence[a]
Tanzania	(12)	5.0 NSI/HCW/year 9.0 MCC/HCW/year
Zambia	(3)	3.0 NSI/surgeon/year
Nigeria	(13)	2.3 NSI/dentist/year 2.3 NSI/surgeon/year 0.6 NSI/nurse/year 0.4 NSI/physician/year
Several African countries	(1)	15.0 NSI/physician/year 12.0 NSI/midwife/year 3.4 NSI/nurse/year
Several African countries	(2)	2.0 NSI/physician/year 1.9 NSI/nurse/year
France	(14) (15)	0.3 NSI/nurse/year 0.1 MCC/nurse/year 9.5 NSI/surgeon/year 28.0 MCC/surgeon/year

[a]NSI indicates needlestick injury; HCW, health care worker; MCC, mucocutaneous contact.

TABLE 2. Factors Determining the Overall Risk of Occupational HIV Infection in African Countries[a]

Factor	Frequency in Africa	Conditions contributing to the frequency
Incidence of ABE	High	Excessive workload, more frequent use of injections (12,17–22), lack of protective and safety devices or sharps containers
Severity of ABE	Variable	Lack of gloves (gloves reduce transferred blood volume [23,24])
Prevalence of bloodborne pathogens in patients	Very high	Very high in the general population; patients who visit care centers tend to be very ill
Pathogen transmission	Variable	HIV-1: 0.3% (9,10), HCV: 3% (25), HBV: 30% (26–28), HIV-2: unknown[b]
Viral load in source patient	High	High prevalence of advanced disease, lack of antiretroviral therapy
Post–ABE management • Prompt response, antisepsis • PEP	Poor	Lack of information, lack of access to free-of-cost PEP

[a]ABE indicates accidental blood exposure; PEP, postexposure prophylaxis.
[b]These data were collected in the United States, Europe, and Japan. Data from Africa are not available.

skin contact with blood (32–34), as well as the blood inoculum present on the surface of a solid-bore suture needle by the time it reaches the skin, should a needlestick occur (23,24).

The likelihood of any given ABE occurring with an HIV-infected source patient is higher in African countries than in many other countries because of the high HIV prevalence in many African populations. This risk is increased further due to the even higher HIV prevalence specifically among patients in African hospitals. Patients with limited resources tend to resort to in-hospital care only when faced with severe medical complications; such complications are frequently the result of HIV or AIDS-related disease, and often in advanced stages. Limited data from Africa show that HIV-1 seroprevalence among patients in some wards has risen dramatically in recent years. For example, in Dakar, Senegal, in 1994, approximately 30% of all inpatients in the infectious disease ward at Fann University Hospital were HIV-infected; by the year 2000, this percentage was higher than 80% (Salif Sow, personal communication, December 15, 2000). Similarly, although HIV seroprevalence in the general population is approximately 32% in KwaZulu Natal, South Africa, the proportion of HIV-positive patients presenting for care at King Edward Hospital in Durban is significantly higher—40% to 50% (Sawera Singh, personal communication, December 16, 2000). Patients at this hospital whose rapid test results are initially HIV-1–negative are then screened using p24 antigen tests and are often found to be undergoing seroconversion for HIV, a process that is associated with a high viremia, and a yet higher risk of transmission.

The vast majority of patients in Africa do not have access to antiretroviral therapy. Without treatment, HIV viral load in African patients at a given stage of disease may be higher than that in patients receiving antiretroviral therapy. Higher viral load further increases viral inoculum and thus the risk of transmission in cases of occupational exposure.

Finally, the overall risk of occupational infection with HIV-1 can be reduced with timely access to PEP. Most HCWs in Africa lack access to PEP (36–38). This is yet another factor that significantly increases the overall risk of occupational infection by HIV-1 in HCWs in Africa.

RISK OF HIV TRANSMISSION FOLLOWING SEXUAL EXPOSURE

Rates of Transmission Per Sexual Act

Estimates of the probability of HIV transmission per sexual act have been generated from studies of HIV-1–discordant couples. These estimates are averages, and the actual probability of transmission may vary widely depending on the presence of risk factors. Table 3 shows published estimates of the probability of HIV transmission per unprotected sexual act from different regions of the world. In the United States and Europe the estimated probability of transmission, regardless of the sex of the infected partner, is 0.1% (39,40). The specific probability of male-to-female transmission is 0.15% and 0.09% for female-to-male transmission (40). A study carried out in Thailand among newly married couples produced an estimate, regardless of sex, of 0.2% (41).

Risk Factors for Sexual Transmission

The probability of HIV infection through sexual contact varies greatly depending on several factors (see Chapters 13 and 14, *this volume*). Factors that increase the probability of HIV transmission include the stage of infection of the host (39,40,43)—infectiousness is increased both during acute primary infection (46,47) and advanced disease in the absence of potent antiretroviral treatment (48–50); the presence of reproductive tract infections in the HIV-infected host and/or the susceptible partner, especially ulcerative infections such as chancroid, syphilis, or herpes (51); cervical ectopy (51); lack of male circumcision (51–54); menstruation (51); and pregnancy (51).

TABLE 3. Published Estimates of the Probability of HIV Transmission Per Unprotected Sexual Act

COHORT			
Type of risk	Study site(s)	Probability of transmission	Reference
Heterosexual couples			
Overall	USA, Europe	0.1%	(39,40)
	Thailand	0.2%	(41)
Receptive vaginal intercourse	Europe	0.05%–0.15%	(40)
Insertive vaginal intercourse	Europe	0.03%–0.09%	(40)
Sex workers' clients			
Intercourse with a female sex worker	Kenya	13%[a]	(42)
	Thailand	3.1%–5.6%	(43)
Men who have sex with men			
Receptive anal intercourse	USA	0.5%–3%	(44)
		0.3%–2.8%	(45)
Insertive anal intercourse	USA	0.03%–0.12%	(45)
Receptive oral sex	USA	0.01%–0.18%	(45)

[a] In men who had contracted an STD from a sex worker.

Of 415 HIV-1–discordant couples followed for 30 months in a recent study conducted in rural Uganda, 90 individuals seroconverted (55). Factors associated with seroconversion were: young age (the highest incidence of HIV infection was measured in 15- to 19-year-olds); lack of circumcision (no seroconversion occurred among 50 circumcised men, while incidence was 16.7 per 100 person-years among 137 uncircumcised men); level of serum HIV-1 RNA (no seroconversions occurred among those whose viral loads were less than 1,500 copies per ml). The rate of male-to-female transmission did not differ from that of female-to-male. History of genital discharge or dysuria in an HIV-1–positive partner increased the rate of transmission, as did the presence of AIDS-defining symptoms or signs in the unadjusted analysis.

The continued rapid expansion of the heterosexual epidemic in sub–Saharan Africa most likely reflects the interaction of several behavioral and biologic factors. Biologic factors that could play a major role in transmission include the higher level of blood and semen HIV-1 RNA in seropositive men in sub–Saharan Africa (56), the fact that most men are uncircumcised (52), and the high prevalence of classic inflammatory or ulcerative STDs in areas where HIV-1 prevalence is high (57).

Specific Factors in Cases of Sexual Assault

The probability of HIV transmission following sexual assault depends on the likelihood that the assailant is infected with HIV, the clinical status of the assailant if HIV-infected, the body fluids and routes of exposure involved in the assault, the number of discrete contacts, the type and severity of physical trauma caused by the assault, and the presence of other STDs in the assailant and/or the victim (58). Moreover, sexual violence is a factor per se which increases the risk of HIV transmission due to resulting mucous membrane lesions.

POSTEXPOSURE PROPHYLAXIS: THE SCIENTIFIC RATIONALE

Animal Models

A large number of animal studies have investigated the preventive effect of antiviral agents following inoculation with a lentivirus. The SIV/primate model most closely resembles HIV-1 in humans in terms of pathophysiologic mechanism, viral and immunologic marker dynamics, and the development of an immunodeficiency syndrome. However, researchers must exercise caution in applying the findings of animal models to humans. The studies that have been conducted are representative only of the specific methodologies and parameters used.

Initial PEP trials were conducted in the late 1980s and yielded encouraging results using a combination of ZDV and interferon-alpha (IFN-α) in a murine viral leukemia model (59). However, a trial with SIV showed no evidence of prevention of infection in rhesus monkeys that were inoculated parenterally with a very high dose of SIV and then treated 3 hours later with ZDV or IFN-α plus ZDV over a 3-week period (60). More encouraging indications of a prophylactic effect of ZDV in primates were obtained in later studies by Van Rompay and others (61,62).

More recent trials were conducted with new nucleoside analogs: (R)-9-(2-phosphonylmethoxypropyl)adenine (PMPA) and 2′,3′-dideoxy-3′-hydroxymethylcitidine (BEA 005). These drugs prevented infection in animals when administered at different times after inoculation. In the first trial using PMPA, conducted by Tsai (63), the 10 cynomolgus monkeys that had been treated at either 4 or 24 hours after inoculation for a total duration of 4 weeks remained uninfected. An equivalent study in macaques yielded similar results and showed that animals receiving PMPA 24 hours after inoculation were not infected, whereas those treated 48 hours after inoculation became infected (64). A shorter, three-day course of treatment initiated 24 hours after inoculation remained ineffective. Tsai et al. conducted another study using PMPA following intravenous inoculation with SIV in macaques, testing regimens that involved different intervals between inoculation and the initiation of PMPA treatment, as well as various durations of treatment (65). None of the macaques that were treated for 28 days beginning 24 hours postinoculation showed evidence of infection at 46 weeks follow-up. Extending the time of treatment initiation from 24 hours to 48 or 72 hours, however, or decreasing the duration of treatment to 10 days, reduced effectiveness in preventing infection. A trial with BEA 005 was instructive, showing that monkeys treated with this drug very early (at 1, 3, or 8 hours) following intravenous and rectal inoculation were not infected. Later initiation of this treatment (24 hours) reduced its preventive effect (66). Although the results of these studies are not conclusive, they do suggest that PEP using nucleoside reverse transcriptase inhibitors (NRTIs) must be administered as early as possible and for a duration of more than 10 days. There is a need for studies in new animal models that more closely resemble HIV infection in humans.

Human Studies

Zidovudine treatment after occupational exposure to HIV has been recommended by national health authorities in many industrialized countries since 1990, despite the lack of data available at the time on the safety and efficacy of ZDV in human victims of such exposures. The risk of seroconversion following a single needlestick exposure is so low (approximately 0.3%) that a randomized trial of PEP efficacy cannot be conducted. In 1994, the CDC undertook an investigation of the risk factors for infection among exposed HCWs, based on a retrospective case-control study carried out in collaboration with researchers from the United Kingdom, France, and Italy (11). This study included 33 cases of occupational infection following percutaneous exposure to HIV-infected blood and 679 controls (cases in which exposure had occurred but had not resulted in seroconversion). Exposures in cases and controls had been documented between 1988 and 1994. Analysis using a logistical regression model identified the following factors associated with the risk of transmission: exposure via a deep injury, visible blood on the device causing injury, injury with a device that had been previously placed in a source patient's vein or artery, and exposure to a source patient in a terminal stage of disease. Having received ZDV was significantly linked to a reduction in the risk of infection (adjusted odds ratio 0.2; 95% CI, 0.1–0.6). The model used in this study indicated that the risk of transmission was reduced by 81% (95% CI, 48%–94%) in HCWs who received ZDV, after the other factors had been taken into account. Despite methodologic biases, the results of this study provide statistical evidence of ZDV's prophylactic efficacy following percutaneous exposures to blood.

Antiretroviral drug use has also been shown to be effective in the prevention of perinatal HIV transmission, and the mother-to-child model is useful in the design of new PEP regimens. A randomized, placebo-controlled trial carried out in 1994 among pregnant women showed that ZDV reduced the risk of transmission by 67% (67). The contributory effect of ZDV on viral load reduction in treated mothers was estimated to be only 16.6%, suggesting that the preventive mechanism of this treatment likely includes a direct prophylactic effect on the infant while he or she is exposed to the mother's virus (68).

More recently, a very short course of nevirapine, a nonnucleoside reverse transciptase inhibitor (NNRTI), during delivery has been shown to be more effective in reducing the rate of mother-to-child HIV transmission than a 10-week regimen of ZDV (69). The long half-life of NNRTIs and the fact that they do not need to be metabolized to become active are two major reasons for considering them for PEP. However, to date they are not used as frequently as NRTIs for PEP.

More efficient PEP regimens are needed. Since 1990, PEP efforts have been observed and studied in industrialized countries, and failures have been documented. For example, in 1997 a case of HIV infection following needlestick injury was documented in the United States, and another in France. Each of these exposures involved a hollow-bore needle containing blood. HIV transmission occurred, despite the use of highly active antiretroviral therapy with three drugs. In the U.S. case, the infecting virus was resistant to lamivudine, which had been used in the therapeutic drug combination (70). In the French case, the virus was wholly sensitive to all three antiviral drugs used. The first dose had been administered within 2 hours of exposure, compliance was good, and the duration of treatment was 28 days without any side effects (71). The fact that transmission occurred in this case shows that although PEP has a prophylactic effect, its efficacy remains incomplete. Prevention of blood exposure remains the safest way to avoid occupational HIV infection. In France, surveillance data of occupational infections show a marked downward trend since 1995 (71), and no occupational HIV infection was identified by active surveillance between 1997 and 2001. This decline in occupational HIV infections among HCWs may be a result of various factors, including the reduction of ABE due to prevention programs, the reduction of viral load in patients with HIV due to effective treatments, and the efficacy of PEP.

PREVENTION OF OCCUPATIONAL HIV INFECTION: COMPREHENSIVE APPROACHES AND POSTEXPOSURE PROPHYLAXIS

Prevention of ABE in all health care settings must remain a priority, regardless of the availability of PEP. Chemoprophylaxis is not 100% effective, and it is expensive, difficult to manage, and does not prevent infection with other bloodborne pathogens such as hepatitis C.

Universal precautions (72) constitute a statutory minimum for all health care institutions: gloves should be worn during any contact with blood or body fluid; hands should be washed immediately after contact with potentially infected fluids; care should be taken in handling sharps; needles and other sharps should be disposed of immediately in a special sealed container and should never be bent or put back in their original holders; needles should never be removed from syringes by hand; used instruments and surfaces soiled by blood should be disinfected immediately with a 1/10 bleach solution or equivalent disinfecting agent.

To reduce occupational HIV infections, health care institutions must put in place numerous protective measures and procedures, including PEP. All health care institutions must incorporate HCW safety into their health care plans. Specific safety measures must be adopted based on analysis of the causes of accidents observed locally and the type of activity at the facility, financial constraints, and the availability of suitable safety equipment. Gloves and safety containers must be constantly supplied in adequate quantities. The use of safety devices should be progressively introduced. Protective measures must be adapted to the local conditions under which each procedure takes place in order to limit the risk of contact with blood and to ensure that universal precautions are observed. A staff member in each facility should be specifically designated to oversee the identification and institution of such measures. Surveillance of ABE must be implemented to support and guide safety policies. All HCWs should be trained in ABE prevention methods. All active HCWs and health professionals in training (medical and nursing students) must be immunized against hepatitis B virus.

Health care worker information, training, and access to gloves, blood-drawing safety devices (73), and blunt suture needles

(31), are safety measures that have been shown to be effective in preventing occupational exposure to HIV. However, should an incident of exposure occur, PEP offers a second line of defense that effectively reduces the risk of occupational HIV infection (74). The following are requirements for health care facilities implementing PEP systems:

- the ability of persons at risk to identify relevant accidents. All HCWs should be trained to recognize incidents of ABE. Students should receive practical training prior to hands-on training with actual patients;
- a well-defined policy of ABE notification;
- a functioning system known to all and accessible at all times for any exposed HCW;
- designated staff members who assist exposed personnel in following the necessary steps;
- the designation of one or more trained physicians to assess the risk of infection, prescribe, and monitor PEP if indicated; or the designation of other centers where PEP will be available for the facility's HCWs and those from surrounding sites;
- PEP drugs that are chosen based on an understanding of the local circulating viruses (for example, nevirapine should not be used in cases of possible HIV-2 infection). Drugs must be available at all times, adequately stocked, and dispensed free of charge by a qualified professional for the full duration of the PEP regimen (three days for nevirapine only, 28 days if other antiretrovirals are used). Drugs in stock must not have expired;
- baseline HIV testing for the exposed HCW within 1 week of an accident, the result of which must remain confidential; pregnancy tests for HCWs in situations where antiretrovirals that are contraindicated in pregnant women may be used;
- serologic monitoring at least at 3 and 6 months after an accident, the results of which must remain confidential;
- HIV testing for the source patient. This should be conducted with his or her informed consent and test results must remain confidential. Should HIV testing of the source patient not be possible, PEP should be discussed on the basis of the severity of exposure and other clinical and epidemiologic considerations;
- the absence of discrimination of HIV-infected HCWs in the workplace;
- antiretroviral treatment free of charge for HCWs who become HIV-infected as a result of documented occupational exposure.

MANAGEMENT OF SEXUAL ASSAULT CASES

Postexposure prophylaxis for HIV after sexual assault should be part of a comprehensive rape treatment program (75,76). Information about clinics where victims of sexual assault may seek care from experienced physicians, or be referred by the police, must be available in the community. Patients presenting at these clinics must be allowed to choose whether to file a report with the police; if they choose not to do so, confidentiality of the data recorded should be maintained.

Patient History and Examination

Patient history and examination should be conducted in a calm and sensitive manner. Injuries requiring immediate attention will take precedence over any other examination. The orifices involved in the assault, the timing of the assault, prior and/or subsequent consenting sexual intercourse, use of condoms by the assailant, and whether ejaculation occurred should be documented. Physical inspection should accurately note any genital or other injuries; the throat should be inspected if there is history of forced oral penetration; anal examination, including proctoscopy, should be conducted if there is history of forced anal penetration, noting any trauma.

Various studies have demonstrated high prevalence of STDs among rape victims (up to 20% of all penetrative rapes of women—mostly trichomoniasis, bacterial vaginosis, chlamydia, or gonorrhea (76,77). A full STD screen at presentation is recommended, including: culture for *Neisseria gonorrhoeae* and tests for *Chlamydia trachomatis* from any sites of penetration; gram stained slides of urethral, cervical, and rectal specimens for microscopy for gonococci; vaginal slides for microscopy for yeasts, bacterial vaginosis, and *Trichomonas vaginalis* (ideally culture should also be performed); and blood for syphilis serology. HIV and hepatitis B testing should be offered as patient may have pre-existing risks of infection.

Treatment, PEP, and Counseling

Antibiotic prophylaxis covering both chlamydia and gonorrhea may be offered in situations where the patient may default a repeat examination. Hepatitis B vaccination should be offered to all victims of sexual assault (up to 3 weeks after the event). If there is a risk of pregnancy, postcoital oral contraception can be issued within 72 hours of the assault.

HIV prophylaxis should be considered if there are risk factors for HIV and if the patient is referred early enough (within 72 hours after assault). There is often a delay in reporting rape, which may limit the effectiveness of prophylactic treatment. Information about perpetrators' HIV status is unavailable in most cases of sexual assault.

The patient must be aware of the limited data on PEP efficacy and the potential toxicity of the treatment. Treatment regimen, duration, and follow up are the same as for health care workers. HIV prophylaxis entails a two- to three-fold increase in the cost of rape treatment and should be offered free of cost to the victim.

Postexposure prophylaxis for HIV following sexual assault must be considered in the overall context of the physical and emotional health of the victim. Sexual assault results in a high incidence of psychologic trauma (78), making it difficult for victims to make informed decisions about whether to initiate PEP. Specific education and support is needed, given the complexity of the treatment and follow-up. Contact with a local victim organization and HIV/AIDS advocacy group should facilitate this. The patient's need for immediate and ongoing counseling should be assessed.

Legal Considerations

Some assault victims claim the right to know their assailants' HIV status and may want to pursue having them tested (78). In some countries, law authorizes compulsory testing of offenders. However, only a small proportion of offenders are actually arrested (18% in the United States in 1990). Furthermore, the average time between arrest and conviction (254 days) necessitates making a decision about victim testing and prophylaxis without knowing the assailant's HIV serostatus (78).

EXPERIENCE WITH THE USE OF POSTEXPOSURE PROPHYLAXIS IN AFRICA

With the notable exception of South Africa, there has been limited experience with postexposure prophylaxis in African countries. Between March 1997 and June 30, 1998, 236 occupational injuries were documented by Dr. Sawera Singh and colleagues in collaboration between the departments of virology and medicine at King Edward Hospital in Durban, South Africa. Overall, 50% of these injuries involved an HIV-positive source. Twenty-three percent of the 236 injuries were sustained by interns, 54% of whom were exposed to HIV-positive source patients and thus took a 30-day course of prophylactic antiretrovirals (AZT and 3TC). Thirty-six (15%) of the total injuries were sustained by registrars, 58% of whom were treated with AZT and 3TC. Fifty percent of 22 sixth-year students were exposed to HIV, as were 4 of 6 exchange students (Sawera Singh, personal communication, December 16, 2000).

Health care teams in Senegal, Mali, and Côte d'Ivoire are leading a joint, collaborative effort with the Groupe d'Etude sur le Risque d'Exposition des Soignants (GERES) to investigate the frequency and conditions of ABE occurrence in West African hospitals (79). The teams of Professor Salif Sow in Senegal, Dr. Aliou Sylla in Mali, and Professor Bissagnene in Côte d'Ivoire have begun gathering experience in initiating PEP. To date, Professor Salif Sow has treated three surgeons and four nurses or nursing students at Fann University Hospital in Dakar. Six ABEs occurred with known HIV-1–infected source patients, while the seventh occurred with a patient carrying HIV-2. All exposed HCWs received AZT, 3TC, and indinavir and completed the four-week regimen. Only one surgeon experienced unwanted side effects.

Other infectious disease and occupational health specialists throughout Africa have undoubtedly accumulated valuable experience in PEP prescription, although an African registry of PEP prescriptions following well-documented ABEs remains to be created. The principal challenge in implementing PEP in resource-poor countries is securing access to free-of-charge and timely PEP and follow-up that is prescribed by physicians who are experienced in the evaluation of risks of infection, and the prescription and monitoring of antiretroviral drugs. In South Africa, PEP for occupational exposure is financed by health workers' health plans and is readily available at most reference centers. In Senegal, the program for increased access to antiretroviral therapy has made provisions for chemoprophylaxis kits containing ZDV, lamivudine, and indinavir to be soon accessible at no cost in health care centers throughout the country.

CONCLUSION

Randomized studies of PEP cannot be carried out for ethical and practical reasons. There are, however, many arguments supporting the use of anti–HIV PEP following ABE or sexual assault. States and health systems in resource-poor countries face the challenge of guaranteeing exposed HCWs and rape victims full-time and free-of-charge access to a physician capable of conducting a risk assessment, PEP drugs, and technical facilities for biologic assessment and serologic monitoring. Nonetheless, the use of HIV PEP in African countries must be supported and increased. Such efforts however, must also include the support and assurance of exposure prevention practices and a reduction in ABE incidence in health care settings. Likewise, efforts to reduce sexual violence worldwide must be stepped up.

While the number of occupationally infected HCWs is not in itself a public health crisis in comparison with the growing number of infections in the general population in Africa, ABE is a public health issue, as is the fear of occupational infection faced by ill-paid, ill-protected, and overworked HCWs in resource-poor countries. Providing prevention training, support, and free access to PEP is an ethical and fair measure that will help support HCWs in Africa in their continuing effort to provide quality care to an increasing number of HIV-infected patients.

REFERENCES

1. Veeken H, Verbeek J, Houweling H, et al. Occupational HIV infection and health care workers in the tropics. *Trop Doct*, 1991;21:28–31.
2. de Graaf R, Houweling H, van Zessen G. Occupational risk of HIV among western health care professionals posted in AIDS endemic areas. *AIDS Care*, 1998;10:441–452.
3. Consten EC, van Lanschot JJ, Henny PC, et al. A prospective study on the risk of exposure to HIV during surgery in Zambia. *AIDS*, 1995;9:585–588.
4. Mann JM, Francis H, Quinn TC, et al. HIV seroprevalence among hospital workers in Kinshasa, Zaire: lack of association with occupational exposure. *JAMA*, 1986;256:3099–3102.
5. N'Galy B, Ryder RW, Bila K, et al. Human immunodeficiency virus infection among employees in an

African hospital. *N Engl J Med*, 1988;319: 1123–1127.
6. Habimana P, Bullterys M, Usabuwera P, et al. A survey of occupational blood contacts and HIV infection among traditional birth attendants in Rwanda. *AIDS*, 1994;8:701–704.
7. Diakhaté M, Diallo I, Sow PS, et al. Risques de transmission du VIH chez les accoucheuses traditionnelles au Sénégal. In: Abstracts of the Xth International Conference on AIDS and STDs in Africa; December 7–11, 1997; Abidjan, Côte d'Ivoire. Abstract B245.
8. Du Plessis R, Webber L, Saymaan G. Bloodborne viruses in forensic medical practice in South Africa. *Am J Forensic Med Pathol*, 1999;20:364–368.
9. Henderson DK, Fahey BJ, Willy M, et al. Risk for occupational transmission of human immunodeficiency virus type 1 (HIV-1) associated with clinical exposures: a prospective evaluation. *Ann Intern Med*, 1990;113:740–746.
10. Public Health Laboratory Service. AIDS and STD at the Communicable Disease Surveillance Centre. Occupational transmission of HIV: Summary of published reports to June 1999. Public Health Laboratory Service, 1999:9–11.
11. Cardo DM, Culver DH, Ciesielski CA, et al. A case-control study of HIV seroconversion in health care workers after percutaneous exposure. Centers for Disease Control and Prevention Needlestick Surveillance Group. *N Engl J Med*, 1997;337: 1485–1490.
12. Gumudoka B, Favot I, Berege ZA, et al. Occupational exposure to the risk of HIV infection among health care workers in Mwanza Region, United Republic of Tanzania. *Bull World Health Org*, 1997;75:133–140.
13. Adegboye AA, Moss GB, Soyinka F, et al. The epidemiology of needlestick and sharp instrument accidents in a Nigerian hospital. *Infect Control Hosp Epidemiol*, 1994;15:27–31.
14. Abiteboul D, Antona D, Fourrier A, et al. GERES. Exposition accidentelle au sang du personnel soignant. Resultats d'un an de surveillance du risque pour les infirmieres dans 17 hopitaux. *Pathol Biol* (Paris), 1992;40:983–989.
15. Johanet H, Antona D, Bouvet E, et le GERES. Risques d'exposition accidentelle au sang au bloc operatoire. Résultats d'une étude prospective multicentrique. *Ann Chir*, 1995;49:403–410.
16. Malachy O. Evaluation of a training workshop on HIV/AIDS for health care workers in Enugu and Anambra States of Nigeria. In: Abstracts of the Xth International Conference on AIDS and STDs in Africa; December 7–11, 1997; Abidjan, Côte d'Ivoire. Abstract B246.
17. Berkley S. Parenteral transmission of HIV in Africa. *AIDS*, 1991;5(Suppl 1):S87–S92.
18. Birungi H. Injections and self-help: risk and trust in Ugandan health care. *Soc Sci Med*, 1998;47: 1455–1462.
19. Sagoe-Moses C, Pearson RD. Risks to health care workers in developing countries. *N Engl J Med*, 2001;345:538–541.
20. Simonsen L, Kane A, Lloyd J, et al. Unsafe injections in the developing world and transmission of bloodborne pathogens: a review. *Bull World Health Org*, 1999;77:789–800.
21. Van de Perre P, Diakhate L, Watson-Williams J. Prevention of blood-borne transmission of HIV. *AIDS*, 1997;11(Suppl B):S89–S98.
22. Wyatt HV. The popularity of infections in the third world: origins and consequences for poliomyelitis. *Soc Sci Med*, 1984;19:911–915.
23. Mast ST, Woolwine JD, Gerberding JL. Efficacy of gloves in reducing blood volumes transferred during simulated needlestick injury. *J Infec Dis*, 1993;168:1589–1592.
24. Bennett NT, Howard RJ. Quantity of blood inoculated in a needlestick injury from suture needles. *J Am Coll Surg*, 1994;178:107–110.
25. Puro V, Petrosillo N, Ippolito G, et al. Update on occupational HCV infection incidence studies. In: Program and Abstracts of the International Colloquium on Bloodborne Infections; June 8, 1995; Paris, France. International Social Security Association Section for Health Services, 1995. Abstract PA8.
26. Alter HJ, Seeff LB, Kaplan PM, et al. Type B hepatitis: the infectivity of blood positive for e antigen and DNA polymerase after accidental needlestick exposure. *N Engl J Med*, 1976;295:909–913.
27. Grady GF, Lee VA, Prince AM, et al. Hepatitis B immune globulin for accidental exposures among medical personnel: final report of a multicenter controlled trial. *J Infect Dis*, 2002;138:625–638.
28. Seeff LB, Wright EC, Zimmerman HJ, et al. Type B hepatitis after needle-stick exposures: Prevention with hepatitis B immune globulin: Final report of the Veteran's Administration Cooperative Study. *Ann Intern Med*, 1978;88:285–293.
29. Gilks CF, Wilkinson D. Reducing the risk of nosocomial HIV infection in British health workers working overseas: role of post-exposure prophylaxis. *BMJ*, 1998;316:1158–1160.
30. Sow PS, Rachline A, Tarantola A, et al. pour les Correspondants du Réseau AES 3 Pays et le GERES. Connaissances et Practiques à Risque d'Accident Exposant au Sang (AES) chez les Soignants en Médecine dans 3 Pays d'Afrique de l'Ouest. Oral Presentation at the 12th International Conference on AIDS and STDs in Africa; December 8–13, 2001; Ouagadougou, Burkina Faso. Abstract 12BT3–4.
31. Centers for Disease Control and Prevention. Evaluation of blunt suture needles in preventing

percutaneous injuries among health care workers during gynecologic surgical procedures—New York City, March 1993–June 1994. *MMWR*, 1997; 46:25–29.

32. Gerberding JL, Littell C, Tarkington A, et al. Risk of exposure of surgical personnel to patients' blood during surgery at San Francisco General Hospital. *N Engl J Med*, 1990;322:1788–1793.
33. Wright J, McGeer AJ, Chyatte D, et al. Mechanisms of glove tears and sharp injuries among surgical personnel. *JAMA*, 1991;266:1668–1671.
34. Matta H, Thompson AM, Rainey JB. Does wearing two pairs of gloves protect operating theater staff from skin contamination? *BMJ*, 1988;297:597–598.
35. Diarra J, Msellati P, Brissac M, et al. SIDA et personnel soignant en Côte d'Ivoire. *Med Trop*, 1996;56:259–263.
36. Russi M, Hajdun M, Barry M. A program to provide antiretroviral prophylaxis to health care personnel working overseas. *JAMA*, 2000;283:1292–1293.
37. N'Dri A, Boka Yao A, Ouattara Y, et al. Les accidents exposant au sang (AES) en milieu de soins: évaluation et prise en charge. In: Abstracts of the Xth International Conference on AIDS and STDs in Africa; December 7–11, 1997; Abidjan, Côte d'Ivoire. Abstract B969.
38. Gamester CF, Tilzey AJ, Banatvala JE. Medical students' risk of infection with bloodborne viruses at home and abroad: questionnaire survey. *BMJ*, 1999;318:158–160.
39. Mastro TD, De Vincenzi I. Probabilities of sexual HIV-1 transmission. *AIDS*, 1996;10(Suppl A): S75–S82.
40. Downs A, De Vincenzi I, and the European study group in heterosexual transmission of HIV. Probability of heterosexual transmission of HIV: relationship to the number of unprotected sexual contacts. *J AIDS*, 1996;11:388–395.
41. Duerr A, Xia Z, Nagachinta T, et al. Probability of male-to-female HIV transmission among married couples in Chiang Maï, Thaïland. In: Abstracts of the Xth International Conference on AIDS; August 7–12, 1994; Yokohama, Japan. Abstract 105C.
42. Cameron DW, Simonsen JN, D'Costa LJ, et al. Female to male transmission of human immunodeficiency virus type 1: risk factors for seroconversion in men. *Lancet*, 1989;ii:403–407.
43. Mastro TD, Satten GA, Nopkesorn T, et al. Probability of female-to-male transmission of HIV-1 in Thailand. *Lancet*, 1994;343:852–853.
44. DeGruttola V, Seage GR, Mayer KH, et al. Infectiousness of HIV between male homosexual partners. *J Clin Epidemiol*, 1989;42:849–856.
45. Vittinghoff E, Buchbinder SP, Judson F, et al. Per-contact risk for transmission of HIV associated with four types of homosexual contact. In: Abstracts of the Vth Conference on Retroviruses and Opportunistic Infections; February 1–5, 1998; Chicago, IL, USA. Abstract 140.
46. Pantaleo G, Graziosi C, Fauci AS. The immunopathogenesis of human immunodeficiency virus infection. *N Engl J Med*, 1993;328:327–335.
47. Tindall B, Evan L, Cunningham P, et al. Identification of HIV-1 in semen following primary HIV-1 infection. *AIDS*, 1992;6:949–952.
48. Saag MS, Crain MJ, Decker WD, et al. High-level viremia in adults and children infected with immunodeficiency virus: relation to disease stage and CD4+ lymphocyte levels. *J Infect Dis*, 1991;164:72–80.
49. Vernazza PL, Eron JJ, Cohen MS, et al. Detection and biologic characterization of infectious HIV-1 in semen of seropositive men. *AIDS*, 1994;8: 1325–1329.
50. Vernazza PL, Gillian BL, Dyer J, et al. Quantification of HIV in semen: correlation with antiviral treatment and immune status. *AIDS*, 1997;11:987–993.
51. Royce RA, Sena A, Cates W, et al. Sexual transmission of HIV. *N Engl J Med*, 1997;15:1072–1078.
52. Halperin DT, Bailey RC. Male circumcision and HIV infection: 10 years and counting. *Lancet*, 1999;354:1813–1815.
53. Weiss H, Quigley M, Hayes R. Male circumcision and risk of infection in sub-Saharan Africa: a systematic review and meta-analysis. *AIDS*, 2000;14: 2361–2370.
54. Buve A. Male circumcision and spread of HIV in sub-Saharan Africa. In: Abstracts of the XIII International AIDS Conference; July 9–14, 2000; Durban, South Africa. Abstract MoOr192.
55. Quinn TC, Wawer MJ, Sewankambo N, et al. Viral load and sexual transmission of human immunodeficiency virus type I. *N Engl J Med*, 2000; 342: 921–929.
56. Dyer JR, Kazembe P, Vernazza PL, et al. High level of human immunodeficiency virus type 1 in blood and semen of seropositive men in sub-Saharan Africa. *J Infect Dis*, 1998;177:1742–1746.
57. Fleming DT, Wasserheit JN. From epidemiological synergy to public health policy and practice: the contribution of other sexually transmitted diseases to sexual transmission of HIV infection. *Sex Transm Infect*, 1999;75:3–17.
58. Bamberger JD, Waldo CR, Gerberding JL, et al. Postexposure prophylaxis for human immunodeficiency virus (HIV) infection following sexual assault. *Am J Med*, 1999;106:323–327.
59. Ruprecht RM, Chou TC, Chipty F, et al. Interferon alpha and 3′ azido-3′ deoxythymidine are highly synergistic in mice and prevent viremia after acute retrovirus exposure. *JAIDS*, 1990;3:591–600.
60. Fazely F, Haseltine WA, Rodger RF, et al. Postexposure chemoprophylaxis with zidovudine or

zidovudine combined with INF-α: failure after inoculating rhesus monkeys with a high dose of SIV. *J AIDS*, 1991;4:1093–1097.

61. Van Rompay KKA, Marthas ML, Ramos RA, et al. Simian immunodeficiency virus (SIV) infection of infant rhesus macaques as a model to test antiretroviral drug prophylaxis and therapy: oral 3′-azido-3′-deoxythymidine prevents SIV infection. *Antimicrob Agents Chemother*, 1992;36:2381–2386.
62. Van Rompay KKA, Otsyula MG, Marthas ML, et al. Immediate zidovudine treatment protects simian immunodeficiency virus infected newborn macaques against rapid onset of AIDS. *Antimicrob Agents Chemother*, 1995;39:125–131.
63. Tsai CC, Follis KE, Sabo A, et al. Prevention of SIV infection in macaques by (R)-9-(2-phosphonylmethoxypropyl) adenine. *Science*, 1995;270: 1197–1199.
64. Lifson JD, Lloyd A, Hirsch V, et al. Clues to primate lentiviral pathogenesis from the study of SIV viral dynamics. Paper presented at: Retroviruses of human AIDS and related animal diseases: XI Colloque des cents gardes; October 27–29, 1997; Paris, France.
65. Tsai CC, Emau P, Follis KE, et al. Effectiveness of postinoculation (R)-9-(2-phosphonylmethoxypropyl) adenine treatment for prevention of persistent simian immunodeficiency virus SIVmne infection depends critically on timing of initiation and duration of treatment. *J Virol*, 1998;72:4265–4273.
66. Bottiger D, Johansson NG, Samuelsson B, et al. Prevention of SIV, SIVsm, or HIV-2 infection in cynomolgus monkeys by pre- and postexposure administration of BEA-005. *AIDS*, 1997;11:157–162.
67. Conner EM, Sperling RS, Gelber R, et al. Reduction of maternal-infant transmission of human immunodeficiency virus type 1 with zidovudine treatment. *N Engl J Med*, 1994;331:1173–1180.
68. Sperling RS, Shapiro DE, Coombs RW, et al. Maternal viral load, zidovudine treatment, and the risk of transmission of human immunodeficiency virus type 1 from mother to infant. *N Engl J Med*, 1996;335:1621–1629.
69. Guay LA, Musoke P, Fleming T, et al. Intrapartum and neonatal single-dose nevirapine compared with zidovudine for prevention of mother-to-child transmission of HIV-1 in Kampala, Uganda: HIVNET 012 randomised trial. *Lancet*, 1999;354:795–802.
70. Perdue B, Wolderufael D, Mellors J, et al. HIV-1 transmission by a needlestick injury despite rapid initiation of four-drug postexposure prophylaxis. In: Abstracts of the 6th Conference on Retroviruses and Opportunistic Infections. January 31–February 4, 1999; Chicago, Illinois, USA. Abstract 210.
71. Lot F, de Benoist AC, Abiteboul D. Infections professionnelles par le VIH en France chez le personnel de santé—le point au 30 juin 1998. *Bull Epid Hebd*, 1999;18:69–70.
72. Centers for Disease Control and Prevention. Guidelines for the Prevention of Transmission of Human Immunodeficiency Virus and Hepatitis B Virus to Health-Care and Public Safety Workers. *MMWR*, 1989;38(Suppl 6):1–37.
73. Centers for Disease Control and Prevention. Evaluation of Safety Devices for Preventing Percutaneous Injuries Among Health Care Workers During Phlebotomy Procedures—Minneapolis-St. Paul, New York City, and San Francisco, 1993–1995. *MMWR*, 1997;46:21–25.
74. Henderson DK. Postexposure chemoprophylaxis for occupational exposures to the human immunodeficiency virus. *JAMA*, 1999;281:931–936.
75. Clinical Effectiveness Group. National guideline for the management of adult victims of sexual assault. *Sex Transm Inf*, 1999;75(Suppl 1):S82–S84.
76. Bottomley CP, Sadler T, Welch J. Integrated clinical service for sexual assault victims in a genitourinary setting. *Sex Transm Inf*, 1999;75:116–119.
77. Jenny C, Hooton TM, Bowers A, et al. STDs in victims of rape. *N Engl J Med*, 1990;322:713–716.
78. Gostin LO, Lazzarini Z, Alexander D, et al. HIV test, counseling, and prophylaxis after sexual assault. *JAMA*, 1994;271:1436–1444.
79. Doumbia S, Tarantola A, Bouvet E for the West African Accidental Blood Exposure Surveillance Network and the GERES. Implementation of prospective accidental blood exposure surveillance systems in three western African countries. In: Abstracts of the XIII International AIDS Conference; July 9–14, 2000; Durban, South Africa. Abstract TuPeD3652.

38

The Need for a Vaccine

Seth Berkley

International AIDS Vaccine Initiative, New York, New York, USA.

Although current HIV prevention efforts can reduce the spread of the virus, and treatment with highly active antiretroviral therapies can prolong the lives of those already infected, only a safe, effective, and widely available preventive vaccine holds any promise of significantly curbing the AIDS epidemic in sub–Saharan Africa. Until recently, HIV vaccines were not considered high priority on political agendas and as a result, have not received adequate funding or attention. However, in recent years, HIV vaccines have begun to receive more attention and the scientific community has made progress that has led to increased optimism. This chapter reviews some of the reasons for making an AIDS vaccine an international priority and endorses the involvement of the public sector in vaccine research since a market failure prevents industry alone from shouldering the burden of vaccine design, development, and delivery. Some of the policy approaches that may be used to accelerate the production of a vaccine are also discussed.

LIMITATIONS OF CURRENT PREVENTION AND TREATMENT METHODS

There are a number of effective strategies for preventing, treating, and mitigating the consequences of HIV infections. None have been fully implemented in any African country and therefore, the potential impact of these different interventions for preventing infections at the population level is unknown. Currently, most prevention programs are pilot projects that often cover much less than 5% of the eligible populations (1); scaling up these programs to become national interventions remains a major challenge. Still, it is clear that none of these programs, even if implemented widely, is a panacea for the extensive problems caused by the AIDS epidemic at national or local levels, and that only a vaccine offers any hope for ultimately ending the epidemic.

Current prevention methods, such as barrier methods, are generally not favored by either male or female users. Attempts to make both male and female condoms more "user friendly" should be a priority. Research toward producing better female-controlled methods should also be supported. These efforts should include creating vaginally active microbicides, with the ultimate goal of producing both spermicidal formulations and formulations that would be safe to use while trying to conceive. Microbicides that can be used rectally must also be a research priority. Finally, simpler and less expensive STD and HIV diagnostics that can provide results more quickly than the current techniques should be developed to allow broad expansion of STD screening, voluntary counseling and testing, and HIV treatment programs in resource-limited countries.

There has been a great deal of advocacy in the area of therapeutics. One outcome of the intense focus on therapy by the industrialized world has been the unprecedented success in creating novel antiretroviral drugs. There are currently 15 licensed antiretroviral drugs in the United States. However, antiretroviral treatment is expensive. Furthermore, because antiretroviral regimens are complex—requiring combinations of multiple medications, stringent dosage schedules, toxicity and resistance monitoring (2), careful prescribing to avoid cross-reactivity with other drugs, and lifetime therapy—it is not clear what role these medications will play in serving the vast numbers of people infected with HIV in the resource-poor countries of sub-Saharan Africa.

THE ROLE OF VACCINES IN CONTROLLING INFECTIOUS DISEASES

Vaccines are among the most cost-effective of all medical interventions (3). They can be implemented in campaign format and often only require a few doses for lifelong protection. Vaccines have been responsible for the eradication of smallpox, the elimination of polio in the Americas, and the control of many other infectious diseases. Although there is no question that vaccines are extremely cost-effective, the funds and commitment required to fully achieve disease control and eradication are substantial. For example, it is estimated that when polio is globally eradicated, at least USD$1.5 billion per year will be released for other purposes (4).

Currently in the Organization for Economic Cooperation and Development (OECD) countries, immunizations are common during childhood; some 11 antigens are given before entering school, amounting to more than 15 injections. There are, however, anti-vaccine movements in some countries that no longer see, and therefore no longer fear, the diseases targeted by many of these vaccines, such as pertussis, hepatitis B, and measles. Some parents, worried about potential side effects and knowing that these diseases are relatively uncommon, choose not to have their children vaccinated. This may not be problematic in the short term, but over time, such a voluntary decrease in vaccine usage will impact public health. For example, the decline in pertussis vaccination in the United Kingdom during the 1970s (from 79% to 31%) resulted in 28 child deaths and 5,000 hospital admissions (4). In countries where high vaccine coverage was maintained, pertussis incidence remained 10 to 100 times lower than in the United Kingdom (5).

The Expanded Programme of Immunization (EPI), initiated by the World Health Organization (WHO) in 1974, aims to immunize 90% of infants in developing countries with the primary immunization series (Bacille Calmette-Guérin [BCG], oral polio vaccine [OPV], diphtheria-pertussis-tetanus [DPT], and measles). As a result of an enormous global push to achieve this goal, immunization rates were increased from less than 5% in 1974 to approximately 80% in 1990, the year of Universal Childhood Immunization (6). This was a major accomplishment that required the cooperation of donors, the international community, and local health care workers. Since 1990, however, immunization rates have declined in many countries and low coverage rates still allow more than 2 million preventable deaths from these diseases in developing countries annually (7).

Public health strategies for sustaining immunization efforts must be improved and expanded. The infrastructure already in place to deliver immunization services will serve as a base for HIV vaccination. However, refinement of this infrastructure will be necessary since an HIV vaccine will not, at first, be delivered to infants and children, the targets of most current vaccination campaigns. Initial HIV immunization is likely to be targeted at high-risk groups such as commercial sex workers, truck drivers, and adolescents. Currently, there are few mechanisms for reaching these groups for vaccination, or for other health interventions. It is therefore critical that strategies to reach these groups be developed and implemented immediately.

IDEAL CHARACTERISTICS OF AN AIDS VACCINE

A preventive AIDS vaccine intended for use in Africa would ideally have all of the technical characteristics listed in Table 1. Although each of these ideals will obviously not be met initially, some of them are more critical (such as simple delivery, temperature stability, and cost) for developing country settings. In fact, an inexpensive vaccine that requires only one dose may be more useful in selected settings, even if it is of slightly lower efficacy than an expensive vaccine that requires numerous inoculations because the infrastructure required to deliver multiple doses is also quite costly.

Although complete safety is the obvious ideal, the vaccine risk-to-benefit ratio, which varies by population, should be considered. In populations at very high risk for HIV infection, particularly those without access to other preventive interventions, the use of a vaccine with a risk-to-benefit ratio that would make it less attractive in lower risk populations may be justified. One example of a vaccine with this type of changing risk-to-benefit ratio is OPV, which was the standard polio vaccine for more than 2 decades in the United States. After naturally occurring polio had been eliminated in the United States, the risk of vaccine-induced paralysis led officials to recommend administering enhanced inactivated polio vaccine for the first two doses instead of OPV. Oral polio vaccine remains, however, the standard in most other populations of the world, where the threat of contracting polio is extant and ease of vaccine administration is of utmost importance.

ECONOMICS OF VACCINES

The Vaccine Industry and Its Role in Vaccine Development and Production

Vaccine manufacture is a complicated procedure that requires elaborate and expensive

TABLE 1. Ideal Characteristics of an HIV Vaccine for Use in Africa

Protection: The vaccine should be able to stimulate the production of a durable, functional, protective immune response against most, if not all, HIV subtypes to which an individual is likely to be exposed, and from all potential routes of exposure.

Safety: The vaccine must be safe in both the short and long term. The vaccine should also be safe to deliver without prior screening for HIV infection (i.e., the vaccine should not induce any adverse reactions when given to HIV-infected individuals) and should be safe in pregnancy so that it can be given to sexually active adolescent girls without pregnancy screening.

Delivery: The vaccine should provide long-lasting protection with a minimum number of doses (preferably one), have a long shelf-life, be heat stable and not require a cold chain, and be simple to administer (preferably oral but if by injection, with an injection gun).

Unambiguous marker for seroconversion: Health care professionals should be provided with a marker that enables seroconversion due to vaccination and seroconversion due to infection to be distinguished rapidly, easily, and affordably.

Cost: The final price of the vaccine should be one that will be affordable for widescale distribution to all people at risk of infection throughout the world, but particularly those in the poorest countries.

Manufacturing: The vaccine should be able to be manufactured in large volume, packaged simply, and ideally, able to be transferred to selected developing country sites for packaging or production.

facilities. Although much of the basic science underlying vaccine development comes from the national research agencies of industrialized countries, it is commercial industry that, until recently, has conducted most of the world's new vaccine product research and development (R&D).

The world's market for preventive vaccines is rather small (approximately USD$4 billion compared with more than $300 billion for the global sales of pharmaceutical drugs). However, vaccines are considered an essential part of public health programs, and some are recommended or required by public policy in virtually all countries. There are over 170 vaccine producers, the vast majority of which are directly under the control of governments. These entities each produce one or more of the six basic EPI vaccines, which are in the public domain. More than 60% of the world's commercially produced vaccine doses are purchased in bulk and sold to multinational organizations. These sales, however, bring in a very small percentage of the industry's profit. For example, approximately 23% of the volume of globally sold vaccines is purchased by the United Nations Children's Fund (UNICEF), but because of their low price, sales to UNICEF account for only 6% of the global revenue (8).

Because vaccine manufacturing is largely a fixed-cost business (approximately 85% of the costs are fixed and only 15% variable) the cost of producing large numbers of vaccine doses is marginal (9). Furthermore, the efficiency of production is increased with large-scale production. When production costs are lower and spread over a larger number of doses, profits per dose in the most profitable market also increase. This can occur as a result of tiering, or differential pricing, a process by which products are offered at different prices in different markets. Tiering for the EPI vaccines has been quite steep; the vaccine pricing spans a very broad range with an average 70-fold price differential between the poorest and wealthiest markets (9). As an overall result, 14% of the total volume of vaccine doses sold in standard commercial markets accounts for 75% to 80% of the market value of these vaccines.

Currently the six leading vaccine-producing companies supply about 70% of the commercial market with vaccines. A few new vaccines that are priced substantially higher than their predecessors and are sold in the OECD countries almost exclusively generate most of these companies' profits. Such large multinational companies are the largest investors in vaccine research, development, and production facilities, and would logically be the organizations to invest heavily in HIV vaccine development.

There are barriers, however, to the involvement of these companies. Vaccine development is becoming increasingly expensive. On average it takes at least 10 to 12 years to develop a new product and bring it to market. Development costs are reported to be in excess of USD$250 million; this amount includes the losses of abandoned and unsuccessful products, opportunity costs, and marketing costs, but does not include tax credits (10). Furthermore, vaccine development is a risky business: only about 22% of vaccines that leave the preclinical stage end up entering the market.

Over the past few decades, the vaccine industry has consolidated and vaccine companies are now subsidiaries of the broader pharmaceutical industry. The pharmaceutical industry is highly profitable. For example, in 1996, the average profit margin of the 10 largest drug firms was 30% (11). As a result of the way these new companies are structured, the vaccine industry—a subset of the pharmaceutical industry—must compete in that marketplace. This is particularly challenging since the life of a patent is only 20 years, and experience has shown that it often takes more than a decade to recoup the R&D costs of a new vaccine.

In the 1970s and 1980s the vaccine market was not particularly attractive to investors. However, during the 1980s, changes were made to resolve the liability crisis in the United States by capping potential damages and creating a fund to provide settlement. Such changes, combined with the advances that were being made in molecular biology, have once again made vaccine development a potentially attractive field for investment.

For HIV vaccines, however, investment has been seen as particularly high risk, and investment for HIV vaccines in Africa a non-priority. There are a number of reasons for this perception. The science is difficult, and there are controversies within the research community as to what potential approaches might be successful. Some members of the HIV activist community have created discomfort for some industry leaders. Furthermore, infection with HIV is still stigmatized. The need for an HIV vaccine is largest in some of the poorest developing countries, as are the inherent opportunity costs for working in these countries. As a result, what started out as a broad-based effort by the pharmaceutical industry has since contracted considerably (although a recent reversal of this trend has occurred with a renewed effort and commitment by Merck). As a recent industry publication noted, "The pharmaceutical industry has virtually turned its back on HIV vaccine research, leaving the biotechnology industry as the gatekeepers of hope for a preventive vaccine, yet the number of biotechnology companies in the field is small and getting smaller" (12).

For industry to invest heavily in HIV vaccine development, research costs will have to be supplemented and/or the vaccine market will have to be made more attractive. If specific vaccines for developing countries are needed, the barriers to industrial investment will be even higher. If vaccines that will only serve those living in the poorest developing countries are needed, then a new mechanism will be required.

Potential Production

Without knowing exactly what technology will ultimately prove effective in an HIV vaccine, it is impossible to know the best mechanism for assuring the production of adequate quantities of the final product. Some speculation, however, is possible. Because a vaccine is a biologic and not a "pure" chemical product, the processes of manufacturing (using good manufacturing practices [GMP]) are very complicated and need to be certified by regulatory agencies, as does the manufacturing plant. The trend in industry is to construct single-use production facilities, although it takes more than 5 to 7 years to plan, build, validate, and certify a vaccine facility. These facilities are expensive to build (USD$50 to $150 million) and run under GMP conditions. Given the sensitivity of vaccine prices to production volume, it is likely that the construction of one or a few large manufacturing plants will be more cost-effective than the construction of a number of smaller plants around the world. As a result, it is likely that one of the large pharmaceutical companies will, at least initially, be the major supplier of an HIV vaccine.

South Africa is the only country in sub–Saharan Africa that has a tradition of vaccine manufacturing. Hypothetically, South Africa could thus enter the market for vaccine production. However, the vaccine production facility in South Africa is relatively antiquated and would require major improvements before it would be an acceptable place for large-scale vaccine production for Africa. Furthermore, South Africa would need to assure that its quality standards would be accepted not only for domestic use but also for export.

Distribution

Vaccines are distributed in sub–Saharan Africa primarily from stationary clinics that usually provide other health care services in addition to immunization. Vaccines are also distributed from mobile clinics designed to reach people living in remote communities. In resource-poor countries, much of this infrastructure is provided by external agencies such as UNICEF and the WHO, governmental development assistance agencies such as DFID, SIDA, CIDA, Danida, Norad, USAID and the Italian Cooperation, as well as nongovernmental agencies.[a]

Vaccination campaigns require different strategies to reach different populations. Many adolescents, for example, can probably best be reached via school-based clinics. However, this approach must be accompanied by outreach mechanisms to provide access to those not attending school, a group that in many resource-poor countries may represent more than half of the targeted population. Nonetheless, the advantages of administering an HIV vaccine through a school-based health care system could be enormous and cost-effective. A trained nurse could provide not only AIDS education and vaccination, but could also create a school-based curriculum on reproductive health, safe motherhood, nutrition, parenting, malaria prevention, and violence and injury protection.

Effective distribution of an AIDS vaccine will also require strategies for reaching soldiers, commercial sex workers, intravenous drug users, truck drivers, and others who are both at high-risk for HIV infection and often mobile. Such strategies must be developed and tested now—well before an HIV vaccine becomes available for use in the general population—so that the benefits of an eventual lifesaving vaccine will not be obstructed or delayed by logistical problems.

The Economics of Regionally Specific Vaccines

There are currently at least 10 distinct genetic subtypes of HIV-1 circulating globally. All of these are found in Africa, some uniquely so. The significance of HIV genetic subtypes for vaccine design, although hotly debated, is currently unknown. As more recombinant strains are being seen around the world, the distinctiveness of the subtypes identified to date will likely become less obvious over time. Nevertheless, antigens from vaccines that are based on cellular immunity are selectively recognized based on the genetic makeup (and major histocompatibility antigens) of a given population. Because people (and their viruses) travel, a globally applicable vaccine is clearly needed. However, it is possible that specific vaccines (made from local circulating strains or based on the genetic makeup of persons in different populations) will be required. If this situation arises, for-profit industry cannot be relied on to bear the resulting costs of research, development, manufacturing, and distribution for the lowest income countries. Alternative mechanisms might include contracting between the private sector and manufacturers for vaccine production, or creating nonprofit vaccine facilities. Such alternatives would require new management and financing procedures to assure the quality, efficiency, and cost-effectiveness of the effort.

ACCESS ISSUES

The world has never successfully deployed a vaccine in the developed and developing world simultaneously. The usual paradigm has been the development and deployment of a vaccine at high prices initially in the developed world to recoup the significant R&D costs. Over time (10 to 15 years), with competition and increases in production efficiency, prices drop and the product begins to trickle into developing countries. Traditionally, African countries have been among the last to receive and administer such vaccines. For example, vaccine coverage for hepatitis B and *Haemophilus influenzae* Type b, both of which are of great public health

[a]DFID indicates Department for International Development (United Kingdom); SIDA, Swedish International Development Corporation Agency; CIDA, Canadian International Development Agency; Danida, Danish International Development Agency; Norad, Norwegian Agency for Development Cooperation; USAID, United States Agency for International Development.

importance, is virtually nonexistent in Africa. Despite the effectiveness of hepatitis B vaccination and the enormous burden of hepatitis and resultant liver cancer in developing countries (1 million deaths annually), the vaccine is still not widely used in most of the world's immunization programs. The first hepatitis B vaccine was licensed in a developed country 17 years ago and its initial offering price has been reduced almost 40-fold to $1.50 per dose. One dollar and a half, however, is still about 1.5 times more costly than a full course of the currently used childhood immunizations (BCG, OPV, DPT, and measles) in developing countries.

Assuring the simultaneous availability of an HIV vaccine in both developed and developing countries will require a series of activities and considerations, all of which have long lead times and therefore, must be started now (13). These considerations are outlined in the following subsections.

Pricing and Global Financing Mechanisms

Differential pricing is the most effective mechanism for ensuring worldwide access to vaccines. Not only does differential pricing lead to a more appropriate use of a product, but it permits a higher level of R&D than would occur under uniform pricing (14). However, differential pricing may be controversial if full political commitment is not obtained in the wealthier countries where people will have to pay many times more than those living in resource-limited countries for the same product. Furthermore, for a differential pricing program to be effective, there can be no parallel trade (the import of the product from another country where it has been priced less). Firm political commitment across the G8 countries will be pivotal in allowing an equity-based pricing system for HIV vaccines to succeed.

Unfortunately, even with steeply differential pricing, some countries will still find the cost of a vaccine too high for local use. In this case, financing from international agencies will be required until the country is able to cover its own costs. Such resources must be in place and expeditiously available as soon as an HIV vaccine is ready for large-scale distribution. Generally, the cost of distributing a vaccine is many times higher than the cost of its manufacture and purchase. For example, the total cost per dose of all six EPI antigens is USD$1, but the delivery costs in Africa are about USD$12 (6). Thus, financing vaccine distribution may be as important as, or more important than financing vaccine purchases.

Demand Estimates and Preparedness for Production Capacity

As mentioned previously, it is expensive and time-consuming to scale up vaccine production. As a result, a potential manufacturer must be secured early-on, and estimates of the number of eventual doses required must be generated, so that an appropriate manufacturing facility can be built. For most new childhood vaccines, the number of doses that are required initially is not very different from the number of children in the birth cohorts that will require vaccination annually thereafter (perhaps 2–4 times greater). By contrast, with an HIV vaccine, there will be an initial period of mass vaccination to cover all potentially sexually active populations (groups from 13 years of age and older). This means that the manufacturer will need to produce an initially vast number of immunizations—a much higher volume than the eventual annual production size—to supply the demand. This may require extra production facilities.

Willingness-to-pay studies must be conducted to understand what people will pay out of their pockets for an HIV vaccine. These studies are notoriously difficult to conduct, and probably particularly so around sensitive topics such as HIV and sexuality. Results from willingness-to-pay studies may thus be only partially useful. It will also be important to determine public perceptions of the need for an HIV vaccine in lower-risk countries, and whether there will be initial demand for such a vaccine—particularly among those who deny their risk of becoming infected.

Appropriate Delivery Systems and Strategies for High-Risk Populations

As mentioned earlier, most vaccines in Africa are delivered through the EPI. This program, with the exception of tetanus toxoid for pregnant women, targets children under 1 year of age for vaccination against childhood diseases. The initial targets of a successful HIV vaccine campaign will be very different populations: adolescents, sexually active adults, truck drivers, commercial sex workers, etc. As a result, cost-effective systems to reach these groups must be created and validated. Routine approaches such as the use of schools, military bases, religious gatherings, etc. will need to be complemented by new delivery approaches that will reach beyond these first-line places.

Sustainable Prevention Strategies to Accompany Vaccine Deployment

It is unlikely that any HIV vaccine will be 100% effective. In fact, in any clinical HIV trial, vaccine efficacy will be measured by comparing incidence among those who receive maximum prevention education alone with that among those who receive both maximum prevention education and the vaccine. The efficacy of a vaccine alone, without prevention interventions, will thus remain unmeasured in trials for ethical reasons. Furthermore, even a fully effective HIV vaccine will not preclude people from risk of other STDs, pregnancy, or other reproductive health problems. As a result, HIV vaccine distribution and use must be accompanied by full, sustained implementation of prevention and behavioral change interventions. These interventions must be created where they are not already in place, validated for use in various communities and populations, and then scaled up.

Harmonization of African Regulatory Systems and Guidelines for Approval

Obtaining regulatory approval for drugs and vaccines in individual countries is a lengthy and expensive process. Harmonizing the regulatory procedures in this process, so that the same application could be submitted to most, if not all, African countries would allow an HIV vaccine to become available to more people in a shorter period of time. The complicated and different systems that are currently in place in individual African countries, may lead industry to apply for registration first in other markets, another obstacle to ensuring early access to the poorest countries.

Increasing the Use of Existing Vaccines to Pave the Way for HIV Vaccines

The current concern and heated debate about ensuring the availability of an eventual HIV vaccine may not be taken seriously, considering the number of other already proven, safe, effective, and inexpensive vaccines that are still not used in African countries today. For arguments about ensuring access to HIV vaccines to be taken more seriously, mechanisms for moving existing vaccines into higher levels of use in developing countries should be pursued aggressively. The new Global Alliance for Vaccines and Immunization and the Global Fund for Children's Vaccines aim to get new vaccines into the 74 poorest countries over the next few years. The benefits of this initiative will go beyond the immediate results of improved child health. Not only will this effort add credibility to the argument that an HIV vaccine must also reach these countries immediately, but it will improve vaccine delivery and management systems, lead to a renewed interest in vaccines, and facilitate the introduction of new vaccines, such as an HIV vaccine, in resource-poor countries.

AFRICAN- SPECIFIC STRATEGIES

As described earlier, it is likely that the participation of both the public and private sectors will be required to assure the development and eventual availability of any HIV vaccine for use in the general population. A number of innovative efforts are underway.

Role of the International AIDS Vaccine Initiative (IAVI)

IAVI was established as an international, private, not-for-profit scientific organization in 1996 in response to the languishing efforts to create an HIV vaccine in the public and private sectors (15). IAVI's work encompasses four strategies: (*i*) to create global demand for a vaccine through advocacy and education; (*ii*) to aggressively accelerate product development; (*iii*) to create incentives for industrial investment and participation in vaccine development; and (*iv*) to help assure access. IAVI currently has five vaccines moving forward for Africa—each made from locally circulating viral strains and designed in collaboration with African scientists from the beginning. IAVI also uses a form of social venture capital investing. Rather than asking companies for a return on investments in the form of profit or intellectual property, the organization instead asks for access for the poor. If manufacturers contracted by IAVI do not provide the eventually successful vaccine in reasonable quantities and at a reasonable cost (cost plus a reasonable profit) to the public sector in developing countries, IAVI reserves the right to transfer production of its vaccine to another manufacturer.

The South African AIDS Vaccine Initiative (SAAVI)

This initiative was established in 1999 to pursue the goal of a safe, effective, affordable and accessible vaccine for South Africa and the Southern African Development Community by 2005. SAAVI supports vaccine development, the development of trial sites and infrastructure, community mobilization and advocacy, and research on ethical issues. SAAVI is based at the Medical Research Council and works with all groups (both internal and external) who are working on AIDS vaccines for South Africa (16).

The African Vaccine Strategy

The UNAIDS/WHO HIV Vaccine Initiative has recently established a working group of African scientists to help strengthen the human and material infrastructure that will be needed for vaccine trials and distribution. This group of African scientists are to pool their expertise and facilities toward the common goal of conducting vaccine trials; this process is facilitated by peer support and information exchange (17).

Political Commitment

Although there is a need for political commitment to all aspects of the AIDS agenda, it is especially critical for vaccine development. At their last meeting in Ouagadougou, Burkina Faso, the Organization of African Unity (OAU) health ministers endorsed the development of an HIV vaccine. Unfortunately, there has been little follow-up or identification of specific ways in which the OAU could help. At the Commonwealth Heads of Government meeting in Durban in 2000, there was also a call for action on HIV vaccines. These political statements need to be turned into plans of action.

There is not enough political advocacy for HIV prevention interventions, particularly for long-term research to develop better prevention tools. Most politicians undervalue the benefit of using limited and precious political capital to promote something that does not have a constituency or immediately visible results. It is thus more attractive to respond to the acute emergency of care for those who are already sick, a response for which there is an enormous and rightfully very vocal community. It is, however, the responsibility of the public sector to stand in when the market is failing—particularly in providing R&D for an international public good such as an HIV vaccine. When more politicians take this brave step, others will likely be called to do the same. Of course, this political advocacy must not compete with, but should rather complement, efforts to scale up prevention interventions, treat those who are infected, and reduce the social consequences of HIV infection. The public must convey to politicians that this epidemic will not fully end without a vaccine and insist that adequate attention and resources be devoted to this effort.

It is particularly a tragedy that, until recently, development agencies and developing countries' governments have not significantly invested in or advocated for HIV vaccine work. The industry's lack of emphasis on developing countries raises legitimate concerns about the ultimate speed with which a vaccine will be developed and provided for those in greatest need. For example, the industry investment in product development has, in general, been targeted at those vaccine approaches that are perceived to be the safest investments, and are based on the subtypes of HIV-1 found in developed countries. Approaches with technical characteristics better suited for use in developing countries, particularly those in Africa, are not being pursued aggressively. The rationale for this approach is that proving the efficacy of the first vaccine should be the priority, and other products will be developed afterward. However, because numerous scientific uncertainties remain about the ultimate approach to HIV vaccine development, the simultaneous design and testing of multiple empirical approaches will be a faster route to safe, effective, and inexpensive vaccines that are appropriate for widespread use. The primary focus of current efforts on the subtypes of HIV-1 found in developed countries may also delay the full evaluation of candidate vaccines by restricting the sites where they can be tested in clinical trials.

CONCLUSION

There is no question that there is a critical global need for an HIV vaccine that can protect all people from the varying HIV viruses circulating around the world. This effort has been woefully underfunded and underprioritized. HIV vaccine development is now beginning to get more of the attention it deserves and resources are slowly following. It is clear that the world should be investing far more in the search for a vaccine and prioritizing the creation of vaccines that will be appropriate for use where the epidemic is spreading most rapidly. Furthermore, it is clear that a system must be put in place to assure that all those who need a vaccine will have access to one, regardless of their economic or social status. The latter relies heavily on international efforts to aggressively move R&D forward and to begin to prepare for success.

REFERENCES

1. Binswanger HP. Scaling up HIV/AIDS programs to national coverage. *Science*, 2000;288:2173–2176.
2. Carr A, Cooper DA. Adverse effects of antiretroviral therapy. *Lancet*, 2000;356:1423–1430.
3. World Health Organization. Ad Hoc Committee on Health Research Relating to Future Intervention Options, Investing in Health Research for Development. TDR/Gen/96.1. Geneva: World Health Organization, 1996.
4. Peltola H. What would happen if we stopped vaccination? *Lancet*, 2000;356(Suppl):s22.
5. Gangarosa EJ, Galazka AM, Wolfe CR, et al. Impact of anti-vaccine movements on pertussis control: The untold story. *Lancet*, 1998;351:356–361.
6. The World Bank. World Development Report 1993; Investing in Health. New York: Oxford University Press, 1993:72–73.
7. Global Alliance for Vaccines and Immunization website. Available at: *www.vaccinealliance.org*. Accessed February 3, 2002.

8. Mercer Management Consulting. A commercial perspective of vaccine supply. New York: Report to UNICEF by Mercer Management Consulting, 1994.
9. Batson A. Win-win interactions between the public and private sectors. *Nat Med*, Vaccine Supplement, 1998;4:487–491.
10. Gregersen, Jens-Peter. Vaccine Development: The Long Road from Initial Idea to Product Licensure. In: Levine M, ed. *New Generation Vaccines*, 2nd Ed. New York: Marcel Dekker, 1997:1165–1177.
11. The Economist. The Pharmaceutical Industry: The alchemists. *The Economist*, Insert, February 21, 1998.
12. Glaser V. Number of biotechnology companies pursuing HIV vaccines begins to dwindle. *Genetic Engineering News*, 1997;17:14,44.
13. The International AIDS Vaccine Initiative. AIDS Vaccines for the World: Preparing now to assure access. July 2000. The International AIDS Vaccine Initiative website. Available at *www.iavi.org*. Accessed February 3, 2002.
14. Danzon PM. The Economics of Parallel Trade. *Pharmacoeconomics*, 1998;13:293–304.
15. International AIDS Vaccine Initiative website. Available at: *www.iavi.org*. Accessed February 3, 2002.
16. Galloway, MR. *The IAVI Report*, 1999:4(5):1,14.
17. Esparza J, Bhamarapravati N. Accelerating the development and future availability of HIV-1 vaccines: why, when, where, and how? *Lancet*, 2000;355:WA15-WA20.

39

HIV Vaccines

Design and Development

Tun-Hou Lee and Vlad Novitsky

Department of Immunology and Infectious Diseases, Harvard School of Public Health, Boston, Massachusetts, USA.

Since the discovery of human immunodeficiency virus (HIV) in the early 1980s and the subsequent delineation of HIV genes and gene products involved in its replication cycle, great strides have been made in disrupting the HIV replication cycle by chemotherapeutic means. Many developing countries, including those in sub–Saharan Africa, have not benefited significantly from this achievement because the resources needed to make antiretroviral therapy sustainable worldwide remain out of reach. A more cost-effective means to address the AIDS epidemic in these developing countries is the development of an efficacious HIV vaccine. In this chapter, candidate HIV vaccines that have been, or will soon be tested in clinical trials will be reviewed, followed by a discussion of a design modality for an HIV vaccine for southern Africa.

WHAT CONSTITUTES PROTECTIVE IMMUNITY IN HIV INFECTION?

The HIV vaccine development effort has gone through three different chronologic phases. In each phase varying degrees of emphasis have been placed on targeting different arms of the immune response with an HIV-1 vaccine. The first phase placed more emphasis on eliciting neutralizing antibodies than on eliciting cytotoxic T-cell (CTL) responses. The next phase aimed at eliciting both the humoral and cellular immune responses, rather than just humoral responses. The most recent phase has placed far more emphasis on eliciting CTL responses than on humoral responses. In addition, eliciting a robust helper T-cell response has also been suggested to be important (1–3). The uncertainty about the best choice of arms of the immune response to target in order to elicit protective immunity by an HIV vaccine is one of the key challenges of HIV vaccine design.

The first phase of HIV vaccine development placed significant emphasis on developing neutralizing antibody by either targeting the third variable (V3) region or the CD4-binding region of the HIV envelope. During this phase, researchers focused on T-cell line adapted (TCLA) HIV strains. The convenience of propagating HIV in immortal T-cell lines, as opposed to primary T-cells derived from HIV-negative donors, led to the disproportionate amount of attention paid to TCLA HIV. It is now recognized that TCLA HIV possesses distinct characteristics that are not shared by HIV strains that are freshly derived from patients and have only been grown in primary T-cells. One such characteristic is the relative ease with which TCLA HIV is neutralized *in vitro* by antibodies directed at V3. The substantial effort that had been devoted to this line of vaccine design and development came to a halt with the realization that the V3 antibodies elicited by candidate vaccines using TCLA HIV do not neutralize primary HIV. There are suggestions that primary HIV has a relatively inaccessible V3, which would preclude it from being a target for neutralizing antibodies. One of the challenges facing scientists in HIV vaccine design is the identification of the means to target V3 since this region of the HIV envelope interacts with the cell chemokine coreceptor during the early stages of viral cell entry.

A similar line of vaccine development was carried out based on the observation that the interaction between TCLA HIV and the primary receptor of HIV, CD4, could be blocked in vitro by antibodies targeting the CD4-binding region of the HIV envelope. This approach garnered enthusiastic support because targeting the more conserved CD4 region was regarded as a better alternative to targeting the more variable regions of V3. Recombinant HIV envelope proteins that lack proper post-translational modifications or that have low solubility in physiologic solutions tend to elicit antibody responses to V3, rather than to the CD4 binding region. Therefore, substantial technologic emphasis was placed on preserving the conformation of the HIV envelope protein gp120 by using expression systems that allowed adequate post-translational modifications to facilitate the folding of recombinant gp120. Despite the advance in eliciting antibody to the CD4-binding region, this approach had the same shortcoming as those targeting the V3: blocking of HIV infection only occurs with TCLA HIV, but not primary HIV. Taken together, this initial phase of HIV vaccine development was characterized by a lack of success in designing a vaccine that could elicit neutralizing antibodies to block primary HIV.

The transition from the initial phase of HIV vaccine development to the next phase was catalyzed by the observation that CTLs appeared to be linked to the clearance of the initial round of virus replication during the acute phase of HIV infection (4,5). A similar observation was also made with SIV (simian immunodeficiency virus), the HIV counterpart in the rhesus macaque model (6,7). In this new phase of HIV vaccine development, more attention was paid to techniques with the potential to elicit CTL responses, with the overall goal of eliciting responses from both arms of the immune system.

The hallmark of this second phase of the HIV vaccine development effort was the design of a new vaccination strategy called "prime-boost." With this approach, the host is first primed with a live vector that has a higher potential to elicit a CTL response due to its ability to express HIV antigens via the MHC class I pathway. The host is subsequently boosted with recombinant subunit proteins to elicit antibodies to HIV envelope. The most-studied live virus vector is canarypox virus, a poxvirus. The properties of this virus vector will be discussed later in this chapter. Based on the studies conducted thus far, it appears that priming with this live vector does elicit a more robust CTL response than recombinant subunit protein-based vaccines. However, the positive CTL response rate is only about 25%, indicating that further optimization of this vector and/or alternative approaches should be seriously considered.

The most-studied recombinant subunit envelope protein is HIV envelope gp120, which is derived from the MN strain. This particular TCLA strain of HIV was chosen primarily because its V3 was more reactive to serum samples collected from HIV-infected subjects than the V3 derived from other HIV strains (8). The implication was that the MN strain was most antigenically representative of all HIV, thus the most appropriate one to include in a vaccine preparation. Despite the seemingly sound rationale for selecting the envelope antigen from the MN strain, antibodies elicited to the envelope protein of TCLA HIV could not neutralize primary HIV, and it remains doubtful that any antibody response elicited will be of benefit.

As more emphasis was gradually placed on eliciting CTL responses, the HIV vaccine development effort began to move into a third phase, focusing almost exclusively on eliciting CTL responses. The vaccine strategy that was most explored during this phase was a derivative of the original "prime-boost" approach. This time, the priming agent deemed most effective was a DNA vaccine, and the most commonly used boosting agent was a live recombinant virus vector. In two recent studies, this new prime-boost approach was found to offer protection against a lethal challenge of SHIV—the hybrid of simian and human immunodeficiency viruses that has been used to study the protective efficacy of candidate vaccines (9,10). In both studies, it appeared that the CTL response alone was sufficient to offer protection against lethal challenges by SHIV. Because this approach has only been studied in experimental animals, it remains to be determined if such an approach will prove to be effective in future clinical trials. Researchers question whether this most recent phase of HIV vaccine development will be as transitional as those preceding it.

Why is the process of developing an HIV vaccine so drawn-out and complicated? The answer to this question lies primarily in the fact that natural immunity does not appear to have a strong impact on the final outcome of HIV infection. In fact, without chemotherapeutic intervention, HIV infection is responsible for an extremely high mortality rate. Because studies of natural infection have not guided scientists in understanding what constitutes protective immunity, it has not yet been possible to identify the critical viral sequences to include in an HIV vaccine.

CANDIDATE HIV VACCINES IN CLINICAL TRIALS

Candidate vaccines for clinical trials can be grouped into four major categories based on the technology involved. These categories include: recombinant subunit proteins, synthetic peptides, recombinant poxviruses, and DNA vaccines. For a detailed listing of HIV clinical trials, please refer to the database compiled by the U.S. National Institutes of Health (11).

Most of the recombinant subunit protein vaccines are the molecular replicas of the HIV envelope proteins gp160 or gp120. Different vectors have been used to produce these recombinant Env proteins: Baculovirus (12), vaccinia virus (13,14), yeast expression vectors (15,16), and other mammalian expression vectors that allow recombinant Env proteins to be stably expressed in CHO cells (17,18). A few other recombinant subunit proteins are the molecular replicas of HIV Gag proteins. These include recombinant p17 and p24, which are expressed by yeast vectors as virus-like particles, and a recombinant p24 that is expressed in CHO cells (11,16). A bacterial expression vector has also been used to express a recombinant subunit protein of the HIV regulatory protein Tat (11). Among these, the recombinant Env protein-based vaccines have been studied most extensively. Currently, large-scale phase III clinical trials are being conducted with recombinant Env proteins derived from both TCLA and primary HIV (11).

Most of the synthetic peptide-based vaccines are monovalent or polyvalent peptides with amino acid sequences corresponding to the V3 of the HIV envelope (19,20). Some of the polyvalent V3 synthetic peptides are presented in two different octameric forms (11). Some synthetic peptides contain a fusion sequence of V3 and C4 (11) or epitopes from *nef*, *gag* and V3 (21). In addition to these, a p17-based synthetic peptide (22) and a *gag*-based lipopeptide have been made (11). Most of the synthetic peptide-based vaccines evaluated in clinical trials have not been found to be particularly immunogenic, whether they were used by themselves, or in combination with other candidate vaccines (11). Although the hybrid V3-C4 synthetic peptides formulated in the Incomplete Freund's Adjuvant appeared to be more immunogenic than other synthetic peptides, the adverse effect of this vaccine preparation observed in some vaccinees limits its usefulness. It is doubtful that an efficacious HIV vaccine will consist exclusively of synthetic peptides, although the inclusion of synthetic peptides in a vaccine remains possible.

In addition to being used as an expression vector to produce recombinant subunit proteins, the recombinant poxvirus has also been used as a live viral vector vaccine. Three types of recombinant poxvirus that have been used for this purpose include recombinant Vaccinia virus (23,24), canarypox virus (25,26) and the so-called MVA (Modified Vaccinia Ankara) strain. The canarypox virus vector was chosen for its inability to reinfect cells of human origin. This property is believed to help avoid some of the types of side effects associated with live recombinant Vaccinia virus. The approach of priming with live recombinant canarypox vector and boosting with recombinant subunit Env protein(s) has been studied in several phase I and phase II clinical trials. Plans are being made to test the efficacy of this vaccine approach in phase III clinical trials. Recently, the MVA strain of the recombinant Vaccinia virus has received increased attention. This strain causes fewer side effects than the more conventional recombinant Vaccinia virus, yet its unimpaired ability to infect human cells allows a higher level of HIV expression that appears to enhance its immunogenicity. For the approach of priming with a DNA vaccine and boosting with a live recombinant viral vector, the MVA is one of the live recombinant viral vectors chosen for phase I clinical trials in the near future. In most of the recombinant poxvirus vectors, the HIV-1 genes incorporated are *gag*, *pol*, and *nef*, and in some instances, *env* as well (11).

The approach of using DNA plasmid vectors as HIV vaccines was a relatively recent development. Introduction of DNA into skin or muscle cells was found to elicit a sufficiently high level of immune response to warrant further exploration of this approach. Two general types of DNA plasmids have been constructed for this purpose. The first one is the more traditional type of mammalian expression vector in which the expression of the HIV gene is directly under the control of a strong promoter (11,27). The second type is the so-called RNA replicon-based DNA vector in which the HIV sequence is expressed from a subgenomic RNA that has undergone multiple rounds of amplification mediated by the replicase complex of the Alphavirus (28–30). The latter type of vector was reported to have enhanced immunogenicity either through a higher level of protein expression and/or through the release of immunostimulatory cytokines from the transfected cells (29,31).

A common modification introduced to the HIV sequences in DNA vaccines is the so-called "codon-optimization" or "humanized" sequence. Replacing HIV codons with those more commonly found in the highly expressed mammalian genes has the net effect of reducing AT content, increasing HIV expression, and making the DNA vaccines that have such modified HIV genes more immunogenic. Although there is no consensus regarding whether more efficient expression of HIV is mechanistically linked to an increase in translational efficiency, codon-optimization does allow HIV genes to be expressed in a *rev*-independent manner. Regardless of the precise mechanism, codon-optimization of HIV genes is a commonly adopted strategy for DNA vaccines.

DNA vaccines have also been designed for use in combination with adjuvants, cytokines, or synthetic polymers to increase their immunogenicity. In addition, the approach of incorporating DNA vaccines into live bacterial vectors to target the mucosal immune system has also been reported (32).

The "prime-boost" approach, using DNA vaccines as the priming agents has been studied quite extensively in the current phase of HIV vaccine development. There is a general perception that DNA vaccines are effective priming agents for inducing immune memory. It is likely that more clinical trials will be conducted with vaccine preparations that include DNA vaccines as a component.

Other Technologies Adopted in the Preclinical Development of HIV Vaccines

Many different viral vectors, besides the poxviruses mentioned earlier, have been proposed as delivery vehicles for HIV-1 vaccines (reviewed in (33)). The expression systems of viral vectors are able to induce high levels of both humoral and cellular immune responses and to induce mucosal immunity, which is believed to be an important component of an effective HIV-1 vaccine. However, the safety issues of viral vectors (especially in immunocompromised recipients) and pre-existing immunity within the population to the vector itself, might pose obstacles to their practical use.

Herpesviridae (34,35), Papovaviridae (36–38), and Adenoviridae (39–47), in addition to poxviridae (26,48–58) have all been used to construct candidate HIV vaccines. Additionally, five RNA viruses—Togaviridae (59–64), Picornaviridae (65–72), Rhabdoviridae (73–80), Orthomyxoviridae (81–84), and Paramyxoviridae (85)—have also been used to construct candidate HIV-1 vaccines. Table 1 summarizes the representative viral vectors and the advantages and disadvantages of each of these viral vectors. With such a large choice of recombinant viral vectors, the problem of eliciting an immune response to the vector itself could be overcome by presenting the same or a related antigen to the immune system by different vectors.

Bacterial vectors expressing HIV antigens can be administered orally and provide effective mucosal immunity. A *Salmonella* vector carrying the *env* gene of HIV-1 was shown to generate Env-specific CTL (86,87)

TABLE 1. DNA and RNA Viral Vectors as Delivery Vehicles for HIV-1 Vaccines

	Advantages	Disadvantages	Representative vectors	References
DNA viruses				
Poxviridae	Multiple large genes; Stable expression; Thermostable; Replication-deficient vectors are safe in humans.	Replication-competent: vectors might not be safe in immunocompromised vaccinees; Replication-deficient vectors induce low immune response; Pre-existing immunity to vaccinia.	Replication Competent vaccinia virus; Replication deficient: Modified vaccinia virus Ankara (MVA), Canarypox virus, and Fowlpox virus.	(26,48–58)
Herpesviridae	Long-term expression; Durable immune response.	Safety is uncertain; Pre-existing immunity.	Herpes simplex virus type 2 (HSV-2).	(34,35)
Papovaviridae	Elicits both humoral and cellular immune responses; Does not elicit response to the vector itself.	Packaging capacity restricts insert size.	Simian virus 40 (SV40).	(36–38)
Adenoviridae	Induction of mucosal immunity; Oral or intranasal administration; Both humoral and cellular immune responses; Long-lasting immune protection.	High doses might be required; Controversial immunogenicity.	Replication-competent adenovirus; Replication-deficient adenovirus.	(39–47)
RNA viruses				
Togaviridae	High level of expression; No pre-existing immunity in humans; Elicits both humoral and cellular immune responses.	Uncertain immunogenicity.	Venezuelan equine encephalitis (VEE); Semliki forest virus (SFV).	(59–64)
Picornaviridae	Safe; Induction of mucosal immunity; Proven immunogenicity.	Pre-existing vector-specific immunity in humans; Restricted cloning capacity; Low genetic stability of constructs.	Polio virus; Hepatitis A virus; Foot and mouth disease (FMDV); Mengo virus; Human Rhino virus (HRV).	(65–72)
Rhabdoviridae	Multiple large genes; Stable expression; Elicits both humoral and cellular immune responses.	Replication-competent vectors might not be safe in immunocompromised vaccines.	Rabies virus (RV); Vesicular stomatitis virus (VSV).	(73–80)
Paramyxoviridae	Under investigation in relation to HIV vaccine.	Safety in humans.	Newcastle disease virus (NDV).	(85)
Orthomyxoviridae	Induction of mucosal immunity.	Small cloning capacity; Pre-existing immunity in humans.	Influenza virus A.	(81–84)

and T-helper responses (88), both in mucosal and systemic lymphoid tissue. *Listeria* is an alternative bacterial vector that can elicit T-cell immunity because it specifically infects monocytes and because natural infection originates in the mucosa. An HIV-1 Gag-expressing hyperattenuated D-alanine-dependent *Listeria monocytogenes* was demonstrated as efficient at stimulating Gag-specific human CTLs in vitro (89–91). Several strains of *Streptococcus gordonii* were successfully tested as vaccine vehicles to induce HIV-specific immune responses in mice and monkeys (92, 93). The recombinant Mycobacterium (BCG)-based vectors were also shown to express several HIV genes and to induce strong humoral and cellular immune responses in experimental animals (94–98). Evaluation of a *Shigella* vector that expressed HIV-1 gp120 in a murine model using intranasal and intramuscular administration demonstrated the inducement of robust $CD8^+$ T-cell responses and antiviral protective immunity (99).

To enhance the immunogenicity of an HIV-1 vaccine, adjuvants, which include a growing number of substances with immunostimulating effects (reviewed in (100,101)), have been tested. Adjuvants could enhance, prolong, or alter the immune response to recombinant subunit proteins and synthetic peptides. Some adjuvants have been physically associated with the antigen (i.e., aluminum salts or emulsions) while others provide immunostimulation through their interaction with antigen-presenting cells and cytokine secretion (100).

In the earlier stages of HIV vaccine development, envelope-based antigens were widely used with aluminum salts or oil-in-water emulsions to induce humoral response (102–107). Iron hydroxide was shown to be a superior adjuvant compared with aluminum hydroxide (108). A number of other emulsions (i.e., MF59, ISCOM, and ISA720) that have adjuvant effects have also been tested in primary or boost immunizations (26, 109–112). The aluminum salts and emulsions are especially useful as booster components in immunization protocols. It is possible that these adjuvants could complement recombinant live vectors to elicit strong antibody and T-helper responses.

Although the immunostimulants saponin QS21 and monophosphoryl lipid A (MPL) could be used as single-component adjuvants, a vaccine formulation that combined them resulted in enhanced induction of both cell-mediated and humoral responses, clearly indicating that QS21 and MPL could complement each other (113,114).

Several other adjuvants were recently studied with HIV antigens, mostly in murine models. Polytuftsin, a synthetic polymer of the natural immunomodulator tuftsin, was shown as a potent enhancer of HIV-1–specific immune response when it was chemically linked to the gp120 and gp41 synthetic peptides (115). HIV-1 antigens that were covalently coupled to aluminum oxide nanoparticles induced strong HIV-1–specific antibodies in mice (116). Liposomes were shown to be efficient delivery vehicles for HIV-1 antigens. In one study, the V3 loop peptides encapsulated into pH-sensitive liposomes, which were composed of phosphatidylethanolamine-beta-oleoyl-gamma-palmitoyl (POPE)/cholesterol hemisuccinate (CHOH)/MPL (mole ratio 7:3:0.1), elicited both antibodies and virus-specific CTL responses, while peptides without liposomes were not as immunogenic (117).

Several approaches have been tested to enhance the immunogenicity of a DNA vaccine. The C3d component of complement was shown to increase the immunogenicity of the DNA vaccines that encoded Env fused to C3d (118). Cationic and anionic microparticles were shown to enhance HIV-1-specific immune responses, especially when applied to DNA constructs and recombinant subunit protein-based vaccines (119–124). The biodegradable cationic microparticles were shown to improve the delivery of adsorbed DNA into antigen-presenting cells, to enhance antibody responses, and to induce potent cytotoxic T-lymphocyte responses after intramuscular injection (125). Mucosal (intranasal) delivery of microparticles with the adsorbed *gag* DNA resulted in the Gag-specific cell- and antibody-mediated responses (126). The vaccine formulation consisting of recombinant gp120 (rgp120) and poly(lactic-co-glycolic) acid microparticles provided a "prime-boost" effect with a single immunization by performing in-vivo pulses of an antigen (127). It was also shown that durable immune responses might be further enhanced by QS21 adjuvant. However, not all microparticles work equally well, as seen when an HIV-1 antigen encapsulated in biodegradable microparticles composed of co-polymers of lactic and glycolic acids and administered by the oral route resulted in no significant humoral, cellular, or mucosal immune responses (128).

DESIGN OF AN HIV VACCINE FOR SOUTHERN AFRICA

Until recently, HIV vaccine development has focused more on HIV viruses prevalent in developed countries than those prevalent in developing countries. A few studies have reported that some antigenic epitopes are shared by HIVs circulating in different parts of the world. However, evidence that such antigenic epitopes by themselves are sufficient to offer protective immunity is lacking. It is therefore imperative to evaluate the possibility that HIV vaccines with antigens that most closely match the HIV circulating in a target population may be more efficacious than those relying on antigenic cross-reactivity. This section deals with an HIV vaccine design approach that is particularly relevant to HIV prevention in southern Africa and illustrates how factors such as the choice of HIV strain and the HLA type of the at-risk population could be taken into consideration when developing an HIV vaccine for southern Africa.

Southern Africa has the most severe AIDS epidemic in the world. An extensive molecular monitoring of the epidemic revealed that, in contrast to the multi-type and multi-subtype HIV epidemics in the West and in central and East Africa, the epidemic in southern Africa and in the horn of Africa is caused predominantly by HIV-1 subtype C (HIV-1C). Representing at least 56% of all circulating group M infections worldwide (129), HIV-1C has evolved as a fast spreading HIV-1 subtype since the mid 1990s, and as the only HIV-1 subtype that accounts for prevalence rates as high as 20% to 40% in the general adult population within the southern African region (130,131).

Molecular characterization of virus is an important part of HIV vaccine design. Nonetheless, until recently, most HIV vaccine designs have been based on sequences derived mostly from HIV-1 subtype B, the virus that predominates in the developed countries. The first nearly full-length genome sequence of HIV-1C was determined in 1996 (132). A number of recent studies (133–140) have led to the generation of an HIV-1C full-length genome sequence database that is comprised, to date, of 73 non-recombinant HIV-1C isolates. Full-length genome sequences have provided valuable information regarding diversity, variability, and consensus sequence and, together with biologic and phenotypic characterization of HIV-1C variants, greatly facilitated the HIV vaccine design effort.

A high degree of HIV-1C diversity (135,139,141) poses a significant challenge for the development of an efficacious HIV vaccine. To address the issue of how to select the most representative HIV antigen to develop into an HIV vaccine for southern Africa, the approach of adopting the consensus HIV sequence was proposed (140). The central hypothesis of this approach is that a higher homology between the vaccine strain and the circulating strain(s) should result in a more efficacious vaccine. In a recent study (140) the questions of (*i*) whether the genetic diversity

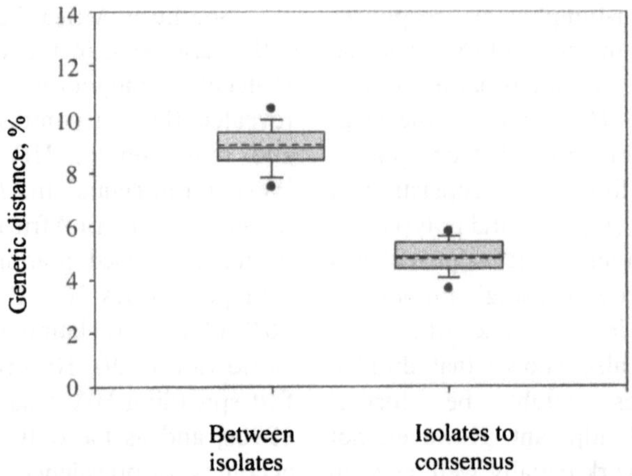

FIGURE 1. Nucleotide distances among the 73 near full-length HIV-1C genomes. "Between samples" distances are compared with distances "to the consensus" sequence. The boundary of the box closest to zero indicates the 25th percentile, a solid line within the box marks the mean value, a dashed line within the box shows the median, and the boundary of the box farthest from zero indicates the 75th percentile. Whiskers above and below the box indicate the 10th and 90th percentiles. Points above and below the whiskers indicate the 5th and 95th percentiles when the sample size permitted these calculations.

of HIV-1C might be overcome by using a consensus sequence as a vaccine candidate instead of any particular viral isolate; and (*ii*) whether the extent of potential vaccine coverage of circulating viral variants would be sufficient for the vaccine efficacy were addressed. As shown in Figure 1, the genetic distances to the consensus sequence could be almost halved as compared to distances between the viral isolates (4.86% versus 8.93%; analysis was performed for 73 near full-length genome sequences). Furthermore, the predictive power of the consensus sequence was found to be high, which supported the argument that a new emerging sequence was unlikely to significantly alter the distribution of distances to the consensus sequence. The result of this analysis suggests that such a consensus sequence could be a better choice than any particular HIV isolate when designing an HIV vaccine for southern African countries.

To incorporate the HLA profiles of the at-risk population living in southern Africa into an HIV vaccine design is an additional attempt to improve and to generate optimal immune responses among the southern African population. Ward (142) and Haynes (143,144) suggested an HIV-1 vaccine design that considers the MHC class I alleles prevalent in the targeted geographic area and includes multiple CTL epitopes restricted by common HLA class I alleles among potential vaccinees. It may be necessary to design HLA-based vaccines for specific geographic locations and perhaps even for specific ethnic groups (143). If common HLA alleles that cover at least 80% to 90% of the target population of potential vaccinees can be identified, then CTL epitopes that are restricted by those HLA alleles could be included in a vaccine construct. Moreover, it has been shown recently that carriers of certain HLA class I alleles mediate better cellular immune responses to HIV-1 vaccines than carriers of other HLA alleles (145). The genetic background of a vaccinee population might restrict the breadth and magnitude of CTL responses through the diversity and frequency of MHC class I HLA alleles within the population in southern Africa. Thus, the profile of HLA class I alleles could be an important determinant of HIV vaccine design, and is valuable information for monitoring post-vaccination response. A systematic identification of HLA alleles and generation of an HLA database for the southern African countries could improve HIV vaccine design, particularly those seeking to elicit CTL responses.

The significant role of HIV-1–specific CTL responses in the control of HIV-1 infection has been shown in several recent studies (4,5, 146–148). Although correlates of protection in HIV-1 infection are still not known, identification of naturally occurring dominant and subdominant CTL responses allows mapping of CTL epitopes that could be targeted by an HIV vaccine (149–152). An ideal HIV vaccine would be one that could contain antigens with both CTL epitopes and T-helper epitopes and could elicit broadly neutralizing antibodies against primary HIV. Identification of CTL-rich regions across the entire viral genome and subsequent fine mapping of CTL epitopes should lead to the design of an HIV vaccine that has better potential to target these CTL epitopes. This is especially the case if the vaccine design also takes into consideration common HLA alleles of the at-risk population and the actual sequences of predominant HIV.

It should be recognized that the vast majority of CTL epitopes identified thus far have been largely based on HIV-1 subtype B sequences (153). It is possible that the genetic properties of the predominant viruses circulating in southern Africa might affect the breadth and magnitude of CTL responses. Thus, CTL studies relevant to vaccine design for southern African countries should pay attention to the specificities and diversity of locally circulating HIV-1C.

Identification of immunodominant CTL regions and fine mapping of CTL epitopes across the viral genome could help to address the issue of clade-specificity vs. cross-clade reactivity vis-à-vis HIV vaccine design. A significant number of CTL epitopes that are located in highly conserved regions of the viral genome and are almost identical between HIV-1 clades appear to account for the observed cross-clade CTL recognition (154–158). However, CTL epitopes that are unique to each HIV-1 subtype are likely to be highly clade-specific (159–161). As shown in a recent study (162), the magnitude of Nef-specific Elispot-based CTL responses to subtype C peptides was higher than responses to subtype B peptides, suggesting that, despite the existence of cross-clade CTL recognition, subtype-specific CTL responses are of a higher magnitude. Demonstrated differences in the profiles of dominant Gag-specific (148,162), and Tat- and Rev-specific (162–164) CTL responses among HIV-1B-infected Caucasians and HIV-1C-infected Africans suggest remarkable differences in the CTL epitope clustering among different ethnic groups infected by different HIV-1 subtypes.

Taken together, the observed differences in CTL responses and in profiles of immunodominant CTL responses among different ethnic groups suggest the possible advantage of adopting an approach that takes into consideration virus diversity, HLA profiles, and naturally occurring CTL responses.

The schematic drawing shown in Figure 2 depicts a candidate HIV vaccine that contains multiple, highly responsive CTL epitopes across the entire viral genome. The identification and the ranking of dominant and subdominant CTL epitopes in the context of predominant virus and common HLA types in a certain geographic area provide the key determinants for such HIV vaccine design. The introduction of multiple copies of dominant viral variants into vaccine constructs has the potential to increase vaccine coverage of naturally occurring viruses in the epidemic. From the perspective of both viral escape and HLA restriction, the inclusion of multiple variants of key immunodominant CTL epitopes in an HIV vaccine could provide a more effective protection.

CONCLUSION

Despite the fact that many technologies have been adopted for HIV vaccine design,

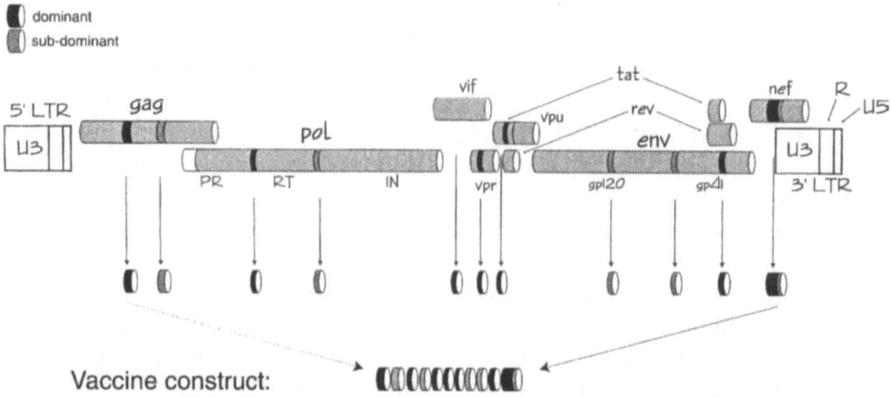

FIGURE 2. Immunodominant regions across HIV-1C.

and many candidate HIV vaccines have entered clinical trials, the prospect of having an efficacious HIV vaccine available in the near future remains uncertain. A lack of knowledge about protective immunity has hindered HIV vaccine development. This obstacle is to some extent offset by the knowledge researchers in the field have gained about HIV diversity, the structure of some key HIV proteins, the events surrounding HIV entry into its target cells, and host responses to HIV antigens. Even though many of these scientific gains have been, and will continue to be translated into HIV vaccine designs, it should be recognized that only through clinical trials will it be possible to evaluate the effectiveness an intended immune response that is elicited by a candidate vaccine. HIV vaccine development needs to be an empirical process, involving repeated rounds of clinical testing of a large array of candidate HIV vaccines. An efficacious HIV vaccine developed from such a process is our best hope of arresting the growing AIDS epidemic both in sub-Saharan Africa and in other regions of the world.

REFERENCES

1. Rosenberg ES, Billingsley JM, Caliedo AM, et al. Vigorous HIV-1-specific CD4+ T cell responses associated with control of viremia. *Science*, 1997; 278:1447–1450.
2. Walker BD. Immune reconstitution and immunotherapy in HIV infection. Available at http://www.medscape.com/Medscape/HIV/ClinicalMgmt/CM.v15/CM.v15/public/CM.v15-toc.html. Accessed: December 13, 2001.
3. Ahlers JD, Belyakov IM, Thomas EK, et al. High-affinity T helper epitope induces complementary helper and APC polarization, increased CTL, and protection against viral infection. *J Clin Invest*, 2001;108:1677–1685.
4. Borrow P, Lewicki H, Hahn BH, et al. Virus-specific CD8+ cytotoxic T-lymphocyte activity associated with control of viremia in primary human immunodeficiency virus type 1 infection. *J Virol*, 1994;68:6103–6110.
5. Koup RA, Safrit JT, Cao Y, et al. Temporal association of cellular immune responses with the initial control of viremia in primary human immunodeficiency virus type 1 syndrome. *J Virol*, 1994;68: 4650–4655.
6. Jin X, Bauer DE, Tuttleton SE, et al. Dramatic rise in plasma viremia after CD8(+) T cell depletion in simian immunodeficiency virus-infected macaques. *J Exp Med*, 1999;189:991–998.
7. Schmitz JE, Kuroda MJ, Santra S, et al. Control of viremia in simian immunodeficiency virus infection by CD8+ lymphocytes. *Science*, 1999;283:857–860.
8. LaRosa GJ, Davide JP, Weinhold K, et al. Conserved sequence and structural elements in the HIV-1 principal neutralizing determinant. *Science*, 1990;249:932–935.
9. Amara RR, Villinger F, Altman JD, et al. Control of a mucosal challenge and prevention of AIDS by a multiprotein DNA/MVA vaccine. *Science*, 2001;292:69–74.
10. Kahn P. Keystone Symposium: New Vaccine Candidates and a Major New Player. *IAVI Report*, 2001;5:1,13.
11. Graham BS. Clinical trials of HIV vaccines. In: Kuiken C, Foley B, Hahn B, Marx P, McCutchan F,

Mellors JW, eds. *HIV Sequence Compendium 2000.* Los Alamos, NM, USA: Theoretical Biology and Biophysics, Los Alamos National Laboratory, 2000:82–105.

12. Kovacs JA, Vasudevachari MB, Easter M, et al. Induction of humoral and cell-mediated anti-human immunodeficiency virus (HIV) responses in HIV sero-negative volunteers by immunization with recombinant gp160. *J Clin Invest*, 1993;92:919–928.
13. Belshe RB, Clements ML, Dolin R, et al. Safety and immunogenicity of a fully glycosylated recombinant gp160 human immunodeficiency virus type 1 vaccine in subjects at low risk of infection. NIAID AIDS Vaccine Evaluation Group Network. *J Infect Dis*, 1993;168:1387–1395.
14. Gorse GJ, McElrath MJ, Matthews TJ, et al. Modulation of immunologic responses to HIV-1MN recombinant gp160 vaccine by dose and schedule of administration. NIAID AIDS Vaccine Evaluation Group. *Vaccine*, 1998;16:493–506.
15. Keefer MC, Graham BS, McElrath MJ, et al. Safety and immunogenicity of Env 2–3, a human immunodeficiency virus type 1 candidate vaccine, in combination with a novel adjuvant, MTP-PE/MF59. NIAID AIDS Vaccine Evaluation Group. *AIDS Res Hum Retroviruses*, 1996;12:683–693.
16. Martin SJ, Vyakarnam A, Cheingsong-Popov R, et al. Immunization of human HIV-seronegative volunteers with recombinant p17/p24:Ty virus-like particles elicits HIV-1 p24-specific cellular and humoral immune responses. *AIDS*, 1993;7: 1315–1323.
17. Schwartz DH, Gorse G, Clements ML, et al. Induction of HIV-1-neutralising and syncytium-inhibiting antibodies in uninfected recipients of HIV-1IIIB rgp120 subunit vaccine. *Lancet*, 1993; 342:69–73.
18. Kahn JO, Sinangil F, Baenziger J, et al. Clinical and immunologic responses to human immunodeficiency virus (HIV) type 1SF2 gp120 subunit vaccine combined with MF59 adjuvant with or without muramyl tripeptide dipalmitoyl phosphatidylethanolamine in non-HIV-infected human volunteers. *J Infect Dis*, 1994;170:1288–1291.
19. Gorse GJ, Keefer MC, Belshe RB, et al. A dose-ranging study of a prototype synthetic HIV-1MN V3 branched peptide vaccine. NIAID AIDS Vaccine Evaluation Group. *J Infect Dis*, 1996;173:330–339.
20. Rubinstein A, Goldstein H, Pettoello-Mantovani M, et al. Safety and immunogenicity of a V3 loop synthetic peptide conjugated to purified protein derivative in HIV-seronegative volunteers. *AIDS*, 1995;9:243–251.
21. Gahery-Segard H, Pialoux G, Charmeteau B, et al. Multiepitopic B- and T-cell responses induced in humans by a human immunodeficiency virus type 1 lipopeptide vaccine. *J Virol*, 2000;74:1694–1703.
22. Sarin PS, Mora CA, Naylor PH, et al. HIV-1 p17 synthetic peptide vaccine HGP-30: induction of immune response in human subjects and preliminary evidence of protection against HIV challenge in SCID mice. *Cell Mol Biol*, 1995;41:401–407.
23. Zagury D, Bernard J, Cheynier R, et al. A group specific anamnestic immune reaction against HIV-1 induced by a candidate vaccine against AIDS. *Nature*, 1988;332:728–731.
24. Corey L, McElrath MJ, Weinhold K, et al. Cytotoxic T cell and neutralizing antibody responses to human immunodeficiency virus type 1 envelope with a combination vaccine regimen. AIDS Vaccine Evaluation Group. *J Infect Dis*, 1998;177:301–309.
25. Pialoux G, Excler JL, Riviere Y, et al. A prime-boost approach to HIV preventive vaccine using a recombinant canarypox virus expressing glycoprotein 160 (MN) followed by a recombinant glycoprotein 160 (MN/LAI). The AGIS Group, and l'Agence Nationale de Recherche sur le SIDA. *AIDS Res Hum Retroviruses*, 1995;11:373–381.
26. Evans TG, Keefer MC, Weinhold KJ, et al. A canarypox vaccine expressing multiple human immunodeficiency virus type 1 genes given alone or with rgp120 elicits broad and durable CD8+ cytotoxic T lymphocyte responses in seronegative volunteers. *J Infect Dis*, 1999;180:290–298.
27. Boyer JD, Cohen AD, Vogt S, et al. Vaccination of seronegative volunteers with a human immunodeficiency virus type 1 env/rev DNA vaccine induces antigen-specific proliferation and lymphocyte production of beta-chemokines. *J Infect Dis*, 2000; 181:476–483.
28. Tubulekas I, Berglund P, Fleeton M, et al. Alphavirus expression vectors and their use as recombinant vaccines: a mini review. *Gene Ther*, 1997;190:191–195.
29. Hariharan MJ, Driver DA, Townsend K, et al. DNA immunization against herpes simplex virus: enhanced efficacy using a Sindbis virus-based vector. *J Virol*, 1998;72:950–958.
30. Herweijer H, Latendresse JS, Williams P, et al. A plasmid-based self-amplifying Sindbis virus vector. *Hum Gene Ther*, 1995;6:1161–1167.
31. Berglund P, Smerdou C, Fleeton MN, et al. Enhancing immune responses using suicidal DNA vaccines. *Nat Biotechnol*, 1998;16:562–565.
32. Sizemore DR, Branstrom AA, Sadoff JC. Attenuated Shigella as a DNA delivery vehicle for DNA-mediated immunization. *Science*, 1995;270: 299–302.
33. Schnell MJ. Viral vectors as potential HIV-1 vaccines. *FEMS Microbiology Letters*, 2001;200: 123–129.
34. Murphy CG, Lucas WT, Means RE, et al. Vaccine protection against simian immunodeficiency virus

by recombinant strains of herpes simplex virus. *J Virol*, 2000;74:7745–7754.

35. Da Costa XJ, Morrison LA, Knipe DM. Comparison of different forms of herpes simplex replication-defective mutant viruses as vaccines in a mouse model of HSV-2 genital infection. *Virology*, 2001;288:256–263.
36. Jayan GC, Cordelier P, Patel C, et al. SV40-derived vectors provide effective transgene expression and inhibition of HIV-1 using constitutive, conditional, and pol III promoters. *Gene Ther*, 2001;8:1033–1042.
37. Strayer DS. SV40-based gene therapy vectors: turning an adversary into a friend. *Curr Opin Mol Ther*, 2000;2:570–578.
38. Strayer DS, Lamothe M, Wei D, et al. Generation of recombinant SV40 vectors for gene transfer. *Methods Mol Biol*, 2001;165:103–117.
39. Prevec L, Christie BS, Laurie KE, et al. Immune response to HIV-1 gag antigens induced by recombinant adenovirus vectors in mice and rhesus macaque monkeys. *J Acquir Immune Defic Syndr Hum Retrovirol*, 1991;4:568–576.
40. Lubeck MD, Natuk RJ, Chengalvala M, et al. Immunogenicity of recombinant adenovirus-human immunodeficiency virus vaccines in chimpanzees following intranasal administration. *AIDS Res Hum Retroviruses*, 1994;10:1443–1449.
41. Lubeck MD, Natuk R, Myagkikh M, et al. Long-term protection of chimpanzees against high-dose HIV-1 challenge induced by immunization. *Nat Med*, 1997;3:651–658.
42. Zolla-Pazner S, Lubeck M, Xu S, et al. Induction of neutralizing antibodies to T-cell line-adapted and primary human immunodeficiency virus type 1 isolates with a prime-boost vaccine regimen in chimpanzees. *J Virol*, 1998;72:1052–1059.
43. Xin KQ, Urabe M, Yang J, et al. A novel recombinant adeno-associated virus vaccine induces a long-term humoral immune response to human immunodeficiency virus. *Hum Gene Ther*, 2001; 12:1047–1061.
44. Guan YJ, Liu HY, Zhu YK, et al. Construction and expression of recombinant adeno-associated HIV-1 virus. *Zhonghua Shi Yan He Lin Chuang Bing Du Xue Za Zhi*, 2000;14:322–324.
45. Buge SL, Murty L, Arora K, et al. Factors associated with slow disease progression in macaques immunized with an adenovirus-simian immunodeficiency virus (SIV) envelope priming-gp120 boosting regimen and challenged vaginally with SIVmac251. *J Virol*, 1999;73:7430–7440.
46. Yoshida T, Okuda K, Xin KQ, et al. Activation of HIV-1-specific immune responses to an HIV-1 vaccine constructed from a replication-defective adenovirus vector using various combinations of immunization protocols. *Clin Exp Immunol*, 2001;124:445–452.
47. Fu TM, Trigona W, Davies ME, et al. Replication-incompetent recombinant adenovirus vector expressing SIV gag elicits robust and effective cellular immune responses in Rhesus Macaques. In: Program of the AIDS Vaccine 2001; Philadelphia, Pennsylvania, USA. September 5–8, 2001. Abstract 37.
48. Seth A, Ourmanov I, Kuroda MJ, et al. Recombinant modified vaccinia virus Ankara-simian immunodeficiency virus *gag pol* elicits cytotoxic T lymphocytes in rhesus monkeys detected by a major histocompatibility complex class I/peptide tetramer. *Proc Natl Acad Sci USA*, 1998;95:10112–10116.
49. Seth A, Ourmanov I, Schmitz JE, et al. Immunization with a modified vaccinia virus expressing simian immunodeficiency virus (SIV) Gag-Pol primes for an anamnestic Gag-specific cytotoxic T-lymphocyte response and is associated with reduction of viremia after SIV challenge. *J Virol*, 2000;74:2502–2509.
50. Barouch DH, Santra S, Kuroda MJ, et al. Reduction of simian-human immunodeficiency virus 89.6P viremia in rhesus monkeys by recombinant modified vaccinia virus Ankara vaccination. *J Virol*, 2001;75:5151–5158.
51. Allen TM, Vogel TU, Fuller DH, et al. Induction of AIDS virus-specific CTL activity in fresh, unstimulated peripheral blood lymphocytes from rhesus macaques vaccinated with a DNA prime/modified vaccinia virus Ankara boost regimen. *J Immunol*, 2000;164:4968–4978.
52. Belyakov IM, Wyatt LS, Ahlers JD, et al. Induction of a mucosal cytotoxic T-lymphocyte response by intrarectal immunization with a replication-deficient recombinant vaccinia virus expressing human immunodeficiency virus 89.6 envelope protein. *J Virol*, 1998;72:8264–8272.
53. Hanke T, Blanchard TJ, Schneider J, et al. Immunogenicities of intravenous and intramuscular administrations of modified vaccinia virus Ankara-based multi-CTL epitope vaccine for human immunodeficiency virus type 1 in mice. *J Gen Virol*, 1998;79(Pt 1):83–90.
54. Hanke T, Neumann VC, Blanchard TJ, et al. Effective induction of HIV-specific CTL by multi-epitope using gene gun in a combined vaccination regime. *Vaccine*, 1999;17:589–596.
55. Hanke T, McMichael AJ. Design and construction of an experimental HIV-1 vaccine for a year-2000 clinical trial in Kenya. *Nat Med*, 2000;6:951–955.
56. Dale CJ, Zhao A, Jones SL, et al. Induction of HIV-1-specific T-helper responses and type 1 cytokine secretion following therapeutic vaccination of macaques with a recombinant fowlpoxvirus co-expressing interferon-gamma. *J Med Primatol*, 2000;29:240–247.

57. Kent SJ, Zhao A, Dale CJ, et al. A recombinant avipoxvirus HIV-1 vaccine expressing interferon-gamma is safe and immunogenic in macaques. *Vaccine*, 2000;18:2250–2256.
58. Radaelli A, Gimelli M, Cremonesi C, et al. Humoral and cell-mediated immunity in rabbits immunized with live non-replicating avipox recombinants expressing the HIV-1SF2 env gene. *Vaccine*, 1994;12:1110–1117.
59. Colmenero P, Berglund P, Kambayashi T, et al. Recombinant Semliki Forest virus vaccine vectors: the route of injection determines the localization of vector RNA and subsequent T cell response. *Gene Ther*, 2001;8:1307–1314.
60. Berglund P, Quesada-Rolander M, Putkonen P, et al. Outcome of immunization of cynomolgus monkeys with recombinant Semliki Forest virus encoding human immunodeficiency virus type 1 envelope protein and challenge with a high dose of SHIV-4 virus. *AIDS Res Hum Retroviruses*, 1997;13:1487–1495.
61. Caley IJ, Betts MR, Davis NL, et al. Venezuelan equine encephalitis virus vectors expressing HIV-1 proteins: vector design strategies for improved vaccine efficacy. *Vaccine*, 1999;17:3124–3135.
62. Caley IJ, Betts MR, Irlbeck DM, et al. Humoral, mucosal, and cellular immunity in response to a human immunodeficiency virus type 1 immunogen expressed by a Venezuelan equine encephalitis virus vaccine vector. *J Virol*, 1997;71:3031–3038.
63. Davis NL, Caley IJ, Brown KW, et al. Vaccination of macaques against pathogenic simian immunodeficiency virus with Venezuelan equine encephalitis virus replicon particles. *J Virol*, 2000;74:371–378.
64. Johnston R, Davis N, Collier M, et al. Intrarectal challenge of macaques immunized with VEE replicon vectors. In: Program of the AIDS Vaccine 2001; September 5–8, 2001; Philadelphia, Pennsylvania, USA. Abstract 41.
65. Crotty S, Miller CJ, Lohman BL, et al. Protection against simian immunodeficiency virus vaginal challenge by using Sabin Poliovirus vectors. *J Virol*, 2001;75:7435–7452.
66. Crotty S, Lohman BL, Lu FX, et al. Mucosal immunization of cynomolgus macaques with two serotypes of live poliovirus vectors expressing simian immunodeficiency virus antigens: stimulation of humoral, mucosal, and cellular immunity. *J Virol*, 1999;73:9485–9495.
67. Anderson MJ, Porter DC, Moldoveanu Z, et al. Characterization of the expression and immunogenicity of poliovirus replicons that encode simian immunodeficiency virus SIVmac239 Gag or envelope SU proteins. *AIDS Res Hum Retroviruses*, 1997;13:53–62.
68. Moldoveanu Z, Porter DC, Lu A, et al. Immune responses induced by administration of encapsidated poliovirus replicons which express HIV-1 gag and envelope proteins. *Vaccine*, 1995;13:1013–1022.
69. Van der Ryst E, Nakasone T, Habel A, et al. Study of the immunogenicity of different recombinant Mengo viruses expressing HIV1 and SIV epitopes. *Res Virol*, 1998;149:5–20.
70. Smith AD, Geisler SC, Chen AA, et al. Human rhinovirus type 14: human immunodeficiency virus type 1 (HIV-1) V3 loop chimeras from a combinatorial library induce potent neutralizing antibody responses against HIV-1. *J Virol*, 1998;72:651–659.
71. Arnold GF, Resnick DA, Smith AD, et al. Chimeric rhinoviruses as tools for vaccine development and characterization of protein epitopes. *Intervirology*, 1996;39:72–78.
72. Halim SS, Collins DN, Ramsingh AI. A therapeutic HIV vaccine using coxsackie-HIV recombinants: a possible new strategy. *AIDS Res Hum Retroviruses*, 2000;16:1551–1558.
73. McGettigan JP, Sarma S, Orenstein JM, et al. Expression and immunogenicity of human immunodeficiency virus type 1 Gag expressed by a replication-competent rhabdovirus-based vaccine vector. *J Virol*, 2001;75:8724–8732.
74. McGettigan JP, Foley HD, Belyakov IM, et al. Rabies virus-based vectors expressing human immunodeficiency virus type 1 (HIV-1) envelope protein induce a strong, cross-reactive cytotoxic T-lymphocyte response against envelope proteins from different HIV-1 isolates. *J Virol*, 2001;75:4430–4434.
75. Schnell MJ, Foley HD, Siler CA, et al. Recombinant rabies virus as potential live-viral vaccines for HIV-1. *Proc Natl Acad Sci USA*, 2000;97:3544–3549.
76. Johnson JE, Schnell MJ, Buonocore L, et al. Specific targeting to CD4+ cells of recombinant vesicular stomatitis viruses encoding human immunodeficiency virus envelope proteins. *J Virol*, 1997;71:5060–5068.
77. Schnell MJ, Johnson JE, Buonocore L, et al. Construction of a novel virus that targets HIV-1-infected cells and controls HIV-1 infection. *Cell*, 1997;90:849–857.
78. Schnell MJ, Buonocore L, Whitt MA, et al. The minimal conserved transcription stop-start signal promotes stable expression of a foreign gene in vesicular stomatitis virus. *J Virol*, 1996;70: 2318–2323.
79. Rose N, Marx P, Luckay A, et al. An effective AIDS vaccine based on live-attenuated vesicular stomatitis virus recombinants. In: Program of the AIDS Vaccine 2001; September 5–8, 2001; Philadelphia, Pennsylvania, USA. Abstract 38.
80. McGettigan J, Foley HD, Sarma S, et al. Rhabdovirus-based vectors expressing HIV-1 Env or Gag induce vigorous cellular responses against HIV-1 and infect efficiently human dendritic cells.

In: Program of the AIDS Vaccine 2001; September 5–8, 2001; Philadelphia, Pennsylvania, USA. Abstract 195.
81. Ferko B, Stasakova J, Sereinig S, et al. Hyperattenuated recombinant influenza A virus nonstructural-protein-encoding vectors induce human immunodeficiency virus type 1 Nef-specific systemic and mucosal immune responses in mice. *J Virol*, 2001;75:8899–8908.
82. Ferko B, Katinger D, Grassauer A, et al. Chimeric influenza virus replicating predominantly in the murine upper respiratory tract induces local immune responses against human immunodeficiency virus type 1 in the genital tract. *J Infect Dis*, 1998;178:1359–1368.
83. Muster T, Ferko B, Klima A, et al. Mucosal model of immunization against human immunodeficiency virus type 1 with a chimeric influenza virus. *J Virol*, 1995;69:6678–6686.
84. Gonzalo RM, Rodriguez D, Garcia-Sastre A, et al. Enhanced CD8+ T cell response to HIV-1 env by combined immunization with influenza and vaccinia virus recombinants. *Vaccine*, 1999;17: 887–892.
85. Huang Z, Krishnamurthy S, Panda A, et al. High-level expression of a foreign gene from the most 3′-proximal locus of a recombinant Newcastle disease virus. *J Gen Virol*, 2001;82(Pt7):1729–1736.
86. Shata MT, Reitz MSJ, DeVico AL, et al. Mucosal and systemic HIV-1 Env-specific CD8(+) T-cells develop after intragastric vaccination with a Salmonella Env DNA vaccine vector. *Vaccine*, 2001;20:623–629.
87. Hone DM, Wu S, Powell RJ, et al. Optimization of live oral Salmonella-HIV-1 vaccine vectors for the induction of HIV-specific mucosal and systemic immune responses. *J Biotechnol*, 1996;44:203–207.
88. Wu S, Pascual DW, Lewis GK, et al. Induction of mucosal and systemic responses against human immunodeficiency virus type 1 glycoprotein 120 in mice after oral immunization with a single dose of a Salmonella-HIV vector. *AIDS Res Hum Retroviruses*, 1997;13:1187–1194.
89. Friedman RS, Frankel FR, Xu Z, et al. Induction of human immunodeficiency virus (HIV)-specific CD8 T-cell responses by Listeria monocytogenes and a hyperattenuated Listeria strain engineered to express HIV antigens. *J Virol*, 2000;74:9987–9993.
90. Rayevskaya MV, Frankel FR. Systemic immunity and mucosal immunity are induced against human immunodeficiency virus Gag protein in mice by a new hyperattenuated strain of Listeria monocytogenes. *J Virol*, 2001;75:2786–2791.
91. Mata M, Paterson Y. Th1 T cell responses to HIV-1 Gag protein delivered by a Listeria monocytogenes vaccine are similar to those induced by endogenous listerial antigens. *J Immunol*, 1999;163:1449–1456.
92. Oggioni MR, Medaglini D, Romano L, et al. Antigenicity and immunogenicity of the V3 domain of HIV type 1 glycoprotein 120 expressed on the surface of *Streptococcus gordonii*. *AIDS Res Hum Retroviruses*, 1999;15:451–459.
93. Di Fabio S, Medaglini D, Rush CM, et al. Vaginal immunization of Cynomolgus monkeys with Streptococcus gordonii expressing HIV-1 and HPV 16 antigens. *Vaccine*, 1998;16:485–492.
94. Aldovini A, Young RA. Humoral and cell-mediated immune responses to live recombinant BCG-HIV vaccines. *Nature*, 1991;351:479–482.
95. Lim EM, Lagranderie M, Le Grand R, et al. Recombinant *Mycobacterium bovis* BCG producing the N-terminal half of SIVmac251 Env antigen induces neutralizing antibodies and cytotoxic T lymphocyte responses in mice and guinea pigs. *AIDS Res Hum Retroviruses*, 1997;13:1573–1581.
96. Honda M, Matsuo K, Nakasone T, et al. Protective immune responses induced by secretion of a chimeric soluble protein from a recombinant *Mycobacterium bovis* Bacillus Calmette-Guerin vector candidate vaccine for human immunodeficiency virus type 1 in small animals. *Proc Natl Acad Sci USA*, 1995;92:10693–10697.
97. Lagranderie M, Winter N, Balazuc AM, et al. A cocktail of *Mycobacterium bovis* BCG recombinants expressing the SIV Nef, Env, and Gag antigens induces antibody and cytotoxic responses in mice vaccinated by different mucosal routes. *AIDS Res Hum Retroviruses*, 1998;14:1625–1633.
98. Lagranderie M, Balazuc AM, Gicquel B, et al. Oral immunization with recombinant *Mycobacterium bovis* BCG simian immunodeficiency virus nef induces local and systemic cytotoxic T-lymphocyte responses in mice. *J Virol*, 1997;71:2303–2309.
99. Shata MT, Hone DM. Vaccination with a shigella DNA vaccine vector induces antigen-specific CD8(+) T cells and antiviral protective immunity. *J Virol*, 2001;75:9665–9670.
100. Voss G, Villinger F. Adjuvanted vaccine strategies and live vector approaches for the prevention of AIDS. *AIDS*, 2000;14(suppl 3):S153–S165.
101. O'Hagan DT, MacKichan ML, Singh M. Recent developments in adjuvants for vaccines against infectious diseases. *Biomol Eng*, 2001;18: 69–85.
102. Gorse GJ, Rogers JH, Perry JE, et al. HIV-1 recombinant gp160 vaccine induced antibodies in serum and saliva. The NIAID AIDS Vaccine Clinical Trials Network. *Vaccine*, 1995;13: 209–214.
103. Gorse GJ, Corey L, Patel GB, et al. HIV-1MN recombinant glycoprotein 160 vaccine-induced cellular and humoral immunity boosted by HIV-1MN recombinant glycoprotein 120 vaccine. NIAID AIDS Vaccine Evaluation Group. *AIDS Res Hum Retroviruses*, 1999;15:115–132.

104. Berman PW, Groopman JE, Gregory T, et al. Human immunodeficiency virus type 1 challenge of chimpanzees immunized with recombinant envelope glycoprotein gp120. *Proc Natl Acad Sci USA*, 1988;85:5200–5204.
105. Berman PW, Huang W, Riddle L, et al. Development of bivalent (B/E) vaccines able to neutralize CCR5-dependent viruses from the United States and Thailand. *Virology*, 1999;265:1–9.
106. Goebel FD, Mannhalter JW, Belshe RB, et al. Recombinant gp160 as a therapeutic vaccine for HIV-infection: results of a large randomized, controlled trial. European Multinational IMMUNO AIDS Vaccine Study Group. *AIDS*, 1999;13: 1461–1468.
107. Sandstrom E, Wahren B. Therapeutic immunisation with recombinant gp160 in HIV-1 infection: a randomised double-blind placebo-controlled trial. Nordic VAC-04 Study Group. *Lancet*, 1999;353: 1735–1742.
108. Leibl H, Tomasits R, Bruhl P, et al. Humoral and cellular immunity induced by antigens adjuvanted with colloidal iron hydroxide. *Vaccine*, 1999; 17:1017–1023.
109. Verschoor EJ, Davis D, van Gils M, et al. Efforts to broaden HIV-1-specific immunity by boosting with heterologous peptides or envelope protein and the influence of prior exposure to virus. *J Med Primatol*, 1999;28:224–232.
110. Verschoor EJ, Mooij P, Oostermeijer H, et al. Comparison of immunity generated by nucleic acid-, MF59-, and ISCOM-formulated human immunodeficiency virus type 1 vaccines in Rhesus macaques: evidence for viral clearance. *J Virol*, 1999;73:3292–3300.
111. Cano CA. The multi-epitope polypeptide approach in HIV-1 vaccine development. *Genet Anal*, 1999;15:149–153.
112. Raya NE, Quintana D, Carrazana Y, et al. A prime-boost regime that combines Montanide ISA720 and Alhydrogel to induce antibodies against the HIV-1 derived multiepitope polypeptide TAB9. *Vaccine*, 1999;17:2646–2650.
113. Mooij P, van der Kolk M, Bogers WM, et al. A clinically relevant HIV-1 subunit vaccine protects rhesus macaques from in vivo passaged simian-human immunodeficiency virus infection. *AIDS*, 1998;12:F15–F22.
114. Moore A, McCarthy L, Mills KH. The adjuvant combination monophosphoryl lipid A and QS21 switches T cell responses induced with a soluble recombinant HIV protein from Th2 to Th1. *Vaccine*, 1999;17:2517–2527.
115. Gokulan K, Khare S, Rao DN. Increase in the immunogenicity of HIV peptide antigens by chemical linkage to polytuftsin (TKPR40). *DNA Cell Biol*, 1999;18:623–630.
116. Frey A, Mantis N, Kozlowski PA, et al. Immunization of mice with peptomers covalently coupled to aluminum oxide nanoparticles. *Vaccine*, 1999;17:3007–3019.
117. Chang JS, Choi MJ, Kim TY, et al. Immunogenicity of synthetic HIV-1 V3 loop peptides by MPL adjuvanted pH-sensitive liposomes. *Vaccine*, 1999;17:1540–1548.
118. Ross T, Green T, Xu Y, et al. Enhanced humoral immune responses elicited by DNA vaccination with HIV gp120-C3d fusion constructs. In: Program of the AIDS Vaccine 2001; September 5–8, 2001; Philadelphia, Pennsylvania, USA. Abstract 181.
119. O'Hagan D, Singh M, Ugozzoli M, et al. Induction of potent immune responses by cationic microparticles with adsorbed human immunodeficiency virus DNA vaccines. *J Virol*, 2001;75:9037–9043.
120. Denis-Mize KS, Dupuis M, MacKichan ML, et al. Plasmid DNA adsorbed onto cationic microparticles mediates target gene expression and antigen presentation by dendritic cells. *Gene Ther*, 2000;7:2105–2112.
121. Kazzaz J, Neidleman J, Singh M, et al. Novel anionic microparticles are a potent adjuvant for the induction of cytotoxic T lymphocytes against recombinant p55 gag from HIV-1. *J Control Release*, 2000;67:347–356.
122. O'Hagan DT, Ugozzoli M, Barackman J, et al. Microparticles in MF59, a potent adjuvant combination for a recombinant protein vaccine against HIV-1. *Vaccine*, 2000;18:1793–1801.
123. Kaneko H, Bednarek I, Wierzbicki A, et al. Oral DNA vaccination promotes mucosal and systemic immune responses to HIV envelope glycoprotein. *Virology*, 2000;267:8–16.
124. Briones M, O'Hagan D, Singh M, et al. Induction of potent immune responses by cationic microparticles with adsorbed HIV DNA vaccines. In: Program of the AIDS Vaccine 2001; September 5–8, 2001; Philadelphia, Pennsylvania, USA. Abstract 183.
125. Singh M, Briones M, Ott G, et al. Cationic microparticles: A potent delivery system for DNA vaccines. *Proc Natl Acad Sci USA*, 2000;97: 811–816.
126. Singh M, Vajdy M, Gardner J, et al. Mucosal immunization with HIV-1 gag DNA on cationic microparticles prolongs gene expression and enhances local and systemic immunity. *Vaccine*, 2001;20:594–602.
127. Cleland JL, Lim A, Daugherty A, et al. Development of a single-shot subunit vaccine for HIV-1. 5. programmable in vivo autoboost and long lasting neutralizing response. *J Pharm Sci*, 1998;87:1489–1495.
128. Lambert JS, Keefer M, Mulligan MJ, et al. A Phase I safety and immunogenicity trial of

UBI microparticulate monovalent HIV-1 MN oral peptide immunogen with parenteral boost in HIV-1 seronegative human subjects. *Vaccine*, 2001;19: 3033–3042.

129. Esparza J, Bhamarapravati N. Accelerating the development and future availability of HIV-1 vaccines: why, when, where, and how? *Lancet*, 2000;355:2061–2066.
130. UNAIDS. *AIDS epidemic update – December 2000.* Geneva, Switzerland: UNAIDS, 2000.
131. UNAIDS, WHO. Global HIV/AIDS & STD Surveillance. Epidemiological fact sheets by country. Available at: http://www.who.int/emc-hiv/fact_sheets/. Accessed: February 7, 2002.
132. Salminen MO, Johansson B, Sonnerborg A, et al. Full-length sequence of an Ethiopian human immunodeficiency virus type 1 (HIV-1) isolate of genetic subtype C. *AIDS Res Hum Retroviruses*, 1996;12:1329–1339.
133. Gao F, Robertson DL, Carruthers CD, et al. A comprehensive panel of near-full-length clones and reference sequences for non-subtype B isolates of human immunodeficiency virus type 1. *J Virol*, 1998;72:5680–5698.
134. Lole KS, Bollinger RC, Paranjape RS, et al. Full-length human immunodeficiency virus type 1 genomes from subtype C-infected seroconverters in India, with evidence of intersubtype recombination. *J Virol*, 1999;73:152–160.
135. Novitsky VA, Montano MA, McLane MF, et al. Molecular cloning and phylogenetic analysis of HIV-1 subtype C: a set of 23 full-length clones from Botswana. *J Virol*, 1999;73:4427–4432.
136. Mochizuki N, Otsuka N, Matsuo K, et al. An infectious DNA clone of HIV type 1 subtype C. *AIDS Res Hum Retroviruses*, 1999;15:1321–1324.
137. Ndung'u T, Renjifo B, Novitsky VA, et al. Molecular cloning and biological characterization of full-length HIV-1 subtype C from Botswana. *Virology*, 2000;278:390–399.
138. Rodenburg CM, Li Y, Trask SA, et al. Near full-length clones and reference sequences for subtype C isolates of HIV type 1 from three different continents. *AIDS Res Hum Retroviruses*, 2001;17:161–168.
139. van Harmelen J, Williamson C, Kim B, et al. Characterization of full length HIV-1 subtype C sequences from South Africa. *AIDS Res Hum Retroviruses*, 2001;17:1527–1531.
140. Novitsky V, Smith UR, Gilbert P, et al. HIV-1 subtype C molecular phylogeny: consensus sequence for an AIDS vaccine design. *J Virol*, 76(11):5435–5451.
141. Choudhury S, Montano MA, Womack C, et al. Increased promoter diversity reveals a complex phylogeny of human immunodeficiency virus type 1 subtype C in India. *J Hum Virol*, 2000;3:35–43.
142. Ward FE, Tuan S, Haynes BF. Analysis of HLA frequencies in population cohorts for design of HLA-based HIV vaccines. In: Korber B, ed. *HIV Molecular Immunology Database*. Los Alamos, NM: 1995: IV-10–IV-16.
143. Haynes BF. HIV vaccines: where we are and where we are going. *Lancet*, 1996;348:933–937.
144. Haynes BF, Yasutomi Y, Torres JV, et al. Use of synthetic peptides in primates to induce high-titered neutralizing antibodies and MHC class I-restricted cytotoxic T cells against acquired immunodeficiency syndrome retroviruses: an HLA-based vaccine strategy. *Trans Assoc Am Physicians*, 1993;106:33–41.
145. Kaslow RA, Rivers C, Tang J, et al. Polymorphisms in HLA class I genes associated with both favorable prognosis of human immunodeficiency virus (HIV) type 1 infection and positive cytotoxic T-lymphocyte responses to ALVAC-HIV recombinant canarypox vaccines. *J Virol*, 2001;75: 8681–8689.
146. Klein MR, van Baalen CA, Holwerda AM, et al. Kinetics of Gag-specific cytotoxic T lymphocyte responses during the clinical course of HIV-1 infection: a longitudinal analysis of rapid progressors and long-term asymptomatics. *J Exp Med*, 1995;181:1365–1372.
147. Goulder PJ, Addo MM, Altfeld MA, et al. Rapid definition of five novel HLA-A*3002-restricted human immunodeficiency virus-specific cytotoxic T-lymphocyte epitopes by Elispot and intracellular cytokine staining assays. *J Virol*, 2001;75: 1339–1347.
148. Goulder PJ, Brander C, Annamalai K, et al. Differential narrow focusing of immunodominant human immunodeficiency virus gag-specific cytotoxic T-lymphocyte responses in infected African and caucasoid adults and children. *J Virol*, 2000;74:5679–5690.
149. Barouch DH, Santra S, Schmitz JE, et al. Control of viremia and prevention of clinical AIDS in rhesus monkeys by cytokine-augmented DNA vaccination. *Science*, 2000;290:486–492.
150. Patterson LJ, Peng B, Abimiku AG, et al. Cross-protection in NYVAC-HIV-1-immunized/HIV-2-challenged but not in NYVAC-HIV-2-immunized/SHIV-challenged rhesus macaques. *AIDS*, 2000; 14:2445–2455.
151. Gallimore A, Hombach J, Dumrese T, et al. A protective cytotoxic T cell response to a subdominant epitope is influenced by the stability of the MHC class I/peptide complex and the overall spectrum of viral peptides generated within infected cells. *Eur J Immunol*, 1998;28:3301–3311.
152. Gallimore A, Dumrese T, Hengartner H, et al. Protective immunity does not correlate with the hierarchy of virus-specific cytotoxic T cell responses to naturally processed peptides. *J Exp Med*, 1998;187:1647–1657.

153. Korber B, Brander C, Haynes B, eds. *HIV Molecular Immunology 2000.* Los Alamos, New Mexico, USA: Los Alamos National Laboratory, Theoretical Biology and Biophysics, 2000.
154. Cao H, Kanki P, Sankale JL, et al. Cytotoxic T-lymphocyte cross-reactivity among different human immunodeficiency virus type 1 clades: implications for vaccine development. *J Virol*, 1997;71:8615–8623.
155. Durali D, Morvan J, Letourneur F, et al. Cross-reactions between the cytotoxic T-lymphocyte responses of human immunodeficiency virus-infected African and European patients. *J Virol*, 1998;72:3547–3553.
156. Betts MR, Krowka J, Santamaria C, et al. Cross-clade human immunodeficiency virus (HIV)-specific cytotoxic T-lymphocyte responses in HIV-infected Zambians. *J Virol*, 1997;71:8908–8911.
157. McAdam S, Kaleebu P, Krausa P, et al. Cross-clade recognition of p55 by cytotoxic T lymphocytes in HIV-1 infection. *AIDS*, 1998;12:571–579.
158. Wilson SE, Pedersen SL, Kunich JC, et al. Cross-clade envelope glycoprotein 160-specific CD8+ cytotoxic T lymphocyte responses in early HIV type 1 clade B infection. *AIDS Res Hum Retroviruses*, 1998;14:925–937.
159. Rowland-Jones SL, Dong T, Fowke KR, et al. Cytotoxic T cell responses to multiple conserved HIV epitopes in HIV-resistant prostitutes in Nairobi. *J Clin Invest*, 1998;102:1758–1765.
160. Dorrell L, Dong T, Ogg GS, et al. Distinct recognition of non-clade B human immunodeficiency virus type 1 epitopes by cytotoxic T lymphocytes generated from donors infected in Africa. *J Virol*, 1999;73:1708–1714.
161. Cao H, Mani I, Vincent R, et al. Cellular immunity to human immunodeficiency virus type 1 (HIV-1) clades: relevance to HIV-1 vaccine trials in Uganda. *J Infect Dis*, 2000;182:1350–1356.
162. Novitsky V, Rybak N, McLane MF, et al. Identification of human immunodeficiency virus type 1 subtype C Gag-, Tat-, Rev-, and Nef-specific Elispot-based cytotoxic T-lymphocyte responses for AIDS vaccine design. *J Virol*, 2001;75:9210–9228.
163. Addo MM, Altfeld M, Rosenberg ES, et al. Analysis of cytotoxic T-lymphocyte (CTL) responses against the regulatory HIV-1 proteins Rev and Tat in HIV-1-infected individuals and identification of novel CTL epitopes. Poster presented at the XIII International Conference on AIDS; July 9–14, 2000; Durban, South Africa.
164. Addo MM, Altfeld M, Rosenberg ES, et al. The HIV-1 regulatory proteins Tat and Rev are frequently targeted by cytotoxic T lymphocytes derived from HIV-1-infected individuals. *Proc Natl Acad Sci USA*, 2001;98:1781–1786.

HIV-1 Vaccine Testing, Trial Design, and Ethics

*Peter B. Gilbert and †José Esparza

*Department of Biostatistics, University of Washington, Seattle, Washington, USA.
†WHO-UNAIDS HIV Vaccine Initiative, World Health Organization, Geneva, Switzerland.

It is likely that widely accessible vaccines to prevent clinically significant HIV-1 infection, used in concert with educational prevention programs will be important for stemming the HIV-1 epidemic in Africa (1). Development of effective HIV-1 vaccines requires global cooperative research in basic science, clinical applied science, and large-scale efficacy trials. In this chapter, scientific and ethical issues in vaccine testing and trial design are discussed with an emphasis on efficacy trials. Scientific issues covered include preclinical and early clinical testing; endpoints for measuring vaccine efficacy (with an emphasis on the use of HIV-1 viral load as a surrogate marker for reduced HIV-1 disease or infectiousness); monitoring clinical, biologic, and behavioral outcomes; evaluating correlates of protective immunity; and evaluating the dependency of vaccine efficacy on genotypic and phenotypic characteristics of HIV-1. Ethical issues are addressed through a discussion of the recommendations contained in the document issued in 2000 by UNAIDS. Issues in the design of HIV-1 vaccine trials in infants (2) or in trials of therapeutic vaccines administered after infection by HIV-1, however, will not be discussed.

PRECLINICAL TESTING

Basic and applied research are both necessary efforts to identify and prepare promising vaccine candidates for clinical testing. Through basic research, scientists discover or design putative protective antigens and construct appropriate expression and delivery systems (3,4). Preclinical applied research aims initially to demonstrate immunogenicity of candidate vaccines in small animals. If a vaccine candidate shows promise, then a reliable and validated process for reproducing stable, highly purified, and well-characterized lots of the vaccine can be established. This process must adhere to good manufacturing practice (GMP) guidelines (4). Next, safety, immunogenicity, and tolerability of the vaccine at high doses must be demonstrated in nonhuman primates. Taken together the latter studies provide the requisite data for applying to regulatory agencies for clearance to begin human testing (5).

Prior to or simultaneous with early human testing, vaccine challenge studies may be conducted in nonhuman primates to evaluate protective efficacy against infection, persistent infection, or disease, as measured by reductions in viral burden in various compartments. The best available nonhuman primate models are rhesus macaques challenged with simian immunodeficiency virus (SIV) or a chimeric simian–human immunodeficiency virus (SHIV) (6–13), and chimpanzees challenged with HIV-1 (14–18). To maximize the relevance of animal experiments for human vaccine development, it is important that study parameters such as the genotype/phenotype and dose of the challenge virus, the schedule of vaccination, the assays for measuring immune response, and the viral-load surrogate endpoints are standardized across trials (19). In addition, studies that use reagents, adjuvants, vaccine products, immune response assays, and exposure routes that are as comparable as possible to those used in early human trials produce data that are most pertinent to vaccine development. For example, an animal study that might be maximally relevant for vaccine development in Africa would use a subtype C vaccine to prevent disease in macaques vaginally challenged repeatedly over a several week period following immunization with a low dose of moderately pathogenic subtype C SHIV with genotypic and phenotypic characteristics matching those of HIV-1 strains found in contemporary African populations. In addition, animal challenge trials of large scope are needed with several vaccines compared in dozens of monkeys followed for 1 to 4 years. Such large studies can provide enough statistical information to usefully rank the candidate vaccines by their potential efficacy to prevent clinical disease (20–22).

Animal challenge experiments are also useful for investigating correlates of protective immunity and the degree to which protective efficacy depends on the genotype and/or phenotype of the challenge virus. Although such correlates analyses are valuable for formulating scientific principles for guiding vaccine design, it is important to recognize that correlates of protection identified in animal studies may not predict efficacy of the same vaccines in human trials (23,24). Only after an efficacy trial shows some level of protection in humans can the validity of animal models for predicting vaccine efficacy in humans be established (25). Furthermore, demonstrating vaccine protection in animal models and elucidating its mechanisms should not be viewed as prerequisites for moving vaccines into efficacy trials in humans, since several efficacious vaccines have been developed without use of a predictive animal model (23,25).

EARLY CLINICAL TESTING

Conventionally, clinical testing of vaccines is divided into three phases (26–28). Involving a small number of healthy adult volunteers at low risk for HIV-1 infection (for example, 10–80 participants), Phase I trials evaluate safety and immune responses of a vaccine candidate(s) that may be administered in a dose-escalating regimen. A preliminary assessment of the optimal immunogen concentration, schedule, and route of administration may also be made. Phase II trials evaluate the same parameters in a larger number of volunteers (for example, 100–500 participants) that includes people at higher risk for HIV-1 infection. If the vaccine appears safe, based on comparisons of rates at which similar adverse events occur among vaccinees and placebo recipients, and prespecified milestones for sufficiently strong vaccine-induced immune responses are met, then the vaccine can be tested in Phase III efficacy trials involving thousands of high-risk volunteers. Demonstration of efficacy in a Phase III trial leads to an application for licensure of the vaccine for distribution. Trials in the three phases have typically taken from 12–18 months, 2 years, and 4 years, respectively. The urgent need for an HIV-1 vaccine suggests that these time schedules should be accelerated (29).

More than 60 candidate HIV-1 vaccines have been studied in Phase I trials, representing 11 immunization strategies and nine HIV-1 antigens (29) (Table 1). Five of these

TABLE 1. HIV-1 Vaccine Approaches that have Undergone Clinical Testing

Vaccince concept	Approach	Phase I trial references (year first published trial)	Phase II trial references (year first published trial)
Envelope protein	Produced in vitro, recombinant protein subunits (e.g., monomeric or oligomeric gp160 and gp120) aim to induce antibody responses and $CD4^+$ T-cells	30–43 (1991)	63–65 (2000)
Synthetic peptide	Produced in vitro, synthetic peptides (e.g., based on the V3 loop sequence) aim to induce immune responses to specific epitopes (e.g., those in conserved regions), in either or both MHC class I or II pathways, and often contain multiple epitopes	34,44–51 (1991)	
Poxvirus	Live recombinant poxvirus vaccines mimic antigen presentation that occurs during natural viral infection, and aim to induce MHC class I-restricted $CD8^+$ CTL responses. Multiple HIV-1 antigens (e.g., gp41, gp120 gag, pol, nef) can be simultaneously expressed in a natural form		
Canarypox	Canarypox is an *Avipoxvirus* that enters mammalian cells to express its gene products, but cannot replicate in non-avian cells (preventing it from spreading beyond the site of inoculation)	52–54 (1995)	
Vaccinia	Vaccinia is the virus used in live attenuated smallpox vaccine, and may spread beyond the site of inoculation, which can potentially cause disease	55–61 (1991)	
Salmonella	Attenuated strains of *Salmonella enterica typhimurium* aim to express HIV-1 antigens that elicit CTL responses and antibody responses, and can stimulate the inductive sites of the mucosal immune system	In progress	
DNA	Recombinant DNA technology produces nucleic acid vectors which allow direct inoculation of DNA for expression of multiple genes encoding vaccine antigens, and aim to induce both antibody and MHC class I-restricted $CD8^+$ CTL responses, as well as mucosal immune responses	In progress	
Pox virus prime plus subunit boost	Priming with a pox virus vaccine and boosting with a subunit aims to optimally induce both $CD8^+$ CTL responses and antibody responses	40,52,54,55,58, 60,62 (1993)	64,66 (2000)
DNA prime plus vector boost	Priming with a DNA vaccine and boosting with a subunit aims to optimally induce $CD8^+$ CTL responses, mucosal immune responses, and antibody responses	In progress	

TABLE 2. HIV-1 Vaccine Candidates that have Undergone Phase II or III Clinical Testing

Vaccine antigen	HIV-1 Subtype	Vaccine developer	Site of study	Trial reference
Phase II				
Envelope protein				
rgp120	B	Genentech	United States	63,64
rgp120	B	Chiron/Biocine	United States	64,65
Pox virus prime plus subunit boost				
vCP205 Canarypox gp120, TM gp41, gag, protease + rgp120	B	Pasteur-Merieux Connaught + VaxGen	United States	64,66
vCP205 Canarypox gp120, TM gp41, gag, protease, nef, pol + rgp120	B	Pasteur-Merieux Connaught + VaxGen	United States	
vCP205 Canarypox gp120, TM gp41, gag, protease, nef, pol + rgp120	B + E	Pasteur-Merieux Connaught + VaxGen	Thailand	
vCP205 Canarypox gp120, TM gp41, gag, protease, nef, pol + rgp120	E	Pasteur-Merieux Connaught + Chiron/Biocine	Thailand	
vCP205 Canarypox gp120, TM gp41, gag, protease, nef, pol + oligomeric rgp140	E	Aventis-Pasteur	Thailand	
vCP205 Canarypox gp120, TM gp41, gag, protease + rgp120	B	Pasteur-Merieux Connaught + VaxGen	Brazil/Haiti/ Trinidad	
vCP205 Canarypox gp120, TM gp41, gag, protease, nef, pol + rgp120	B	Pasteur-Merieux Connaught + VaxGen	Brazil/Haiti/ Trinidad	
Phase III				
Envelope protein				
rgp120 bivalent	B + B	VaxGen	United States	In progress
rgp120 bivalent	B + E	VaxGen	Thailand	In progress

candidates have undergone Phase II testing, and two are currently in Phase III (Table 2). Given the number of vaccine immunogens and expression/delivery approaches under development and the possibility of combined vaccines, there could be a considerable number of potentially efficacious vaccine candidates available for testing in clinical trials. This suggests that comparative, head-to-head Phase I and II trials of several vaccine candidates—using standardized assays, reagents, and protocols—are needed to rapidly screen and prioritize candidates for efficacy trials. Vaccines that induce the strongest, broadest, and most durable immune responses relevant to a certain population (for example, relevant for heterosexual exposure and for local HLA haplotypes and HIV-1 variants), and are sufficiently safe and practical, would move into efficacy trials.

Uncertainties about the clinical significance of immune response assays should not unduly inhibit the rate at which vaccines enter Phase II and III testing. Until data from prior efficacy trials show some protective efficacy of a similar vaccine, any determinations of milestones for the quality and quantity of immune responses needed to trigger efficacy trials are somewhat arbitrary. Consequently, it may be unwarranted to set the immunogenicity hurdles at the levels elicited by natural HIV-1 infection. Weaker levels, as well as responses of a different kind and duration from those seen in natural infection, may suffice; there are many examples of vaccines that are protective despite failing on one or more of these criteria (25). Furthermore, many efficacious vaccines (for example, those for influenza, pertussis, gastroenteritis, and typhoid fever) have been found without knowledge of an immune response correlate. In addition, failure to detect the targeted level of an immune response may reflect the limited sensitivity of the employed assay rather than the lack of induction of a protective immune response (67,68). Since the capability of laboratory assays to predict protection is unknown until efficacy trials are conducted, results from such assays should not unduly inhibit the progression to efficacy testing for vaccine candidates (63).

VACCINE PREPAREDNESS STUDIES

Before an efficacy trial can begin, vaccine preparedness studies (VPSs) are conducted to identify feasible HIV-1 vaccine trial sites and to establish the needed infrastructure. Carrying out Phase I and II trials in regions within Africa could facilitate this process and accelerate the development of an HIV-1 vaccine specific for the epidemic on this continent. Objectives of a VPS conducted within any given region include measuring the incidence and genotype and/or phenotype of HIV-1, measuring the frequencies of HLA haplotypes, assessing the willingness of high-risk individuals to participate and the factors affecting this decision, assessing the population's knowledge of concepts associated with vaccine trials (a prerequisite for proper informed consent), the feasibility of and strategies for recruiting and retaining volunteers, and assessing the risk behavior in the population before and after educational and counseling processes are in place (69–76). In addition to rating favorably on the above criteria, a region suitable for inclusion in a vaccine trial must have adequate infrastructure in terms of clinical, laboratory, and data management facilities and administrative and communication structures. Furthermore, many nonscientific issues, including garnering political commitment and community involvement and ensuring the protection of human rights and the maintenance of ethical standards, must receive attention in the planning stages. To expedite vaccine development, VPSs should be ongoing in many regions within Africa, regardless of whether a candidate vaccine is nearing readiness for efficacy testing. Within Africa, VPSs have taken place (or are taking place) in Botswana, Côte d'Ivoire, Ethiopia, Kenya, Senegal, South Africa, Tanzania, Uganda, Zambia, and Zimbabwe, and, hopefully, will begin soon in other African nations with relatively high HIV-1 incidence.

SCIENTIFIC ISSUES IN HIV-1 VACCINE EFFICACY TRIALS

In classically designed Phase III efficacy trials, thousands of volunteers at high risk for HIV-1 infection are randomized to receive vaccine or placebo and are monitored for HIV-1 infection at regular intervals for 2–6 years. Randomization and blinding ensure that known and unknown factors associated with the risk for HIV-1 infection and disease will be balanced, on average, between individuals assigned vaccine and individuals assigned placebo. These mechanisms are vital because they allow observed differences among the groups to be attributed to the vaccine, which is critical for the results of trials to be widely accepted, and for licensure of vaccines that show efficacy.

Study Population

For efficacy trials planned for Africa, it is useful to first consider some general criteria for the selection of the study population before discussing potential African vaccine trial cohorts. First, efficacy trials should be conducted in populations within which the vaccine will be used once efficacy is shown. Second, the trial should be in populations with high incidence of HIV-1 infection, to minimize the required number of volunteers. Third, a population that can be reliably followed for a minimum period of 3 to 5 years after the last immunization is needed (77). This will minimize bias in the assessment of vaccine efficacy and maximize statistical power. Possible cohorts for efficacy trials in Africa include commercial sex workers, members of the military, attendees of sexually transmitted disease (STD) clinics, truck drivers, and young employees of large companies.

Sample Size

The calculation of sample size depends primarily on the incidence of the primary endpoint measuring vaccine efficacy, the duration of study-follow-up, the rate of retention of trial participants, and the minimum level of vaccine efficacy that the investigators wish to detect. Vaccine efficacy is calculated as one minus the ratio of the rates of endpoint occurrence among the vaccine and placebo groups (78–80). A first step in calculating the sample size is determining the minimum value of the lower 95% confidence limit about the "true" vaccine efficacy parameter that makes the trial result useful. "Useful" could be defined by framing a decision-rule for applying for vaccine licensure, or by allowing sufficiently precise evaluations of correlates of vaccine protection. For instance, a vaccine with minimum 30% vaccine efficacy to prevent persistent HIV-1 infection may be worth licensing in some African countries (81), and a minimum 10% to 20% vaccine efficacy can be enough for correlates analyses to be well powered.

Figure 1 shows the sample size per group needed to detect a 30% or a 10% lower 95% confidence limit for the specified level of vaccine efficacy, given a 5% or 15% annual loss to follow-up rate. For example, assuming a 1-year recruitment period, 3 years of follow-up, 5% of volunteers lost to follow-up per year, and a 3% annual HIV-1 incidence in the placebo group, 2,500 participants are needed to detect a minimum 60% vaccine efficacy with 30% lower 95% confidence bound. The first Phase III trial in a developing country (Thailand), ongoing at the time of this writing, was designed approximately with these characteristics (63).

Education of communities and counseling of volunteers about high-risk behaviors imply that the observed HIV-1 incidence in a vaccine trial may be less than expected from the initial sample-size calculation. This is true also because the heterogeneity in biologic susceptibility and in exposure to HIV-1 among trial participants imply that a relatively large number of infections is expected to occur early during the vaccination series, before maximal vaccine-induced immunity is conferred. To accommodate the possibility of underestimating the sample size, the monitoring of trials should allow for the enrollment of additional sites (perhaps in multiple countries) and/or an extension of the follow-up period.

Endpoints

Ideally, analysis of the study endpoints of an efficacy trial provides an unequivocal indication of the clinical impact the vaccine will have in a public health program. To meet this objective, study endpoints must be carefully chosen. Thus, it is useful to consider the main outcome measures sought in Phase III trials and issues relevant to their selection.

Safety Outcomes

Vaccine trial participants are regularly monitored for clinical and laboratory evidence of vaccine reactogenicity (82), and all safety data are monitored periodically by an independent data and safety monitoring

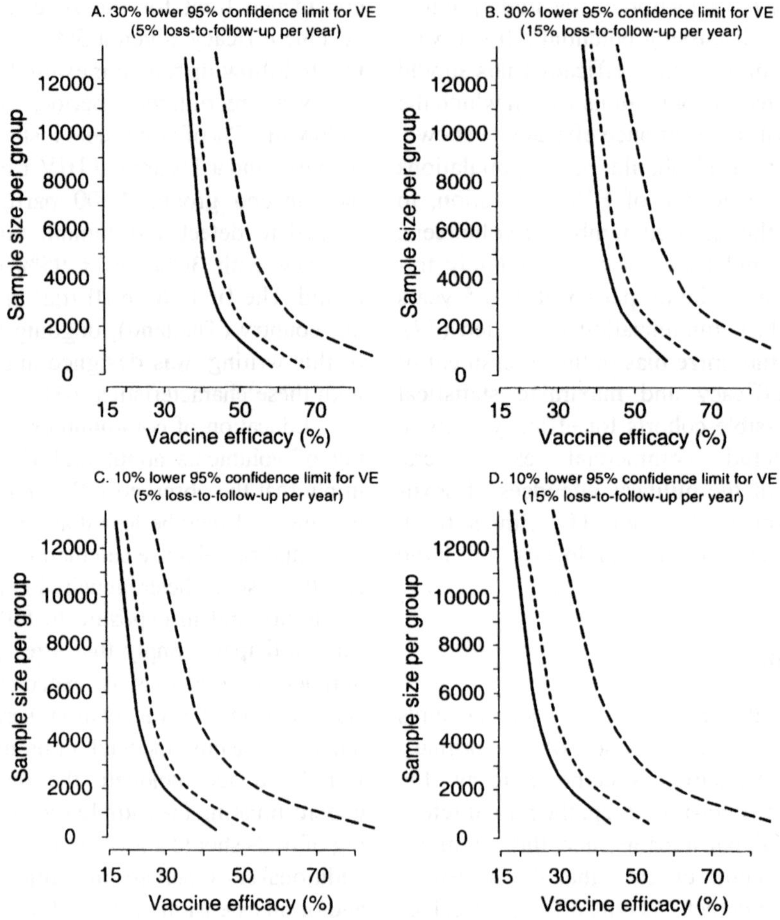

FIGURE 1. Sample size requirement versus the level of vaccine efficacy (VE) to prevent persistent HIV-1 infection, for a classically designed Phase III efficacy trial with two groups (vaccine versus placebo), a 1-year recruitment period, and a 3-year follow-up period. If the estimated VE equals the value given on the *x*-axis, then the lower 95% confidence limit for the true VE is 30% in A and B, and 10% in C and D. A and C assume 5% of volunteers are annually lost to follow-up, while B and D assume 15% of volunteers are annually lost to follow-up. For each graph, the solid curve represents a 5% increase in HIV-1 infections per year, the short-dash curve represents a 3% increase in HIV-1 infections per year, and the long-dash curve represents a 1% increase in HIV-1 infections per year.

board (83). Long-term follow-up for safety outcomes is important (for a minimum of 5 years after volunteers receive the last immunization or, ideally, for a lifetime). In addition to following a uniform list of safety measures, including clinical exams, systemic and local vaccine reactions, and laboratory measures such as $CD4^+$ T-cell counts and levels of serum alanine aminotransaminase (ALT) and creatine, adverse outcomes that may arise connected with particular features of the vaccine should be monitored (22). For example, because in-vitro assays have suggested that vaccines based on envelope proteins could theoretically enhance susceptibility to HIV-1 infection through antibody-dependent enhancement (ADE), it is important that the presence of ADE and its possible association with disease be assessed in trials such as VaxGen's current Phase III trials of bivalent envelope vaccines (84–91). Because of human and viral genetic heterogeneity, it may be important to conduct safety testing for some vaccines in the location of the planned efficacy trial as well as in the country where the vaccine was initially developed.

HIV-1 Infection

In each of the two ongoing Phase III trials, the primary endpoint is HIV-1 infection, measured by enzyme-linked immunosorbent assay (ELISA) and immunoblot (63). The risk of an HIV-1–uninfected volunteer testing positive on HIV-1 serologic tests is minimal. This follows because (*i*) only a small fraction of recipients of the tested vaccines have been found to test positive on the most commonly used commercial ELISA assays, due to the limited ability of the assays to detect anti-gp120 antibodies, and (*ii*) for those who do test positive on an ELISA assay, the required confirmatory immunoblot will not be scored positive unless bands other than for gp120 are shown (63). Since vaccine-induced immunity may increase as more doses are administered over a several-month vaccination period or may wane toward the end of the follow-up period as a result of loss of immunity or changes in antigenic characteristics of the circulating HIV-1 variants, the level of vaccine efficacy to prevent HIV-1 infection may change over time. Therefore, it is important to estimate how vaccine efficacy changes over time, a demand that can be satisfied using available statistical methods (92,93).

Since there is no precedent for effective viral vaccines that prevent initial infection [although some effective vaccines prevent persistent infection by eliminating virus within a short period after the initial infection (22)], persistent infection may be a more realistically preventable endpoint than initial infection. Furthermore, some observations suggest that it may be easier to develop an HIV-1 vaccine that prevents disease and/or reduces secondary transmission than to develop a vaccine to prevent persistent infection. Historically, most effective vaccines have worked by allowing persistent infection but preventing disease and/or reducing secondary transmission (25,94–97). HIV-1's biologic properties include the maintenance of function (for example, the ability to infect cells and replicate) even though it undergoes a large number of mutations and recombinations, an ability to evade immune responses by establishing latent infection, and the progressive destruction of the $CD4^+$ T-cells it infects (98). In addition, a recent survey of 20 vaginal and intrarectal pathogenic challenge studies of nonlive attenuated vaccines in macaques showed a 0% (0 of 34) rate of protection against infection and a 38% (13 of 34) rate of protection against disease, as measured by reductions in viral load (99). These animal studies support that vaccines that reduce viral load may be more readily developed than vaccines that prevent infection, though it should be recognized that most of the experiments used highly infectious challenge doses which seriously limited their utility as models for evaluating protection against infection. Nevertheless, the above factors strongly argue the importance of considering postinfection endpoints that measure efficacy against disease progression and/or infectiousness.

Viral Load

To evaluate definitively the effects of a vaccine on HIV-1 disease progression, it would be necessary to compare clinical endpoints such as AIDS-defining illnesses and death between vaccinees and placebo recipients, which would require at least 5–10 years of follow-up. Given the length of this interval, and other complicating factors that will be described, it may be more practical to base inferences on a biologic marker (for example, viral load or $CD4^+$ T-cell count) that is an approximate "surrogate" for clinical disease outcomes. The two ongoing Phase III trials use plasma RNA viral load as the surrogate marker for disease progression (63). Lower levels of viral load in plasma, lymph, or other compartments may imply that the vaccine slows or arrests the progression of HIV-1 disease to AIDS (100–102). There are, however, at least three qualifications to drawing this inference from viral load data. One qualification would be that a vaccine effect to reduce viral load levels may not predict a vaccine effect to reduce the rate of clinical progression (103–105). This problem, common to many clinical trials in many diseases (104–115), may occur if the vaccine effect on clinical progression is mediated through biologic mechanisms other than the suppression of virus levels as measured by the employed assay. Another qualification to drawing conclusions from viral load data would be that some trial participants may receive antiretroviral therapy shortly after a diagnosis of HIV-1 infection. The therapy will likely suppress virus levels in many recipients and may modulate the interaction between viral replication and immune responses, thereby complicating the evaluation of the vaccine's effect on viral load (116,117). For infected participants who receive antiretroviral therapy, it should be possible to obtain at least two viral-load measurements prior to the initiation of therapy. In trials where antiretroviral therapies are commonly received, it may be prudent to focus analyses on these measurements (as the ongoing trials do), rather than on longitudinal viral-load determinations that are influenced by suppressive antiretroviral therapy. Where viral-load trajectories are analyzed, the confounding and biasing influences of antiretroviral therapies can be minimized by using a combined disease endpoint defined by either viral load above a failure threshold or prior initiation of antiretroviral therapy (2).

A third qualification to deriving too much from viral load data alone pertains to the potential for selection bias in comparisons of viral-load distributions of infected vaccinees and infected placebo recipients. Because comparison groups are selected by the postrandomization event of HIV-1 infection, such comparison is prone to selection bias, with a key potential source the partial efficacy of the vaccine to prevent infection. If the vaccine is completely ineffective at reducing the susceptibility to HIV-1 infection, then no selection bias is expected, as the event HIV-1 infection does not select subjects differentially in the two groups. However, if the vaccine prevents HIV-1 infections in a fraction of trial participants, then the two groups are no longer comparable. For example, the vaccine may confer some protection against mildly virulent strains but allow infections with highly virulent viruses which establish relatively high viremia levels. As a result, highly virulent viruses will be overrepresented in infected vaccinees relative to infected placebo recipients. The effect will be a selective shifting upwards of the viral load distribution in vaccinees, which could incorrectly suggest that the vaccine causes enhanced viremia. If this potential selection bias is not appreciated, then a partially efficacious vaccine with no adverse effects could mistakenly be thought to increase viral burden. This false conclusion could slow or destroy continued development of a safe, partially efficacious vaccine. Sensitivity analyses may be useful for distinguishing between selection bias and a true vaccine effect on viral load.

Levels of HIV-1 RNA in cervicovaginal secretions or in seminal plasma may also be useful surrogate endpoints for measuring vaccine efficacy to reduce secondary transmission. This assessment is one of the most important objectives of an efficacy trial, since a vaccine that induces herd immunity by interrupting the chain of transmission may have the most dramatic effect on infection rates in a community, as is the case for vaccines against *Haemophilus influenzae* type B, hepatitis B, measles, poliovirus, and rubella (67).

It is difficult to measure vaccine effects on secondary transmission directly, because it requires the monitoring of individuals exposed to vaccinees who become infected. This can be accomplished by augmenting classic Phase III designs by enrolling steady sexual partners of infected trial participants and monitoring them for HIV-1 infection. These "augmented partners" designs are of value because they permit an estimation of the vaccine's efficacy to reduce susceptibility to infection and to reduce infectiousness (97, 118,119). The challenge to implementing these designs is recruiting enough steady sexual partners to achieve high statistical power. In situations where the HIV-1 infection rate from infected participants to their partners is 30% or greater, these designs may be feasible, requiring enrollment of steady partners of at least one-third of the infected participants (119). Cluster-randomized trials, in which groups of individuals, such as villages, factories, or STD clinic attendees, are randomized to receive vaccine or placebo, provide a second approach to obtaining direct information on vaccine efficacy to reduce infectiousness (97,118,120). Although these designs potentially enjoy advantages of administrative convenience, simplifications of ethical considerations, and improved compliance, they are challenging to carry out because a much larger total sample size is required than for a classic individual-level randomized trial (2). Feasibility evaluations within VPSs are needed to identify locations and cohorts where these innovative designs can be feasibly employed.

Because more resources are required for augmented partners and cluster-randomized designs, classic designs that can only study vaccine effects on infectiousness indirectly through surrogate markers have received more attention. A viral load surrogate endpoint can be defined as the time from infection until virus levels rise above a prespecified failure threshold. To the extent possible, the selected threshold should reflect knowledge about predictiveness for clinical progression and/or secondary transmission. For example, data from a discordant-couples study in Uganda suggested that suppression of plasma viral load to a level below 1,500 copies/ml dramatically reduces the risk of secondary transmission (121). Because the predictiveness of a chosen threshold can only be partially validated, it is important to conduct sensitivity analyses that consider a range of threshold definitions (122).

In classically designed efficacy trials, the use of antiretroviral therapies and the need for long-term follow-up make it difficult to assess the validity of surrogate markers. However, observations of significant vaccine effects on viral-load endpoints in classic trials could prompt subsequent Phase III augmented partners or cluster-randomized trials that can confirm surrogate markers (123).

Behavioral Outcomes

For interpreting trial results, it is important to measure types and frequencies of risk behavior prior to, at initiation, and during the trial (73). In addition to questionnaire data, risk-behavior information can potentially be measured through more objective markers such as the incidence of STDs. Risk behavior data are useful for calculating vaccine efficacy in risk-group strata (for example, women exposed by heterosexual contact or men exposed by sex with men), and for adjusting vaccine efficacy estimates for the mode and quantity of risk behavior.

Vaccination may modify risk behavior, either by increasing it (for example, by instilling in vaccine recipients an unvalidated belief in its protectiveness) or by decreasing it (for example, as a result of risk behavior counseling provided to vaccinees). Since behavioral effects of vaccination can strongly affect the overall public health impact of a partially biologically efficacious vaccine, it is important to evaluate the effect of vaccination on vaccinees' risk behavior (124). The aggregate biologic and behavioral effects of an HIV-1 vaccine could be assessed directly in an open-label trial, but this design would not give an estimate of biologic vaccine efficacy. A four-arm trial with arms blinded vaccine, placebo, open-label vaccine, and nothing (or an open-label control, such as a vaccine for a different disease) would facilitate simultaneous evaluation of a vaccine's biologic and behavioral effects (2).

Immune Responses

Humoral, cellular, and mucosal immune responses of trial participants are monitored periodically throughout an efficacy trial, with the timing of sampling designed to study the kinetics of responses to each immunization. Measured humoral responses include antibodies to HIV-1 proteins or neutralization of viral infection (125) and measured cellular responses include the proliferation of T-cells and the induction of $CD8^+$ T-lymphocytes against target cells expressing HIV-1 antigens (126). The immune response assays should be sensitive, quantitative, practical, reproducible, and applicable to stored samples.

Matching the Vaccine to Local Viruses

Although the ultimate goal is to develop broadly protective vaccines, many individuals involved in HIV-1 vaccine development think that the vaccine immunogen(s) should be matched to local predominant HIV-1 genotypes and phenotypes as closely as possible, to provide the best chance of conferring protection. In sub-Saharan Africa, this means that vaccines based on the highly prevalent subtype C, and secondly on subtypes A and D (and perhaps on intersubtype recombinants), should be prioritized. This approach would be valid even in places like Uganda or Kenya where few subtype C viruses have yet been found, since recent migratory patterns of subtype C suggest that its prevalence may increase in these places (127,128). Ultimately, trials that simultaneously test a matched vaccine and a mismatched vaccine may be required to determine finally whether matching is necessary.

Most HIV-1 vaccines that have undergone clinical testing are designed with subtype B antigens (Table 2). It is encouraging to note that during the past 2 years several candidate vaccines against subtypes found in Africa have begun development (29). It should be borne in mind that genetic subtype may not be the most immunologically relevant classification system; it may be more important to match vaccine immunogens on other aspects of HIV-1 variation. For example, a vaccine could be designed to contain the dominant CTL epitopes of a local population, taking into account the distribution of HLA types (129). Alternatively, the genetic sequence of the immunogen could be selected as the consensus sequence observed in a sample of local viruses from recent seroconvertors.

Correlates of Vaccine Protection

An important objective of vaccine efficacy trials is to assess why a vaccine fails to confer protection in some participants, as this knowledge would guide reformulation efforts (130–132). Possible reasons for vaccine failure include an exposure prior to receipt of all immunizations or by a route different than the targeted one, the need for a more potent adjuvant, the absence of an immune response, or an exposure to an HIV-1 strain antigenically divergent from an immunogen represented in the vaccine. This section addresses the latter two possibilities.

Correlates of Protective Immunity

A correlate of protective immunity can be identified as an immune response that is overrepresented in participants who are vaccinated but are uninfected or undiseased as compared against its representation among participants who are vaccinated but are infected or diseased. The analysis can be conducted efficiently by matching 2–6 uninfected vaccinees to each infected vaccinee (123). For a correlate to provide clues about protective mechanisms, it is necessary to see some degree of protective efficacy. There are several caveats of analyses to identify correlates of protective immunity. As examples, the correlates for one HIV-1 vaccine may not be correlates for other HIV-1 vaccines (133–136), the increased presence of an immune response in uninfected or undiseased vaccinees may be a marker for intrinsic susceptibility but not have a causal relationship with protection (33, 124), and multiple immune responses may be needed to confer protection. Since a single assay may not be able to measure a multifaceted protective immune response, multiple assays and multivariate analysis techniques may be needed to identify multifactorial correlates of protective immunity.

Viral Correlates of Vaccine Protection (Sieve Analysis)

An important question guiding vaccine formulation is whether, and if so, how, vaccine protection against infection and disease varies with genotypic and phenotypic characteristics of HIV-1. Analysis of this question by comparing characteristics of HIV-1 isolates between infected vaccinees and infected placebo recipients has been called "sieve analysis" (130,137). These analyses provide guides to the selection of the appropriate strain or strains to incorporate in a vaccine and to whether a multivalent vaccine is needed. High dimensional data statistical techniques can be used to search for viral genotypes or phenotypes that predict differential vaccine efficacy to prevent infection or decrease viral load (138,139). In such exploratory analyses, there are a large number of ways to classify genotypic or phenotypic HIV-1 variation into categories that are potentially meaningful immunologically. Examples include HIV-1 subtype, R4 or R5 CD4 coreceptor use phenotype, serotype defined by binding or neutralizing antibody titers to the vaccine strain(s), and CTL epitopes, defined by HLA-restricted dissimilarity in CTL epitopes between the infecting strain and the vaccine strain. If differential protection by a viral determinant is detected, it is of interest to assess possible modulating host factors. Age, risk group, nutritional status, HLA type, or the absence of a particular immune response may help explain the observed selective vaccine protection.

It is important to carry out both exploratory and confirmatory correlates analyses. The main purpose of exploratory analyses is to use data on protective efficacy rates to guide the choice of viral attributes on which to focus vaccine design. These analyses are especially helpful since alternative guides—animal data, laboratory data from humans, or scientific theory—are not based directly on empirical clinical data for humans (137,140). Immune responses and viral features found to be most associated with protective efficacy in exploratory analyses are identified as putative correlates of protection, which can be further investigated through animal challenge trials, basic laboratory research, and iterative vaccine trials in humans. In this light, correlates analyses in efficacy trials are seen to be integral to the entire process of vaccine development. The capability of efficacy trials to identify correlates drives the interest in carrying them out even when only low levels of vaccine efficacy may be anticipated.

Prespecified hypotheses about correlates of protective immunity or immunotypic HIV-1 classification factors can be confirmed or rejected in efficacy trials. When earlier studies show a reasonably sensitive assay or a viral determinant to be predictive of protection (as indicated by better reactivity against homologous viruses than against viruses divergent in the particular viral feature), it may be appropriate to design a trial specifically for confirming the potential correlate of protection.

ETHICAL ISSUES IN HIV-1 VACCINE EFFICACY TRIALS

The ethical issues surrounding the conduct of HIV-1 vaccine trials have been the subject of recent intense debates (141), resulting in a guidance document issued by UNAIDS (142). The document presents 18 points on the critical elements that must be considered when planning and implementing HIV-1 vaccine trials.

General recommendations include a recognition of the ethical responsibility of the international community to promote the development of a much needed HIV-1 vaccine, using collaborative partnerships between the different players and leading to capacity building in host countries where many of the trials will be conducted—and where future vaccines urgently need to be deployed. The document emphasizes the importance of good science and appropriate research protocols and indicates that "countries may choose, for valid scientific and public health reasons, to conduct any phase (I, II or III) within their populations, if they are able to ensure sufficient scientific infrastructure and sufficient ethical safeguards." This approach requires the existence of appropriate mechanisms to conduct independent and competent scientific and ethical review, with strategies in place to overcome conditions that could result in the exploitation of vulnerable populations.

The UNAIDS guidance document strongly recommends involving community representatives, early and in a sustained manner, in the design, development, implementation, and distribution of research results. Leadership from medical, religious, and other local groups will likely be key to the successful conduct of vaccine trials.

Independent and informed consent should be obtained from each individual while he or she is being screened for eligibility to participate in an HIV-1 vaccine trial and before he or she is actually enrolled in a trial. Appropriate risk reduction counseling and access to prevention methods should be provided to all vaccine trial participants, and a plan to monitor the adequacy of the informed consent process and of risk-reduction interventions should be integral parts of the trial design.

Care and treatment for HIV-1 and AIDS and its associated complications should be provided to participants who become infected during the trial, with the ideal response being to provide the "best proven therapy" and the minimum response being to provide the highest level of care attainable in the host country within the context of the research project. A comprehensive care package should be agreed upon through a host/community/sponsor dialogue that reaches consensus prior to the initiation of the trial. It has been argued that the availability of treatment for infected volunteers may have not only ethical but also scientific benefits, by helping ensure long-term follow-up of infected participants. Use of a uniform treatment regimen would aid comparability of clinical, immunologic, and virologic outcomes across vaccinees and placebo recipients.

Last, but not least, any vaccine demonstrated to be safe and effective should be made available as soon as possible to all participants in the trial in which it was tested, as well as to other populations at high risk of HIV-1 infection. Plans should be developed at the initial stages of HIV-1 vaccine development to ensure such availability.

CONCLUSION

To minimize the time until practical and efficacious HIV-1 vaccines are widely distributed in Africa, it is important to continually conduct vaccine preparedness studies and standardized, comparative Phase I and II screening trials of multiple vaccines in many cohorts and geographic locations, and to move the most promising candidates rapidly into efficacy trials. Efficacy trials are needed to assess vaccine effects on susceptibility to HIV-1 infection, infectiousness, disease progression, and behavior, as well as to identify immune and viral correlates of vaccine protection. Since evaluations of vaccine efficacy on infectiousness and disease will rely to some degree on unvalidated surrogate markers such as viral load, it is important to follow HIV-1–infected participants long enough to observe clinical outcomes. Given the differences among populations in many factors including host and viral genetics and routes of exposure, it is also important to carry out multiple, parallel efficacy trials in several high-incidence regions and populations in Africa and elsewhere (67). The success of these trials should be judged not by demonstration of efficacy but by the contribution they make toward the identification of efficacious vaccines (29,123). The ethical validity of an HIV-1 vaccine trial will ultimately depend on the balance of risks and benefits of the proposed research and on its relevance to its intended population, including access to a vaccine that has been shown to be safe and effective.

REFERENCES

1. Esparza J, Bhamarapravati N. Accelerating the development and future availability of HIV-1 vaccines: why, when, where, and how. *Lancet*, 2000; 355:2061–2066.
2. Gilbert PB. Some statistical issues in the design of HIV-1 vaccine and treatment trials. *Stat Meth Med Res*, 2000;9:207–229.
3. Anonymous. Stages of vaccine development. In: Mitchell VS, Philipose NM, and Sanford JP, eds. *The Children's Vaccine Initiative Achieving the Vision*. Washington DC: National Academy Press, 1993:109–127.
4. Gregersen JP. Vaccine development: The long road from initial idea to product licensure. In: Levine MM, Woodrow GC, Kaper JB, and Cobon GS, eds. *New Generation Vaccines*. New York: Marcel Dekker, Inc., 1997:1165–1177.
5. Folkers GK, Fauci AS. The role of US government agencies in vaccine research and development. *Nat Med*, 1998;4(Suppl):491–494.
6. Schultz AM, Hu SL. Primate models for HIV-1 vaccines. *AIDS*, 1993;7(Suppl 1):S161–S170.
7. Li J, Lord CI, Haseltine W, et al. Infection of cynomolgus monkeys with a chimeric HIV-1/SIVmac virus that expresses the HIV-1 envelope glycoproteins. *J Acquir Immune Defic Syndr*, 1992;5:639–646.
8. Almond N, Heeney JL. AIDS vaccine development in primate models. *AIDS*, 1998;12(Suppl A): S133–S140.
9. Hulskotte EGJ, Geretti AM, Osterhaus AD. Towards an HIV-1 vaccine: lessons learned from studies in macaque models. *Vaccine*, 1998;16:904–915.
10. Heeney J, Akerblom L, Barnett S, et al. HIV-1 vaccine induced immune responses which correlate with protection from SHIV-1 infection: Compiled preclinical efficacy data from trials with 10 different HIV-1 vaccine candidates. *Immunol Lett*, 1999;66:189–195.
11. Mascola JR, Lewis MG, Stiegler G, et al. Protection of Macaques against pathogenic simian/human immunodeficiency virus 89.6PD by passive transfer of neutralizing antibodies. *J Virol*, 1999;73: 4009–4018.
12. Barouch DH, Santra S, Schmitz JE, et al. Control of viremia and prevention of clinical AIDS in Rhesus monkeys by cytokine-augmented DNA vaccination. *Science*, 2000;290:486–492.
13. Mascola JR, Stiegler G, VanCott TC, et al. Protection of macaques against vaginal transmission of a pathogenic HIV-1/SIV chimeric virus by passive infusion of neutralizing antibodies. *Nat Med*, 2000;6:207–210.
14. Alter JH, Eichberg JW, Masur H, et al. Transmission of HTLV-III infection from human plasma to chimpanzees: an animal model for AIDS. *Science*, 1984;226:549–552.
15. Francis DP, Feorino PM, Broderson JR, et al. Infection of chimpanzees with lymphadenopathy associated virus. *Lancet*, 1984;11:1276–1277.
16. Gadjusek DC, Amyx HL, Gibbs CR Jr, et al. Transmission experiments with human T-lymphotropic retroviruses and human AIDS tissue. *Lancet*, 1984;1:1415–1416.
17. Murthy KK, Cobb EK, Rouse SR, et al. Correlates of protective immunity against HIV-1 infection in immunized chimpanzees. *Immunol Lett*, 1996; 51:121–124.
18. Murthy KK, Cobb EK, Rouse SR, et al. Active and passive immunization against HIV type 1 infection in chimpanzees. *AIDS Res Hum Retroviruses*, 1998;14(Suppl 3):S271–S276.
19. Graham BS, Sawyer LA, Walker MC, et al. Interface between animal models and clinical Phase I trials workshop: Conference summary. *AIDS Res Hum Retroviruses*, 1995;11:1305–1306.
20. Rida W, Meier P, Stevens C. Design and implementation of HIV vaccine efficacy trials: a working group summary. *AIDS Res Hum Retroviruses*, 1993;9:S59–S63.
21. Hirsch VM, Goldstein S, Hynes NA, et al. Prolonged clinical latency and survival of macaques given a whole inactivated simian immunodeficiency virus vaccine. *J Infect Dis*, 1994;170: 51–59.
22. Graham BS, Karzon DT. AIDS vaccine development. In: Merigan TC Jr., Bartlett JG, Bolognesi D,

eds. *Textbook of AIDS Medicine, Second Edition.* Baltimore: Williams and Wilkins, 1998:689–724.

23. Offit PA. Rotaviruses: Immunological determinants of protection against infection and disease. *Adv Virus Res*, 1994;44:161–202.
24. Corey L, Ashley R, Sekulovich R, et al. Lack of efficacy of a vaccine containing recombinant gD2 and gB2 antigens in MF59 adjuvant for the prevention of genital HSV-2 acquisition. In: 37th Interscience Conference on Antimicrobial Agents and Chemotherapy; 1997; Toronto. LB-28.
25. Clements-Mann ML. Lessons for AIDS vaccine development from non-AIDS vaccines. *AIDS Res Hum Retroviruses*, 1998;14(Suppl 3):S197–S203.
26. Fast PE, Walker MC. Human trials of experimental AIDS vaccines. *AIDS*, 1993;7(Suppl 1):S147–S159.
27. Belshe RB, Clements ML, Keefer MC, et al. Interpreting serodiagnostic test results in the 1990s: social risks of HIV vaccine studies in uninfected volunteers. *Ann Intern Med*, 1994;121:584–589.
28. Karzon DT. Preventive vaccines. In: Broder S, Merigan TC Jr, Bolognesi D, eds. *Textbook of AIDS medicine.* Baltimore: Williams and Wilkins, 1994: 667–692.
29. International AIDS Vaccine Initiative. Scientific blueprint 2000: Accelerating global efforts in AIDS vaccine development. July, 2000. Available at: www.iavi.org. Accessed: February 2, 2002.
30. Dolin R, Graham BS, Greenberg SB, et al. The safety and immunogenicity of a human immunodeficiency virus type 1 (HIV-1) recombinant gp160 candidate vaccine in humans: NIAID AIDS Vaccine Clinical Trials Network. *Ann Intern Med*, 1991;114:119–127.
31. Schwartz DH, Gorse G, Clements ML, et al. Induction of HIV-1-neutralising and syncytium-inhibiting antibodies in uninfected recipients of HIV-1IIIB rgp120 subunit vaccine. *Lancet*, 1993;342:69–73.
32. Berman PW. Development of bivalent rgp120 vaccines to prevent HIV type 1 infection. *AIDS Res Hum Retroviruses*, 1998;14(Suppl 3):S277–S289.
33. Berman PW, Huang W, Riddle L, et al. Development of bivalent (B/E) vaccines able to neutralize CCR5-dependent viruses from the United States and Thailand. *Virology*, 1999;265:1–9.
34. Kahn JO, Sinangil F, Baenziger J, et al. Clinical and immunologic responses to human immunodeficiency virus (HIV) type 1 (SF2) gp120 subunit vaccine combined with MF59 adjuvant with or without muramyl tripeptide dipalmitoyl phosphatidylethanolamine in non-HIV-infected human volunteers. *J Infect Dis*, 1994;170:1288–1291.
35. Belshe RB, Graham BS, Keefer MC, et al. Neutralizing antibodies to HIV-1 in seronegative volunteers immunized with recombinant gp120 from the MN strain of HIV-1: NIAID AIDS Vaccine Clinical Trials Network. *JAMA*, 1994;272: 475–480.
36. Keefer MC, Graham BS, Belshe RB, et al. Studies of high doses of a human immunodeficiency virus type 1 recombinant glycoprotein 160 candidate vaccine in HIV type 1-seronegative humans. *AIDS Res Hum Retroviruses*, 1994;10:1713–1723.
37. Keefer MC, Graham BS, McElrath MJ, et al. Safety and immunogenicity of Env 2–3, a human immunodeficiency virus type 1 candidate vaccine, in combination with a novel adjuvant, MTP-PE/MF59. *AIDS Res Hum Retroviruses*, 1996;12:683–693.
38. Kovacs JA, Vasudevachari MB, Easter M, et al. Induction of humoral and cell-mediated anti-human immunodeficiency virus (HIV) responses in HIV sero-negative volunteers by immunization with recombinant gp160. *J Clin Invest*, 1993;92: 919–928.
39. Gorse GJ, Rogers JH, Perry JE, et al. HIV-1 recombinant gp160 vaccine induced antibodies in serum and saliva. *Vaccine*, 1995;13:209–214.
40. Corey L, McElrath J, Weinhold K, et al. Cytotoxic T cell and neutralizing antibody responses to human immunodeficiency virus type 1 envelope with a combination vaccine regimen. *J Infect Dis*, 1998;177:301–309.
41. Gorse GJ, McElrath MJ, Matthews TJ, et al. Modulation of immunologic responses to HIV-1 MN recombinant gp160 vaccine by dose and schedule of administration. *Vaccine*, 1998;16:493–506.
42. Salmon-Ceron D, Excler JL, Sicard D, et al. Safety and immunogenicity of a recombinant HIV type 1 glycoprotein 160 boosted by a V3 synthetic peptide in HIV-negative volunteers. *AIDS Res Hum Retroviruses*, 1995;11:1479–1486.
43. Wintsch J, Chaignat CL, Braun DG, et al. Safety and immunogenicity of a genetically engineered human immunodeficiency virus vaccine. *J Infect Dis*, 1991;163:219–225.
44. Sarin PS, Mora CA, Naylor PH, et al. HIV-1 p17 synthetic peptide vaccine HGP-30: induction of immune response in human subjects and preliminary evidence of protection against HIV challenge in SCID mice. *Cell Mol Biol*, 1995;41:401–407.
45. Kahn JO, Stites DP, Siliciano J, et al. A phase I study of HGP-30, a 30 amino acid subunit of the human immunodeficiency virus (HIV) p17 synthetic peptide analogue sub-unit vaccine in seronegative subjects. *AIDS Res Hum Retroviruses*, 1992;8:1321–1325.
46. Naylor PH, Sztein MB, Wada S, et al. Preclinical and clinical studies on immunogenicity and safety of the HIV-1 p17-based synthetic peptide AIDS vaccine: HGP-30-KLH. *Int J Immunopharmacol*, 1991;13(Suppl 1):117–127.
47. Gorse GJ, Keefer MC, Belshe RB, et al. A dose-ranging study of a prototype synthetic HIV-1 MN

V3 branched peptide vaccine. *J Infect Dis*, 1996;173:330–339.

48. Li D, Forrest BD, Li Z, et al. International clinical trials of HIV vaccines. II. Phase I trial of an HIV-1 synthetic peptide vaccine evaluating an accelerated immunization schedule in Yunnan, China. *Asian Pac J Allergy Immunol*, 1997;15:105–113.
49. Kelleher AD, Emery S, Cunningham P, et al. Safety and immunogenicity of UBI HIV-1 (MN) octameric V3 peptide vaccine administered by subcutaneous injection. *AIDS Res Hum Retroviruses*, 1997;13:29–32.
50. Phanuphak P, Teeratakulpixrn S, Sarangbin S, et al. International clinical trials of HIV vaccines. I. Phase I trial of an HIV-1 synthetic peptide vaccine in Bangkok, Thailand. *Asian Pac J Allergy Immunol*, 1997;15:41–48.
51. Rubinstein A, Goldstein H, Pettoello-Mantovani M, et al. Safety and immunogenicity of a V3 loop synthetic peptide conjugated to purified protein derivative in HIV-seronegative volunteers. *AIDS*, 1995; 9:243–251.
52. Pialoux G, Excler JL, Riviere Y, et al. A prime-boost approach to HIV preventive vaccine using a recombinant canarypox virus expressing glycoprotein 160 (MN) followed by a recombinant glycoprotein 160 (MN/LAI). *AIDS Res Hum Retroviruses*, 1995;11:373–381.
53. Fleury B, Janvier G, Pialoux G, et al. Memory cytotoxic T lymphocyte responses in human immunodeficiency virus type 1 (HIV-1)-negative volunteers immunized with a recombinant canarypox expressing gp160 of HIV-1 and boosted with a recombinant gp160. *J Infect Dis*, 1996;174:734–738.
54. Clements-Mann ML, Weinhold K, Matthews TJ, et al. Immune responses to human immunodeficiency virus (HIV) type 1 induced by canarypox expressing HIV-1 MN gp120, HIV-1 SF-2 recombinant gp120, or both vaccines in seronegative adults. *J Infect Dis*, 1998;177:1230–1246.
55. Graham BS, Matthews TJ, Belshe RB, et al. Augmentation of human immunodeficiency virus type 1 neutralizing antibody by priming with gp160 recombinant vaccinia and boosting with rgp160 in vaccinia-naïve adults: the NIAID AIDS Vaccine Clinical Trials Network. *J Infect Dis*, 1993;167: 533–537.
56. Zagury D, Bernard J, Cheynier R, et al. A group specific anamnestic immune reaction a gainst HIV-1 induced by a candidate vaccine against AIDS. *Nature*, 1988;332:728–731.
57. Cooney EL, Collier AC, Greenberg PD, et al. Safety of and immunological response to a recombinant vaccinia virus vaccine expressing HIV envelope glycoprotein. *Lancet*, 1991;337:567–572.
58. Cooney EL, McElrath MJ, Corey L, et al. Enhanced immunity to human immunodeficiency virus (HIV) envelope elicited by a combined vaccine regimen consisting of priming with a vaccinia recombinant expressing HIV envelope and boosting with gp160 protein. *Proc Natl Acad Sci USA*, 1993;90: 1882–1886.
59. Graham BS, Belshe RB, Clements ML, et al. Vaccination of vaccinia-naive adults with human immunodeficiency virus type 1 gp160 recombinant vaccinia virus in a blinded, controlled, randomized clinical trial: the AIDS Vaccine Clinical Trials Network. *J Infect Dis*, 1993;166:244–252.
60. Graham BS, Gorse GJ, Schwartz DH, et al. Determinants of antibody response after recombinant gp160 boosting in vaccinia-naive volunteers primed with gp160-recombinant vaccinia virus. *J Infect Dis*, 1994;170:782–786.
61. Stanhope PE, Clements ML, Siliciano RF. Human $CD4^+$ cytolytic T lymphocyte responses to a human immunodeficiency virus type 1 gp160 subunit vaccine. *J Infect Dis*, 1993;168:92–100.
62. Evans TG, Keefer MC, Weinhold KJ, et al. A canarypox vaccine expressing multiple human immunodeficiency virus type 1 genes given alone or with rgp120 elicits broad and durable $CD8^+$ cytotoxic T lymphocyte responses in seronegative volunteers. *J Infect Dis*, 1999;180:290–298.
63. Francis DP, Gregory T, McElrath MJ, et al. Advancing AIDSVAX to phase 3: safety, immunogenicity, and plans for phase 3. *AIDS Res Hum Retroviruses*, 1998;14(Suppl 3):S325–S331.
64. McElrath JM, Corey L, Montefiori D, et al. A Phase II study of two HIV type 1 envelope vaccines, comparing their immunogenicity in populations at risk for acquiring HIV type 1 infection. *AIDS Res Hum Retroviruses*, 2000;16:907–919.
65. Nitayaphan S, Khamboonruang C, Sirisophana N, et al. A phase I/II trial of HIV SF2 gp120/MF59 vaccine in seronegative Thais. AFRIMS-RIHES Vaccine Evaluation Group. Armed Forces Research Institute of Medical Sciences and the Research Institute for Health Sciences. *Vaccine*, 2000;18: 1448–1455.
66. Belshe RB, Stevens C, Gorse GJ, et al. Safety and immunogenicity of a canarypox-vectored human immunodeficiency virus type 1 vaccine with or without gp120: a phase 2 study in higher- and lower-risk volunteers. *J Infect Dis*, 2001;183:1343–1352.
67. Clements ML. Clinical trials of human immunodeficiency virus vaccines. In: DeVita VT Jr., Hellman S, Rosenberg SA, eds. *AIDS, Etiology, Diagnosis, Treatment and Prevention, Fourth ed.* New York: Lippincott-Raven, 1997:617–626.
68. Berman PW, Murthy KK, Wrin T, et al. Protection of MN-rgp120 immunized chimpanzees from heterologous infection with a primary isolate of human immunodeficiency virus type 1. *J Infect Dis*, 1996;173:52–59.

69. Esparza J, Osmanov S, Kallings LO, et al. Planning for HIV vaccine trials: the World Health Organization perspective. *AIDS*, 1991;5:S159.
70. Hoff R. Preparations of HIV vaccine trials: Moving from baseline studies to efficacy trials. *AIDS Res Hum Retroviruses*, 1994;10:S191–S193.
71. Hoth DF, Bolognesi DP, Corey L, et al. HIV vaccine development: A progress report. *Ann Intern Med*, 1994;121:603.
72. Sheon AR. Overview: HIV vaccine feasibility studies. *AIDS Res Hum Retroviruses*, 1994;10(Suppl 2): S195–S196.
73. Temoshok LR. Behavioral research contributions to planning and conducting HIV vaccine efficacy studies. *AIDS Res Hum Retroviruses*, 1994;10(Suppl 2): S277–S280.
74. Vermund SH, Schultz AM, Hoff R. Prevention of HIV with vaccines. *Curr Opin Infect Dis*, 1994;7:82–94.
75. Hoff R, Lawrence DN. Preparation for HIV vaccine efficacy trials. *Antibiot Chemother*, 1996;48: 155–160.
76. Koblin BA, Heagerty P, Sheon A, et al. Readiness of high-risk populations in the HIV Network for Prevention Trials to participate in HIV vaccine efficacy trials in the United States. *AIDS*, 1998; 12:785–793.
77. Hayes R. Design of human immunodeficiency virus intervention trials in developing countries. *J R Stat Soc [Ser A]*, 1998;161(Part 2):251–263.
78. Smith PG, Rodrigues LC, Fine PEM. Assessment of the protective efficacy of vaccines against common diseases using case-control and cohort studies. *Int J Epidemiol*, 1984;13:87–93.
79. Hoff R, Barker LF. Trial objectives and end points for measuring the efficacy of HIV vaccines. *Infect Agents Dis*, 1995;4:95–101.
80. Rida WN, Lawrence DL. Prophylactic HIV vaccine trials. In: Finkelstein DM, Schoenfeld DA, eds. *AIDS clinical trials: Guidelines for design and analysis*. New York: Wiley-Liss, 1995:319–348.
81. Anderson RM, Garnett GP. Low-efficacy HIV vaccines; potential for community-based intervention programmes. *Lancet*, 1996;348:1010–1013.
82. Keefer MC, Belshe R, Graham B, et al. Phase I/II trials of preventive HIV vaccine candidates. Safety profile of HIV vaccination: first 1000 volunteers of the AIDS Vaccine Evaluation Group. *AIDS Res Hum Retroviruses*, 1994;10:S139.
83. DeMets DL, Fleming TR, Whitley RJ, et al. The Data and Safety Monitoring Board and Acquired Immune Deficiency Syndrome (AIDS) clinical trials. *Cont Clin Trials*, 1995;16:408–421.
84. Robinson WE, Montefiori DC, Mitchell WM. Antibody-dependent enhancement of human immunodeficiency virus type 1 infection. *Lancet*, 1988;1:790–794.
85. Matsuda S, Gidlund M, Chiodi F, et al. Enhancement of human immunodeficiency virus (HIV) replication in human monocytes by low titres of anti-HIV antibodies in vitro. *Scand J Immunol*, 1989;30:425–434.
86. Takeda A, Tuazon CU, Ennis FA. Antibody-enhanced infection by HIV-1 via Fc receptor-mediated entry. *Science*, 1989;242:580–583.
87. Homsy J, Meyer M, Levy JA. Serum enhancement of human immunodeficiency virus (HIV) infection correlates with disease in HIV-infected individuals. *J Virol*, 1990;64:1437–1440.
88. Tremblay M, Meloche S, Sekaly RP, et al. Complement receptor 2 mediates enhancement of HIV-1 infection in Epstein-Barr virus-carrying B cells. *J Exper Med*, 1990;171:1791–1796.
89. Montefiori DC, Lefkowitz LB Jr, Keller RE, et al. Absence of a clinical correlation for complement-mediated, infection-enhancing antibodies in plasma or sera from HIV-1-infected individuals. *AIDS*, 1991;5:413–417.
90. Burke DS. Human HIV vaccine trials: Does antibody-dependent enhancement pose a genuine risk? *Perspect Biol Med*, 1992;35:511–530.
91. Mascola JR, Mathieson BJ, Zack PM, et al. Summary report: workshop on the potential risks of antibody-dependent enhancement in human HIV vaccine trials. *AIDS Res Human Retroviruses*, 1993;9:1175–1184.
92. Schoenfeld D. Partial residuals for the proportional hazards regression model. *Biometrika*, 1982;69: 239–241.
93. Durham LK, Longini IM, Halloran ME, et al. Estimation of vaccine efficacy in the presence of waning: application to cholera vaccines. *Am J Epidemiol*, 1998;147:948–959.
94. Fine P. Herd immunity: History, theory, practice. *Epidemiol Rev*, 1993;15:265–302.
95. Murphy BR, Chanock RM. Immunization against virus disease. In: Fields BN, Knipe DM, Howley PM, Chanock RM, Melnick JL, Monath TP, Roizman B, Straus SE, eds. *Fields Virology*. Philadelphia: Lippincott-Raven, 1996:467–497.
96. Clemens JD, Naficy A, Rao MR. Long-term evaluation of vaccine protection: Methodological issues for phase 3 trials and phase 4 studies. In: Levine MM, Woodrow GC, Kaper JB, Cobon GS, eds. *New Generation Vaccines*. New York: Marcel Dekker, Inc., 1997:47–67.
97. Halloran ME, Struchiner CJ, Longini IM. Study designs for evaluating different efficacy and effectiveness aspects of vaccines. *Am J Epidemiol*, 1997;146:789–803.
98. Shen X, Siliciano RF. AIDS: Preventing AIDS but not HIV-1 infection with a DNA vaccine. *Science*, 2000;290:463–465.
99. Warren JT, Levinson MA. AIDS preclinical vaccine development: biennial survey of HIV, SIV, and

SHIV challenge studies in vaccinated nonhuman primates. *J Med Primatol*, 1999;28:249–273.
100. O'Brien TR, Blattner WA, Waters D, et al. Serum HIV-1 RNA levels and time to development of AIDS in the Multicenter Hemophilia Cohort Study. *JAMA*, 1996;276:105–110.
101. Mellors JW, Rinaldo CR Jr., Gupta P, et al. Prognosis in HIV-1 infection predicted by the quantity of virus in plasma. *Science*, 1996;272: 1167–1170.
102. Mellors JW, Munoz A, Giorgi JV, et al. Plasma viral load and $CD4^+$ lymphocytes as prognostic markers of HIV-1 infection. *Ann Intern Med*, 1997;126:946–954.
103. Prentice RL. Surrogate endpoints in clinical trials: Definition and operational criteria. *Stat Med*, 1989;8:431–440.
104. Fleming TR. Evaluation of active control trials in AIDS. *JAIDS*, 1990;3:S82–S87.
105. Fleming TR. Evaluating therapeutic interventions (with Discussion and Rejoinder). *Stat Science*, 1992;7:428–456.
106. Fleming TR, DeMets DL. Surrogate endpoints in clinical trials: Are we being misled? *Ann Intern Med*, 1996;125:605–613.
107. Effects of encainide, flecainide, imipramine and moricizine on ventricular arrhythmias during the year after acute myocardial infarction: the CAPS. The Cardiac Arrhythmia Pilot Study (CAPS) Investigators. *Am J Cardiol*, 1988;61:501–509.
108. Preliminary report: Effect of encainide and flecainide on mortality in a randomized trial of arrhythmia suppression after myocaridial infarction. The Cardiac Arrhythmia Suppression Trial (CAST) Investigators. *N Engl J Med*, 1989;321: 406–412.
109. A controlled trial of interferon gamma to prevent infection in chronic granulomatous disease. The International Chronic Granulomatous Disease Cooperative Study Group. *N Engl J Med*, 1991; 324:509–516.
110. Choi S, Lagakos SW, Schooley TT, et al. $CD4^+$ lymphocytes are an incomplete surrogate marker for clinical progression in persons with asymptomatic HIV-1 infection taking zidovudine. *Ann Intern Med*, 1993;118:674–680.
111. DeGruttola V, Wulfsohn M, Fischl M, et al. Modeling the relationship between survival and $CD4^+$ lymphocytes in patients with AIDS and AIDS-related complex. *J Acquir Immune Defic Syndr*, 1993;6:359–365.
112. Lin DY, Fischl MA, Schoenfeld DA. Evaluating the role of CD4-lymphocyte counts as surrogate endpoints in HIV-1 clinical trials. *Stat Med*, 1993;12:835–842.
113. Fleming TR. Surrogate markers in AIDS and cancer trials. *Stat Med*, 1994;13:1423–1435.
114. Hughes MD, Daniels MJ, Fischl MA, et al. CD4 cell count as a surrogate endpoint in HIV-1 clinical trials: A meta-analysis of studies of the AIDS Clinical Trials Group. *AIDS*, 1998;12:1823–1832.
115. HIV Surrogate Marker Collaborative Group. Human immunodeficiency virus type 1 RNA level and CD4 count as prognostic markers and surrogate endpoints: A meta-analysis. *AIDS Res Hum Retroviruses*, 2000;16:1123–1133.
116. Carpenter CC, Fischl MA, Hammer SM, et al. Antiretroviral therapy for HIV-1 infection in 1998: updated recommendations of the International AIDS Society-USA Panel. *JAMA*, 1998;28:78–86.
117. Guidelines for the use of antiretroviral agents in HIV-infected adults and adolescents. *MMWR*, 1998;47(RR-4):1–43.
118. Halloran ME, Struchiner CJ. Study designs for dependent happenings. *Epidemiology*, 1991;2: 331–338.
119. Longini IM, Susmita D, Halloran ME. Measuring vaccine efficacy for both susceptibility to infection and reduction in infectiousness for prophylactic HIV-1 vaccines. *J Acquir Immune Defic Syndr and Hum Retrovirology*, 1996;13:440–447.
120. Donner A, Birkett N, Buck C. Randomization by cluster: sample size requirements and analysis. *Am J Epidemiol*, 1981;114:906–914.
121. Quinn TC, Wawer MJ, Sewankambo N, et al. Viral load and heterosexual transmission of human immunodeficiency virus type 1. *New Engl J Med*, 2000;342:921–929.
122. Scharfstein DO, Rotnitzky A, Robins JM. Adjusting for nonignorable drop-out using semiparametric nonresponse models. *J Am Stat Assoc*, 1999;94:1096–1146.
123. Rida W, Fast P, Hoff R, et al. Intermediate-sized trials for the evaluation of HIV vaccine candidates: a workshop summary. *J Acquir Immune Defic Syndr*, 1997;16:195–203.
124. Schaper C, Fleming T, Self S, et al. Statistical issues in the design of HIV-1 vaccine trials. *Ann Rev Pub Health*, 1995;16:1–22.
125. Dolin R. Human studies in the development of human immunodeficiency virus vaccines. *J Infect Dis*, 1995;172:1175–1183.
126. Carruth LM, Greten TF, Murray CE, et al. An algorithm for evaluating human cytotoxic T lymphocyte responses to candidate AIDS vaccines. *AIDS Res Hum Retroviruses*, 1999;15:1021–1034.
127. Renjifo B, Chaplin B, Mwakagile D, et al. Epidemic expansion of HIV type 1 subtype C and recombinant genotypes in Tanzania. *AIDS Res Hum Retroviruses*, 1998;14:635–638.
128. Renjifo B, Gilbert P, Chaplin B, et al. Emerging recombinant human immunodeficiency viruses: uneven representation of the envelope V3 region. *AIDS*, 1999;13:1613–1621.

129. Novitsky V, Rybak N, McLane MF, et al. Identification of human immunodeficiency virus type 1 subtype C Gag-, Tat-, Rev-, and Nef-specific Elispot-based CTL responses for AIDS vaccine design. *J Virol*, 2001;75:9210–9228.
130. Berman PW, Gray A, Wrin T, et al. Genetic and immunologic characterization of viruses infecting MN-rgp120-vaccinated volunteers. *J Infect Dis*, 1997;176:384–397.
131. Graham BS, McElrath MJ, Connor RI, et al. Analysis of intercurrent HIV-1 infections in phase I and II trials of candidate AIDS vaccines. *J Infect Dis*, 1998;177:310–319.
132. Connor RI, Korber BTM, Graham BS, et al. Immunological and virological analyses of persons infected by human immunodeficiency virus type 1 while participating in trials of recombinant gp120 subunit vaccines. *J Virol*, 1998;72:1552–1576.
133. Kilbourne ED, Chanock RM, Coppin PW, et al. Influenza vaccines: Summary of influenza workshop V. *J Infect Dis*, 1974;129:750–771.
134. Clements ML, Betts RF, Tierney EL, et al. Serum and nasal wash antibodies associated with resistance to experimental challenge with influenza A wild-type virus. *J Clin Microbiol*, 1986;24:157–160.
135. Edwards KM, Dupont WD, Westrich MK, et al. A randomized controlled trial of cold-adapted and inactivated vaccines for the prevention of influenza A disease. *J Infect Dis*, 1994;169:68–76.
136. Levine MM. Typhoid fever vaccines. In: Plotkin SA, Mortimer EA Jr., eds. *Vaccines, Second Edition*. Philadelphia: WB Saunders Company, 1994:597–633.
137. Gilbert PB, Self SG, Ashby MA. Statistical methods for assessing differential vaccine protection against human immunodeficiency virus types. *Biometrics*, 1998;54:799–814.
138. Breiman L, Friedman JH, Olshen RA, et al. *Classification and regression trees*. London: Wadsworth, 1984.
139. Zhang H, Singer B. *Recursive partitioning in the health sciences*. New York: Springer-Verlag, 1999.
140. Sugaya N, Nerome K, Ishida M, et al. Efficacy of inactivated vaccine in preventing antigenically drifted influenza type A and well-matched type B. *JAMA*, 1994;272:1122–1126.
141. Guenter D, Esparza J, Macklin R. Ethical consideration in international HIV vaccine trials: summary of a consultative process conducted by the Joint United Nations Programme on HIV/AIDS. *J Med Ethics*, 2000;26:37–43.
142. UNAIDS: Ethical considerations in HIV-1 preventive vaccine research. Geneva: UNAIDS, 2000.

41

Regional Variations in the African Epidemics

*Max Essex and †Souleymane Mboup

*Harvard AIDS Institute and the Department of Immunology and Infectious Diseases, Harvard School of Public Health, Boston, Massachusetts, USA.
†LeDantec Université, Cheikh Anta Diop, Dakar, Senegal.

Sub–Saharan Africa, home to only about 10% of the world's population, accounts for more than 70% of the HIV infections in the world (1). In sub–Saharan Africa as a whole, about 8.4% of adults were estimated to be HIV-infected as of 2001 (2). This percentage is at least 10-fold higher than that of any other region of the world, except perhaps for the Caribbean if taken separately from North and South America (1). However, the distribution of HIV on the African continent has been uneven. For example, the HIV prevalence rates of North Africa and the island countries are among the lowest in the world (1).

The first evidence of the existence of HIV in Africa came from Central Africa, where at least one sample was found to be positive as early as 1959 (3,4). The samples studied were from a population of tuberculosis patients and the virus reactivity appeared to be most closely related to HIV-1B and HIV-1D.

Most evidence suggests that the first expansion of an HIV-1 epidemic in Africa took place in the early 1980s, at about the same time the disease was first recognized in the United States (5,6). Some of the first HIV infections and AIDS cases described in Africa were in individuals from Central Africa (7,8). A retrospective analysis suggests that the first plateauing of a regional epidemic occurred in the region of Brazzaville and Kinshasa, where HIV prevalence rates appear to have stabilized at 5%–7% (1) (Figure 1). In the mid-to-late 1980s, Kinshasa was the center of much international attention by researchers and public health officials who were working to better understand and prevent HIV infection. Many of these efforts were phased out in the early 1990s, due in part to political instability, but there is no evidence that HIV rates in the region have increased. In contrast, Southern Africa, the last region in sub–Saharan Africa to experience the epidemic, has had the highest rates of HIV infection (1) (Figure 2).

Except perhaps for North Africa and the island countries, the vast majority of HIV infections in adults in Africa are believed to be acquired by heterosexual exposure. Women have slightly higher rates than men, especially at younger ages, and so rates of infant infections are often also very high.

Both the smaller island countries, such as Comoros, and the larger island countries, such as Madagascar, are reported to have very low rates of HIV infection (1). It seems logical that this could be related to their relative isolation, but similarly low rates are also

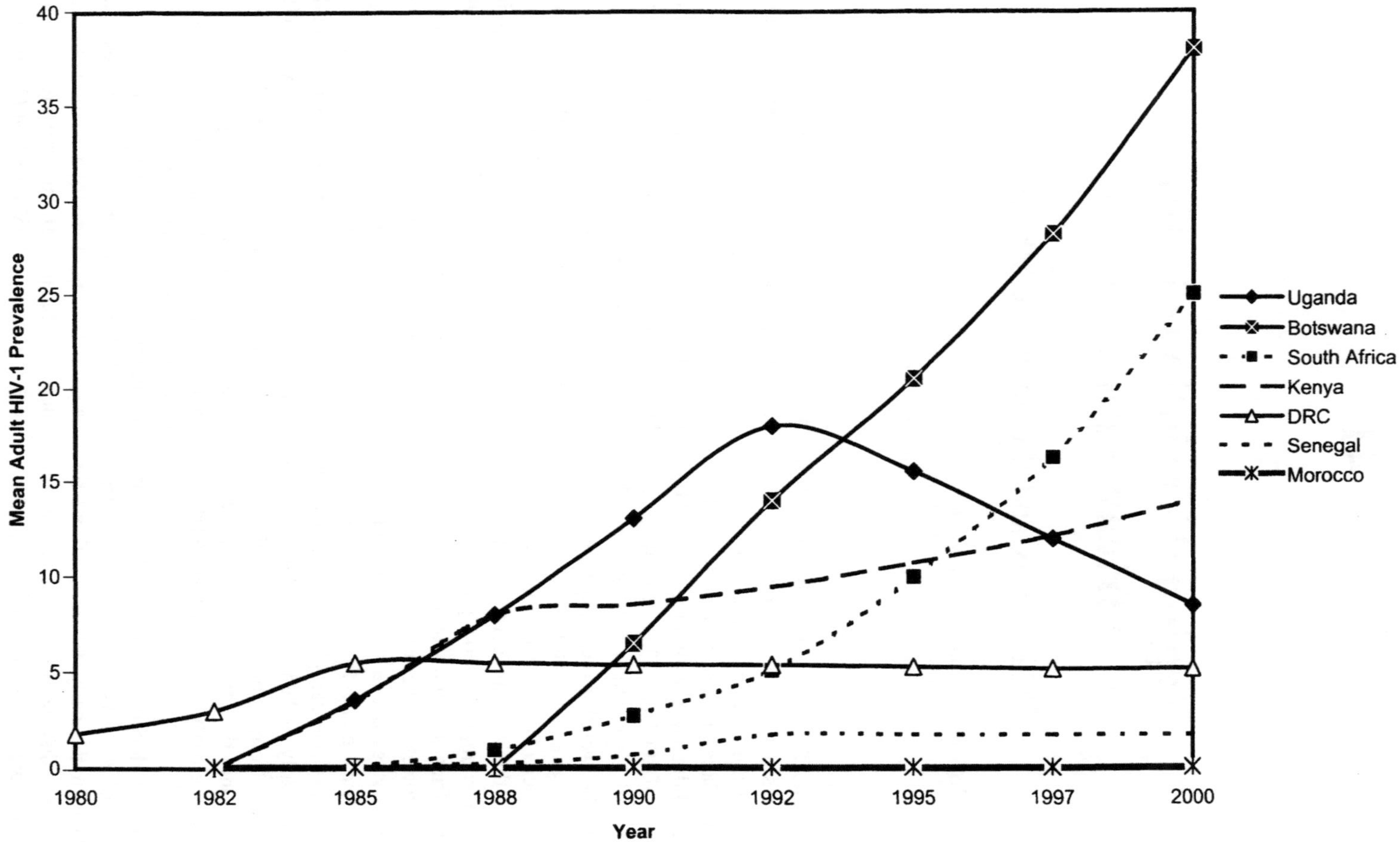

FIGURE 1. Schematic representation of trends for mean adult HIV-1 prevalence rates for different countries of Africa. DRC indicates Democratic Republic of Congo.

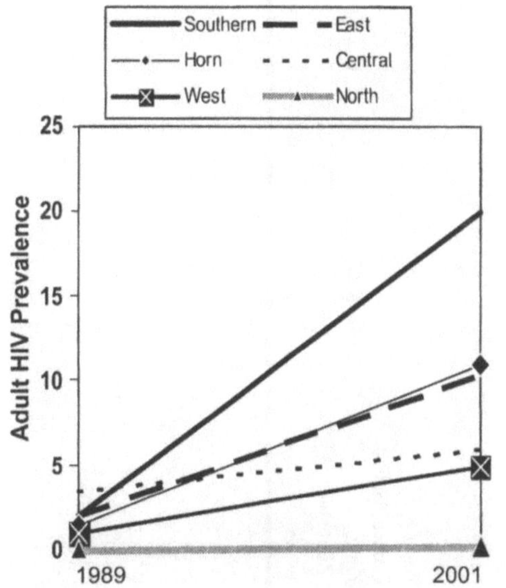

FIGURE 2. Estimates of trends in mean adult HIV prevalence rates for different regions of Africa.

seen in North Africa where the populations are not isolated.

NORTH AFRICA

The population of North Africa is the second largest on the continent (Table 1). Mean life expectancy is higher and infant mortality rates are lower than for other regions of Africa. Mean per capita income is higher than that of most other regions, except for Southern Africa. Sudan and Algeria represent two of the largest African countries with respect to total land mass. More than half of the people of North Africa live in cities. French and Arabic are the most common official languages, and Islam is the dominant religion.

In all countries of North Africa except Sudan, rates of HIV infection are among the lowest in the world. Sudan, which is the southern-most country often grouped with North Africa, has an adult HIV prevalence rate of about 1%, while none of the other countries of the region appear to have rates above 0.1% (1). Virtually all of the samples analyzed from the coastal countries of North Africa have been HIV-1B (9). This suggests that the epidemic of the region is related to virus that originally moved from Europe. HIV-1B is prevalent in southern European countries such as Spain (9), but it is rare in sub–Saharan Africa (10).

The vast majority of the people in North Africa are Muslim, and most adult men are circumcised—both factors that have been associated with low rates of HIV infection (see Chapter 31, *this volume*). It is not evident that classic programs for the prevention of HIV infection, such as condom distribution or education, have been very active in this region. In large cities such as Cairo in Egypt or Casablanca and Marrakech in Morocco, international and national travel clearly occurs at significant rates. While HIV prevalence rates in North Africa have been remarkably low, it is not clear why they are so low, and thus the possibility that higher rates may occur in the future must be considered.

WEST AFRICA

West Africa is the region of sub–Saharan Africa with the largest number of people (Table 1). This is in part because it includes Nigeria, which has a population of about 110 million. About 30% to 40% of the people of West Africa live in cities. French is the official language of the majority of countries in the region, although English, Portuguese, and numerous tribal languages are spoken in some countries. Islam is the most common religion, covering a large fraction of the people in countries such as Senegal, Niger, Mali, Gambia, and Guinea. However, a large fraction of the population in countries such as Benin, Côte d'Ivoire, and Guinea Bissau practice traditional religions.

The overall prevalence of HIV infection in adults in West Africa is about 5%. The populations of most countries in this region became exposed to HIV later than those of the countries in Central and East Africa (11).

TABLE 1. Estimated Mean Adult Prevalence and Predominant HIV-1 Subtypes for Different Regions of Africa

Region of Africa	Estimated populations (thousands)	% of total African population[a]	Countries	Estimated mean adult HIV-1 prevalence	Predominant HIV-1 subtypes
North	170,800	22.8	Algeria, Egypt, Libya, Morocco, Sudan, Tunisia	0.2	B
West	217,400	29.0	Benin, Burkina Faso, Côte d'Ivoire, Gambia, Ghana, Guinea, Guinea-Bissau, Liberia, Mali, Mauritania, Niger, Nigeria, Senegal, Sierra Leone, Togo	5.0	A/G
Horn	73,400	9.8	Djibouti, Eritrea, Ethiopia, Somalia	11.0	C
East	97,700	13.0	Burundi, Kenya, Rwanda, Tanzania, Uganda	10.5	A, D
Central	81,000	10.8	Cameroon, Central African Republic, Chad, Congo, Democratic Republic of Congo, Equitorial Guinea, Gabon	6.0	A/G, A
Southern	109,400	14.6	Angola, Botswana, Lesotho, Malawi, Mozambique, Namibia, South Africa, Swaziland, Zambia, Zimbabwe	20.0	C
All	749,700	100	All	6.5	

[a]Excluding island countries.

The first country in West Africa to experience very high rates of HIV infection was Côte d'Ivoire, which had an estimated adult prevalence of 11% in 2000 (1). The country with the next highest rates is Burkina Faso, and recent reports suggest that the epidemic has not yet peaked there (12,13).

Countries of West Africa that lie primarily within the Sahara desert have the lowest rates of HIV-1 prevalence in the region, such as Mauritania (0.5%) and Niger (1.35%) (1). Senegal also has a relatively low prevalence rate (1.8%) (1), which has been attributed to early action by governmental and academic leaders (14).

HIV-1 CRF02, which is an A/G recombinant (see Chapter 16, *this volume*), accounts for two-thirds to three-fourths of all HIV infections in West Africa (Table 1). Most of the CRF02 viruses were originally reported as HIV-1A (15). The next most common virus is HIV-1G, which appears to have spread after CRF02 (16,17). In Nigeria, a geographic localization has been reported, with HIV-1G more common in the north (18). Most of the subtypes of the main subgroup of HIV-1 have been detected in Senegal, even though the overall rates of infection there are low (19,20).

Guinea Bissau has apparently had the highest prevalence of HIV-2 in the world (21, 22). HIV-2 has also been found in other countries of the region such as Burkina Faso (23), Côte d'Ivoire (24), Gambia (25), and Senegal (23). HIV-2 probably only accounts for less than one million infections in the world, but most of them are in West Africa.

HORN

The Horn of Africa represents a very poor region of about 73 million people, most of them living in Ethiopia. The region does not appear to have been impacted by the HIV epidemic as early as Central or East Africa. For example, in 1991 only 1% of female sex workers were reported to be HIV-infected in Mogadishu, Somalia (26), and only 2.6% of Ethiopian military recruits were reported to be infected (27). HIV prevalence rates have recently risen very rapidly in the region (28).

Only about 20% of the people in the Horn of Africa live in cities. About half are Muslim. Infant mortality rates are high, and literacy rates and mean life expectancy are low, even for sub–Saharan Africa.

The estimated mean HIV prevalence for adults in the Horn of Africa is 11%, and the predominant subtype causing the epidemic is HIV-1C (29,30). Little is known about the natural history of HIV-1 infections in Ethiopians. However, one report has claimed that the coreceptor CCR5 is expressed at higher levels in Ethiopian cells, implying that the genetics of the population might allow the virus to be more virulent (31). HIV-1C viruses, more than any other subtypes, appear to show preference for cell entry through the CCR5 coreceptor (32,33).

EAST AFRICA

Most of the countries of East Africa showed evidence of an expanding HIV epidemic in the early to mid-1980s, with countries such as Uganda, Rwanda, and Burundi showing the earliest rise in prevalence (34–36). East Africa has a population of about 98 million people, accounting for approximately 13% of the people in Africa (Table 1). Only about one-quarter of the people live in urban areas. The most common religion is Roman Catholicism. Indicators of development such as infant mortality rates, literacy, mean life expectancy, and mean per capita income are average or below average for African countries.

HIV-1 subtypes A and D coexist in large segments of the population in East Africa (9,37,38). More recently HIV-1C has also been expanding in the region, presumably because of the northward spread of the virus from the more recent epidemic in Southern Africa (38). HIV-1C is also starting to emerge in

Uganda (39). In addition to the increasing numbers of people becoming infected with HIV-1C, an increasing number appear to be infected with multiple subtypes, generating a large number of intersubtype recombinants (38).

The estimated mean adult HIV prevalence in East Africa is 10.5%, with Uganda and Tanzania somewhat below this level, even though Uganda apparently once had the highest rates in Africa (40). Since the mid-1990s HIV-1 rates in Uganda have been falling (41) (Figure 1). Rates in Tanzania may also be falling (42,43). Rates in Kenya continue to be very high, but there are suggestions that even there the epidemic is stabilizing, with lowest rates in the eastern regions of the country (44). Uganda, like Senegal, is a country in which political leaders have been credited with helping to curb the epidemic through active policies for AIDS education (45).

CENTRAL AFRICA

Central Africa has about 81 million people, most of whom live in the Democratic Republic of Congo. The region was perhaps the first in Africa to be impacted by HIV. About 35% to 45% of the people of the region live in cities. Roman Catholicism is the most commonly practiced religion, and French is the official language in most countries. Infant mortality rates are generally high; mean life expectancy and literacy rates are about average for Africa. Mean per capita income is also about average for Africa, with Gabon as a notable exception. Due in part to natural resources, Gabon has the highest per capita income in Africa.

The overall rate of HIV infection in the region is 6%, and the most common viruses are HIV-1 CRF02_AG and HIV-1A. The highest prevalence rates are found in the Central African Republic (1). The countries that experienced the earliest expansion of the HIV epidemic were the Democratic Republic of Congo (Figure 1) and the Central African Republic (46,47). However, HIV prevalence in the Democratic Republic of Congo appeared to plateau at 5%–6% by the late 1980s (48,49), whereas in the Central African Republic it did not (50). The dominant virus in the Central African Republic was initially HIV-1 CRF01_AE, but prevalence of this virus seems to have been decreasing in proportion to the increasing prevalence of HIV-1A (50).

The epidemic appeared to take longer to develop in Cameroon and Congo, but rates continue to increase in these countries (51,52). Central Africa, including Equatorial Guinea and Gabon as well as Cameroon, the Democratic Republic of Congo, and Congo, has been characterized by having a wide variety of HIV-1 subtypes (49,53–58). These subtypes include those in the O and N groups of HIV-1 as well as the M group (58–61).

SOUTHERN AFRICA

Southern Africa has about 110 million people. The Republic of South Africa has about 40 million, Mozambique about 20 million, and Angola, Zimbabwe, Malawi, and Zambia about 10 million each. Most of the other countries in the region have only 1–2 million people. This region was the last in Africa (excluding North Africa) to have a major HIV epidemic. In the Republic of South Africa about 60% of the people live in cities. In most of the other countries only 20% to 30% of the population live in cities. For much of the region English is the official language, and Christianity is the most common religion.

In Malawi, Mozambique, and Angola, infant mortality rates are high, and literacy, mean life expectancy, and mean per capita income are low. Conversely, Botswana, Namibia, and the Republic of South Africa have had relatively low infant mortality rates, and relatively high mean life expectancy, at least until very recently when AIDS deaths started to escalate. These three countries also have mean per capita incomes that are among the highest in Africa.

For the region of Southern Africa as a whole, about 20% of all adults are infected with HIV (Table 1). Angola has a relatively low prevalence rate of 3% (62), but all the other countries of the region have at least 13% infected, and Namibia, Republic of South Africa, Botswana, Lesotho, Swaziland, Zambia, and Zimbabwe all have rates of 20% or above (1,63–65). Malawi and Zambia, in the north of the region, were apparently the first countries to experience the epidemic (66–69). Zimbabwe then began to experience higher rates of HIV in the early 1990s (70,71).

Although the rates in Botswana, Mozambique, Namibia, and the Republic of South Africa are very high now, these countries experienced relatively low rates until the early 1990s (63,72–75). In the Republic of South Africa, Caucasians in the cities were the first to be infected in the 1980s, presumably from partners in the United States or Europe, and with the subtype HIV-1B. At that time South African mine workers had very low rates of HIV infection (72,75). By the early 1990s rates began to rise rapidly among mine workers, presumably due to the southern migration of people from Central Africa (76). By 1995 and later, both rural and urban prevalence rates had become very high in the Republic of South Africa (65,77–79) (Figure 1). Almost all infections in Southern Africa are HIV-1C (9,80,81). This subtype now accounts for the majority of infections in the world (Figure 3), and appears to evolve even faster than the other major subtypes (80).

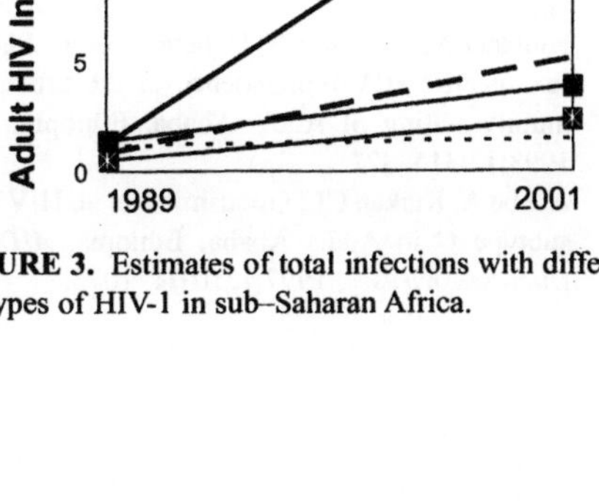

FIGURE 3. Estimates of total infections with different subtypes of HIV-1 in sub–Saharan Africa.

CONCLUSION

About 6.5% of adults in Africa are infected with HIV. Because rates in North Africa are very low, the overall HIV prevalence rate for sub–Saharan Africa is 8.4%. The HIV epidemic was initially noticed in Central Africa, although HIV prevalence in countries of that region such as the Democratic Republic of Congo appears to have plateaued by the late 1980s (Figure 1). Southern Africa has the most severe epidemic. In this region prevalence rates average about 20% in adults and the major expansion of the epidemic did not begin until the 1990s. Prevalence rates are about 5% in West Africa and 10%–11% in the Horn of Africa and East Africa. Most of the countries with extremely high rates are in Southern Africa—countries such as Botswana, Zimbabwe, Swaziland, and the Republic of South Africa. As countries with strong leadership, Senegal was able to initially prevent the expansion of HIV prevalence beyond about 2%, and Uganda was able to substantially reduce prevalence in the late 1990s.

Different HIV-1 subtype viruses are associated with the different epidemics: HIV-1C in Southern Africa and the Horn of Africa, HIV-1 CRF02_AG predominating in West and Central Africa, and HIV-1A and HIV-1D in East Africa. A wide variety of subtypes and/or recombinants have been observed in Cameroon in west Central Africa and Tanzania in East Africa. Most HIV-2 infections occur in West Africa.

REFERENCES

1. UNAIDS. Report on the Global HIV/AIDS Epidemic. Geneva: UNAIDS, 2000.
2. UNAIDS/WHO. AIDS Epidemic Update. Geneva: UNAIDS and the WHO, December 2001.
3. Nahmias AJ, Weiss J, Yao X, et al. Evidence for human infection with an HTLV III/LAV-like virus in Central Africa, 1959. *Lancet*, 1986;1:1279–1280.
4. Zhu T, Korber BT, Nahmias AJ, et al. An African HIV-1 sequence from 1959 and implications for the origin of the epidemic. *Nature*, 1998;391:594–597.
5. Gottlieb MS, Schroff R, Schanker HM, et al. Pneumocystis carinii pneumonia and mucosal candidiasis in previously healthy homosexual men: evidence of a new acquired cellular immunodeficiency. *N Engl J Med*, 1981;305:1425–1431.
6. Siegal FP, Lopez C, Hammer GS, et al. Severe acquired immunodeficiency in male homosexuals, manifested by chronic perianal ulcerative herpes simplex lesions. *N Engl J Med*, 1981;305: 1439–1444.
7. Coddy-Zitsamele R. Lutte contre le SIDA en République Populaire du Congo. *OCEAC Bull*, April–June 1989;88:
8. Nzilambi N, De Cock KM, Forthal DN, et al. The prevalence of infection with human immunodeficiency virus over a 10-year period in rural Zaire. *N Engl J Med*, 1988;318:276–279.
9. Burke DS, McCutchan FE. Global distribution of HIV-1 clades. In: DeVita VT, Hellman S, Rosenberg SA, Curran J, Essex M, Fauci AS, ed. *AIDS Etiology, Diagnosis, Treatment and Prevention*. 4th ed. Philadelphia: Lippincott Co., 1997:119–128.
10. Essex M. Human immunodeficiency viruses in the developing world. *Adv Virus Res*, 1999;53:71–88.
11. Romieu I, Marlink R, Kanki P, et al. HIV-2 link to AIDS in West Africa. *J Acquir Immune Defic Syndr*, 1990;3:220–230.
12. Meda N, Zoundi-Guigui MT, van de Perre P, et al. HIV infection among pregnant women in Bobo-Dioulasso, Burkina Faso: comparison of voluntary and blinded seroprevalence estimates. *Int J STD AIDS*, 1999;10:738–740.
13. Sangare L, Meda N, Lankoande S, et al. HIV infection among pregnant women in Burkina Faso: a nationwide serosurvey. *Int J STD AIDS*, 1997;8:646–651.
14. UNAIDS. Acting to Prevent AIDS: The Case of Senegal. Geneva: UNAIDS, June 1999.
15. Montavon C, Toure-Kane C, Liegeois F, et al. Most env and gag subtype A HIV-1 viruses circulating in West and West Central Africa are similar to the prototype AG recombinant virus IBNG. *J Acquir Immune Defic Syndr*, 2000;23:363–374.
16. Ellenberger DL, Pieniazek D, Nkengasong J, et al. Genetic analysis of human immunodeficiency virus in Abidjan, Ivory Coast reveals predominance of HIV type 1 subtype A and introduction of subtype G. *AIDS Res Hum Retroviruses*, 1999;15:3–9.
17. Davies FJ, d'Almeida O, Timmers E, et al. Molecular genotyping of HIV-1 in 61 patients with AIDS from Lome, Togo. *J Med Virol*, 1999;57:25–30.
18. Peeters M, Esu-Williams E, Vergne L, et al. Predominance of subtype A and G HIV type 1 in Nigeria, with geographical differences in their distribution. *AIDS Res Hum Retroviruses*, 2000;16: 315–325.
19. Toure-Kane C, Montavon C, Faye MA, et al. Identification of all HIV type 1 group M subtypes in Senegal, a country with low and stable seroprevalence. *AIDS Res Hum Retroviruses*, 2000;16: 603–609.
20. Kanki PJ, Hamel DJ, Sankale JL, et al. Human immunodeficiency virus type 1 subtypes differ in disease progression. *J Infect Dis*, 1999;179:68–73.
21. Poulsen AG, Aaby P, Jensen H, et al. Risk factors for HIV-2 seropositivity among older people in Guinea-Bissau. A search for the early history of HIV-2 infection. *Scand J Infect Dis*, 2000;32:169–175.
22. Larsen O, da Silva Z, Sandstrom A, et al. Declining HIV-2 prevalence and incidence among men in a community study from Guinea-Bissau. *AIDS*, 1998;12:1707–1714.
23. Kanki P, M'Boup S, Marlink R, et al. Prevalence and risk determinants of human immunodeficiency virus type 2 (HIV-2) and human immunodeficiency virus type 1 (HIV-1) in west African female prostitutes. *Am J Epidemiol*, 1992;136:895–907.
24. De Cock KM, Adjorlolo G, Ekpini E, et al. Epidemiology and transmission of HIV-2. Why there is no HIV-2 pandemic. *JAMA*, 1993;270: 2083–2086.
25. Del Mistro A, Chotard J, Hall AJ, et al. HIV-1 and HIV-2 seroprevalence rates in mother–child pairs living in The Gambia (west Africa). *J Acquir Immune Defic Syndr*, 1992;5:19–24.
26. Ahmed HJ, Omar K, Adan SY, et al. Syphilis and human immunodeficiency virus seroconversion during a 6-month follow-up of female prostitutes in Mogadishu, Somalia. *Int J STD AIDS*, 1991;2: 119–123.
27. Mehret M, Khodakevich L, Zewdie D, et al. Progression of human immunodeficiency virus epidemic in Ethiopia. *Ethiop J Health Dev*, 1990;4: 183–190.
28. Fontanet AL, Messele T, Dejene A, et al. Age- and sex-specific HIV-1 prevalence in the urban community setting of Addis Ababa, Ethiopia. *AIDS*, 1998;12:315–322.
29. Abebe A, Kuiken CL, Goudsmit J, et al. HIV type 1 subtype C in Addis Ababa, Ethiopia. *AIDS Res Hum Retroviruses*, 1997;13:1071–1075.

30. Hussein M, Abebe A, Pollakis G, et al. HIV-1 subtype C in commerical sex workers in Addis Ababa, Ethiopia. *J Acquir Immune Defic Syndr*, 2000;23: 120–127.
31. Kalinkovich A, Weisman Z, Leng Q, et al. Increased CCR5 expression with decreased beta chemokine secretion in Ethiopians: relevance to AIDS in Africa. *J Hum Virol*, 1999;2:283–289.
32. Tscherning C, Alaeus A, Fredriksson R, et al. Differences in chemokine coreceptor usage between genetic subtypes of HIV-1. *Virology*, 1998;241: 181–188.
33. Ping LH, Nelson JA, Hoffman IF, et al. Characterization of V3 sequence heterogeneity in subtype C human immunodeficiency virus type 1 isolates from Malawi: underrepresentation of X4 variants. *J Virol*, 1999;73:6271–6281.
34. Standaert B, Kocheleff P, Kadende P, et al. Acquired immunodeficiency syndrome and human immunodeficiency virus infection in Bujumbura, Burundi. *Trans R Soc Trop Med Hyg*, 1988;82: 902–904.
35. Rwandan HIV Seroprevalence Study Group. Nationwide community-based serological survey of HIV-1 and other human retrovirus infections in a central African country. *Lancet*, 1989;1:941–943.
36. Berkley S, Okware S, Naamara W. Surveillance for AIDS in Uganda. *AIDS*, 1989;3:79–85.
37. Rayfield MA, Downing RG, Baggs J, et al. A molecular epidemiologic survey of HIV in Uganda. HIV Variant Working Group. *AIDS*, 1998;12: 521–527.
38. Renjifo B, Chaplin B, Mwakagile D, et al. Epidemic expansion of HIV type 1 subtype C and recombinant genotypes in Tanzania. *AIDS Res Hum Retroviruses*, 1998;14:635–638.
39. Downing R, Pieniazek D, Hu DJ, et al. Genetic characterization and phylogenetic analysis of HIV-1 subtype C from Uganda. *AIDS Res Hum Retroviruses*, 2000;16:815–819.
40. Serwadda D, Mhalu F, Karita E, et al. HIVs and AIDS in East Africa. In: Essex M, Mboup S, Kanki P, Kalengaye M, ed. *AIDS in Africa*. 1st ed. New York: Raven Press, 1994: 669–690.
41. Kamali A, Carpenter LM, Whitworth JA, et al. Seven-year trends in HIV-1 infection rates, and changes in sexual behaviour, among adults in rural Uganda. *AIDS*, 2000;14:427–434.
42. Kwesigabo G, Killewo J, Godoy C, et al. Decline in the prevalence of HIV-1 infection in young women in the Kagera region of Tanzania. *J Acquir Immune Defic Syndr Hum Retrovirol*, 1998;17:262–268.
43. Kwesigabo G, Killewo JZ, Urassa W, et al. Monitoring of HIV-1 infection prevalence and trends in the general population using pregnant women as a sentinel population: 9 years experience from the Kagera region of Tanzania. *J Acquir Immune Defic Syndr*, 2000;23:410–417.
44. Jackson DJ, Ngugi EN, Plummer FA, et al. Stable antenatal HIV-1 seroprevalence with high population mobility and marked seroprevalence variation among sentinel sites within Nairobi, Kenya. *AIDS*, 1999;13:583–589.
45. UNAIDS. A Measure of Success in Uganda. Geneva: UNAIDS, May 1998.
46. Georges-Courbot MC, Merlin M, Josse R, et al. Seroprevalence of HIV-I is much higher in young women than men in Central Africa. *Genitourin Med*, 1989;65:131–132.
47. Ryder RW, Nsa W, Hassig SE, et al. Perinatal transmission of the human immunodeficiency virus type 1 to infants of seropositive women in Zaire. *N Engl J Med*, 1989;320:1637–1642.
48. Mulanga-Kabeya C, Nzilambi N, Edidi B, et al. Evidence of stable HIV seroprevalences in selected populations in the Democratic Republic of the Congo. *AIDS*, 1998;12:905–910.
49. Mokili JL, Wade CM, Burns SM, et al. Genetic heterogeneity of HIV type 1 subtypes in Kimpese, rural Democratic Republic of Congo. *AIDS Res Hum Retroviruses*, 1999;15:655–664.
50. Muller-Trutwin MC, Chaix ML, Letourneur F, et al. Increase of HIV-1 subtype A in Central African Republic. *J Acquir Immune Defic Syndr*, 1999;21:164–171.
51. Durand JP, Musi S, Josse R, et al. Prevalence of carriers of antibodies against human immunodeficiency virus (HIV-1 and HIV-2) in South Cameroon. Results of attempts to isolate retroviruses. *Med Trop (Mars)*, 1988;48:391–395.
52. Lallemant M, Lallemant-Le-Coeur S, Cheynier D, et al. Mother-child transmission of HIV-1 and infant survival in Brazzaville, Congo. *AIDS*, 1989; 3:643–646.
53. Bikandou B, Takehisa J, Mboudjeka I, et al. Genetic subtypes of HIV type 1 in Republic of Congo. *AIDS Res Hum Retroviruses*, 2000;16:613–619.
54. Tscherning-Casper C, Dolcini G, Mauclere P, et al. Evidence of the existence of a new circulating recombinant form of HIV type 1 subtype A/J in Cameroon. The European Network on the Study of In Utero Transmission of HIV-1. *AIDS Res Hum Retroviruses*, 2000;16:1313–1318.
55. Roques P, Menu E, Narwa R, et al. An unusual HIV type 1 env sequence embedded in a mosaic virus from Cameroon: identification of a new env clade. European Network on the study of *in utero* transmission of HIV-1. *AIDS Res Hum Retroviruses*, 1999;15:1585–1589.
56. Mboudjeka I, Zekeng L, Takehisa J, et al. HIV type 1 genetic variability in the northern part of Cameroon. *AIDS Res Hum Retroviruses*, 1999;15: 951–956.
57. Takehisa J, Zekeng L, Ido E, et al. Various types of HIV mixed infections in Cameroon. *Virology*, 1998;245:1–10.

58. Delaporte E, Janssens W, Peeters M, et al. Epidemiological and molecular characteristics of HIV infection in Gabon, 1986–1994. *AIDS*, 1996;10:903–910.
59. Hunt JC, Golden AM, Lund JK, et al. Envelope sequence variability and serologic characterization of HIV type 1 group O isolates from Equatorial Guinea. *AIDS Res Hum Retroviruses*, 1997;13: 995–1005.
60. Mauclere P, Loussert-Ajaka I, Damond F, et al. Serological and virological characterization of HIV-1 group O infection in Cameroon. *AIDS*, 1997;11:445–453.
61. Fonjungo PN, Dash BC, Mpoudi EN, et al. Molecular screening for HIV-1 group N and simian immunodeficiency virus cpz-like virus infections in Cameroon. *AIDS*, 2000;14:750–752.
62. Santos-Ferreira MO, Cohen T, Lourenco MH, et al. A study of seroprevalence of HIV-1 and HIV-2 in six provinces of People's Republic of Angola: clues to the spread of HIV infection. *J Acquir Immune Defic Syndr*, 1990;3:780–786.
63. Botswana 2000 HIV Sero-Prevalence and STD Syndrome Sentinel Survey. Gaborone: National AIDS Coordinating Agency (NACA) in collaboration with AIDS/STD Unit, District Health Teams WHO and CDC, December 2000.
64. Fylkesnes K, Musonda RM, Kasumba K, et al. The HIV epidemic in Zambia: socio-demographic prevalence patterns and indications of trends among childbearing women. *AIDS*, 1997;11: 339–345.
65. Stuart JM, Irlam JH, Wilkinson D. Routine reporting or sentinel surveys for HIV/AIDS surveillance in resource-poor settings: experience in South Africa, 1991–97. *Int J STD AIDS*, 1999;10: 328–330.
66. Chiphangwi J, Liomba G, Ntaba HM, et al. Human immunodeficiency virus infection is prevalent in Malawi. *Infection*, 1987;15:363.
67. Meeran K. Prevalence of HIV infection among patients with leprosy and tuberculosis in rural Zambia. *BMJ*, 1989;298:364–365.
68. Miotti PG, Dallabetta GA, Chiphangwi JD, et al. A retrospective study of childhood mortality and spontaneous abortion in HIV-1 infected women in urban Malawi. *Int J Epidemiol*, 1992;21:792–799.
69. Kachapila L. The HIV/AIDS epidemic in Malawi. *Int Nurs Rev*, 1998;45:179–181.
70. Mertens T, Tondorf G, Siebolds M, et al. Epidemiology of HIV and hepatitis B virus (HBV) in selected African and Asian populations. *Infection*, 1989;17:4–7.
71. Mahomed K, Kasule J, Makuyana D, et al. Seroprevalence of HIV infection amongst antenatal women in greater Harare, Zimbabwe. *Cent Afr J Med*, 1991;37:322–325.
72. Dusheiko GM, Brink BA, Conradie JD, et al. Regional prevalence of hepatitis B, delta, and human immunodeficiency virus infection in southern Africa: a large population survey. *Am J Epidemiol*, 1989;129:138–145.
73. Sheller JP, Pedersen NS, Kvinesdal BB, et al. HIV infection, syphilis and genital diseases in Maun, Botswana. *Ugeskr Laeger*, 1990;152:1441–1443.
74. Mencarini P, De Luca A, Ghirga P, et al. Human immunodeficiency virus type 1 infection in a community of southern Mozambique. *Trop Geogr Med*, 1991;43:39–41.
75. Tshibangu NN. HIV infection in Bophuthatswana. Epidemiological surveillance 1987–1989. *S Afr Med J*, 1993;83:36–39.
76. Abdool Karim Q, Abdool Karim SS, Singh B, et al. Seroprevalence of HIV infection in rural South Africa. *AIDS*, 1992;6:1535–1539.
77. Coleman RL, Wilkinson D. Increasing HIV prevalence in a rural district of South Africa from 1992 through 1995. *J Acquir Immune Defic Syndr Hum Retrovirol*, 1997;16:50–53.
78. Kustner HG, Swanevelder JP, van Middelkoop A. National HIV surveillance in South Africa—1993–1995. *S Afr Med J*, 1998;88:1316–1320.
79. Wilkinson D, Abdool Karim SS, Williams B, et al. High HIV incidence and prevalence among young women in rural South Africa: developing a cohort for intervention trials. *J Acquir Immune Defic Syndr*, 2000;23:405–409.
80. Novitsky VA, Montano MA, McLane MF, et al. Molecular cloning and phylogenetic analysis of human immunodeficiency virus type 1 subtype C: a set of 23 full-length clones from Botswana. *J Virol*, 1999;73:4427–4432.
81. Batra M, Tien PC, Shafer RW, et al. HIV type 1 envelope subtype C sequences from recent seroconverters in Zimbabwe. *AIDS Res Hum Retroviruses*, 2000;16:973–979.

42

Human Rights and HIV/AIDS

*Sofia Gruskin and †Miriam Maluwa

*Harvard School of Public Health, Boston, Massachusetts, USA.
†Joint United Nations Programme on HIV/AIDS, Geneva, Switzerland.

In sub–Saharan Africa people concerned with the prevention and treatment of HIV and AIDS initially became interested in human rights because they saw that discrimination against HIV-infected people and people living with AIDS was counterproductive to public health efforts. It has now become increasingly recognized that lack of respect for human rights at personal and societal levels is also closely linked to individual and collective risk of infection, and to access to care and support once infected. Preventing HIV transmission, providing good care for people who are already infected, and adequately supporting individuals and communities affected by the HIV epidemic requires attention to human rights on the part of policy makers, program managers, researchers, and activists. These leaders must make a conscious effort to address the adverse impact of discrimination on groups considered vulnerable to HIV and AIDS, including women, members of racial, ethnic, linguistic, and sexual minority groups, people with disabilities, and those who are economically disadvantaged.

The HIV epidemic has had an increasing impact on the lives of adults and children in sub–Saharan Africa (1). Women, men, and children may be infected, affected and/or vulnerable to HIV infection and AIDS. People infected with HIV continue to face marginalization and discrimination, as well as violations of many of their rights to health, education, and social services (2,3,4).

People are affected by HIV/AIDS when their close or extended families, their communities, or more broadly, the structures and services that exist for their benefit are strained by the consequences of the epidemic. The impact on communities has been extreme, particularly in places where high rates of infection have resulted in increased demand for health services and a simultaneous loss of health care workers (5). The impact on education has also been devastating: many families can no longer afford to pay the fees for their children to go to school, and teachers are among those who are losing their lives to AIDS in increasing numbers (5,6). Children are especially affected when their immediate family environment and support system is challenged by the sickness, disability, and premature death of one or both of their parents (7,8,9,10). Additional burdens on affected children include impoverishment as a result of their caregivers being unable, or less able, to sustain livelihoods and the stigma that may be associated with the death of their parents (5,11).

Young people are particularly vulnerable to HIV; the majority of new infections occur in this age group. In addition, in many societies, the unequal social status of women makes them unable to refuse unwanted or unprotected sexual intercourse, thereby increasing their vulnerability to HIV (12,13). In sub–Saharan Africa in particular, low intensity and open conflicts, massive flows of refugees, migration, population displacement, and austere circumstances also contribute to the vulnerability of individuals to HIV infection and AIDS (5,14,15,16).

This chapter addresses some of the major concepts relevant to human rights thinking and practice in sub–Saharan Africa, highlights official documents relevant to these concepts, and provides examples of the ways in which human rights have been considered in relation to HIV/AIDS in the region.

WHAT ARE HUMAN RIGHTS?

The basic characteristics of human rights are that they inhere in individuals because they are human; they apply to people everywhere in the world; and they are principally concerned with the relationship between the individual and the state. In practical terms, international human rights law is about defining what governments can do to us, cannot do to us, and should do for us. The language of human rights, however, may be used differently by activists, government officials, health professionals, and researchers, depending on the reasons that human rights are being invoked. Thus, it is important to clarify the ways in which this language is used and interpreted. Human rights and even the documents outlining them have been used differently for advocacy, for analysis, for accountability, or as a framework for designing, implementing, or evaluating policies and programs. Human rights are generally invoked as they relate to the responsibility and accountability of governments, and not with respect to the specific actions of individual physicians, researchers, or corporations. Unless explicitly stated otherwise, the basic frame of reference used here is of human rights as understood by governments and others interested in their use for policy and program design.

The United Nations (UN) Charter establishes general obligations that apply to all its member states, including respect for human rights and dignity (17). Under the auspices of the UN, more than 20 multilateral human rights treaties exist which create legally binding obligations for the nations that have ratified them (18). In addition, the Organization of African Unity has in place its own regional human rights treaty, which is open for signature and ratification to all countries in Africa (19). Countries that become party to international human rights treaties accept certain procedures and responsibilities, including periodic submission of reports on their compliance with the substantive provisions of the texts to international treaty monitoring bodies. Table 1 details the status of human rights commitments by the nations of sub–Saharan Africa.

Governments are responsible not only for not directly violating rights, but also for ensuring conditions that enable individuals to realize their rights as fully as possible. This responsibility is understood as an obligation to respect, protect, and fulfill rights. Governments are legally responsible for complying with the range of obligations for each right in every human rights document they have ratified (20) (Table 2).

Resource and other constraints can make it difficult or impossible for any government to fulfill all rights immediately and completely. A genuine commitment to the right to health, for example, requires much more than the passing of a law. Such a commitment requires financial resources, trained personnel, facilities, and most importantly, a sustainable infrastructure. Therefore, realization of rights is generally understood to be a process of "progressive realization" by making steady progress towards a goal (21,22). The principle of progressive realization is fundamental to the achievement of human rights. It is a critical principle for resource-poor

TABLE 1. Ratifications by African States (55)

Country	African Charter	ICESCR	ICCPR	CERD	CRC	CEDAW	CAT	CRSR
Angola	1990	1992	1992	—	1990	1986	—	1981
Benin	1986	1992	1992	1967s	1990	1992	1992	1962
Botswana	1986	—	2000	1974	1995	1996	2000	1969
Burkina Faso	1984	1999	1999	1974	1990	1987	1999	1980
Burundi	1989	1990	1990	1997	1990	1992	1993	1963
Cameroon	1989	1984a	1984a	1971	1993	1994	1986	1961d
Cape Verde	1987	1993	—	1979	1992	1980	1992	—
Central African Republic	1986	1981	1981	1971	1992	1991	—	1962d
Chad	1986	1995	1995	1977	1990	1995	1995	1981
Comoros	1986	—	—	2000s	1993	1994	2000s	—
Congo	1982	1983	1983	1988	1993	1982	—	1962d
Côte d'Ivoire	1992	1992	1992	1973	1991	1995	1995	1961d
Djibouti	1991	—	—	—	1990	1998	—	1997d
Equatorial Guinea	1986	1987	1987	—	1992	1984	—	1986
Eritrea	1999	—	—	—	1994	1995	—	—
Ethiopia	1998	1993	1993	1976	1991	1981	1994	1969
Gabon	1986	1983	1983	1980	1994	1983	2000	1964
Gambia	1983	1978	1979	1978	1990	1993	1985s	1966d
Ghana	1989	2000	2000	1966	1990	1986	2000	1963
Guinea	1982	1978	1978	1977	1990	1982	1989	1965d
Guinea-Bissau	1985	1992	2000	2000	1990	1985	2000	1976
Kenya	1992	1972	1972	—	1990	1984	1997	1966
Lesotho	1992	1992	1992	1971	1992	1995	—	1981
Liberia	1982	1967s	1967s	1976	1993	1984	—	1964
Madagascar	1992	1971	1971	1969	1991	1989	—	1967
Malawi	1989	1993	1993	1996	1991	1987	1996	1987
Mali	1981	1974	1974	1974	1990	1985	1999	1973d
Mauritania	1986	—	—	1988	1991	—	—	1987
Mauritius	1992	1973	1973	1972	1990	1984	1992	—
Mozambique	1989	—	1993	1983	1994	1997	1999	1983
Namibia	1992	1994	1994	1982	1990	1992	1994	1995
Niger	1986	1986	1986	1967	1990	1999	1998	1961d
Nigeria	1983	1993	1993	1967	1991	1985	1988s	1967
Rwanda	1983	1975	1975	1975	1991	1981	—	1980
Sao Tome & Principe	1986	1995s	1995s	2000s	1991	1995s	2000s	1978
Senegal	1982	1978	1978	1972	1990	1985	1986	1963d
Seychelles	1982	1992	1992	1978	1990	1992	1992	1980
Sierra Leone	1983	1996	1996	1967	1990	1988	1985s	1993d
Somalia	1985	1990	1990	1975	—	—	1990	1978
South Africa	1996	1994s	1998	1998	1995	1995	1998	1996
Sudan	1982	1986	1976	1977	1990	—	1986s	1974
Swaziland	1995	—	—	1969	1995	—	—	2000
Togo	1982	1984	1984	1972	1990	1983	1987	1994d
Uganda	1986	1987	1995	1980	1990	1985	1986	1976
United Rep. of Tanzania	1984	1976	1976	1972	1991	1985	—	1964
Zaïre	1987	1976	1976	1976	1990	1986	1996	1985
Zambia	1984	1984	1984	1972	1991	1985	1998	1969d
Zimbabwe	1986	1991	1991	1991	1990	1991	—	1981

African Charter, The African [Banjul] Charter on Human and People's Rights; ICESCR, International Covenant on Economic, Social and Cultural Rights; ICCPR, International Covenant on Civil and Political Rights; CERD, International Convention on the Elimination of All Forms of Racial Discrimination; CRC, Convention on the Rights of the Child; CEDAW Convention on the Elimination of All Forms of Discrimination Against Women; CAT, Convention Against Torture and other Cruel, Inhuman or Degrading Treatment or Punishment; CRSR, Convention Relating to the Status of Refugees. Year given is ratification date; — indicates not listed as having signed or ratified; s, signature date; d, succession date.

TABLE 2. Respecting, Protecting, and Fulfilling Human Rights

Respecting the right means a state cannot violate the right directly. A government violates its responsibility to respect the right to health when it is immediately responsible for providing medical care to certain populations, such as prisoners or the military, and its decisions to withhold care can be found to be arbitrary or discriminatory.
Protecting the right means a state has to prevent violations of rights by non-state actors and offer some sort of redress that people know about and can access, if a violation does occur. This means the state would be responsible for making it illegal to automatically deny insurance or health care to people on the basis of a health condition, and for making sure some system of redress exists that people know about and can access should a violation occur.
Fulfilling the right means a state has to take all appropriate measures—including but not limited to legislative, administrative, budgetary, and judicial—towards fulfillment of the right, including the obligation to promote the right in question. A state could be found to be in violation of the right to health if it fails to incrementally allocate sufficient resources to meet the public health needs of the communities within its borders.

countries that are responsible for striving towards human rights goals to the maximum extent possible. It is, however, also of relevance to wealthier countries because they are responsible for respecting, protecting, and fulfilling human rights not only within their own borders, but also through their engagement in international assistance and cooperation (23).

A major human rights problem in the context of HIV/AIDS is discrimination against those known or perceived to be HIV-infected and those affected by HIV/AIDS, as well as discrimination against others that leads to denial of access to entitlements and services and increases vulnerability to HIV and AIDS (24–27). Each of the major human rights treaties specifically sets out the principle of nondiscrimination with respect to certain categories such as race, color, sex, language, political or other opinion, national or social origin, property, birth, and, as it is called, "other status." Adverse discrimination ensues when a distinction is made against a person that results in their being treated unfairly and unjustly on the basis of their belonging, or being perceived to belong, to one of these categories. The principle of nondiscrimination is central to human rights thinking and practice. The prohibition of discrimination does not mean that differences should not be acknowledged, only that different treatment must be based on reasonable and objective criteria (28).

LINKING HIV/AIDS WITH HUMAN RIGHTS

The importance of protecting human rights has been acknowledged from the very beginning of the international response. Starting in 1987, the World Health Organization (WHO) Global Programme on AIDS incorporated human rights into its global AIDS strategy and its guidelines on a range of issues including HIV testing, travel and immigration policies, blood safety, prison health, mother-to-child transmission, and employment.

National AIDS Plans

By 1990, every country in sub–Saharan Africa had a national AIDS program (NAP) in place. The focus of these programs tended to be almost exclusively on prevention (29). Human rights issues were given little attention, except in relation to some aspects of privacy and freedom of movement. A review of NAPs from 24 sub–Saharan African countries conducted a decade later in November 2000, revealed that 20 of the 24 plans make explicit reference to human rights (30) (Table 3). However, the content and the

TABLE 3. Approaches to Human Rights Issues in African National AIDS Programs[a]

Human rights issues	Country
Protection of rights of PLWHA in general and in specific circumstances/cases (employment, education, in jail, in eating places, in public facilities, for children, for mentally challenged people)	Angola, Benin, Botswana, South Burundi, Cameroon, CAR, Chad, Côte d'Ivoire, DRC, Eritrea, Ethiopia[b], Ghana, Malawi, Nigeria, South Africa, Uganda, Zimbabwe
Prevention of mandatory testing as a condition of employment, education, etc.	Angola, DRC, Ghana, Nigeria, Zimbabwe
Appropriateness of mandatory testing for college students, immigrants, prisoners, ANC patients, TB patients, CT scan patients, and patients in surgery to be determined	Namibia
Focus on confidentiality/shared confidentiality	Namibia
Direct access for sexual partners to information on the serostatus of their partners if the partner refuses to disclose test results	Ethiopia, Zimbabwe
Provision for health professionals to be able to inform third parties of the HIV status of persons who refuse to disclose their serostatus	Zimbabwe
Mandatory testing of persons charged with a sexual offense	Zimbabwe
Protection of victims of sexual violence	South Africa
No restriction of travel, but questions raised as to immigration policy	Ghana
Punitive measures for reckless transmission	Ethiopia
Provision of education, workshops, and information on the rights of PLWHA to reduce stigma, discrimination	Botswana, DRC, Eritrea, Kenya, Malawi, Namibia, South Africa, Tanzania, Uganda, Zimbabwe
Support networks/organizations/legal assistance for the rights of PLWHA and the rights of people affected by HIV/AIDS	Botswana, Côte d'Ivoire, DRC, Malawi, Mozambique, South Africa, Tanzania, Uganda
Guidelines on medical confidentiality and informed consent to be put in place	Botswana, DRC, Eritrea, Ghana, Nigeria, Zimbabwe
Regular meetings of legal/ethical group must be ensured	Senegal
Legal and policy protection for those infected and affected by HIV and AIDS, with special attention to families	Côte d'Ivoire, Eritrea, Malawi, Nigeria, South Africa, Uganda, Zimbabwe
Reduction of stigma against people affected by HIV	Kenya
Rights of spouses of infected individuals to counseling, and to make choices about personal safety and safety of unborn children	Eritrea
Rights of orphans to basic needs, including education, social and medical support	Eritrea
Identification of legal and ethical problems linked to HIV status to be determined	Cameroon, DRC
Legislation and/or ethical review of any HIV-related research, including clinical trials in humans to be ensured	DRC, Ethiopia
Recognition of the necessity to determine why stigma is high despite awareness/assessment of human rights needs/documentation of human rights abuses	Tanzania, Uganda

[a]PLWHA indicates people living with HIV or AIDS; CAR, Central African Republic; DRC, Democratic Republic of Congo; ANC, antenatal clinic; TB, tuberculosis; CT, computerized tomography.
[b]Protection for children only.

interpretation of the relevance of these rights vary greatly in each plan, highlighting once again the very different ways human rights can be described even by the same actors. For example, in some cases the words "human rights" are used to promote the interests of people infected or affected by HIV and AIDS and, in other cases, to promote the interests of others *against* the rights of those infected. Finally, while care and support are given some attention in the plans, there is yet to be established a concrete link between the need for care and support and the provision of care and support in relation to human rights.

The lack of attention to care and support for HIV-infected people became apparent as the impact of HIV on the lives of individuals put increasing demands on families, communities, and health systems in countries throughout the continent (5,31). The need to devise strategies for the care of HIV-infected people has become progressively clearer, even though such strategies require a level of financial expenditure that may not be immediately available or accessible (32–34). As stated earlier, governments that have ratified human rights documents have an obligation to take steps toward the progressive realization of rights even if they require resources, such as the right to access health and social services. For sub–Saharan African countries, this can be understood as an obligation to make efforts progressively to implement care and support strategies, including the provision of access to antiretroviral drugs. Wealthier states, according to the call for "international assistance and cooperation" found in the relevant documents, should cooperate in this effort (22).

Regional Declarations and Policy Statements

Since the start of the epidemic in sub–Saharan Africa, activists and government officials have made a number of declaratory statements linking human rights to HIV/ AIDS prevention, care, and research (Table 4). The strategy document for the International Partnership Against AIDS in Africa (IPAA) is the most comprehensive regional policy document to link HIV with human rights in recent years. The IPAA, which brings together African governments, the United Nations, donors, the private sector, and the community sector, was established to help "curtail the spread of HIV, and to reduce sharply the impact of AIDS on human suffering and on the development of human, social, and economic capital in Africa." The IPAA strategy document outlines eight principles that are meant to form the basis of all efforts to respond to HIV/AIDS within the continent. The fourth principle is noteworthy here in that its specific language concerns "respect, protection, and fulfillment of human rights, compassion, and active opposition to all forms of stigma and exclusion of people living with HIV/AIDS" (35,36). One of the specific concerns of the IPAA is the support of effective national strategic plans, under government leadership. Thus the specific inclusion of human rights in the IPAA guiding principles provides a framework for ensuring specific attention to human rights in all aspects of national plans.

Government Reports to the Human Rights Monitoring System

Over the past several years, sub–Saharan African governments have devoted increasing attention to HIV/AIDS in their reporting of progress on implementing their human rights obligations to relevant human rights bodies. All of the human rights treaty monitoring bodies have expressed concern over the impact of increasing rates of HIV infection in relation to human rights on the lives of people living in Africa. Since 1997, treaty monitoring bodies have discussed HIV/AIDS in the context of human rights with the governments of Benin, Burkina

TABLE 4. Chronology of Selected Regional Documents Relevant to the Human Rights Aspects of HIV and AIDS in Africa

Year	Document
1990	Ethical and Social Aspects of AIDS in Africa, a background paper for a meeting of Representatives of Member States, Lusaka, Zambia.
1990	Maputo Statement on HIV and AIDS in Southern Africa, Fourth International Conference on Health in Southern Africa, Maputo, Mozambique, April 1990.
1992	Declaration of the AIDS Epidemic in Africa, Organization of African Unity, Dakar, Senegal, 1992.
1994	Tunis Declaration on AIDS and the Child in Africa, Organization of African Unity, Tunis, Tunisia, 13–15 June, 1994, AHG/Dec. 1.
1994	Proceedings of the Intercountry Consultation, African Network on Ethics, Law and HIV, UNDP, Dakar, Senegal, June 27–July 1, 1994.
1994	Dakar Declaration, African Network on Ethics, Law and HIV, Dakar, Senegal, July 1, 1994.
1995	Brazzaville Declaration, "Rights, Responsibilities and Principles for Action in the Response to the HIV Pandemic" Brazzaville, 2 December, 1995.
1999	Education for All: A Framework for Action in Sub–Saharan Africa: Education for African Renaissance in the Twenty-First Century Adopted by the Regional Conference on Education for all for Sub–Saharan Africa, Johannesburg, South Africa, 1999.
1999	African Declaration and Regional Plan of Action Adopted by the Sixth African Regional Conference on Women, Beijing, China, 1999.
2000	The Ouagadougou Declaration of the 5th Pan African Conference, Ouagadougou, Burkina Faso, 21–25 September, 2000.
2000	The African Consensus and Plan of Action: Leadership to Overcome HIV/AIDS, African Development Forum, 3–7 December, 2000.
2001	Abuja Declaration on HIV/AIDS, Tuberculosis and Other Related Infectious Diseases.
2001	Lome Declaration adopted at the 3rd Regional Conference of the African National Human Rights Institutions for the Protection and Promotion of Human Rights, Lome, Togo, 14–16 March, 2001.

Faso, Burundi, Cameroon, Central African Republic, Comoros, Congo, Côte d'Ivoire, Democratic Republic of Congo, Djibouti, Equatorial Guinea, Ethiopia, Gambia, Ghana, Guinea, Lesotho, Libya, Mali, Mauritius, Namibia, Nigeria, Senegal, Sierra Leone, South Africa, Sudan, Togo, Uganda, and Zimbabwe (37). Of the treaty bodies interacting with African governments, the Committee on the Rights of the Child and the Committee on the Elimination of Discrimination Against Women have been the most active in this regard, both in their questions about HIV/AIDS in relation to human rights and in the responses they have elicited.

A primary focus of these discussions has been on the need for governments to use a human rights framework to enact strategies for HIV prevention, care, and impact mitigation that are realistically targeted to the needs of impacted populations. These strategies should allow for providing information and education, ensuring care and support for people living with HIV and AIDS, and taking steps to reduce the social and economic consequences of the disease. In their interactions with some countries, treaty monitoring bodies have focused specifically on laws and policies they believe might increase rates of infection; with other countries, they have focused more on the impact of harmful practices. In Benin, for example, this meant attention both to the 1920 law that prohibits the use of contraceptives, and to the lack of health care facilities available to adolescents without parental consent. Likewise, in dialogue with Cameroon, it was stated that health services should not be denied to sex workers and, in addition, that poverty alleviation programs should be designed so that adolescent girls do not have to resort to prostitution for their livelihoods. Treaty bodies' formal comments and observations on the degree of compliance with human rights provisions by individual African governments in relation to HIV/AIDS may provide useful points of reference for those concerned with HIV/AIDS prevention and care in the region.

THE GAP BETWEEN HIV/AIDS COMMITMENTS TO HUMAN RIGHTS AND REALITY

In spite of governmental commitments and increased attention to human rights, government policies and actions relevant to HIV/AIDS fail to adequately protect human rights in many ways. There is a contradiction between many international and national commitments to human rights and HIV/AIDS and actual legal and policy implementation and practice.

Most of the human rights issues that were identified in relation to the lives of HIV-infected people at the start of the HIV epidemic are still with us (38). People living with HIV continue to be rejected by their families and communities. The threat of this ostracism results in people not wanting to know their HIV status, or, if aware of their infection, not wanting to disclose this information to their families or partners (2). In fact, stigma was recently identified as *the* key challenge to current prevention and care efforts in Africa (39).

The current interest of some governments in compulsory testing and involuntary disclosure of HIV status is of concern. When disclosure is not voluntary, potential benefits associated with HIV testing must be weighed against potential adverse consequences to the individual, and to their families, when test results become known. For example, when test results are given to family members, employers, and others without an individual's consent, not only has the individual's right to privacy been violated, he or she might also be denied housing, health care, employment, scholarships or educational opportunities (4,40–44). The recent interest of a number of governments in the Southern African Development Community (SADC), such as Namibia and South Africa, in instituting mandatory named reporting and partner notification for people who test HIV-positive is thus of concern. Fear of such policies may explain the underutilization of the limited voluntary testing and counseling sites that do exist. For example, in Botswana where some services are available, preliminary data show that stigma and discrimination, including fear of test results, has kept people away (45). It is estimated that in sub–Saharan Africa, two-thirds of people living with HIV do not even know they are infected (5).

The language of human rights in relation to HIV/AIDS has been raised in unexpected and, at times, contradictory ways in some countries. For example, while making increasing efforts to bring traditional healers into HIV prevention efforts, the Namibian government has recently invoked human rights in ordering the arrest of those traditional healers thought to be encouraging HIV-infected individuals to have sex with minors who are believed to be virgins in order to treat HIV infection (46). Likewise, in Zimbabwe and Botswana, questions concerning the criminalization of HIV transmission have placed some women's groups at odds with some HIV/AIDS groups: some women's groups have demanded the mandatory testing of men accused of rape and sexual offenses to protect the rights and health of women, while some HIV/AIDS groups argue that to do so prior to conviction would violate the rights of the accused (5). In each case, these groups have used the language and power of human rights discourse to advocate their views. These examples illustrate that while attention to human rights does not in and of itself resolve debates, it does provide a language in which these issues can be discussed.

The lack of access to appropriate therapies for HIV-infected people living in Africa, and the inadequacy of the health infrastructure and systems needed to deliver such therapies is increasingly being framed as a human rights issue. Interestingly, African governments and activists are increasingly speaking together in human rights terms as they focus on the actions of international entities, including multinational pharmaceutical companies and governments of the North, such as the United States. This is most apparent in the coming together of the government of South Africa with treatment action groups to claim access to therapies as a human rights issue. Although such claims are being made primarily with respect to pharmaceutical companies, which technically fall outside the system of accountability provided by the human rights framework, these recent developments represent a change in the understanding of human rights, as well as the actors willing to stand together to claim them.

Finally, the range of human rights considerations for women, both in approaches to reducing perinatal transmission and in access to antiretroviral therapies and other forms of care, merits some discussion. The issue of access to drugs for women remains largely focused on mother-to-child transmission. There is increasing rhetorical attention to the fact that life-saving drugs should not be given to women only in order to protect the health of their infants, but there has been little programmatic change toward increasing women's access to antiretrovirals outside of the perinatal prevention effort (47). Gender-based discrimination must receive more attention in the research and conceptual and strategic approaches that are used over the next few years to begin to ensure the availability of HIV treatment in Africa. Once drugs are available within a community, attention must be given to the impact of gender-based discrimination on the ability of women to access them.

STRATEGIES FOR ACTION

The usefulness of governmental commitments, both political and legal, is ultimately dependent on the ability of individuals and communities to hold their governments accountable. A community's ability to bring the effects of HIV under control is directly impacted by the extent to which people living with HIV/AIDS are aware of their rights and feel they have the support and tools at their disposal to fight for them. Without information and education, individuals and communities may be unable to hold their governments accountable or to work toward changing the policies and practices that make them vulnerable to HIV and AIDS.

Expanded partnerships between governments, nongovernmental organizations (NGOs), and AIDS support groups and service organizations within countries and at regional levels have the potential to make human rights a greater priority and provide a crucial link between the promotion and protection of public health and human rights for individuals and communities. A number of organizations in recent years have either incorporated human rights into their HIV/AIDS work, or conversely, brought HIV/AIDS into their legal support work and advocacy. For example, AfriCASO, the regional secretariat of the International Council of AIDS Service Organizations has explicitly taken on a human rights framework for its work, and the AIDS Law Project (ALP) based in South Africa focuses on social, legal, and human rights issues for people living with HIV and with AIDS (48, 49).

Following international consultative meetings under the auspices of UNDP, in Accra, Ghana in 1992 and Dakar, Senegal in 1994, national networks on human rights, ethics and law were established in many parts of Africa with the objectives, *inter alia*, of: (*i*) enabling persons and organizations and national networks to share experiences, resources, and information on HIV/AIDS; (*ii*) promoting human rights and empowering persons to develop guidelines; and (*iii*) collaborating with existing networks and strengthening existing and emerging networks.

By the year 2000 national networks were in place in Burundi, Central African Republic, Côte d'Ivoire, Ghana, Kenya, Rwanda, Senegal, South Africa, Uganda, the Democratic Republic of Congo, and Zambia. The Uganda Legal and Ethical Network (UGANET) was established in 1994, following a series of in-country consultations and an international consultation. UGANET is a registered NGO and has an established permanent secretariat with an elected chairperson and secretary. By early 1999, UGANET had approximately 70 member organizations, a task force of 19 people to oversee activities, and a salaried six-person secretariat (although funding remains precarious). Membership is broad, comprising organizations and individuals representing the law, medicine, health, people living with HIV or AIDS, HIV/AIDS-related NGOs, human rights organizations, religious bodies, academia, governmental structures, and traditional practitioners. The task force meets approximately once a month and operates primarily through six subcommittees focusing respectively on: program development, editorial, advocacy, finance, research, and international public relations. The focus of UGANET has been capacity-building in the area of human rights and HIV/AIDS through workshops at district levels. By the year 2000 workshops had been held in 20 districts and a number of newsletters had been produced and distributed. A number of government partners also interact with UGANET, including the Uganda AIDS Commission (UAC), the Uganda Human Rights Commission, and the Uganda National AIDS Control Programme.

The Kenyan Legal and Ethical Network (KELIN) has collaborated with a range of stakeholders to analyze the human rights issues raised by the HIV epidemic in Kenya and has produced a paper under the auspices of the Ministry of Health to enable the government to make progress in this area. Although the paper has not yet been passed by Parliament, KELIN and others continue to urge that the paper's recommendations be implemented. KELIN's current efforts are focused principally on promoting legally sound national HIV/AIDS policies and legislation and on building resource networks of lawyers at provincial levels to carry out community education on human rights issues in the context of HIV/AIDS.

Another important area bringing together HIV/AIDS and human rights issues in sub–Saharan Africa concerns the development of codes of conduct in relation to employment practices. A best practice example with implications for much of the region is the South African HIV/AIDS Employment Code of Conduct, which was developed between 1994 and 1996. The code was drafted by the AIDS Law Project and the Consortium on Legal Rights and AIDS in a process that brought together the input of trade unions, employers, and government. The process included intensive advocacy and lobbying efforts, the widespread dissemination of consultation drafts of the code (5,000 of each of the several drafts, and publication in a national business newspaper with a circulation of 40,000), and seminars and workshops around the country. The final provisions of the code focus on the rights of HIV-infected employees (including potential or past employees), the responsibilities of employers, and the use of the workplace for targeted prevention programs. The fundamental principle underpinning the code is that HIV/AIDS should be treated like other comparable life-threatening diseases. It covers issues such as discrimination, informed consent to testing, confidentiality, access to benefits, sick leave, compensation, dispute resolution, grievance, and disciplinary procedures. In May 1997, 10 out of 11 Ministers of Labor in SADC countries adopted this code as a regional guideline (50). In September 1997 the code was formally endorsed by the 15 heads of government from SADC countries, and the process of national implementation is currently under way. It has also been adopted by a number of local councils and private companies, some of which have adapted it as their own policy document.

A critical element to improving the lives of people living with HIV or AIDS in the region is increased collaboration between law and human rights organizations and others concerned with HIV prevention, treatment and impact reduction in mutually strengthening ways (51,52). Recent interest in the ongoing problem of HIV/AIDS–related discrimination in sub–Saharan Africa has resulted in the creation of an email forum exclusively focused on issues of HIV/AIDS stigma, denial, shame, and discrimination. While just started, this forum promises to be a useful avenue for the exchange of information and strategies by many different actors to reduce the effects of stigma and discrimination within communities and institutions (53).

CONCLUSION

The importance of bringing HIV/AIDS policies and programs in line with human rights law is generally acknowledged (54). The course of the AIDS epidemic has shown that public health efforts to prevent and control the spread of HIV/AIDS are more likely to succeed when policies and programs promote and protect human rights. Those involved in policy and decision-making, as well as implementation within each sector of the government, must be made aware of the commitments made by their representatives in both national and international forums, as these commitments are often neglected or overlooked. Enhanced community participation in the implementation of strategies relevant to HIV/AIDS will help ensure attention to human rights concerns and improve their effectiveness. National level mechanisms concerned with HIV/AIDS and human rights must be strengthened and recognized as forming an integral part of the response to the HIV epidemic. Information, education, and advocacy in the context of a human rights framework continues to provide an opportunity to ensure that public health efforts will positively impact the response to the HIV/AIDS epidemic in the next century.

REFERENCES

1. Tarantola D, Schwartländer B. HIV/AIDS in Africa: status, trends (stable, declining) projections, newly affected areas. *AIDS*, 1997;11(Suppl B): S5–S21.
2. UNAIDS. *HIV and AIDS-related stigmatization, discrimination and denial: forms, contexts and determinants.* Research studies from Uganda and India, Best Practice Collection. Geneva: UNAIDS, 2000.
3. Amnesty International. *Human Rights Abuses in the Context of HIV/AIDS Relevant to the Mandate.* Chicago: Amnesty International, 1994.
4. Human Rights Internet. *Human rights and HIV/AIDS: Effective Community Responses.* Ottawa: International Human Rights Documentation Network, 1998.
5. UNAIDS. *Report on the global HIV/AIDS epidemic.* Geneva: UNAIDS, 2000.
6. UNICEF: *The Progress of Nations*, 2000. New York: UNICEF, 2000.
7. Levine C, ed. *The White Oak Report.* A report from a workshop held at the White Oak Conservation Center; October 1–4, 1998; Yulee, Florida, USA.
8. USAID. *Children on the Brink: Strategies to Support a Generation Isolated by HIV/AIDS.* Health Technical Services Project for USAID. Washington DC: USAID, 1997.
9. UNICEF. *AIDS and Orphans in Africa.* New York: United Nations, 1991.
10. Hunter SS, Williamson J. *Developing strategies and policies for support of HIV/AIDS infected and affected children.* Washington, DC: USAID, 1997.

11. Ayieko MA. *From single parents to child-headed households: The case of children orphaned by AIDS in Kisimu and Siaya districts*. University of Illinois, Department of International Program and Studies. New York: UNDP, 1997.
12. Albertyn C. *Prevention, treatment and care in the context of human rights*. Expert Group meeting on the HIV/AIDS Pandemic and its Gender Implications; November 13–17, 2000; Windhoek, Namibia. Full paper available at: http://www.un.org/womenwatch/daw/csw/hivaids/albertyn.html. Accessed February 9, 2002.
13. UNAIDS. *Women and AIDS*. Geneva: UNAIDS Best Practice Collection, 1997.
14. Decosas J. Migration et sida en Afrique de L'Ouest. *Le Journal du Sida*, 1996;86–87:97–100.
15. World Bank. *Intensifying Action Against HIV/AIDS in Africa. Responding to a Development Crisis*. Washington, DC: World Bank, 1999.
16. UNHCR. *UNHCR policy and guidelines regarding refugee protection and assistance and the acquired immune deficiency syndrome (AIDS)*. Geneva: UNHCR, 1988.
17. Charter of the United Nations, signed at San Francisco on 26 June 1945, *entry into force 24 October 1945*, in accordance with Article 110. [See, in particular, Preamble and articles 1, 2, 7, 13, 55, 56, 62, 73, 74, and 75–85]. Available at: http://www.unhchr.ch/html/intlinst.htm. Accessed January 11, 2002.
18. United Nations. International Human Rights Instruments. [See in particular, International Covenant on Civil and Political Rights (ICCPR), G.A. Res. 2200 (XXI), UN GAOR, 21st Sess., Supp. No. 16, at 49, UN Doc. A/6316 (1966); International Covenant on Economic, Social and Cultural Rights (ICESCR), G.A. Res. 2200 (XXI), UN GAOR, 21st Sess., Supp. No. 16, at 49, UN Doc. A/6316 (1966); Convention on the Elimination of All Forms of Racial Discrimination, UN G.A. Res. 2106A (XX) (1965); Convention on the Elimination of All Forms of Discrimination Against Women, G.A. Res. 34/180, UN GAOR, 34th Sess., Supp. No. 46, at 193, UN Doc. A/34/46 (1979); Convention on the Rights of the Child (CRC), G.A. Res. 44/25, UN GAOR, 44th Sess., Supp. No. 49, at 166, UN Doc. A/44/25 (1989)]. Available at: http://www.unhchr.ch/html/intlinst.htm. Accessed January 11, 2002.
19. African [Banjul] Charter on Human and Peoples' Rights, adopted 27 June 1981, OAU Doc. CAB/LEG/67/3 rev. 5, 21 I.L.M. 58 (1982), *entered into force* Oct. 21, 1986. Available at: http://www.itcilo.it/english/actrav/telearn/global/ilo/law/africahr.htm. Accessed January 11, 2002.
20. Eide A. Economic, social and cultural rights as human rights. In: Eide A, Krause C, Rosas A, eds. *Economic, Social and Cultural Rights: a Textbook*. Dordrecht: Martinus Nijhoff, 1995:21–40.
21. Alston P, Quinn G. The nature and scope of state parties' obligations under the international covenant and economic, social and cultural rights. *Human Rights Quarterly*, 1987;9:165–66.
22. International Covenant on Economic, Social and Cultural Rights, G.A. Res. 2200 (XXI), U.N. GAOR, 21st Sess., Supp. NO. 16, at 49 [U.N. Doc. A/6316 (1966), Article 2]. Available at: http://www.unhchr.ch/html/intlinst.htm. Accessed January 11, 2002.
23. United Nations. Progressive development of the principles and norms of international law relating to the new international economic order: Report of the Secretary General; 1984; G.A., Sess. 39 [UN Doc. A/39/504/Add. 1].
24. United Nations Human Rights Commission. Non-discrimination in the field of health. United Nations resolution 1989/11; March 2, 1989.
25. Mann J. Human rights and AIDS: the future of the pandemic. *The John Marshall Law Review*, 1996;30:195–206.
26. Tarantola D. Reducing HIV/AIDS risk, impact and vulnerability. Editorial in: Special Theme—Immunization Safety. *Bulletin of the World Health Organization*, 2000;78(2):236–237.
27. International Federal of Red Cross and Red Crescent Societies (IFRCRC) and François-Xavier Bagnoud Center for Health and Human Rights (FXBC). The public health—human rights dialogue. In: *AIDS, health and human rights: an explanatory manual*. Geneva and Boston: IFRCRC, 1995.
28. Gruskin S, Hendricks A, Tomaševski K. Human rights and responses to HIV/AIDS. In: Mann J, Tarantola D, eds. *AIDS in the World II*. New York: Oxford University Press, 1996:326–340.
29. Mann J, Tarantola D, Netter T. National AIDS plans. In: Mann J, Tarantola D, Netter T, eds. *AIDS in the World*. Cambridge, MA: Harvard University Press, 1992:297.
30. Harvard AIDS Institute. African priorities for HIV and AIDS: A Summary Document from the National AIDS Plans of Several Sub-Saharan Countries. Paper presented at *Africa Now*! A Leadership Summit to Define African Priorities for AIDS; November, 2000; Boston, MA.
31. Tarantola D. Grandes et petites histories des programmes sida. Le Journal du SIDA, 1996; 86–87:109–116.
32. The Panos Institute. *Beyond our means? The cost of treating HIV/AIDS in the developing world*. The Panos Institute, London, 2000.
33. Coates T, Sangiwa G, Balmer D, et al. Voluntary HIV counseling and testing reduces risk behavior in developing countries: results from the voluntary HIV-1 counseling and testing efficacy study.

12th World AIDS Conference Update on CD-ROM, 1998. [133/33269].

34. UNAIDS. *HIV/AIDS prevention in the context of new therapies*. Geneva: UNAIDS, 1999.
35. International Partnership Against AIDS in Africa. *Working in Partnership: Intensifying National and International Responses to AIDS in Africa. A Framework for Action*. Geneva: UNAIDS, 1999.
36. International Partnership Against AIDS in Africa. Available from the UNAIDS web site, http://www.unaids.org/africapartnership/background.html. Accessed January 11, 2002.
37. Documents by treaty. Available from the United Nations High Commissioner for Human Rights web site: http://www.unhchr.ch/tbs/doc.nsf. Accessed January 11, 2002.
38. Gruskin S, Wakhweya A. A human rights perspective on HIV/AIDS in sub-Saharan Africa. *AIDS*, 1997;11(suppl B):S159–S167.
39. Statement from the 1st Regional Conference on Community Home Based Care; March 5–8 2001; Gaborone, Botswana.
40. Gruskin S, Hendricks A, Tomaševski K. Human rights and responses to HIV/AIDS. In: Mann J, Tarantola D, eds. *AIDS in the World II*. New York: Oxford University Press, 1996:336–337.
41. Appendix E. Laws and practices in the context of HIV: a survey of Government National AIDS Program managers. In: Mann J, Tarantola D, eds. *AIDS in the World II*. New York: Oxford Univesrity Press, 1996:578–587.
42. Gruskin S and Tarantola D. Discrimination and Human Rights: HIV/AIDS and Human Rights Revisited. *Canadian HIV/AIDS Policy and Law Review*, 2001;6(1/2):24–29.
43. Human Rights Watch. *World Report 2001*. New York: Human Rights Watch, 2001.
44. AIDS Law Project. *Annual report 1999*. Johannesburg: AIDS Law Project, 1999.
45. UNICEF, UNAIDS, WHO, UNFPA. Report from the African Regional Meeting on Pilot Projects for the Prevention of Mother to Child Transmission of HIV; March 2000; Gabarone, Botswana.
46. Ahmad K. Namibian government to prosecute healers. *The Lancet*, 2001;357:371.
47. Gruskin S. Some thoughts while attending AIDS 2000. *Women's Health Project Newsletter*, 2000;35:6.
48. Available from the AFRICASO web site at: http://www.africaso.org. Accessed January 11, 2002.
49. Available from the AIDS Law Project web site at http://www.hri.ca/partners/alp. Accessed January 11, 2002.
50. HIV/AIDS and the Law: A Resource Manual. AIDS Law Project and Lawyers for Human Rights, University of Witwatersrand, South Africa, May 1997, Appendix 2.
51. O'Malley J. Nongovernmental organizations. In: Mann J, Tarantola D, eds. *AIDS in the World II*. New York: Oxford University Press, 1996:341–361.
52. Cosmas C, Schmidt-Ehry B. Human rights and health in developing countries: barriers to community participation in public health in Cameroon. *Health and Human Rights*, 1995;1:244–254.
53. France N, Anderson S, Manchester J. Stigma, denial and shame in Africa: barriers to community and home-based care for people infected and affected by HIV/AIDS. Plenary presentation on stigma, delivered at the 1st Regional Home and Community-Based Care Conference; March 2001; Gaborone, Botswana.
54. UNAIDS. Framework for global leadership on HIV/ AIDS: Report of the Third Ad Hoc Thematic Meeting of the Programme Coordinating Board of UNAIDS; Rio de Janeiro: UNAIDS, 2000.
55. Available from the United Nations High Commissioner for Human Rights web site at: http://www.unhchr.ch/. Accessed April 17, 2001.

43

Gender and HIV/AIDS

Sheila D. Tlou

Department of Nursing Studies, University of Botswana, Gaborone, Botswana.

Sub–Saharan Africa is unique in that it is the only region in the world where more women than men are infected with HIV. Not only are women in Africa disproportionately infected, but HIV infection in women often places them at particularly increased risk of rejection, loss of security, stigma, and violence (1). The main argument of this chapter is that while both women and men in Africa are vulnerable to HIV infection and AIDS, women are more vulnerable and are more severely impacted because of their status, roles, and limited rights in society. The differential sociocultural and economic vulnerability of women and men will be explored, and recommendations will be made for reducing vulnerability to HIV and AIDS in order to work toward an AIDS-free generation in the future.

UNAIDS estimates that over 13 million women in Africa are living with HIV, compared to 11 million men. AIDS is the leading cause of death for women aged 19 to 40, and infant mortality rates have increased as a result of perinatal HIV transmission (2). A gender-based approach to the analysis of the risk factors and impact of HIV infection helps to explain why a virus that infects both men and women is affecting women and girls in an increasingly disproportionate manner.

BIOLOGIC VULNERABILITY

Most African women become infected with HIV through unprotected vaginal intercourse, and male-to-female sexual transmission of HIV is generally more efficient—up to four times more efficient according to UNAIDS (2)—than female-to-male transmission. The major factors responsible for this differential in transmission efficiency are the large mucosal surface area exposed to the virus in women, and the greater viral concentration in semen compared with vaginal secretions (see Chapter 13, *this volume*). Some of the other cofactors that have been found to increase women's vulnerability to HIV infection include: contaminated blood and blood products, general poor health, and the presence of sexually transmitted diseases (STDs), especially ulcerative infections such as chancroid, syphilis, and herpes. While it is relatively easy to diagnose and treat STDs in men, most women with STDs are asymptomatic and therefore may be unaware that they need to seek health care. This situation impedes early detection and timely treatment of STDs in women, thus increasing their chances of contracting HIV (see Chapter 14, *this volume*).

SOCIOCULTURAL AND ECONOMIC VULNERABILITY

The biologic factors that differentiate men and women's susceptibility to HIV are greatly overshadowed by the sexual and economic subordination that increases women's vulnerability to HIV infection. African women's relative lack of power over their bodies and their sexual lives, a situation that is reinforced by social and economic inequality, makes them more vulnerable to HIV infection and the consequences of the epidemic.

Social and economic inequality, traditional gender roles, attitudes toward fertility, lack of access to information about sexual and reproductive health, traditional practices and beliefs about HIV and AIDS, gender-based violence, and limited political will and commitment to change inequitable conditions, are among some of the culturally and socioeconomically constructed gender-bound factors that increase women and men's vulnerability to HIV infection and AIDS.

Economic Inequality

The legal systems and cultural norms of many African countries reinforce gender inequality by giving men control over productive resources such as land, through, for example, marriage customs that subordinate wives to their husbands, and inheritance customs that make males the principal beneficiaries of family property. For example, in Botswana, a woman married in community of property cannot access credit without her husband's permission (3). Such restrictions have far-reaching consequences for the rights of women, the achievement of national development, and the transmission and rapid spread of HIV.

Young women face discrimination in employment and in economic opportunities in virtually every African society, resulting in a feminization of poverty, and perpetuating women's economic subordination to men. Women often lack access to technical assistance and training. Furthermore, there are laws that limit women's ability to enter into independent contracts or to obtain credit in their own names. These and other inequitable conditions impede women's ability to control income and property (4,5). Economic dependence on men further limits women's sexual negotiating power and makes it difficult for them to refuse unsafe sex even when they know that their male partners are involved in risky sexual behaviors that could predispose them to HIV infection.

The current economic crises in many of the less developed African countries have affected the profitability of the overcrowded informal sector in which a majority of young women are engaged in activities such as petty trade, food preparation, gardening, sewing, domestic service, hairdressing, midwifery, and beer brewing. As economic conditions worsen, many young women, especially in urban areas, are compelled to barter sex for survival and to seek occasional sexual partners to help meet their cash needs. Some women also become engaged in commercial sex work, for which there is demand in urban settings, in order to avoid poverty for themselves and their families (1,5). In an environment of reduced educational and economic opportunities, coupled with denial of the dangers of HIV infection, young women may become easy targets for the advances of older, rich, and increasingly higher risk "sugar daddies"—men who provide money and goods in exchange for extramarital relationships with younger women who are presumably at lower risk for being HIV-infected. Also, schoolgirls and students are often required to provide sexual services to teachers in order to avoid having low grades (6,7).

Men and HIV/AIDS

Prevention programs have traditionally neglected the role that heterosexual African men play in the transmission of HIV. Until recently, men have been almost invisible as part of the solution to the HIV epidemic even though it has been obvious that their socialization and resultant behaviors often determine when, how, and to whom the virus is transmitted (7–9). It is only in the year 2000 that for World AIDS Day many stakeholders realized that men could be enlisted to role model appropriate and constructive masculine behaviors.

The same gender roles and relationship dynamics that increase women's vulnerability to HIV infection also increase the risks for men. Dominant ideologies of masculinity encourage men to be aggressive and to demonstrate their sexual prowess or virility by having multiple partners, and by consuming alcohol and other substances that predispose them to violent behavior and sexual risk taking. Research indicates that some men tend to think that it is acceptable to have extramarital affairs, but that they are not necessarily keen on using condoms and would use them only when they do not trust their partners (for example in casual sex) (8,9). Such attitudes and behaviors are the root of the growing AIDS epidemic and need urgent intervention. What is also apparent is that even though men generally assume the knowledgeable, aggressive, and directive role in sexual encounters with women, they often lack the necessary information to make healthy choices. For example, studies in Botswana have found that a significant number of men are not aware that STDs enhance HIV transmission or that they could benefit from clinical treatment of STDs (6,10). They prefer to consult traditional doctors or get over-the-counter treatment, and some of them may thus not be getting adequate treatment for STDs.

There is still a denial of the rights of gay men in most African countries. In fact "sodomy" is considered a criminal offense and some African heads of state have openly declared a "war" against gay communities. Because of these sanctions, men who have sex with men may be hesitant to publicly declare their sexual orientation, but this does not mean that they do not exist in African countries, or that they are not sexually active. Worse still, since society expects them to be heterosexual, some are likely to date girls and even marry under pressure, but secretly continue their sexual activities with other men. This predisposes them and potentially their families to unnecessary psychologic trauma, and it predisposes them and their partners to HIV infection. It also deprives men who have sex with men of their right to be guided and informed about safer sex in the same manner as heterosexual men.

Attitudes toward Fertility

Most Africans generally believe that a person becomes immortal or "leaves something of oneself behind after death" by procreating. Men prove their virility by making a woman or women pregnant. For women, motherhood is the passport to womanhood and the only way a woman can prove that she is fertile. A married woman's infertility has major social and psychologic consequences: she can be blamed for her past sexual behavior, isolated, scorned by relatives or in-laws, divorced by her husband, or forced to accept and even raise her husband's children with other women. Thus, sexuality and fertility are treated as synonymous and a woman's status is closely tied to her reproductive roles as mother and wife. In some cases a husband may insist on more children even when he or his wife is known to be HIV-infected and the wife must comply or risk a broken marriage (10–12).

Many women are therefore eager to bear children for their male partners to "cement" the relationship or to encourage marriage. Condoms do not feature in such relationships, thus increasing the risk of HIV infection for both partners.

Access to Sexual and Reproductive Health Care and Information

The special vulnerability of girls and young women to HIV infection has been documented in many studies and discussed at various forums of the United Nations. While most African states agree that all young people have the right to develop their capacities, to access a range of services and opportunities, to live, learn, and earn in a safe and supportive environment, and to participate in decisions and actions that affect them, social institutions such as schools, NGOs, the media, the private sector, and the government are doing very little to support these rights. This is partly because of strong cultural prohibitions against discussing sexual matters and the expectation that virgins should be ignorant about sex, sexuality, and even HIV and AIDS (13, 14). Access to information relating to sexual health for girls and boys is still a controversial issue despite extensive research showing that school-based life skills education empowers youth and does not increase their sexual activity.

Parents are often conspicuously absent in the sexual education of their children. Research on intergenerational communication (5,6,15,16) has shown that fathers and mothers are constrained by a culture that forbids them to talk to their sons and daughters about sex. While a few mothers do give their daughters instructions on menstruation and personal hygiene, most of them feel unable to broach any topic related to sex, other than the admonition to "stay away from boys". Girls, in turn, feel embarrassed about discussing these matters with their mothers and rely on friends or older sisters for information. Boys receive even less instruction on how to make responsible sexual decisions. In fact, some boys have reported being pressured by peers and older brothers and cousins to become sexually active since having sex is seen as achievement of proper masculinity (8,9).

Boys and girls, therefore, lack access to sexual and reproductive health information in a social context in which the majority of adult women face male control over sexual information and decision-making. Unplanned pregnancies and STDs that can lead to infertility and HIV acquisition are among the consequences for young girls and boys who engage in early sexual activity in the absence of sexuality education.

Cultural Beliefs and Practices Relating to HIV/AIDS

Public health campaigns have generally created high levels of awareness and concern about HIV and AIDS among Africans. However, the major problem in most countries is still the translation of this concern into responsible sexual behavior. This gap between awareness and action results partly from cultural beliefs and myths. African youth grow up hearing about HIV and AIDS from older adults who share stories and myths that may render all prevention messages useless. This misinformation may lead youth to adopt fatalistic behaviors. For example, a young person who believes that HIV can be transmitted by mosquitoes is likely to see no point in abstaining from sex or using a condom.

Some traditional doctors also claim that they can cure AIDS and cite stories of how their clients were healed and went on to live an AIDS-free life (3,17). What seems to happen, is an alleviation of some symptoms such that the client believes he or she has been cured, not an actual eradication of HIV in the body. Such clients, believing they are HIV-free, are not likely to practice safer sex, and thus transmit HIV to their partners.

Beliefs about HIV transmission and AIDS are also rooted in cultural perceptions of disease being a result of witchcraft or the breaking of social norms and taboos. For example, in Botswana (18), many older people believe that AIDS is not a new disease, but an epidemic resulting from noncompliance with the sexual taboos relating to widowhood, or *boswagadi*. *Boswagadi* is a state of widowhood whereby one whose spouse has died must undergo ritual cleansing and observe several taboos, the major one being sexual abstinence for a period of one year. The purpose of these rituals is to dissolve the physical and spiritual unity between the living and the dead spouse that was established at marriage and at subsequent births of children. At the end of a year, only a traditional doctor can perform the purification rituals and declare the widow or widower free to live as a single person (i.e., have sexual relations, remarry, etc.). It is believed that failure to partake in the rituals and abstain from sex can result in disease and ultimately, the death of the widower or widow, or any person who has sex with him or her. The term *boswagadi* is also used to name the disease that is believed to result from failure to observe the prescribed rituals, the symptoms of which are the same as those attributed to AIDS— weight loss, diarrhea, swollen limbs, multiple infections, etc. Thus, AIDS is seen as an epidemic of *boswagadi* brought about by young "modern" people who refuse to observe sexual taboos and end up spreading disease. An interesting point is that traditional doctors can prescribe herbs to enable widowers to break abstinence before the year-long period is over but the same treatment is believed to be ineffective for widows.

Among the practices that increase risk for HIV infection, one of the most worrying is the use of vaginal desiccating agents because of the belief that "dry sex" enhances male pleasure and strengthens emotional bonds. Vaginal drying practices, in which herbs, aluminium hydroxide powder, stones, and other agents are inserted into the vagina, are widely reported in African countries (1,5,17,19). Many of these agents are reported to cause inflammation and irritation of the vaginal mucosa which can increase the likelihood of heterosexual HIV transmission.

Gender-Based Violence

Gender-based violence is a major violation of human rights and a constraint to national development in Africa. In most countries women continue to experience severe beating, rape, socioeconomic abuse, as well as verbal and emotional abuse. The perpetrators of violence are usually husbands/partners and male acquaintances, as well as male family members, indicating that the home environment may not necessarily be as safe for many women and girls as is often assumed. In addition to the psychologic consequences of sexual violence, survivors experience physical injuries, unwanted pregnancies, and STDs. Practices such as female genital mutilation, and acts of rape and coercive sex, especially in young women and girls, result in damage to the genital mucosa and facilitate HIV transmission. Young women who are forced to have unprotected sex by their partners often cannot insist on condom use for fear of violence (20–22).

Violence against women is deeply rooted in stereotypical gender beliefs and roles. Physical violence, the threat of violence, and fear of abandonment act as significant barriers for women who want to negotiate the use of a condom, discuss fidelity with their partners, or leave relationships that they perceive to be risky. Those who are at special risk of violence are women known or suspected to be HIV-positive, young women and girls, sex workers, trafficked women, street children, and children orphaned by AIDS. Fear of violence also inhibits women from living positively with HIV. For example, a study in Kinshasa, Democratic Republic of Congo found that about 97% of women with HIV were unwilling to inform their sexual partners of their HIV status for fear of violence, physical harm, or even murder (12, 19).

Sexual exploitation of girls in Africa takes the form of males expecting sexual relationships with any females that receive their financial support, forced early marriages, males seeking partners in younger age groups that are perceived to have lower HIV prevalence, and erroneous prescriptions by traditional healers that sex with a virgin can cure AIDS (5,19). Because of these practices, increasing numbers of young girls are having sex at early ages and becoming predisposed to HIV infection.

The trafficking of girls into prostitution and sexual slavery is another form of violence against young women in Africa, which is fueled by widespread poverty, international sex tourism, and the forces of globalization. Because many of these girls and women enter receiving countries illegally and are in settings where commercial sex work is illegal, they are not protected by the law, experience greater social stigma as foreign sex workers, and have even less access to social services than other women (1,5).

Wars and other conflicts increase the vulnerability of women and girls to HIV infection, particularly through systematic rape and other war crimes. UNAIDS has noted that most countries with severe AIDS epidemics have experienced some civil conflict (22). Conflict increases local and regional insecurity, increases poverty, and can lead to the breakdown of social services and infrastructure and a lack of food, shelter, medicines, and health care workers. Conflicts also result in large portions of limited resources being allocated to military spending rather than to social services.

THE GENDER-SPECIFIC IMPACT OF HIV/AIDS

The impact of HIV and AIDS on African communities, economies, and social structures has been extensively covered in this book. However, there are some particularly gender-bound consequences of HIV and AIDS that deserve mention here.

Women often discover their HIV status, or suspect that they are infected, by chance; a woman's spouse or child may be symptomatic, or she may be pregnant and therefore counseled on HIV testing at an antenatal clinic. HIV diagnosis may be the first indication that a woman or her spouse has had another partner, and this disclosure is usually very traumatic.

Women are also often wrongly accused of having brought HIV infection into the family. This is especially true if a woman goes for testing first or develops noticeable symptoms earlier than her partner does. Fear of social stigma, physical harm, isolation and loneliness, and/or abandonment by loved ones, family, and friends often compel women to keep their HIV diagnosis a secret until the very last hour (23). In a recent study conducted by researchers in Botswana and Zambia in collaboration with researchers from the International Centre for Research on Women, both men and women expressed concern for women who test HIV-positive because they felt that men would be likely to abandon an HIV-positive partner. On the other hand, it was expected that women would initially get angry with an HIV-positive partner, but ultimately accept him (24).

The diagnosis of HIV infection has been seen to take a serious emotional toll on men. While women might confide in a mother, a sister, or a friend about their HIV status and receive the needed support, men may be less likely, because their socialization, to do so. The resultant lack of emotional support for men, exacerbates their isolation and self-pity, and may even predispose them to committing suicide (25,26).

HIV-related illness affects male-headed and female-headed households differently. Death of the male in a male-headed household usually results in a reduction of disposable household income. In cultures where women are the primary providers of food for the household, female illness or death is likely to contribute to problems with food security for other family members (3,26,27).

Women and the Burden of Care

The provision of care to sick family members has traditionally been seen as a woman's rather than a man's responsibility, and AIDS caregiving is no exception. Caring for people living with AIDS has been shown to be physically and psychologically stressful. Studies on home-based care (18,20,27) indicate that elderly women and girls are the major caregivers for people living with HIV or AIDS, yet they tend to have little access to resources such as good nutrition, transport, and professional support. Furthermore, they often have less access to care and support when they themselves are infected. Very few men and boys share domestic responsibilities, so the burden of providing respite for female adult carers falls on girls. They are expected to help with caregiving and other chores immediately after school, which has a negative effect on their ability to do homework and school work in general. School grades are affected and most girls end up not performing as well as boys, resulting in more and more girls being absent from the natural science careers, for example, and being channeled into the less-paying social science careers, such as nursing and teaching. Some girls are even withdrawn from school to assist with household chores or to engage in income generating activities, including sex work, to augment family incomes. If the situation of girls is not improved, it will be impossible for Africa to ever attain gender equality in education, employment, and economic empowerment.

RECOMMENDATIONS FOR AN AIDS-FREE GENERATION

In general, African governments do recognize that gender inequality is one of the determinants of HIV transmission and that strategies to reduce HIV transmission thus include: supporting and strengthening women's NGOs, supporting a review of policies and laws that disadvantage women, supporting enforcement of Children's Acts to protect girl children, ensuring equal access to education and health, initiating income generating activities to reduce women's economic dependency on men, and empowering women and girls with safer sex negotiation skills. The major problem is that very few of the above strategies have actually been implemented. Gender inequality persists, and it is fueling the HIV epidemic.

Africa's response to the epidemic must be comprehensive and address both the prevention of HIV infection and the impact of HIV and AIDS on young men and women. In addition to mainstreaming a gender perspective into all policies, programs, and activities for youth, the following strategies are recommended for African governments, the private sector, donor agencies, and civil society.

Institute Legal and Policy Reforms

An important way of reducing vulnerability to HIV is to catalyze equitable social and economic development. A major part of this effort should include addressing factors that limit young women's access to productive resources and economic opportunities by eliminating all laws and cultural practices that discriminate against women, as stated in the United Nations Convention on the Elimination of All Forms of Discrimination Against Women (CEDAW), a convention that most African countries have ratified. Public policy and legal reforms need to be geared toward the promotion of human rights, protection against violence, stigma and discrimination, as well as equitable access to information, health, education, property, and credit facilities.

Governments should take concrete measures to eradicate all forms of violence against boys and girls, including in conflict situations, through gender-sensitive economic, legal, and social services and programs.

Ensure Political Will and Commitment

The issues of HIV and AIDS should by now be on each country's national agenda because of the many U.N. sessions at which governments, U.N. agencies, and civic society have discussed and adopted resolutions and documents for further actions, particularly on issues concerning women, gender, and HIV and AIDS. Some of the documents from these sessions are: The Beijing Platform for Action (23), which came out of the Fourth World Conference on Women; and the Programme of Action of the International Conference on Population and Development, which calls for a holistic life cycle approach to women's health care with emphasis on increased allocation of resources for the sexual health and reproductive rights of all women, provision of affordable health care, health promotion and disease prevention, and prevention and treatment of STDs and HIV/AIDS. Resolutions were also made at the 43rd, 44th, and 45th sessions of the U.N. Commission on the Status of Women when member states resolved to ensure greater protections of women from HIV infection, including access to female-controlled HIV prevention methods. These resolutions were reiterated at the Special Session of the General Assembly of HIV/AIDS (UNGASS) in June 2001, which was attended by Heads of State from all over the world. Each political leader must put these resolutions into action and allocate the necessary resources for programs and activities. Sub–Saharan Africa needs to adopt a human rights approach to the AIDS epidemic; such an approach entrenches the principle that governments should be accountable to their people. Each time a woman is unable to negotiate safer sex, it is a violation of her civil rights because it indicates her lack of autonomy to decide on matters relating to her sexual and reproductive health, and such situations cannot continue. Women and men should be able to access affordable treatment for HIV and AIDS, including antiretrovirals and prophylactic treatment for opportunistic infections.

There is concrete evidence that peer group interventions, combined with the social marketing of condoms, mass media campaigns, high level political commitment, and other structural changes, have reduced new infections in countries such as Thailand and in Uganda, where sexual activity among young people has declined (1,22).

Mainstream HIV/AIDS Activities into Research and Development Programs

Linkages must be made between HIV/AIDS prevention, other activities that aim to alleviate the impact of the epidemic, and development programs, such as poverty alleviation, tourism, health, education, labor, lands allocation, immigration, agriculture, and manufacturing and industry. For example, for the health sector, integrating HIV and AIDS prevention services into existing primary health care services would make them more accessible to youth, and would reduce fears of the social stigma associated with premarital sex.

Research on gender and HIV/AIDS issues should inform and drive policy; therefore, there should be forums for interaction between researchers, policy makers, and implementers of programs. The value of policy-oriented research and evidence-based practice of HIV/ AIDS cannot be overemphasized.

Fund and Promote Research on HIV Vaccines and Female-Controlled HIV Prevention Methods

Ethical guidelines have already been developed for the conduct of HIV vaccine trials, and communities, especially women's networks, need to be mobilized to participate in such trials. An HIV vaccine would be a prevention strategy available to all, regardless of gender. Of major importance is the urgent promotion of female-controlled methods, such as female condoms and microbicides. Female condoms are discussed elsewhere (see Chapter 32, *this volume*). However, it is worth noting that any condom use requires the cooperation of the male partner. African men have been shown to express anxiety about female condoms because of a presumed lack of control over female partners who use female condoms (24,28). Microbicides are currently being tested for their effectiveness in the prevention of HIV transmission and other STDs. For young women who can neither insist on condom use nor quit relationships that put their health at risk, microbicides are ideal because they are safe, inexpensive, easy to store, and can be used discretely without the male partner's knowledge. For youth, the ideal microbicide would also have contraceptive properties to avoid teenage pregnancy.

Promote Life Skills among Young People, with Parental Involvement

Empowerment of young boys and girls with sexual and reproductive health information long before they are sexually active should include discussions on gender roles, gender-based violence, sexuality, relationships, and shared responsibilities for HIV prevention and care of people living with HIV and AIDS. Life skills education, embracing sexual and reproductive health and the rights of both boys and girls, would reinforce already existing moral and religious attitudes and values, and could be fully integrated into the primary and secondary school curricula. To reinforce the school curricula, parents need to be empowered with knowledge and skills to help with homework and to talk to their children about responsible sexual behavior. In Botswana and Zimbabwe, for example, pilot projects have been initiated by UNICEF and the respective Ministries of Health to equip parents and teachers with skills to communicate with youth on sexual and reproductive health matters (3). Such efforts need to be replicated throughout Africa to complement other HIV/AIDS prevention strategies for young women and men.

People living with HIV/AIDS must be involved as educators, carers, and counselors in their communities. They should also be involved in making and implementing sound and humane public health decisions that would ensure a better quality of life and care for themselves and others living with HIV. Young men should be involved in national and international activities relating to HIV prevention, impact alleviation, and care of people living with HIV/AIDS. Situating HIV/AIDS campaigns in places where men frequently gather, such as at sports events, or beer shebeens and other drinking places, has also been shown to be effective, especially when men are persuaded to protect themselves so that they can protect their children and families (25,26).

Provide Access to Voluntary Counseling and HIV Testing Centers

An important element of any prevention and care strategy is access to information about one's HIV status. However, most African countries have very few voluntary counseling and testing centers. More viable centers need to be set up in each country so that people are able to access information about their HIV status, get the counseling and information they need, and receive support to either maintain a negative HIV status or to live positively with HIV. In addition, it is only through voluntary counseling and testing that vertical transmission of HIV can be reduced.

CONCLUSION

In most sub–Saharan African countries, women and girls are more vulnerable to HIV and AIDS because of economic and social inequalities that diminish women's abilities to make choices that promote their overall health status. The HIV epidemic threatens African women's full enjoyment of their basic human rights and fundamental freedoms. It threatens all the progress made toward the advancement of women's rights and their status, particularly the rights of young girls, as they become the primary caregivers. In many instances girls are forced to drop out of school and are deprived of their right to basic education. Women and young girls are also subject to pressure to provide for their families, and at times resort to exploitative occupations such as sex work. The epidemic also exacerbates the impact of harmful social norms, beliefs, and practices, and has caused a tremendous setback in maternal mortality and women's overall life expectancy.

It is, therefore, imperative to eliminate the social, economic, and political inequalities that make women vulnerable to HIV in order to create an environment for change toward gender equality, an environment in which an expanded response to the epidemic could ensure the protection of both men and women, the continued development of African nations, and hopefully, an AIDS-free generation in the future.

REFERENCES

1. UNAIDS. *Gender and HIV/AIDS: Taking Stock of Research and Programmes*. Geneva: United Nations, 1999.
2. UNAIDS. *Men and AIDS-a gender approach.* 2000 World AIDS Campaign. New York: UNAIDS, 2000.
3. Botswana Government and UNAIDS. *Human Development Report:* Gaborone: UNAIDS, 2001.
4. Schoepf BG. AIDS action-research with women in Kinshasa, Zaire. *Social Science and Medicine*, 1993;37:1401–1413.
5. Ankrah EM, Mhloyi M, Nduati R, et al. Women, Children and AIDS. In: Essex M, Mboup S, Kanki P, and Kalengayi M, eds. *AIDS in Africa.* New York: Raven Press, 1993:533–546.
6. Norr K, Tlou SD, McElmurry B. AIDS prevention for women: A Community-based approach. *Nursing Outlook*, 1993;40:250–256.
7. Rao Gupta G. Gender, sexuality and HIV/AIDS: The what, the why, and the how. Plenary. *The World Bank Research Observer*, 1994;9:203–240.
8. Panos. *AIDS and Men: Old Problem, New Angle.* London: Panos, 1998.
9. Palai IY. *Men, sex and AIDS*. Gaborone: the Government printer, 1997.
10. Nogobe KD. Experiences of infertility among Botswana women. Unpublished PhD thesis. Gaborone: University of Botswana, 1998.
11. Weiss E, Rao Gupta G. *Bridging the Gap: Addressing Gender and Sexuality in HIV Prevention.* Washington, DC: International Centre for Research on Women, 1998.
12. Measring H, Sibanda R. Condoms, family planning and living with HIV in Zimbabwe. *Reproductive Health Matters*, 1995;5:56–67.
13. Weiss E, Whelan D, Rao Gupta G. *Vulnerability and opportunities: adolescents and HIV/AIDS in the developing world.* Washington DC, International Centre for Research on Women, 1996.
14. Weiss ED, Whelan D, Rao Gupta G. Gender, Sexuality and HIV: Making a Difference in the Lives of Young Women in Developing Countries. *Sexual and Relationship Therapy*, 2000;15:233–245.
15. Agyei WKA, Epepma E. Adolescent Fertility in Kampala, Uganda: Knowledge, Perceptions and Practice. *Biol Soc,* 1991;7:203–214.
16. Mhloyi MM. Perceptions on Communication and Sexuality in Zimbabwe. In: *Therapy: Women's Mental Health in Africa*. London: Haworth, 1990.
17. Parker R, Easton D, Klein CH. Structural Barriers and Facilitators in HIV Prevention: A Review of International Research. *AIDS*, 2000;14(Suppl 1): 22–32.
18. Tlou SD. Empowering Older Women in AIDS Prevention and Care. *Southern African Journal of Gerontology*, 1996;92:27–32.
19. Schoepf BG. AIDS, sex and condoms: African healers and the reinvention of tradition in Zaire. *Medical Anthropology*, 1992;14:225–242.
20. Tlou SD. The girl child and HIV/AIDS. In: Program and abstracts of the XIII International Conference on AIDS; July 9–14, 2000; Durban, South Africa. Abstract ThOrD690.
21. UNAIDS. *Women and AIDS: A point of view.* Geneva: UNAIDS, 1997.
22. UNAIDS. Women, the girl child and HIV/AIDS. Paper presented at the 45th session of the United Nations Commission on the status of women; March 6–16, 2001; New York.
23. United Nations. Report of the Fourth World Conference on Women, Beijing, September 1995. New York: United Nations, 1995.
24. Heise L, Elias C. Transforming AIDS Prevention to Meet Women's Needs. A Focus on Developing Countries. *Social Science and Medicine*, 1995;40: 933–943.
25. Nyblade L, Field ML. *Women, Communities, and the Prevention of Mother-to-Child Transmission of HIV: Issues and Findings from Community Research in Botswana and Zambia.* Washington, DC: International Center for Research on Women, 2000.
26. Tlou SD, Nyblade L, Field M, et al. Men's perspectives on initiatives to prevent mother to child transmission of HIV in Botswana. In: Abstracts of the XIII International AIDS Conference; July 9–14, 2000; Durban, South Africa. Abstract MoOrD204.
27. Tlou SD. Caring for people living with AIDS: Experiences and needs of rural older women in Botswana. In: Abstracts of the Fourth International Conference on Home and Community Care for People Living with HIV/AIDS; December 5–8, 1999; Paris, France. Page 53.
28. de Brayn M. Women and AIDS in developing countries. *Soc Sci Med*, 1992;343:249–262.

44

The Orphan Crisis

*Geoff Foster and †Stefan Germann

*Mutare Provincial Hospital, Mutare, Zimbabwe.
†Masiye Camp, Bulawayo, Zimbabwe.

Some human catastrophes begin with unmistakable fury: natural disasters like earthquakes, hurricanes, and volcano eruptions; technological disasters like the nuclear meltdown at Chernobyl, Ukraine; political and military disasters like the murder and expulsion of civilians in Rwanda, Kosovo, and East Timor; and biologic disasters like the rapid spread of the Ebola virus in Africa (1). But others begin slowly and subtly, often imperceptibly, their full impact shrouded until they seem too large and complex to be addressed. This has been the case with AIDS.[a]

More than 20 years have passed since the first deaths from this previously unknown condition occurred. Although the past two decades have seen progress made on many scientific fronts, the impact of the epidemic on children and families has proven to be particularly hard to quantify, analyze, and confront—and even harder to put on the agendas of policymakers, philanthropic agencies, and political and scientific leaders (2). The media's focus is on instant impact disasters rather than on slowly evolving catastrophes such as the orphan crisis. The focus of clinicians, researchers, and service organizations is on people who are ill and dying while that of public health officials is on preventing HIV transmission. Children's issues are seen mainly in the context of mother-to-child transmission and pediatric AIDS, certainly a compelling part—but only a part—of the picture.

[a]This section includes material first published in (1).

This chapter charts the dimensions of the orphan crisis, drawing attention to the social, economic, and psychologic effects of the epidemic that combine to increase the vulnerability of African children. It concludes with a sign of hope: in the midst of this event's legacy of overwhelming human suffering, there is a remarkable proliferation of community-based support initiatives for orphans and vulnerable children.

SOCIAL IMPACT

In the past, the sense of duty and responsibility among extended families in Africa was almost without limit. Even when a family did not have sufficient resources to care for its existing members, orphans were taken in. This was the basis for the assertion that traditionally, "there is no such thing as an orphan in Africa" (3). Africa is home to 95% of the children orphaned by AIDS (4). Paradoxically, the effectiveness by which the African extended family has absorbed millions of vulnerable children has contributed to the complacency of external agencies concerning the emerging orphan crisis.

Families cope with relatives' deaths by ensuring that orphans receive care from a substitute caregiver. The extended-family support network functions through changes in household composition; relatives move into households to care for children who survive their parents, or orphans move into households of one or more relatives in response to the overwhelming demands of the epidemic. The extended family remains the predominant caregiving unit for orphans in communities in Africa with severe epidemics (5–7). But the extended family is not a social sponge with an infinite capacity to soak up orphans. This traditional safety net is becoming saturated, overwhelmed, and weakened by a combination of three factors: a huge increase in the number of orphans, a significant decrease in the number of prime-age caregivers, and a systemic change to the social structure that underpins the traditional safety net.

Orphan Prevalence is Increasing Dramatically

Estimates for 26 African countries suggest that the number of children losing a father (paternal orphans) or mother (maternal orphans) from any cause will more than double between 1990 and 2010. Within the same period, the number of children who will have lost both mother and father (double orphans) will increase 8-fold throughout all of Africa, with a staggering 17-fold increase (from 0.2 to 3.4 million) in southern Africa, the worst affected region in the world (Figure 1). By 2010, 15% of the children in these 26 countries will have lost one or both parents, with the greatest changes expected in Botswana (37%), Zimbabwe (34%), Swaziland and Namibia (32%), South Africa and Central African Republic (31%) (8). Even if rates of new HIV infections in adults were to fall in the next few years, the virus' long incubation period means parental mortality rates would not plateau until 2020. Thus, the percentage of orphans is expected to remain unusually high throughout the first half of the twenty-first century.

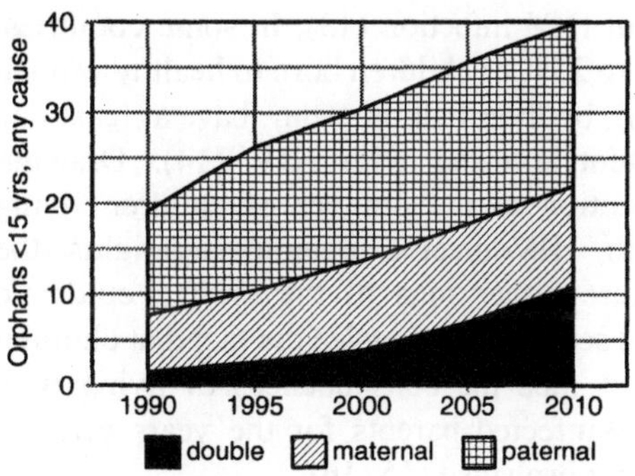

FIGURE 1. Orphans (millions) for 26 African countries. Data derived from (8).

As staggering as these figures appear, they fail to reveal the true extent of the number of children affected by HIV and AIDS. These estimates exclude children between the ages of 15 and 17, a group with the highest orphan rate. This exclusion effectively underestimates total orphan numbers by 25% to 35% (9). In addition, many children in Africa do not live with their biologic parents but are instead fostered by relatives even though the children's parents may be alive. According to household surveys carried out in 19 African countries in the past decade, between 12% and 35% of older children were fostered (10). In Tanzania, 12% of children were not living with either parent and 34% were living with only one parent, yet only 1% of children were double orphans and only 8% had lost one parent (11). Given this fostering tradition, the social, economic, and psychologic impact of the loss of guardians on fostered children may be as great as that which they experience with the loss of their natal parents. Finally, an unknown number of children live with parents with HIV-related symptoms; many more live with asymptomatic HIV-infected parents. In Thailand, for every child maternally orphaned by AIDS, there are 12 children living with mothers who are infected with HIV (12). In Brazil, for every orphan whose mother has died of AIDS, there are 3 children with mothers living with AIDS and 12 with mothers living with HIV infection (13). In some countries, up to 25% of children born to healthy women will, by their fifth birthday, have at least one parent infected with HIV (14). Drawing attention to the number of children living with HIV-infected parents highlights the future dimensions of the orphan epidemic and serves to emphasize the fact that children must face the consequences of living with HIV-infected parents for the years prior to being orphaned (15, 16).

The Number of Prime-Age Caregivers is being Reduced

Life expectancy in many countries has declined as a result of AIDS. In most countries in southern Africa, life expectancy in 2000 was between 37 and 40 years and was still declining. The epidemic is distorting the structure of populations in Africa. Instead of the familiar "population pyramid," AIDS is producing a new demographic structure, the "population chimney" (see Figure 2 in Chapter 17, *this volume*; Table 1). The total number of children has dropped because of HIV-related child mortality, premature maternal death, and reduced fertility. Distortion of the pyramid occurs 10 to 15 years after the age at which people become sexually active, when those infected with HIV early in their sexual lives begin to die. The population of women beyond their early 20s and men beyond their early 30s will shrink in affected countries leading to fewer middle-aged people. The epidemic takes a greater toll on women than men; women become infected with HIV at younger ages and die earlier. In Botswana, the country with the highest HIV prevalence, reversal of the male-to-female gender ratio will occur with more men than women for all ages between 20 and 50 (17, 18).

A shortage of prime-age adults has consequences for the next generation. Increasingly, instead of being cared for by uncles and aunts, a minority of orphans will grow up in households headed by elderly or adolescent caregivers. Many households will be large and will include orphans from more than one family. In the future, the profile of many extended families will include several "skip-generation" households headed by elderly relatives. The shortage of older adults will continue for decades and will worsen as adults over 60 are not replaced because of the AIDS-related depletion of the ranks of middle-aged adults. Child-headed households, which started to be seen in the 1990s, will become commonplace as boys, as well as girls, are forced to assume caregiving roles. As well as being potential caregivers, prime-age relatives are also important sources of financial and material support to their extended families. Their loss impoverishes not just the immediate family but the whole clan.

The Safety Net is Unraveling as a Result of Social Change

The extended family in Africa was the traditional social security system, and its members were responsible for the protection

TABLE 1. Changes in Population in Botswana, 2000 and 2025 (Thousands) (18)

Age range	2000			2025			% Change	
(years)	Male	Female	Total	Male	Female	Total	Male	Female
0–19	418	413	831	273	266	538	−35	−36
20–39	226	242	468	277	230	506	+22	+5
40–59	83	103	186	45	47	93	−46	−54
60+	39	53	92	33	69	102	−15	+30
Total	**766**	**811**	**1577**	**628**	**612**	**1240**	**−18**	**−25**

of the vulnerable, the care of the poor and sick, and the transmission of social values. Extended families involve a large network of connections among people representing varying degrees of relationship including multiple generations and reciprocal relations. In recent years, changes such as labor migration, the cash economy, demographic change, formal education, and urbanization have weakened extended families. In general, where traditional values are maintained, such as in rural communities, the extended-family safety net is better preserved. But where communities are more urbanized, safety nets are weakened. In the few countries where formal, government-supported, social safety nets do exist, they have been ineffective, generally, in delivering services to the destitute and marginalized, especially those living in impoverished or remote rural communities (19). Moreover, social welfare systems had started to weaken prior to the impact of AIDS as a result of economic mismanagement, corruption, and the imposition of structural adjustment programs. The largest increases in orphan numbers are occurring in the countries in southern Africa that have high rates of urbanization and weakened extended-family safety nets.

Various factors reflect the strength of the extended-family safety net (3). Where traditional bride price and widow inheritance are practiced, orphan inheritance is common. Purposive fostering is the practice whereby children are fostered outside the natal family; in cultures where purposive fostering is practiced, those same relatives who have a right to claim a child have an obligation to foster that child at times of crisis (20). Where contact with relatives is maintained, orphans are more likely to be fostered. Conversely, orphaned children of migrant workers and commercial sex workers, groups that often have little contact with relatives, are at risk of being abandoned.

Children Who Slip Through the Safety Net

The combination of increased orphan numbers, reduced numbers of prime-age caregivers, and weakened extended families means many orphans slip through society's overstressed safety net. Their care is falling to the poor and elderly, especially to women. In Kenya, most families that agree to take in foster children live below the poverty line; wealthier relatives usually maintain few links with orphaned family members (21). With fewer uncles and aunts to serve as caregivers, grandparents are recruited, often as a last resort and, in many cases, after other relatives refuse the role (3,22). In some cases, where the elderly seem to be providing childcare, the situation is actually one of mutual support with increasingly frail grandparents being cared for by grandchildren.

Families often separate siblings following the death of the parents so as to share more easily the burden of care. Adolescent girls may be "pawned," sent to a relative or neighbor to work in return for money paid to the fostering family (21). Children, especially those under five, may be fostered, while older siblings are left to live by themselves (23).

Children who slip through the safety net often end up in a variety of vulnerable situations. Rising numbers of households headed by orphans sometimes as young as 11 or 12 years old are a recent phenomenon (23). Rising numbers of orphaned children living on the street, working children, and children removed from school to provide caregiving or labor are all indicators of stress on the safety net (3,24).

ECONOMIC IMPACT

The economic impact of AIDS on families and communities must be understood within the context of declining gross domestic products within most of sub–Saharan Africa, much of which predates the macroeconomic effects of AIDS. Household resilience to the economic and social impact of an unusually high death rate among prime-age adults is considerable (25,26). In many AIDS-affected communities, the mechanism that keeps families and households from destitution comprises material relief, labor, and emotional support provided by community members. Seeking relief from family, friends, and neighbors is a common response to economic crises that result from disasters (27). At times of distress such as bereavement, all community members are obliged to participate and to contribute toward funeral costs (28). The widespread and progressive economic impact of AIDS is leading to adverse impacts upon communities and families.

Orphan Households are Often Impoverished

Economic factors are crucial to determining how the extended family will provide care for its orphans. The death of a father within a household often has deleterious economic consequences for children because of high treatment costs, the loss of income, funeral costs, and often, the loss of family property as a result of property grabbing (16). When there are no other sources of income, a poor household will sell off vital assets to provide desperately needed revenue even if their sale will jeopardize the household's long-term development (29). In Uganda, per capita income in orphan households was 15% less than in non-orphan households (30). In rural Zimbabwe, only 3% of orphan households had a member who was a breadwinner in employment (19). The situation for children in child-headed households is particularly dire. In Zimbabwe, average monthly income in child-headed households is $8 compared with a $21 monthly average in non-orphan households (31).

The economic safety net provided by families and communities is being further weakened because the reserves of better-off families are being depleted as a result of answering the need of relatives affected by AIDS. These families are becoming less able to contribute in cash, in needed materials, or in the provision of work to destitute families. Although seemingly evident, it is important to note that as the number of households falling from poverty into destitution increases, the amount of relief that can be provided per destitute household decreases. In Tanzania, it is reported that less than one-quarter of orphans receive support from a surviving parent and less than 10% receive support from other relatives or elsewhere (11). In addition, assistance from government or nongovernmental organizations was considerably less than that received from community members (16).

Orphans Experience Migration and Child Labor

Economic factors also drive decisions to migrate. Urban–rural relocation is often spurred by the onset of serious illness, in the so-called going-home-to-die syndrome (32). Children affected by AIDS are particularly likely to be relocated before or following a parent's death (6). Rural–urban migration, in contrast, occurs when widows migrate to towns in search of work or partners (33). Reports indicate that children from child-headed households were considerably more likely to have moved within a two-year period than were children of adult-headed households (31). Such intrarural or intraurban migration of orphans has been shown to lead to a clustering of orphan households in poor areas (34).

Mobility is common among adolescents affected by AIDS (23). In order to generate an income, adolescents leave orphan households to seek work, as agricultural laborers for more prosperous farmers or, in towns, as domestic laborers. Some girls become involved in commercial sex work or enter into marriage as girl brides to provide for the needs of younger children in their household. In addition, young relatives from rural areas may be recruited as caregivers for orphans in urban households so as to allow the urban relatives to continue their education (35).

Children who live on the streets are significantly more likely to be orphans; the numbers of street children have increased as a result of the epidemic (36,37). Children of HIV-infected commercial sex workers are especially likely to end up on the streets or working for other people. A study of the fate of the children of 11 female sex workers in Kenya showed that, at the time of the mother's death, 8 out of 39 children were living on the street, 3 of 39 were commercial sex workers, 2 of 39 were casual laborers, and 1 of 39 had become a girl bride. The other 25 orphans were taken in by relatives with whom the mothers had re-established contact prior to their deaths (38).

One less obvious economic impact of the epidemic has been an increase in child labor, sometimes involving children as young as five (29). The additional workload for children affected by HIV or AIDS begins to increase when parents become sick, and peaks with orphanhood. In fact, within one household, the workload of orphans may be greater than that of the non-orphans, especially true if the orphan is female (39). Orphans may be co-opted into agricultural activities or may work as virtual slaves for domestic chores.

Education of Orphans is Often Disrupted

A study of households in Uganda found most were so financially strained that they could not raise funds to send their own children to school (40). Likewise, the education of children in households with parents weakened by HIV disease may be disrupted if the children take over household and caregiving chores. When families need to generate cash, boys, who have more earning power, may be removed from school. Among children between the ages of 15 and 19 whose parents had died, only 29% continued their schooling without disruption, 25% lost school time, and 45% dropped out of school altogether. School-age children with the greatest chance of continuing their education were those who lived with a surviving parent, while those fostered by grandparents had the least chance (15).

Other studies confirm lower enrollment rates in orphans compared with non-orphans and identify certain risk factors as increasing the likelihood that an orphan will fail to continue school. These factors are: being a female orphan, losing both parents, losing a parent or parents to AIDS, being from a rural or poor household, and living in a household headed by a man (11,16,30,41,42). Even where orphans manage to continue their schooling, their performance is often poorer than their non-orphaned counterparts (43).

Child Health and Nutrition are Adversely Affected

There is a close correlation between the quality of parenting and child morbidity (44). Studies of fostered children in West Africa found these children had higher mortality rates than other children, usually the result of poorer care, malnutrition, and reduced access to modern medicine (45,46). Elderly and adolescent caregivers, in particular, may be uninformed about good nutrition, oral rehydration treatment for diarrhea, or about the symptoms of serious illness (47).

A four-year follow-up study of orphans in Uganda found a higher, though not significantly higher, mortality rate among children under the age of five, compared to non-orphans (41). Likewise, younger orphans in rural Zambia were more likely to have frequent illnesses than were non-orphans (48). However, no difference in morbidity was found in Zaire or in mortality in Tanzania between orphans and non-orphans (11,49).

The epidemic interferes with a family's ability to feed its members. Reductions of between 37% and 61% in marketed outputs of maize and other crops was noted in AIDS-affected households in Zimbabwe (50). In an urban slum in Nairobi, Kenya, orphans were significantly more malnourished than non-orphans (51). Orphans in Zambia and Tanzania were more likely to be stunted in their growth than non-orphans, but not more likely to be wasted (52,53). Malnutrition in orphans may result from the effects of parental illness and household death on childrearing practices rather than from shortage of food (16).

PSYCHOSOCIAL IMPACT

Where basic needs are not met, it is difficult for agencies to concentrate on addressing psychologic needs, which may not be as obvious as physical needs and may seem less pressing. In fact, in some contexts, a blanket and food may be more appropriate than counseling (54). In developing countries, the severe social and economic effects of AIDS on children overshadow concerns about the psychologic consequences of the epidemic. The effect that parental illness and death have on a child's mental health and ability to cope are complex and depend upon the child's development, resilience, and culture. Consequently, psychologic effects are less obvious and often go unnoticed or neglected. Changed behavior may be dismissed as a mere transitional stage, a temporary disorder that will pass, rather than as an indicator of psychologic trauma with possible long-term implications (55). The impact of AIDS on households leads to the sequential trauma associated with continuous traumatic stress syndrome (56). Many children suffer multiple losses—a father, mother, siblings, grandparents, uncles, aunts, and other relatives. In addition, because of migration or poverty, many children lose friends, familiar surroundings, schooling, their hopes for the future, and their remaining childhoods. Separation of siblings is a major factor contributing to psychologic distress among orphans; this underlines the importance of providing support to orphans in ways that go beyond traditional psychologic interventions (48).

The impact of AIDS on children in developing and developed countries is essentially without difference, with most children showing psychologic reactions to parental illness and death. A child's psychologic health depends to a large extent upon the status of his or her parents. Signs of a mother's depression, guilt, anger, or fear may be realized though not understood and may then become reflected in children as changed behavior. When asked, orphans most often say they miss the love of their parents and their families; in many ways, the trauma they experience is similar to that experienced by children of war and violence (57). A study in Zambia found that 82% of those caring for children noted changes in their behavior during parental illness. Parents noted that children became worried and sad, and that they tried to help more in the home and stopped playing so as to stay nearby. Children in households affected by HIV or AIDS were more likely to become solitary, to appear miserable or distressed, and to be fearful of new situations than were children in households not affected by the epidemic (52). Stigmatization, discrimination, social isolation, dropping out of school, moving away from friends, and bearing an increased workload in the home all heighten the stress and trauma that accompanies the death of a parent. Stigmatization based on orphan status or poverty rather than parental HIV status is common and is also associated with adverse mental health (39,58).

In a study in Uganda, children expressed feelings of hopelessness or anger when their parents became sick and feared that their parents would die. Most who were orphaned were depressed and had lower expectations about the future. Compared with non-orphans, few orphans expected to get a job, wanted to get married, or wanted children. Depression was highest among those between the ages of 10 and 14. Children showing these symptoms were more likely to be living with a widowed father than with a widowed mother, suggesting that the loss of a mother is more distressing than the loss of a father (15). Orphans were found to internalize behavior changes, such as depression, anxiety, and decreased self-esteem, rather than to exhibit acting out or sociopathic behavior such as stealing, truancy, aggression, and running away (52,59).

It is imperative that psychologic support be strategically integrated into programs for orphans and vulnerable children. Low cost, culturally appropriate interventions have been shown to improve the resilience and coping capacity of affected children. Such interventions include support to overcome grief and trauma, self-esteem strengthening, and life skills education to increase goal setting and decision making (60).

It is difficult to predict the long-term consequences of AIDS-related trauma for children in Africa; there are no longitudinal studies of the psychologic impact of this epidemic. Among children in developed countries, continuous traumatic stress, even of a mild form, is known to have long-term developmental consequences (61,62). Affected individuals may withdraw, resign, and isolate themselves from society. If similar effects are found in children in Africa, the orphan crisis of this epidemic may produce large numbers of adults with chronic traumatic stress syndromes (63). A second generation of problems, including alcohol and drug abuse, severe depression, violent behavior, suicide, and HIV infection may occur. The failure to help children overcome the psychologic impacts of AIDS will, therefore, undoubtedly have a long-term negative impact on society and produce unpredictable societal changes.

VULNERABILITY TO HIV INFECTION

The social, economic, and psychologic impacts of the epidemic combine to increase the vulnerability of children affected by AIDS with a range of consequences including illiteracy, poverty, child labor, unemployment, sexual abuse and exploitation, and HIV, the subject of the next section. Children on the margins of society—refugees, migrants, and residents of urban slums, remote rural areas, or the street—have increased risk for HIV infection (64). Preventing HIV infection is not a priority among people whose main concern is meeting basic day-to-day needs. In a study of street children in Accra, Ghana, most were sexually active and had had their first sexual experience on the streets and with commercial sex workers, and most had misconceptions about AIDS and were doing little to protect themselves from contracting HIV (65).

Children from households affected by HIV or AIDS lack adult protection from sexual exploitation by relatives in their homes or by males in their communities. Susceptibility to such exploitation increases during parental illness or after parental death because of the increased frequency of male visitors to affected households. Male relatives often move into orphaned households to provide supervision or because these relatives need a place to live in urban areas.

Breakdown of social cohesion within communities as a result of AIDS weakens traditional restraints on promiscuity. As a result, rape and forced or coerced sexual abuse of children is increasing in these communities. Girls may be taken in by male relatives because of the economic value of their bride price, or they may be exploited through domestic service masquerading as foster care and then subjected to unfettered sexual abuse (57). In general, the movement of children out of their parental home reduces community-based child protection mechanisms and increases the children's vulnerability.

In a study in Uganda, 30% of 12-year-old orphaned girls and 85% of 18-year-old orphaned girls were sexually active. The reasons for their becoming sexually active included economic need, peer pressure, discovery, lack of parental supervision, and rape by strangers, relatives, or teachers (66). Although most orphans were aware of the existence of AIDS, few knew how to protect themselves from HIV (67).

Failure to prevent HIV infection in this increasingly large group of children has implications for future generations. Orphans represent a pool of at-risk children and youth who have an increased likelihood of contributing to the HIV/AIDS epidemic. When orphaned adolescents or adults contract HIV infection and become ill, they have no mothers to nurse them during their terminal illness. When orphaned adults die, there will be no grandmothers alive to care for their children. This second generation of the AIDS epidemic has already begun with increasing numbers of grandparent-less "orphans of orphans" being left without adult caregivers. Lack of middle-aged grandparents leads to failure of the alternate safety net and increases the dimensions of the orphan crisis.

Care and support programs for orphans are ideal entry points for HIV-prevention activities. Youth involvement in the provision of care and psychosocial support to orphans is an effective youth HIV prevention strategy (68). Perhaps nowhere is the need to link care and support activities with HIV prevention more imperative than in programs for orphaned children (69).

COMMUNITY RESPONSES

The realization that extended families are under stress has led some outside agencies to assume that their principal response should be to develop alternatives such as institutions, children's villages, and adoptive placements. External organizations frequently establish child-support programs that bypass community ownership, decision making, and contributions (70). Such programs often fail to reach the most vulnerable children and may collapse or falter when outside support is withdrawn. Institutional responses do not meet children's cultural and psychosocial needs and may be viewed as inappropriate by community members who recognize their potential to undermine existing community coping mechanisms (71).

Child support programs must be owned by communities if they are to be successful and sustainable. There is growing recognition that mobilizing and strengthening community-based initiatives is as urgent as preventing the further spread of HIV. The groups best placed to strengthen family and community capacity are small grass-roots organizations supported by nongovernmental organizations (72,73). Community-based child support programs have demonstrated their ability to target small amounts of material support to large numbers of destitute orphan households (74,75).

In the past decade, the response of communities to the impact of AIDS upon their children has been striking. In contrast to the belated recognition of the orphan crisis by national and international agencies and the isolated responses of communities to the needs of people dying from AIDS, thousands of community initiatives to address this crisis have been established throughout Africa. People living in communities overburdened by AIDS are responding to the plight of children with ingenuity (74). Community initiatives often result from the concern of small groups of women who take part in activities such as identifying the poorest and most vulnerable children in the community, regularly visiting vulnerable households, raising money for school fees and essential material needs of the poorest children, and increasing community ownership and involvement in activities to support vulnerable children (76).

Though promising, community initiatives are limited in relation to the magnitude of the orphan problem. Not all communities have developed programs. Those that have are scattered. Even where communities are responding, efforts typically do not match the level of need; they are only able to marginally improve the material well-being of orphans. With more resources, made available appropriately and committed for the long term, communities could do much more. Scaling up orphan and vulnerable children responses demands that resources be made available, especially to train NGO personnel in community mobilization and capacity building skills (76).

There is need for better understanding of the nature, diversity, and capacity of community initiatives. Those planning interventions must understand existing norms and practices and must seek to strengthen family and community capacities to protect and care for vulnerable children before developing large-scale child support programs (74). There is a danger that poorly designed programs could jeopardize fledgling community initiatives and dampen initiatives being spearheaded by affected communities to support orphans and vulnerable children.

Many communities in Africa are organizing their responses and molding them into coordinated child support programs. For the most part, these initiatives, programs, and emerging community organizations are unknown outside their immediate locale because they have not been documented. Few organizations or networks have sought to partner grass-roots clusters or support their development, yet community initiatives along with extended families represent the front-line response for increasing numbers of children affected by AIDS. Extraordinarily, the evidence up to now is that traditional fostering systems in Africa will at least meet the basic needs for a majority of orphans created by the AIDS epidemic (25). The hope is that appropriate external support will be provided to enable communities to provide for increasingly large numbers of vulnerable children who slip through the extended-family safety net.

ACKNOWLEDGMENT

The authors gratefully acknowledge the generous and helpful comments of John Williamson in the preparation of this manuscript.

REFERENCES

1. Levine C, Foster G. *The White Oak Report: Building International Support for Children Affected by AIDS.* New York: The Orphan Project, 2000.
2. Foster G. Orphans. *AIDS Care*, 1997;9:82–87.
3. Foster G. The capacity of the extended family for orphans in Africa. *Psychology, Health & Medicine*, 2000;5:55–62.
4. UNAIDS/WHO. *AIDS Epidemic Update.* Geneva: UNAIDS, 1999.
5. Ankrah EM. The impact of HIV/AIDS on the family and other significant relationships: the African clan revisited. *AIDS Care*, 1993;5:5–22.
6. Foster G, Shakespeare R, Chinemana F, et al. Orphan prevalence and extended family care in a peri-urban community in Zimbabwe. *AIDS Care*, 1995;7:3–17.
7. Ntozi JPM. AIDS morbidity and the role of the family in patient care in Uganda. *Health Transit Rev*, 1997;7(Suppl):1–22.
8. Hunter S, Williamson J. *Children on the Brink: Executive Summary: Updated Estimates & Recommendations for Intervention.* Washington: USAID, 2000.
9. Foster G, Williamson J. Impact of HIV/AIDS on children in Africa: a review of current knowledge. *AIDS*, 2000;14(Suppl 3):S275–S284.
10. Ayad M, Barrere B, Otto J. *Demographic and Socioeconomic Characteristics of Households: Demographic and Health Comparative Studies No. 26.* Calverton, Maryland: Macro International, 1997.
11. Urassa M, Boerma T, Ng'weshemi JZL, et al. Orphanhood, child fostering and the AIDS epidemic in rural Tanzania. *Health Transit Rev*, 1997;7(Suppl 2):141–153.
12. Brown T, Sittitrai W. *The Impact of HIV on Children in Thailand.* Bangkok: Program on AIDS, Thai Red Cross Society, 1995.
13. UNAIDS. Global orphan project, Boston & Brasilia estimates. In: *Children living in a world with AIDS media briefing.* Geneva: UNAIDS, 1997.
14. Palloni A, Lee YJ. Some aspects of the social context of HIV and its effects on women, children and families. *Population Bulletin of the United Nations*, 1992;33:64–87.
15. Sengendo J, Nambi J. The psychological effect of orphanhood: a study of orphans in Rakai district. *Health Transit Rev*, 1997;7(Suppl):105–124.
16. World Bank. *Confronting AIDS: Public priorities in a global epidemic.* New York: Oxford University Press, 1997.
17. UNAIDS. *Report on the Global HIV/AIDS Epidemic: June, 2000.* Geneva: UNAIDS, 2000.
18. US Bureau of the Census. *HIV/AIDS surveillance data base.* Population Division. Washington: US Bureau of the Census, 2000.
19. Drew RS, Foster G, Chitima J. Poverty—a major constraint in the community care of orphans: A study from the North Nyanga District of Zimbabwe. *SafAIDS News*, 1996;4:14–16.
20. Goody E. *Parenthood and social reproduction: Fostering and occupational roles in West*

Africa. Cambridge: Cambridge University Press, 1982.

21. Saoke P, Mutemi R, Blair C. Another song begins: children orphaned by AIDS. In: *AIDS in Kenya: socio-economic impact and policy implications*. Washington: USAID/AIDSCAP/Family Health International, 1996:45–64.
22. McKerrow N. *Responses to orphaned children: a review of the current situation in the Copperbelt and Southern Provinces of Zambia*. Research Brief No. 3. Lusaka: UNICEF Lusaka, 1997.
23. Foster G, Makufa C, Drew R, et al. Factors leading to the establishment of child-headed households: the case of Zimbabwe. *Health Transit Rev*, 1997;7(Suppl 2):155–168.
24. Veale AM. Dilemmas of "community" in post-emergency Rwanda. *Community, Work & Family*, 2000;3:233–239.
25. Caldwell JC. The impact of the African AIDS epidemic. *Health Transit Rev*, 1997;7(Suppl. 2): 169–188.
26. Carey F. AIDS and orphans. *Africans on Africa*, 1995;3:18–22.
27. Donahue J. *Community-based economic support for households affected by HIV/AIDS*. Discussion papers on HIV/AIDS care and support no. 6. Arlington, VA: Health Technical Services (HTS) Project for USAID, 1998.
28. Tibaijuka AK. AIDS and the economic welfare in peasant agriculture: Case studies from Kagabiro Village, Kagera Region, Tanzania. *World Development*, 1997;25.
29. Rugalema G. It is not only the loss of labour: HIV/AIDS, loss of household assets and household livelihood in Bukoba District, Tanzania. In: Mutangadura G, Jackson H, Mukurazita D, eds. *AIDS and African Smallholder Agriculture*. Harare: Southern Africa AIDS Information Dissemination Service, 1999:41–52.
30. Konde-Lule JK, Ssengonzi R, Wawer M, et al. The HIV epidemic and orphanhood, Rakai District, Uganda. In: Program and abstracts of the IXth International Conference on AIDS and STD in Africa; December 1995; Kampala, Uganda. Abstract TuD670.
31. Foster G. HIV and AIDS: Orphans and sexual vulnerability. In: Kilbourn P, McDermid M, eds. *Sexually Exploited Children: Working to Protect and Heal*. Monrovia: MARC, 1998:216–232.
32. Foster S. *ADZAM—a Study of Adult Diseases in Zambia—Final Report*. London: Overseas Development Agency, 1995.
33. Ntozi JPM. Widowhood, remarriage and migration during the HIV/AIDS epidemic in Uganda. *Health Transit Rev*, 1997;7(Suppl):125–144.
34. McKerrow N. *Responses to orphaned children*. Lusaka: UNICEF Lusaka, 1996.
35. Robson E. Invisible carers: young people in Zimbabwe's home-based health care. *Area*, 2000;32:59–69.
36. Haworth A, Mulenga M, Mwewa L, et al. On being an orphan on the streets of Lusaka, Zambia. In: Program and abstracts of the Xth International Conference on AIDS and STD in Africa; December 1997; Abidjan, Cote d'Ivoire. Abstract C346.
37. Lungwangwa G, Macwan'gi M. *Street Children in Zambia: A Situation Analysis*. Lusaka: UNICEF, 1996.
38. Njoroge M, Ngugi E, Waweru A. Female sex workers (FSWs) AIDS orphans multi prolonged problem in Kenya: a case study. In: Program and Abstracts of the XII International Conference on AIDS; July 1998; Geneva. Abstract 60116.
39. Foster G, Makufa C, Drew R, et al. Perceptions of children and community members concerning the circumstances of orphans in rural Zimbabwe. *AIDS Care*, 1997;9:391–406.
40. Muller O, Abbas N. The impact of AIDS mortality on children's education in Kampala Uganda. *AIDS Care*, 1990;2:77–80.
41. Kamali A, Seeley JA, Nunn AJ, et al. The orphan problem: experience of a sub-Saharan Africa rural population in the AIDS epidemic. *AIDS Care*, 1996;8:509–515.
42. Rossi MM, Reijer P. Prevalence of orphans and their education status. Research report, 1995. Quoted in: *Situation Analysis of Orphans in Zambia, Volume 1, Bibliography: An Annotated Review of Literature Relevant to the Situation of Orphans & Vulnerable Children in Zambia*. Lusaka: Joint USAID/UNICEF/SIDA/Study Fund Project, 1999.
43. Conroy R, Tomkins A, Landsdown R, et al. *Identifying emerging needs among AIDS orphans in Kenya*. Annual Scientific Review. Nairobi: University of Nairobi, 2000.
44. Ware H. Effects of maternal education, women's roles and child care on child mortality. *Population Development Review*, 1984;10(Suppl):191–214.
45. Bledsoe CH, Ewbank DC, Isiugo-Abanihe UC. The effect of child fostering on feeding practices and access to health services in rural Sierra Leone. *Soc Sci Med*, 1988;27:627–636.
46. Oni JB. Fostered children's perception of their health care and illness treatment in Ekita Yoruba households, Nigeria. *Health Transit Rev*, 1995; 5:21–34.
47. Foster G. Today's children—challenges to child health promotion in countries with severe AIDS epidemics. *AIDS Care*, 1998;10(Suppl 1):S17–S23.
48. Nampanya-Serpell N. *Children orphaned by HIV/AIDS in Zambia: risk factors from premature parental death and policy implication*. Doctoral Dissertation. Baltimore: University of Maryland, 1998.

49. Ryder RW, Kamenga M, Nkusu M, et al. AIDS orphans in Kinshasa, Zaire: incidence and socioeconomic consequences. *AIDS*, 1994;8:673–679.
50. USAID. *HIV/AIDS in Southern Africa: Background, Projections, Impacts and Interventions*. The POLICY Project for Bureau for Africa, Office of Sustainable Development. Washington: United States Agency for International Development, 2000.
51. Nduati RW, Muita JW, Olenja J, et al. A survey of orphaned children in Kibera Urban Slum, Nairobi. In: Program and Abstracts of the IXth International Conference on AIDS; July 1993; Berlin. Abstract WS-D26-4.
52. Poulter C. *A psychological and physical needs profile of families living with HIV/AIDS in Lusaka, Zambia*. Research Brief No. 2. Lusaka: UNICEF Lusaka, 1997.
53. Semali I, Ainsworth M. The impact of adult deaths on the nutritional status and growth of young children. In: Program and Abstracts of the IX International Conference on AIDS and STDs in Africa; 1995; Kampala, Uganda. Abstract MoD066.
54. Ankrah EM. AIDS: A research problematic. *Soc Sci Med*, 1989;293:265–279.
55. Humuliza. *Manual: Psycho-social support for orphans*. Basel: Terre Des Hommes, 1999.
56. Straker G. *Phases of Revolution; The psychological effects of violence in townships in South Africa*. Johannesburg: David Phillips, 1992.
57. Hunter S. *Reshaping societies: HIV/AIDS and social change*. New York: Hudson Run Press, 2000.
58. Naerland V. *AIDS-learning to be more helpful*. Kampala: Redd Barna, 1993.
59. Kirya SK. AIDS-related parental death and its effect on orphaned children's self-esteem and sociability at school. In: Program and Abstracts of the XI International Conference on AIDS; July 7–12, 1996; Vancouver. Abstract Th.D. 4871.
60. UNAIDS. *Investing in Our Future: Psychosocial Support for Children Affected by HIV/AIDS: A Case Study in Zimbabwe and the United Republic of Tanzania*. UNAIDS Case Study. Geneva: UNAIDS, July 2001.
61. Silvermann P, Worden JW. Child Bereavement Study. *Omega—Journal of Death and Dying*, 1996; 33:91.
62. Worden JW. *Children and Grief*. New York: Guilford Publications, 1996.
63. Germann S. HIV/AIDS and social change: Child-headed households in urban Bulawayo, Zimbabwe. Draft Doctoral Dissertation. Pretoria: University of South Africa, 2000.
64. Richter LM, Swart-Kruger J. AIDS-risk among street children and youth: Implications for intervention. *South African Journal of Psychology*, 1995;25:31–38.
65. Anarfi J. Vulnerability to sexually transmitted disease: street children in Accra. *Health Transit Rev*, 1997;7(Suppl):281–306.
66. Sharpe U, Ssentongo R, Ssenyonga A, et al. Orphans sexual behaviour in Masaka diocese, Uganda. In: Program and abstracts of the IXth International Conference on AIDS; 1993; Berlin, Germany. Abstract WS-D26-5.
67. Ministry of Labour & Social Affairs, & UNICEF (Uganda). *Operational Research on the Situation of Orphans within Family and Community Contexts in Uganda*. Kampala: Ministry of Labour & Social Affairs & UNICEF, 1993.
68. Lee T. *FOCUS Evaluation Report: Report of a participatory self-evaluation of the FACT Families, Orphans and Children Under Stress (FOCUS) programme*. Mutare: Family AIDS Caring Trust, 1999.
69. Schietinger H. *Psychosocial Support for People Living with HIV/AIDS: Discussion Papers on HIV/AIDS Care and Support*. No. 5. Arlington, VA: Health Technical Services (HTS) Project for USAID, 1998.
70. Verhoef HS. Seeing Beyond the Crisis: What International Relief Organizations are Learning from Community-Based Childrearing Practices. In: Lerner R, Jacobs F, and Wertlieb D, eds. *Promoting positive child, adolescent, and family development: A handbook of program and policy innovations*. Volume 3. Thousand Oaks, California: Sage, 2002.
71. Rutayuga JBK. Assistance to AIDS orphans within the family/kinship system and local institutions: a program for east Africa. *AIDS Educ Prev*, 1992;4(Suppl):57–68.
72. Drew RS, Makufa C, Foster G. Strategies for providing care and support to children orphaned by AIDS. *AIDS Care*, 1998;10(Suppl):S9–S15.
73. WHO/UNICEF. *Action for children affected by AIDS – programme profiles and lessons learned*. New York: World Health Organisation/United Nations Children Fund, 1994.
74. Foster G, Makufa C, Drew R, et al. Supporting children in need through a community-based orphan visiting programme. *AIDS Care*, 1996;8:389–403.
75. Foster G. Responses in Zimbabwe to children affected by AIDS. *SafAIDS News*, 2000;8:2–7.
76. Phiri SN, Foster G, Nzima M. *Expanding and strengthening community action: A study to explore ways to scale up effective, sustainable community mobilization interventions to mitigate the impact of HIV/AIDS on children and families*. Washington: Displaced Children and Orphans Fund of USAID, 2001.

45

The Economics of AIDS in Africa

Amar A. Hamoudi and Jeffrey D. Sachs

Center for International Development, Harvard University, Cambridge, Massachusetts, 02138, USA.[a]

This chapter focuses on the effects of AIDS on economic activity at all levels, and the economics of HIV and AIDS interventions. Financing challenges for AIDS interventions, and specific needs for mobilizing international donor support for Africa will also be discussed.

THE EFFECTS OF AIDS ON ECONOMIC ACTIVITY IN AFRICA

Assessments of the economic effects of AIDS may be considered *static* or *dynamic*. Static assessments focus on the comprehensive costs of AIDS for an economy at a given point in time. A dynamic assessment focuses on potential changes in time paths of key economic variables—GNP, savings, household formation, school enrollment, unemployment, food production, and so on—as a consequence of AIDS. Both types of assessments can help answer questions such as, What percentage of its GNP should a government spend on AIDS control? and How should governments and international donor agencies balance their efforts in AIDS control against other social investments, such as education, road building, and the like? These calculations are also useful for planning by macroeconomic authorities and by enterprises, families, and communities.

Measuring the Costs of AIDS

Economists, health specialists, and philosophers have not sorted out the precise economic costs of disease on a single individual, much less on a national economy. Much can be assumed about the financial losses that follow HIV infection, but the complex interaction between the various consequences of these losses can be difficult to quantify. Take the case of an African man, a husband and father of young children, who earns a market income, and who becomes infected with HIV. He is likely to experience several years of declining market income due to absenteeism from work and reduced labor productivity before suffering a premature death. He will incur increasingly heavy out-of-pocket costs on medical care, perhaps including visits to traditional healers, and will likely sell assets and perhaps borrow at very high interest rates to get even minimal access to palliative care. He will not have access to most modern medical treatments, given the existing policy environment. His children may be sent away to live with relatives or a foster family either before or after his death. His funeral expenses will also require several months of wages, potentially leaving his family in debt.

[a] For more information on the economics of AIDS and related topics, visit the Center for International Development's website: http://www.cid.harvard.edu.

How then, to measure the economic costs of the infection? The narrowest approach would be to compare the man's wage income while HIV-infected with an estimate of the income that he would have earned if he had never been infected. A more comprehensive approach would also consider his expenditures on health care. A still more comprehensive approach would take account of the value of the man's lost leisure time, his pain and suffering due to the disease, and his loss of well-being due to a shortened life span. The economic effects of the man's disease on others—the so-called "external effects"—which are felt by his wife, children, other family members, his employer's enterprise, the community, and others in his social network could also be considered.

There are major philosophical and practical problems in carrying out these measurements. The first involves what to include in the calculation, and how to value things like pain and suffering or lost leisure time. To measure individual costs, the economist's preferred measure is known as the *equivalent variation* (EV) of income due to disease. The EV is a number that answers the question, How much would it be worth for the man to avoid the HIV infection in the first place or to cure the disease? The disease is going to rob the man of purchasing power (due to both lost income and health care outlays), leisure time, general health, and of course future life-years. If properly informed and fully aware of the lifetime consequences, he would presumably be willing to pay a substantial flow of current and future income to avoid the HIV infection or to cure the disease. In addition to the amount the individual would be willing to pay, there would in principle be additional sums that would be paid by others to avoid the external effects of the man's HIV-infection. Of course, such calculations are rarely made. Hypothetical questions about willingness to pay to avoid a disease are extremely hard to frame in ways that elicit meaningful answers. Still less is known about the willingness to pay by others (family, neighbors, enterprise) in an individual's social network.

To estimate the scale of effects caused by disease, health economists have often resorted to making a crude calculation of the economic value of a "representative" lifetime, or an additional life-year, and then multiplying this value by the number of lives or life-years that are lost due to a disease. The value of a representative life-year is considered to be a very rough estimate of a representative individual's willingness to pay for a life-year. Consider the effect of losing one year of working life. The individual loses the value of consumption of both goods and leisure time during that working year. If the annual market income is $1,000, which can buy $1,000 of consumption goods, the combined value of consumption plus leisure will be higher than $1,000. The added value of leisure is sometimes estimated to equal the value of consumption spending, in which case the full value of the life-year would be measured as $2,000, or twice the annual market income. There is also the lost utility of longevity itself; even for a given lifetime, income and leisure must be crowded into fewer years when longevity is shortened. On top of the $2,000 lost per life-year and the economic costs of shortened longevity, an economist would add in the estimated outlays for health care to get a crude calculation of the cost of the disease to the individual. This cost, in very rough terms, would be consistent with a willingness-to-pay estimate.

This estimate of the cost of a life-year can be used to get a very crude idea of the scale of the cost of AIDS in Africa. Let's assume for now that each lost life-year should be valued at twice the per capita income of a representative infected individual in Africa. Many economists routinely value a life-year at three times annual income, so we are being conservative. We will assume, also conservatively, that this amounts to about US$833.[b] South Africa accounts for around one-sixth of

[b] All monetary estimates in this chapter are referred to in U.S. dollars.

the total AIDS burden (1), and has an average income for blacks of around $1,000 per year (2,3). People in other African countries earn an average income of around $300 per year (2). Therefore, each life-year lost could be valued at $2 \times [(1/6) \times \$1{,}000 + (5/6) \times \$300]$, which equals $833. This is a conservative estimate, considering that the individuals suffering from HIV/AIDS tend to be in the prime years of their working lives, with incomes typically higher than the national average. The World Health Organization (WHO) estimates that about 74 million life-years are lost each year in Africa due to disability or death caused by HIV and AIDS (4). This suggests that the economic costs of HIV and AIDS are around $61 billion ($\$833 \times 74{,}000{,}000$), an amount roughly 19% of sub–Saharan Africa's total 1999 GNP.

Now, let's add an equally rough estimate of medical outlays. Schwartländer and others estimate that affected households spend about one-third of a year's income on medical care during the final two years of life of a person suffering from AIDS (5). We will assume that on average, outlays for all other HIV-infected individuals amount to about one-tenth of yearly income. These estimates include outlays for formal health care as well as informal or traditional health care. Based on estimates of the number of people living with HIV or AIDS and these household costs, health spending would be equal to the average income of around $(4.4/3 + 21/10)$ million people, or roughly $2.9 billion in total. The combination of the value of illness, death, and health expenditure due to HIV/AIDS would then amount to an annual loss to Africa of $63.9 billion, an amount equivalent to approximately 20% of African GNP in 1999. Even though these calculations are exceedingly crude and they only consider a small piece of the total cost, they do highlight the stunning magnitude of the economic losses associated with the pandemic at this stage.

The calculations made thus far in this chapter have been based on the valuation of healthy life years, in this case measured as the number of DALYs (disability-adjusted life-years) saved. However, the costs of AIDS are more conventionally measured in terms of reduced GNP. Gross national product is, roughly speaking, the sum of market incomes earned by a nation's residents during one year. When an individual is HIV-infected or dies of AIDS, the respective reduction or loss of his or her market income is captured by a corresponding reduction of aggregate GNP. The additional losses due to lost leisure time, increased medical outlays, and pain and suffering, are not captured in the reduction of GNP; note that each lost life-year was earlier assumed to be equal to *twice* the average market income.

Although GNP per capita is sometimes used as an indicator of average economic well-being in a country, changes in GNP per capita do not properly capture the economic costs of disease because only the well-being of survivors is measured. Obviously, the economic costs of the epidemic ought to include its effects on those who die. This point bears repeating since many casually measure the effect of the pandemic with regard to changes (or lack thereof) in GNP per capita.

Accounting for the Specific Economic Effects of AIDS

The effects of disease on economic activity are pervasive and often subtle. There are obvious direct effects caused by the absenteeism and premature death of workers and increased medical expenditures, but there are much more subtle effects as well on enterprise productivity, foreign investment patterns, macroeconomic stability, educational and health status of orphans, age structure of the population, household saving propensities, and so on. Health economics evaluations have not comprehensively assessed the impact of AIDS on economic structure and performance in ways that take all of these effects into account. Nonetheless, it is useful to think about the impact of AIDS on economic performance as falling into the following seven distinct categories, even if not all of them can be quantified at this point.

> *1. Human Capital*
> AIDS reduces worker productivity, increases absenteeism, reduces household income, and leads to premature death of skilled workers including teachers and doctors. The young children of HIV-infected adults are also harmed, through reduced caregiving and access to schooling, health care, and nutrition.
> *2. Enterprise Capital*
> AIDS increases the costs of business by creating high employee turnover, increasing search costs for new workers, reducing enterprise morale, reducing incentives for training, and reducing specialization within a firm and between firms. These effects not only reduce enterprise profits but also the rate of investment by both foreign and domestic enterprises.
> *3. Social Capital*
> AIDS undermines social trust, and in some instances leads to charges of malevolence. AIDS increases poverty, which may in turn lead to increased crime. Increased personal risks (due to crime or accidental HIV infection as a result of contaminated blood transfusion, for example) and fear of exposure cause increased emigration as well as reduced tourism and foreign contacts.
> *4. Macroeconomic Stability*
> AIDS puts strains on national budgets by reducing economic growth and government revenues, and increasing the budgetary costs of health care and community support (e.g. care of orphans).
> *5. Health Costs*
> AIDS strains household budgets by reducing working incomes while simultaneously raising out-of-pocket health expenditures. Many families are thrown into poverty from which they never recover.
> *6. Saving and Investment*
> With a shorter life expectancy of HIV-infected individuals, households reduce their accumulation of financial capital and human capital, the latter often through reduced investments in education and on-the-job training.
> *7. Demographics*
> Overall population growth is reduced (or even turned negative) by increased mortality. The age structure of the population may change dramatically, as AIDS reduces the proportion of the population at working ages and increases the proportions of the young and the very old.

There has been, as yet, no comprehensive assessment of these effects that projects the longer-term economic impact of AIDS on African economies. Furthermore, surprisingly little is known about the total expenditures by households, business, and government as a result of the AIDS pandemic.

AIDS, Household Income, and Human Capital

AIDS reduces household income by reducing the earnings of HIV-infected individuals, and by reducing or eliminating the number of adults in the labor force due to premature death. The magnitude of these effects, surprisingly, has not been studied in detail. A few large-scale longitudinal studies have been undertaken in Africa to examine the effect of the death of an economically active adult on household income and wealth. These studies include those conducted in Rakai district, Uganda, in Côte d'Ivoire, in the Kagera region of Tanzania, and in Zimbabwe (6–11). These studies demonstrated that HIV infection in the household contributes to a measurable reduction in the income and wealth of the household, and has long-term negative effects on survivors, including for example, malnutrition and reduced school attendance among surviving children. Due to time and resource constraints, these studies cannot capture the more subtle effects of adult illness on household income and consumption. The true magnitude of the impact of adult illness on household income and wealth is likely to be much greater than these studies indicate. Nonetheless, these household-level studies provide important insights into the economic impact of HIV and AIDS and highlight the need for longer-term and larger-sample longitudinal research.

Adult HIV infections impact children's human capital in many ways. Even for the majority of children who do not acquire HIV infection during gestation, childbirth, or nursing, the consequences of adult illness can be severe. Foster caregivers are less likely than biological parents to be informed about tools for proper child health care including oral rehydration, immunization, the diagnosis of serious illness, and the proper use of primary health care (12–14). Empirical studies confirm that adult illness and death in the household increases the risk to orphaned children of stunting and wasting (9,10,14). Older children who have lost their mothers or other female caregivers are less likely to attend school than their non-orphan peers (9,15). These and other less direct effects on child health and well-being due to the loss of a family member are only vaguely understood.

Childhood morbidity and mortality also impose large costs on households. In addition to the emotional distress caused by the loss of a child, households suffer economic losses when children fall ill and die. When a child dies, not only do parents lose the life of a loved one, they lose the time and resources they had invested in raising and caring for the child (16, 17). Since HIV-infected children are usually born to HIV-infected adults, childhood HIV-related illness often follows adult illness, exacerbating economic hardship (18). When infected children outlive their parents, their foster parents may be forced to divert resources away from uninfected siblings in order to pay for their care.

In addition to the effects of HIV- and AIDS-related morbidity and mortality on the productivity of individual workers, the loss of trained personnel may have important effects on the present and future capacity of the economy to increase production. For example, a recent study in Zambia suggested that teachers were unusually likely to die of AIDS compared with the general adult population (19). Together, the decline in the transfer of skills, norms, and values from one generation to the next may be expected to have effects on economic and human development in the long run.

AIDS and Enterprise Capital

The direct effect of AIDS-related morbidity on the productivity of each worker is manifested in reduced labor income. However, there may be additional effects on the productivity of business enterprises beyond the loss of the productive contributions of each individual employee. In general, enterprises have an economic value in excess of the invested physical capital: workers have been trained, sorted according to skills and abilities to cooperate, and invested with firm-specific modes of teamwork that are costly to replace or reproduce. This extra value of the firm, which is built up over time through ongoing investments in workforce training, sorting, and placement, is known as "enterprise capital." It is reduced by the high rate of absenteeism and premature mortality of the firm's labor force.

The effect of HIV and AIDS on enterprise capital shows up in many ways. There may be "low productivity" employees who function at production bottlenecks or who are important sources of institutional memory; the morbidity or mortality of these employees will have downstream effects far exceeding the loss of their individual market wages. Similarly, if mistakes in any of the tasks in a production chain have downstream productivity effects, then the loss of a few skilled workers will incur costs more than proportional to their productivity (20). There are also likely to be severe losses of staff morale resulting from sustained high levels of morbidity and mortality among colleagues within firms. However, this loss of morale has not been analyzed empirically.

There are also likely to be labor productivity effects that operate at an economy-wide scale. For example, if the relative wage paid to skilled workers increases sharply, firms in hard-hit countries that rely on skilled workers might find themselves less able to compete in world markets. Furthermore, an increase in the relative wage of skilled workers may worsen disparity in income distribution. Conversely, if a "critical mass" of skilled workers is necessary for the operation of skill-based enterprises, then the epidemic—by wiping out this "critical mass"—may actually *reduce* the relative wage paid to those who survive. This may reduce incentives for future generations to invest in developing their skills, and even induce more of Africa's most skilled workers to emigrate. As the probability of infection increases, so does the risk to individuals and firms associated with investments in on-the-job training. If these risks increase sufficiently, investments may become sufficiently expensive to affect the rate of skill formation in the economy as a whole. These types of effects are likely to be particularly destructive in contexts where the availability of specialized labor is the limiting factor in economic production.

The loss of skills, reduced productivity of enterprises, changes in local demand for certain goods and services, and increased operating costs resulting from the epidemic will also affect the profitability of foreign investment. The role of disease in Africa's isolation from global networks of trade and investment has only recently begun to be acknowledged (21); the HIV epidemic will tend to exacerbate this isolation.

AIDS and Social Capital

In addition to the losses of individual productivity and enterprise capital, other potential social effects of the epidemic might include increased crime rates, paranoia, and a loss of social cohesion. HIV infection might be particularly pernicious in this regard, not only because of the scale of the epidemic, but also because the disease clusters in geographic space and is intertwined with social mores regarding sexuality. Ashforth has carefully documented how HIV is interpreted in Soweto as a manifestation of witchcraft, so that each case of HIV illness has a double effect: the direct loss of well-being of the affected individual, and a loss of trust within the community (22). Such negative social effects will be exacerbated by the sharp shift in age structure of the population towards a high proportion of youth, and also by the likely rise in crime and acts of violence that results from a sharp drop in incomes. The CIA-sponsored Task Force on State Failure found that mortality rates (probably a proxy for a high disease burden in general) are strong predictors of future collapse of the state due to coups, assassinations, and other forms of internal violence (23). There is probably an important causal chain running from disease burden to political disarray.

AIDS and Macroeconomic Stability

High levels of government spending and recurrent fiscal deficits have economic consequences in the medium- and long-run, including high rates of price inflation, vulnerability to economic crisis, or diversion of resources away from social priorities in favor of debt service. The epidemic will increase demand for publicly supported services, including, for example, health services (and, in South Africa and a few other countries, welfare grants). In addition, it will increase the costs of all government activity, as the supply of skilled labor decreases due to the deaths of teachers, health care providers, civil servants, and so on. At the same time, countries that rely primarily on domestic taxation for government revenue will see a shrinking tax base. The structure of government spending may thus become unsustainable in the face of the epidemic, and the adjustments that will be required may be difficult and costly.

AIDS and Saving and Investment

Those in the young adult age group, which has historically seen the lowest mortality risks, are most likely to die of AIDS (24).

This increased risk is likely to fundamentally alter the savings and investment behavior of adults in high-prevalence areas. There has been little empirical or theoretical research into the effects of these behavioral changes. Kalemli-Ozcan and others however, have recently offered a theoretical model that explores the effect of shorter time horizons on investments in schooling (25). Bloom, Canning, and Malaney provide some econometric evidence that high disease burden reduces household saving rates (26). Because reduced household saving rates are generally accompanied by wider government budget deficits (and reduced government saving) national saving rates will also decline.

AIDS and Demographics

AIDS will have a powerful effect on population growth and age structure, through both its direct impact on age-specific mortality, and the indirect effects that behavior changes will have on fertility. Declining risk of age-specific mortality has been observed generally to lead to a decline in fertility behavior: households can choose to have fewer children with the confidence that these children will survive into adulthood. However, for a number of reasons, the relationship between mortality rates, fertility rates, and AIDS is more difficult to predict. Among these reasons are the age and gender distribution of the risk of AIDS death, the effects of risk-reducing behavior change on fertility, the biologic effects of HIV on fecundity, and the effects of orphan fostering on household demographic composition (27–31).

A few empirical studies have been undertaken to elucidate the relationship between HIV infection and household fertility behavior. One study conducted in rural Zimbabwe used in-depth household surveys to examine the relationship between the HIV epidemic and a few proximate determinants of fertility (28). The study concluded that the HIV epidemic was likely to lead to a modest acceleration of the overall fertility decline already underway, as a result of reduced fecundity among HIV-infected women, changes in sexual behavior and contraceptive use in response to risk of HIV infection, and increased mortality among women of reproductive age. These findings were supported by a prospective cohort study in rural Uganda (30), which found that reduced fertility among HIV-infected women resulted in a decline in cohort total fertility rate. Specifically, they found that the average level of fertility among HIV-infected women was only 75% the level among uninfected women.

Ainsworth, Filmer, and Semali used census data and the results of household surveys in the Kagera region of Tanzania to test the effect of HIV risk and other factors on the likelihood of a childbirth in a household in the 12 months preceding the survey (27). The results pointed to a modest decline in total fertility associated with the epidemic, and specifically a decreased likelihood of childbearing among surviving women in households that had experienced a recent adult female death. However, although adult deaths in the household and community were correlated with reduced fertility behavior, child deaths were associated with increased fertility. Therefore, the overall effect of the epidemic on fertility behavior will be difficult to estimate.

Changes in fertility and adult mortality together will determine the impact of the epidemic on population structure. These changes are likely to lead to a greater number of children and elderly who are dependent on each economically active person. The balance of fertility and adult mortality will also determine whether the overall number of orphans in each community increases or decreases. Furthermore, population structure changes will determine the level of national saving, the stresses on social capital, the educational investments made per child, and other community-level effects. Research into the demographic effects of the epidemic receives far too little attention.

Putting the Pieces Together in a Macroeconomic Framework

In principle, the seven channels through which AIDS specifically affects the economy could be incorporated into a general equilibrium simulation model of an overall economy. The effects of the various channels would be allowed to interact to produce a "bottom line" estimate of the effect of AIDS on economic growth. This technique of using a series of computable equations to simulate the interaction of economic actors under a variety of scenarios is known as Computable General Equilibrium (CGE) modeling. However, no CGE model has been designed or described in the economics literature that captures all of the effects of the AIDS epidemic outlined here. The challenge in creating such a model would be to generate sensible quantitative estimates of the various effects, and to use a sufficiently formulated overall model of the economy to trace the disease impacts with numerical accuracy.

Mead Over, of the World Bank, pioneered the first macroeconomic models of HIV/AIDS in 1992 (32). The models incorporated simple assumptions about the effects of AIDS on worker productivity and household and government saving, and excluded many of the other areas of impact described in this chapter. Based on these assumptions and the prevalence rates at the time, Over's original paper estimated that GNP growth would decline by about 0.3% per year in the countries with the most advanced epidemics.

A fairly recent application of the CGE approach builds on a model of the South African economy that is routinely employed by the government in economic planning (33). The baseline simulation assumes that the economy will continue to perform as it has in the recent past. In contrast, the AIDS simulation incorporates increased morbidity and mortality of workers, increased household and government spending for health, and declining labor productivity. The difference between the with-AIDS and without-AIDS simulations is reported as the economy-wide cost of AIDS. The GNP growth rates diverge steadily between the two scenarios, with the gap reaching up to 2.6 percentage points in the growth rate of aggregate GNP. After taking into account the loss of population to the epidemic, the simulations predict a 7% reduction in the level of per capita income due to AIDS by 2010.

These results notwithstanding, economic models tend to show sizeable declines in total GNP, but much smaller declines (if any) in GNP per capita as a result of HIV and AIDS. As discussed, GNP per capita is not dramatically affected in most simulations because the adverse effects on income that follow HIV infection are mostly incurred by those who die. Furthermore, none of the models described in the economics literature attempt to quantify the "external" effects of an individual's infection, particularly the spillover effects on children of HIV-infected parents, communities, and enterprises.

Rather than relying on simulations of macroeconomic change in the presence and absence of AIDS, two studies have employed statistical regression techniques to estimate the effect of AIDS empirically. In one of these studies, Rene Bonnel created a three-equation "structural model," in which the rate of growth of average GNP per person was taken to be a function of several variables (34). A few of these, in turn, were modeled as a function of other variables, including HIV prevalence. Finally, HIV prevalence was modeled as a function of socioeconomic and cultural variables. Using standard cross-country growth regression techniques, Bonnel's findings suggest that on average, the rate of growth of real per capita GNP in Africa would have been 0.7 % points higher per year if not for HIV. In a country with relatively high HIV prevalence (with 30% of the adult population infected), Bonnel's results suggest that the epidemic has slowed growth rates of GNP per capita by 1.4 percentage points per year.

An earlier study by David Bloom and Ajay Mahal, also using cross-country growth regression techniques, failed to detect a statistically significant effect of the epidemic on subsequent economic growth of GNP per capita (35). The differences between these results and those of Bonnel may be due in part to differences in data sources. More importantly, Bloom and Mahal modeled GNP growth as a function of a number of variables, including the prevalence of AIDS cases in the population, and AIDS cases were modeled as a function of HIV prevalence and other variables.

THE ECONOMICS OF INTERVENTIONS TO CONTROL HIV/AIDS

HIV and AIDS interventions can be targeted to prevent transmission of HIV or to provide treatment and care for those already infected. In addition to the ongoing support of such interventions, public priorities include research aimed at improving the efficiency of existing intervention techniques and technologies, as well as the development of new ones. Economic evaluation of interventions most often involves assessments of "value for money," or cost-effectiveness. However, the discipline of economics has much more to offer to the design of optimal intervention strategies. AIDS and other sexually transmitted diseases are unlike many other communicable diseases in that their incidence is largely determined by behavioral choices. To the extent that these choices are made in response to incentives, economic tools can be used to analyze them. This analysis, in turn, may improve the design and implementation of effective interventions.

The Economics of Preventive Interventions

Although large parts of Africa have been neglected, interventions to prevent HIV infections have been underway in much of the world for about two decades, and there have been a few successes and many failures that could inform future intervention design (36,37). Thailand, Senegal, Uganda, and, most recently, the Indian state of Tamil Nadu, have often been cited as regions that have implemented successful preventive intervention programs (37–40). Intervention programs target several types of transmission, including heterosexual, homosexual, parenteral, and mother-to-child.

Intervention strategies that have been effective have been informed by an understanding of the underlying dynamics of each epidemic, and targeted at important "epidemiologic pumps," or transmitter core groups. Mathematical epidemiologic modeling was extremely useful in indicating the importance of identifying and targeting these groups (41–43). Furthermore, descriptive epidemiologic studies in different contexts are essential to identify these groups.

Targeting effective behavioral change is an essential component of preventive interventions (36). Individual behavior choice is central to the spread of sexually transmitted infections, including HIV. Most often, preventive interventions are designed to encourage people to change their behavior in order to reduce their risk of infection.[c] In the early stages of the epidemic, individuals may have chosen behaviors without being aware of HIV or its mode of transmission. In such a context, information campaigns could be effective in helping people to minimize risks (19,44). However, current studies indicate that people in many high-prevalence settings have accurate knowledge of the causes of AIDS and the modes of transmission of HIV. Therefore, information alone is not likely to be sufficient to cause a change in behavior (36,45–47).

Why do risky behaviors continue, despite awareness of AIDS? What can be done to further reduce such behaviors? Just as mathematical models of the dynamics

[c]Exceptions include, for example, male circumcision or the proper management of ulcerative STDs, which are designed to reduce transmission without necessarily effecting a change in behavior.

of disease transmission have been essential to the design of epidemiologically targeted interventions, a model to answer these questions is essential to the design of behaviorally targeted interventions. The discipline of economics has been described as the study of choice, and as such it has an important role to play in examining these questions. Economic models assume that choices are made in response to incentives and in the face of constraints. In many cases, individuals, most often women, are coerced into engaging in risky behavior (48). However, power asymmetries alone are not sufficient to explain why coercive partners engage in risky behaviors themselves, despite the dangers of their own illness and death. A few economists have begun to incorporate theories of behavioral choice into epidemiologic models of the spread of HIV (49, 50). These models assume that individuals who choose to engage in risky behavior derive some pleasure from these behaviors, and perceive this pleasure to outweigh the risks of illness and death. Of course, we must allow for the fact that even when individuals "know" about the risks of transmission, they might underestimate the true risks by interpreting AIDS in a nonscientific or irrational context.

A few economists have begun to examine empirically the relationship between socioeconomic factors and the prevalence of risk-taking behavior and disease (51, 52). These analyses consistently demonstrate that economic inequality is an important determinant of disease prevalence. Other factors identified to predict risky behavior and AIDS illness include population mobility, residence in urban areas, and lower levels of education.

Jha and others consider several prevention strategies in a model of HIV transmission. While they do not model behavior changes, they do make close links between intervention strategies and the underlying epidemiology of transmission, which is assumed to be heavily driven by high-risk groups such as commercial sex workers. The most cost-effective interventions were as low as $10 per DALY saved (36).

Full-scale integrated programs of preventive interventions have not been attempted in most African countries; therefore, the cost of such programs is difficult to estimate. John Stover used computer simulation models to estimate the costs and cost-effectiveness of an integrated national-scale HIV prevention program in a hypothetical country representative of those in East Africa (53). He estimates the cost of such a program, if effectively targeted, could be as low as $70 per case averted. However, such a program would require resources up to 35 times greater than the current levels of expenditure on AIDS in Africa. UNAIDS has recently estimated that comprehensive prevention programs would require $1.4–2.3 billion per year in sub–Saharan Africa (54).

Modeling exercises like these represent the best attempts at estimating the costs and cost-effectiveness of fully scaled intervention programs. However, their usefulness for policy makers is limited for several reasons. First, they usually draw on cost estimates of specific interventions from case studies and pilot projects, the costs of which may be highly context-specific. Furthermore, the nature and extent of interaction between the costs of various interventions are difficult to estimate, and often these interactions are assumed not to exist. Finally, the effectiveness of fully scaled intervention programs is extremely difficult to estimate. Even the crudest assessments, however, indicate that the level of resources required for effective HIV prevention programs across Africa is at least one order of magnitude greater than current spending, and that many such prevention programs would be more cost-effective (in terms of dollars per DALY averted) than many routinely employed health programs.

The Economics of Therapeutic Interventions

Medical care for persons living with HIV and AIDS can include palliative care, treatment and prevention of opportunistic infections, and antiretroviral therapy. In recent years, the accessibility and affordability of care to residents of the poorest countries has become an increasingly pressing issue (55). In industrialized countries, treatment with highly active antiretroviral therapy (HAART) has significantly extended and improved life with HIV infection, at a cost of $10,000 to $20,000 per person per year—far too expensive for most of the residents of African countries to afford. Many treatments for opportunistic infections such as meningitis, shingles, and tuberculosis (TB) are also priced beyond reach for people in much of Africa (56).

Across much of the developing world, the most important opportunistic infections associated with HIV/AIDS are cryptococcal meningitis and TB. Cryptococcal meningitis may affect up to a third of HIV-positive patients in some parts of sub–Saharan Africa, causing enormous morbidity and mortality (57,58). A combination regimen of fluconazole and another antibiotic has recently been shown to be effective in improving the prognosis of cryptococcal meningitis patients in Uganda (59). However, since its introduction in 1983, fluconazole has been under patent in most of the world, except for a few countries, such as India, where patents on pharmaceuticals were not granted at the time. In sub–Saharan Africa, a day's worth of fluconazole for secondary prophylaxis costs about $10, roughly equivalent to total government health expenditure per person per year (60). Accordingly, in most of Africa, antifungal agents for the management of cryptococcal meningitis are omitted from national formularies. In response to increasing pressure in recent years, the U.S. pharmaceutical firm Pfizer, owner of the fluconazole patent, offered to make the drug available for free to qualifying patients in South Africa.

Tuberculosis is the most lethal opportunistic infection associated with HIV and AIDS, accounting for about 15% of AIDS deaths worldwide according to the WHO (61). In sub–Saharan Africa, HIV-infected patients with TB are at increased risk of death, even after they have been successfully treated (62,63). In recognition of this, there has been increasing interest in providing preventive therapy, including secondary prophylaxis. In one study, a secondary prophylactic regimen of isoniazid and sulfadoxine-pyrimethamine significantly reduced the risk of relapse of TB, as well as other opportunistic infections, although its effects in terms of prolonged life were statistically insignificant. The cost of the regimen, however, was about $50 per patient per year (62). Therefore, given existing technologies, interventions to reduce excess mortality associated with TB infection in HIV/AIDS patients is beyond the reach of many African societies, even though the interventions are highly cost-effective.

Most attention to drug pricing, however, has been devoted to issues surrounding the pricing of antiretroviral drugs. The costs of procurement, distribution, and administration of HAART treatment exceed by several orders of magnitude the African GNP per person. In the face of uncontrolled HIV spread, and in response to the enormous expense of therapeutic interventions, some have argued that public provision of antiretrovirals represents an inefficient drain on resources that ought to be committed to prevention (64,65). However, these arguments gloss over two important facts—first, that therapeutic and preventive interventions may be complementary; and second, that treatment need not come at the expense of prevention.

The proper question is not whether resources should be diverted away from prevention in favor of treatment, but rather how much public provision of antiretroviral care in Africa would be included in the welfare maximizing allocation of global resources. In a recent study examining the clinical and pecuniary benefits of HAART protocols in the United States, Freedberg and others found that these protocols compare favorably with HIV prevention activities and standard clinical interventions against other diseases in the United States. Given the enormous differences between Africa and the United

States in terms of drug prices, infrastructure, disease environment, and the genetic profile of the virus, similar studies must be undertaken in Africa; a few are underway.

There are very strong reasons to believe that antiretroviral therapy, backed by donor assistance, should be included in AIDS prevention and control programs in sub–Saharan Africa. First, the costs of antiretroviral therapy have come down significantly, to around $1,000 per year or less, including both the drugs and the related medical care. This is around twice the per capita income of HIV-infected individuals in Africa (or less if we take into account that such individuals are disproportionately of prime working age). It is quite reasonable, indeed conventional, to accept an intervention if the cost per DALY is at least twice the per capita income.[d] Moreover, the benefits of antiretroviral therapy extend to many individuals, far beyond those receiving treatment. Evan Wood and others found that provision of antiretroviral treatment for 25% of HIV-infected individuals in South Africa between 2000 and 2005 could prevent enough adult deaths as of 2005 to avert the loss of 3.1 years of life expectancy (66). Mitigating the demographic shift caused by AIDS would improve dependency ratios, and may avert some of the macroeconomic effects of the epidemic. Furthermore, averting adult deaths could dramatically reduce the number of orphans, with all of the concomitant social and economic benefits.

One of the most important epidemiologic benefits of widespread access to treatment will derive from changes in individual decision-making. The prevailing structure of incentives and constraints in most African settings strongly discourages infected people from learning and disclosing their HIV serostatus, since HIV-positive status marks them for certain early death and likely ostracism. According to UNAIDS and the WHO, the vast majority of Africans infected with HIV are not aware of their HIV status (67). One's decision to remain ignorant about his or her serostatus generates powerful costs to others. The availability of HAART is likely to encourage individuals to come forward for testing, which will have multiple social benefits.

Another potential epidemiologic benefit of therapeutic interventions is the reduction in the transmission of HIV and opportunistic infections. For example, persons living with HIV may be a transmitter core group of TB. Proper treatment and secondary prophylaxis in this subpopulation may reap epidemiologic benefits for the population as a whole. Clinicians have begun to examine whether patients receiving HAART treatment are as infectious to others as untreated patients (68–72). Although conclusive results have yet to emerge, research lends strong support to the contention that HAART reduces the likelihood of sexual transmission of HIV in any single encounter (73). Widespread use of HAART could therefore have population-wide consequences directly from the reduction of likelihood of transmission by individuals under treatment, provided that treatment qualification criteria are not substantially more restrictive than the criteria used in industrialized countries.

There are, however, some countervailing considerations. To the extent that HAART prolongs life and vigor, it is possible that it results in a sufficient increase in the number of possible transmissions to offset any protective effect (74). Furthermore, virus particles that are transmitted from patients receiving HAART may be more likely to be resistant to antiretroviral treatments (75,76). Low compliance with treatment protocols can foster the spread of resistant strains, reducing the effectiveness of treatment in the overall population (73,77). These epidemiologic risks

[d] In the U.S., twice per capita income is $70,000. A conventional cutoff point for interventions is $100,000 per DALY. Similarly, twice per capita income in the U.K. is £30,000, which is the conventional cutoff point for interventions recommended for the National Health Service.

deserve close analysis, and support the argument that the introduction of HAART into Africa must be very carefully supervised, with substantial monitoring of patient adherence and the emergence of drug resistance (78).

The Economics of Research and Development for HIV/AIDS in Africa

Existing intervention techniques and technologies in Africa are sorely underused and underevaluated. A greater research effort is needed to improve the effectiveness of existing interventions and to develop new technologies. For example, ongoing interventions must be tailored to local circumstances through constant monitoring and evaluation; the costs and effectiveness of alternative drug administration protocols and medical procedures must be compared; the social, socioeconomic, and biologic correlates of infectiousness and susceptibility must be better understood, especially the structure of sexual networks in various regions; topical microbicides are needed, which will allow women to protect themselves from infection; and a vaccine is desperately needed in order to reduce the risk of transmission on a population-wide basis. All of these activities and the many others necessary to the future response to the HIV epidemic require substantial resource investment.

Most research and development (R&D) in response to the African epidemic, including clinical trials of new techniques and technologies, must take place in Africa. In the absence of strong research infrastructure and physical and human capital, the recurrent costs of this research will be extremely high. Therefore, donors should support a much greater effort on a continent-wide basis (79). However, the usefulness of the results of this research will be limited unless the research effort is sustained, conducted in a standardized way over time and across countries and regions, and widely disseminated for use in the monitoring and design of other interventions. The development of physical and human resources is also essential in order to provide the necessary infrastructure to support disease surveillance, operational research, and intervention monitoring and evaluation in the long run (80).

Research into alternative uses of the tools and technologies that are standard in industrialized countries is necessary to improve their effectiveness in African settings. Research is needed to assess whether modifications to these tools and technologies offer cost savings that are justified by therapeutic results. For example, optimized protocols in Africa might involve alternative drug cocktails to reduce risks of toxicity or to economize on costs, or structured interruption of therapy (81–83).

New technologies are also needed including, most importantly, an effective vaccine and effective microbicides. A number of important economic barriers slow the development of these and other tools. Private firms, where most novel medical technologies are developed, are discouraged from investing in projects targeted at African populations because of high costs and low expected returns to investment. The social benefit of HIV preventive tools is almost certain to outweigh the costs of their development. However, a market failure results from the fact that a private firm will be unable to capture this benefit. Policies to correct this market failure can be aimed at either reducing the costs of development, or increasing the market return.

Research and development efforts for HIV/AIDS prevention and treatment in industrialized countries, in both the preclinical and clinical phases, receive substantial public support. Virtually all HIV and AIDS R&D activities in Africa, including a few trials of candidate vaccines and microbicides, have been funded by industrialized country governments or nongovernmental organizations, but the total effort is currently only slightly greater than $50 million, a pittance compared to what is needed (84,85).

Public-sector funding tends to mostly support basic science rather than product development, which is carried out by private-sector, profit-maximizing firms. New approaches will be needed to shepherd the results of basic science through to product development, including the applied product research and the expensive rounds of clinical testing. In order to encourage an optimal level of participation by biotechnology firms, pharmaceutical firms, and other private-sector actors, policy instruments are needed to increase the expected private return to investment in HIV/AIDS product development. Despite the enormous burden of disease, private sector investment in the development of new vaccines and microbicides has been very low (86). Firms avoid investing in the development of vaccines, microbicides, and other tools of particular use in less developed countries because the markets for these products are subject to a number of failures. Not only is the potential market quite small, but firms rightly fear that once they have incurred the high costs of successful R&D, they will be pushed by public opinion to provide their products at marginal production cost rather than at a cost that could recover the prior investments in R&D.

One way, therefore, to address these failures is to ensure that firms will be able to reap a reasonable profit if they produce technology that is useful for prevention and control of HIV in Africa. For example, donor governments could pre-commit to purchase qualifying technologies at a profitable price (87). The Vaccines for the New Millennium Act, introduced in the U.S. Congress in March 2000, sought to address these market failures by offering a tax credit of up to $1 billion to pharmaceutical firms for sales of effective vaccines against malaria, TB, and HIV (S.2132, 106th Congress, 2nd Session; H.R.3812, 106th Congress, 2nd Session). While the bill was not enacted into legislation, a similar bill may well be introduced at another time. The U.K. government has endorsed a similar commitment mechanism.

ORGANIZING THE INTERNATIONAL DONOR EFFORT

The African AIDS epidemic takes place in a context of extreme material deprivation. In the year 1999, Africa's 642 million people produced goods and services worth the equivalent of about US$321 billion, or $500 per person.[e] In addition to about four million new HIV infections, each year the continent is burdened by hundreds of millions of clinical cases of malaria, 1.5 million new cases of TB, and hundreds of millions of episodes of diarrheal disease, respiratory disease, and other devastating infectious diseases (88). Africa lacks the financial resources to manage the HIV epidemic on its own. Current public health spending in sub–Saharan Africa, excluding South Africa, averages about 2% of GNP, or around $6 per person per year.

Africa must therefore look to donor support in order to meet its basic health needs. Donor support, however, has so far been negligible, amounting to less than $1.30 per African for *all* health programs. For AIDS specifically, donor support has amounted to less than $0.17 per African (89). The WHO estimates that the total spent in sub–Saharan Africa (excluding South Africa) in 1999 on prevention programs was $165 million from all sources, domestic and international. This was about one-tenth of the amount that UNAIDS estimated to be necessary for prevention programs across the continent (5).

It is conceivable that sub–Saharan Africa could mobilize as much as 6% of its own GNP each year in effective health care spending. This would require a massive mobilization of political will, and debt relief in order to free up fiscal revenues for public health. Note, however, that this would still leave an enormous gap between the amount mobilized

[e]South Africa is much richer than the average, with a per capita income of $3,200. The rest of sub–Saharan Africa has an average income of around $310.

and the resources needed to meet the health needs of the population, and especially to fight AIDS and other epidemic diseases.

The WHO Commission on Macroeconomics and Health has recently estimated the size of this gap.[f] The Commission set targets for coverage of interventions against HIV/AIDS, malaria, and TB, and estimated the costs that can be covered with domestic resources. Rough estimates suggest that by 2007 Africa would need about $24 billion per year more than is currently spent, of which $19 billion would have to come from donor support. Around three-fourths of this would be targeted at HIV/AIDS (including both treatment and prevention interventions), and the rest at malaria and TB.

The most difficult political challenge in reaching this target will be to mobilize global donor support for such a substantial increase in international assistance. However, in view of the $25 trillion combined GNP of the high-income countries, which can be expected to reach at least $30 trillion by 2007, assistance of $14 billion a year is quite modest. Another political challenge will be to make good use of the increased funds. Current donor efforts are plagued by multiple shortcomings that extend beyond the insufficiency of funding. Donor efforts tend to be highly fragmented, since more than 20 agencies of donor countries manage separate national donor programs, often picking their own small-scale pet projects rather than collaborating in activities at necessary scale. These efforts tend to be underinformed by scientific evidence, since donor agencies typically operate without much contact with scientific or medical communities. Finally, donor efforts are rarely subject to independent professional review and evaluation.

Recent proposals by the United Nations, the WHO, and donor governments to establish a Global Trust Fund to fight HIV/AIDS, malaria, and TB, mark a promising step in improving the effectiveness of donor assistance. The Global Fund should be urged to reverse the proliferation of small, atomized, and often contradictory donor-supported efforts, be driven by proposals designed in recipient countries (not donor agencies), engage civil society, and include independent review by expert scientists.

[f]This chapter was written before the completion of the Commission's report, released December 2001. The final report (Macroeconomics and Health: Investing in Health for Economic Development. WHO, 2001) may be found at http://www.cmhealth.org.

CONCLUSIONS AND FUTURE RESEARCH

The AIDS pandemic is not only causing cataclysmic suffering throughout Africa, it is producing manifold adverse consequences for economic development. AIDS impacts the economy at the level of households (reduced saving and investment, loss of skills, dissolution of families, descent into poverty), enterprises (worker turnover, reduced on-the-job training, loss of worker morale), government (fiscal crisis), and society at large (loss of trust, increased crime). The costs of AIDS morbidity and mortality alone may already reach around 20% of African GNP. These costs will be multiplied through a sharp reduction in economic growth in the coming years.

However, the economics of AIDS at the levels of African households and enterprises is still poorly elucidated. How AIDS affects fertility choices, childrearing, children's health and education, and financial and career choices, are areas for future research, as are the effects of AIDS on enterprise behavior and the location of investments.

Effective interventions exist to control AIDS, though new technologies, especially a preventive vaccine and new microbicides, are still sorely needed. It is possible that prevention and treatment are synergistic, working best when combined together. Highly active antiretroviral therapy, which has led to a sharp drop in mortality from AIDS in the rich countries, should now be introduced in a careful and scientifically monitored manner in the poorest countries as well.

The costs of interventions are often very low for each life-year that is saved. Yet, given the extraordinarily meager economic base of sub–Saharan African countries, it is clear that AIDS control will require donor assistance of several billion dollars per year. Scaling up donor assistance involves not only the mobilization of resources, but also the translation of resources into effective programs. The newly proposed Global Fund to Fight HIV/AIDS, Tuberculosis, and Malaria is a highly promising innovation in this regard.

Targeted prevention programs must build upon knowledge of sexual networks and modes of HIV transmission, as well as on a clear view of the economic and social incentives facing individuals in high-prevalence countries. There is a powerful case for ensuring that scaled-up interventions are combined with extensive operational research to ensure that delivery protocols are optimized to local conditions. There is, simultaneously, a strong need to bolster market incentives for longer-term product development, especially in the area of microbicides and vaccines appropriate for use in Africa. A Vaccine Purchase Fund, through which donor countries would commit to buy at a reasonable price an effective vaccine for use in Africa, could spur financial incentives for private-sector R&D in vaccine research.

REFERENCES

1. UNAIDS. *AIDS Epidemic Update 2001*. Available at: http://www.unaids.org/epidemic_update/report_dec01/index.html. Accessed February 17, 2002.
2. World Bank. *World Development Indicators* [CD Rom]. Washington, DC: World Bank, 2001.
3. Budlender D. Earnings and inequality in South Africa, 1995–98. In: Hirschowitz R, ed. *Measuring Poverty in South Africa, Pretoria: Statistics South Africa*. Available at: http://www.statssa.gov.za.
4. World Health Organization. *World Health Report 2001*. Available at: http://www.who.int/whr/2001/. Accessed February 17, 2002.
5. Schwartlander B, Stover J, Walker N, et al. Resource needs for HIV/AIDS. *Science*, 2001; 292:2434–2436.
6. Menon R, Wawer MJ, Konde-Lule JK, et al. The economic impact of adult mortality on households in Rakai District, Uganda. In: Ainsworth M, Fransen L, Over M, eds. *Confronting AIDS: Evidence from the Developing World*. Brussels: World Bank and European Commission, 1998: Chapter 15.
7. Béchu N. The impact of AIDS on the economy of families in Côte d'Ivoire: changes in consumption among AIDS-affected households. In: Ainsworth M, Fransen L, Over M, eds. *Confronting AIDS: Evidence from the Developing World*. Brussels: World Bank and European Commission, 1998: Chapter 16.
8. Over M. The economic impact of adult illnesses from AIDS and other causes in sub–Saharan Africa. Abstract in: *Abstracts of Current Studies*. Washington, DC: World Bank, 1998.
9. Lundberg M, Over M. Transfers and Household Welfare in Kagera. International AIDS Economic Network discussion paper. Available at: http://www.iaen.org. Accessed: January 17, 2002.
10. Mutangadura G. Household welfare impacts of mortality of adult females in Zimbabwe: implications for policy and program development. Paper presented at: The AIDS and Economics Symposium; July 7–8, 2000; Durban, South Africa. Available at: http://www.iaen.org. Accessed: January 17, 2002.
11. Ngula J, Urassa M, Ng'weshemi J, et al. Msuya S. Medical care utilization and household consequences of adult mortality in the era of AIDS: evidence from rural Tanzania. In: Abstracts of the XIII International Conference on AIDS; July 9–14, 2000; Durban, South Africa. Abstract WeOrD566.
12. Foster G. Today's children—challenges to child health promotion in countries with severe AIDS epidemics. *AIDS Care*, 1998;10(Suppl 1):S17–S23.
13. Foster G, Shakespeare R, Chinemana F, et al. Orphan prevalence and extended family care in a peri-urban community in Zimbabwe. *AIDS Care*, 1995;7:3–17.
14. Ainsworth M, Semali I. Impact of Adult Deaths on Children's Health in Northwestern Tanzania. International AIDS Economic Network discussion paper. Available at: http://www.iaen.org. Accessed: January 17, 2002.
15. Nyirenda C. The Impact of HIV on Families and Children. HIV and Development Program Issue Paper Number 22, 1996. Available at: http://www.undp.org/dpa/publications/hiv.html. Accessed: January 17, 2002.
16. Reher D. Wasted investments: some economic implications of childhood mortality patterns. *Popul Stud*, 1995;49:36–56.

17. Becker GS. A theory of the allocation of time. In: Schultz TP, ed. *Economic Demography*. Volume 1. Northampton: Elgar, 1998:311.
18. Cohen D. Poverty and HIV/AIDS in Sub–Saharan Africa. HIV and Development Program issue paper number 27, 1998. Available at: http://www.undp.org/dpa/publications/hiv.html. Accessed: January 17, 2002.
19. Bazargan M, Kelly EM, Stein JA, et al. Correlates of HIV risk-taking behaviors among African-American college students: the effect of HIV knowledge, motivation, and behavioral skills. *J Natl Med Assoc*, 2000;92:391–404.
20. Kremer M. The O-ring theory of economic development. *Q J Econ*, 1993;108:75.
21. Gallup JL, Sachs JD. The Economic Burden of Malaria. Center for International Development working paper number 52, July 2000. Available at: http://www.cid.harvard.edu/cidwp/. Accessed: January 17, 2002.
22. Ashforth A. *AIDS, Witchcraft, and the Problem of Public Power in Post-Apartheid South Africa*. Princeton, New Jersey: Institute for Advanced Study, 2001.
23. State Failure Task Force. State Failure Task Force Report: Phase II Findings. In: *Environmental Change and Security Project Report*, Issue 5, Summer 1999. Washington, DC: Woodrow Wilson Center, 1999:49–72. Available at: http://ecsp.si.edu/. Accessed February 17, 2002.
24. Way PO, Stanecki K. *The Impact of HIV/AIDS on World Population*. Washington, DC: U.S. Bureau of the Census, 1994.
25. Kalemli-Ozcan S, Ryder HE, Weil DN. Mortality decline, human capital investment, and economic growth. *Journal of Development Economics*, 2000; 62:1–23.
26. Bloom DE, Canning D, Malaney P. Population Dynamics and Economic Growth: The Great Debate Revisited. CAER II discussion paper number 46. Cambridge: Harvard University, 2000.
27. Ainsworth M, Filmer D, Semali I. The impact of AIDS mortality on individual fertility: evidence from Tanzania. In: Montgomery MR, Cohen B, eds. *From Death to Birth: Mortality Decline and Reproductive Change*. Washington, DC: National Academy Press, 1997: Chapter 5.
28. Gregson S, Zhuwau T, Anderson RM, et al. HIV and fertility change in rural Zimbabwe. *Health Trans Rev*, 1997;7:89–112.
29. Desgrees du Lou A, Msellati P, Yao A, et al. Impaired fertility in HIV-1-infected pregnant women: a clinic-based survey in Abidjan, Cote d'Ivoire, 1997. *AIDS*, 1999;13:517–521.
30. Carpenter LM, Nakiyingi JS, Ruberantwari A, et al. Estimates of the impact of HIV infection on fertility in a rural Ugandan population cohort. *Health Trans Rev*, 1997;7(Suppl 2):141–153.
31. Shearer WT, Langston C, Lewis DE, et al. Early spontaneous abortions and fetal thymic abnormalities in maternal-to-fetal HIV infection [review]. *Acta Paediatrica*, 1997;421(Suppl):60–64.
32. Over M. *The Macroeconomic Impact of AIDS in Sub–Saharan Africa*. Washington, DC: World Bank, 1992.
33. Arndt C, Lewis JD. The Macro Implications of HIV/AIDS in South Africa: A Preliminary Assessment. International AIDS Economics Network discussion paper, 2001. Available at, http://www.iaen.org. Accessed: January 17, 2002.
34. Bonnel R. HIV/AIDS: Does it Increase or Decrease Economic Growth in Africa? International AIDS Economic Network discussion paper. Available at: http://www.iaen.org. Accessed: January 17, 2002.
35. Bloom DE. Does the AIDS Epidemic Really Threaten Economic Growth? Working paper W5148. Cambridge, Massachusetts: National Bureau of Economic Research, June 1995.
36. Jha P, Nagelkerke JD, Ngugi EN, et al. Public health: reducing HIV transmission in developing countries. *Science*, 2001;292:224–225.
37. Schwartlander B, Garnett G, Walker N, et al. AIDS in a new millennium. *Science*, 2000;289:64–66.
38. Auerbach JD, Coates TJ. HIV prevention research: accomplishments and challenges for the third decade of AIDS. *Am J Public Health*, 2000;90: 1029–1032.
39. Meda N, Ndoye I, M'Boup S, et al. Low and stable HIV infection rates in Senegal: natural course of the epidemic or evidence for success of prevention? [see comments]. *AIDS*, 1999;13:1397–1405.
40. UNAIDS. *Relationships of HIV and STD Declines in Thailand to Behavioral Change: A Synthesis of Existing Studies*. UNAIDS/98.2. Geneva: UNAIDS Best Practice Collection, 1998.
41. Stigum H, Falck W, Magnus P. The core group revisited: the effect of partner mixing and migration on the spread of gonorrhea, chlamydia, and HIV. *Math Biosci*, 1994;120:1–23.
42. Hethcote HW, Yorke JA. Gonorrhea: Transmission dynamics and control. In: *Lecture Notes in Biomathematics 56*. New York: Springer-Verlag, 1984:32–45.
43. Moses S, Plummer FA, Ngugi EN, et al. Controlling HIV in Africa: effectiveness and cost of an intervention in a high-frequency STD transmitter core group. *AIDS*, 1991;5:407–411.
44. Raffaelli M, Siqueira E, Payne-Merritt A, et al. HIV-related knowledge and risk behaviors of street youth in Belo Horizonte, Brazil. The Street Youth Study Group. *AIDS Educ Prev*, 1995;7:287–297.
45. Sallah ED, Grunitzky-Bekele M, Bassabi K, et al. Sexual behavior, knowledge and attitudes to AIDS and sexually transmitted diseases of students at the University of Benin (Togo) [in French]. *Sante*, 1999;9:101–109.

46. Momas I, Helal H, Pretet S, et al. Demographic and behavioral predictors of knowledge and HIV seropositivity: results of a survey conducted in three anonymous and free counselling and testing centers. *Eur J Epidemiol*, 1997;13:255–260.
47. Morris M, Pramualratana A, Podhisita C, et al. The relational determinants of condom use with commercial sex partners in Thailand [see comments]. *AIDS*, 1995;9:507–515.
48. Van der Straten A, King R, Grinstead O, et al. Couple communication, sexual coercion and HIV risk reduction in Kigali, Rwanda. *AIDS*, 1995;9:935–944.
49. Kremer M. Integrating behavioral choice into epidemiological models of AIDS. *Q J Econ*, 1996; 111:549–573.
50. Philipson TJ, Posner RA. *Private Choices and Public Health: The AIDS Epidemic in an Economic Perspective.* Cambridge: Harvard University Press, 1993.
51. Filmer D. The socioeconomic correlates of sexual behaviour: a summary of results from an analysis of DHS data. In: Ainsworth M, Fransen L, Over M, eds. *Confronting AIDS: Evidence from the Developing World*, Brussels: World Bank and European Commission, 1998: Chapter 7.
52. Stillwaggon E. Economic Variables and HIV Transmission in Africa and Latin America. International AIDS Economic Network discussion paper. Available at: http://www.iaen.org. Accessed: January 17, 2002.
53. Stover JO. The impact of interventions on reducing the spread of HIV in Africa: results from computer simulations. Paper presented at: Population Association of America; April 1995; San Francisco, California, USA.
54. Hecht R. Mobilizing resources for AIDS: new opportunities. Presentation at OAU Health Ministers Meeting on HIV/AIDS; May 8–9, 2000; Ouagadougou, Burkina Faso.
55. Cochrane J. Narrowing the gap: access to HIV treatments in developing countries. A pharmaceutical company's perspective [Review]. *J Med Ethics*, 2000;26:47–50.
56. Roach JO. VSO launches campaign to increase access to AIDS drugs. *Br Med J*, 2000;321:1038.
57. Heyderman RS, Gangaidzo IT, Hakim JG, et al. Cryptococcal meningitis in human immunodeficiency virus-infected patients in Harare, Zimbabwe [see comments]. *Clin Infect Dis*, 1998;26:284–289.
58. Maher D Mwandumba H. Cryptococcal meningitis in Lilongwe and Blantyre, Malawi. *J Infect*, 1994;28:59–64.
59. Mayanja-Kizza H, Oishi K, Mitarai S, et al. Combination therapy with fluconazole and flucytosine for cryptococcal meningitis in Ugandan patients with AIDS. *Clin Infect Dis*, 1998;26: 1362–1366.
60. Sachs JD, Botchwey K, Cuchra M, et al. *Implementing Debt Relief for the HIPCs.* Cambridge: Harvard University, 1999.
61. World Health Organization. Tuberculosis: Fact Sheet no. 104. Geneva: World Health Organization, 2000. Available at: http://www.who.int/inf-fs/en/fact104.html. Accessed February 18, 2002.
62. Haller L, Sossouhounto R, Coulibaly IM, et al. Isoniazid plus sulphadoxine-pyrimethamine can reduce morbidity of HIV-positive patients treated for tuberculosis in Africa: a controlled clinical trial. *Chemotherapy*, 1999;45:452–465.
63. De Cock KM, Binkin NJ, Zuber PL, et al. Research issues involving HIV-associated tuberculosis in resource-poor countries. *JAMA*, 1996;276: 1502–1507.
64. Ainsworth M, Teokul W. Breaking the silence: setting realistic priorities for AIDS control in less-developed countries [see comments]. *Lancet*, 2000;356:55–60.
65. Farmer PF, Over MA. Donor agencies are too focused on prevention and pay insufficient attention to the social and economic impacts of the epidemic. Debate at: XIII International Conference on AIDS; July 10, 2000; Durban, South Africa.
66. Wood E, Braitstein P, Montaner JS, et al. Extent to which low-level use of antiretroviral treatment could curb the AIDS epidemic in sub-Saharan Africa [see comments]. *Lancet*, 2000;355:2095–2100.
67. World Health Organization. Global situation of the HIV/AIDS pandemic, end 2001. *Weekly Epidemiological Record*. 2001;76:381–388.
68. Kashuba AD, Dyer JR, Kramer LM, et al. Antiretroviral-drug concentrations in semen: implications for sexual transmission of human immunodeficiency virus type 1 [see comments]. *Antimicrob Agents Chemother*, 1999;43:1817–1826.
69. Vernazza PL. Sexual transmission of HIV: effect of potent antiretroviral therapy [Review in German]. *Therapeutische Umschau*, 1998;55:285–288.
70. Vernazza PL, Troiani L, Flepp MJ, et al. Potent antiretroviral treatment of HIV-infection results in suppression of the seminal shedding of HIV. The Swiss HIV Cohort Study. *AIDS*, 2000;14:117–121.
71. Liuzzi G, Chirianni A, Bagnarelli P, et al. A combination of nucleoside analogues and a protease inhibitor reduces HIV-1 RNA levels in semen: implications for sexual transmission of HIV infection. *Antivir Ther*, 1999;4:95–99.
72. Gray RH, Brookmeyer R, Wawer MJ, et al. The probability of HIV-1 transmission per coital act in monogamous HIV-discourdant couples, Rakai, Uganda. In: Abstracts of the VIII Conference on Retroviruses and Opportunistic Infections; February 4–8, 2001; Chicago, Illinois, USA. Abstract 266.
73. Blower SM, Gershengorn HB, Grant RM. A tale of two futures: HIV and antiretroviral therapy in San

Francisco [see comments]. *Science*, 2000;287: 650–654.
74. Garnett GP, Anderson RM. Antiviral therapy and the transmission dynamics of HIV-1. [Review]. *J Antimicrob Chemother*, 1996;37(Suppl B):135–150.
75. Taylor S, Back D, Drake S, et al. Antiretroviral drug concentrations in semen of HIV infected men: differential penetration of indinavir (IDV), ritonavir (RTV), and saquinavir (SQV). In: Abstract of the VII Conference on Retroviruses and Opportunistic Infections; January 30–February 2, 2000; Chicago, Illinois, USA. Abstract 318.
76. Eron JJ, Vernazza PL, Johnston DM, et al. Resistance of HIV-1 to antiretroviral agents in blood and seminal plasma: implications for transmission. *AIDS*, 1998;12:F181–F189.
77. Gershengorn HB, Blower SM. Impact of antivirals and emergence of drug resistance: HSV-2 epidemic control [Review]. *AIDS Patient Care STDS*, 2000;14:133–142.
78. Harvard Faculty. Consensus Statement on Antiretroviral Treatment for AIDS in Poor Countries. April 4, 2001. Available at: www.cid.harvard.edu. Accessed: January 17, 2002.
79. UNAIDS. Towards Improved Monitoring and Evaluation of HIV Prevention, AIDS Care, and STD Control Programs. Workshop Report; November 1998; Nairobi, Kenya: UNAIDS, 1998.
80. Office of AIDS Research National Institutes of Health. *Global AIDS Research Initiative and Strategic Plan*. Bethesda: National Institutes of Health, 2000.
81. Friedrich MJ. HAART stopping news: experts examine structured therapy interruption for HIV. *JAMA*, 2000;283:2917–2918.
82. Lederman MM. Is there a role for immunotherapy in controlling HIV infection? [Review]. *AIDS Reader*, 2000;10:209–216.
83. Soriano V, Dona C, Rodriguez-Rosado R, et al. Discontinuation of secondary prophylaxis for opportunistic infections in HIV-infected patients receiving highly active antiretroviral therapy. *AIDS*, 2000;14:383–386.
84. Cohen J. Africa boosts AIDS vaccine R&D. *Science*, 2000;288:2165–2167.
85. Cohen J. Major AIDS research collaborations. *Science*, 2000;288:2156.
86. Wechsler J. Access a global concern. *Pharmaceutical Executive*, 2000;20:26–30.
87. Kremer M. Papers on Commitments to Purchase New Vaccines. 2001. Available at: http://post.economics.harvard.edu/faculty/kremer/vaccine.html. Accessed February 25, 2002.
88. World Health Organization. Scaling up the response to infectious diseases: a way out of poverty. Available at: http://www.who.int/infectious-disease report/2002/index.html. Accessed February 25, 2002.
89. Attaran A, Sachs J. Defining and refining international donor support for combating the AIDS pandemic [see comments]. *Lancet*, 2001;357:57–61.

46

International Cooperation and Mobilization

*Keith E. Hansen and †Debrework Zewdie

*AIDS Campaign Team for Africa, Africa Region, The World Bank, Washington, DC, USA.
†Human Development Network, The World Bank, Washington, DC, USA.

1992: For the sake of our common survival, we must act with courage and urgency. With every passing day, HIV claims thousands of lives. The only possible answer to the new AIDS challenge lies in global solidarity. (1)

1991: Perhaps because of the combined effects of a lack of spectacular successes in AIDS control and a growing international disinterest in the development of Africa, signs of discouragement and complacency are emerging. Warding off complacency and securing international and national support will be the major challenges for AIDS control and prevention in Africa in the 1990s. (2)

A decade later, these passages seem as poignant as they were prescient. What made them prescient was their recognition that after the explosion of activity in the 1980s, the global response to AIDS could easily flag in the 1990s, as it did. Despite dire and accurate forecasts in the 1980s, not until 1998 would the international community finally begin to mobilize a response commensurate with the scope of the crisis. What makes the passages poignant is that the intervening years of inaction have made their urgent call even more pressing today than it was then.

The story of the HIV epidemic is a chronicle of a disaster foretold. By the early 1990s, the scope of the emergency had become clear. The World Health Organization (WHO) had deemed AIDS a threat of "extraordinary scale and extreme urgency" (3) and been waging an aggressive campaign for years. Experts were projecting between 30 million and 110 million HIV infections worldwide by the year 2000—a wide range, but a catastrophe by any measure (4). The U.S. Central Intelligence Agency (CIA), in both classified and unclassified documents, had pointed to projected double-digit drops in life expectancy and had highlighted the epidemic as a security threat (5). Although press coverage was infrequent, leading U.S. newspapers had all published prominent and ominous warnings of the course AIDS could run in Africa (6–8).

The building blocks of an effective response were equally clear. Lessons from the first decade had shown the importance of focusing on core groups, blood safety, sexually transmitted disease management, voluntary counseling and testing, communication for behavior change, and community care and support and had highlighted the central role nongovernmental organizations (NGOs) should play in the response. Drawing on this experience, the WHO's 1992 "Global AIDS Strategy" (1) set out a plan of action that remains the nucleus of good strategy, emphasizing national leadership, multisectoral action, partnerships with the private sector and NGOs, human rights, women's status, a supportive environment for behavior change, and a dramatic increase in resources.

During the next several years, many governments, bilateral and multilateral agencies, and international NGOs expanded their actions on these bases. Efforts grew in research, capacity building, advocacy, and implementation. Cooperation deepened between some African governments and their partners. Support increased to international NGOs working in Africa and to African NGOs, which in many countries began to lead the response to the epidemic. Some work validated previous insights; other work brought forth new tools and techniques that have since become part of the standard package for HIV and AIDS programs. Dissemination of knowledge grew as various stakeholders shared experience. Each of these efforts contributed in some important way to bolstering the response in Africa.

On the whole, however, the international community failed throughout the first decade to convert these individual initiatives into a comprehensive, strategic venture. The failure was both of scale and of substance. The fact that so many of the individual efforts were succeeding but that none were being scaled up made the larger failure all the more tragic. In substance, the international community failed to convert what was largely a public health strategy into a multisectoral strategy. As UNAIDS and its cosponsors concluded in early 1999, "External support remains too small, slow, and disjointed to have a critical impact." (9). As a result, HIV continued to spread. When WHO's strategy was published in 1992, roughly 7 million Africans were living with HIV or AIDS. A decade on, that number has grown four-fold.

Yet during the past three years, a new chapter has opened. AIDS has been catapulted to the center of the international development agenda, buoyed by growing evidence that it is as much an economic and security threat as it is a public health challenge. African leaders have begun to address the epidemic publicly and to advocate more external support. Bilateral and multilateral commitments have swelled and a multitude of formal international partnerships have emerged, including a vast global trust fund. Pressure has intensified to make antiretroviral medications more accessible to more people in Africa. In 2000–01 alone, a host of leading global and regional bodies, multilateral organizations, and national parliaments devoted extraordinary special sessions to the issue of AIDS in Africa. This may at last be the makings of a global solidarity against the epidemic, something for which the AIDS community has long appealed.

This chapter will review the first decade of the response, its impact on Africa, its discrete successes, and its overarching failure. It will then discuss the recent groundswell of global activity, its origins, and its prospects. It will close with recommendations for ensuring effective and sustained collaboration.

INTERNATIONAL COOPERATION AND MOBILIZATION DURING THE FIRST DECADE (1986–96)

Expansion and Stagnation

The WHO produced the first global strategy for AIDS in 1986. The strategy was endorsed by the World Health Assembly and the UN General Assembly the next year, and in early 1988 by more than 100 health ministers at a world summit (1). By that time, the Global Programme on AIDS (GPA) was already the WHO's most dynamic activity, and the organization used the strategy to lead a global push for national programs, greater international funding, and the expansion of key interventions. Although this strategy was still heavily health oriented, the mobilization paid dividends. By 1991, each of more than 40 African countries had set up a national AIDS control program (NACP) and had mobilized support for a first medium-term plan (MTP).

Key bilaterals, such as Sweden and the United States, took a consciously strategic view of the epidemic and channeled resources to help establish and strengthen NACPs. Whatever their weaknesses, NACPs provided a locus for strategic planning, capacity building, and external support. Many technical and program officers honed their skills in this period as a benefit of the concerted approach. NACPs also took the lead in making projections and mounting advocacy campaigns.

With help from the WHO and others, core interventions and indicators were developed for local adaptation, enabling a certain degree of cross-country consistency and comparability. The most ambitious undertaking in the period was USAID's AIDSCAP project. AIDSCAP provided vast collaborative support through a network of subcontractors such as Population Services International and JSI International, and academic institutions such as the Center for AIDS Prevention Studies at the University of California at San Francisco. During its seven years (1991–97), AIDSCAP supported design and implementation of broad HIV and AIDS programs in nine countries and targeted programs in several others. The efforts it sponsored helped validate the efficacy of the syndromic approach, social marketing, and peer education, and enhanced the capacity of tens of thousands of African AIDS workers (10).

Within a few years, however, the strategic push had stagnated. The leadership role that GPA previously had exercised began to decline, and many donor governments started relationships directly with countries. The global response began to fragment. Despite the early concerted effort, virtually no MTPs had been funded or implemented in full and as the epidemic spread, the health sector limitations of the approach and the lack of leadership became more disabling. Few programs devoted attention to factors beyond the health sector or to the links between AIDS and development, since these areas fell outside the competence of most NACPs. As dependents of health ministries, NACPs were politically weak and had little influence except within the health agenda. Therefore, as calls for a broader response grew, most governments found it convenient to continue delegating all AIDS issues to NACPs without bolstering the programs' capacities or scope. Although increasingly burdened by the demands of the spreading epidemic, NACPs had diminishing latitude on issues beyond those originally mandated. For donors working with NACPs, therefore, efforts remained primarily limited to the health sector despite growing evidence that AIDS posed a serious development threat.

With a few notable exceptions, African leaders also failed to address the epidemic strategically. Few would speak openly about AIDS and even fewer elevated it to a policy level. Organization of African Unity (OAU) declarations in 1992 (11) and 1994 (12) had called for full political commitment, for social mobilization, and for making AIDS a high priority for resource allocation. An OAU delegation visited four African leaders in 1995 to assess progress toward these goals. But denial, stigma, and despair prevented all but the most courageous leaders from taking bold action.

At about the same time, international support began to dissipate. In donor countries, the stabilization of HIV incidence, promising new therapies, and a disbelief concerning the worsening epidemiologic projections blunted the sense of urgency that had motivated rapid action in the late 1980s. In some key agencies, skepticism about the importance of AIDS began to grow—sometimes fueled by issue parochialism—and attention shifted to priorities that seemed both more visible and more tractable (13). The persistence of denial and the lack of concrete successes in Africa also bred doubt among donors that more money could, or would, be effective in slowing the epidemic. Although resources for AIDS in Africa gradually grew throughout this period, many donors turned away from governments and multilaterals and began focusing more on discrete programs and interventions, many with NGOs. GPA resident advisers were withdrawn, and donor agencies began hiring away many of the key staff from NACPs, an action that had deleterious effects on national capacity.

As the public sector faltered, civil society took on increasing responsibility for the response in Africa. Almost as if mirroring the creation of antibodies, a vast number of NGOs, community- and faith-based organizations sprang up in those countries hit by the epidemic, each piloting and providing prevention and/or care services. Often focusing on socially stigmatized individuals, these organizations worked with important core groups that most public programs could not, or would not, reach. In so doing, they not only filled critical gaps in national responses but also pioneered many of the interventions that would later be recognized as "best practice." As the AIDS epidemic grew, civil society bore the brunt of the burden of care and support. Some of these undertakings received substantial donor support from organizations such as the Royal Tropical Institute in the Netherlands. Many others were self-sustaining. Among their other accomplishments, these efforts helped demonstrate the pivotal role of communities in shaping and implementing effective local responses to the epidemic (14).

But neither private nor public initiatives alone could succeed against the epidemic. Only concerted, multisectoral action led by governments and based on strong partnerships between the public, private, and civil sectors would suffice. Yet by the mid-1990s, such cooperation remained out of reach. The international effort, in particular, was actually less coordinated or strategic than it had been at the start of the decade.

It was also starved for funds. Annual global resources for AIDS had nearly quadrupled in the first years of the global strategy, from $44 million in 1986 to $165 million in 1990 (15). Then, along with the rest of the international effort, growth in funding began to stagnate. By 1996, total global resources had leveled off at about $300 million per year, two-thirds of which came from only three donor countries. This was, by any measure, insufficient. Globally, it represented less than three-fourths of 1% of the more than $40 billion in annual global development aid. In Africa, the $150 million available each year met only 10% of the continent's minimum estimated annual need of $1.5 billion. Moreover, a significant share of external support for AIDS flowed to firms and consultants in donor countries, rather than directly to the countries most affected by the epidemics.

Several forces joined in this period to keep funding below needed levels. First, AIDS programs suffered from the worldwide falloff in development aid. Between 1992 and 1997, net overseas development assistance dropped 23% in real terms, reaching a new low as a share of donor gross domestic products (GDPs). Second, the combination of complacency and skepticism among donors weakened the bargaining position of AIDS advocates as aid cuts were absorbed. Third, even for the resources on offer, demand was low. Most African governments showed scant interest in using development aid to combat the epidemic and even less interest in spending national resources (which were estimated to total only $15 million as late as 1998). The World Bank, for example, provided more than $1 billion for AIDS programs around the world in the 1990s, which included support to more than 20 African countries. Yet in this time only three African countries asked the World Bank for $10 million or more for the crisis. Other donors encountered a similar reluctance by African nations to seek aid against the epidemic, and, in some cases, ultimately had to reprogram resources they had originally set aside for AIDS programs.

Little Lasting Impact

Although the global effort of the first decade helped produce important knowledge

(10, 16), it failed to convert this knowledge into results in Africa. Of the many programs that proved effective, virtually none was implemented on the scale necessary to turn back the epidemic. Despite the level of advocacy, few African leaders, except those in Senegal and Uganda, took on AIDS as a strategic issue. Research remained largely confined to the health sector. Even today, the dearth of rigorous economic or social studies on the impact of AIDS remains a bottleneck to faster progress. Support for research conducted by developing countries was particularly scarce (17), while efforts to build capacity in other areas were rife but narrow. In sum, 10 years after the first global strategy was published, both Africa and its partners had managed to achieve little sustained effect on policy, behavior, or capacity and, therefore, virtually no effect on the ongoing spread of the epidemic.

RESTRUCTURING AND REVIVAL (1996–2001)

The Formation of UNAIDS

As HIV spread, so did alarm over the global failure. As Jonathan Mann and Daniel Tarantola wrote in 1996 (18), "Constrained by inadequate policies, insufficient financial support, and weakly coordinated programs, the scope, quality and impact of existing HIV/AIDS prevention and control efforts have remained inadequate." In the same year, authors Trussell and Cohen warned that the plateau in the global effort was exacting "enormous costs, in both human and economic terms." (17).

This concern led in 1996 to the founding of UNAIDS, a joint, multisectoral venture of six (now eight) UN agencies whose mandates span the breadth of the development landscape: the International Labour Organization (ILO), the UN International Drug Control Programme (UNDCP), the UN Development Programme (UNDP), the UN Educational, Scientific, and Cultural Organization (UNESCO), the UN Population Fund (UNFPA), the UN Children's Fund (UNICEF), the WHO, and the World Bank. Virtually without precedent in UN history, the program was established explicitly to harness the special expertise of each agency so as to maximize the effect of the UN system contribution. Its overall goals are to strengthen national capacities and to lead, strengthen, and support an expanded response across the globe, with special attention to Africa and other hard-hit regions. In recognition of the pluralistic nature of the crisis, the UNAIDS Programme Coordinating Board was created. It includes representatives from 22 governments (donors and recipients), the eight cosponsors, and 5 NGOs and is the first UN program to include NGOs in its governing board. Global UNAIDS activities are coordinated by a Secretariat in Geneva, which also provides seed money for select initiatives, but the primary responsibility for the partnership rests with the cosponsors. In developing countries, UNAIDS operates through the country-based staff of the cosponsors, who meet together as the UN Theme Group on HIV/AIDS. In many countries, a Secretariat staff member is resident, serving as Country Programme Adviser in support of Theme Group operations.

UNAIDS has four primary, mutually reinforcing, roles:

- **coordination** of the contributions of the cosponsors and other supporters;
- **advocacy**, especially at the global level, using authoritative data and projections, to stimulate an expanded response;
- **policy development and research**, including dissemination of best practices in principles, policies, strategies and implementation; and
- **technical support**, primarily in the form of operational support to build on what countries have in place.

UNAIDS was designed to overcome the sectoral and bureaucratic limitations that had thwarted GPA from stimulating a truly multidimensional and global response. To this end, each agency committed to stepping up its work within its area of expertise, in greater collaboration with other cosponsors and partners. ILO focused on the workplace; WHO on health and surveillance systems; UNDP on capacity building in the public sector; UNICEF on the health of infants and youth; UNFPA on integrating HIV in reproductive health; UNESCO on integrating HIV and AIDS into education; the World Bank on assessing and addressing the economic, sectoral and developmental aspects of HIV and AIDS, and UNDCP on integrating HIV and AIDS concerns into programs to control illicit drugs. Most of the cosponsors had been supporting HIV and AIDS work for years but without the scale or the coordination necessary to make a decisive difference.

Despite some early friction among the cosponsors, UNAIDS soon established itself as the hub of the global AIDS campaign. Working with the various cosponsors, the Secretariat began raising the profile of the epidemic through regular updates and emerging information, which it widely publicized, and media and policymaker attention began to grow. However, the global response remained sluggish.

The turning point came in 1998, with the conjunction of two influential UNAIDS publications: the 1997 estimates of global HIV infections (19) and the assessment of global resource levels for HIV and AIDS, which was published in 1999 but widely circulated in draft form in 1998 (20). The HIV numbers were perhaps the more important. Estimates of global HIV infection published three years earlier by GPA, had to rely on sketchy information from many countries and, consequently, presented only global figures (19). By contrast, for the 1997 estimates the WHO, UNAIDS, and national epidemiologists had both more data and a better understanding of the natural history of HIV. As a result, UNAIDS was able to publish for the first time a country-by-country analysis. The report showed that prevalence rates among populations in several African countries exceeded 25% and that the epidemic was advancing rapidly. On its opening page it stated bluntly "there is worse to come" and implicitly castigated leaders for the inadequacy of the response. The report sparked front-page press coverage around the world.

To this picture of a runaway epidemic, the financing data then added the dimension of an international effort that was too small and too slow to keep pace (20). Aside from noting inadequate levels of spending by both developed and developing countries, the report pointed to the lack of strategic orientation or adequate monitoring mechanisms in current spending. Together, the two reports galvanized renewed attention to the epidemic, particularly at the strategic level. The HIV estimates proved crucial in changing political attitudes around the world, and the resource estimates were widely quoted as indicators of the insufficiency of the global effort (21).

The Growth of New Initiatives

Beginning in 1998, this revived concern began to translate into new action. Virtually every agency and donor, as well as a range of foundations, firms, academic institutions, and NGOs, began to revitalize their efforts. The scale of finance enlarged markedly. Even more important, the focus on collaboration and partnerships was revived. As of this writing, the response remains so dynamic that new initiatives are still coming forth on a regular basis, making it impossible to provide a comprehensive review of the state of global activity. The following discussion helps illustrate the accelerating trend during the past three years.

One of the broadest initiatives was the formation of the International Partnership Against AIDS in Africa (IPAA). In January 1999, the UNAIDS cosponsors and Secretariat resolved to create the IPAA and build it into a global coalition of governments,

NGOs, bilateral and multilateral agencies, the private sector, and the UN system (9). The IPAA aims to bring all major actors together to mobilize an Africa-wide response to the epidemic. Since its formal launch in December 1999, the IPAA has enlisted new partners from all sectors, increased African political support, and mobilized more resources for the continent. IPAA has also helped Ghana introduce the female condom, Burkina Faso and Côte d'Ivoire to set up national solidarity funds, and Ethiopia to develop five-year national and regional AIDS plans.

The United Nations system as a whole took on AIDS as a global issue, sometimes in unprecedented ways. In July 1999, General Assembly members committed themselves for the first time to time-bound specific targets for reducing HIV infection rates. In January 2000, the Security Council devoted a special session to AIDS, the first time it had addressed a development issue. Later that year, the Council passed two resolutions, one drawing a link between the spread of HIV and maintenance of security (22) and another calling on member states to incorporate HIV and AIDS into training programs for security forces and on the Secretary-General to provide such training for civilian personnel in UN peacekeeping operations. (23). The capstone of UN efforts came in the June 2001 General Assembly Special Session on HIV/AIDS. Led by the UN Secretary-General, member states unanimously approved a framework for national and international accountability in the Declaration of Commitment on HIV/AIDS, which included comprehensive benchmark targets for funding and action (24).

The UNAIDS Secretariat accelerated its production of strategic guidelines, case studies, technical updates, policies, and best practices (25–31). At the same time, several UNAIDS cosponsors increased their efforts. The World Bank issued a sweeping new strategy for its work in Africa, calling AIDS "the foremost threat to development" in the region and committing itself to including a response to the epidemic in all its work (32). The Bank also publicized influential research findings (33) and undertook new economic work that demonstrated that AIDS would likely have significant effects at both micro- and macroeconomic levels in Africa. With the International Monetary Fund, the World Bank put AIDS on the international development agenda during their joint spring 2000 meeting of world finance ministers (34).

UNICEF undertook an extensive reorientation of its programs in Africa in five areas: advocacy, parent-to-child transmission, youth, children orphaned by AIDS, and AIDS in the UN workplace. It drew particular attention to the plight of orphans (35) and played a lead role in supporting peer education programs among youth in countries such as Zambia. The WHO increased technical support to Africa at country and district levels and stepped up its efforts to strengthen health systems and to promote evidence-based prevention and care. It also played a lead role in negotiating greater access to antiretroviral drugs in Africa. UNDP began integrating AIDS policies into all sectors and poverty reduction strategies. It also launched the Alliance of Mayors and Municipal Leaders on HIV/AIDS in Africa, comprising officials from dozens of municipalities in nearly 20 countries. UNFPA issued updated guidelines on reproductive health and increased its attention to health information and service programs for youth. In addition, other UN organizations such as the Food and Agriculture Organisation began to develop strategies to contribute to the global response (36).

Bilateral programs also began to grow. The United States had long been the largest bilateral funder of AIDS efforts, but its funding had flattened out during the 1990s. In 1998, the administration of then-President Bill Clinton began an intensive campaign to step up the effort by the United States, including presidential "summits" on AIDS with the private sector, labor, and religious organizations. The White House AIDS policy adviser made several high-profile trips to Africa in 1998 and 1999. Subsequent visits by President Clinton, cabinet secretaries, and members of Congress roused bipartisan resolve to increase U.S. support. This enabled the U.S. government to launch the Leadership and Investment in Fighting an Epidemic initiative in 1999, adding $100 million to its global contribution.

In 2000, the United States used its last days as rotating chair of the UN Security Council to call for the special session on AIDS, which Vice President Al Gore addressed. Following that session, the White House officially designated AIDS a threat to national security, supported in part by a new CIA intelligence report (37) forecasting weakened militaries, slower socioeconomic development, and international friction arising from disease-related restrictions on global trade, travel, and immigration. In May 2000, President Clinton issued Executive Order 13155, protecting African governments from U.S. trade sanctions if they used parallel imports or compulsory licensing for antiretroviral drugs.

The new momentum generated growing U.S. appropriations for AIDS. In fiscal year 2000, USAID's budget for AIDS in Africa surpassed $100 million for the first time. The following year it reached $145 million, roughly three-fold the annual U.S. efforts during the previous several years. By late 2001, several bills authorizing global allocations in the hundreds of millions of dollars were pending in Congress.

U.S.-supported programs also generated valuable analytic work in this period. The POLICY Project (led by Futures Group International in conjunction with the Research Triangle Institute and the Centre for Development and Population Activities) produced important guidelines, software, and advocacy tools for ministries to use in formulating AIDS policies (38).

The United Kingdom, historically one of the top funders of AIDS programs worldwide, has also progressively been expanding its response. The Department for International Development has supported reproductive health programs and health sector strengthening in nine African countries and the development of national HIV and AIDS plans in several more. The UK was also the first country to contribute to the International AIDS Vaccine Initiative (IAVI). It committed in 2000 to produce a comprehensive new HIV and AIDS strategy. The Netherlands, another of the larger funders, also announced major new contributions in 2000, including NLG 45 million to IAVI.

During the 1990s, Canada supported regional AIDS training networks in western and in eastern and southern Africa, as well as research into reducing parent-to-child transmission. It was also instrumental in the creation of UNAIDS and is a supporter of IAVI. In July 2000, Canada announced a substantial expansion of its efforts, expected to triple annual spending by fiscal year 2003 (39). It also committed itself to taking a more strategic approach by linking Canadian International Development Agency (CIDA)-supported projects directly to national HIV and AIDS programs and to incorporating HIV prevention in other sectoral work. Canada committed itself to capitalizing on partnerships with NGOs and to devoting greater attention to gender equality, youth, education, reproductive health, care and support (especially for children), and monitoring and evaluation.

Several other countries are also in the course of expanding their commitment. Following a drop-off in the mid-1990s, Sweden announced a renewed program in July 1999, focusing on building capacity, support to strategy development, and sponsorship of national research. The Swedish development agency has also set up a task force to integrate HIV and AIDS into its programs wherever possible. Norway, already the most generous contributor to AIDS programs, based on its contributions as a share of its GDP, is in the midst of a three-year expansion of support, including direct funding for national programs in several countries, support to UNAIDS for joint programs, and a grant to support development and implementation of the World Bank's new strategy for Africa. Japan has committed ¥90 billion to core social services in Africa with particular attention to AIDS and has assigned AIDS high priority in its new medium-term policy on development aid. Japan also focused the Second Tokyo International Conference on African Development (TICAD II) meetings of October 1998 on an agenda for action on AIDS in Africa. The European Union (EU) has announced a common stand against AIDS, tuberculosis, and malaria in conjunction with the United States, UNAIDS, and the WHO and has convened a high-level roundtable to begin designing an ambitious new program. The EU has also supported the production of toolkits to guide the integration of AIDS into various sectoral programs.

In addition to the increased scale of contributions, the revival has brought renewed commitment to partnerships. Many donor countries contribute directly to UNAIDS as a whole or to its cosponsors, and new members join the IPAA on a regular basis. Collaboration was also vital in creating two path-breaking partnerships on vaccines: IAVI and the Global Alliance for Vaccines and Immunization (GAVI).

Development of vaccines for the developing world has historically been grossly inadequate, hampered by a number of market and political obstacles. Only collective global action could overcome these barriers. IAVI was created in 1996 to accelerate scientific progress and mobilize funding for an AIDS vaccine. It has developed a global strategy to guide accelerated vaccine development, invested nearly $20 million in partnerships to bring promising vaccines to clinical testing, and negotiated intellectual property agreements to ensure vaccines quickly become available in developing countries. IAVI receives support from several governments, foundations, and pharmaceutical firms, as well as from UNAIDS and the World Bank.

GAVI has a similar but broader mandate. Created in 1999, GAVI works to improve access to immunizations of all types, to speed research and development on new vaccines needed in developing countries, and to raise the profile of immunization in international development. GAVI is made up of national governments, bilateral agencies, the vaccine industry, research and public health institutions, technical agencies, foundations, UNICEF, the World Bank, and the WHO. Many of these organizations were traditionally unable to work easily with the private sector. The alliance has made such cooperation possible. By mid-2000, GAVI was making its first disbursements to countries.

Philanthropic efforts have also expanded rapidly, often in conjunction with the private sector. As early as 1994, the Rockefeller Foundation had laid the groundwork for the creation of IAVI, and today supports both it and GAVI. The Bill and Melinda Gates Foundation contributed $750 million to launch GAVI, is a partner in IAVI, and is supporting a host of other initiatives, including Hope for African Children, a partnership of development and relief agencies designed to deliver support and services to children. The Gates Foundation also joined with Merck & Co. to fund the $100 million African Comprehensive HIV/AIDS Partnership, Botswana, which will strengthen primary health care, health system management, and facilitate the distribution of antiretroviral drugs. By the end of 2000, the United Nations Foundation had committed more than $20 million to prevention and care projects in several countries in southern Africa.

The private sector has increasingly taken on HIV and AIDS both in the workplace and in global advocacy. Dozens of corporations such as Chevron Oil in Nigeria, Anglo American and Eskom in South Africa, and Rio Tinto in Zimbabwe have put in place workplace activities. ING-Barings of South Africa has published reports on the likely demographic and economic impact of AIDS in South Africa. The Global Business Council on HIV/AIDS, a confederation of business interests, has supported the formation of national associations such as the Kenya Business Council on HIV/AIDS. Such councils help stimulate contributions to the AIDS effort and support partnership between the private and public sectors. On the labor side, several unions in Africa have activities in place, and the Organisation of African Trade Union Unity (OATUU) has issued guidelines for company interventions on HIV and AIDS. At a July 2000 meeting, the OATUU, the ILO, and UNAIDS agreed to work jointly to further develop labor-based strategies.

The pharmaceutical industry has launched several initiatives in the past two years. Facing withering criticism from ACT UP, other AIDS activists, the public health community, and consumer groups, in early 2000 the five major manufacturers of HIV and AIDS drugs, with assistance from the UNAIDS Secretariat and UNAIDS cosponsors, agreed to make these drugs more accessible and affordable in developing countries. While antitrust laws prohibit the firms from discussing prices with one another, Boehringer Ingelheim, Bristol–Myers Squibb, F. Hoffman–La Roche, Glaxo Wellcome, and Merck & Co., have individually pursued price reductions with various countries. In late 2000, several of the firms agreed with the governments of Senegal and Uganda to reduce prices by as much as 90% for some of the most common ARV medications. Talks in other countries are proceeding. Boehringer Ingelheim also announced that it would provide Viramune™ (nevirapine) free for five years to developing countries to prevent parent-to-child transmission. Other firms have taken similar steps.

Besides these drug initiatives and their participation in GAVI, companies have mounted other programs. Bristol–Myers Squibb started Secure the Future™, a $100 million partnership with five southern African countries to find sustainable ways of managing the impact of AIDS, with particular focus on women, children, and communities.

Academic and research institutions have also intensified their efforts. The largest global research training program remains the AIDS International Training and Research Program at the Fogarty International Center, dedicated to collaborative work between U.S. and international researchers. Established in 1988, the program has built capacity in more than a dozen African countries through epidemiologic research, clinical trials, and prevention programs. In January 1998, the Harvard AIDS Institute and the Merck Company Foundation founded the Enhancing Care Initiative. Designed to support the creation of multidisciplinary teams of local experts, the initiative is now operating in five countries, two of them in Africa: Senegal and South Africa. In the same month, the University of Natal opened a Health Economics and HIV/AIDS Research Division. Working with South African provincial governments, this division has generated a substantial body of operations research in AIDS economics and public and private sector AIDS policies, as well as issuing a series of sectoral guidelines for addressing the epidemic. In May 2000 the International Association of Physicians in AIDS Care, comprising 6,800 physicians in 43 countries, launched the I-Med exchange, a two-way medical education program using the worldwide web.

Most recently, renewed collaboration has given rise to a potentially far-reaching initiative: the Global Fund to Fight AIDS, Tuberculosis, and Malaria (Global Fund). Following calls by the G-8 nations and the UN Secretary-General, the Global Fund was created in 2001 and within a few months had attracted $1.7 billion in pledges from governments, foundations, private firms, and individuals. Its aim is to raise and disburse funds for the three diseases on an unprecedented scale. As the most affected region, Africa is expected to benefit substantially.

The Promise of the New Approach

What, if anything, sets this upsurge of activity apart from the mobilization of the late 1980s? Is there reason to believe that this time the global effort will endure and succeed? History counsels against overconfidence, but there do seem to be grounds for optimism.

Four promising factors stand out. First, and most important, African governments are increasingly showing the necessary leadership. Inadequate political commitment had long been the missing link in Africa's response. As late as mid-1999, not one African head of state appeared at the 11th International Conference on AIDS and STDs in Africa, held in Lusaka, Zambia. Since then, however, leaders in all parts of Africa, including Nigeria and Ethiopia, the two largest nations, have declared AIDS a national emergency and mounted national programs to address it. African countries and regional organizations such as the OAU hosted four major international conferences within 12 months—including the "XIII International AIDS Conference" in Durban, South Africa in July 2000—where participating leaders acknowledged the threat of the epidemic and the scope of prior failings.

Most notable among these was the OAU Special Summit in Abuja, Nigeria, in April 2001. In the resulting Abuja Declaration, leaders endorsed the strongest and most candid statements to date about HIV and AIDS, took personal responsibility for leading comprehensive national efforts, and pledged to set a target of allocating at least 15% of national budgets to strengthen health systems (40).

Second, the new approach is more strategic, comprehensive, and collaborative than its predecessors. Led by UNAIDS, the renewed response is paying more attention to the overall strategic and policy framework within which programs are implemented. Specifically, governments, agencies, and other entities now share a broad consensus that the global response must:

- be guided by national strategies and led by national AIDS authorities;
- build capacity in Africa for research, policymaking, program implementation, and monitoring and evaluation;
- be multisectoral in design and implementation;
- build on partnership with all interested actors from the public and private sectors and from civil society, especially persons living with HIV or AIDS; and
- directly support local, community-led actions.

In designing their programs, nearly all donors and agencies have now committed to work through national authorities and to coordinate with one another in a cluster of common efforts, including UNAIDS, GAVI, IAVI, the IPAA, and the new Global Fund. This commitment and coordination distinguishes recent efforts from the narrow, uncoordinated, enclave projects that typified much external support in the 1990s. Key analytic work has focused on supporting the development of strategy and on evaluating program outcomes (26, 41). All donor governments have also adopted the strategic targets set by the UN General Assembly in 2001, providing further cohesion.

Third, the new commitment is being matched by new funding on a large scale. In late 2000, the World Bank launched its Multi-Country AIDS Program for Africa, which set aside $500 million in concessional funds to support national programs. Within a little more than a year, nearly all the money had been committed to more than a dozen African governments, and the World Bank had replenished the fund. Bilateral donors are also enlarging their assistance. As noted earlier, the United States has increased its funding dramatically during the past three years, and several other governments are budgeting larger contributions. The Global Fund could provide significant new resources (depending on how it is divided among regions and diseases). Under the Highly Indebted Poor Countries initiative (a collective effort of the World Bank, the International Monetary Fund, and the international financial community), donor and recipient governments have agreed to channel savings from debt relief to fund HIV and AIDS programs. And as more African countries build national programs, domestic funding for HIV and AIDS has also begun to grow.

In total, estimates suggest that funding for Africa in 2000 and 2001 may have exceeded $700 million. This still falls short of the minimum needed and has drawn criticism from activists as inadequate. But as the most significant increase since the 1980s, it is a measure of the sincerity of the new commitment and a sign that resource constraints soon may no longer number among the main impediments to an effective response.

Fourth, efforts of the past three years have been driven by a far broader understanding of the epidemics, both in the professional AIDS community and among the general public. In the professional sphere, experience has proven numerous replicable means of preventing HIV and of caring for those living with HIV or AIDS. It has also shown what does not work against the epidemics. This has enabled policymakers to act with greater confidence and on a larger scale.

Perhaps even more important has been the growth in public awareness. During the past three years, AIDS has commanded public attention in Africa, Europe, and the Americas. From 1998 through 2000, major U.S. newspapers ran roughly three-fold as many stories on AIDS in Africa as in the 10 years preceding. Some of this surge has resulted from the sheer shock of the numbers. As infections and deaths have multiplied, AIDS has routinely been likened to the Black Death, the 1918 influenza epidemic, and even the two World Wars. Numbers alone, however, do not guarantee adequate coverage, as the 1990s proved. What has changed most in the past few years—and helped prompt the swell of attention—is the quality of advocacy by the UNAIDS Secretariat and cosponsors and by AIDS activists. Major UNAIDS reports have been geared for general audiences (19) and have typically generated several days of coverage, frequently including editorials. For their part, AIDS activists have targeted high-profile events (such as international conferences and the launch of Al Gore's campaign for president) to call attention to the inadequacy of the global response. The result has been far wider awareness of the issue and growing political support in donor countries to take action. The breadth of the response described in the section above is a testament to the breadth of understanding that now prevails.

Two technologic advances have also played a part. The rapid development of the Internet over the past five years has enabled instant, mass, global communication on an affordable scale. This has accelerated and expanded the flow of information between Africa and donor countries, bringing the epidemics to light in a more immediate and sustained way. The other vital advance has been in antiretroviral therapies. As these drugs have gradually made HIV a manageable disease, the disparity between developed and developing countries has grown all the more striking.

FUTURE OR FAILURE?

In the first edition of *AIDS in the World*, Mann, Tarantola, and Netter (4) discerned four phases in the story of AIDS: silent spread (1970s–81), discovery and response (1981–85), global mobilization (1985–90), and what they feared would become a sustained plateau beginning in 1990. History confirmed their fears. The plateau would ultimately persist for the better part of a decade. Only as of 1998 did a fifth phase, revival, definitively open.

This latest chapter will write the future of Africa. However overstated that may seem, it should be remembered that AIDS has thrived by repeatedly breaching the bounds of incredulity. The projections that once seemed too terrible to be true in short order proved too optimistic. Had the world followed through on the first mobilization, Africa might have confined HIV from spreading and been able to concentrate its resources on helping the several million already infected. But now the continent faces two vastly greater challenges: saving the next generation from an HIV epidemic that is fast becoming ubiquitous, and helping the tens of millions of the current generation who are already infected and affected by AIDS. Even in the absence of AIDS, meeting the developmental needs of the next generation would stretch Africa's resources to the limit. Without sustained, substantial support from the global community, Africa will simply be unable to keep pace with the epidemic and still lay the foundations for its future.

What will it take to make revival the final and decisive chapter? No one can say for certain. That much, at least, the world has learned from 20 years of experience. But three lessons from the initial phases bear heeding. First, the international community must ensure that Africa has the capacity to carry out and sustain its own response. In the past, too little capacity was built, sustained, or retained. Capacity means more than trained personnel. It means strong systems supporting health, education, nutrition, social welfare, and community support, among other things. HIV has preyed on weaknesses in these core systems, and on the inequality, poverty, and social exclusion they generate. If these root causes are not addressed, Africa will remain ever vulnerable to HIV and to other unforeseeable ills. If they are addressed, the effort against AIDS could bring beneficial spin-offs in a wide range of related areas.

Second, the global response must remain vigilant against the most resistant viruses—denial and complacency. Although denial of the epidemic is rapidly subsiding in Africa, denial that anything can be done may recur there and elsewhere. The struggle against HIV and AIDS will likely be long. Setbacks are inevitable. The virus may take turns for the worse, as may whole societies in the countries most affected. It is vital for global partners to prepare themselves and their constituents for a protracted effort. A retreat to denial or "Afro-pessimism" would amount to a reprise of the retreat of the 1990s, with catastrophic consequences. Equally worrisome is complacency. Successful local efforts against HIV in both developed and developing countries have often been followed by diminished resolve or even a resurgence of risky behavior. The arrival of new therapies is especially likely to abate the sense of urgency and to create an impression that the problem is well in hand. The global community needs to make clear that no magic bullet is likely for years, if ever, and that perseverance is the only lasting solution.

Finally, Africa and its partners would do well to take note of Mann and Tarantola's (42) maxim that "how a problem is defined determines what we believe can be done about it, and from there what is actually done to address it." Africans need to see HIV as something they have already begun to overcome through thousands of local successes across the continent. The world needs to learn of those successes and to see AIDS not as an African problem but as a global threat about which Africa has the most to teach the world. So conceived, the problem would offer the first great opportunity for collective action in the new millennium.

In many ways, the 1990s ushered in an era of hope for Africa. Politics opened up; economies resurged; apartheid died; the Cold War ended. Not since the time of independence had so many African countries seen such auspicious prospects for the future. Talk of an "African Renaissance" became commonplace.

Now Africa has entered the 21st century watching many of its gains of the past century evaporate. Yet its promise remains real. If the global community can complete the job it started more than a decade ago, Africa can cope with AIDS while still beginning to live out its potential in full. Whether it does so will depend on how well Africans lead and how well the world responds. Writing his staff after the AIDS conference in Durban, the World Bank's Vice President for Africa, Callisto Madavo (43) summed up the challenge concisely: "AIDS has been Africa's tragedy long enough. It could yet become Africa's triumph. Are we doing enough?"

ACKNOWLEDGMENTS

The authors gratefully acknowledge the substantial assistance of Robert Ritzenthaler in preparing this chapter.

REFERENCES

1. World Health Organization. *The Global AIDS Strategy*. Geneva: WHO, 1992.
2. Piot P, Kapita BM, Were JBO, et al. AIDS in Africa: the first decade and challenges for the 1990s. *AIDS*, 1991;5:S1–S5.
3. World Health Organization. *Guidelines for the Development of a National AIDS Prevention Programme*. Geneva: WHO, 1988.
4. Mann J, Tarantola DJM, Netter TW, eds. *AIDS in the World*. Cambridge: Harvard University Press, 1992.
5. U.S. Central Intelligence Agency. The Global AIDS Disaster. Interagency Intelligence Memorandum 91-10005. Washington, DC: CIA, 2000.
6. Hoagland J. Africa Faces the AIDS Threat. *The Washington Post*, 27 January 1989.
7. Eckholm E, Tierny J. AIDS in Africa: A Killer Rages On. *The New York Times*, 16 September 1990.
8. Hiltzik MA. AIDS Spells Disaster for Africa. *Los Angeles Times*, 28 December 1991.
9. Annapolis Resolution to Create and Support the International Partnership Against HIV/AIDS in Africa. Meeting of the UNAIDS Cosponsoring Agencies and Secretariat; January 19–20, 1999; Annapolis, MD, USA. Available at: http://www.unaids.org/africapartnership/files/FN561.html. Accessed February 21, 2002.
10. U.S. General Accounting Office. *HIV/AIDS: USAID and U.N. Response to the Epidemic in the Developing World*. Washington, DC: GAO/NSIAD-98-202, 1998.
11. Organization of African Unity. *Dakar Declaration on the AIDS Epidemic in Africa*. Dakar, Senegal: Organization of African Unity, 1992.
12. Organization of African Unity. Tunis Declaration on AIDS and the Child in Africa. Declaration No. AHG/Decl.1 (XXX) of 15 June 1994. In: Abdulqawi A. Yusuf, ed. *African Yearbook of International Law*, Volume 3. Martinus Nijhoff, 1995.
13. Gellman B. The Global Response to AIDS in Africa: World Shunned Signs of the Coming Plague. *The Washington Post*, 5 July 2000, p. A1.
14. Ng'weshemi J, Boerma T, Bennett J, Schapnik D, eds. *HIV prevention and AIDS care in Africa: A district level approach*. Amsterdam: Royal Tropical Institute, 1997.
15. UNAIDS. *Level and flow of international resources for the response to HIV/AIDS: 1998 Update*. Geneva: UNAIDS, 2000.
16. Bastos C. *Global Responses to AIDS: Science in Emergency*. Bloomington: Indiana University Press, 1999.
17. Trussell J, Cohen B, eds. *Preventing and Mitigating AIDS in Sub-Saharan Africa: Research and Data Priorities for the Social and Behavioral Sciences*. Washington, DC: National Academy Press, 1996.
18. Mann J, Tarantola D, eds. *AIDS in the World II: Global Dimensions, Social Roots, and Response*. New York: Oxford University Press, 1996.
19. UNAIDS, World Health Organization. *Report on the global HIV/AIDS epidemic: June 1998*. Geneva: UNAIDS/WHO, 1998.
20. UNAIDS, Harvard School of Public Health. *Level and flow of national and international resources for the response to HIV/AIDS, 1996–1997*. Geneva: UNAIDS, 1999.
21. Altman L. In Africa, a Deadly Silence About AIDS Is Lifting. *The New York Times*, 13 July 1999.
22. UN Security Council. UN Security Council Resolution 1308, 2000.
23. UN Security Council. UN Security Council Resolution 1325, 2000.
24. UN General Assembly. UN General Assembly Resolution A/RES/S-26/2, 2001.
25. UNAIDS. Cost-effectiveness analysis and HIV/AIDS, Technical Update. Geneva: UNAIDS, 1998.
26. UNAIDS. Guide to the strategic planning process for a national response to HIV/AIDS: Strategic plan formulation. Geneva: UNAIDS, 1998.
27. UNAIDS. Developing HIV/AIDS treatment guidelines. Geneva: UNAIDS, 1999.
28. UNAIDS. *Handbook for Legislators on HIV/AIDS, Law and Human Rights*. Geneva: UNAIDS/Inter-Parliamentary Union, 1999.

29. UNAIDS. Acting early to prevent AIDS: The case of Senegal. Geneva: UNAIDS, 1999.
30. UNAIDS. Costing Guidelines for HIV Prevention Strategies. Geneva: UNAIDS, 2000.
31. UNESCO, UNAIDS. *Migrant Populations and HIV/AIDS.* Paris and Geneva: UNESCO/UNAIDS, 2000.
32. World Bank. *Intensifying Action Against HIV/AIDS in Africa: Responding to a Development Crisis.* Washington, DC: World Bank, 2000.
33. World Bank. *Confronting AIDS: Public Priorities in a Global Epidemic.* New York: Oxford University Press, 1997.
34. Aid for AIDS. *The Economist*, 29 April 2000, p. 76.
35. UNICEF. *Children orphaned by AIDS: Front-line responses from eastern and southern Africa.* New York: UNICEF, 1999.
36. UN Food and Agriculture Organization, UNAIDS. *Sustainable Agricultural/Rural Development and Vulnerability to the AIDS Epidemic.* Geneva: UNAIDS, 1999.
37. U.S. Central Intelligence Agency. The Global Infectious Disease Threat and Its Implications for the United States (National Intelligence Estimate 99-17D). Washington, DC: CIA, 2000.
38. POLICY Project. *The Art of Policy Formulation: Experiences from Africa in Developing National HIV/AIDS Policies.* Washington, DC: The POLICY Project, 1999.
39. Canadian International Development Agency. *CIDA's HIV/AIDS Action Plan*, 2nd ed. Hull, Quebec: Canadian International Development Agency; 2000.
40. Organization of African Unity. *Abuja Declaration on HIV/AIDS, Tuberculosis and Other Related Infectious Diseases.* In: Proceedings of the OAU Special Summit on HIV/AIDS, Tuberculosis and Other Related Infectious Diseases; April 26–27, 2001; Abuja, Nigeria.
41. UNAIDS. *National AIDS Programmes: A Guide to Monitoring and Evaluation.* Geneva: UNAIDS, 2000.
42. Mann J, Tarantola D. Responding to HIV/AIDS: A Historical Perspective. *Health and Human Rights: An International Quarterly Journal*, 1998;2:5–8.
43. Madavo C. Reflections from Durban: Are We Doing Enough? Memorandum. World Bank, July 10, 2000.

Index

MIX
Papier aus verantwortungsvollen Quellen
Paper from responsible sources
FSC® C105338

If you have any concerns about our products,
you can contact us on
ProductSafety@springernature.com

In case Publisher is established outside the EU,
the EU authorized representative is:
Springer Nature Customer Service Center GmbH
Europaplatz 3, 69115 Heidelberg, Germany

Printed by Libri Plureos GmbH
in Hamburg, Germany